PRECLINICAL DEVELOPMENT HANDBOOK

ADME and Biopharmaceutical Properties

PRECLINICAL DEVELOPMENT HANDBOOK

ADME and Biopharmaceutical Properties

SHAYNE COX GAD, PH.D., D.A.B.T.
Gad Consulting Services
Cary, North Carolina

WILEY-INTERSCIENCE
A JOHN WILEY & SONS, INC., PUBLICATION

Published by John Wiley & Sons, Inc., Hoboken, New Jersey
Published simultaneously in Canada

For general information on our other products and services or for technical support, please contact
our Customer Care Department within the United States at (800) 762-2974, outside the United States
at (317) 572-3993 or fax (317) 572-4002.

Wiley also publishes its books in a variety of electronic formats. Some content that appears in print
may not be available in electronic formats. For more information about Wiley products, visit our web
site at www.wiley.com.

Library of Congress Cataloging-in-Publication Data is available.

ISBN: 978-0-470-24847-8

Printed in the United States of America

10 9 8 7 6 5 4 3 2 1

CONTRIBUTORS

Adegoke Adeniji, Philadelphia College of Pharmacy, University of the Sciences in Philadelphia, Philadelphia, Pennsylvania, *Chemical and Physical Characterizations of Potential New Chemical Entity*

Adeboye Adjare, Philadelphia College of Pharmacy, University of the Sciences in Philadelphia, Philadelphia, Pennsylvania, *Chemical and Physical Characterizations of Potential New Chemical Entity*

Zvia Agur, Institute for Medical Biomathematics (IMBM), Bene-Ataroth, Israel; Optimata Ltd., Ramat-Gan, Israel, *Mathematical Modeling as a New Approach for Improving the Efficacy/Toxicity Profile of Drugs: The Thrombocytopenia Case Study*

Melvin E. Andersen, The Hamner Institutes for Health Sciences, Research Triangle Park, North Carolina, *Physiologically Based Pharmacokinetic Modeling*

Joseph P. Balthasar, University of Buffalo, The State University of New York, Buffalo, New York, *Pharmacodynamics*

Stelvio M. Bandiera, Faculty of Pharmaceutical Sciences, University of British Columbia, Vancouver, British Columbia, Canada, *Cytochrome P450 Enzyme*

Ihor Bekersky, Consultant, Antioch, Illinois, *Bioavailability and Bioequivalence Studies*

Marival Bermejo, University of Valencia, Valencia, Spain, *How and Where Are Drugs Absorbed?*

Jan H. Beumer, University of Pittsburgh Cancer Institute, Pittsburgh, Pennsylvania, *Mass Balance Studies*

Prasad V. Bharatam, National Institute of Pharamaceutical Education and Research (NIPER), Nagar, India, *Modeling and Informatics in Drug Design*

Deepa Bisht, National JALMA Institute for Leprosy and Other Myobacterial Diseases, Agra, India, *Accumulation of Drugs in Tissues*

Scott L. Childs, SSCI, Inc., West Lafayette, Indiana, *Salt and Cocrystal Form Selection*

Harvel J. Clewell III, The Hamner Institutes for Health Sciences, Research Triangle Park, North Carolina, *Physiologically Based Pharmacokinetic Modeling*

Brett A. Cowans, SSCI, Inc., West Lafayette, Indiana, *Salt and Cocrystal Form Selection*

Dipankar Das, University of Alberta, Edmonton, Alberta, Canada, *Protein–Protein Interactions*

A. G. de Boer, University of Leiden, Leiden, The Netherlands, *The Blood–Brain Barrier and Its Effect on Absorption and Distribution*

Pankaj B. Desai, University of Cincinnati Medical Center, Cincinnati, Ohio, *Data Analysis*

Merrill J. Egorin, University of Pittsburgh Cancer Institute, Pittsburgh, Pennsylvania, *Mass Balance Studies*

Julie L. Eiseman, University of Pittsburgh Cancer Institute, Pittsburgh, Pennsylvania, *Mass Balance Studies*

Moran Elishmereni, Institute for Medical Biomathematics (IMBM), Bene-Ataroth, Israel, *Mathematical Modeling as a New Approach for Improving the Efficacy/ Toxicity Profile of Drugs: The Thrombocytopenia Case Study*

Dora Farkas, Tufts University School of Medicine, Boston, Massachusetts, *Mechanisms and Consequences of Drug–Drug Interactions*

Sandrea M. Francis, National Institute of Pharamaceutical Education and Research (NIPER), Nagar, India, *Modeling and Informatics in Drug Design*

Shayne Cox Gad, Gad Consulting Services, Cary, North Carolina, *Regulatory Requirements for INDs/FIH (First in Human) Studies*

P. J. Gaillard, to-BBB Technologies BV, Leiden, The Netherlands, *The Blood–Brain Barrier and Its Effect on Absorption and Distribution*

Srinivas Ganta, University of Auckland, Auckland, New Zealand, *Permeability Assessment*

Sanjay Garg, University of Auckland, Auckland, New Zealand, *Permeability Assessment*

Isabel Gonzalez-Alvarez, University of Valencia, Valencia, Spain, *How and Where Are Drugs Absorbed?*

Eric M. Gorman, The University of Kansas, Lawrence, Kansas, *Stability: Physical and Chemical*

Luis Granero, University of Valencia, Valencia, Spain, *Absorption of Drugs after Oral Administration*

David J. Greenblatt, Tufts University School of Medicine, Boston, Massachusetts, *Mechanisms and Consequences of Drug–Drug Interactions*

Ken Grime, AstraZeneca R&D Charnwood, Loughborough, United Kingdom, *Utilization of* In Vitro *Cytochrome P450 Inhibition Data for Projecting Clinical Drug–Drug Interactions*

William L. Hayton, The Ohio State University, Columbus, Ohio, *Allometric Scaling*

William W. Hope, National Cancer Institute, National Institutes of Health, Bethesda, Maryland, *Experimental Design Considerations in Pharmacokinetics Studies*

Eugene G. Hrycay, Faculty of Pharmaceutical Sciences, University of British Columbia, Vancouver, British Columbia, Canada, *Cytochrome P450 Enzymes*

Teh-Min Hu, National Defense Medical Center, Taipei, Taiwan, *Allometric Scaling*

Subheet Jain, Punjabi University, Patiala, Punjab, India, *Dissolution*

Izet M. Kapetanovic, NIH NCI Division of Cancer Prevention, Chemoprevention Agent Devleopment Research Group, Bethesda, Maryland, *Analytical Chemistry Methods: Developments and Validation*

Kamaljit Kaur, University of Alberta, Edmonton, Alberta, Canada, *Protein–Protein Interactions*

Jane R. Kenny, AstraZeneca R&D Charnwood, Loughborough, United Kingdom, *Utilization of* In Vitro *Cytochrome P450 Inhibition Data for Projecting Clinical Drug–Drug Interactions*

Masood Khan, Covance Laboratories Inc., Immunochemistry Services, Chantilly, Virginia, *Method Development for Preclinical Bioanalytical Support*

Smriti Khanna, National Institute of Pharamaceutical Education and Research (NIPER), Nagar, India, *Modeling and Informatics in Drug Design*

Yuri Kheifetz, Institute for Medical Biomathematics (IMBM), Bene-Ataroth, Israel, *Mathematical Modeling as a New Approach for Improving the Efficacy/ Toxicity Profile of Drugs: The Thrombocytopenia Case Study*

Yuri Kogan, Institute for Medical Biomathematics (IMBM), Bene-Ataroth, Israel, *Mathematical Modeling as a New Approach for Improving the Efficacy/Toxicity Profile of Drugs: The Thrombocytopenia Case Study*

Niels Krebsfaenger, Schwarz Biosciences, Monheim, Germany, *Species Comparison of Metabolism in Microsomes and Hepatocytes*

Thierry Lave, F. Hoffman-LaRoche Ltd., Basel, Switzerland, *Physiologically Based Pharmacokinetic Modeling*

Albert P. Li, In Vitro ADMET Laboratories, Inc., Columbia, Maryland, In Vitro *Evaluation of Metabolic Drug–Drug Interactions: Scientific Concepts and Practical Considerations*

Charles W. Locuson, University of Minnesota, Minneapolis, Minnesota, *Metabolism Kinetics*

Alexander V. Lyubimov, University of Illinois at Chicago, Chicago, Illinois, *Analytical Chemistry Methods: Developments and Validation; Dosage Formulation; Bioavailability and Bioequivalence Studies*

Dermot F. McGinnity, AstraZeneca R&D Charnwood, Loughborough, United Kingdom, *Utilization of In Vitro Cytochrome P450 Inhibition Data for Projecting Clinical Drug–Drug Interactions*

Peter Meek, University of the Sciences in Philadelphia, Philadelphia, Pennsylvania, *Computer Techniques: Identifying Similarities Between Small Molecules*

Donald W. Miller, University of Manitoba, Winnipeg, Manitoba, Canada, *Transporter Interactions in the ADME Pathway of Drugs*

Mehran F. Moghaddam, Celegne, San Diego, California, *Metabolite Profiling and Structural Identification*

Guillermo Moyna, University of the Sciences in Philadelphia, Philadelphia, Pennsylvania, *Computer Techniques: Identifying Similarities Between Small Molecules*

Eric J. Munson, The University of Kansas, Lawrence, Kansas, *Stability: Physical and Chemical*

Ann W. Newman, SSCI, Inc., West Lafayette, Indiana, *Salt and Cocrystal Form Selection*

Mohammad Owais, Aligarh Muslim University, Aligarh, India, *Accumulation of Drugs in Tissues*

Brian E. Padden, Schering-Plough Research Institute, Summit, New Jersey, *Stability: Physical and Chemical*

Sree D. Panuganti, Purdue University, West Lafayette, Indiana, *Drug Clearance*

Jayanth Panyam, University of Minnesota, Minneapolis, Minnesota, *Distribution: Movement of Drugs through the Body*

Yogesh Patil, Wayne State University, Detroit, Michigan, *Distribution: Movement of Drugs through the Body*

James W. Paxton, The University of Auckland, Auckland, New Zealand, *Interrelationship between Pharmacokinetics and Metabolism*

Olavi Pelkonen, University of Oulu, Oulu, Finland, *In Vitro Metabolism in Preclinical Drug Development*

Vidmantas Petraitis, National Cancer Institute, National Institutes of Health, Bethesda, Maryland, *Experimental Design Considerations in Pharmacokinetics Studies*

Ana Polache, University of Valencia, Valencia, Spain, *Absorption of Drugs after Oral Administration*

Elizabeth R. Rayburn, University of Alabama at Birmingham, Birmingham, Alabama, *Linkage Between Toxicology of Drugs and Metabolism*

Micaela B. Reddy, Roche Palo Alto LLC, Palo Alto, California, *Physiologically Based Pharmacokinetic Modeling*

Robert J. Riley, AstraZeneca R&D Charnwood, Loughborough, United Kingdom, *Utilization of* In Vitro *Cytochrome P450 Inhibition Data for Projecting Clinical Drug–Drug Interactions*

Sevim Rollas, Marmara University, Istanbul, Turkey, In Vivo *Metabolism in Preclinical Drug Development*

Bharti Sapra, Punjabi University, Patiala, Punjab, India, *Dissolution*

Richard I. Shader, Tufts University School of Medicine, Boston, Massachusetts, *Mechanisms and Consequences of Drug–Drug Interactions*

Dhaval Shah, University of Buffalo, The State University of New York, Buffalo, New York, *Pharmacodynamics*

Puneet Sharma, University of Auckland, Auckland, New Zealand, *Permeability Assessment*

Beom Soo Shin, University of Buffalo, The State University of New York, Buffalo, New York, *Pharmacodynamics*

Meir Shoham, Optimata Ltd., Ramat-Gan, Israel, *Mathematical Modeling as a New Approach for Improving the Efficacy/Toxicity Profile of Drugs: The Thrombocytopenia Case Study*

Mavanur R. Suresh, University of Alberta, Edmonton, Alberta, Canada, *Protein–Protein Interactions*

Craig K. Svensson, Osmetech Molecular Diagnostics, Pasadena, California, *Drug Clearance*

A. K. Tiwary, Punjabi University, Patiala, Punjab, India, *Dissolution*

Ari Tolonen, Novamass Analytical Ltd., Oulu, Finland; University of Oulu, Oulu, Finland, In Vitro *Metabolism in Preclinical Drug Development*

Timothy S. Tracy, University of Minnesota, Minneapolis, Minnesota, *Metabolism Kinetics*

Miia Turpeinen, University of Oulu, Oulu, Finland, In Vitro *Metabolism in Preclinical Drug Development*

Jouko Uusitalo, Novamass Analytical Ltd., Oulu, Finland, In Vitro *Metabolism in Preclinical Drug Development*

Vladimir Vainstein, Institute for Medical Biomathematics (IMBM), Bene-Ataroth, Israel; Optimata Ltd., Ramat-Gan, Israel, *Mathematical Modeling as a New Approach for Improving the Efficacy/Toxicity Profile of Drugs: The Thrombocytopenia Case Study*

Krishnamurthy Venkatesan, National JALMA Institute for Leprosy and Other Myobacterial Diseases, Agra, India, *Accumulation of Drugs in Tissues*

Lisa L. von Moltke, Tufts University School of Medicine, Boston, Massachusetts, *Mechanisms and Consequences of Drug–Drug Interactions*

Jayesh Vora, PRTM Management Consultants, Mountain View, California, *Data Analysis*

Thomas J. Walsh, National Cancer Institute, National Institutes of Health, Bethesda, Maryland, *Experimental Design Considerations in Pharmacokinetics Studies*

Naidong Weng, Johnson & Johnson Pharmaceutical Research & Development, Bioanalytical Department, Raritan, New Jersey, *Method Development for Preclinical Bioanalytical Support*

Randy Zauhar, University of the Sciences in Philadelphia, Philadelphia, Pennsylvania, *Computer Techniques: Identifying Similarities Between Small Molecules*

Ruiwen Zhang, University of Alabama at Birmingham, Birmingham, Alabama, *Linkage Between Toxicology of Drugs and Metabolism*

Yan Zhang, Drug Metabolism and Biopharmaceutics, Incyte Corporation, Wilmington, Delaware, *Transporter Interactions in the ADME Pathway of Drugs*

Irit Ziv, Optimata Ltd., Ramat-Gan, Israel, *Mathematical Modeling as a New Approach for Improving the Efficacy/Toxicity Profile of Drugs: The Thrombocytopenia Case Study*

CONTENTS

PREFACE

This *Preclinical Development Handbook: ADME and Biopharmaceutical Properties* continues and extends the objective behind the entire *Handbook* series: an attempt to achieve a through overview of the current and leading-edge nonclinical approaches to evaluating the pharmacokinetic and pharmacodynamic aspects of new molecular entity development for therapeutics. The 38 chapters cover the full range of approaches to understanding how new molecules are absorbed and distributed in model systems, have their biologic effects, and then are metabolized and excreted. Such evaluations provide the fundamental basis for making decisions as to the possibility and means of pursuing clinical development of such moieties. Better performance in this aspect of the new drug development process is one of the essential keys to both shortening and increasing the chance of success in developing new drugs.

The volume is unique in that it seeks to cover the entire range of available approaches to understanding the performance of a new molecular entity in as broad a manner as possible while not limiting itself to a superficial overview. Thanks to the persistent efforts of Mindy Myers and Gladys Mok, these 38 chapters, which are written by leading practitioners in each of these areas, provide coverage of the primary approaches to the problems of understanding the mechanisms that operate in *in vivo* systems to transfer a drug to its site of action and out.

I hope that this newest addition to our scientific banquet is satisfying and useful to all those practitioners working in or entering the field.

1

MODELING AND INFORMATICS IN DRUG DESIGN

Prasad V. Bharatam,* Smriti Khanna, and Sandrea M. Francis

National Institute of Pharmaceutical Education and Research (NIPER), S.A.S. Nagar, India

Contents

*Corresponding author.

Preclinical Development Handbook: ADME and Biopharmaceutical Properties,
edited by Shayne Cox Gad
Copyright © 2008 John Wiley & Sons, Inc.

1.1   INTRODUCTION

Modeling and informatics have become indispensable components of rational drug design (Fig. 1.1). For the last few years, chemical analysis through molecular modeling has been very prominent in computer-aided drug design (CADD). But currently modeling and informatics are contributing in tandem toward CADD. Modeling in drug design has two facets: modeling on the basis of knowledge of the drugs/leads/ligands often referred to as ligand-based design and modeling based on the structure of macromolecules often referred to as receptor-based modeling (or structure-based modeling). Computer-aided drug design is a topic of medicinal chemistry, and before venturing into this exercise one must employ computational chemistry methods to understand the properties of chemical species, on the one hand, and employ computational biology techniques to understand the properties of biomolecules on the other. Information technology is playing a major role in decision making in pharmaceutical sciences. Storage, retrieval, and analysis of data of chemicals/biochemicals of therapeutic interest are major components of pharmacoinformatics. Quite

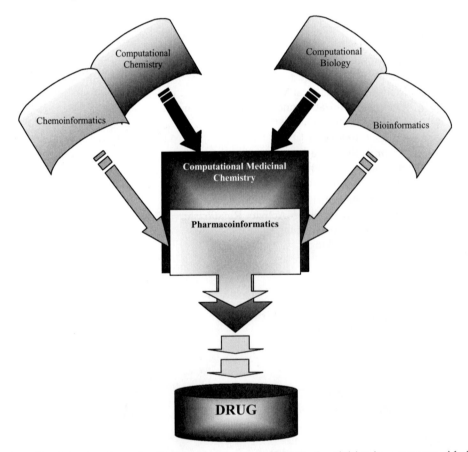

FIGURE 1.1   A schematic diagram showing a flowchart of activities in computer aided drug development. The figure shows that the contributions from modeling methods and informatics methods toward the drug development are parallel and in fact not really distinguishable.

often, the efforts based on modeling and informatics get thoroughly integrated with each other, as in the case of virtual screening exercises. In this chapter, the molecular modeling methods that are in vogue in the fields of (1) computational chemistry, (2) computational biology, (3) computational medicinal chemistry, and (4) pharmacoinformatics are presented and the resources available in these fields are discussed.

1.2 COMPUTATIONAL CHEMISTRY

Two-dimensional (2D) structure drawing and three-dimensional (3D) structure building are the important primary steps in computational chemistry for which several molecular visualization packages are available. The most popular of these are ChemDraw Ultra and Chem3D Pro, which are a part of the ChemOffice suite of software packages [1]. ACD/ChemSketch [2], MolSuite [3], and many more of this kind are other programs for the same purpose. Refinement has to be carried out on all the drawings and 3D structures so as to improve the chemical accuracy of the structure on the computer screen. Structure refinement based on heuristic rules/cleanup procedures is a part of all these software packages. However, chemical accuracy of the 3D structures still remains poor even after cleanup. Further refinement can be carried out by performing energy minimization using either molecular mechanical or quantum chemical procedures. By using these methods, the energy of a molecule can be estimated in any given state. Following this, with the help of first and second derivatives of energy, it can be ascertained whether the given computational state of the molecules belongs to a chemically acceptable state or not. During this process, the molecular geometry gets modified to a more appropriate, chemically meaningful state – the entire procedure is known as geometry optimization. The geometry optimized 3D structure is suitable for property estimation, descriptor calculation, conformational analysis, and finally for drug design exercise [4–6].

1.2.1 Ab Initio Quantum Chemical Methods

Every molecule possesses internal energy (U), for the estimation of which quantum chemical calculations are suitable. Quantum chemical calculations involve rigorous mathematical derivations and attempt to solve the Schrödinger equation, which in its simplest form may be written as

$$H\Psi = E\Psi \tag{1.1}$$

$$\hat{H}_{el} = \sum \left(-\frac{1}{2}\nabla_i^2\right) - \sum_i \sum_a \frac{Z_a}{|r_i - d_a|} + \frac{1}{2}\sum_i \sum_{j \neq i} \frac{1}{|r_i - r_j|} + \frac{1}{2}\sum_a \sum_{b \neq a} \frac{Z_a Z_b}{|d_a - d_b|} \tag{1.2}$$

where ψ represents the wavefunction, E represents energy, ∇ represents the kinetic energy operator for electrons, r_i defines the vector position of electron i with vector components in Bohr radii, Z_a is the charge of fixed nucleus a in units of the elementary charge, and d_a is the vector position of nucleus a with vector components in Bohr radii.

Exact solutions to Schrödinger equation cannot be provided for systems with more than one electron. Several *ab initio* molecular orbital (MO) and *ab initio* density functional theory (DFT) methods were developed to provide expectation value for the energy. This energy can be minimized and thus the geometry of any molecule can be obtained, with high confidence level, using quantum chemical methods. During this energy estimation, the wavefunctions of every molecule can be defined, which possess all the information related to the molecule. Thus, properties like relative energies, dipole moments, electron density distribution, charge distribution, electron delocalization, molecular orbital energies, molecular orbital shapes, ionization potential, infrared (IR) frequencies, and chemical shifts can be estimated using *ab initio* computational chemistry methods. For this purpose, several quantum chemical methods like Hartree–Fock (HF), second order Moller–Plesset perturbation (MP2), coupled cluster (CCSD), configuration interaction (QCISD), many-body perturbation (MBPT), multiconfiguration self-consistent field (MCSCF), complete active space self-consistent field (CASSCF), B3LYP, and VWN were developed. At the same time to define the wavefunction, a set of mathematical functions known as *basis set* is required. Typical basis sets are 3-21G, 6-31G*, and 6-31+G*. Combination of the *ab initio* methods and basis sets leads to several thousand options for estimating energy. For reliable geometry optimization of drug molecules, the HF/6-31+G*, MP2/6-31+G*, and B3LYP/6-31+G* methods are quite suitable. When very accurate energy estimation is required, G2MP2 and CBS-Q methods can be employed. Gaussian03, Spartan, and Jaguar are software packages that can be used to estimate reliable geometry optimization and very accurate energy estimation of any chemical species. In practice, quantum chemical methods are being used to estimate the relative stabilities of molecules, to calculate properties of reaction intermediates, to investigate the mechanisms of chemical reactions, to predict the aromaticity of compounds, and to analyze spectral properties. Medicinal chemists are beginning to take benefit from these by studying drug–receptor interactions, enzyme–substrate binding, and solvation of biological molecules. Molecular electrostatic potentials, which can be derived from *ab initio* quantum chemical methods, provide the surface properties of drugs and receptors and thus they offer useful information regarding complementarities between the two [7–10].

1.2.2   Semiempirical Methods

The above defined *ab initio* methods are quite time consuming and become prohibitively expensive when the drugs possess large number of atoms and/or a series of calculations need to be performed to understand the chemical phenomena. Semiempirical quantum chemical methods were introduced precisely to address this problem. In these methods empirical parameters are employed to estimate many integrals but only a few key integrals are solved explicitly. Although these calculations do not provide energy of molecules, they are quite reliable in estimating the heats of formation. Semiempirical quantum chemical methods (e.g., AM1, PM3, SAM1) are very fast in qualitatively estimating the chemical properties that are of interest to a drug discovery scientist. MOPAC and AMPAC are the software packages of choice; however, many other software packages also incorporate these methods. Qualitative estimates of HOMO and LUMO energies, shapes of molecular orbitals, and reaction mechanisms of drug synthesis are some of the applications of semiempirical analysis [5, 10]. When the molecules become much larger, especially in the case of macromolecules like proteins, enzymes, and nucleic acids, employing these semiempirical methods becomes impractical. In such cases, molecular mechanical methods can be used to estimate the heats of formation and to perform geometry optimization.

1.2.3   Molecular Mechanical Methods

Molecular mechanical methods estimate the energy of any drug by adding up the strain in all the bonds, angles, and torsions due to the energy of the van der Waals and Coulombic interactions across all atoms in the molecule. It reflects the internal energy of the molecule; although the estimated value is nowhere close to the actual internal energy, the relative energy obtained from these methods is indicative enough for chemical/biochemical analysis. It is made up of a number of components as given by

$$E_{mm} = E_{bonds} + E_{angles} + E_{vdw} + E_{torsion} + E_{charge} + E_{misc} \qquad (1.3)$$

Molecular mechanical methods are also known as force field methods because in these methods, the electronic effects are estimated implicitly in terms of force fields associated with the atoms. In Eq. 1.3, the energy (E) due to bonds, angles, and torsional angles can be estimated using the simple Hooke's law and its variations, whereas the van der Waals (vdw) interactions are estimated using the Lennard-Jones potential and the electrostatic interactions are estimated using Coulombic forces. The energy estimation, energy minimization, and geometry optimization using these methods are quite fast and hence suitable for studying the geometries and conformations of biomolecules and drug–receptor interactions. Since these methods are empirical in nature, parameterization of the force fields with the help of available spectral data or quantum chemical methods is required. AMBER, CHARMM, UFF, and Tripos are some of the force fields in wide use in computer-aided drug development [5, 10].

1.2.4   Energy Minimization and Geometry Optimization

Drug molecules prefer to adopt equilibrium geometry in nature, that is, a geometry that possesses a stable 3D arrangement of atoms in the molecule. The 3D structure of a molecule built using a 3D builder does not represent a natural state; slight modifications are required to be made on the built 3D structure so that it represents the natural state. For this purpose, the following questions need to be addressed: (1) Which minimal changes need to be made? (2) How much change needs to be made? (3) How does one know the representation at hand is the true representation of the natural state? To provide answers to these questions we can depend on energy, because molecules prefer to exist in thermodynamically stable states. This implies that if the energy of any molecule can be minimized, the molecule is not in a stable state and thus the current representation of the molecule may not be the true representation of the natural state. This also implies that we can minimize the energy and the molecular structure in that energy minimum state probably represents a true natural state. Several methods of energy minimization have been developed by computational chemists, some of which are nonderivative methods (simplex method) but many of which are dependent on derivative methods (steepest descent, Newton–Raphson, conjugate gradient, variable metrics, etc.) and involve the estimation of the gradient of the potential energy curve [4–6]. The entire procedure of geometry modification to reach an energy minimum state with almost null gradient is known as geometry optimization in terms of the structure of the molecule and energy minimization in terms of the energy of the molecule. All computational chemistry software packages are equipped with energy minimization methods—of which a few incorporate energy minimization based on *ab initio* methods while most include the semiempirical and molecular mechanics based energy minimization methods.

1.2.5 Conformational Analysis

Molecules containing freely rotatable bonds can adopt many different conformations. Energy minimization procedures lead the molecular structure to only one of the chemically favorable conformations, called the local minimum. Out of the several local minima on the potential energy (PE) surface of a molecule, the lowest energy conformation is known as the global minimum. It is important to note all the possible conformations of any molecule and identify the global minimum before taking up a drug design exercise (Fig. 1.2). This is important because only one of the possible conformations of a drug, known as its bioactive conformation, is responsible for its therapeutic effect. This conformation may be a global minimum, a local minimum, or a transition state between local minima. As it is very difficult to identify

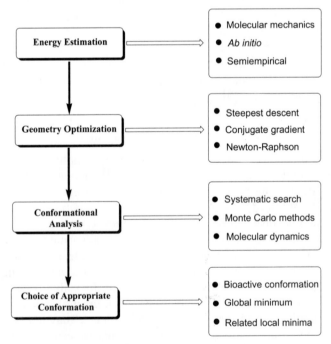

FIGURE 1.2 Flowchart showing the sequence of steps during molecular modeling of drug molecules.

the bioactive conformation of many drug molecules, it is common practice to assume the global minima to be bioactive. The transformation of drug molecules from one conformer to another can be achieved by changing the torsional angles. The computational process of identifying all local minima of a drug molecule, identifying the global minimum conformation, and, if possible, identifying the bioactive conformation is known as conformational analysis. This is one of the major activities in computational chemistry.

Manual conformational search is one method where the chemical intuition of the chemist plays a major role in performing the conformational analysis. Here, a chemist/modeler carefully chooses all possible conformations of a given drug molecule and estimates the energy of each conformation after performing energy minimization. This procedure is very effective and is being widely used. This approach allows the application of rigorous quantum chemical methods for the conformational analysis. The only limitation of this method arises from the ability and patience of the chemist. There is a possibility that a couple of important conformations are ignored in this approach. To avoid such problems, automated conformational analysis methods were introduced.

Various automated methods of conformational analysis include systematic search, random search, Monte Carlo simulations, molecular dynamics, genetic algorithms, and expert systems (Table 1.1) [4, 5]. The systematic conformational search can be performed by varying systematically each of the torsion angles of the rotatable bonds of a molecule to generate all possible conformations. The step size for torsion angle change is normally 30–60°. The number of conformations across a C—C single bond would vary between 6 and 12. With an increase in the number of rotatable bonds, the total number of conformations generated becomes quite large. The "bump check" method reduces the number of possibilities; still, the total number of conformations generated can be in the tens of thousands for drug molecules. Obviously, most of the conformations are chemically nonsignificant.

The random conformational search method employs random change in torsional angle across rotatable bonds and performs energy minimization each time; thus, a handful of chemically meaningful conformations can be generated [11–18].

Molecular dynamics is another method of carrying out conformational search of flexible molecules. The aim of this approach is to reproduce time-dependent motional behavior of a molecule, which can identify bound states out of several possible

TABLE 1.1   Different Methods of Conformational Analysis

Methods for Conformational Analysis	Remarks
Systematic search	Systematic change of torsions
Random search	Conformations picked up randomly
Monte Carlo method	Supervised random search
Molecular dynamics	Newtonian forces on atoms and time dependency incorporated in conformational search
Genetic algorithm	Parent–child relationship along with survival of the fittest techniques employed
Expert system	Heuristic methods based on rules and facts employed

states. The user needs to define step size, time of run, and the temperature supplied to the system at the beginning of the computational analysis. A simulated annealing method allows "cooling down" of the system at regular time intervals by decreasing the simulation temperature. As the temperature approaches 0 K, the molecule is trapped in the nearest local minimum. It is used as the starting point for further simulation and the cycle is repeated several times [19].

1.3 COMPUTATIONAL BIOLOGY

Computational biology is a fast growing topic and it is really not practical to distinguish this topic from bioinformatics. However, we may broadly distinguish between the two topics as far as this chapter is concerned. Molecular modeling aspects of computational biology, which lead to structure prediction, may be discussed under this heading, whereas the sequence analysis part, which leads to target identification, may be discussed under the section of pharmacoinformatics. Structure prediction of biomolecules (often referred to as "structural bioinformatics") adopts many aspects of computational chemistry. For example, energy minimization of protein receptor structure is one important step in computational biology. Molecular mechanics, molecular simulations, and molecular dynamics are employed in performing conformational analysis of macromolecules.

A rational drug design approach is very much dependent on the knowledge of receptor protein structures and is severely limited by the availability of target protein structure with experimentally determined 3D coordinates. Proteins exhibit four tiered organization: (1) primary structure defining the amino acid sequence, (2) secondary structure with α-helical and β-sheet folds, (3) tertiary structure defining the folding of secondary structure held by hydrogen bonds, and (4) quaternary structure involving noncovalent association between two or more independent proteins. Methods for identifying the primary amino acid sequence in proteins are now well developed; however, this knowledge is not sufficient enough to understand the function of the proteins, the drug–receptor mutual recognition, and designing drugs. Various experimental techniques like X-ray crystallography, nuclear magnetic resonance, and electron diffraction are available for determining the 3D coordinates of the protein structure; however, there are many limitations. It is not easy to crystallize proteins and even when we succeed, the crystal structure represents only a rigid state of the protein rather than a dynamic state. Thus, the reliability of the experimental data is not very high in biomolecules. Computational methods provide the alternative approach—although with equal uncertainty but at a greater speed. Homology modeling and *ab initio* methods are being employed to elucidate the tertiary structure of various biomolecules. The 3D structures of proteins are useful in performing molecular docking, *de novo* design, and receptor-based pharmacophore mappings. The computational methods of biomolecular structure prediction are discussed next (Fig. 1.3) [20, 21].

1.3.1 Ab Initio Structure Prediction

This approach seeks to predict the native conformation of a protein from the amino acid sequence alone. The predictions made are based on fundamental understanding of the protein structure and the predictions must satisfy the requirements of free-

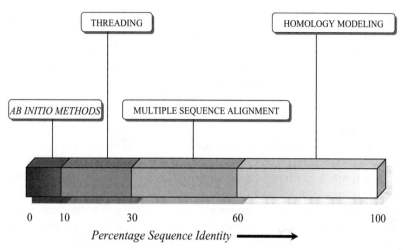

FIGURE 1.3   A list of computer-aided structure prediction methods with respect to their suitability to the available sequence similarity.

energy function associated with lowest free-energy minima. The detailed representation of macromolecules should include the coordinates of all atoms of the protein and the surrounding solvent molecules. However, representing this large number of atoms and the interactions between them is computationally expensive. Thus, several simplifications have been suggested in the representations during the *ab initio* structure prediction process. These include (1) representation of side chains using a limited set of conformations that are found to be prevalent in structures from the Protein Data Bank (PDB) without any great loss in predictive ability [22] and (2) restriction of the conformations available to the polypeptides in terms of phi–psi (ϕ–ψ) angle pairs [23]. Building the protein 3D structure is initiated by predicting the structures of protein fragments. Local structures of the protein fragments are generated first after considering several alternatives through energy minimization. A list of possible conformations is also extracted from experimental structures for all residues. Protein tertiary structures are assembled by searching through the combinations of these short fragments. During the assembling process, bump checking and low energy features (hydrophobic, van der Waals forces) should be incorporated. The final suggested structure is subjected to energy minimization and conformational analysis using molecular dynamics simulations. *Ab initio* structure prediction can be used to guide target selection by considering the fold of biological significance. The *ab initio* macromolecular structure prediction methods, if successful, are superior to the widely used homology modeling technique because no *a priori* bias is incorporated into the structure prediction [24].

1.3.2   Homology Modeling

Homology or comparative modeling uses experimentally determined 3D structure of a protein to predict the 3D structure of another protein that has a similar amino acid sequence. It is based on two major observations: (1) structure of a protein is uniquely determined by its amino acid sequence and (2) during evolution, the structure is more conserved than the sequence such that similar sequences adopt practically identical structure and distantly related sequences show similarity in folds. Homology modeling is a multistep method involving the following steps: (1) obtaining the sequence of the protein with unknown 3D structure, (2) template identification for comparative analysis, (3) fold assignment based on the known chemistry and biology of the protein, (4) primary structure alignment, (5) backbone generation, (6) loop modeling, (7) side chain modeling, (8) model optimization, and (9) model validation.

The methodology adopted in homology modeling of proteins can be described as follows. The target sequence is first compared to all sequences reported in the PDB using sequence analysis. Once a template sequence is found in the data bank, an alignment is made to identify optimum correlation between template and target. If identical residues exist in both the sequences, the coordinates are copied as such. If the residues differ, then only the coordinates of the backbone elements (N, Cα, C, and O) are copied. Loop modeling involves shifting all insertions and deletions to the loops and further modifying them to build a considerably well resembling model. Modeling the side chains involves copying the conserved residues, which also includes substitution of certain rotamers that are strongly favored by the backbone. Model optimization is required because of the expected differences in the 3D structures of the target and the template. The energy minimizations can be performed using molecular mechanics force fields (either well defined and/or self-parameterizing force fields). Molecular dynamic simulations offer fast, more reliable 3D structure of the protein. Model validation is a very important step in homology modeling, because several solutions may be obtained and the scientific user should interfere and make a choice of the best generated model. Often, the user may have to repeat the process with increased caution [20, 24].

1.3.3   Threading or Remote Homology Modeling

Threading (more formally known as "fold recognition") is a method that may be used to suggest a general structure for a new protein. It is mainly adopted when pairwise sequence identity is less than 25% between the known and unknown structure. Threading technique is generally associated with the following steps: (1) identify the remote homology between the unknown and known structure; (2) align the target and template; and (3) tailor the homology model [24].

1.4   COMPUTATIONAL MEDICINAL CHEMISTRY

Representation of drug molecular structures can be handled using computational chemistry methods, whereas that of macromolecules can be handled using computational biology methods. However, finding the therapeutic potential of the chemical species and understanding the drug–receptor interactions *in silico* requires the following well developed techniques of computational medicinal chemistry.

1.4.1   Quantitative Structure–Activity Relationship (QSAR)

QSAR is a statistical approach that attempts to relate physical and chemical properties of molecules to their biological activities. This can be achieved by using easily

TABLE 1.2   Different Dimensions in QSAR

1D QSAR: Affinity correlates with pK_a, log P, etc.
2D QSAR: Affinity correlates with a structural pattern.
3D QSAR: Affinity correlates with the three-dimensional structure.
4D QSAR: Affinity correlates with multiple representations of ligand.
5D QSAR: Affinity correlates with multiple representations of induced-fit scenarios.
6D QSAR: Affinity correlates with multiple representations of solvation models.

calculatable descriptors like molecular weight, number of rotatable bonds, and log P. Developments in physical organic chemistry over the years and contributions of Hammett and Taft in correlating the chemical activity to structure laid the basis for the development of the QSAR paradigm by Hansch and Fujita. Table 1.2 gives an overview of various QSAR approaches in practice. The 2D and 3D QSAR approaches are commonly used methods, but novel ideas are being implemented in terms of 4D–6D QSAR. The increased dimensionality does not add any additional accuracy to the QSAR approach; for example, no claim is valid which states that the correlation developed using 3D descriptors is better than that based on 2D descriptors.

2D QSAR   Initially, 2D QSAR or the Hansch approach was in vogue, in which different kinds of descriptors from the 2D structural representations of molecules were correlated to biological activity. The basic concept behind 2D QSAR is that structural changes that affect biological properties are electronic, steric, and hydrophobic in nature. These properties can be described in terms of Hammett substituent and reaction constants, Verloop sterimol parameters, and hydrophobic constants. These types of descriptors are simple to calculate and allow for a relatively fast analysis.

Most 2D QSAR methods are based on graph theoretical indices. The graph theoretical descriptors, also called the molecular topological descriptors, are derived from the topology of a molecule, that is, the 2D molecular structure represented as graphs. These topological connectivity indices representing the branching of a molecule were introduced by Randíc [25] and further developed by Kier and Hall [26, 27]. The graph theoretical descriptors include mainly the Kier–Hall molecular connectivity indices (chi) and the Weiner [28, 29], Hosoya [30], Zagreb [31], Balaban [32], kappa shape [33], and information content indices [32]. The electrotopological state index (E-state) [34] combines the information related to both the topological environment and the electronic character of each skeletal atom in a molecule. The constitutional descriptors are dependent on the constitution of a molecule and are numerical descriptors, which include the number of hydrogen bond donors and acceptors, rotatable bonds, chiral centers, and molecular weight (1D) [35]. Apart from that, several indicator descriptors, which define whether or not a particular indicator is associated with a given molecule, are also found to be important in QSAR. The quantum chemical descriptors include the molecular orbital energies (HOMO, LUMO), charges, superdelocalizabilities, atom–atom and molecular polarizabilities, dipole moments, total and binding energies, and heat of formation. These are 3D descriptors derived from the 3D structure of the molecule and are electronic in nature [36]. These parameters are also often clubbed with the 2D QSAR analysis.

Statistical data analysis methods for QSAR development are used to identify the correlation between molecular descriptors and biological activity. This correlation may be linear or nonlinear and accordingly the methods may be divided into linear and nonlinear approaches. The linear approaches include simple linear regression, multiple linear regression (MLR), partial least squares (PLS), and genetic algorithm–partial least squares (GA-PLS). Simple linear regression develops a single descriptor linear equation to define the biological activity of the molecule. MLR is a step ahead as it defines a multiple term linear equation. More than one term is correlated to the biological activity in a single equation. PLS, on the other hand, is a multivariate linear regression method that uses principal components instead of descriptors. Principal components are the variables found by principal component analysis (PCA), which summarize the information in the original descriptors. The aim of PLS is to find the direct correlation not between the descriptors and the biological activity but between the principal component and the activity. GA-PLS integrates genetic algorithms with the PLS approach. Genetic algorithms are an automatic descriptor selection method that incorporates the concepts of biological evolution within itself. An initial random selection of descriptors is made and correlated to the activity. This forms the first generation, which is then mutated to include new descriptors, and crossovers are performed between the equations to give the next generation. Equations with better predictability are retained and the others are discarded. This procedure is continually iterated until the desired predictability is obtained or the specified number of generations have been developed. The nonlinear approaches include an Artificial Neural Network (ANN) and machine learning techniques. Unlike the linear approaches, nonlinear approaches work on a black box principle; that is, they develop a relation between the descriptors and the activity to predict the activity, but do not give the information on how the correlation was made or which descriptors are more contributing. The ANN algorithm uses the concept of the functioning of the brain and consists of three layers. The first layer is the input layer where the structural descriptors are given as an input; second is the hidden layer, which may be comprised of more than one layer. The input is processed in this part to give the predicted values to the third output layer, which gives the result to the user. The user can control the input given and the number of neurons and hidden layers but cannot control the correlating method [37–40].

The QSAR model developed by any statistical method has to be validated to confirm that it represents the true structure–activity relationship and is not a chance correlation. This may be done by various methods such as the leave-one-out and leave-multiple-out cross-validations and the bootstrap method. The randomization test is another validation approach used to confirm the adequacy of the training set. Attaching chemical connotation to the developed statistical model is an important aspect. A successful QSAR model not only effectively predicts the activity of new species belonging to the same series but also should provide chemical clues for future improvement. This requirement, as well as the recognition that the 3D representation of the chemicals gives more detailed information, led to the development of 3D QSAR.

3D QSAR   3D QSAR methods are an extension of the traditional 2D QSAR approach, wherein the physicochemical descriptors are estimated from the 3D structures of the chemicals. Typically, properties like molecular volume, molecular shape, HOMO and LUMO energies, and ionization potential are the properties that can be calculated from the knowledge of the 3D coordinates of each and every atom of the molecules. When these descriptors of series of molecules can be correlated to the observed biological activity, 3D QSAR models can be developed. This approach is different from the traditional QSAR only in terms of the descriptor definition and, in a sense, is not really 3D in nature.

Molecular fields (electrostatic and steric), which can be estimated using probe-based sampling of 3D structure of molecules within a molecular lattice, can be correlated with the reported numeric values of biological activity. Such methods proved to be much more informative as they provide differences in the fields as contour maps. The widely used CoMFA (comparative molecular field analysis) method is based on molecular field analysis and represents real 3D QSAR methods [41]. A similar approach was adopted in developing modules like CoMSIA (comparative molecular similarity index analysis) [42], SOMFA (self-organizing molecular field analysis) [43], and COMMA (comparative molecular moment analysis) [44]. Utilization and predictivity of CoMFA itself has improved sufficiently in accordance with the objectives to be achieved by it [45]. Despite the formal differences between the various methodologies, any QSAR method must include some identifiers of chemical structures, reliably measured biological activities, and molecular descriptors. In 3D QSAR, alignment (3D superimposition) of the molecules is necessary to construct good models. The main problems encountered in 3D QSAR are related to improper alignment of molecules, greater flexibility of the molecules, uncertainties about the bioactive conformation, and more than one binding mode of ligands. While considering the template, knowledge of the bioactive conformation of any lead compound would greatly help the 3D QSAR analysis. As discussed in Section 1.2.5, this may be obtained from the X-ray diffractions or conformation at the binding site, or from the global minimum structure. Alignment of 3D structures of molecules is carried out using RMS atoms alignment, moments alignment, or field alignment. The relationship between the biological activity and the structural parameters can be obtained by multiple linear regression or partial least squares analysis. Given next are some details of the widely used 3D QSAR approach CoMFA.

CoMFA (Comparative Molecular Field Analysis)   DYLOMMS (dynamic lattice-oriented molecular modeling system) was one of the initial developments by Cramer and Milne to compare molecules by aligning in space and by mapping their molecular fields to a 3D grid. This approach when used with partial least squares based statistical analysis gave birth to the CoMFA approach [46]. The CoMFA methodology is a 3D QSAR technique that allows one to design and predict activities of molecules. The database of molecules with known properties is suitably aligned in 3D space according to various methodologies. After consistently aligning the molecules within a molecular lattice, a probe atom (typically carbon) samples the steric and electrostatic interactions of the molecule. Charges are then calculated for each molecule using any of the several methods proposed for partial charge estimation. These values are stored in a large spreadsheet within the module (SYBYL software) and are then accessed during the partial least squares (PLS) routine, which attempts to correlate these field energy terms with a property of interest by the use of PLS with cross-validation, giving a measure of the predictive power of the model.

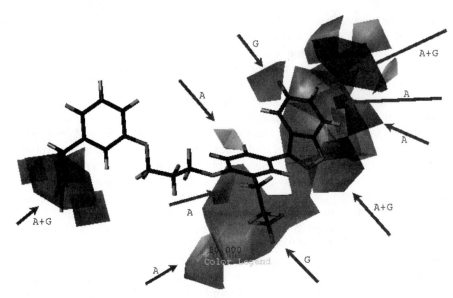

FIGURE 1.4   Steric and electrostatic contour map for the dual model showing the contributions from each model. "A" depicts the contributions made by the α-model and "G" depicts the contributions made by the γ- and model. (Reproduced with permission from The American Chemical Society; S. Khanna, M. E. Sobhia, P. V. Bharatam *J Med Chem* 2005;48:3015.)

Electrostatic maps are generated, indicating red contours around regions where high electron density (negative charge) is expected to increase activity, and blue contours where low electron density (partial positive charge) is expected to increase activity. Steric maps indicate areas where steric bulk is predicted to increase (green) or decrease (yellow) activity [41, 45]. Figure 1.4 shows a typical contour map from CoMFA analysis. CoMSIA [42], CoMMA [44], GRID [47], molecular shape analysis (MSA) [48], comparative receptor surface analysis (CoRSA) [49], and Apex-3D [50] are other 3D QSAR methods that are being employed successfully.

4D QSAR   4D QSAR analysis developed by Vedani and colleagues incorporates the conformational alignment and pharmacophore degrees of freedom in the development of 3D QSAR models. It is used to create and screen against 3D-pharmacophore QSAR models and can be used in receptor-independent or receptor-dependent modes. 4D QSAR can be used as a CoMFA preprocessor to provide conformations and alignments; or in combination with CoMFA to combine the field descriptors of CoMFA with the grid cell occupancy descriptors (GCODs) of 4D QSAR to build a "best" model; or in addition to CoMFA because it treats multiple alignments, conformations, and embedded pharmacophores, which are limitations of CoMFA [51].

5D QSAR   The 4D QSAR concept has been extended by an additional degree of freedom—the fifth dimension—allowing for multiple representations of the topology of the quasi-atomistic receptor surrogate. While this entity may be generated using up to six different induced-fit protocols, it has been demonstrated that the simulated evolution converges to a single model and that 5D QSAR, due to the fact that model selection may vary throughout the entire simulation, yields less biased results than 4D QSAR, where only a single induced-fit model can be evaluated at a time (software Quasar) [52, 53].

6D QSAR   A recent extension of the Quasar concept to sixth dimension (6D QSAR) allows for the simultaneous consideration of different solvation models [54]. This can be achieved explicitly by mapping parts of the surface area with solvent properties (position and size are optimized by the genetic algorithms) or implicitly. In Quasar, the binding energy is calculated as

$$E_{\text{binding}} = E_{\text{ligand-receptor}} - E_{\text{desolvation,ligand}} - T\ \Delta S - E_{\text{internal strain}} - E_{\text{induced fit}} \qquad (1.4)$$

1.4.2 Pharmacophore Mapping

A pharmacophore may be defined as the spatial arrangement of a set of key features present in a chemical species that interact favorably with the receptor leading to ligand–receptor binding and which is responsible for the observed therapeutic effect. It is the spatial arrangement of key chemical features that are recognized by a receptor and are thus responsible for biological response. Pharmacophore models are typically used when some active compounds have been identified but the 3D structure of the target protein or receptor is unknown. It is possible to derive pharmacophores in several ways, by analogy to a natural substrate, by inference from a series of dissimilar biologically active molecules (active analogue approach) or by direct analysis of the structure of known ligand and target protein.

A pharmacophoric map is a 3D description of a pharmacophore developed by specifying the nature of the key pharmacophoric features and the 3D distance map among all the key features. Figure 1.5 shows a pharmacophore map generated from the DISCO software module of SYBYL. A pharmacophore map may be generated from the superimposition of the active compounds to determine their common features. Given a set of active molecules, the mapping of a pharmacophore involves two steps: (1) analyzing the molecules to identify pharmacophoric features, and (2) aligning the active conformations of the molecules to find the best overlay of the corresponding features. Various pharmacophore mapping algorithms differ in the way they handle the conformational search, feature definition, tolerance definition, and feature alignment [55]. During pharmacophore mapping, generation and optimization of the molecules and the location of ligand points and site points (projections from ligand atoms to atoms in the macromolecule) are carried out. Typical ligand and site points are hydrogen bond donors, hydrogen bond acceptors, and hydrophobic regions such as centers of aromatic rings. A pharmacophore map identifies both the bioactive conformation of each active molecule and how to superimpose and compare, in three dimensions, the various active compounds. The mapping technique identifies what type of points match in what conformations of the compounds.

Besides ligand-based automated approaches, pharmacophore maps can also be generated manually. In such cases, common structural features are identified from a set of experimentally known active compounds. Conformational analysis is carried out to generate different conformations of the molecules and interfeature distances

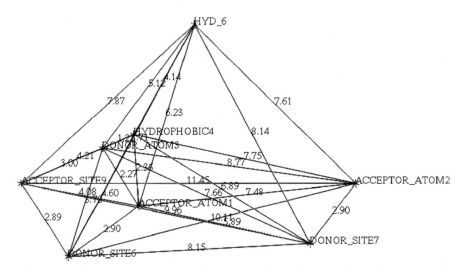

FIGURE 1.5   A pharmacophore map developed from a set of GSK3 inhibitors. The pharmacophore features include hydrogen bond acceptor atoms, hydrogen bond donor atoms, hydrogen bond donor site, hydrogen bond acceptor site, and hydrophobic centers. This 3D picture also shows the distance relationship between various pharmacophoric features present in the map.

are inferred to develop the final models. The receptor mapping technique is also currently in practice to develop pharmacophore models. The important residues required for binding the pharmacophores are identified, which are employed for generating the receptor-based pharmacophores. The structure of protein can be used to generate interaction sites or grids to characterize favorable positions for ligands.

After a pharmacophore map has been derived, there are two ways to identify molecules that share its features and thus elicit the desired response. First is the *de novo* drug design, which seeks to link the disjoint parts of the pharmacophore together with fragments in order to generate hypothetical structures that are chemically novel. Second is the 3D database searching, where large databases comprising 3D structures are searched for those that match to a pharmacophoric pattern. One advantage of the second method is that it allows the ready identification of existing molecules, which are either easily available or have a known synthetic route [56, 57]. Pharmacophore mapping methods are described next.

Distance Comparison Method (DISCO)   The various steps involved in DISCO-based generation of a pharmacophore map are conformational analysis, calculation of the location of the ligand and site points, finding potential pharmacophore maps, and graphics analysis of the results. In the process of conformational search, 3D structures can be generated using any building program like CONCORD, from crystal structures, or from conformational searching and energy minimization with any molecular or quantum mechanical technique. Comparisons of all the duplicate conformations are excluded while comparing all the conformations. If each corresponding interatomic distance between these atoms in the two conformations is less than a threshold (0.4 Å), then the higher energy conformation is rejected. DISCO calculates the location of site points, which can be the location of ligand atoms, or other atom-based points, like centers of rings or a halogen atom, which are points of potential hydrophobic groups. The other point is the location of the hydrogen bond acceptors or donors. The default locations of site hydrogen bond donor and acceptor points are based on literature compilations of observed intermolecular crystallographic contacts in proteins and between the small molecules. Hydrogen bond donors and acceptors such as OH and NH_2 groups can rotate to change the locations of the hydrogen atom.

During the process of performing pharmacophore mapping in DISCO, the user may input the tolerance for each type of interpoint distance. The user may direct the DISCO algorithm to consider all the potential points and to stop when a pharmacophore map with a certain total number of points is found. Alternatively, the user may specify the types of points, and the maximum and minimum number of each, that every superposition must include. It can also be directed to ignore specific compounds if they do not match a pharmacophore map found by DISCO. The user may also specify that only the input chirality is used for certain molecules and that only certain conformations below a certain relative energy should be considered.

The DISCO algorithm involves finding the reference molecule, which is the one with the fewest conformations. The search begins by associating the conformations of each molecule with each other. DISCO then calculates the distances between points in each 3D structure. Then it prepares the corresponding tables that relate interpoint distances in the current reference conformation and distances in every other 3D structure. Distances correspond if the point types are the same. These distances differ by no more than the tolerance limits. The clique-detection algorithm then identifies the largest clique of distances common between the reference XYZ set and every other 3D structure. It then forms union sets for the cliques of each molecule. Finally, the sets with cliques that meet the group conditions are searched [58, 59].

CATALYST   According to the pharmacophore mapping software CATALYST, a conformational model is an abstract representation of the accessible conformational space of a ligand. It is assumed that the biologically active conformation of a ligand (or a close approximation thereof) should be contained within this model. A pharmacophore model (in CATALYST called a hypothesis) consists of a collection of features necessary for the biological activity of the ligands arranged in 3D space, the common ones being hydrogen bond acceptor, hydrogen bond donor, and hydrophobic features. Hydrogen bond donors are defined as vectors from the donor atom of the ligand to the corresponding acceptor atom in the receptor. Hydrogen bond acceptors are analogously defined. Hydrophobic features are located at the centroids of hydrophobic atoms. CATALYST features are associated with position constraints that consist of the ideal location of a particular feature in 3D space surrounded by a spherical tolerance. In order to map the pharmacophore, it is not necessary for a ligand to possess all the appropriate functional groups capable of simultaneously residing within the respective tolerance spheres of the pharmacophoric features. However, the fewer features an inhibitor maps to, the poorer is its fit to them and the lower is its predicted affinity [60–63].

1.4.3 Molecular Docking

There are several possible conformations in which a ligand may bind to an active site, called the binding modes. Molecular docking involves a computational process of searching for a conformation of the ligand that is able to fit both geometrically and energetically into the binding site of a protein. Docking calculations are required to predict the binding mode of new hypothetical compounds. The docking procedure consists of three interrelated components—identification of the binding site, a search algorithm to effectively sample the search space (the set of possible ligand positions and conformations on the protein surface), and a scoring function. In most docking algorithms, the binding site must be predefined, so that the search space is limited to a comparatively small region of the protein. The search algorithm effectively samples the search space of the ligand–protein complex. The scoring function used by the docking algorithm gives a ranking to the set of final solutions generated by the search. The stable structures of a small molecule correspond to minima on the multidimensional energy surface, and different energy calculations are needed to identify the best candidate. Different forces that are involved in binding are electrostatic, electrodynamic, and steric forces and solvent related forces. The free energy of a particular conformation is equal to the solvated free energy at the minimum with a small entropy correction. All energy calculations are based on the assumption that the small molecule adopts a binding mode of lowest free energy within the binding site. The free energy of binding is the change in free energy that occurs upon binding and is given as

$$\Delta G_{\text{binding}} = G_{\text{complex}} - (G_{\text{protein}} + G_{\text{ligand}}) \tag{1.5}$$

where G_{complex} is the energy of the complexed protein and ligand, G_{protein} is the free energy of noninteracting separated protein, and G_{ligand} is the free energy of noninteracting separated ligand.

The common search algorithms used for the conformational search, which provide a balance between the computational expense and the conformational search, include molecular dynamics, Monte Carlo methods, genetic algorithms, fragment-based methods, point complementary methods, distance geometry methods, tabu searches, and systematic searches [64].

Scoring functions are used to estimate the binding affinity of a molecule or an individual molecular fragment in a given position inside the receptor pocket. Three main classes of scoring functions are known, which include force field-based methods, empirical scoring functions, and knowledge-based scoring functions. The force field scoring functions use molecular mechanics force fields for estimating binding affinity. The AMBER and CHARMM nonbonded terms are used as scoring functions in several docking programs. In empirical scoring functions, the binding free energy of the noncovalent receptor–ligand complex is estimated using chemical interactions. These scoring functions usually contain individual terms for hydrogen bonds, ionic interactions, hydrophobic interactions, and binding entropy, as in the case of SCORE employed in DOCK4 and Böhm scoring functions (explained in detail in Section 1.4.4) used in FlexX. In empirical scoring functions, less frequent interactions are usually neglected. Knowledge-based scoring functions try to capture the knowledge about protein–ligand binding that is implicitly stored in the Protein Data Bank by means of statistical analysis of structural data, for example, PMF and

DrugScore functions, Wallqvist scoring function, and the Verkhivker scoring function [5, 37, 65–67]. Various molecular docking software packages are available, such as FlexX [68], Flexidock [58], DOCK [69], and AUTODOCK [70].

FlexX   FlexX is a fragment-based method for docking which handles the flexibility of the ligand by decomposing the ligand into fragments and performs the incremental construction procedure directly inside the protein active site. It allows conformational flexibility of the ligand while keeping the protein rigid. The base fragment or the ligand core is selected such that it has the most potential interaction groups and the fewest alternative conformations. It is placed into the active site and joined to the side chains in different conformations. Placements of the ligand are scored on the basis of protein–ligand interactions and ranked after the estimation of binding energy. The scoring function of FlexX is a modification of Böhm's function developed for the *de novo* design program LUDI. Figure 1.6 shows details of the interaction between a ligand and a receptor, obtained from FlexX molecular docking.

DOCK   DOCK is a simple minimization program that generates many possible orientations of a ligand within a user selective region of the receptor. DOCK is a program for locating feasible binding orientations, given the structures of a "ligand" molecule and a "receptor" molecule [69]. DOCK generates many orientations of one ligand and saves the best scoring orientation. The docking process is handled

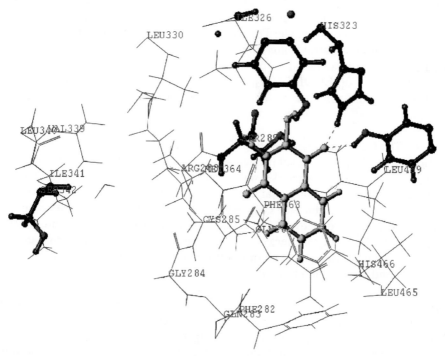

FIGURE 1.6   The result of docking a ligand in the active site of PPARγ. The ligand has a hydrogen bonding interaction with histidine and tyrosine.

in four stages—ligand preparation, site characterization, scoring grid calculation, and finally docking. Site characterization is carried out by constructing site points, to map out the negative image of the active site, which are then used to construct orientations of the ligand. Scoring grid calculations are necessary to identify ligand orientations. The best scoring poses may be viewed using a molecular graphics program and the underlying chemistry may be analyzed.

There are many other widely used molecular docking software packages, like Flexidock (based on genetic algorithm), Autodock (based on Monte Carlo simulations and annealing), MCDOCK (Monte Carlo simulations), FlexE (ensemble of protein structures to account for protein flexibility), and DREAM++ (to dock combinatorial libraries).

1.4.4 De Novo Design

De novo design is a complementary approach to molecular docking: whereas in molecular docking already known ligands are employed, in *de novo* design, ligands are built inside the ligand binding domain. This is an iterative process in which the 3D structure of the receptor is used to build the putative ligand, fragment by fragment, within the receptor groove. Two basic types of algorithms are being widely used in *de novo* design. The first one is the "outside-in-method," in which the binding site is first analyzed to determine which specific functional groups might bind tightly. These separated fragments are then connected together with standard linker units to produce the ligands. The second approach is the "inside-out-method," where molecules are grown within the binding site so as to efficiently fit inside. *De novo* design is the only method of choice when the receptor structure is known but the lead molecules are not available. This method can also be used when lead molecules are known but new scaffolds are being sought. There are several programs developed by various researchers for constructing ligands *de novo*. GROW [71], GRID [72], CAVEAT [73], LUDI [74–77], LEAPFROG [58], GROUPBUILD [78], and SPROUT [79] are some of the *de novo* design programs that have found wide application.

GRID The GRID program developed by Goodford [72] is an active site analysis method where the properties of the active site are analyzed by superimposition with a regular grid. Probe groups like water, methyl group, amine nitrogen, carboxyl oxygen, and hydroxyl are placed at the vertices of the grid and its interaction energy with the protein is calculated at each point using an empirical energy function that determines which kind of atoms and functional groups are best able to interact with the active site. The array of energy values is represented as a contour, which enables identification of regions of attractions between the probe and the protein. It is not a direct ligand generation method but positions simple fragments.

LUDI LUDI, developed by Böhm [74–77], is one of the most widely used automated programs available for *de novo* design. It uses a knowledge-based approach based on rules about the energetically favorable interaction geometries of nonbonded contacts like hydrogen bonds and hydrophobic contacts between the functional groups of the protein and ligand. In LUDI the rules derived from statistical analysis of crystal packings of organic molecules are employed. LUDI is fragment based and works in three steps. It starts by identifying the possible hydrogen bonding donors and acceptors and hydrophobic interactions, both aliphatic and aromatic, in the binding site represented as interaction site points. The site points are positions in the active site where the ligand could form a nonbonded contact. A set of interaction sites encompasses the range of preferred geometries for a ligand atom or functional group involved in the putative interaction, as observed in the crystal structure analyses. LUDI models the H-donor and H-acceptor interaction sites and the aliphatic or aromatic interaction sites. The interaction sites are defined by the distance R, angle α, and dihedral angle ω. The fragments from a 3D database of small molecules are then searched for positioning into suitable interaction sites such that hydrogen bonds can be formed and hydrophobic pockets filled with hydrophobic groups. The suitably oriented fragments are then connected together by spacer fragments to the respective link sites to form the entire molecule. Figure 1.7 shows LUDI generated fragment interaction sites inside the iNOS substrate binding domain.

An empirical but efficient scoring function is used for prioritizing the hit fragments given by LUDI. It estimates the free energy of binding (ΔG) based on the

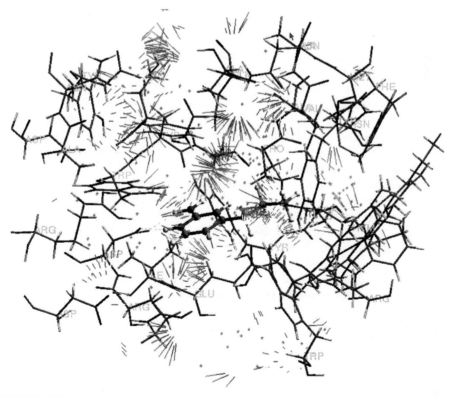

FIGURE 1.7 An example of *de novo* design exercise. In the substrate binding domain of inducible nitric oxide synthase, the stick representation shows the protein structure; ball-and-stick representation belongs to the designed ligand, and the gray sticks point out the interaction sites.

hydrogen bonding, ionic interactions, hydrophobic contact areas, and number of rotatable bonds in the ligand. The LUDI scoring function is given as

$$\Delta G = \Delta G_o + \Delta G_{hb} \sum f(\Delta R)f(\Delta \alpha) + \Delta G_{ion} \sum f(\Delta R)f(\Delta \alpha)$$
$$+ \Delta G_{lipo} A_{lipo} + \Delta G_{rot} NR + \Delta G_{aro/aro} \Delta N_{aro/aro} \qquad (1.6)$$

ΔG_o represents the constant contribution to the binding energy due to loss of translational and rotational entropy of the fragment. ΔG_{hb} and ΔG_{ion} represent the contributions from an ideal neutral hydrogen bond and an ideal ionic interaction, respectively. The ΔG_{lipo} term represents the contribution from lipophilic contact and the ΔG_{rot} term represents the contribution due to the freezing of internal degrees of freedom in the fragment. NR is the number of acyclic sp^3-sp^3 and sp^3-sp^2 bonds.

1.5   PHARMACOINFORMATICS

Information technology provides several databases, data analysis tools, and knowledge extraction techniques in almost every facet of life. In pharmaceutical sciences, several successful attempts are being made under the umbrella of pharmacoinformatics (synonymously referred to as pharmainformatics) (Fig. 1.8). The scope and limitations of this field are not yet understood. However, it may be broadly defined as the application of information technology in drug discovery and development. It encompasses all possible information technologies that eventually contribute to drug discovery. Chemoinformatics and bioinformatics contribute directly to drug discovery through virtual screening. Topics like neuroinformatics, immunoinformatics, vaccine informatics, and biosystem informatics contribute indirectly by providing necessary inputs for pharmaceutical design in this area. Topics like metabolomics, toxicoinformatics, and ADME informatics are contributing to this field by providing information regarding the fate of a NCE/lead *in vitro* and *in vivo* conditions. In this chapter some important aspects of these topics are presented. It is not easy to offer a comprehensive definition of this field at this stage owing to the fact that several bold attempts are being made in this field and initial signals related to a common platform are only emerging. *Drug Discovery Today* made initial efforts in this area by bringing out a supplement on this topic in which it was mainly treated as a scientific discipline with the integration of both bioinformatics and chemoinformatics [80, 81]. Recent trends in this area include several service-oriented themes including healthcare informatics [82], medicine informatics [83], and nursing informatics [84]. Here we present an overview of the current status.

1.5.1   Chemoinformatics

Chemoinformatics deals with information storage and retrieval of chemical data. This has been pioneered principally by the American Chemical Society and Cambridge Crystallographic Databank. However, the term chemoinformatics came into being only recently when methods of deriving science from the chemical databases was recognized. The integration of back-end technologies (for storing and representing chemical structure and chemical libraries) and front-end technologies (for assessing and analyzing the structures and data from the desktop) provides

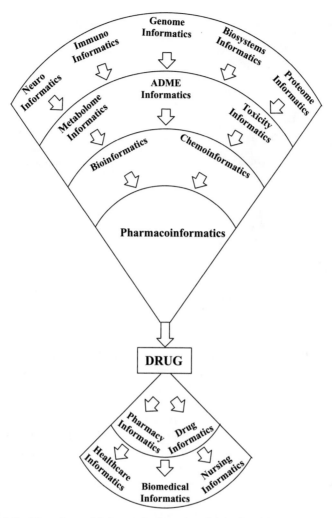

FIGURE 1.8   Flowchart of informatics-based activities in pharmaceutical sciences.

opportunities in chemoinformatics. Virtual screening and high-throughput (HTS) data mining are some of the important chemoinformatics methods.

Chemical data is mostly considered as heuristic data, because it deals with names, properties, reactions, and so on. However, chemoinformatics experts devised many ways of representing chemical data (Fig. 1.9). (1) One-dimensional information of the chemicals can be represented in terms of IUPAC names, molecular formulas, Wiswesser line notation (WLN), SMILES notation, SYBYL line notation (SLN), and so on in addition to numerical representation of physicochemical parameters like molecular weight, molar refractivity, surface area, log P, and pK_a. (2) Two-dimensional chemical information consists of the chemical structural drawings, corresponding hashing, hash codes, connectivity tables, bond matrix, incidence matrix, adjacency matrix, bond-electron matrix, and so on. Graph theoretical procedures are extensively employed in this approach. To get a unique representation of

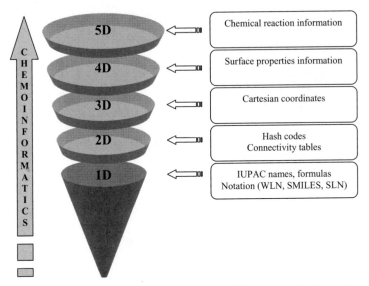

FIGURE 1.9   Information flowchart in chemistry. In this context the dimensionality is not a geometrical dimensionality but an information complexity dimensionality.

chemicals, several algorithms (e.g., Morgan algorithm) were devised, which are found to be extremely important while performing chemical data mining. (3) Three-dimensional representation of structures involves the definition of the Cartesian coordinates of each and every element in the molecule. Along with connection tables, distance matrix, bond angle matrix, and torsional angle matrix, the representations of chemical 3D structures are being made in the form of formatted flat files like .mol and .sdf. (4) Fourth-dimensional information of chemicals is also available in the form of surface properties (e.g., Connolly surface, solvent accessible surface, electron density surfaces, molecular electrostatic potential (MESP), internal structure representation (molecular orbitals)). (5) Fifth-dimensional information about the chemical reactions is of course the most important information about chemical species. This involves defining chemical reaction parameters like inductive effect, resonance effect, polarizability effect, steric effect, and stereochemical effect, on the one hand, and chemical bond formation representations like Hendrickson scheme, Ugi scheme, and InfoChem scheme on the other. Some of the useful chemoinformatics databases include CAS, CSD, STN, MARPAT, UNITY-3D, MACCS-3D, CONCORD, MAYBRIDGE, NCI, and CASReact, which include chemical data in all the possible dimensions as discussed earlier [6, 10, 85–88].

Searching chemical data also requires distinctive methodologies. Search based on hash codes, graph theoretical indices (e.g., Weiner index), charge-related topological indices, Tanimoto coefficients, Carbo coefficient, Hamming distances, Euclidean distance, clique detection, and pharmacophore map searching are some of the important techniques uniquely required in chemoinformatics. Virtual generation of synthesizable chemicals is an important component of this technique. The principles of similarity and diversity need to be employed simultaneously while performing this exercise. Virtual screening is often considered under chemoinformatics, which is discussed in Section 1.5.3 as the most important topic of pharmacoinformatics.

Chemical reaction informatics involves the exploration of synthetic pathways and the designing of new experiments. About 15–20 million reactions are currently available in chemical reaction databases (CASReact, ChemReact, CrossFire Plus, etc.). The chemical reaction informatics would essentially assist the chemist in giving access to reaction information, deriving knowledge, predicting the course and outcome of chemical reactions, and designing syntheses. The main tasks include (1) storing information on chemical reactions, (2) retrieving the information, (3) comparing and analyzing sets of reactions, (4) defining the scope and limitations of a reaction type, (5) developing models of chemical reactivity, (6) predicting the course of the reactions, (7) analyzing reaction networks, and (8) developing methods for the design of syntheses. Chemical reaction databases consist of the following information: (1) reactants and products; (2) atom mapping, which allows you to determine which atom becomes which product atom through the reaction; (3) information regarding reacting center(s); (4) the catalyst used; (5) the atmosphere, including temperature, pressure, and composition; (6) the solvent used; (7) product yield; (8) optical purity, and (9) references to literature.

1.5.2 Bioinformatics

The area of bioinformatics encompasses various fields of molecular biology requiring data handling like genomics, proteomics, sequence analysis, and regulatory networks. Results of the Human Genome Project have triggered several activities in bioinformatics as a result of the complete sequencing of the human genome consisting of approximately 30,000 genes. The data generated in the biology laboratories is being stored in data banks like GenBank (United States), EMBL (Europe), DDBJ (Japan), and Swiss-Prot, as primary data sources. Secondary data banks like PROSITE, Profiles, and Pfam contain the fruits of analyses of the sequences in the primary databases (Table 1.3). These databases are available on the Web as well as on some specialized networks like EMBnet and NCBInet. Apart from the sequence data, data related to gene expression, gene products, and protein interactions are also available, whose management, analysis, and storage are the objectives of bioinformatics. Sequence analysis is the most important aspect of bioinformatics. There are many sequence analysis packages available like the Genetics Computing Group (GCG) package from Accelrys and the EMBOSS suite (European Molecular Biology Open Software Suite) from European Molecular Biology Laboratory (EMBL). Pairwise and multiple alignment algorithms were developed for determining the similarity between the sequences. Dotplot, which gives a dot matrix plot of any two sequences with respect to the amino acid comparison, is the simplest pairwise sequence analysis tool. Sequence identity, if present, becomes evident along diagonal areas in a dotplot. Dynamic programming methods like the Needleman–Wunsch algorithm (global alignment) and Smith–Waterman algorithm (local alignment) provide additional information after inserting necessary gaps. The sequence alignment program GAP from the GCG software and NEEDLE from EMBOSS are for global alignment, whereas BESTFIT from GCG and WATER from EMBOSS are for local alignment. Dynamic programming techniques provide optimal alignment between the amino acid sequences defined by the highest score. The number of matched pairs, mismatched pairs, and gaps can be used in estimating the score of a given pairwise comparison of two sequences. Percent Accepted Mutation matrix

TABLE 1.3   Some Important Bioinformatics Resources

Category	Name	Description	Source
Sequence databases	GenBank	Genetic sequence database	National Center for Biotechnology Information http://www.ncbi.nlm.nih.gov
	EMBL	Nucleic acid and protein databases	European Molecular Biology Laboratory http://www.ebi.ac.uk/embl/index.html
	DDBJ	Nucleic acid database	http://www.ddbj.nig.ac.jp
	UniProt/Swiss-Prot	Protein database	http://www.uniprot.org
	PIR	Protein Information Resource	http://pir.georgetown.edu/pirwww/
Genome databases	dbEST	Expressed Sequence Tags database	http://www.ncbi.nlm.nih.gov/dbEST/index.html
	GDB	Human Genome Database	http://www.gdb.org/
	Ensembl	Genome database	http://www.ensembl.org/index.html
Secondary protein databases	Pfam	Protein family database with multiple sequence alignments and hidden Markov models	http://www.sanger.ac.uk/Software/Pfam/
	Prodom	Protein family and domain database	http://protein.toulouse.inra.fr/prodom/current/html/home.php
	PROSITE	Protein family and domain database	http://us.expasy.org/prosite/details.html
Protein interaction databases	BIND	Biomolecular Interaction Network Database	http://www.bind.ca
	DIP	Database of Interacting Proteins	http://dip.doe-mbi.ucla.edu/
	HPRD	Human Protein Reference Database	http://www.hprd.org/

250 (PAM250) or the BLOsum SUbstitution Matrix 62 (BLOSUM62) for protein sequences are the well accepted scoring matrices. The word k-tuple method is also a widely used sequence search tool, with heuristic algorithms like BLAST (Basic Local Alignment Search Tool) and FASTA. Multiple Sequence Alignment (MSA) methods like CLUSTALW and PILEUP have also been developed for alignment of three or more sequences. Highly conserved regions can be identified from such types of alignments, which is important for identifying members of the same protein family or for studying evolutionary relationships. Most of these tools are available

from the National Center for Biotechnology Information (NCBI) website (http://www.ncbi.nlm.nih.gov). An efficient search engine, ENTREZ, is also provided by NCBI for searching sequences or the related literature. The sequences are stored in various formats like GenBank, EMBL, Swiss-Prot, FASTA, and PIR. Some commercial software packages like the GCG Wisconsin package incorporate the databases and analysis tools, which can be customized for the purpose of end users [89].

Proteomics involves a detailed study of all the proteins present in a cell, their expression, post-translational modifications, interactions with drugs and proteins, and so on. Major technologies in the field of proteomics are mass spectrometry and gel electrophoresis. Proteome informatics deals with the application of informatic tools for proteome analysis. Several databases are available that contain information about the interactions between the proteins—for example, Database of Interacting Proteins (DIP) [90], the General Repository for Interaction Datasets (GRID) [91], the Biomolecular Interaction Network Database (BIND) [92], and the Human Protein Reference Database (HPRD) [93]. The general methods for extracting interaction information from the literature are natural language processing (NLP), naïve Bayes [94], decision trees [95], neural networks, nearest neighbor, and support vector machine (SVM). The prediction of protein functions can also be carried out by a comparative genome analysis. Domain fusion studies, chromosomal proximity studies, and phylogenetic profiling are some methods attempted in the postgenomic scenario to take the sequence information beyond, to the annotation of the proteome. In genome informatics, tools for genome comparison like PipMaker and Artemis Comparison Tool (ACT) and tools from NCBI like HomoloGene and LocusLink are included. Databases that integrate different computational methods to predict functional associations have also been developed, like STRING [96, 97] and POINT [98].

Target identification and target validation are the two major aspects of modern bioinformatics which are relevant to drug discovery. A relatively small number of targets (200–500) have been considered until now for the development of drugs. The traditional target identification process follows the path: assay observation → identification of the key protein → cloning of its gene. This process was bogged down by the dearth of information on several fronts, for example, structural data of proteins. With the recent advances in protein crystallography combined with the 2D- and 3D-NMR experiments, the available structural data improved drastically. This is further supplemented by the *ab initio* fold prediction from the primary sequence data. Thousands of structures can now be determined on an industrial scale. The trends in target identification made a paradigm shift in the recent past from a "deductive" approach involving assay-to-genes path to an "inductive" approach involving genes-to-assay path. The greatest challenge in bioinformatics is to facilitate this paradigm shift by providing automated tools for the identification of new genes as potential targets. Target validation involves the identification of the function of targets in disease states, such that "drugable" targets can be recognized. Experimental efforts in this context can be effectively complemented by computational methods by understanding drug–target interactions. For example, the identification of PPARγ as a target for insulin resistance could be carried out with the effective integration of the results from experimental, computational biology and bioinformatics methods. Initially, a model of *trans*-retinoid acid receptor (RXR) was built on the basis of available crystal structures. Multiple sequence alignment was then carried out on two human retinoic acid receptors and three human PPAR subtypes. Secondary structure prediction and homology modeling were carried out to understand the structure and binding characteristics of PPARγ. Several computational techniques like pattern recognition, artificial neural networks, genetic algorithms, and alignment techniques are being employed in analyzing the data stored in databases. The advances in the area of bioinformatics should lead to an explosion in the number of available target molecules, and contribute tremendously to pharmacoinformatics.

1.5.3   Virtual Screening

Virtual screening is one of the most important technologies of pharmacoinformatics. It employs the databases and analysis tools discussed in the previous sections and pharmacophore mapping and molecular docking discussed under computational medicinal chemistry. This topic is considered under pharmacoinformatics because this technology is being heavily used for hit/lead identification through data search rather than studying molecular interactions and chemical principles. Virtual screening (also called *in silico* screening) provides a fast and cost effective tool for computationally screening compound databases in the search for novel drug leads. Various changes have occurred in the methods of drug discovery, the major ones taking place in the field of high throughput synthesis and screening techniques. The basic goal of virtual screening is the reduction of the huge chemical space of synthesized/virtual molecules and to screen them against a specific target protein virtually. Thus, the field of virtual screening has become an important component of drug discovery programs. Substantial efforts in this area have been made by large pharmaceutical companies. However, there are no well defined standards in virtual screening as yet [37].

Virtual Libraries   Two types of virtual libraries can be generated. One is produced by computational design, with the basic idea to design synthesizable compounds computationally. The other is a virtual library of compounds that are already synthesized. It is possible to extract millions of compounds from these sources and create databases. Virtual libraries are useful in the absence of knowledge about specific drug targets for virtual screening. Focused virtual libraries are important sometimes to save resources as the hit rate is higher in such cases [62].

Various Approaches of Virtual Screening   Virtual screening methods can be roughly divided into target structure-based and small molecule-based approaches, as shown in Table 1.4. When no structural information about the target protein is given, pharmacophore models can be used as filters for screening. These are mostly used when a set of active compounds is known that bind in a similar way to the protein. A pharmacophore capturing these features should be able to identify novel compounds with a similar pattern from the database. These pharmacophores may be generated manually or by automated software packages like CATALYST (HipHop, HypoGen) or DISCO, as described earlier. If the 3D structure of the receptor is known, a pharmacophore model can be derived based on the receptor active site. Usually all the pharmacophore searches are done in two steps: first the

TABLE 1.4   Computational Methods and Tools for Virtual Screening

Target structure-based approaches
   Protein–ligand docking
   Active site-directed pharmacophores
Molecule-based queries
   2D substructures
   3D pharmacophores
   Complex molecular descriptors (e.g., electrotopological)
   Volume- and surface-matching algorithms
Molecular fingerprints
   Keyed 2D fingerprints (each bit position is associated with a specific chemical feature)
   Hashed 2D fingerprints (properties are mapped to overlapping bit segments)
   Multiple-point 3D pharmacophore fingerprints
Compound classification techniques
   Cluster analysis
   Cell-based partitioning (of compounds into subsections of n-dimensional descriptor
     space)
   3D/4D QSAR models
Statistical methods
   Binary QSAR/QSPR
   Recursive partitioning

software confirms whether or not the screened compound has the required atom types or functional groups, and then it checks whether the spatial arrangement of these elements matches the query. In actual practice, receptor-based and small molecule-based approaches can be used in combination, taking into account as much information as possible.

Structure based virtual screening is carried out by docking and scoring techniques. Database of thousands of compounds can be screened against the specific target protein. FlexX [68], Flexidock [58], DOCK [52], and AUTODOCK [70] are the various docking programs employed. Molecular fingerprinting is another technique for performing virtual screening. These search tools consist of varying numbers of bits and encode different types of molecular descriptors and their values. Calculation of descriptors for a given molecule produces a characteristic bit pattern that can be quantitatively compared to others, applying a similarity metric [37].

Various filters can be used during the screening process which improves the chances of obtaining reliable hits. One such filter is the substructure filter. The database may contain certain functional groups in molecules that interact at unwanted sites and are "false positives." Many of these features are called as the substructures that are used to filter datasets. Other filters applied are the molecular weight, the number of rotatable bonds, and the calculated log P. All these considerations have led to the formulation of *Lipinski's rule of five* [99]. These rules suggest whether or not a molecule is going to be absorbed. The criteria for choosing better absorbed molecules are: (1) molecular weight <500, (2) log P < 5, (3) hydrogen bonds donors <5, and (4) hydrogen bond acceptors <10. The rule of five has been derived following a statistical analysis of known drugs. More sophisticated computational models of "drug-likeness" have been developed by employing the techniques of artificial neural networks, decision trees, and genetic algorithms [6].

It is important to realize that virtual screening is expected to produce hits, not leads. The identification of nanomolar inhibitors by database mining is an extremely rare probability. Lead optimization should be taken up to further modulate the structural features. A virtual screening exercise cannot distinguish the agonists; also, in several cases, the inactives are picked up. Hence it is better not to be very narrow toward the end of any virtual screening procedure [62, 63].

Virtual screening can be applied to target-based subset selection from the databases. Statistical approaches like binary QSAR or recursive partitioning can be applied to process HTS results and develop predictive models of biological activity. The developed models can then be employed to select candidate molecules from databases. Similarly, hits from HTS are used in fingerprint searches or compound classification analysis to identify sets of similar molecules. Based on these results, a few compounds are selected for additional testing. Many assumptions are made in virtual screening, and a positive outcome cannot be guaranteed every time. However, the overall process is extremely cost effective and fast. Virtual screening has the ability to produce leads that otherwise may not have been identified. Hence, virtual screening is emerging as a major component of pharmacoinformatics.

1.5.4 Neuroinformatics

Neuroinformatics may be defined as the organization and analysis of neuroscientific data using the tools of information technology. The information sources in neuroinformatics include behavioral sciences (psychological description) and medicinal (including drugs and diagnostic images) and biological (membranes, neurons, synapses, genes, etc.) aspects. The aim of neuroinformatics is to unravel the complex structure–function relationship of the brain in an integrative effort. Neuroscientists work at multiple levels and are producing enormous amounts of data. Distributed databases are being prepared and novel analytical tools are being generated with the help of information technology. Producing digital capabilities for web-based information management systems is one of the major objectives of neuroinformatics. Apart from data sharing, computational modeling of ion channels, neurons and neural networks, second messenger pathways, morphological features, and biochemical reaction are also often included in neuroinformatics. The initial ideas on neuroinformatics can be traced to the work of Hodgkin and Huxley, who initiated computational neuronal modeling. Current efforts in the direction include studies related to modeling the neuropsychological tests, neuroimaging, computational neuroscience, brain mapping, molecular neuroimaging, and magnetic resonance imaging.

Important Databases in Neuroinformatics A probabilistic atlas and reference system for human brain is being developed as a neuroinformatics and neuroscience tool. Such a system is required because of the vast variance observed in the structure, function, and organization of human brain. It is a data source of digital images of human brain along with information on racial and ethnic conditions, education, handedness, personal traits, habits, and so on. It allows one to examine the relationship and distribution of the macro- and microscopic structure and function of human brain [100, 101]. Surface management system (SuMS) is another database that mainly deals with studies of the structure and function of cerebral cortex. All the data generated during reconstruction of cerebral cortex and subsequent flattening procedures is included in this database. SuMS (1) provides a systematic framework for classification and storage, (2) serves as a version control system for the surface and volume datasets, (3) is an efficient data retrieval module, and (4) acts as a service request broker [102, 103]. Similarly, there are many other database systems with data analysis tools available in this field, a few of which are listed in Table 1.5.

TABLE 1.5   Selected List of Important Neuroinformatics Tools and Databases

Databases	Brief Description	URL
Brain Architecture Management System (BAMS)	Repository of brain structure information; contains to date around 40,000 connections	http://brancusi.usc.edu/bkms/
BrainMap	For meta-analysis of human functional brain-mapping literature	http://brainmap.org/
BrainInfo	Information about the brain and its functions	http://braininfo.rprc.washington.edu/
Brede Database	Neuroimaging data	http://hendrix.imm.dtu.dk/services/jerne/brede/
Surface Management System (SuMS)	A surface-based database to aid cortical surface reconstruction, visualization and analysis	http://sumsdb.wustl.edu/sums/index.jsp
fMRIDC	Functional neuroimaging (fMRI) data (fMRI Data Center)	http://www.fmridc.org
LGICdb	Ligand Gated Ion Channel database	http://www.ebi.ac.uk/compneursrv/LGICdb/
ModelDB	Neuronal and Network Models	http://senselab.med.yale.edu/senselab/ModelDB
CoCoMac	Collation of Connectivity data on the Macaque brain	http://cocomac.org/home.htm
L-Neuron	Computational Neuroanatomy Database	http://www.krasnow.gmu.edu/LNeuron
NeuroScholar	MySQL Database frontend with management of bibliography, histological and tracing data	http://www.neuroscholar.org
Catacomb	Components and Tools for Accessible Computer Modeling in Biology (Modeling Software for Neuroscience)	http://www.compneuro.org/catacomb/index.shtml
GENESIS	Neural Simulator	http://www.genesissim.org/GENESIS/
Channel Lab	Single channel modeling program	http://www.synaptosoft.com/Channelab/index.html
NEURON	Simulation of individual neurons and networks of neurons	http://www.neuron.yale.edu
HHsim	Graphical Hodgkin–Huxley Simulator	http://www.cs.cmu.edu/~dst/HHsim/
NEOSIM	Neural Open Simulation—for modeling of networks	http://www.neosim.org/
NANS	Neuron and Network Simulator	http://vlsi.eecs.harvard.edu/research/nans.html
SNNAP	Simulator for Neural Networks and Action Potentials	http://snnap.uth.tmc.edu/

Several software tools have been made available over the past few years in the field of neuroinformatics. Neuroscholar [104] allows scientists to interact with information in the literature in a modular fashion. This tool permits the user to isolate fragments of data from a source and then bring them together to prepare a fact base for analysis and interpretation in a knowledge base environment. GENESIS (General Neural Simulation System) is a tool that helps in the simulation of neurosystems including subcellular components, biochemical reactions, single neurons, large neural networks, and system level models.

The Human Brain Project is one of the major initiatives under neuroinformatics. This is a broad based effort by neuroscientists and information scientists whose objective is to produce interoperable databases and analysis tools. This project included several tools for modeling simulation, information retrieval from multidisciplinary data, graphical interfaces, and integration of data analysis tools through electronic collaboration [105].

1.5.5   Immunoinformatics

Immunoinformatics is another major area in biomedical research where computational and informational technologies are playing a major role in the development of drugs and vaccines. This field is still in its infancy and it covers both modeling and informatics of the immune system and is the application of informatics technology to the study of immunological macromolecules, addressing important questions in immunobiology and vaccinology. Data sources for immunoinformatics include experimental approaches and theoretical models, both demanding validation at every stage. Major immunological developments include immunological databases, sequence analysis, structure modeling, modeling of the immune system, simulation of laboratory experiments, statistical support for immunological experimentation, and immunogenomics [106, 107]

There are many databases of relevance to immunologists, some of which are given in Table 1.6. IMGT, the international ImMunoGeneTics information system created in 1989, is one of the important ventures in immunoinformatics and is a knowledge resource comprising databases, tools, resources on immunoglobulins, T cell receptors, major histocompatibility complex (MHC), and related proteins of the immune system. IMGT includes sequence and genome databases with different interfaces, 3D structure database, web resources, and interactive tools for sequence and genome analysis. IMGT ONTOLOGY, which is a semantic specification of the terms to be used in immunogenetics and immunoinformatics, is available for IMGT users in the IMGT Scientific chart formalized in IMGT-ML (XML) schema [108–114]. The HIV Molecular Immunology Database is a database containing sequence and epitope maps of HIV-1 cytotoxic and helper T-cell epitopes.

Computer-aided vaccine design (CAVD) or computational vaccinology is another application of immunoinformatics involving prediction of immunogenicity. Immune interactions can be modeled using artificial neural networks (ANNs), hidden Markov models, molecular modeling, binding motifs, and quantitative matrices, of which ANN models have proved to be superior for the prediction of MHC-binding peptides [115–117]. Table 1.6 also gives a list of some of the tools for predicting whether or not a peptide would bind to a major histocompatibility complex. In addition to immunoinformatics, theoretical immunology is another related discipline and is the

TABLE 1.6   Some Selected Immunoinformatics Databases and Tools

Databases and Tools	Brief Description	URL
IMGT, the international ImMunoGeneTics information system	A sequence, genome, and structure database for immunogenetics data	http://imgt.cines.fr
HIV Molecular Immunology Database	A database of HIV-specific B-cell and T-cell responses	http://www.hiv.lanl.gov/content/ immunology/index.html
MHCBN	Comprehensive database of MHC-binding, nonbinding peptides and T-cell epitopes	http://bioinformatics.uams.edu/ mirror/mhcbn/
MHCPEP	Database of MHC-binding peptides	http://wehih.wehi.edu.au/ mhcpep/
ADABase (Mutation Registry for Adenosine Deaminase Deficiency)	Contains information on diseases and mutations associated with adenosine deaminase	http://bioinf.uta.fi/ADAbase/
BCIPep	Database of B-cell epitopes	http://bioinformatics.uams.edu/ mirror/bcipep/
FIMM	Database of Functional Immunology	http://research.i2r.a-star.edu.sg/ fimm/
IPD (Immuno Polymorphism Database)	Database for the study of polymorphism in genes of the immune system	http://www.ebi.ac.uk/ipd/
DHR (The Database of Hypersensitive Response)	Definition, source, and sequence of hypersensitive response (HR) proteins, etc.	http://sdbi.sdut.edu.cn/hrp/
VBASE2	Database of variable genes from the immunoglobulin loci	http://www.vbase2.org/
BIMAS	Bioinformatics and Molecular Analysis Section (MHC peptide-binding prediction)	http://bimas.dcrt.nih.gov/ molbio/hla_bind/
SYFPEITHI	Database and prediction server of MHC ligands	http://www.syfpeithi.de/
ProPred	MHC Class I and II Binding Peptide Server	http://www.imtech.res.in/ raghava/propred/ http://www.imtech.res.in/ raghava/propred1/
nHLAPred	A neural network-based MHC Class I Binding Peptide Prediction Server	http://bioinformatics.uams.edu/ mirror/nhlapred/
NetMHC	Peptide-binding prediction using artificial neural networks (ANNs) and weight matrices	http://www.cbs.dtu.dk/services/ NetMHC/
MHCPred	Predict binding affinity for MHC I and II molecules	http://www.jenner.ac.uk/ MHCPred/

application of mathematical modeling to diverse aspects of immunology ranging from T-cell selection in the thymus to the epidemiology of vaccination. The results from immunoinformatics are being heavily employed in defining another emerging science called Artificial Immune Systems (immunological computation or immuno-computing). The AIS computation is also of interest in modeling the immune system and solving immunological problems [118].

1.5.6   Drug Metabolism Informatics

An understanding of the pharmacokinetics of a drug can play a major role in reducing the probability of bringing a new chemical entity (NCE) with inappropriate ADME/Toxicity profile to the market. Drug metabolism and toxicity in the human body are primarily assessed during clinical trials, and preclinical assessment of the same involves study on *in vivo* and *in vitro* systems. *In silico* models for predicting pharmacokinetic properties based on the experimental results can greatly reduce the cost and time required for the experiments. These methods range from modeling approaches such as QSARs, to similarity searches as well as informatics methods like ligand–protein docking and pharmacophore modeling. Several ADME properties can be explained by simple molecular descriptors derived from the 2D chemical structure and can be used for the development of QSAR models. Such *in silico* prediction methods help chemists in judging whether or not a potential candidate may continue in the drug discovery pipeline. Metabolic biotransformation of any NCE may profoundly affect the bioavailability, activity, distribution, toxicity, and elimination of a compound; the effects of probable metabolism are now considered in the early stages of drug discovery with the help of computer-aided methods.

In silico prediction of metabolic biotransformation occurring at the liver cytochrome enzymes (CYP450 enzymes) are being studied [119]. Many databases and software systems are available in this field for the early prediction of substrates of CYP450 enzymes. Some of the databases and predictive systems for metabolic information of drugs are given in Table 1.7. The Human Drug Metabolism Database (hDMdb) project is a nonprofit, internet database of xenobiotic metabolic transformations that are observed in humans [120]. Other databases like MDL Metabolite contain xenobiotic transformation information that can also be linked to a toxicity database like MDL Toxicity database. Thus, it can give toxicity, if present, in the metabolite shown by the database. The predictive systems available for metabolism are mainly expert systems based on experimental data representing the metabolic effects (database) and/or rules derived from such data (rule-base). The rules may either be induced rules, which are quantitative, derived from a statistical analysis of the metabolic data, or knowledge-based rules derived from expert judgment. Some of the expert systems are MetabolExpert, METEOR, and META, as given in Table 1.7. These can also be linked to the corresponding toxicity prediction modules. METEOR covers both phase I and phase II biotransformation reactions and can analyze mass spectrometry data from metabolism studies. It can be linked to the DEREK software for toxicity prediction of the metabolites. Likewise, Metabol-Expert can be linked to HazardExpert and META can be interfaced with MULTI-CASE, both of which are toxicity prediction modules. MetabolExpert is an open knowledge base, where the user can add his/her own rules. The META program operates from dictionaries of transformation operators, created by experts to rep-

TABLE 1.7 Databases and Tools for Metabolism Informatics

Databases and Tools	Brief Description	URL
Human Drug Metabolism Database (hDMdb)	IUPAC project for a web-based model database for human drug metabolism information	http://www.iupac.org/projects/2000/2000-010-1-700.html
MDL Metabolite	Comprised of a database, registration system, and browsing interface	http://www.mdl.com/products/predictive/metabolite/index.jsp
Accelrys' Metabolism Database	Biotransformations of organic molecules in a variety of species	http://www.accelrys.com/products/chem_databases/databases/metabolism.html
Biofrontier/P450	Human cytochrome P450 information and predictive system	http://www.fqs.pl/
Metabolism and Transport Drug Interaction database	Database developed by University of Washington	http://www.druginteractioninfo.org/
MetabolExpert (CompuDrug, Inc.)	Predictive system for metabolic fate of a drug	http://www.compudrug.com/
MEXAlert (CompuDrug, Inc.)	Rule-based prediction for first-pass metabolism	http://www.compudrug.com/
META (Multicase, Inc.)	Uses dictionaries to create metabolic paths of query molecules	http://www.multicase.com/products/prod05.htm
METEOR (LHASA Ltd., Leeds, UK)	Predictions presented as metabolic trees	http://www.lhasalimited.org/

resent known metabolic paths, and is capable of predicting the sites of potential enzymatic attack and the metabolites formed [121].

1.5.7 Toxicoinformatics

Early prediction of toxicological parameters of new chemical entities (NCEs) is an important requirement in the drug discovery strategy today. This is being emphasized in the wake of many drug withdrawals in the recent past. Computational methods for predicting toxicophoric features is a cost effective approach toward saving experimental efforts and saving animal life. Current efforts in toxicoinformatics are mainly based on QSTR (quantitative structure–toxicity relationships) and rule-based mechanistic methods [122–125]. QSTR is a statistical approach, in which a correlation is developed between structural descriptors of a series of compounds and their toxicological data. In this approach, a model can be trained with the help of a set of known data, validated using many approaches, and then used for the prediction of toxicological parameters. The only limitation of this approach is that the predictive power of these models gets reduced when chemicals belonging to a class outside the series of molecules is used for the construction of the model. Toxicity prediction tools using this approach include TOPKAT and CASE/M-CASE.

TOPKAT mainly employs electrotopological descriptors based on graph theory for the development of QSTR models. TOPKAT uses linear free-energy relationships in statistical regression analysis of a series of compounds. In this software, the continuous/dichotomous toxicity end points are correlated to the structural features like electronic topological descriptors, shape descriptors, and substructure descriptors. CASE (Computer Automated Structure Evaluation) and M-CASE are toxicoinformatics software packages that have the capability to automatically generate predictive models. A hybrid QSTR artificial expert system-based methodology is adopted in CASE-based systems. A linear scale called "CASE units" is defined, which segregate the given set of molecules as active/inactive/marginally toxic species. Molecular fragments are classified in terms of biophores (fragments associated with activity) and biophobes (fragments associated with inactivity). One advantage of these packages is that they also include experimental data that is not released by the FDA, which increases the applicability of this set of packages.

Toxicity prediction tools based on "mechanistic approaches" are knowledge based-systems, where a fact base and rule base can be effectively analyzed to give qualitative information regarding the toxicity of chemical species. The expert rules included in the knowledge base are generally derived from the molecular mechanism of the drug action and hence they are known as "mechanistic approaches." Well known software packages in this category are DEREK (Deductive Estimation of Risk from Existing Knowledge), HazardExpert, and Oncologic. DEREK is a widely used toxicity prediction system. This program not only predicts the potential toxicity of a query chemical but also provides details of the logical process that leads to the predicted results. Table 1.8 gives a list of known resources in toxicoinformatics.

1.5.8   Cancer informatics

Application of information technology has been extended to specific subtopics of pharmaceutical sciences like cancer, diabetes, and AIDS. One important example, wherein information technology is being extensively used, is cancer informatics. The necessity of such focused subtopics of pharmacoinformatics was required because of the overflow of information and lack of integrated data formats. Major cancer informatics initiatives are being undertaken by the National Cancer Institute Center for Bioinformatics (NCICB), National Institutes of Health (United States), National Cancer Research Institute (NCRI) (United Kingdom), and the National Cancer Center (NCC) (Japan).

A web-based environment called CaCORE (Cancer Common Ontologic Reference Environment) was established, which helps in the management, redistribution, integration, and analysis of data arising from studies involving cell and molecular biology, genomics, histopathology, drug development, and clinical trials. The structural and functional components of CaCORE include (1) Enterprise Vocabulary Services (EVS), which provide terminology development, dictionary, and thesaurus services like the description-logics based NCI Thesaurus and the NCI Metathesaurus, which is a collection of biomedical vocabularies based on National Library of Medicine (NLM) and the Unified Medical Language System (UMLS); (2) The Cancer Data Standards Repository (CaDSR), which is a metadata registry for

TABLE 1.8 Toxicoinformatics Tools

Tools	Description	URL	Predicted Endpoints
TOPKAT	QSAR	Accelrys http://www.accelrys.com/ products/topkat	Mutagenicity, carcinogenicity, mammalian acute and chronic toxicities, developmental toxicities
M-CASE, CASE, ToxAlert, Casetox	Hybrid QSAR and expert system	Multicase Inc. http://www.multicase. com	Carcinogenicity, mutagenicity, teratogenicity, mammalian acute and chronic toxicities
DEREK	Knowledge based, structural rules	Lhasa Limited http://www.lhasalimited. org/	Mutagenicity, carcinogenicity, teratogenicity/ developmental toxicity, skin sensitization, acute toxicity, etc.
OncoLogic	Knowledge based	www.oncologic.net	Carcinogenicity
HazardExpert	Knowledge based	CompuDrug http://www.compudrug. com	Carcinogenicity, mutagenicity, teratogenicity, membrane irritation, neurotoxicity
COMPACT	QSAR; mechanistic supported by molecular modeling studies	Surrey	Cytochrome P450 metabolism

common data elements that have been identified to simplify and standardize the data collection requirements and eligibility/exclusion criteria; and (3) the Cancer Bioinformatics Infrastructure Objects (CaBIO) module, which provides the data interface architecture [126–128].

Apart from the web-based facilities, several machine learning techniques like artificial neural networks and decision trees are also being utilized for cancer detection and diagnosis and more recently for prediction and prognosis. Several bioinformatics resources that are helpful in gene function prediction, in protein structure and function predictions, and in studies of protein–protein interactions are being employed in cancer informatics as well [129]. Several specific databases like PDQ, CGED, and FaCD (Table 1.9) are being heavily used by cancer informatics specialists. The NCI chemical databank is a source of all the chemicals tested for anticancer effects.

TABLE 1.9   Cancer Informatics Resources

Databases	Brief Descvription	URL
PDQ (Physician Data Query)	NCI's Comprehensive Cancer Database	http://www.cancer.gov/ cancertopics/pdq/ cancerdatabase
CGED (Cancer Gene Expression Database)	Database of gene expression profile and accompanying clinical information	http://cged.hgc.jp/
Mouse Retroviral Tagged Cancer Gene Database	Retroviral and transposon insertional mutagenesis in mouse tumors	http://rtcgd.ncifcrf.gov
The Familial Cancer Database (FaCD)	Assists in the differential diagnosis in familial cancer	http://facd.uicc.org/
International Agency for Research on Cancer (IARC) p53 Mutation database	Information on TP53 gene mutations	http://www.iarc.fr/p53/
The Tumor Gene Database	Information on genes that are targets for cancer-causing mutations	http://condor.bcm.tmc. edu/oncogene.html
SNP500Cancer Database	Central Resource for Sequence verification of SNPs	http://snp500cancer. nci.nih.gov

1.6   FUTURE SCOPE

The field of computer-aided drug development has undergone a paradigm shift in the past five years. Earlier, this subject was dominated by chemistry and physics of drug discovery, mainly through molecular modeling, QSAR. A dramatic increase has been noted in these two topics—several practical solutions are being offered and novel concepts are being introduced. At the same time an additional component is emerging in CADD through informatics. The current status of CADD includes both modeling and informatics with equal and synergistic contributions. Although a lot has been done in this area over the past twenty years, there is still a lot of scope left for future growth. First and foremost is winning the confidence of the experimental colleague, who is still skeptical about the value of these efforts. Second is the proper integration of modeling efforts and informatics efforts. Although virtual screening has proved to be highly successful, the methodologies being adopted lack common elements. Often the methods adopted in CADD are considered as technological components, although several fundamentals exist. In fact, the fundamentals of the field of drug discovery are only emerging. CADD methods should strongly contribute in establishing these fundamentals; efforts should be concentrated in this direction.

REFERENCES

1. http://www.cambridgesoft.com.
2. http://www.acdlabs.com/download/chemsk.html.

3. http://www.chemsw.com.

4. Goodman JM. *Chemical Applications of Molecular Modeling.* Cambridge, UK: Royal Society of Chemistry; 1998.

5. Holtje HD, Sippl W, Rognan D. *Molecular Modeling Basic Principles and Applications,* 2nd ed. Weinheim: Wiley-VCH Verlag GmbH; 2003.

6. Leach AR, Gillet VJ. *An Introduction to Chemoinformatics.* Dordrecht: Kluwer Academics; 2003.

7. Levine IN. *Quantum Chemistry,* 4th ed. Englewood Cliffs, NJ: Prentice-Hall; 1991.

8. Szabo A, Ostlund S. *Modern Quantum Chemistry.* New York: MacMillan; 1982.

9. Foresman JB, Frisch AE. *Exploring Chemistry with Electronic Structure Methods,* 2nd ed. Pittsburgh: Gaussian Inc.; 1995.

10. Gasteiger J, Engel T. *Chemoinformatics: A Textbook.* Weinheim: Wiley-VCH Verlag GmbH; 2003.

11. Howard AE, Kollman PA. An analysis of current methodologies for conformational searching of complex molecules. *J Med Chem* 1998;31:1669–1675.

12. Lipton M, Still WC. The multiple minimum problem in molecular modeling. Tree searching internal coordinate conformational space. *J Comput Chem* 1988;9:343–355.

13. Dammkoehler RA, Karasek SF, Shands EF, Marshall GR. Constrained search of conformational hyperspace. *J Comput Aided Mol Des* 1989;3:3–21.

14. Saunders M. Stochastic exploration of molecular mechanics energy surfaces. Hunting for the global minimum. *J Am Chem Soc* 1987;109:3150–3152.

15. Saunders M. Stochastic search for the conformations of bicyclic hydrocarbons. *J Comput Chem* 1989;10:203–208.

16. Ferguson DM, Raber DJ. A new approach to probing conformational space with molecular mechanics: random incremental pulse search. *J Am Chem Soc* 1989;111:4371–4378.

17. Chang G, Guida WC, Still WC. An internal-coordinate Monte Carlo method for searching conformational space. *J Am Chem Soc* 1989;111:4379–4386.

18. Saunders M, Houk KN, Wu YD, Still WC, Lipton M, Chang G, Guida, WC. Conformations of cycloheptadecane. A comparison of methods for conformational searching. *J Am Chem Soc* 1990;112:1419–1427.

19. Lybrand TP, Computer simulation of biomolecular systems using molecular dynamics and free energy perturbation methods, in *Reviews in Computational Chemistry.* Hoboken, NJ: Wiley-VCH; 1990, pp 295–320.

20. Bourne PE, Weissig H. *Structural Bioinformatics (Methods of Biochemical Analysis).* Hoboken, NJ: Wiley-Liss; 2003.

21. Clote P, Backofen R. Computational *Molecular Biology: An Introduction.* Hoboken, NJ: Wiley; 2000.

22. Dunbrack RL Jr, Karplus M. Conformational analysis of the backbone-dependent rotamer preferences of protein sidechains. *Nat Struct Biol* 1994;1:334–340.

23. Park BH, Levitt M. The complexity and accuracy of discrete state models of protein structure. *J Mol Biol* 1995;249:493–507.

24. Sternberg MJE. *Protein Structure Prediction: A Practical Approach (The Practical Approach Series).* New York: Oxford University Press; 1997.

25. Randíc M. Characterization of molecular branching. *J Am Chem Soc* 1975;97: 6609–6615.

26. Kier LB, Hall LH. *Molecular Connectivity in Chemistry and Drug Research.* New York: Academic Press; 1976.

27. Kier LB, Hall LH. *Molecular Connectivity in Structure–Activity Analysis*. Hoboken, NJ: Wiley; 1986.

28. Müller WR, Szymanski K, Knop JV, Trinajstic N. An algorithm for construction of the molecular distance matrix. *J Comput Chem* 1987;8:170–173.

29. Wiener H. Structural determination of paraffin boiling points. *J Am Chem Soc* 1947;69:17–20.

30. Hosoya H. Topological index. A newly proposed quantity characterizing the topological nature of structural isomers of saturated hydrocarbons. *Bull Chem Soc Jpn* 1971;44:2332–2339.

31. Bonchev D. *Information Theoretic Indices for Characterization of Chemical Structures*. Hoboken, NJ: Wiley; 1983.

32. Balaban AT. Highly discriminating distance-based topological index. *Chem Phys Lett* 1982;89:399–404.

33. Kier LB. A shape index from molecular graphs. *Quant Struct-Activity Relat* 1985;4: 109–116.

34. Kier LB, Hall LH, Frazer JW. An index of electrotopological state for atoms in molecules. *J Math Chem* 1991;7:229–241.

35. Todeschini R, Consonni V. *Handbook of Molecular Descriptors*. Weinheim: Wiley-VCH Verlag GmbH; 2000.

36. Karelson M, Lobanov VS, Katritzky AR. Quantum-chemical descriptors in QSAR/QSPR studies. *Chem Rev* 1996;96:1027–1044.

37. Abraham DJ. *Burger's Medicinal Chemistry & Drug Discovery*, 6th ed. Hoboken, NJ: Wiley-Interscience; 2003.

38. Hansch C, Leo A, Heller SR. *Exploring QSAR: Volume 1: Fundamentals and Applications in Chemistry and Biology*. Washington DC: American Chemical Society; 1995.

39. Kubinyi H, QSAR: Hansch analysis and related approaches. In *Methods and Principles in Medicinal Chemistry*. Weinheim: VCH; 1993.

40. Kubinyi H, *QSAR In Drug Design. Theory, Methods and Applications*. Leiden: ESCOM; 1993.

41. Cramer RDI, Patterson DE, Bunce JD. Comparative molecular field analysis (CoMFA). 1. Effect of shape on binding of steroids to carrier proteins. *J Am Chem Soc* 1988;110:5959–5967.

42. Klebe G, Abraham U, Meitzner T. Molecular similarity indices in a comparative analysis (CoMSIA) of drug molecules to correlate and predict their biological activity. *J Med Chem* 1994;37:4130–4146.

43. Robinson DD, Winn PJ, Lyne PD, Richards WG. Self-organizing molecular field analysis: a tool for structure–activity studies. *J Med Chem* 1999;42:573–583.

44. Silverman BD, Platt DE. Comparative molecular moment analysis (CoMMA): 3D-QSAR without molecular superposition. *J Med Chem* 1996;39:2129–2140.

45. Kubinyi H. Comparative molecular field analysis (CoMFA), in *The Encyclopedia of Computational Chemistry*. Chichester: Wiley; 1998, pp 448–460.

46. Wise M, Cramer RD, Smith D, Exman I. Progress in three-dimensional drug design: the use of real-time colour graphics and computer postulation of bioactive molecules in DYLOMMS. In *Quantitative Approaches to Drug Design*. Amsterdam: Elsevier; 1983, pp 145–146.

47. Pastor M, Cruciani G, Watson KAA. Strategy for the incorporation of water molecules present in a ligand binding site into a three-dimensional quantitative structure–activity relationship analysis. *J Med Chem* 1997;40:4089–4102.

48. Polanski J, Walczak B. The comparative molecular surface analysis (COMSA): a novel tool for molecular design. *Comput Chem* 2000;24:615–625.

49. Ivanciuc O, Ivanciuc T, Cabrol-Bass D. Comparative receptor surface analysis (CoRSA) model for calcium channel antagonists. *SAR QSAR Environ Res* 2002;12:93–111.

50. Hariprasad V, Kulkarni VM. A proposed common spatial pharmacophore and the corresponding active conformations of some peptide leukotriene receptor antagonists. *J Comput Aided Mol Des* 1996;10:284–292.

51. Vedani A, Briem H, Dobler M, Dollinger H, McMasters DR. Multiple-conformation and protonation-state representation in 4D-QSAR: the neurokinin-1 receptor system. *J Med Chem* 2000;43:4416–4427.

52. Vedani A, Dobler M, Dollinger H, Hasselbach KM, Birke F, Lill MA. Novel ligands for the chemokine receptor-3 (CCR3): a receptor-modeling study based on 5D-QSAR. *J Med Chem* 2005;48:1515–1527.

53. Vedani A, Dobler M. 5D-QSAR: the key for simulating induced fit? *J Med Chem* 2002;45:2139–2149.

54. Vedani A, Dobler M, Lill MA. Combining protein modeling and 6D-QSAR. Simulating the binding of structurally diverse ligands to the estrogen receptor. *J Med Chem* 2005;48:3700–3703.

55. Martin YC, Bures M, Dahaner, E. A fast approach to pharmacophore mapping and its applications to dopaminergic and benzodiazepine agonists. *J Comput Aided Mol Des* 1993;7:83–102.

56. Marriott DP, Dougall IB, Meghani P, Liu Y-J, Flower DR. Lead generation using pharmacophore mapping and three-dimensional database searching: application to muscarinic M(3) receptor antagonists. *J Med Chem* 1999;42:3210–3216.

57. Sutter J, Güner OF, Hoffmann R, Li H, Waldman M. *Pharmacophore, Perception Development and Use In Drug Design*. La Jolla, CA: International University Line, 2000, pp 504–506.

58. *SYBYL7.0*, Tripos Inc, 1699 South Hanley Rd, St Louis, MO 631444, USA. http://www.tripos.com.

59. Gardiner EJ, Artymiuk PJ, Willett P. Clique-detection algorithms for matching three-dimensional molecular structures. *J Mol Graph Model* 1997;15:245–253.

60. Sprague PW. Automated chemical hypothesis generation and database searching with CATALYST. In *Perspectives in Drug Discovery and Design*. Leiden: ESCOM Science; 1995, pp 1–20.

61. *CATALYST4.10*, Biosyn-MSI, San Diego, CA, USA, 2005. http://www.accelrys.com.

62. Bajorath J. Virtual screening in drug discovery: methods, expectations and reality. *Curr Drug Discov* 2002, pp 24–28.

63. Klebe G. *Virtual Screening: An Alternative or Complement to High Throughput Screening?* Berlin: Springer; 2000.

64. Leach AR. *Molecular Modelling: Principles and Applications*, 2nd ed. Boston: Addison Wesley Longman, Harlow; 1996.

65. Cohen N. *Guidebook on Molecular Modeling in Drug Design*. San Drego, CA: Academic Press; 1996.

66. Charifson PS. *Practical Application of Computer-Aided Drug Design*. New York: Marcel Dekker; 1997.

67. Schneider G, Bohm H-J. Virtual screening and fast automated docking methods. *Drug Discov Today* 2002;7:64–70.

68. Rarey M, Kramer B, Lengauer T, Klebe G. A fast flexible docking methods using an incremental construction algorithm. *J Mol Biol* 1996;261:470–489.

69. Kuntz ID, Blaney JM, Oatley SJ, Langridge R, Ferrin TE. A geometric approach to macromolecule–ligand interactions. *J Mol Biol* 1982;161:269–288.

70. Morris GM, Goodsell DS, Huey R, Olson AJ. Distributed automated docking of flexible ligands to proteins: parallel applications of AutoDock2.4. *J Comput Aided Mol Des* 1996;10:293–304.

71. Moon JB, Howe WJ. Computer design of bioactive molecules: a method for receptor-based *de novo* ligand design. *Proteins* 1991;11:314–328.

72. Goodford PJ. A computational procedure for determining energetically favorable binding sites on biologically important macromolecules. *J Med Chem* 1985;28:849–857.

73. Lauri G, Bartlett PA. CAVEAT: a program to facilitate the design of organic molecules. *J Comput Aided Mol Des* 1994;8:51–66.

74. Böhm HJ. LUDI: rule-based automatic design of new substituents for enzyme inhibitor leads. *J Comput Aided Mol Des* 1992;6:593–606.

75. Böhm HJ. The computer program LUDI: a new method for the *de novo* design of enzyme inhibitors. *J Comput Aided Mol Des* 1992;6:61–78.

76. Böhm HJ. A novel computational tool for automated structure-based drug design. *J Mol Recognit* 1993;6:131–137.

77. Böhm HJ. The development of a simple empirical scoring function to estimate the binding constant for a protein–ligand complex of known three-dimensional structure. *J Comput Aided Mol Des* 1994;8:243–256.

78. Rotstein SH, Murcko MA. GroupBuild: a fragment-based method for *de novo* drug design. *J Med Chem* 1993;36:1700–1710.

79. Gillet V, Johnson AP, Mata P, Sike S, Williams P. SPROUT: a program for structure generation. *J Comput Aided Mol Des* 1993;7:127–153.

80. Gund P, Sigal N. Applying information systems to high-throughput screening and analysis. In *Pharmainformatics: A Trend Guide. Drug Discor Today 1999; (Suppl)*, 25–29.

81. Bharatam PV. Pharmacoinformatics: IT solutions for drug discovery and development, *CRIPS (Current Research and Information on Pharmaceutical Sciences)*, 2003;4:2–5.

82. Hanson CW. *Healthcare Informatics.* New York: McGraw-Hill Professional; 2005.

83. Goodman KW. *Ethics, Computing, and Medicine: Informatics and the Transformation of Health Care*, 1st ed. Cambridge, UK: Cambridge University Press; 1998.

84. Saba VK, McCormick KA. *Essentials of Nursing Informatics*, 4th ed. New York: McGraw-Hill Medical; 2005.

85. Gadre SR, Shirsat RN. *Electrostatics of Atoms and Molecules.* Hyderabad: Universities Press (India) Limited; 2000.

86. Oprea TI. Chemoinformatics in drug discovery. In *Methods and Principles in Medicinal Chemistry*, Vol 23. Weinheim: Wiley-VCH Verlag GmbH; 2005.

87. Gasteiger J. Handbook on chemoinformatics: from data to knowledge, In *Representation of Molecular Structures.* Hoboken, NJ: Wiley; 2003.

88. Bajorath J. Chemoinformatics: concepts, methods, and tools for drug discovery. In *Methods in Molecular Biology.* Totowa, NJ: Humana Press; 2004.

89. Mount DW. *Bioinformatics: Sequence and Genome Analysis.* Cold Spring Harbor, NY: Cold Spring Harbor Laboratory Press; 2001.

90. Xenarios I, Salwinski L, Duan XJ, Higney P, Kim SM, Eisenberg D. DIP, the Database of Interacting Proteins: a research tool for studying cellular networks of protein interactions. *Nucleic Acids Res* 2002;30:303–305.

91. Breitkreutz BJ, Stark C, Tyers M. The GRID: the General Repository for Interaction Datasets. *Genome Biol* 2003;4:R23.

92. Bader GD, Betel D, Hogue CW. BIND: the Biomolecular Interaction Network Database. *Nucleic Acids Res* 2003;31:248–250.

93. Peri S, Navarro JD, Kristiansen TZ, Amanchy R, Surendranath V, Muthusamy B, Gandhi TK, Chandrika KN, Deshpande N, Suresh S, Rashmi BP, Shanker K, Padma N, Niranjan V, Harsha HC, Talreja N, Vrushabendra BM, Ramya MA, Yatish AJ, Joy M, Shivashankar HN, Kavitha MP, Menezes M, Choudhury DR, Ghosh N, Saravana R, Chandran S, Mohan S, Jonnalagadda CK, Prasad CK, Kumar-Sinha C, Deshpande KS, Pandey A. Human protein reference database as a discovery resource for proteomics. *Nucleic Acids Res* 2004;32:D497–501.

94. Marcotte EM, Xenarios I, Eisenberg D. Mining literature for protein–protein interactions. *Bioinformatics* 2001;17:359–363.

95. Wilcox A, Hripcsak G. Classification algorithms applied to narrative reports. Proc AMIA Symp 1999;455–459.

96. *STRING*, http://string.embl.de/.

97. von Mering C, Huynen M, Jaeggi D, Schmidt S, Bork P, Snel B. STRING: a database of predicted functional associations between proteins. *Nucleic Acids Res* 2003;31:258–261.

98. Tien AC, Lin MH, Su LJ, Hong YR, Cheng TS, Lee YC, Lin WJ, Still IH, Huang CY. Identification of the substrates and interaction proteins of aurora kinases from a protein–protein interaction model. *Mol Cell Proteomics* 2004;3:93–104.

99. Lipinski CA, Lombardo F, Dominy BW, Feeney PJ. Experimental and computational approaches to estimate solubility and permeability in drug discovery and development settings. *Adv Drug Deliv Rev* 1997;23:3–25.

100. Mazziotta J, Toga A, Evans A, Fox P, Lancaster J, Zilles K, Woods R, Paus T, Simpson G, Pike B, Holmes C, Collins L, Thompson P, MacDonald D, Iacoboni M, Schormann T, Amunts K, Palomero-Gallagher N, Geyer S, Parsons L, Narr K, Kabani N, Le Goualher G, Boomsma D, Cannon T, Kawashima R, Mazoyer B. A probabilistic atlas and reference system for the human brain: International Consortium for Brain Mapping (ICBM). *Philos Trans R Soc Lond B Biol Sci* 2001;356:1293–1322.

101. Mazziotta J, Toga A, Evans A, Fox P, Lancaster J, Zilles K, Woods R, Paus T, Simpson G, Pike B, Holmes C, Collins L, Thompson P, MacDonald D, Iacoboni M, Schormann T, Amunts K, Palomero-Gallagher N, Geyer S, Parsons L, Narr K, Kabani N, Le Goualher G, Feidler J, Smith K, Boomsma D, Hulshoff Pol H, Cannon T, Kawashima R, Mazoyer B. A four-dimensional probabilistic atlas of the human brain. *J Am Med Inform Assoc* 2001;8:401–430.

102. Dickson J, Drury H, Van Essen DC. The surface management system (SuMS) database: a surface-based database to aid cortical surface reconstruction, visualization and analysis. *Philos Trans R Soc Lond B Biol Sci* 2001;356:1277–1292.

103. Van Essen DC. Windows on the brain: the emerging role of atlases and databases in neuroscience. *Curr Opin Neurobiol* 2002;12:574–579.

104. Burns GA. Knowledge management of the neuroscientific literature: the data model and underlying strategy of the NeuroScholar system. *Philos Trans R Soc Lond B Biol Sci* 2001;356:1187–1208.

105. Shepherd GM, Mirsky JS, Healy MD, Singer MS, Skoufos E, Hines MS, Nadkarni PM, Miller PL. The Human Brain Project: neuroinformatics tools for integrating, searching and modeling multidisciplinary neuroscience data. *Trends Neurosci* 1998;21:460–468.

106. Rammensee HG. Immunoinformatics: bioinformatic strategies for better understanding of immune function. Introduction. *Novartis Found Symp* 2003;254:1–2.

107. Brusic V, Zeleznikow J, Petrovsky N. Molecular immunology databases and data repositories. *J Immunol Methods* 2000;238:17–28.

108. Robinson J, Waller MJ, Parham P, de Groot N, Bontrop R, Kennedy LJ, Stoehr P, Marsh SG. IMGT/HLA and IMGT/MHC: sequence databases for the study of the major histocompatibility complex. *Nucleic Acids Res* 2003;31:311–314.

109. Lefranc MP. IMGT, the international ImMunoGeneTics database. *Nucleic Acids Res* 2003;31:307–310.

110. Giudicelli V, Lefranc MP. Ontology for immunogenetics: the IMGT-ONTOLOGY. *Bioinformatics* 1999;15:1047–1054.

111. Petrovsky N, Schonbach C, Brusic V. Bioinformatic strategies for better understanding of immune function. *In Silico Biol* 2003;3:411–416.

112. Lefranc MP. IMGT, The international ImMunoGeneTics Information System. *Methods Mol Biol* 2004;248:27–49.

113. Lefranc MP, Giudicelli V, Ginestoux C, Bosc N, Folch G, Guiraudou D, Jabado-Michaloud J, Magris S, Scaviner D, Thouvenin V, Combres K, Girod D, Jeanjean S, Protat C, Yousfi-Monod M, Duprat E, Kaas Q, Pommie C, Chaume D, Lefranc G. IMGT-ONTOLOGY for immunogenetics and immunoinformatics. *In Silico Biol* 2004;4:17–29.

114. Lefranc MP. IMGT-ONTOLOGY and IMGT databases, tools and Web resources for immunogenetics and immunoinformatics. *Mol Immunol* 2004;40:647–660.

115. Brusic V, Zeleznikow J. Artificial neural network applications in immunology, in *Proceedings of the International Joint Conference on Neural Networks*, 1999;5:3685–3689.

116. De Groot AS, Bosma A, Chinai N, Frost J, Jesdale BM, Gonzalez MA, Martin W, Saint-Aubin C. From genome to vaccine: *in silico* predictions, *ex vivo* verification. *Vaccine* 2001;19:4385–4395.

117. De Groot AS, Sbai H, Aubin CS, McMurry J, Martin W. Immuno-informatics: mining genomes for vaccine components. *Immunol Cell Biol* 2002;80:255–269.

118. de Castro LN, Timmis JI. Artificial immune systems: a novel paradigm to pattern recognition. In *Artificial Neural Networks in Pattern Recognition*. Paisley, UK: University of Paisley; 2002, pp 67–84.

119. Korolev D, Balakin KV, Nikolsky Y, Kirillov E, Ivanenkov YA, Savchuk NP, Ivashchenko AA, Nikolskaya T. Modeling of human cytochrome P450-mediated drug metabolism using unsupervised machine learning approach. *J Med Chem* 2003;46:3631–3643.

120. Erhardt PW. A human drug metabolism database: potential roles in the quantitative predictions of drug metabolism and metabolism-related drug–drug interactions. *Curr Drug Metab* 2003;4:411–422.

121. Langowski J, Long A. Computer systems for the prediction of xenobiotic metabolism. *Adv Drug Deliv Rev* 2002;54:407–415.

122. Barratt MD, Rodford RA. The computational prediction of toxicity. *Curr Opin Chem Biol* 2001;5:383–388.

123. Pearl GM, Livingston-Carr S, Durham SK. Integration of computational analysis as a sentinel tool in toxicological assessments. *Curr Top Med Chem* 2001;1:247–255.

124. Dearden JC, Barratt MD, Benigni R, Bristol DW, Combes RD, Cronin MTD, Judson PN, Payne MP, Richard AM, Tichy M, Worth AP, Yourick JJ. The development and validation of expert systems for predicting toxicity. *ATLA* 1997;25:223–252.

125. Schultz TW, Cronin MTD, Walker JD, Aptula AO. Quantitative structure–activity relationships (QSARs) in toxicology: a historical perspective. *J Mol Structure (Theochem)* 2003;622:1–22.

126. Covitz PA, Hartel F, Schaefer C, De Coronado S, Fragoso G, Sahni H, Gustafson S, Buetow KH. caCORE: a common infrastructure for cancer informatics. *Bioinformatics* 2003;19:2404–2412.

127. Silva JS, Ball MJ, Douglas JV. The Cancer Informatics Infrastructure (CII): an architecture for translating clinical research into patient care. *Medinfo* 2001;10:114–117.

128. Hubbard SM, Setser A. The Cancer Informatics Infrastructure: a new initiative of the National Cancer Institute. *Semin Oncol Nurs* 2001;17:55–61.

129. Kihara D, Yang YD, Hawkin T. Bioinformatics resources for cancer research with an emphasis on gene function and structure prediction tools. *Cancer Informatics* 2006; pp 25–35.

2

COMPUTER TECHNIQUES: IDENTIFYING SIMILARITIES BETWEEN SMALL MOLECULES

PETER MEEK, GUILLERMO MOYNA, AND RANDY ZAUHAR

University of the Sciences in Philadelphia, Philadelphia, Pennsylvania

Contents

Preclinical Development Handbook: ADME and Biopharmaceutical Properties,
edited by Shayne Cox Gad
Copyright © 2008 John Wiley & Sons, Inc.

2.1 INTRODUCTION

In this chapter, current computational methodologies available for the comparison of structurally similar compounds are presented and analyzed in detail. Problems encountered throughout these types of endeavors are summarized first, giving particular emphasis to the suitability of *in silico*, or computer-based, methods for evaluating molecular similarity among members of large compound libraries. The chapter then concentrates on the description of different techniques, starting from the simplest ones, then more complex, and finishing with emerging approaches. Salient examples of a technique application found in the literature are discussed, and brief guidelines for readers interested in employing these computational tools are outlined.

2.2 COMPUTER-AIDED DRUG DESIGN (CADD)

Implementing CADD techniques depends heavily on what molecular information is provided or accessible. However, of equal or even greater importance is how the information that is searched and utilized is organized and constructed. These, of course, are the databases containing the small molecules. The format of how a molecular entry is recorded and stored is pivotal and dictates what transformations of the entries are required before any kind of search or CADD application can be performed. In fact, this chapter might be described as a series of illustrations of the different ways in which molecules can be represented in a computer, each with its potential benefits and drawbacks.

2.3 HARVESTING DATA FROM SMALL MOLECULES

Over the past few decades there has been an unprecedented explosion of information in the chemical and life sciences. Development of new biological and chemical tools has been documented and new pharmaceutical agents are discovered with ever-increasing frequency year by year [1]. At the same time, it has become more and more difficult to gain regulatory approval of new chemical entities [2] due to new and stricter legislation. There are millions of molecules that are now known to possess bioactivity against one or more targets, or to be useful as reagents in academic and industrial research. Before any computer-based technique can be implemented, these vast numbers of isolated and synthesized molecules need to be organized. As might be expected, the need to catalog this abundant information was recognized early on, and many molecules are organized into indexes (e.g., CAS system) and/or are held in commercial [3–6], industrial [7, 8], or public [9–11] databases. Given the vast volume of "chemical space" that has already been explored, it is to the advantage of the investigator to consult these knowledge bases before planning a new synthesis, and at the outset of any efforts to identify new therapeutic or bioactive compounds. In particular, synthesizing a new compound often represents an enormous effort in the laboratory, work carried out in vain if the target compound (or one similar to it) is already available from a commercial source.

Given the sheer volume of information, there is considerable need to employ computers to carry out these investigations as few human minds past, present, or future can compare one molecule to a previously memorized database of 10,000,000 molecules. Harnessing computer power is not without drawbacks; we discuss here the importance and careful considerations required to represent chemical structures. Chemical database storage and searching relies on electronic definitions of chemical structures, and the details of the methodology used are vital to defining and measuring similarity between molecules.

2.4   REPRESENTING MOLECULES FOR INTERPRETATION BY COMPUTERS

Molecules are represented based on their constituent parts and the way in which these constituent parts are connected. The components of a small molecule are atoms, which are minimally identified by element type, but which may be characterized by a number of additional descriptors, including but not limited to van der Waals radius, valence, and/or charge state. The next step beyond simply enumerating the atoms in a molecule is to provide detailed connectivity information, typically in terms of a list of bonds of recognized chemical type; in this way the molecule is defined mathematically as a graph, with the atoms as vertices and the bonds as edges of specified type. The atom and bond definitions act as the building blocks of molecules that can be represented in one of three major forms: one-dimensional (1D), two-dimensional (2D), or three-dimensional (3D). Over the years several standard computer file formats have been developed for each dimension class (Table 2.1), and these have steadily evolved to allow incorporation of additional data types. For instance, many applications require a detailed distribution of partial atomic charges (as opposed to simply specifying ionization state); such charges are required by some force fields, such as MMFF94 [19], and are routinely computed using rapid semiempirical methods (Gasteiger [20] and Gastegier and Huckel [21]). This information is readily included in many molecular file formats, including the structure data file sdf [22] and mol2 [14] specifications. In addition, some current formats (such as sdf) admit the possibility of "tagging" a molecule with arbitrary data, a boon in the sense of providing open-ended flexibility, but a peril in that descriptors may not be added uniformly across a database, and/or the additions may not be clearly annotated.

2.4.1   Importance of Continuity Within Molecular Representations

One of the most critical issues when applying various molecular databases is to recognize the varying levels of faithfulness between the representation of the molecule in the computer and the actual material available to the investigator. This is a function of both the database and the source of the compound. For example, suppose that a sample of a potentially bioactive compound is available in the form of a purified enantiomer. Many molecular databases store connectivity (bonding) information but do not distinguish between different stereoisomers. If the database entry corresponding to this compound is used to generate a molecular model with

TABLE 2.1   Representation of the Small Molecule β-D-Glucopyranose

1D[a]

SMILES string representation of β-D-glucopyranose (@ = S, @@ = R):

[H][C@@]1(O)O[C@]([H])(CO)[C@@]([H])(O)[C@]([H])(O)[C@@]1([H])O

SLN string representation of β-D-glucopyranose:

O[1]CH(CH(CH(CH(CH@1OH)OH)OH)OH)CH2OH

2D[b]	*3D*[c]
MarvinSketch representation of β-D-glucopyranose	SYBYL representation of β-D-glucopyranose

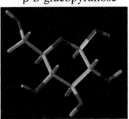

[a]Two examples: a SMILE string notation [12] and the SLN (SYBYL Line Notation [13], by Tripos [14]).
[b]Representation using the classic bond-wedge diagram (MarvinSketch [15]).
[c]The image of β-D-glucopyranose created from a mol2 file (SYBYL by Tripos). The 2D and 3D structures are collapsible to linear notation and converted into a required file format by CORINA [16]; stereoisomers are generated with STERGEN [17] and tautomers with TAUTOMER [18].

detailed atomic positions, the resulting model may not correspond to the material sample. Conversely, the investigator may have a racemic mixture, whereas the database entry assumes a specific enantiomeric form. In either case, incorrect predictions may result, since biological activity is often remarkably sensitive to the details of 3D molecular structure.

Generally, it is often the case that small changes in chemical structure or physicochemical properties can have profound implications for the specificity and magnitude of the biological effects associated with a compound. Speaking first to the effects of structural variations, we can identify classic examples of chemical isomerism, including chiral, cis/trans (*E/Z*), functional group, and positional isomerism. Small variations such as substitution of atoms and/or isomeric rearrangements can have an important impact on both molecular shape and physical properties (e.g., dipole moment, hydrophobicity) that are a function of 3D structure. Hence, it is imperative for the investigator to be aware of the details in the information stored in a database, particularly when data is absent (e.g., no representation of stereoisomerism) as well as when data is present but may not correspond to the state of the physical sample (e.g., *R* chiral form where *S* is found in the material sample, or a neutral database entry corresponding to a molecule that may be ionized at the pH of interest). It is therefore imperative to use, derive, and develop uniform molecular representation systems meticulously, without which predictions or application of *in silico* techniques would be impossible.

(a) Similarity of atomic arrangements of carbon, nitrogen, and phosphorus

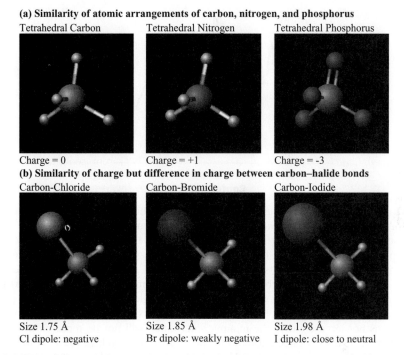

Tetrahedral Carbon   Tetrahedral Nitrogen   Tetrahedral Phosphorus

Charge = 0   Charge = +1   Charge = -3

(b) Similarity of charge but difference in charge between carbon–halide bonds

Carbon-Chloride   Carbon-Bromide   Carbon-Iodide

Size 1.75 Å   Size 1.85 Å   Size 1.98 Å
Cl dipole: negative   Br dipole: weakly negative I dipole: close to neutral

FIGURE 2.1   (**a**) Depiction of three tetrahedral atom arrangements: (**left**) the central **carbon** in methane, (**center**) the central protonated **nitrogen** in ammonium, and (**right**) the **phosphorus** in phosphate all look similar but carry different charges. (**b**) Atomic arrangements of a tetrahedral carbon bonded with a single halide of increasing size: (**left**) chloromethane, (**center**) bromomethane, and (**right**) iodomethane. All molecule constructions were created with MarvinSketch [15].

To highlight this concept further, we present some examples of small molecular frameworks that are at first glance similar but that in fact differ significantly (Fig. 2.1). Certain atoms have similar sizes and the same bond orientation (e.g., tetrahedral carbon, phosphorus, and protonated nitrogen, Fig. 2.1a) yet the molecular charge distribution is considerably different. In contrast, substituting one halide for another at a specified location in a framework has a small effect on total dipole moment, and yet these atoms differ significantly in size, with the largest, iodine, occupying about the same volume as a methyl group (Fig. 2.1b). This raises the question: When similarity is measured, what governs how similar an atom is to another atom? In other words, how similar is O to S, or N to P or C, or an atom to a small group (e.g., I to CH_3)? The answer depends heavily on the context of the atom or group in question. Moreover, it is important to recognize that the physical influences of atom or small group in determining molecular properties depend on its context; such factors include hybridization state and the local chemical environment, an insight first proposed by Hammet [23] and Hansch et al. [24]. These researchers developed mathematical representations for predicting molecular properties on the basis of structure.

Yet more complexity arises if we introduce the possibility of molecular flexibility. Most molecules of biological interest admit some degree of flexibility, including bonds about which free rotation is possible and saturated ring systems that can

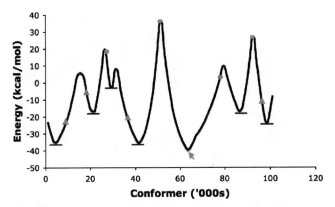

FIGURE 2.2   Graph of molecular conformation versus energy. An energy profile plot is shown for each possible conformation of a hypothetical molecule in 3D space. The troughs denote local energy minima (short gray lines) and the global energy minimum (gray arrow). When exploring molecular space, finding the global energy minimum is not guaranteed. For example, if the four starting points were the gray triangles, the output would not detect the global energy minimum, but maybe five local energy minima at best. Using the start points with the gray circles would almost certainly guarantee the global energy minima and possibly all the local minima too. The problem is inherent to all experimental investigations: if the sample size is not large enough, the minima determined will not be representative of the whole. Likewise, in energy calculations if the energy barrier is too high to climb, the pockets or valleys over the hills cannot be entered into and located. This is why small molecules bound to their targets are highly sought after; a more active molecule will have a bound structure not too dissimilar to its gas phase global minima.

adopt alternate conformations (e.g., chair vs. boat forms for six-membered rings, various classes of puckering observed in pyranoses). This leads to the possibility of multiple conformers for a molecule, each representing a local minimum on the energy surface of the compound. While a molecule will often have a single global energy minimum representing the conformation most favored in terms of energy, there may be other important minima of similar energy (Fig. 2.2), and there is no guarantee that the global minimum corresponds to the form of the molecule that is active against a particular biological target [25]. A number of techniques are available to identify low energy conformers [14, 26]. Although many databases include a representative low energy conformer for each compound, detailed considerations of molecular flexibility are usually relegated to the final stages of analysis, after a relatively small set of interesting molecules have been identified. Nonetheless, consideration of flexibility is often critical for rationalizing differences in activity among a panel of bioactive molecules.

2.5   DEFINING SIMILARITY

Defining similarity between molecules is an inherently ambiguous undertaking. What makes two molecules similar? Should we focus on the volumes occupied by molecules, their patterns of chemical bonding, the presence of particular functional

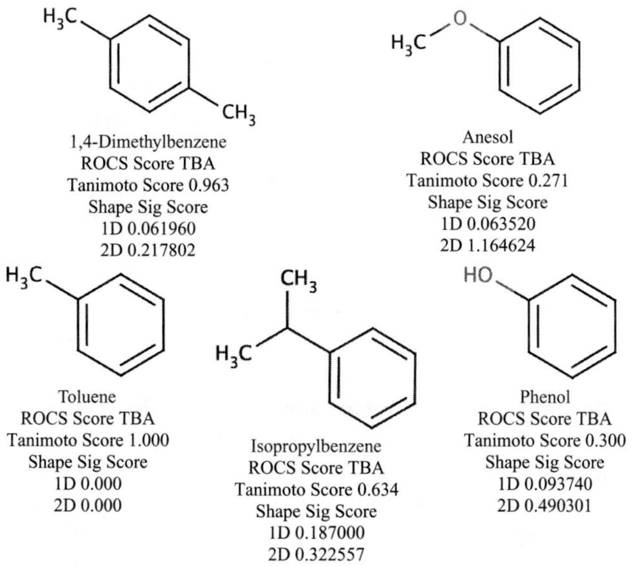

FIGURE 2.3 A simple similarity example using different comparison methods. A collection of five benzene derivatives is displayed and an assessment is made of their similarity to a toluene reference using Tanimoto index [27], 1D Shape Signatures, (shape comparison), and 2D Shape Signatures (shape and mean electrostatic potential comparison) [28–30]. All three types of comparison required 3D coordinate input files (mol2). A Tanimoto score of 1.000 implies a perfect match, with 0.000 implying a complete mismatch; a Shape Signatures score of 0.000 is a perfect match and 2.000 is a complete mismatch.

groups, ionization state, hydrophobicity, dipole moment, or any or all of a host of other topological and physicochemical descriptors? In most cases the desire is to find molecules that "look like" a particular query molecule, or that are compatible with a chemical/spatial pattern (corresponding perhaps to a pharmacophore model). Note that we are not typically interested in stringent criteria; rather, the goal is to cast a fairly wide net and identify molecules that have the potential to interact with a particular target of interest. Examples of comparisons (Fig. 2.3) demonstrate that different tools, each employing its own valid approach to defining molecular similarity, can produce very different results. This is not in itself surprising but does highlight the need for care and caution when applying *in silico* methods to scan chemical databases for lead compounds. It is important to understand what features a particular method is "looking for," and it is just as critical to recognize what the method ignores! Similarity is itself an arbitrarily defined concept (with appreciable overlaps between techniques) and will depend entirely on the tool(s) used.

Essentially, *in silico* search techniques prove most useful when the similarity measurement (scoring index) reliably returns molecules with the same desired characteristics as the query. Such a technique will take a large dataset of unrelated molecules and reduce it to a smaller set, but with proportionally more molecules similar to the query. This process is called *enrichment*. Methods are available to quantitate enrichment [29, 31], and a measure of enrichment may provide a useful figure of merit when comparing and assessing computational search tools.

2.5.1   Why Do We Wish to Compare Molecules?

In the context of drug development (or identification of bioactivity in general), there are two motivations for comparing molecules. One is to locate molecules in a database that are similar to a known active, which might also be active against the target, and furthermore could conceivably provide better compounds as determined by any number of measures (e.g., activity, bioavailability, ease of synthesis). The second is to rationalize the efficacy of a set of known active compounds, to identify the features that are directly related to activity, and thus to determine how existing compounds can be improved. Of course, the two motivations can be combined: one might first use a library search to locate interesting lead compounds and then improve the leads by making modifications in line with established models that relate structure to activity. Clearly, at the very least, the database search component of this strategy needs to be automated, since humans do a poor job of scanning through hundreds of structures, let alone the hundreds of thousands that are available in contemporary libraries. But the central point is that drug design methods that employ measures of molecular similarity have the potential to rapidly locate lead compounds, to support the finetuning of structures to improve activity and other critical features, and to dramatically reduce costs by identifying compounds that may be readily available or easily modified.

Similarity searching is not a straightforward task: small alterations of a molecule (e.g., *cis/trans* stereoisomerism (Fig. 2.4a) and chirality (Fig. 2.4b)) can have a profound and marked effect on activity. Indeed, the protonation state of the molecule

-- ➤

FIGURE 2.4   (**a**) Shape and *cis/trans* isomerism. This part demonstrates how a subtle change in the arrangement of a carbon–carbon double bond (sp^2＝sp^2) can dramatically affect the appearance of a molecule. The bond (black dot) is either in the *cis* conformation (same side), (**i**) and (**iii**), or the *trans* conformation (opposite sides), (**ii**) and (**iv**). One should take paticular note that as small molecules are usually designed to biological targets, it is inevitable that *cis/trans* isomerism can dramatically affect the activity of a potential drug, and consequently is a major headache in chemical synthesis. (**b**) Shape and chiral isomerism. Controlling chirality poses a huge challenge for synthetic chemists. There are several chiral centers in this molecule; the only differing one is marked with an arrow, being S on the isomer to the left and R on the one to the right. Usually one optical isomer, or enantiomer, will have activity against a biological target (known as the eutomer), while the other lacks the desired activity. Due to the expense associated with the separation or enantiomers from a mixture, chirality is of paramount importance when searching molecular databases. (**c**) Shape and distribution of charge. Shown are two representations of aspartic acid—an amino acid: (**left**) the fully protonated amino acid and (**right**) the fully deprotonated amino acid. Usually the nitrogen is tetrahedral at physiological pH and the C terminus and side chain (connected to the Cα-carbon) are deprotonated. The state of the proton donors and acceptors modifies the local charge and overall shape of the molecule; hence, the small molecule being investigated needs to mimic the donor and acceptor sites to be truly similar. As a general rule, the termini are not involved in donor and acceptor sites on a protein, as the vast majority are lost in the peptide bond formation. The side chains dictate the number of donor and acceptor sites.

can affect the structure and surface charge distribution (Fig. 2.4c), with flexibility and rotation further complicating the matter. Hence, one could define this problem as akin to a box of left-threaded and right-threaded nuts and bolts. The different classes of bolts may have many properties in common, such that even a trained eye might sort them together, yet they have distinct and incompatible functions. This paradigm is clearly evident in the biological context and highlighted with respect to

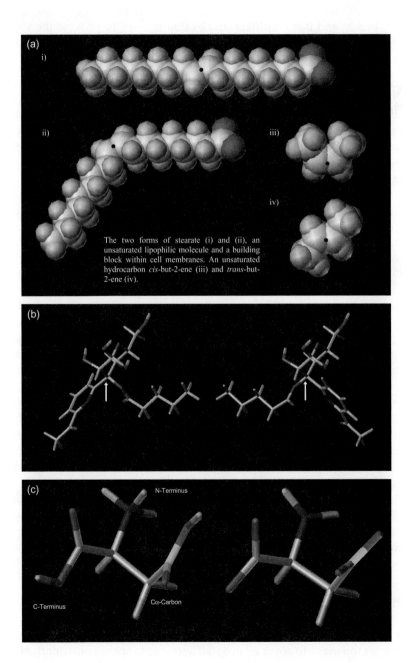

(a)
i)
ii)
iii)
iv)

The two forms of stearate (i) and (ii), an unsaturated lipophilic molecule and a building block within cell membranes. An unsaturated hydrocarbon *cis*-but-2-ene (iii) and *trans*-but-2-ene (iv).

(b)

(c)
N-Terminus
C-Terminus
Cα-Carbon

enantiomer specificity (HIV serine proteases made of exclusively either D or L amino acids) [32] and the toxic effects observed with thalidomide [33].

Consequently, while attempts to measure similarity between molecules have an objective basis, the evaluations depend heavily on the algorithms employed, sometimes leading to the appearance of subjectivity (the results obtained depend on the specific tools selected). That said, it has been evident for a long while that molecular similarity provides the foundation for rational drug design. As far as the choice of tools and algorithms is concerned, these are of course ultimately evaluated at the laboratory bench, and it is empirical studies that in the end provide the validation of existing approaches, and point out new directions for improvement and development on the computational side.

2.5.2   Utilizing External Sources of Information

As discussed earlier, several scenarios admit the use of similarity searching. In some cases, a relatively small set of molecules are compared, but in others the goal is to scan a potentially enormous library of compounds. To a large extent, the form of the investigation will be determined by the molecular descriptors maintained in the target database. These vary considerably from one database to another; for example, many commonly used compound databases (National Cancer Institute [10]) include only chemical formulas in the form of SMILES strings [12], with no 3D structures. On the other hand, these same libraries may be offered by other vendors with atomic coordinates appended (Tripos version of NCI), and furthermore a number of fast tools are available to generate coordinates from SMILES strings (CORINA [16], CONCORD [34]), so this data can be added by the end user. Some databases include a range of molecular descriptors for each entry, such as $\log P$, molar refractivity, molecular weight, or custom topological descriptors (e.g., chemical fingerprints [35]). Again, these descriptors, when missing, can sometimes be added by third-party tools (MOE [36], DayLight [37]). At the same time, whether these newly added atomic coordinates and/or descriptors can readily be used with available search software is a question that needs to be addressed at the outset; if a tool requires a proprietary database format, it is an open question as to whether any modifications can be introduced by the end user. An extreme case is found when the database is accessible only via a website maintained by a company or academic laboratory, and the raw data is inaccessible except through the supplied interface. The most attractive approach, rarely realized, is to maintain a flexible database format and something akin to a relational database that can be used to construct arbitrary queries of the information held in the library.

Databases for use in similarity searching are difficult to procure or expensive to obtain [3–8]. Recently, several have become available that are utilizable and relevant to small molecule comparison [9–11]. The research conducted at the University of the Sciences in Philadelphia aims to provide a readily searchable database to the global academic community (see Section 2.6.6).

2.6   DETECTING SIMILARITY WITH *IN SILICO* TECHNIQUES

There is a vast expanse of *in silico* techniques that "detect" similarity between small molecules, far too many to cover all in detail here due to space constraints. However, the aim is to give a flavor of techniques that are in common use and applied in contemporary research. We begin with established techniques that are the least complex and require the least amount of input data and move through to more complicated data intensive methods and finally emerging technologies.

2.6.1 HQSAR

HQSAR (hologram quantitative structure–activity relationships) is a powerful approach that can claim important advantages over many of the traditional QSAR (quantitative structure–activity relationship) techniques we will describe later. This is especially true when little is known about the receptor target of interest. A key advantage of HQSAR is that it requires only 2D chemical structures combined with experimental binding data; there is no need to generate atomic coordinates or alignments of structures, as is required by some 3D methods like CoMFA (comparative molecular field analysis, discussed in Section 2.6.5). At the same time, predictions from HQSAR can be combined with other methods to sometimes improve the overall accuracy of predicted activities. Models of high statistical quality and predictive value can be rapidly and easily generated by HQSAR and can often be used in conjunction with chemical databases to select molecules with superior biological activity, providing the model is robust. HQSAR can be used to rapidly scan chemical libraries but is also useful with small datasets.

HQSAR requires a set of training molecules in order to construct predictive models. As with any machine learning algorithm, the reliability of the model generated is largely a function of the quality of the training set; it is imperative that the training molecules be well characterized, with a common binding site and accurate IC_{50} measurements.

HQSAR Application HQSAR is a rapid and inexpensive means to test compounds using a computer algorithm. The computer "learns" from the input provided from real data derived from actual experiments and generates a model (Fig. 2.5a). This model in turn serves as the basis for predicting the activity of compounds that have been proposed as new leads, or for scanning a chemical library for compounds likely to be active (Fig. 2.5b). While we will describe the HQSAR methodology in more detail below, the basic idea is straightforward. It is usually true that a biologically active compound has three or four groups that are crucial to activity, and these are held at specific distances by a skeleton/backbone structure. HQSAR aims to identify these groups and to correlate the arrangement of these key components with activity.

HQSAR: A Computational Perspective To understand HQSAR, an appreciation of the computational algorithm is required, and for this we need to consider the underlying representation of the data. Linear notation (more specifically SLN) is utilized to represent molecules (Table 2.1), [12, 13, 38], but the molecule is finally represented as a fingerprint [35]. The key importance of HQSAR fingerprint representations (Fig. 2.6) is that fragments are generated based on the chemical structure of each compound and need not correspond to a predefined list of functional groups and structural components. This flexibility leads to more robust database

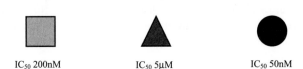

a) Known bioactive molecules and associated IC_{50} values

IC_{50} 200nM	IC_{50} 5μM	IC_{50} 50nM

b) HQSAR predictions for theoretical compound designs based on input data

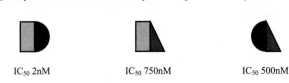

IC_{50} 2nM	IC_{50} 750nM	IC_{50} 500nM

FIGURE 2.5 Simplified representation of HQSAR with a small molecule training and test set. The methodology behind HQSAR consists of (**a**) the training set of known molecules and (**b**) the predictions for theoretically designed molecules. The points at the very extremities of the shapes can be considered as active groups, and the overall shape as a molecular skeleton. When an HQSAR run is conducted, the molecules in the training set (**a**) define whether particular groups contribute to or negate activity in the HQSAR model (in this case experimentally derived IC_{50} values are used). Theoretical compounds incorporating variations in the component parts (**b**) are then tested with this HQSAR model. In many incidences results make sense (**lower center** and **lower right**) being between the IC_{50} values of the two component parts. There are cases where the IC_{50} can appear to be greater than the sum of the component parts (**lower left**), and in this case it is in a more favorable direction: 2 nM while previously the best molecule was 50 nM (**upper right**).

Fingerprint	0	0	1	1	0	1	0	0	0	1	1	1	1	0	0	0
Hologram	0	0	2	5	0	9	0	0	0	1	3	8	7	0	0	0

$\Sigma = 35$

FIGURE 2.6 An example of a fingerprint and a hologram. The chemical structure has 35 fragments. In the case of the hashed fingerprint, the representation is purely binary, whereas in the case of the hologram, the bins contain information about the number of fragments hashed into each bin and its contribution (positive, negative, or otherwise to biological activity).

screening [37], and more effective 2D and/or similarity searches, than a structural key approach [39]. The package used [14], however, provides the capabilities of each approach.

Conventional QSARs can identify critical relationships between the properties—the geometric and the chemical characteristics of a molecular system of interest. In QSAR, the measured bioactivity of a set of compounds is correlated with structural descriptors to determine trends and predict the bioactivity of related, untested compounds. HQSAR (like combined QSAR and CoMFA) works by identifying substructural features in sets of molecules that are relevant to biological activity. A key advantage of HQSAR is the relative simplicity of the required input, which in the training phase consists of chemical (2D) structures and their experimental activity (i.e., relative binding affinity, LD_{50} or IC_{50}).

The underlying principle of HQSAR is simply stated: since the structure of the molecule is encoded within its 2D fingerprint and that structure is a key determinant of all molecular properties including biological activity, then it should be possible to predict the activity of a molecule from its fingerprint, which implicitly encodes the structure. Molecular fingerprints (Fig. 2.6) are strings of 1's and 0's (binary) that indicate the presence or absence of a particular fragment (e.g., a carbonyl, hydroxyl, or halide). The fingerprint is therefore a shorthand list of the fragments present in a structure. A *molecular hologram* extends this concept to incorporate both *branched fragments* and *counts* of the fragments that are present. These additions are important as the inclusion of branched fragments helps distinguish hybridization states, and the counting function differentiates between compounds with (for example) one, two, or more carbonyls. Thus, a hologram is a list of integers, not a bit string, and is therefore a fingerprint. In summary, a molecular hologram contains all possible molecular fragments within a molecule, including overlapping fragments, and maintains a count of the number of times each unique fragment occurs. This process of incorporating information about each fragment, and each of its constituent subfragments, implicitly encodes 3D structural information. These fragments are arranged into (or hashed) a linear array of numbers (the hologram, Fig. 2.6). Note that the hashing algorithm guarantees that a particular fragment will always hash to the same numerical value but does not guarantee that different fragments will always have unique hash values. If different fragments, all important for determining biological activity, should hash to the same bin positions in the hologram, it will not be possible to distinguish their effects using a partial least squares analysis (or any other approach for that matter). This phenomenon is called fragment collision and results in poor models with little predictive validity. Using holograms of different lengths (*L*) can prevent fragments that are responsible for biological activity from being hashed to the same bin.

When the various lengths of holograms are chosen at even intervals, the chances of resolving bad collisions are reduced. For example, if fragment collisions occur with the length set at 400, these collisions will not be resolved at length 200 (nor 100, 50, or 25 as these are all factors of 400). Since the 400 bin hologram is simply folded over to produce the 200 bin hologram, the colliding fragments will still end up in the same bin. For this reason, the default values for the hologram lengths are all prime numbers. This reduces the chances of seeing the same bad collisions at the various lengths. It is wise to use all available lengths so that the best model can be generated in a single HQSAR run.

Despite the fundamental simplicity of HQSAR, there are many options and much terminology connected with the application of the method, only a portion of which is described here. Each molecule in the training set is broken down into structural fragments whose size falls within a specified range; here we will denote the lower limit for the number of atoms in a fragment as *M*, and the upper limit as *N*. The parameters *M* and *N* are user-defined (typically with $M = 4$–7 and $N = 7$–9), as is the length (*L*) of the molecular hologram into which the fragments are hashed. Given the length *L* of the hologram, a fragment with a particular chemical structure always hashes to the same well-defined bin. However, the hashing function can be adjusted to ignore certain molecular features; for example, the user controls whether or not fragments with the same chemical structure but opposite chirality hash into the same or different hologram bins.

The calculation of a set of molecular holograms for a training set of structures yields a data matrix of dimension $n \times L$, where *n* is the number of compounds in the dataset and *L* is the length of the molecular hologram. The partial least squares technique is then employed to generate a statistical model that relates the descriptor variables (occupancy numbers of the bins in the hologram) to an observable property, for example, the biological activity expressed as $-\log IC_{50}$. The selection of the hologram length leading to the "best" HQSAR is based on the PLS analysis that gives either the highest cross-validated q^2 or the lowest standard error associated with the cross-validation analysis. The predictive power of the model is determined by using statistical cross-validation, the default approach being the leave-one-out (LOO) method.

An important role of a QSAR model, besides predicting the activities of untested molecules, is to provide hints about what molecular fragments may be important contributors to activity. This information is of great value to the synthetic chemist. Such information can be combined with knowledge of the maximal common structure (MCS) between compounds to get ideas for the synthesis of new molecules that might lead to suitable drug candidates. Clearly, the HQSAR method, which focuses directly on elements of chemical structure (rather than derived properties such as dipole moment or hydrophobicity), is well suited to proposing changes in chemical structure that are likely to improve activity.

The contributions of individual atoms to activity can be assessed through their representation in the hologram hash bins and can be used to color code the atoms of each molecule. Atoms that contribute positively to activity are colored toward the blue end of the spectrum; atoms that contribute negatively are colored toward the red end, and atoms that do not significantly affect activity (usually constituting the backbone or skeleton of the molecule) are colored white.

An important feature of HQSAR is the capability to recognize the maximal substructure common to the training compounds and to remove this substructure from consideration when constructing holograms. It is usually the case that a series of active molecules will share a significant common framework, and the predictive power of the method is enhanced by excluding portions of the molecule that are shared across the training set, and thus cannot be correlated with activity. Using this maximum common substructure (MCS) feature also allows the user to exclude in a consistent way molecules that lie too far outside the predictive space of the model. Moreover, identifying the MCS allows the user to better rationalize the relationship between structure and activity, and provides a template for proposing new compounds with activity that is likely to be accurately predicted by the HQSAR model. An MCS must contain at minimum seven connected atoms and is calculated purely by the molecules that constitute the training dataset; it is possible for good models to be derived without an MCS, but this is of less use when establishing and developing biological theories and of course for a centralized chemical synthesis route.

Once a HQSAR model has been calculated, the next step is to validate the model quality; the preferred method being the leave-one-out method (this is covered in detail in the next section). After model validation, proposed synthetics or other candidate theory molecules may be tested using the model. Often a search of chemical databases for molecules similar to those in the training set is conducted. Predictions of their activities, based on the model, are organized with the predicted activities in descending order. In a typical application, the database is first prescreened using a fast measure of similarity, such as the Tanimoto index, with a user-selected value for the minimum similarity cutoff (the default threshold for this index is 0.85). The results of the Tanimoto screen, which is effectively a 2D similarity search, is carried out, and the hits found from the search are entered onto a spreadsheet. The activities of the compounds are calculated from the HQSAR model. Compounds are sorted according to their predicted measured variable (usually IC_{50}). These findings can be presented in simple bar charts with test compound versus predicted variable. Using the Tanimoto coefficient is not absolutely essential, but can aid in reducing the size of larger databases. Frequently a database including only those molecules proposed by medicinal chemists is used.

Successful HQSAR requires a minimum of five molecules in the training set, but preferably more than ten. These should be structurally different molecules, but with some similarity. The model should not be used to predict the activity of compounds that are structurally very different from those in the training set.

HQSAR Example   Vacuolar ATPase is an ATP-dependent proton pump that is important in many biological processes by acidifying specialized cell compartments. Of particular interest is the implication of V-ATPase in bone resorption by osteoclasts. Excessive bone resorption by osteoclasts and failure of osteoblasts laying down new bone are indicative of osteoporosis. The structural defects that accumulate and weaken the bones are primarily due to demineralization of the bone (removal of Ca^{2+} and PO^{3-}). Approximately one in three postmenopausal women and one in twelve older men suffer from osteoporosis. Currently, treatment of osteoporosis is via two methods—bisphosphonates and selective estrogen receptor modulators, the latter not being the favored treatment for men. Current therapies are useful in two respects. First, the bisphosphonates rapidly increase bone mineral density by forming a dead end complex; hence, bone resorption is impaired. Second, estrogenic molecules have the beneficial effect of mimicking endogenous hormones promoting remineralization, but increase in bone density is poor compared to bisphosphonates. Estrogenics do offer a considerable advantage in that bone integrity is maintained, whereas with bisphosphonates microfractures tend to accumulate. To date, V-ATPase inhibitors are not suitable because of poor selectivity toward the osteoclast form of the enzyme and because of their more potent effect on kidney, liver, and neural forms. Structures and IC_{50} data from literature sources incorporating medicinal chemistry to improve selectivity [40–45] were used to aid design of new V-ATPase inhibitors. The data was organized in a manner so HQSAR could specifically assess and augment compound activity against desired V-ATPase species (osteoclast), yet decrease activity against undesired V-ATPases (liver and kidney). HQSAR models with high predictive quality were produced and tested, and a selection of proposed compounds were synthesized and evaluated *in silico*.

All compounds from the source papers were entered into a SYBYL database and transferred to a spreadsheet manually and checked for absolute stereochemistry. While constructing HQSAR models is a straightforward process, producing a model that will be robust and have high predictive value requires care in the selection and processing of activity data. The quality of models is assessed using *cross-validation*. In this approach, subsets of the training data are selected at random, and removed. An HQSAR model is constructed using the observations that remain and is used to predict the activities of the points removed. There are different protocols for carrying out this procedure; in the "leave-one-out" technique, every element of the training set is removed, and its activity is predicted based on all the remaining observations. Whatever the protocol, the measure of the quality of the model is the cross-validated r^2, denoted q^2, which measures the error when the points predicted are excluded when constructing the model. Cross-validation is critical not only for HQSAR but for any method that potentially uses a large number of descriptors, and where there is high probability of finding "random" variation in the attributes of the training molecules that will closely match any pattern of activity presented.

In the present case, the quality of the models (as measured by both q^2 and standard error) was improved by two means: normalizing IC_{50} data relative to one compound of the set, or predicting differences between activity against different targets to produce a selectivity index (e.g., activity against chicken osteoclast cOc minus activity measured using bovine chromaffin granules bCG). An ideal set of compounds would contain IC_{50} values that cover a wide range of activity (10–15 orders of magnitude or more) and also a diverse collection of functional groups, so that the resulting model is valid over a large chemical space. In particular, compounds that include large, complex groups (e.g., an Fmoc group, see Compound 4 in [40]) will be poorly predicted if underrepresented in the training set.

With the goal of the study to create, detect, and evaluate new compounds selective for osteoclast V-ATPase inhibition, some HQSAR results (Figs. 2.7–2.9) illustrate a few the best models produced. These were measured by achieving a cross-validated $q^2 > 0.5$ and a standard deviation < 1 between the training dataset (experimentally derived measured variable) and the predicted dataset (HQSAR model-derived measured variable) (Table 2.2). Within the figures the y-axis scale was calculated relative to bafilomycin A_1; in essence, this compound serves as a reference value for the HQSAR algorithm, to which all other compounds were compared (i.e., bafilomycin has an inhibitory selective index of 1 for chicken osteoclast

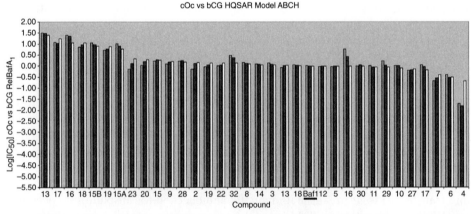

FIGURE 2.7   Selection of HQSAR results I. Actual data (**light gray bars**) $\log IC_{50}$ cOc − $\log IC_{50}$ bCG of a compound measured relative to bafilomycin A_1 V-ATPase phosphate assay from original data [40, 44], versus predicted $\log IC_{50}$ according to HQSAR (**dark gray bars**), versus the cross-validated HQSAR prediction (**white bars**). The graph is sorted in decreasing order of the cross-validated prediction relative to bafilomycin A_1 specificity. The graph suggests a strong correlation between the actual measured values of cOc/bCG selectivity and the predicted values (small difference between actual and predicted data). Hence, the model is likely to be of strong predictive value. To summarize, any compound left of bafilomycin A_1 (**Baf1**) has an increased specificity for cOc; any compound to the right has a decreased specificity for cOc.

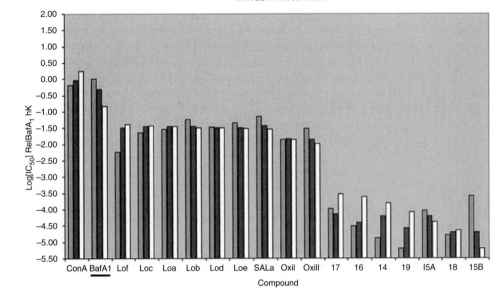

FIGURE 2.8 Selection of HQSAR results II. Actual data (**light gray bars**) log IC$_{50}$ hK of a compound measured relative to bafilomycin A$_1$ V-ATPase phosphate assay (**BafA1**) from original data [41, 44], versus predicted according to HQSAR (**dark gray bars**), versus the cross-validated HQSAR prediction (**white bars**). The graph is sorted in decreasing order of the cross-validated prediction and has a relatively strong predictive power. This data could provide a reasonable model for predicting the action of potential lead compounds against hK toxicity.

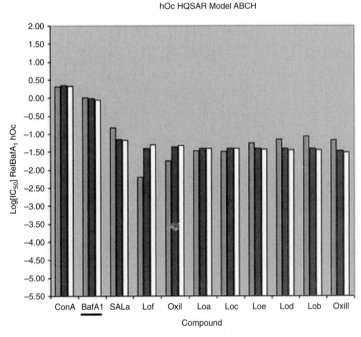

FIGURE 2.9 Selection of HQSAR results III. Actual data (**light gray bars**) log IC$_{50}$ hOc of a compound measured relative to bafilomycin A$_1$ V-ATPase phosphate assay (**BafA1**) from original data [41], versus predicted according to HQSAR (**dark gray bars**), versus the cross-validated HQSAR prediction (**white bars**). Despite the small size of this group, the HQSAR model was of high quality and may provide an indication of the activity of the potential lead compounds on hOc.

TABLE 2.2 HQSAR Models[a]

Parameter	Model	ApF	q^2	STD_ERR	CVSTD_ERR	Length	Components	MCS	Pred-r^2
hOc	ABC	4 to 7	0.672	0.384	0.437	401	1	N	D2S
hOc	ABCH	4 to 7	0.708	0.365	0.412	401	1	N	D2S
hOc	ACDo	4 to 7	0.606	0.413	0.478	401	1	N	D2S
hOc	ACHDo	4 to 7	0.645	0.395	0.454	401	1	N	D2S
hK	ABC	4 to 7	0.857	0.516	0.681	199	2	N	D2S
hK	ABCH	4 to 7	0.831	0.472	0.766	97	3	N	D2S
hK	ACDo	4 to 7	0.890	0.469	0.598	61	2	N	D2S
hK	ACHDo	4 to 7	0.968	0.189	0.295	59	3	N	D2S
cOc/bCG	ABC	5 to 8	0.819	0.148	0.279	59	5	N	0.7371
cOc/bCG	ABCH	5 to 8	0.766	0.130	0.323	83	6	N	0.8109
cOc/bCG	ABCCh	5 to 8	0.817	0.124	0.286	97	6	N	0.8219
cOc/bCG	ABCHCh	5 to 8	0.719	0.115	0.355	353	6	N	0.8204
cOc/bCG	ACChDo	5 to 8	0.775	0.121	0.311	83	5	N	0.8829
cOc/bCG	ACDo	5 to 8	0.766	0.158	0.317	97	5	N	0.8335
cOc	ABC	5 to 8	0.413	0.572	0.904	53	5	N	D2S
cOc	ABCCh	5 to 8	0.449	0.370	0.890	199	6	N	D2S
cOc	ACChDo	5 to 8	0.490	0.381	0.857	353	6	N	0.3572
cOc	ACDo	5 to 8	0.461	0.452	0.881	61	6	N	D2S
bCG	ABC	4 to 7	0.577	0.634	0.895	59	5	N	D2S
bCG	ABCH	4 to 7	0.525	0.650	0.948	401	5	N	D2S
bCG	ABCCh	4 to 7	0.589	0.563	0.882	199	5	N	0.3111
bCG	ACChDo	4 to 7	0.633	0.360	0.849	257	6	N	0.5615
bCG	ACDo	5 to 8	0.568	0.513	0.921	307	6	N	D2S

[a]The HQSAR model accuracy was assessed by linear regression. The predictive power of the HQSAR model was calculated for each compound dataset (Pred-r^2), where some compounds were omitted in the HQSAR model construction. D2S = Dataset too Small for HQSAR model validation. An $r^2 > 0.35$–0.4 is good, with a value of 1.0 being perfect. The Parameter column is the dataset used and constitutes the dependent variable (i.e., IC$_{50}$ relative to bafilomycin A$_1$), the Model column specifies the flags used. The Atoms per Fragment (ApF) column indicates the optimum number of atoms per fragment to generate the best q^2 value. STD_ERR = Standard Error, and CVSTD_ERR = Cross-Validated Standard Error. Length is the optimal holographic length; in each case all available hologram lengths were used (53, 59, 61, 71, 83, 97, 151, 199, 257, 307, 353, 401). Components are the fragments that were calculated to be potentially of greatest interest to modulate activity of the ligand (the larger the number, the better and more informative the model). The maximal common structure (MCS) was only effective when comparing the plecomacrolides.

over bovine chromaffin granules). The cOc versus bCG compares the selectivity ratio of bafilomycin A_1 against the two biological targets (computed as the difference of $\log_{10}$ values), and then subtraction of the result from itself. The value is 0 because

$$\text{bafilomycin } A_1 \text{ selectivity (on cOc/bCG)} - \text{bafilomycin } A_1 \\ \text{selectivity (on cOc/bCG)} = 0$$

For compounds with greater selectivity toward cOc, the value will be >0 (*positive*) and those with less selectivity to cOc, the value will be <0 (*negative*).

The data (Fig. 2.7) classically demonstrates a good quality HQSAR model (relative to bafilomycin A_1); Indole 3 (**I3**) was the most selective experimentally derived compound for cOc versus bCG (38-fold). The predicted value from the HQSAR model also indicated **I3** as the most selective because it had the greatest magnitude. Likewise, the most nonselective compound for cOc over bCG was concanamycin derivative 4 (**4**), which had correspondingly the greatest negative magnitude. The cross-validated values indicate the predicted actvity of omitted compounds and can improve the quality of the model (by making q^2 closer to 1, and standard deviation closer to 0), but in these results the cross-validation impaired the quality. The quality of HQSAR models can be assessed directly by leaving out bioactive molecules that have known IC_{50} data. It is advisable to select molecules over the majority of the measured data range to ensure a fair test. An HQSAR model is constructed as usual with these selected molecules omitted from the training set. The HQSAR model was then used to evaluate the predicted IC_{50} of these omitted molecules. Plotting the known IC_{50} versus the predicted IC_{50} values should produce a graph of $y = x$, with an ideal graph having the points plotted close to the $y = x$ line. Applying linear regression evaluates the quality of the predicted activities against their known values and hence is a direct measure of the quality of an HQSAR model(s). A linear regression score (r^2) close to 1 is ideal with 0 being the worst possible model. If the predicted r^2 value is close to 1, it adds confidence to the HQSAR model (Table 2.2), although datasets can be too small to apply such a technique and one must rely on the HQSAR model alone (Fig. 2.10). When evaluating proposed new chemical inhibitors (Figs. 2.11–2.13), researchers prefer a predictive r^2 value of around 0.35–0.40 (or greater) when considering candidates for chemical synthesis or chemical modification.

HQSAR has been used for investigations into several other ligand classes [46–52], but while computational output is exciting and valid, links with *wet* experiments and subsequent success are pressing issues and hence such techniques often evade academic interest.

2.6.2   QSAR

In the last ten years, QSAR has become an important tool that is used by nearly every pharmaceutical, agrochemical, and biotechnology company to increase the efficiency of lead discovery. The value of the QSAR approach is that it may be used either in the absence of detailed receptor site knowledge (i.e., binding site structural information) or in conjunction with such information if it is available. A QSAR model is a multivariate mathematical relationship between a set of physicochemical

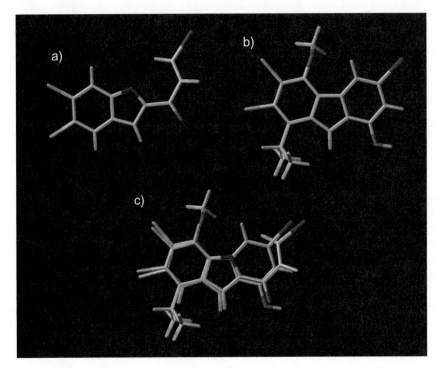

FIGURE 2.10 Two small molecules that at first glance look very different (**a** and **b**). When superimposed (**c**), the fused ring structure of the second molecule (**b**) does not appear too different from the nonfused ring structure (**a**). Only by careful alignment by eye can overlaps such as these be accomplished. Slowly, computers are improving in performing these tasks.

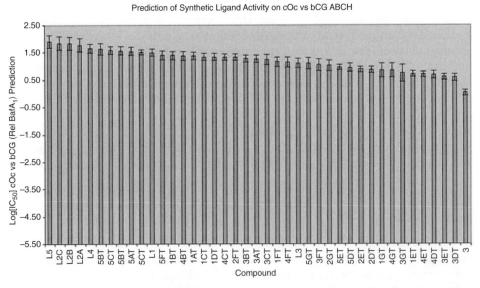

FIGURE 2.11 Application of HQSAR model predictions for *in silico* ligand database assessment I. Evaluation of the database of proposed synthetic ligands for selective action on cOc over bCG V-ATPase. Database compounds of significant interest lie to the left of the graph.

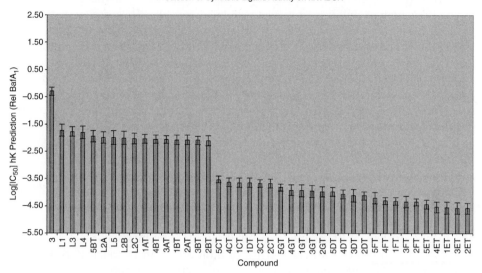

FIGURE 2.12 Application of HQSAR model predictions for *in silico* ligand database assessment II. Evaluation of the database of proposed synthetic ligands sorted by IC_{50} for hK V-ATPase phosphate assay. Database compounds of significant interest lie to the right of the graph.

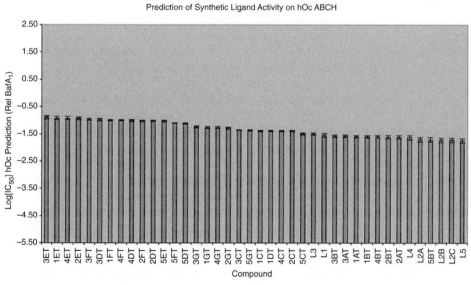

FIGURE 2.13 Application of HQSAR model predictions for *in silico* ligand database assessment III. Evaluation of the database of proposed synthetic ligands sorted by IC_{50} for hOc V-ATPase phosphate assay. Database compounds of significant interest lie to the left of the graph.

properties (*descriptors*) and a property of the system being studied, such as the biological activity, solubility, or mechanical behavior. QSARs correlate with cogeneric series of compounds, affinities of ligands to their binding sites, inhibition constants, rate constants, and other biological activities, either with certain structural features (e.g., Free Wilson analysis) or with atomic, group, or molecular properties, such as lipophilicity, polarizability, and electronic and steric properties (e.g., Hansch analysis). QSAR models have proved to be reliable tools for speeding up lead discovery [53–55] and have had an important place in molecular informatics throughout the world for at least two decades.

QSAR, like HQSAR, is based on measuring molecular similarity, but in the case of "classical" QSAR that similarity is based on characteristics, such as charge distribution and hydrophobicity, that derive from but are clearly secondary to molecular structure. While it is possible to rely exclusively on descriptors derived from experimental data, it is often the case that the molecular descriptors used in a QSAR study are directly computed from chemical structure; for example, a number of accurate algorithms are available to estimate $\log P$ from molecular structure [56], and likewise the electrostatic properties of molecules can be calculated using *ab initio* quantum chemical methods [57–62]. So, even if molecular structure is not immediately related to function by a QSAR model, it lies close in the background of these studies. In fact, this has become increasingly the case as the chemical libraries being used have increased in size, and it has become less likely that experimental data will be uniformly available for all the compounds being considered.

The elements of a QSAR model are the training data, consisting of selected physicochemical properties, a method for generating a predictive regression model from the training data, and a set of validation data (which are usually removed from the initial training set at the beginning). A variety of mathematical techniques are available to generate predictive models, which map a set of values for the molecular descriptors to a predicted activity. The simplest is classical multivariate linear regression, but this approach becomes less satisfactory as the number of descriptors increases, and it becomes likely that some of the descriptors will be highly correlated. More satisfactory approaches include principal components analysis (PCA) [63] and partial least squares (PLS) [64], which despite some differences in mathematical approach have the same function of automatically generating "aggregate" variables that are linear combinations of descriptors and building regression models based on these. Models constructed using PCA or PLS are less complex and more robust than those based on straightforward regression. They provide the added benefit of highlighting just those descriptors that are important for explaining the activity to be predicted, and effectively dropping those that are uncorrelated with the activity to be explained. Cross-validation is critical, especially when many descriptors are in use, and is performed just as was described in the context of HQSAR (Section 2.6.1).

The goal of QSAR is to derive a function that relates to biological activity with some parameter(s) describing a feature of the molecule. Analyzing the correlation between biological activity and molecular parameters for a series of molecules that have already been tested forms the QSAR relationship. The concept is based on the assumption that the difference in the physical and chemical properties of molecules, whether experimentally measured or computed, accounts for the difference in their observed biological or chemical properties. Thus, in general, the QSAR method deals with identifying and describing important structural features of molecules that are relevant to explaining variations in biological or chemical properties. The QSAR indicates the descriptors that are most statistically significant in determining the property, and studies can be focused on the molecular characteristics that those descriptors represent. QSARs thus help to make maximum use of data, whether that data is from experiment, simulation, or a database search.

QSAR is often carried out in the context of a *congeneric series*, a collection of molecules that share a common framework, but with significant variation of attached functional groups. Such a series comprises "variations on a theme," and it is this scenario that is most likely to lead to a robust, useful predictive model. While this might be seen as a drawback for classical QSAR, in that only molecules of a specified class are considered, the approach is very much compatible with most drug design methodologies where one begins with a framework that is amenable to variation using well-understood synthetic routes. The goal in this case is to develop a QSAR that rationalizes changes in activity with respect to structure, and to use this as a guide in proposing additional modifications that will further improve activity.

The "series" (a library of molecules with a shared characteristic) will consist of a common molecular framework with variance only in physicochemical descriptors such as hydrophobic constants, electronic parameters, or individual atoms. These physicochemical adaptations explain why individual molecules in a series have different biological activities. Relationships between activity and physicochemical characteristics can then be postulated, and the postulated relationship can be tested by generation of new compounds with predicted properties. The methods used to establish the equation that best describes the relationship between the property and the descriptors include regression techniques, PCA, and genetic algorithms. The expressed QSAR takes the form of either a search query or a predictive model, which can then be used to select new molecules with the specified activity from a database, or to predict the activity of individual molecules of interest. QSAR thus provides invaluable knowledge of which interactions are important to activity. This understanding provides the basis to formulate new active compounds that possess better overall therapeutic profiles, for example, compounds with increased functionality or that are more orally active. In fact, any biological or chemical activity that can be measured or derived from measurements can potentially be used as input for QSAR.

It should also be remembered that *in vitro* activity data only produce a QSAR that selects molecules that satisfy the *tested biological assay*, and do not necessarily indicate *in vivo* activity. The quality of the assay is therefore important. It has become increasingly important to conduct QSAR using more than one measured activity variable, such as adding a bioavailability measure to the activity data. The addition of *in vivo* data is difficult, as often many variables may exist that affect activity (primarily metabolism and excretion that are not tailored for), but this should be considered as an important development of QSAR.

2.6.3 Superimposition

One of the most compelling similarity techniques is not automated, can be time consuming, but is always done to get the point across clearly and effectively to a reader or critic. Usually after several techniques have been employed to narrow down the best matches to a particular query molecule, potential candidates can be compared for similarity by 2D superimposition. The coordinates of one molecule (the query) is taken and mapped onto another molecule (the candidate) to assess how similar the two molecules are. However, the drawback is that so far only we humans can deduce where to appropriately overlay them (Fig. 2.10). Therefore, it is hard to implement superimposition until there is a short list of molecules: a list of thousands is not appropriate for evaluation by this method. Ultimately, this technique convinces medicinal chemists that the candidate molecule is indeed similar to another, and they will commence synthesis (providing there are not too many chiral centers, *E/Z* isomers, or complex heterocyclic ring structures).

2.6.4 Program Suites

UNITY is a program suite offered by Tripos [14], which contains a combination of techniques and methods to represent small molecules and identify potential molecules for biological trials via similarity. Another such suite available for purchase is CATALYST [65] offered by the commercial vendor Accelrys [66].

Identifying Molecules Via Behavioral Similarities   The principles governing the biological activity of many chemical entities used as drugs are usually due to particular groups and core structure within the molecule. These physicochemical descriptors are usually unique to a particular class of molecule. For instance, a hydrogen bond donor (or acceptor) could interact favorably with the biological target and be crucial for activity; often coordinated water molecules are critical in such cases (e.g., estrogens 1ERR [67]). Maximizing contact between the molecule and the target via van der Waals interactions is the driving force for ligand binding (i.e., a good fit), releasing water used in solvation and increasing the entropy of the system. To employ UNITY, the user needs strong biological understanding of the active ligands known and, if possible, should have an available protein structure.

Before searching large databases, it is imperative to design a robust representation of the parts of the molecule responsible for the drug class activity. This simplified representation is called a *pharmacophore*; it incorporates the features of as many drugs within the class as possible (deemed crucial for activity). If the design is of good quality, the pharmacophore will return the molecules known to be active and thus validate itself. Once the pharmacophore is designed suitably and holds well by returning other molecules within the drug class, the next step can be taken.

Large databases of molecules are available at cost and also without charge (Section 2.5.2) and are an excellent resource to find if there are compounds already similar to the pharmacophore. The goal is to find subtly different molecules that contain the groups and structural features essential for activity. Even if the molecule is not ideal, it may be available and amenable to medicinal chemistry.

In UNITY the procured molecular databases must be processed into a recognizable format for use by the program and often requires expertise. One must be exceptionally careful when building the database and when relying on prepared databases that the compounds are indeed represented correctly. CORINA [16] and STERGEN [17] are among the best tools for this particular job, but naming compounds uniquely is the most imperative and difficult task to accomplish. On construction of UNITY databases, unique names for each molecule are responsible for most of the observed errors reported back. There are more sinister examples of errors such as the interpretation of molecules by SYBYL itself. One needs to be very vigilant with molecules having double bonds and conjugated aromatic and cyclized compounds. It is often the case that subtle changes can occur and the user is oblivious to these mistakes. A particularly good example is Raloxifene from the WDI database being interpreted incorrectly. Many PDB files contain mistakes and can also be interpreted incorrectly. When the database in constructed, it is important to note that 2D fingerprints and 2D macroscreens can be included in the database build. Often incorporating this into the UNITY database design increases the build time dramatically; but on the upside, all the searches will be considerably faster and nonmatching molecules are rapidly evaluated in a prescreen first.

These shortcomings aside, UNITY is still a powerful and reproducible means to search for similar molecules with many extra features, including the possibility of using key amino acids interacting with the ligand for structure-based drug design. What is sadly lacking is a score of how well the hits from the database fit the pharmacophore to describe the quality of the hit itself. This is rectified using an inbuilt feature to obtain Tanimoto coefficients for the returned hits: pitching these molecules against the best known drug molecules and implementing a cutoff to similarity.

Designing New ACE Inhibitors   Angiotensin converting enzyme (ACE) inhibitors are an excellent means to demonstrate pharmacophore design, not to mention their significant economic and medicinal importance. Heart disease affects approximately 65+ million Americans. The costs incurred via healthcare bills, lost revenue, and sick days are a serious nationwide medical and financial concern. The prime contributor to heart disease is hypertension (high blood pressure); 95% of cases are diagnosed as "essential hypertension." Blood pressure higher than 140/90 mmHg is considered seriously hypertensive and requires treatment.

ACE inhibitors work by preventing the final cleavage step of the rennin–angiotensin system; at this step angiotensin I is converted to angiotensin II by the enzyme ACE. Angiotensin II is the most potent endogenous vasoconstrictor known and increases peripheral reistance to blood flow by reducing the bore of arterioles. Inhibition of ACE would logically follow with a reduction in blood pressure and reduce the strain on the heart and circulatory system.

Recently, the crystal structure of lisinopril (Zestril by AstraZeneca) has been solved (PDB file 1O86) [68] and is considerably useful since potential molecules can be evaluated via docking into the active site of the receptor. Several ACE inhibitors combined with known IC_{50} data are available [69], as are pharmacophore designs [70, 71]. To highlight the use of such information and data, we demonstrate how UNITY can be used by incorporating pharmacophore designs for database screening. Our example is somewhat simpler than that presented in the literature for clarity and ease of understanding.

The pharmacophore designed is more simplistic but serves an important purpose in orienting the mind to appreciate that pharmacophores do not need to be overly complex to be effective. As each feature is added and the pharmacophore is built up, it adds further complexity to the screening process, unlike a macroscreen or fingerprint comparison that is rapid; a spatial or distance constraint between atoms requires a lot more computational time. Hence, a pharmacophore with one defined feature is a 1-point pharmacophore and can be identified very rapidly. Two defined features constitute a 2-point pharmacophore, and so on; typically, a pharmacophore has between 4 and 6 points, with some being very complex indeed [71]. As more points are added, the complexity of the calculations increases exponentially, so when screening, simple pharmacophores followed by a more complex one will save time in investigations. To screen a library of approximately 6 million molecules, it took approximately two weeks (in computer time) to create and screen the UNITY databases with incorporation of 2D macroscreens via fingerprints. This was six weeks in real time to manipulate and screen and modify the residual hit list data. Figure 2.14 shows the simple pharmacophore used incorporating the fragments conserved between all the ACE inhibitors [69], the three-carbon chain, and nitrogen in the five-membered ring. The features of this 2-point pharmacophore (Fig. 2.14a) were rapidly identified by the 2D Macro function and the matches were easily recognized by 1D comparisons. The 3-point pharmacophore (Fig. 2.14b), however, includes distance and spatial constraints, consequently requiring a lot more computational time. Thus, in screening a large library one would almost certainly conduct the search using the 2-point pharmacophore followed by the second. When testing the pharmacophores sequentially, all but one of the 23 known ACE inhibitors were returned, thus validating the pharmacophore design. The pharmacophores were used to screen an NCI database containing all possible stereoisomers of each entry and the residual dataset was organized using the Tanimoto coefficient. The top 4000

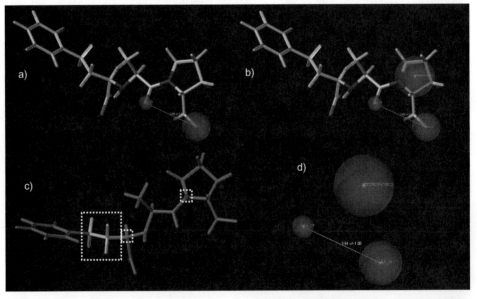

FIGURE 2.14   Three pharmacophores were used in a similarity search: (**a**) 2 points + distant constraint, (**b**) 3 points + distant constraint, (**c**) fragment-based pharmacophore with four hydrogens and 3 carbons (large box) and one nitrogen (small box); (**d**) what the computer sees for (**b**).

hits against lisinopril were docked into the PDB file 1O86 with the GOLD algorithm [72]. A comprehensive study of this investigation is currently under way.

UNITY Summary   UNITY demonstrates that robust design of a molecular template as a pharmacophore can prove insightful for identifying similar molecules. Although investment is required in software and expertise, it is not a particularly difficult technique to become adept with. Probably the biggest concern is maintenance and networking issues requiring specialized staff capable of system administration. This example merely scratches the surface of what UNITY can do: it is most relevant in identifying similar molecules.

2.6.5   Comparative Molecular Field Analysis (CoMFA) and Related Approaches

Comparative molecular field analysis (CoMFA) [73, 74], a proprietary method developed and marketed by Tripos, Inc. [14], is one of the most popular approaches to constructing quantitative models that link structure and activity [75–78]. Unlike conventional QSAR approaches, which use descriptors that describe the entire molecule (dipole moment, log P, topological indices, etc.), CoMFA is a 3D method that correlates a measured activity (e.g., log IC_{50}) with variations in electrostatic and steric properties for an aligned series of molecules. Since CoMFA identifies regions of the aligned structures that are important for determining activity, it allows the synthetic chemist to focus on sites of an exisiting molecular framework where variations are likely to be most productive. In favorable circumstances, a CoMFA can be thought of as an inverse model of the target receptor, since positive variations in activity require changes in the steric and electrostatic properties of the ligand that are compatible with (complementary to) those of the host receptor site. A CoMFA model can be generated to rationalize the activities of a series of ligands already characterized, and can then be used in predictive mode to estimate the activities of new molecules being proposed. CoMFA is one of a number of techniques that implicitly measure molecular shape by superimposing a regular grid on a collection of molecules.

The prerequisite for CoMFA is an aligned training set of ligands with known activities. This condition is most easily met by a congeneric series, since the shared molecular scaffold provides an immediate means to align the members of the set. In situations where a common framework is not available, CoMFA still requires that the molecules being analyzed can be superimposed in a meaningful way. One approach to this is *molecular field-fit*, where each molecule is positioned on a grid so as to maximize overlap with a preexisting set of field values (steric or electrostatic) computed on the grid vertices [79]. This approach can be used to construct a progressive alignment, where one or more seed molecules are used to generate a field on the grid, and successive molecules are aligned to the existing grid. As molecules are added to the alignment, their fields can be added to the vertices, potentially reinforcing the alignment field. Other methods that rely on a molecular field representation to carry out alignment include SEAL [80], FLUFF [81], and FIGO [82] (which combines a minimization procedure with 3D descriptors generated by the program GRID [83]).

A simple and effective approach for collections of structurally dissimilar molecules is to align them using their principal moments of inertia [84]—a procedure that aligns molecules based on their distributions of mass. Yet another approach, applicable when a structure is available for the target protein receptor, is to dock the molecules into the common receptor site, thus aligning them [85–87]. At first this might seem an ideal approach, since the molecules will be aligned with biologically relevant conformations; however, owing to inevitable perturbations in the conformations and positions of the docked ligands, even when the molecules exhibit very similar docking modes, this procedure tends to produce CoMFA models that are inferior to those generated using a receptor-free alignment [88]; but on occasion improvements are evident [89].

Once an alignment has been constructed using an appropriate set of training molecules, the next step is to embed the aligned set in a cubical grid and to compute the interactions of a probe atom with the aligned molecules. The default probe is a carbon atom (with van der Waals parameters appropriate for a tetrahedral carbon) with a charge of +1. The probe is positioned at each vertex of the grid, and its steric (van der Waals 6–12) and electrostatic (Coulomb's law) interactions are computed separately with each of the molecules in the alignment. (It should be pointed out that the choice of probe is flexible, and a number of novel modifications have been introduced, including probes that measure hydrophobicity through the HINT potential [90–92], and use of an orientable water molecule as a probe, to measure local hydrogen-bonding potential [93].) The grid spacing is an important parameter in determining the performance of the resulting CoMFA model, and there is also some influence due to the position and orientation of the aligned molecules with respect to the grid. The importance of these factors can be evaluated by adjusting the grid spacing as well as the orientation of the aligned molecules. In addition, a grid "focusing" procedure is available, which can be used to automatically refine the grid by identifying those grid vertices on which changes in potential are highly correlated with activity [73, 74, 94]; those portions of the grid most important for creating a robust predictive model can then be refined by subdivision, effectively increasing the density of vertices in the regions of the alignment with greatest predictive importance.

The final step in the construction of a CoMFA model is the application of partial least squares (PLS) regression, a method already discussed, to generate a quantitative relationship between the field values computed on the grid and measured activity (although the technique SOMFA shows new and promising advantages [95]). In CoMFA, each vertex of the grid gives rise to at least one descriptor (a steric or electrostatic field value for each molecule in the alignment). Since these typically number in the hundreds or thousands, there is the danger that the PLS procedure will pick out vertices with potential values that correlate well with activity merely by chance. In fact, it is almost always the case that CoMFA will produce a model that predicts the activities of the training molecules with a very favorable r^2. To ensure that the model is robust and applicable outside the training set, it is an absolute requirement to apply cross-validation. This is usually accomplished using the leave-one-out approach discussed previously (although more sophisticated techniques are available). As a rule of thumb, CoMFA models with a cross-validated r^2 (q^2) of 0.5 or better are considered to be useful as predictive models. As with all established techniques, CoMFa is subject to evaluation [96] and improvement [95, 97].

2.6.6 Shape Signatures

Shape Signatures is a new method for detecting molecular similarity recently developed in our laboratory [98]. The fundamental motivation of the method is to generate compact descriptors that capture the features of molecular shape and polarity while avoiding details of chemical structure. By maintaining a focus on shape, our approach emphasizes those characteristics of molecules important for biological activity, making it much easier to scan chemical libraries for compounds that may be both bioactive and of novel structure.

The key feature of Shape Signatures is our approach for exploring and encoding shape and polarity information. We have adapted the method of ray tracing, widely used in computer animation and presentation graphics, as a probe of molecular geometry. To do this, we initiate a ray in the interior of a molecule, which is bounded by a triangulated representation of the solvent-accessible molecular surface (Fig. 2.15a), and allow the ray to propagate by the laws of optical reflection (Fig. 2.15b,c). Probability distributions are derived from the ray, and it is these distributions, stored as histograms, which we denote as Shape Signatures. The signatures are independent of the orientation of the molecule and can be compared very quickly using simple metrics below:

$$L_1^{1D} = \sum_i |H_i^1 - H_i^2|$$

$$L_1^{2D} = \sum_i \sum_j |H_{i,j}^1 - H_{i,j}^2|$$

The simplest signature is the probability distribution of ray-trace segment lengths, where a segment is the portion of the trace between two successive reflections. We call this a one-dimensional (1D) signature, as the domain of the distribution is one dimensional (Fig. 2.15e). Shape Signatures of higher dimension can easily be generated by combining ray-trace segment length with properties measured on the molecular surface; for example, by computing the joint probability distribution for observing a particular sum of segment lengths on either side of a reflection point, combined with the molecular electrostatic potential (MEP) measured at the reflection, we produce a "2D-MEP" signature with two-dimensional domain (length + electric potential), which encodes both shape and polarity information (Fig. 2.15f).

Although not as well developed as the ligand-based approach just described, it is also possible to apply the Shape Signatures method in *receptor-based* mode. Here, the ray-trace operation is carried out in the volume exterior to a protein receptor site, with Shape Signature histograms accumulated in the same way as in the ligand-centered approach. In this case, a match between the signatures for a potential ligand and the receptor indicates shape complementarity between the small molecule and the shape of the receptor-site volume. While harder to apply than the ligand-based method (primarily because of ambiguities in defining the binding-site volume), the receptor-based approach offers the exciting prospect of scanning chemical libraries for potential bioactive compounds on the basis of shape, without the bias of using specific chemical structure queries, and without the computational expense of database docking.

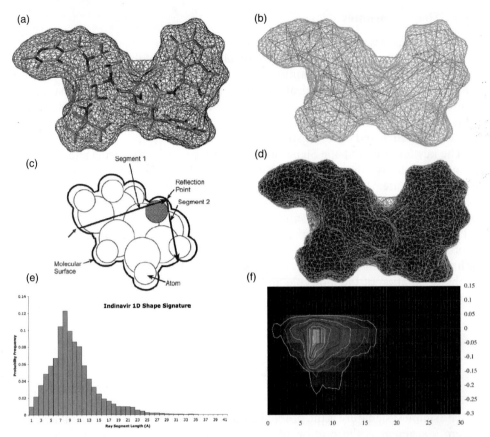

FIGURE 2.15 Process of Shape Signature generation. (**a**) The structure of Indinavir enclosed in the triangulated solvent-accessible surface is generated using SMART [41]. (**b**) Propagation of a ray trace around the inside of the triangulated molecular surface. Propagation of the ray trace around the Indinavir molecule with (**c**) 100 ray-trace segments and (**d**) 10,000 ray-trace segments is shown. On completion of a Shape Signature, the generated trace (**d**) is illustrated by (**e**), a histogram denoting the probability distribution (ordinate) of ray-trace segment lengths (abscissa), a "1D Shape Signature." A Shape Signature trace defined by ray-trace segment lengths and a mean electrostatic potential (MEP) is shown by (**f**) a contour plot, a "2D Shape Signature." It is these data stored as text files that are compared when performing a database screen.

Although the method is in its infancy, Shape Signatures similarity comparisons have already been shown to be very effective for biological application [28–30, 98–100]. A current area of intensive research in our laboratory is to develop further ways of applying Shape Signatures for multiple conformers and stereoisomers, and to further develop the receptor-based strategy along with the existing ligand-based approach. It is clear that it is not unreasonable to expect to be able to carry out well over a thousand million comparisons a day on a single processor (Table 2.3)— numbers that are not easily attainable by other techniques. The method is trivial to

TABLE 2.3 Comparison Between Speeds for Database Construction and Screening

Technique	Number of Molecules/Time Unit					CPU + RAM Computer Specifications
	Minute	Hour	Day	Month	Year	
Database Construction						
Shape Signatures (Ray Tracing)						
	5.6	3.3×10^2	8.0×10^3	2.4×10^5	2.9×10^6	$1 \times 3.5\,GHz$ Intel Pentium 4, 2 GB
	1.1×10^4	2.1×10^4	5.1×10^5	1.5×10^7	1.9×10^8	$32 \times$ Opteron 2.6 GHz, 0.5 GB
Raptor Model (Generation)						
	4.5	2.7×10^2	6.5×10^3	1.9×10^5	2.4×10^6	$1 \times 1.8\,GHz$ Pentium 4
Database Screening						
Shape Signatures (Screening)						
	1×10^6	6.0×10^7	1.4×10^9	4.3×10^{10}	5.3×10^{11}	$1 \times 3.5\,GHz$ Intel Pentium 4, 2 GB
	6.4×10^7	3.8×10^9	9.2×10^{10}	2.8×10^{12}	3.4×10^{13}	$32 \times$ Opteron 2.6 GHz, 0.5 GB
ROCS (Rapid Overlay of Chemical Structures)						
	7.6×10^2	4.6×10^5	1.1×10^7	3.3×10^8	4.0×10^9	$1 \times 3.5\,GHz$ Intel Pentium 4, 2 GB
UNITY (Pharmacophore)						
3pt	81.6	4.9×10^3	1.2×10^5	3.5×10^6	4.3×10^7	$1 \times$ RG14000 MIPS SGI $1 \times 500\,mHz$, 1 GB
4pt	68.9	4.1×10^3	9.9×10^4	3.0×10^6	3.6×10^7	
5pt	56.6	3.4×10^3	8.2×10^4	2.4×10^6	3.0×10^7	
Docking GOLD 2.2						
	0.6	34.7	8.3×10^2	2.5×10^4	3.0×10^5	$2 \times 3.0\,GHz$ Intel Xeon, 4 GB
Raptor (Molecule Evaluation)						
	8.0	4.8×10^2	1.2×10	3.5×10^5	4.2×10^6	$1 \times 1.8\,GHz$ Pentium 4

parallelize: both database generation and comparison—hence submission of queries via the Internet—could be implemented and accomplished in the near future. The data returned dramatically reduces the initial database size, a vital part of any successful CADD strategy [101]. Furthermore, Shape Signatures also achieves the second important quality of CADD: enrichment of molecules from the same class as the query [28–30, 98, 99]. Initial successes with Shape Signatures and estrogenic molecules (Fig. 2.16) were supported with experimental findings [99]. A potential novel molecule involved in analgesia has been discovered using Shape Signatures and offers considerable benefits over current compounds in this class [100]. Many groups [102–104] have previously used similar techniques for virtual-spatial recognition, but they have not been used in biological applications (with the exception of Ankerst and colleagues [105]). The Shape Signatures method is distinct from these

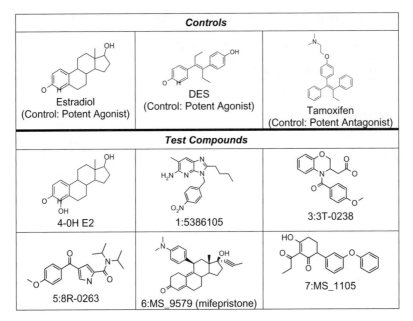

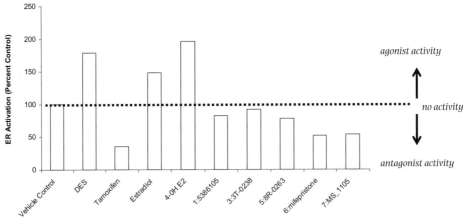

other previous attempts that use histogram comparisons for recognition of objects [102–104] or for lead discovery [105]. The Shape Signatures technique is rotationally invariant, meaning that it does not require, nor depend on, the orientation of the ligand or receptor site to obtain a reproducible histogram profile [103, 107].

As an example of the application of the Shape Signatures method, the query molecule WHI-P131 [106, 107], a tyrosine kinase inhibitor of interest as a therapeutic against several diseases (including leukemia and amyotrophic lateral sclerosis), is shown along with the top Shape Signatures hits located in the NCI database (Table 2.4) (were clarified by superimposition, see Section 2.6.3). Note the clear shape similarity between query and hits that nonetheless differ significantly in details of chemical structure. Finding these matches by other CADD methods would entail either generating a large set of structural queries based on the molecule of interest, or generating a pharmacophore model for the inhibitor. In either case, there

FIGURE 2.16 Examples of molecules selected by Shape Signatures demonstrating estrogenic activity on human estrogen receptor (ER) based on known controls. Three known estrogenic compounds (**top**)—estradiol, diethylbesterol, and tamoxifen—are all known to interact with human ER control. Using these as query molecules to screen an in-house database (1.2×10^6 molecules), the returned molecules (**middle**) were tested via assay [48]. Taking each of the selected "hits" from the search in turn, a 25 μM sample was tested using the NR peptide ERα ELISA kit (Active Motif, Carlsbad, CA) according to manufacturer's instructions. 17β-estradiol and tamoxifen were included as part of the kit. Briefly, a precoated 96-well plate was supplied with an optimized peptide containing the consensus binding motif of ERα coactivator SRC-1. Each compound was incubated for 1 hour with MCF-7 nuclear extract and the coactivator peptide in each well. The ligand-activated ERα was first detected using primary antibody specific for ERα and further with HRP-conjugated secondary antibody. The ER competitive binding assays used a gel filtration displacement assay for estrogen receptor alpha (ERα) and was employed to assess competitive binding by selected ER antagonists among the hit compounds. Estrogen receptor binding assays were conducted in duplicate in 50 mM Tris-HCl, pH 7.5, 1 mM EDTA, 20% glycerol, and 1 mM DTT buffer. Radioligands that were used included [6,7-³H]estradiol (specific activity 44 Ci/mmol, Amersham Biosciences). Binding assays were conducted on ice in a volume of 1 mL with 10 ng of purified full-length ERα and 25 nM ³H-estradiol in final concentration; 10 μM 17α-estradiol was used to define specific binding. Following a 1-hour incubation, assays were terminated by filtration through Whatman GF/B filters. Filters were soaked in Ecoscint liquid scintillation mixture (National Diagnostics, Somerville, NJ) and filter bound radioactivity was counted using a Beckman LS 1071 counter. (**Bottom**) One molecule was strongly agonistic (4-OH E2), while two were strongly antagonistic (6:mifepristone and 7:MS_1105). The other three molecules were only marginally antagonistic.

◀————————————————————————————

would be the presumption of specialized knowledge to construct the queries actually used to scan the database, and a small omission in constructing that query could mean missing important hits. In contrast, the ligand-based Shape Signatures search is very easy to carry out; the investigator need only present the single compound of interest as the query.

There is one potential drawback of Shape Signatures that must be addressed up front. Because the method collapses a great deal of chemical space onto very compact descriptors, it is inevitable that a Shape Signatures search will turn up false

TABLE 2.4 Shape Signatures Search of the NCI Database with WHI-P131

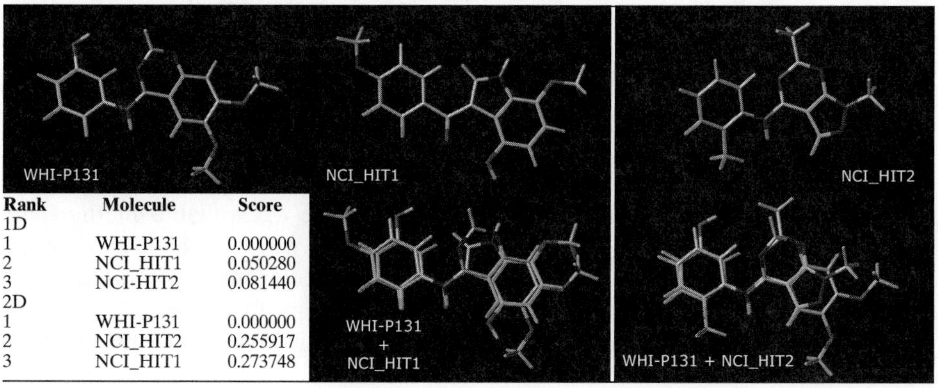

Rank	Molecule	Score
1D		
1	WHI-P131	0.000000
2	NCI_HIT1	0.050280
3	NCI-HIT2	0.081440
2D		
1	WHI-P131	0.000000
2	NCI_HIT2	0.255917
3	NCI_HIT1	0.273748

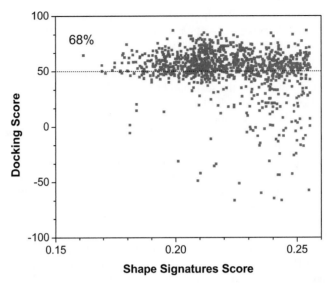

FIGURE 2.17 Evaluation of Shape Signatures with the GOLD algorithm. The plot indicates Shape Signatures score (abscissa) versus GOLD (ordinate) with the dashed line at 50 indicating a good GOLD docking hit.

positives in the hit list. To test how significant this issue might be, an independent assessment of the quality of the hits produced by a Shape Signatures search with the ACE inhibitor Enalapril was established. First, docking of known ACE inhibitors that have measured IC_{50} data [69] into ACE (PDB code 1O86) [68] was carried out using GOLD [72], producing a significant correlation between inhibitor pIC_{50} and the GOLD score, with scores for the known actives ranging from 50 to 87. In the second phase of our study, we identified the top 250 hits produced by a Shape Signatures search for the single query, Enalapril, conducted on an in-house database of 423 drugs and the NCI database [10] of over 250,000 compounds. The hit compounds were extracted from the database and docked into the active site of ACE using GOLD. Not only did our search, conducted using a single query, immediately identify 11 of the 20 well-characterized ACE inhibitors, but the fitness scores by GOLD evaluation of all 250 hits gave >75 for 4%, and >50 for 70% of the hits (Fig. 2.17). Assuming that the correlation between the experimental IC_{50} and the GOLD score holds, the Shape Signatures method is shown to readily identify known actives and interesting lead molecules, and with a modest proportion of false positives.

2.7   CONCLUSION

In this chapter we have merely scratched the surface of available methods to measure molecular similarity, focusing on methods with which we have experience and omitting any number of popular methods. In particular, there are a large and steadily growing body of 3D methods that are similar in spirit to CoMFA, but which nonetheless incorporate variations and refinements. In this context we must mention approaches that use descriptors generated using GRID [83] and first-cousins to CoMFA, such as COMSIA [108]. We hope that this chapter has provided an introduction to the spirit of molecular similarity methods and will serve as a foundation for further exploration by the interested reader.

ACKNOWLEDGMENTS

We kindly acknowledge Dr. Zhiwei Liu at the University of the Sciences in Philadelphia for her efforts in providing us with Fig. 2.16 for this chapter. We also extend gracious thanks to Ching Y. Wang and her supervisor, Professor William Welsh, at the University of Medicine and Dentistry of New Jersey for their efforts in constructing Fig. 2.15.

REFERENCES

1. Center for Drug Evaluation and Research, 2004, Report to the Nation: Improving Public Health Through Human Drugs. (http://www.fda.gov/cder/reports/rtn/2004/rtn2004. htm).

2. Mullin R. Tufts report anticipates upturn; cites drugmakers' actions to accelerate drug development. *Chem Eng News* 2006;84:9.

3. Newman DJ, et al. Natural products as sources of new drugs over the period 1981–2002. *J Nat Prod.* 2003;66:1022–1037.

4. Laatsch H. AntiBase 2007: The Natural Product Identifier. Hoboken, NJ: John Wiley & Sons; 2007.

5. Pauli A. AmicBase 2005. Hoboken, NJ: John Wiley & Sons; 2005.

6. Thomson Scientific World Drug Index. http://www.scientific.thomson.com/products/wdi (accessed July 2006).

7. GlaxoSmithKline, Plc. http://www.gsk.com (accessed July 2006).

8. Pfizer, Inc. http://www.pfizer.com (accessed July 2006).

9. Irwin JJ, Shoichet BK. ZINC—a free database of commercially available compounds for virtual screening. *J Chem Inf Model* 2005;45:177–182. (http://zinc.docking.org).

10. NCI Database. http://cactus.nci.nih.gov/ncidb2/download.html (accessed July 2006).

11. ChemBank Database (1.1 million entries). http://chembank.broad.harvard.edu/.

12. Weininger D. SMILES, a chemical language and information system. 1. Introduction to methodology and encoding rules. *J Chem Inf Comput Sci* 1988;28:31–36.

13. Ash S, et al. SYBYL Line Notation (SLN): a versatile language for chemical structure representation. *J Chem Inf Comput Sci* 1997;37:71–79.

14. Tripos, Inc. http://www.tripos.com (accessed July 2006).

15. MarvinSketch. http://www.chemaxon.com/marvin (accessed July 2006).

16. CORINA. http://www.mol-net.de/software/corina/index.html (accessed July 2006).

17. STERGEN. http://www.mol-net.de/software/stergen/index.html (accessed July 2006).

18. TAUTOMER. http://www.mol-net.de/software/tautomer/index.html (accessed July 2006).

19. Halgren TA. Merck molecular force field. III. Molecular geometries and vibrational frequencies for MMFF94. *J Comp Chem* 1995;17:553–586.

20. Gasteiger J, Marsili M. A new model for calculating atomic charges in molecules. *Tetrahedron Lett* 1978;34:3181–3184.

21. Gasteiger J, Saller H. Calculation of the charge distribution in conjugated systems by a quantification of the resonance concept. *Angew Chem Int Ed Engl* 1985;24:687–689.

22. Dalby A, et al. Description of several chemical-structure file formats used by computer-programs developed at Molecular Design Limited. *J Chem Inf Comput Sci.* 1992;32: 244–255.

23. Hammett LP. *Physical Organic Chemistry*, 1st and 2nd eds. New York: McGraw Hill; 1940, 1970. Hammond GS. A correlation of reaction rates. J Am Chem Soc 1955;77:334–338.

24. Hansch C, et al. *Substituent Constants for Correlation Analysis in Chemistry and Biology.* Hoboken, NJ: Wiley; 1979. Leo A, et al. Partition coefficients and their uses. Chem Rev 1971;71:525–554.

25. ROTATE. http://www.mol-net.de/software/rotate/index.html (accessed July 2006).

26. Example of energy minimization algorithm. http://www.chemsoc.org/exemplarchem/entries/pkirby/exemchem/mmmintro.html (accessed July 2006).

27. Weininger D, inventor; Daylight Chemical Information Systems, Inc, assignee. Method and apparatus for designing molecules with desired properties by evolving successive populations. US patent US5434796, 1995.

28. Zauhar RJ, et al. Shape Signatures: a new approach to ligand- and receptor-based molecular design. *J Med Chem.* 2003;46:5674–5690.

29. Nagarajan K, et al. Enrichment of ligands for the serotonin receptor using the Shape Signatures approach. *J Chem Inf Model* 2005;45:49–57.

30. Meek PJ, et al. Shape Signatures: speeding up computer aided drug discovery. *Drug Discov Today* 2006;11:895–904.

31. Nordling E, Homan E. Generalization of a targeted library design protocol: application to 5-HT7 receptor ligands. *J Chem Inf Comput Sci* 2004;44:2207–2215.

32. Milton RC, et al. Total chemical synthesis of a D-enzyme: the enantiomers of HIV-1 protease show reciprocal chiral substrate specificity. *Science* 1992;256:1403–1404. Errantum, *Science* 1992;257(Jul):147.

33. Thalidomide toxicity information. http://www.k-faktor.com/thalidomide (accessed July 2006).

34. CONCORD. http://www.tripos.com/index.php?family=modules,SimplePage,,,&page=sybyl_concord (accessed July 2006).

35. Barnard JM, et al. Use of Markush structure analysis techniques for descriptor generation and clustering of large combinatorial libraries. *J Mol Graph Model* 2000;18:452–463.

36. Molecular Operating Environment (MOE). http://www.chemcomp.com/software.htm (accessed July 2006).

37. James CA, Weininger D. *Daylight Theory Manual.* Daylight Chemical Information Systems, Inc; 1995.

38. Smith EG, et al. The Wiswisser line-formula chemical notation (WLN). Cheery Hill, NJ: Chemical Information Management; 1975.

39. MACCS-II. San Leandro, CA: MDL Limited; 1992.

40. Dröse S, et al. Semisynthetic derivatives of concanamycin A and C, as inhibitors of V- and P-type ATPases: structure–activity investigations and developments of photoaffinity probes. *Biochemistry* 2001;40:2816–2825.

41. Boyd MR, et al. Discovery of a novel antitumor benzolactone enamide class that selectively inhibits mammalian vacuolar-type (H$^+$)-atpases. *J Pharmacol Exp Ther* 2001;297:114–120.

42. Farina C, et al. Novel bone antiresorptive agents that selectively inhibit the osteoclast V-H$^+$-ATPase. *Farmaco* 2001;56:113–116.

43. Gagliardi S, et al. 5-(5,6-Dichloro-2-indolyl)-2-methoxy-2,4-pentadiamides: novel and selective inhibitors of the vacuolar H$^+$-atpase of osteoclasts with bone antiresorptive activity. *J Med Chem* 1998;41:1568–1573.

44. Gagliardi S, et al. Synthesis and structure–activity relationships of bafilomycin A1 derivatives as inhibitors of vacuolar H$^+$ATPase. *J Med Chem* 1998;41:1883–1893.

45. Nadler G, et al. (2Z,4E)-5-(5,6-dichloro-2-indolyl)-2-methoxy-N-(1,2,2,6,6- pentamethylpiperidin-4-yl)-2,4-pentadienamide, a novel, potent and selective inhibitor of the osteoclast V-ATPase. *Bioorg Med Chem Lett* 1998;8:3621–3626.

46. Chen D, et al. Holographic QSAR of selected esters. *Chemosphere* 2004;57:1739–1745.

47. Zhang H, et al. CoMFA, CoMSIA, and molecular hologram QSAR studies of novel neuronal nAChRs ligands—open ring analogues of 3-pyridyl ether. *J Chem Inf Model* 2005;45:440–448.

48. Zhu W, et al. QSAR analyses on ginkolides and their analogues using CoMFA, CoMSIA, and HQSAR. *Bioorg Med Chem* 2005;13:313–322.

49. Castilho MS, et al. Two- and three-dimensional quantitative structure–activity relationships for a series of purine nucleoside phosphorylase inhibitors. *Bioorg Med Chem* 2006;14:516–527.

50. Honorio KM, et al. Hologram quantitative structure–activity relationships for a series of farnesoid X receptor activators. *Bioorg Med Chem Lett* 2005;15:3119–3125.

51. Doddareddy MR, et al. Hologram quantitative structure–activity relationship studies on 5-HT6 antagonists. *Bioorg Med Chem* 2004;12:3815–3824.

52. Pungpo P, et al. Hologram quantitative structure–activity relationships investigations of non-nucleoside reverse transcriptase inhibitors. *Curr Med Chem* 2003;10:1661–1677.

53. Lohray BB, et al. 3D QSAR studies of *N*-4-arylacryloylpiperazin-1-yl-phenyl-oxazolidinones: a novel class of antibacterial agents. *Bioorg Med Chem Lett* 2006;16: 3817–3823.

54. Desai PV, et al. Identification of novel parasitic cysteine protease inhibitors by use of virtual screening. *J Med Chem* 2006;49:1576–1584.

55. Allan GM, et al. Modification of estrone at the 6, 16, and 17 positions: novel potent inhibitors of 17beta-hydroxysteroid dehydrogenase type 1. *J Med Chem* 2006;49: 1325–1345.

56. Eros D, et al. Reliability of log*P* predictions based on calculated molecular descriptors: a critical review. *Curr Med Chem* 2002;9:1819–1829.

57. Goller AH, et al. *In silico* prediction of buffer solubility based on quantum-mechanical and HQSAR- and topology-based descriptors. *J Chem Inf Model* 2006;46:648–658.

58. Ermondi G, et al. A combined *in silico* strategy to describe the variation of some 3D molecular properties of beta-cyclodextrin due to the formation of inclusion complexes. *J Mol Graph Model* 2006;25:296–303.

59. Clark M. Generalized fragment–substructure based property prediction method. *J Chem Inf Model* 2005;45:30–38.

60. Votano JR, et al. New predictors for several ADME/Tox properties: aqueous solubility, human oral absorption, and Ames genotoxicity using topological descriptors. *Mol Divers* 2004;8:379–391.

61. Holm R, Hoest J. Successful *in silico* predicting of intestinal lymphatic transfer. *Int J Pharm* 2004;272:189–193.

62. Lobell M, Sivarajah V. *In silico* prediction of aqueous solubility, human plasma protein binding and volume of distribution of compounds from calculated pK_a and A log$P$98 values. *Mol Divers* 2003;7:69–87.

63. Introduction of Principal Components Analysis (PCA). http://www.statsoft.com/ textbook/stfacan.html (accessed July 2006).

64. Introducton of Partial Least Squares (PLS). http://www.statsoft.com/textbook/stpls.html (accessed July 2006).

65. CATALYST. http://www.accelrys.com/products/catalyst (accessed July 2006).

66. Accelrys, Inc. http://www.accelrys.com/products (accessed July 2006).

67. Brzozowski AM, et al. Molecular basis of agonism and antagonism in the oestrogen receptor. *Nature* 1997;389:753–758.

68. Natesh R, et al. Crystal structure of the human angiotensin-converting enzyme–lisinopril complex. *Nature* 2003;421:551–554.

69. Kamenska V, et al. The COREPA approach to lead generation: an application to ACE-inhibitors. *Eur J Med Chem* 1999;34:687–699.

70. Tzakos AG, Gerothanassis IP. Domain-selective ligand-binding modes and atomic level pharmacophore refinement in angiotensin I converting enzyme (ACE) inhibitors. *Chem Biochem* 2005;6:1089–1103.

71. Sutherland JJ, et al. Pruned receptor surface models and pharmacophores database searching. *J Med Chem* 2004;47:3777–3787.

72. Jones G, et al. Development and validation of a genetic algorithm for flexible docking. *J Mol Biol* 1997;267:727–748.

73. Cramer RD III, et al. Comparative molecular field analysis (CoMFA). 1. Effect of shape on binding of steroids to carrier proteins. *J Am Chem Soc* 1988;110:5959–5967.

74. CoMFa. http://www.tripos.com/index.php?family=modules,SimplePage,,,&page=sybyl_ qsar_with_comfa

75. Sheng C, et al. Structure-based optimization of azole antifungal agents by CoMFA, CoMSIA, and molecular docking. *J Med Chem* 2006;49:2512–2525.

76. Menezes IR, et al. Three-dimensional models of non-steroidal ligands: a comparative molecular field analysis. *Steroids* 2006;71:417–428.

77. Demyttenaere-Kovatcheva A, et al. Identification of the structural requirements of the receptor-binding affinity of diphenolic azoles to estrogen receptors alpha and beta by three-dimensional quantitative structure–activity relationship and structure–activity relationship analysis. *J Med Chem* 2005;48:7628–7636.

78. Aguirre G, et al. New potent 5-nitrofuryl derivatives as inhibitors of *Trypanosoma cruzi* growth. 3D-QSAR (CoMFA) studies. *Eur J Med Chem* 2006;41:457–466.

79. Dixon S, et al. QMQSAR: utilization of a semiempirical probe potential in a field-based QSAR method. *J Comput Chem* 2005;26:23–34.

80. Kearsley SK, Smith GM. An alternative method for the alignment of molecular structures: maximizing electrostatic and steric overlap. *Tetrahedron Comput Methodol* 1990;3:615–633.

81. Korhonen SP, et al. Comparing the performance of FLUFF-BALL to SEAL-CoMFA with a large diverse estrogen data set: from relevant superpositions to solid predictions. *J Chem Inf Model* 2005;45:1874–1883.

82. Melani F, et al. Field interaction and geometrical overlap: a new simplex and experimental design based computational procedure for superposing small ligand molecules. *J Med Chem* 2003;46:1359–1371.

83. Goodford PJA. Computational procedure for determining energetically favorable binding sites on biologically important macromolecules. *J Med Chem* 1985;28:849–857. (GRID, version 19; Molecular Discovery Ltd, Mayfair, London, England, 2001.)

84. Collantes ER, et al. Use of moment of inertia in comparative molecular field analysis to model chromatographic retention of nonpolar solutes. *Anal Chem* 1996;68: 2038–2043.

85. Gallardo-Godoy A, et al. Sulfur-substituted alpha-alkyl phenethylamines as selective and reversible MAO-A inhibitors: biological activities, CoMFA analysis, and active site modeling. *J Med Chem* 2005;48:2407–2419.

86. Thaimattam R, et al. 3D-QSAR CoMFA, CoMSIA studies on substituted ureas as Raf-1 kinase inhibitors and its confirmation with structure-based studies. *Bioorg Med Chem* 2004;12:6415–6425.

87. Iskander MN, et al. Optimization of a pharmacophore model for 5-HT4 agonists using CoMFA and receptor based alignment. *Eur J Med Chem* 2006;41:16–26.

88. Kamath S, Buolamwini JK. Receptor-guided alignment-based comparative 3D-QSAR studies of benzylidene malonitrile tyrphostins as EGFR and HER-2 kinase inhibitors. *J Med Chem* 2003;46:4657–4668.

89. Datar PA, Coutinho EC. A CoMFA study of COX-2 inhibitors with receptor based alignment. *J Mol Graph Model* 2004;23:239–251.

90. Abraham DJ, Leo AJ. A program has recently become available that provides a functionality long missing from the molecular modeling world. HINT is a program that performs approximations of atom-based hydrophobicity based on the hydrophobic fragment work of Hansch and Leo. *Proteins* 1987;2:130–152.

91. Kellogg GE, et al. HINT—a new method of empirical hydrophobic field calculation for CoMFA. *J Comput Aided Mol Des* 1991;5:545–552.

92. Huey R, et al. Olson grid-based hydrogen bond potentials with improved directionality. *Lett Drug Des Discov* 2004;1:178–183.

93. Kim KH, et al. Use of the hydrogen bond potential function in a comparative molecular field analysis (CoMFA) on a set of benzodiazepines. *J. Comput Aided Mol Des* 1993;7:263–280.

94. Stuti G, et al. CoMFA and CoMSIA studies on a set of benzyl piperazines, piperadines, pyrazinopyridoindoles, pyrazinoisoquinolines and semi rigid analogs of diphenhydramine. *Med Chem Res* 2004;13:746–757.

95. Korhonen SP, et al. Improving the performance of SOMFA by use of standard multivariate methods. *SAR QSAR Environ Res* 2005;16:567–579.

96. Cavalli A, et al. Linking CoMFA and protein homology models of enzyme-inhibitor interactions: an application to non-steroidal aromatase inhibitors. *Bioorg Med Chem* 2000;8:2771–2780.

97. Moitessier N, et al. Combining pharmacophore search, automated docking, and molecular dynamics simulations as a novel strategy for flexible docking. Proof of concept: docking of arginine-glycine-aspartic acid-like compounds into the alphavbeta3 binding site. *J Med Chem* 2004;47:4178–4187.

98. Zauhar RJ, et al. Shape Signatures: a new approach to computer-aided ligand- and receptor-based drug design. *J Med Chem* 2003;46:5674–5690.

99. Wang CY, et al. Identification of previously unrecognized antiestrogenic chemicals using a novel virtual screening approach. *Chem Res Toxicol* 2006;19:1595–1601.

100. Zhang Q. et al. Discovery of novel triazole-based opioid receptor antagonists. *J Med Chem* 2006;49:4044–4047.

101. Zeman SP. Charting chemical space: finding new tools to explore biology. *Nature* 1–3. The 4th Horizon Symposium, Black Point Inn, Maine, USA, 20–22 May 2004.

102. Liu X, et al. *Proceedings of the 2003 IEEE Computer Society Conference on Computer Vision and Pattern Recognition* (CVPR'03); 2003, pp 1–8.

103. Osada R, et al. Matching 3D models with shape distributions. *Shape Model Int* 2001;May:154–166.

104. Ohbuchi R, et al. Shape-similarity search of 3D models by using enhanced shape functions. *Int J Comput Appl Tech* 2005;23:70–85.

105. Ankerst M, et al. Nearest neighbor classification in 3D protein databases. In *Proceedings of the 7th Conference on Intelligent Systems for Molecular Biology* (ISMB'99); 1999, pp 34–43.

106. Amin HM, et al. Inhibition of JAK3 induces apoptosis and decreases anaplastic lymphoma kinase activity in anaplastic large cell lymphoma. *Oncogene* 2003;22: 5399–5407.

107. Jilek RJ, et al. Lead hopping method based on topomer similarity. *Chem Inf Comput Sci* 2004;44:1221–1227.

108. Klebe G. Comparative molecular similarity indices: CoMSIA. In *Kubinyi H, Folkers G, Martin YC, Eds. 3D QSAR in Drug Design*. London: Kluwer Academic Publishers; 1998, Vol 3, p 87.

3

PROTEIN–PROTEIN INTERACTIONS

Kamaljit Kaur, Dipankar Das, and Mavanur R. Suresh
University of Alberta, Edmonton, Alberta, Canada

Contents

3.1 INTRODUCTION

Living organisms are almost exclusively comprised of four classes of molecules, namely, proteins, nucleic acids, polysaccharides, and lipids. Of these, barring lipids, all other classes can be regarded as macromolecules that are built from a limited number of building blocks or monomers. In the case of proteins, such building blocks are amino acids. Proteins are formed by polymerization of essentially twenty

Preclinical Development Handbook: ADME and Biopharmaceutical Properties,
edited by Shayne Cox Gad
Copyright © 2008 John Wiley & Sons, Inc.

"standard" amino acids. Yet, the myriad of proteins and their diverse functions, ranging from basic metabolism to structural and reproductive functions, can be astounding and constitute the very basis of life on Earth. For instance, an *Escherichia coli* bacterium contains over 4000 different proteins participating in virtually every life sustaining function of the cell.

The Greek root of the word protein, *proteios*, meaning *of first importance*, identifies the paramount role of this class of macromolecules in eukaryotes. It is perhaps discernible that twenty amino acids can be combined in different manners to yield virtually innumerable proteins, with a variety of functions. It is, however, interesting to note that even a slight alteration of the amino acid sequence can significantly alter the structure and function of a protein molecule. A well known example is the modification of hemoglobin in sickle cell anemia. Normal hemoglobin (HbA) contains a Glu at the sixth position of each β-chain, which is replaced by Val in the sickle cell hemoglobin (HbS). This single substitution causes aggregation of HbS into stiff filaments, leading to the deformation of the red blood cells into elongated "sickled" shapes, and the consequent symptoms of sickle cell anemia.

Being macromolecules, proteins predominantly interact with other molecules, including other proteins, via weak long-range interactions. These are also referred to as nonbonded interactions and are of two types, van der Waals and electrostatic. As two interacting proteins approach very close to each other, stronger specific bonds can be formed between them. For instance, the strongest specific interaction between two proteins occurs in the form of a covalent bond in the so-called disulfide linkage. Hydrogen bonds, less strong than covalent bonds, are more common forms of specific interactions exhibited by proteins. The four common types of interactions observed are listed in Fig. 3.1. A second factor that modifies long-range interactions is the tertiary structure of proteins. Proteins or peptides with defined secondary structural elements like helices, strands, and coils fold into three-dimensional arrangements, which give them a tertiary structure. For example, an α-helix, a β-sheet, and a coil region in the three-dimensional solution structure of an antibacterial peptide are highlighted in Fig. 3.2. Sequences with less than 50 amino acids are generally considered as peptides and more than 50 amino acids are called proteins.

Protein–protein interactions are key to several biological pathways and thus are attractive targets for therapeutic intervention. Such approaches are frequently based on a sound assessment of the strong and weak interactions and the protein's secondary or tertiary structures. The modulation or disruption of protein–protein inter-

Interactions	
Long-Range/Weak	Short-Range/Strong
Electrostatic (5 kcal/mol)	Covalent bonds (40 kcal/mol)
van der Waals (< 1 kcal/mol)	Hydrogen bonds (3-7 kcal/mol)

FIGURE 3.1 Long-range and short-range interactions between biomolecules. The energy values in parentheses are approximate.

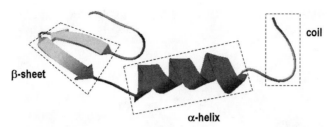

FIGURE 3.2   Tertiary structure of an antibacterial peptide (leucocin A) displaying secondary structure elements, namely, α-helix, β-sheet, and coil. The figure was generated from the 1CW6 Protein Data Bank coordinates [1].

actions has been difficult owing to their large surface areas of interaction. For several extracellular protein complexes, antibodies and other proteins have been identified as successful antagonists. The main rationale for this being that large macromolecules can readily disrupt the interaction between two proteins. From a cursory glance, this appears to be an attractive therapeutic option. However, a closer inspection of the problem indicates that large proteins are generally not orally bioavailable or cell permeable. Thus, these cannot be particularly effective for targeting intracellular protein–protein interactions. In light of this, one might presume that small molecules will provide more attractive therapeutic intervention options. However, such small molecules have been less successful in this regard, since they cannot provide specific recognition needed for a large protein surface. Protein surfaces do not often present deep indentations for small molecules to bind, and affinity is achieved through summing up several weak interactions.

Recent studies report several protein complexes as targets for drug design, with some of these targets amenable to small molecule inhibition [2–7]. Here we review the interactions between some of the important protein–protein pairs, followed by the recent successes in developing peptides, peptidomimetics, or small organic molecules as inhibitors of these interactions. This field is still in its infancy as most of the compounds identified are still in preclinical stages. Recent developments made in this broad field that have pharmaceutical and clinical implications will be discussed in this chapter.

3.2   PROTEIN–PROTEIN INTERACTIONS AND HUMAN PATHOGENESIS

3.2.1   Oncogenesis

Interaction between specific regions in a protein has been found to be essential for all stages of development and homeostasis. Subsequently, many human diseases occur by either loss of essential protein–protein interaction or through the formation of a protein complex at an inappropriate time or location. Several such interactions have been found to be responsible for the onset of oncogenesis and have been well studied [4, 8]. In the following, interactions between some of the well known protein pairs that lead to oncogenesis are discussed.

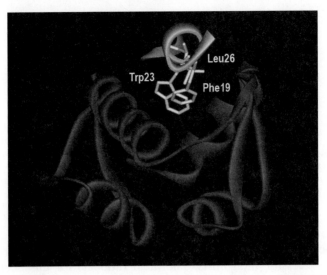

FIGURE 3.3   The ribbon representation of the MDM2–p53 complex (PDB entry 1YCR [10]) displaying the hydrophobic cleft of MDM2 where the p53 peptide binds as an amphipathic α-helix. The hydrophobic side chains of Phe19, Trp23, and Leu26 of p53 inserting deep into the MDM2 cleft are shown.

HDM2-p53   The tumor suppressor protein p53 is involved in the maintenance of the genomic integrity of the cell. It coordinates the cellular response to DNA damage by binding to specific DNA sequences and activating genes responsible for growth arrest or apoptosis. The inactivation of p53 by the binding of the cellular oncoprotein HDM2 (human double minute 2) has been identified as an important step in tumorigenesis [9]. In normal cells, HDM2 and p53 form a negative feedback loop that helps to limit the growth-suppressing activity of p53. The identification of this key negative regulator HDM2 provided a great opportunity to manipulate the levels of the tumor suppressor p53 in cancer cells.

The mouse homolog MDM2 binds the N terminus of p53, thereby interfering with the transcriptional ability of p53. The crystal structure of the amino terminal domain of MDM2 bound to a small region on the N terminus of p53 displayed the specific interaction between a hydrophobic cleft in the MDM2 protein and an amphipathic α-helix of p53 [10]. Several van der Waals contacts augmented by two intermolecular hydrogen bonds were found at the interface. The MDM2 cleft lined with hydrophobic and aromatic amino acids interacts with the hydrophobic face of p53 amphipathic helix. As shown in Fig. 3.3, the side chains of Phe19, Trp23, and Leu26 from the p53 α-helical region nestle deep inside the hydrophobic pocket of MDM2. Since residue Leu22 and Trp23 of p53 are critical for its transcriptional activity, p53 is rendered transcriptionally inactive after binding to MDM2. Inhibitors of the MDM2–p53 interaction have thus been found as attractive targets to gain activity of p53 in tumor cells [11].

Bcl-2/Bcl-X_L-BH3   The proteins in the Bcl-2 family regulate apoptosis by maintaining a fine balance between the pro- and antiapoptotic proteins within the cell

[12–14]. Proapoptotic members of Bcl-2 family such as Bax, Bak, Bid, and Bad, and antiapoptotic members such as Bcl-2 and Bcl-X_L exist as homodimers or mixed heterodimers. The nature of dimerization between these proteins dictates how a cell will respond to an apoptotic signal. Antiapoptotic proteins, Bcl-2, Bcl-X_L, or both, are overexpressed in the majority of human cancers and may play a vital role in cancer development. Therefore, inhibition of Bcl-2/Bcl-X_L activity is gaining recognition for the development of potent therapeutics as anticancer drugs. Several strategies have been employed to target these proteins, including inhibition of expression levels using antisense oligonucleotides and identification of peptide ligands that affect protein–protein association [15, 16].

The antiapoptotic function of Bcl-2 and Bcl-X_L is partially attributed to their ability to heterodimerize with proapoptotic members and antagonize their proapoptotic function. Three regions of the antiapoptotic proteins, namely, the Bcl-2 homology 1 (BH1), BH2, and BH3 binding sites, participate in their death-inhibiting activity and heterodimerization with the proapoptotic protein. However, only the BH3 binding site of the Bcl-2 and Bcl-X_L proteins is found critical for the ability to antagonize apoptosis. Small, truncated peptides derived from the BH3 region of Bak (16 mer) and Bad (25 mer) have been found necessary and sufficient both for promoting cell death and binding to Bcl-X_L [17, 18]. Furthermore, a synthetic cell permeable BH3 peptide derived from proapoptotic Bad has been shown to induce apoptosis *in vitro* and to have *in vivo* activity in human myeloid leukemia growth in severe combined immunodeficient mice [19].

The NMR solution structures of Bcl-2 and Bcl-X_L alone [20, 21] and Bcl-X_L in complex with Bak or Bad BH3 peptides [17, 18] have provided detailed information about the binding interactions of these proteins to the BH3 peptides (Fig. 3.4). The three-dimensional structures illustrate the formation of a hydrophobic cleft (the BH3 binding site) by the three BH domains of Bcl-2 and Bcl-X_L in which the Bak or Bad BH3 domain binds. The overall binding motif of Bcl-X_L/Bak and Bcl-X_L/Bad

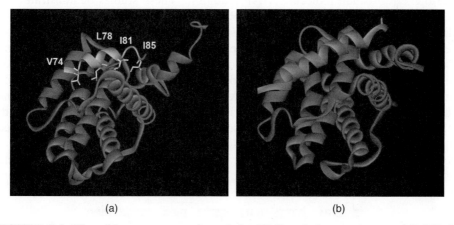

(a)   (b)

FIGURE 3.4 The ribbon representation of the NMR solution structures of Bcl-X_L in complex with (a) Bak BH3 peptide and (b) Bad BH3 peptide derived from the PDB codes 1BXL [17] and 1G5J [18], respectively. Bak and Bad BH3 peptides bind in the hydrophobic cleft of the Bcl-X_L protein. The hydrophobic side chains Val74, Leu78, Ile81, and Ile85 of Bak BH3 peptide inserting into the Bcl-X_L cleft are highlighted as a stick model.

complex was found to be very similar with only a few differences at the protein–peptide interface. The Bcl-X$_L$/Bak structure shows that the hydrophobic side chains of the Bak peptide (Val74, Leu78, Ile81, and Ile85) point into the hydrophobic cleft (BH3 binding site) of Bcl-X$_L$ and stabilize complex formation. Several electrostatic interactions between the oppositely charged residues of Bcl-X$_L$ (Glu129, Arg139, and Arg100) and the Bak peptide (Arg76, Asp83, and Asp84, respectively) were also present. Similar interactions were also found between the Bcl-X$_L$ and 25 mer Bad peptide. However, the longer Bad peptide makes additional contact at the two ends of the BH3 binding site, forming a tighter complex (K_d 0.6 nM) as compared to the Bcl-X$_L$/Bak 16 mer complex (K_d 480 nM). These observations suggest that the BH3 binding pocket of Bcl-X$_L$ as well as Bcl-2 is essential for its antiapoptotic function, and small molecules that bind to the BH3 binding pocket of Bcl-X$_L$/Bcl-2 can block the interaction between Bcl-X$_L$/Bcl-2 and proapoptotic proteins such as Bak, Bax, and Bad.

XIAP-Caspase   Inhibitors of apoptosis proteins (IAPs) are important but incompletely understood negative regulators of apoptosis. Among other mechanisms, IAPs selectively bind and inhibit caspases-3, -7, and -9, but not caspase-8. Currently, there are eight members of the IAP family. Of these members, X-linked inhibitor of apoptosis protein (XIAP) is upregulated in many cancers and has thus garnered the most attention as a drug discovery target [22].

XIAP is a 57 kDa protein with three zinc-binding baculovirus IAP repeat domains (BIR1–3) and a really interesting new gene (RING)-finger that binds and inhibits caspases with nanomolar affinity (Fig. 3.5). The BIR2 domain inhibits caspases-3 and -7, whereas BIR3 domain inhibits caspase-9. The function of the BIR1 domain has not yet been determined. The RING finger contains an E3 ubiquitin ligase. The proapoptotic protein SMAC is an endogenous human IAP antagonist that binds and inhibits XIAP, thereby releasing caspases and reactivating apoptosis. Structural studies map the interaction between XIAP and SMAC and provide a basis for the development of small molecule XIAP inhibitors. These studies demonstrate that SMAC binds to both the BIR3 and BIR2 domains of XIAP. Crystal structure of BIR3 domain of XIAP in complex with caspase-9 [23] and SMAC [24] illustrates the key interactions between the complexes. The N terminus of the small subunit of caspase-9 binds the same shallow groove on BIR3 as the N terminus of SMAC (Fig. 3.6). The N-terminal 4–7 amino acids of active SMAC are necessary and sufficient for binding the BIR3 pocket of XIAP and preventing XIAP from binding and inhibiting caspase-9. A 4 mer peptide, Ala-Val-Pro-Ile, derived from SMAC binds to XIAP with ~500 nM affinity [25]. These results indicate that small molecules that

XIAP

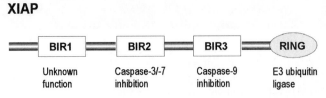

FIGURE 3.5   Schematic representation of XIAP showing different domains and their functions.

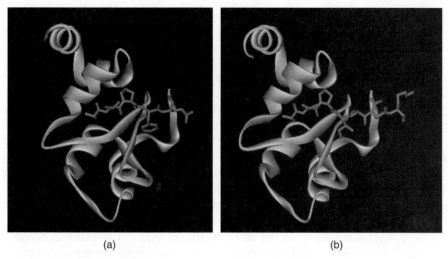

(a)   (b)

FIGURE 3.6 The three-dimensional structures of XIAP-BIR3 domain in complex with (a) N terminus of the small subunit of caspase-9 (Ala316, Thr317, Pro318, Phe319, and Gln320 shown as stick model) and (b) N terminus of SMAC (Ala1, Val2, Pro3, Ile4, Ala5, Gln6, and Lys7 shown as stick model). Both caspase-9 and SMAC bind in the same pocket of BIR3 as illustrated by the crystal structures of the complexes (PDB accession codes 1NW9 [23] and 1G73 [24], respectively).

mimic the actions of SMAC could be identified, providing an opportunity for a structure-based approach to the design of BIR3 inhibitors.

Stat3 Dimerization   Signal transducer and activator of transcription 3 (Stat3) is a cytoplasmic transcription factor that is activated in response to cytokines and growth factors. Upstream regulators of Stat3 constitute JAKs, Src, and EGF receptors and downstream targets include antiapoptotic and cell cycling genes such as Bcl-X_L and cyclin D1. Stat3 is overactivated in a surprisingly large number of cancers including head and neck, breast, brain, prostate, lung, leukemia, multiple myeloma, lymphoma, and pancreas and has therefore been identified as a potential target for cancer drug development [26].

Stat3 is composed of several domains, namely, an oligomerization domain (N terminal), a coiled coil domain, a DNA-binding domain, a linker domain, a Src homology 2 (SH2) domain, a critical tyrosine at position 705 (C-terminal end), and a C-terminal transactivation domain. On activation, JAK kinase-2 phosphorylates the tyrosine residues of its coreceptor, thereby facilitating the binding of Stat3 to specific phosphotyrosine residues of JAK-2 through its SH2 domain. This leads to phosphorylation of Tyr705 on the C terminus of Stat3, followed by Stat3 dimerization by the reciprocal interaction between the SH2 domain of one monomer and the phosphorylated tyrosine of the other. The activated dimers translocate to the nucleus, where they bind to specific DNA sequences and activate gene expression. These observations have pointed out Stat3 inhibition, such as inhibition of JAK-2/Stat3 interaction and Stat3 dimerization, as a novel molecular target for the advancement of a broad anticancer therapy. The X-ray elucidation of three-dimensional structure of the Stat3 homodimer bound to DNA reveals some details about the interaction between the two monomers and may facilitate the development of Stat3 inhibitors [27].

Rac1-GEF   Rho family GTPases, such as Rac1, control signaling pathways that are involved in cell adhesion, cell migration, and other cellular processes. Over-expression or upregulation of Rho GTPases has been discovered in many human tumors, including colon, breast, lung, myeloma, and head and neck squamous-cell carcinoma [28]. They can be activated through specific interaction with guanine nucleotide exchange factor (GEF) proteins that catalyze the exchange of GDP for GTP. One strategy to control tumor spreading is the selective inhibition of Rho GTPase activation by its GEF TrioN or Tiam1. Trio is a large multifunctional domain molecule with the amino-terminal module (TrioN) displaying the Rac1-specific GEF activity. Similarly, Tiam1, the T-cell invasion and metastasis gene product of the Dbl family, is shown to be an active GEF for Rac1. The three-dimensional structures of GEF–Rho protein complexes discern the specific interactions between GEFs and Rho GTPases needed for the signaling specificity mediated by Rho proteins. The cocrystal structure of Rac1/Tiam1 complex [29] shows that a domain of Tiam1, mainly dominated by α-helices, binds a shallow groove of Rac1, suggesting the presence of a small-molecule binding site (Fig. 3.7). A micromolar inhibitor of Rac1/TrioN interaction that selectively inhibits Rac1/Tiam1 and Rac1/TrioN versus related complexes and inhibits Rac1 activation in cells has been reported [30]. This study indicates that inhibition of the Rac1–GEF protein–protein interaction is possible, and such interactions have cellular consequences.

Integrin $\alpha_v\beta_3$ – Fibronectin   Another well studied example of cell adhesion proteins is the integrins. Integrins are the cell-surface receptors that act as molecular recognition sites for other proteins (for cell–cell and cell–extracellular matrix inter-

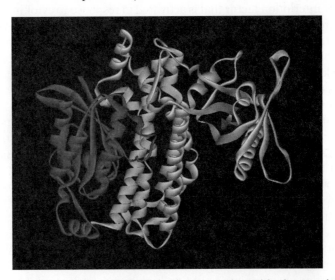

FIGURE 3.7   Crystal structure of Rac1 (left) in complex with the guanine nucleotide exchange region of Tiam1 (right) determined by Worthylake et al. [29] (PDB code 1FOE). The extensive interface of the complex buries over $3000\,\text{Å}^2$ of primarily hydrophobic surface area.

actions) as well as signaling molecules transferring ligand-binding information to the cytoplasm. Integrins are heterodimeric proteins consisting of α and β subunits and typically have a high molecular mass of ~300 kDa. At least, 25 $\alpha\beta$ integrin heterodimers have been reported and six of them are currently being evaluated in clinical trials for cancer [31]. Integrin $\alpha_v\beta_3$ has received particular attention as a potential target for anticancer drug design. The expression of $\alpha_v\beta_3$ is significantly increased on vascular cells in human tumors, but is weakly expressed on normal or quiescent endothelial cells. Since this integrin is relatively limited in its normal distribution, inhibition of its action is considered as an effective means of depriving tumors of nascent blood vessels without involving normal tissues.

Integrin recognition of the extracellular matrix ligands, such as fibronectin, collagen, and vitronectin, relies on the concerted binding of both the α and β subunits to regions of the ligand containing the Arg-Gly-Asp (RGD) sequence [32]. The RGD motif was the first integrin binding motif discovered. Several new motifs have been found since then that bind to a specific class of integrins [33]. Studies on RGD sequence have led to the discovery of cyclic pentapeptide Arg-Gly-Asp-{D-Phe}-{N-methyl-Val} or cyclo RGDf{NMe}V that specifically binds and inhibits integrin $\alpha_v\beta_3$ [34].

3.2.2   Pathogen–Host Interaction

Some viruses and bacteria enter eukaryotes by attachment to specific cell-surface receptors or cell-surface receptor-binding proteins. Viruses infect higher eukaryotes to reproduce themselves, whereas bacterial pathogens invade primarily to gain protection against the host immune system. Pathogens have always "enjoyed" invading human cells and have coevolved with their hosts to enable efficient entry, replication, and exit during their infectious cycles. An excellent review by Dimitrov [35] describes in depth the different virus entry mechanisms at the molecular level and opportunities for therapeutic intervention by inhibiting these processes. In this section, interaction between specific proteins of virus or bacteria and the target cell that facilitates pathogen entry into the target cell are discussed.

Papillomavirus E2 Protein   Infection by papillomavirus causes benign lesions that can lead to cervical cancer and other tumors [36, 37]. Papillomaviruses are small DNA viruses that infect higher eukaryotes by invading the basal layer of epithelial cells where they replicate successfully. Viral E2 protein has been found essential for replication and survival. E2 protein contains two conserved domains, the C-terminal viral DNA binding domain and the N-terminal transactivation domain that binds the viral E1 protein. Molecules that can bind these two domains of E2, thereby inhibiting the E2/DNA or E1/E2 interaction, are attractive targets for the development of therapeutics to prevent or treat papillomavirus infections. The three-dimensional structure of E1 bound to E2 reveals some important contact points between the complex [38]. The interaction surface, comprised of three helices from the N-terminal domain of E2, buries ~940 Å^2 surface area per protomer on E1–E2 complex formation (Fig. 3.8).

HCV-Envelope Protein 2   Hepatitis C virus (HCV) infection, another important target for antiviral drug design, causes severe medical problems, including chronic hepatitis, cirrhosis, and hepatocellular carcinoma. HCV genome is composed of a

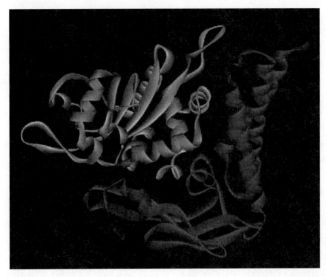

FIGURE 3.8   The X-ray structure of papillomavirus E1 helicase (upper structure) in complex with its molecular partner E2 (lower structure). PDB accession code: 1TUE [38].

single-stranded positive sense RNA of approximately 9600 nucleotides that are translated into a polyprotein precursor of about 3000 amino acids. The HCV polyprotein precursor is processed by host and viral proteases to yield structural and nonstructural proteins, which are essential for replication and assembly of new viral particles. The viral envelope E2 protein initiates the infection by association with specific cell-surface receptor(s). Many groups have demonstrated that the truncated soluble versions of E2 bind specifically to hepatocytes [39, 40]. This glycoprotein is found to interact with CD81, scavenger receptor class B type 1 (SR-B1), and dendritic cell-specific intracellular adhesion molecule 3-grabbing nonintegrin (DC-SIGN). Such findings suggest that these proteins may act as receptors for HCV on the cell surface. Therefore, inhibition of interaction between E2 and the cell-surface receptors, such as CD81, has been identified as a possible target for designing anti-HCV molecules [41, 42].

SARS-Angiotensin Receptor   SARS-CoV is a member of the Coronaviridae, a family of positive strand RNA virus that have long been known to cause severe acute respiratory syndrome in many animals and more recently in humans. Similar to other known coronaviruses, SARS-CoV is an enveloped virus containing four structural proteins, namely, the membrane (M), envelope (E) glycoprotein, spike (S) glycoprotein, and nucleocapsid (NP) proteins [43]. The spike protein of SARS-CoV is a large type I glycoprotein and is made up of two domains, the S1 near the N terminus and the S2 near the C terminus. Unlike other coronaviruses, the spike protein of SARS-CoV is not posttranslationally cleaved in virus producing cells. The S1 and S2 domains form the globular head and the stalk of the spike protein and play an important role in specific receptor recognition and cell fusion. The S1 domain mediates receptor association whereas the S2 domain is membrane associated and likely undergoes structural rearrangements. This conformational change initiates the

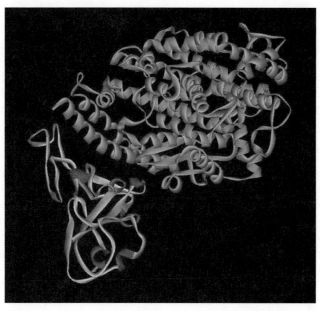

FIGURE 3.9   Crystal structure of SARS-CoV spike protein RBD (lower ribbon structure) in complex with human receptor ACE2 (upper structure). PDB accession code 1AJF [47].

fusion of the virus and host cell membrane, allowing for entry of the virus. The first step in viral infection is the binding of viral proteins to certain host cell receptors. The spike protein of coronavirus is considered as the main site of viral attachment to the host cells. It has been demonstrated that a metallopeptidase, angiotensin converting enzyme 2 (ACE2) isolated from Vero E6 cells, efficiently binds the S1 domain of the SARS-CoV spike protein [44]. A discrete receptor binding domain (RBD) of the spike protein has been defined at residues 318–510 of the S1 domain [45] and this receptor binding domain is the critical determinant of virus receptor interaction and thus of viral host range and tropism. It has been demonstrated that this RBD binds ACE2 with higher affinity than does the full length S1 domain [46]. The crystal structure (Fig. 3.9) of SARS-CoV RBD complexed with ACE2 receptor at 2.9 Å shows that the RBD presents a gentle concave surface, which cradles the N-terminal lobe of the peptidase [47].

Bacterial Fibronectin-Binding Proteins   One of the mechanisms by which bacterial pathogens invade cells is by displaying fibronectin-binding proteins (FBPs) on their surface. This approach to internalize into the host cell has been adopted by some pathogenic gram-positive bacteria. FBPs contain tandem arrays of intrinsically disordered repeat sequences that bind fibronectin–integrin complexes. The NMR solution structure of a complex comprising a peptide fragment of a streptococcal fibronectin-binding protein bound to the first two domains of human fibronectin reveals the tandem β-zipper interactions between the two fragments [48]. The tandem β-zipper is created by the β-strand conformation of the repeat sequences of FBP peptide fragment that extends existing antiparallel β-sheets in both directions upon binding to fibronectin. The binding affinity of these complexes is relatively weak but increases significantly when additional domains of both proteins are present. For example, the binding affinity (K_A) of two FBP repeats to pairs of fibronectin domains is ~$10^6 M^{-1}$. The tandem β-zipper interaction is a common phenomenon found in several pathogenic gram-positive bacteria, such as *Staphylococcus aureus, Streptococcus pyogenes*, and *Borrelia burgdorferi*, and may prove to be a widespread mechanism for bacterial foray of host cells [49–51]. Molecules that disrupt these β-zipper interactions may prove to be useful therapeutics for bacterial infections.

3.2.3   Loss of Normal Protein–Protein Interaction

Modular protein–protein interactions mediated by the tandem β-zipper have also been observed in eukaryotes [52, 53]. The LIM domains, found only in eukaryotes, are proteins with diverse functions such as transcription factors and protein kinases [54]. They are known to mediate specific protein–protein interactions through their LIM domains. Human genome encodes four LIM-only (LMO) and 12 LIM-homeodomain (LIM-HD) proteins each with a pair of tandem LIM domains at their N terminus (Fig. 3.10a). Three out of four LMO proteins have been implicated in oncogenesis. The LIM domains of all LMO and LIM-HD proteins bind the LIM domain-binding protein, Ldb1, through the 30 residue LIM interaction domain (LID) of this protein. Ldb1 is a ubiquitously expressed protein that contains an N-terminal dimerization domain, LID, and several other binding domains and is an

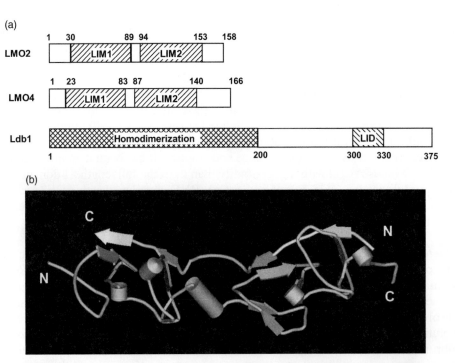

FIGURE 3.10   (a) Schematic representation of different domains of LMO2, LMO4, and Ldb1 proteins. (b) The schematic of LMO4 in complex with the Ldb1-LID domain displaying the "tandem β-zipper" interaction (PDB code 1RUT) [52]. The β-strand conformation of the peptide extends the existing β-structure in the partner protein in a modular fashion.

essential cofactor that plays diverse roles in the development of complex organisms. Since LMO proteins bind the same region of Ldb1 (LID) as the LIM-HD, LMO proteins can regulate the transcriptional activity of LIM-HD by competing for binding to Ldb1. The displacement of endogenous LMO4 by ectopically expressed LMO2, as the normal binding partner for Ldb1, has been directly linked with the overexpression of LMO2 in T cells and the onset of T-cell acute lymphoblastic leukemia in children [55].

The three-dimensional structures of the complexes comprising LIM domains and Ldb1-LID present that the intrinsically disordered Ldb1-LID forms a "tandem β-zipper" upon binding to LIM domains (Fig. 3.10b) [52]. In the complex, the four β-strands of Ldb1-LID extend across one face of LMO4 and remain in continuous contact with the LIM domains, mainly by backbone–backbone hydrogen bonds, burying a total surface area of $3800\,\text{Å}^2$. Ldb1 is known to interact with LMO and LMO-HD proteins only and not with any other LIM domain containing proteins. Recent studies [52, 53], highlight the specific features of the interaction between Ldb1 and the LMO2 or LMO4 proteins. Structural, mutagenesis, and yeast two hybrid analysis are used to identify the key binding determinants for the complex formation. The differences in the binding interaction between the two protein complexes suggest that molecules that could bind specifically to LMO2 or LMO4 may have potential uses in the treatment of neoplastic disorders.

The protein complexes discussed above are a few examples of interaction pairs that have been identified as possible drug design targets where the interactions have been mapped at the atomic level. A wide variety of approaches are utilized in the identification of these protein–protein interaction pairs and their inhibitors. Some of the most popular approaches are discussed in the following section.

3.3 SCREENING OF PROTEIN–PROTEIN INTERACTION INHIBITORS

Several approaches have been utilized in the identification of protein–protein interaction inhibitors with the aim of developing therapies for a variety of human diseases [6, 56, 57]. An analysis of current strategies employed for the identification of lead molecules demonstrates that a search for competitors of a known binder is the basis of traditional screening as well as more modern approaches. In the following sections, some of these approaches are described in detail.

3.3.1 Structure–Activity Relationship

A common approach relies on the experimentally determined (NMR or X-ray) structure of the protein complex. In this approach, one attempts to disrupt the interfacial interactions between the two proteins by developing mimics of the interface amino acid residues (peptide fragment) for one of the binding partners. The structure of the interface peptide fragment is modified using computer docking and molecular dynamics simulations to obtain peptidomimetics or small organic molecules [3]. The resulting peptides or peptide analogues present the interacting functional groups in similar spatial orientations as the interface amino acid residues. Peptidomimetic or small molecule inhibitors have higher affinity, better selectivity, and often better pharmacokinetic properties than the parent peptide. A second approach involves screening of a huge library of compounds using computer docking to find molecules with high affinity toward one of the binding partners of the protein complex. The lead structures identified using the above procedures are further optimized for potency and selectivity by structure–activity relationship (SAR) studies [58]. The SAR methods utilize experimental techniques, like nuclear magnetic resonance (NMR) spectroscopy, or computation methods, such as docking studies, and provide a structural perspective throughout the discovery and optimization of a lead molecule.

3.3.2   Genetic Screening Systems and Phage Display

The new library methodologies, such as phage display, allow generation of a large number of molecules with a fast screening and selection procedure to identify the most interesting lead candidates. Phage display technology has proved to be a very powerful *in vitro* technique for generating libraries containing millions of different peptides, proteins, or small molecules. Using the same technique, these libraries have been screened to identify ligands for peptide receptors, to define epitopes for monoclonal antibodies, to select substrates for enzymes, and to screen cloned antibody repertoires [59, 60].

In the phage display technique, filamentous virus is used as a platform for cloning of a DNA library (a library of genes or gene segments) encoding millions of variants of certain ligands into the phage genome and is fused to the gene encoding the phage coat or tail protein. Upon expression in the *E. coli* host in the presence of helper phage, the fusion protein (e.g., Coat protein-scFv) is incorporated into new phage particles that are assembled in the periplasmic space of the bacterium. Expression of the target gene fusion product and its subsequent incorporation into the mature phage coat results in the ligand being presented on the phage surface, while its genetic material resides within the phage genome. The proteins that are encoded by the library are expressed on the surface of phage and can be selected on the immobilized target molecule by biopanning. This interaction allows selection of high affinity binders for a variety of biomedical applications. Phages that bind the target molecule contain the gene for the protein and have the ability to replicate while nonadherent phages are washed away. This method can be used to efficiently clone genes encoding proteins with particular binding characteristics. In antibody phage display, the Fab or single chain fragment of IgG variable proteins is displayed on phage. This approach for antibody development offers advantages over immunization of animals and hybridoma technology [61]. Phage display can produce antibodies more quickly in a cost effective manner than traditional approaches. Additionally, antibody phage display techniques can potentially isolate antibodies to molecules that are not immunogenic in animals due to tolerance mechanism. Phage selection is not limited to the isolation of antibodies or short peptides. This approach has also been instrumental in studies and manipulation of a variety of other biologically active molecules and their designer variants [62].

3.3.3   Yeast Two Hybrid System and Intracellular Antibodies

Cell-based assays that monitor the intracellular behavior of target molecules, rather than binding or catalytic activity of purified proteins, are also being used in high throughput screening of protein interaction inhibitors. These assays offer an opportunity to discover entirely new classes of compounds, molecules that act primarily by modulating protein interactions in living cells.

The yeast two hybrid system is a cell-based genetic selection assay that has been successfully used to identify protein–protein interactions *in vivo*. The model originally developed by Fields and Song [63] exploits the fact that transcription factors are comprised of two domains, a DNA binding domain and a transactivation domain. As an example, GAL4 protein of yeast (*Saccharomyces cerevisiae*) is a transcriptional activator required for the expression of genes encoding enzymes of galactose utilization. The native GAL4 protein contains two domains: an N-terminal domain that binds to specific DNA sequences but fails to activate transcription; and the C-terminal acidic domain that is necessary to activate transcription but cannot initiate function without the N-terminal domain. The basic strategy of the two hybrid system involves two proteins of interest that are expressed as two different fusion proteins. One fusion protein, known as the bait, is fused to the DNA binding domain to bind at specific sites upstream of the reporter gene. The second fusion protein, known as prey, is fused to the transactivation domain. If a physical interaction occurs between the two proteins, it brings the GAL4 domain in sufficient proximity to activate the GAL4-dependent transcription of a reporter gene. There will be no expression of the reporter gene if the two proteins do not interact in the intracellular milieu.

The two hybrid system may not be a useful tool for all protein–protein interactions. The limitation of the technique includes where the protein of interest is able to initiate GAL4-dependent transcription. Toxicity of the expressed protein or misfolding of the chimeric protein inside the cell might result in a limited activity or inaccessibility of binding site to the other protein. Furthermore, some protein–protein interactions depend on posttranslational modification (S–S bond, glycosylation, and phosphorylation) that may not appropriately occur in yeast. Two hybrid systems need the fusion protein to be targeted to the yeast nucleus and it might be a disadvantage for extracellular proteins. Weak and transient interactions are often the most interesting in signaling cascades. These are more rapidly detected in the two hybrid system in view of the significant amplification of the reporter gene in this system.

Intracellular antibodies are antibody fragments that are targeted and expressed inside the cells for interaction with cellular target antigens. This strategy can inhibit the regular function or in some cases mediate cell killing following antigen binding. Specific activity of certain intracellular proteins has been blocked by microinjection of full length antibodies [64, 65] or of hybridoma mRNA [66, 67] into the cytoplasm of various cell types. Recent advances in DNA technology and antibody engineering have allowed the development of specific, high affinity antibodies to target antigens. These probes could be targeted intracellularly as unique nontoxic therapeutics. Recombinant antibody reductants that provide many of the essential features of antibodies are suitable forms to be expressed *in vivo* or internalized efficiently inside the cells. The recombinant single chain Fv fragment (scFv) has been the most widely used for intracellular antibodies [68]. Intracellular single domain antibodies have also been isolated from yeast libraries with good antigen binding affinities [69].

The first step of intracellular antibody isolation is the derivation of the V regions of the heavy and light chains of a high affinity monoclonal antibody against a target antigen. The VH and VL sequences could be amplified by RT-PCR of mRNA isolated from the hybridoma cells, assembled and cloned as a scFv [70]. Alternatively, one of the *in vitro* display systems, such as phage display [60], yeast display [71], or ribosome display [72] techniques, could be employed to generate the scFv libraries from immunized mouse spleen total mRNA and screen scFv libraries with the desired antigen to select specific scFv clones. Intracellular antibody capture technology [73, 74] has also been developed for *in vivo* screening of scFv libraries for a target antigen. This involves *in vitro* biopanning of diverse scFv libraries developed by phage display, followed by *in vivo* screening of antigen–antibody interaction using the yeast two hybrid system. The coding sequences of the antigen are cloned in one of the two hybrid vectors expressing the GAL4 DNA binding domain–antigen fusion protein. The coding sequence of scFv is cloned in the other two hybrid vector resulting in expression of GAL4 activation domain–scFv fusion protein. Yeast cells cotransformed with both the vectors will result in the expression of the reporter gene if the antigen and scFv interact with each other. There will be no reporter gene expression if the antibody fragment does not functionally interact with the antigen inside the yeast cells. By this technology it is possible to select and isolate intracellular antibodies, which could widely interact with the target protein inside the cells to alter or affect the protein function. Such induced intracellular protein–protein interactions could be an efficient pathogen neutralizing strategy for several viral and bacterial diseases [68, 75].

3.4   INHIBITORS OF PROTEIN–PROTEIN INTERACTIONS

As mentioned earlier, a large number of protein interaction complexes are emerging as potential targets for developing therapeutic agents. However, a big portion of these are ruled out at the onset due to the intricacies involved at the interaction site such as innate mutations and the atomic details of the binding site. The binding site may not present particular indentations, or if a pocket is present, its dimensions may be too small, or its geometry may be too shallow. Such features do not support tight binding of a drug-like molecule. Some of the above issues can be handled and a drug can be produced by generating antibodies against the target. In fact, therapeutic antibodies, including chimeric, humanized, and multivalent antibodies, and antibody fragments have been utilized in several instances and comprise over 30% of biopharmaceuticals currently undergoing clinical trials [76]. Several monoclonal antibodies against growth factors or their receptors are found effective in the treatment of solid tumors [77]. Antibodies tend to bind their targets with both high affinity and specificity and therefore block protein–protein interactions efficiently. However, antibodies are incompatible for intracellular targets, encountering problems such as poor delivery due to their relatively large size and lower stability of their disulfide-bonded structure in the reducing environment of the cell. Peptide inhibitors provide a much smaller substitute for *in vitro* inhibition of protein–protein interactions but are often not stable *in vivo* to be successful drugs. More stable variants, such as crosslinked peptides, peptide mimetics, and small molecule inhibitors, may prove to be better blocking agents for both intracellular and extracellular protein–protein interactions.

3.4.1 Peptide and Peptidomimetic Inhibitors

Specific recognition needed for a large protein surface seeks at least ~6 nm^2 area buried at the interface. The unique spatial distribution of the charged, polar, and hydrophobic residues at the interface are deemed important for recognition. Despite being conceptually simple, mimetics of the large interfacial area required for specific recognition remains a challenging endeavor. Nonetheless, steady progress has been made in the discovery of compounds that mimic protein surface and function.

A variety of peptide inhibitors have been reported over the last decade for blocking the MDM2–p53 association [11]. These peptides have been helpful in mapping out the interaction between the two proteins. The key interactions between MDM2 and p53 involve a relatively small area represented by three amino acids, namely, Phe19, Trp23, and Leu26 of p53. Optimization of peptides has led to the discovery of several low nanomolar inhibitors of MDM2 that have recently been reviewed by Fotouhi and Graves [11]. Peptide mimetics have also been explored in order to increase the metabolic and proteolytic stability over α-peptide inhibitors. Schepartz and colleagues [78] targeted the HDM2–p53 interaction with a 14-helical structure made of beta amino acids to display the functional groups of Phe19, Trp23, and Leu26 in the same spatial orientation as found in p53. These synthetic β^3-peptides exhibited significant helical character in aqueous buffer and one of the oligomers, **1** (Fig. 3.11), selectively inhibited HDM2 interaction with nanomolar affinity. Similarly, Hamilton and associates [79] have utilized terphenyl scaffold to mimic one face of α-helical peptides. Substitution of the three ortho positions of the scaffold projected one side of the molecule analogous to the i, i + 4, and i + 7 residues of an α-helix. A terphenyl derivative with three hydrophobic side chains, compound **2** (Fig. 3.11), was found to bind specifically at the p53 binding site of HDM2 and exhibited a K_i of 182 nM. More recently, α-helical peptidomimetics with the terphenyl scaffold and more soluble terephthalamide scaffold inhibited the Bak BH3–Bcl-X$_L$ interactions in the low micromolar range [80, 81].

Verdine and co-workers [82] targeted the BID/ Bcl-X$_L$ interaction by synthesizing hydrocarbon stapled helices to mimic the amphipathic α-helix BH3 domain of BID. These molecules, for example, **3** (Fig. 3.11), with constraint helix became proteolytically stable, cell permeable, and bound Bcl-X$_L$ with nanomolar affinity. In a cell-based assay, these compounds induced apoptosis and in an *in vivo* experiment inhibited the growth of human leukemia xenografts. Gellman and co-workers [83] generated chimeric (α/β + α)-peptides that mimic the α-helical display of BH3 domain of Bak. These peptides are tight binders and therefore potent inhibitors (K_i = 0.7 nM) of Bak/ Bcl-X$_L$ interaction.

RGD motif present in the extracellular matrix ligands, such as fibronectin, was the first integrin binding motif identified. Since then, development of RGD mimetics that bind selectively to a single integrin has been a subject of intense research [33]. Studies have primarily focused on four integrins—$\alpha_4\beta_1$, $\alpha_5\beta_1$, $\alpha_v\beta_3$, and $\alpha_{IIb}\beta_3$—that bind RGD containing ligands and are thought to have the most clinical significance. An important RGD containing molecule that emerged out of these efforts is cyclo RGDf{NMe}V pentapeptide [34]. This cyclic peptide specifically inhibits integrin $\alpha_v\beta_3$ with an IC$_{50}$ of 0.6 nM and is in Phase II clinical trials as an anticancer drug under the name cilengitide. The crystal structure (Fig. 3.12) of the cyclic peptide bound to the extracellular segment of $\alpha_v\beta_3$ integrin in the presence of Mn^{2+} metal

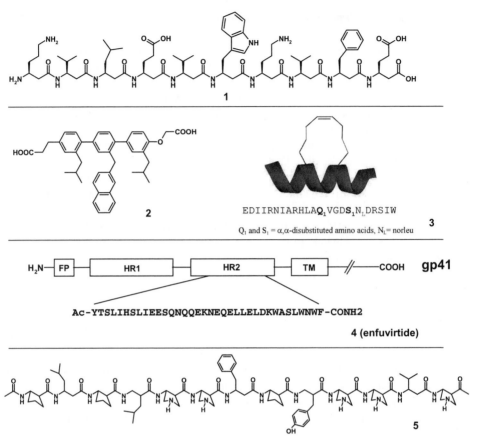

FIGURE 3.11 Structure of peptide or peptidomimetic inhibitors of protein–protein interactions.

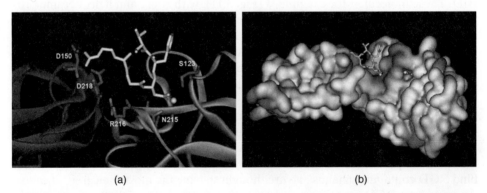

(a)   (b)

FIGURE 3.12 (a) Crystal structure of cyclo RGDf{NMe}V peptide (stick model) bound in the active site of integrin $\alpha_v\beta_3$ (PDB accession code 1L5G [84]). The Asp side chain carboxyl of the cyclic peptide interacts with one of the Mn^{2+}. The interacting residues (stick model) from integrin $\alpha_v\beta_3$ are derived from both the α and β subunits. (b) Surface representation of the two subunits of integrin $\alpha_v\beta_3$ bound to the cyclic peptide (stick model).

cation reveals important binding interactions in the complex [84]. The peptide binds at the major interface between the α_v and β_3 subunits burying about 45% (355 Å^2) of its total surface area. The RGD sequence makes the main contact with the integrin subunits. The availability of the complex structure has prompted search of nonpeptide antagonists of $\alpha_v\beta_3$ integrin using detailed computer docking experiments.

Peptides have also been exploited in the design of antiviral agents [85]. A successful example in this case is the HIV antiviral drug Fuzeon (**4**), enfuvirtide, or T-20, Fig. 3.11) [86]. Fuzeon is a 36 amino acid α-peptide that was introduced in 2003 into the clinics as a potent HIV entry inhibitor [87]. HIV entry into the target cells takes place in several steps, beginning with the binding of viral envelope protein gp120 to CD4 receptors on the target cells, followed by the exposure of the buried transmembrane fusion protein gp41 and conformational changes for the assembly of the hexameric six-helix bundle gp41 that allows the fusion to take place. As depicted in Fig. 3.11, the gp41 is made of an N-terminal fusion peptide (FP), two heptad repeat regions HR1 and HR2, and a transmembrane region. Fuzeon (**4**) is a small peptide derived from the HR2 region of gp41 that competitively inhibits the last step of the viral fusion. Peptidomimetics of the HR2 region would serve as good alternate inhibitors of the HIV fusion, perhaps with better pharmacokinetic profile than the α-peptide. Hamilton and co-workers [88] have utilized the terphenyl derivatives to mimic the helical HR2 domain. The most potent molecule with hydrophobic side chains at the ortho position of the three phenyl rings efficiently inhibits HIV-1 infection in a cell fusion assay (IC$_{50}$ 15.7 µg/mL). Furthermore, *in vivo* studies of these molecules as anti-HIV agents are in progress.

Nozaki et al. [89] discovered that a small peptide fragment from the milk glycoprotein human lactoferrin is able to block the entry of hepatitis C virus (HCV) particles into the hepatocytes. Virus entry inhibitors act extracellularly by blocking the binding of the virus to the host cell and this process of shielding the virus from attachment to the target cells seems more facile compared to targeting other intracellular sites that require exacting precision. The authors demonstrated that the mechanism of action of this peptide fragment is by binding to the E2 protein of HCV, thereby blocking its entry into the host cell, rather than binding to the host cell-surface receptors. Peptide mimics of this 33 amino acid fragment that can resist proteolysis and are metabolically stable will be of great clinical interest, as there is no vaccine for HCV and current therapeutic strategies yield roughly 40% response rates. English et al. [90] have attempted to construct peptidomimetic entry inhibitors of human cytomegalovirus (HCMV). The authors have prepared and tested several β-peptides, oligomers of β-amino acid, as entry inhibitors of HCMV. The most potent β-peptide, **5** (Fig. 3.11), inhibited HCMV infection in a cell-based assay with an IC$_{50}$ ≈ 30 µM.

The above examples reveal the prospect of peptides and peptidomimetics as potential therapeutics for various diseases. Currently, there are more than 40 marketed peptides worldwide and about 670 peptides are in either clinical or advanced preclinical phases. Several different classes of peptidomimetics are also entering the preclinical stages. Peptidomimetics like β-peptides, peptoids, and azapeptides are receiving particular attention as these unnatural oligomers, also called foldamers, fold into a conformationally ordered state in solution, like the natural biopolymers. These unnatural oligomers do not have disadvantageous peptide characteristics and therefore may generate viable pharmaceuticals. They are protease resistant, resistant to metabolism, and may have reduced immunogenicity relative to peptide analogues.

3.4.2 Small-Molecule Inhibitors

A broad range of screening initiatives has helped identify several protein–protein complexes that are amenable to inhibition by small molecules. Several compounds have been identified that help characterize proteins such as MDM2, Bcl-2, and XIAP as drug targets. Additionally, small-molecule antagonists have recently been described for several new targets, including Rac1–Tiam1, β-catenin–T cell factor, and Sur-2-ESX. Several of these small molecule protein–protein inhibitors are virtually at the threshold of becoming therapeutics.

Fotouhi and Graves [11] have reviewed some interesting new scaffolds and leads as MDM2 inhibitors. Among several reported molecules, only a series of compounds termed Nutlins (**6**, Fig. 3.13) possessed *in vivo* activity and therefore drug-like properties [58]. The Nutlins with a core imidazoline mimic the α-helical structure of the p53 backbone. The three aryl rings on the imidazoline are presented in the same space as the side chains of Phe19, Trp23, and Leu26 of p53. Furthermore, it was demonstrated by 2D NMR spectroscopy that they bind to MDM2 at the p53-binding site. The specific interaction of Nutlins with MDM2 indeed translated to the selective growth inhibition of cells containing wild-type p53 ($IC_{50} \approx 1.5\,\mu M$) and showed 10–20-fold selectivity for cells with active versus mutated p53. Compound **6** was well tolerated, orally bioavailable, and inhibited the growth of an MDM2-overexpressing tumor in mice. It achieved a high steady-state concentration during the study, indicating good pharmacokinetic properties.

Bad and Bak proteins bind to Bcl-2 and Bcl-X_L by inserting ~20 residue long α-helical Bad/Bak BH3 peptide into a hydrophobic groove [91]. Isolated BH3-like peptides also bind in this groove, suggesting the existence of a small-molecule binding site. There has been significant progress in developing compounds that bind in this groove on Bcl-2 and/or Bcl-X_L and thereby augment cell death [15, 16]. Recently, several molecules, such as **7** [92], **8** [93], and **9** [94] (Fig. 3.13), have been developed and are moving into clinical trials. GX15-070, a small-molecule inhibitor from Gemin X, is specifically designed to inhibit all of the antiapoptotic members of the Bcl-2 protein family and is the first such small-molecule inhibitor tested in clinical trials. Phase I clinical trials of GX15-070 in patients with refractory solid tumors and lymphomas showed promising results, advancing GX15-070 into Phase II clinical trials.

Small molecules that inhibit the BIR domains of XIAP have been found to be promising candidates for the development of therapeutic XIAP inhibitors [4, 22]. Molecules have been developed to specifically target BIR2 and BIR3 regions of XIAP. This is due to the difference in the mechanism of caspase inhibition by the BIR2 and BIR3 domains and their ability to inhibit different caspases. The structural data available for the interaction between the BIR3 domain of XIAP and caspase-9 suggests that small molecules binding the BIR3 pocket of XIAP could mimic the action of SMAC and inhibit the interaction between XIAP and caspase-9. These structural studies have facilitated several research groups toward the discovery of cell-active ligands for XIAP. Tripeptide inhibitors, such as **10** and **11** (Fig. 3.13) with

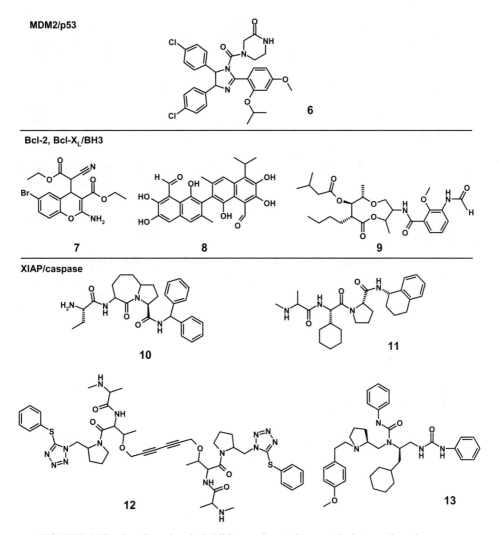

FIGURE 3.13   Small-molecule inhibitors of protein–protein interactions in cancer.

unnatural amino acids were identified and tested for their binding to the BIR3 domain of XIAP by NMR spectroscopy and fluorescent polarization assay [95–97]. These molecules bound to the BIR3 domain at SMAC binding site with nanomolar affinity. Unlike **10**, the BIR3 ligand **11** could activate apoptosis in a caspase-dependent manner in the absence of additional stimuli. Li et al. [98] used computer-aided drug design to mimic SMAC peptide. Lead compound identified included a tetrazoyl thioether moiety and was modified to form a C_2-symmetric diyne. The compound **12** (Fig. 3.13) bound the BIR3 domain of XIAP with an affinity similar to SMAC peptides and also bound cIAP-1 and cIAP-2 in cells. The proposed bivalent binding mechanism of **12** to XIAP resembled the wild-type SMAC, interacting simultaneously with the BIR2 and BIR3 domains of XIAP. SMAC is a dimer and interacts with the BIR2 and BIR3 domains at the same time to inhibit XIAP.

Compounds with polyphenylurea pharmacophore were identified by screening a large combinatorial library for activation of caspase-3 in the presence of XIAP [99]. Compound **13** (Fig. 3.13) was found to be selective for caspases-3 and -7 over caspase-9 and did not inhibit the SMAC-XIAP interaction. The polyphenylurea inhibitors were toxic to a wide spectrum of malignant cell lines and demonstrated preferential toxicity to primary malignant cells over normal cells. In xenograft models, these compounds were found to delay the growth of tumors of the prostate, breast, and colon carcinoma cells without any unpleasant toxicity to the mice. The above examples of XIAP inhibitors clearly suggest additional studies are required to discern the feasibility of small-molecule XIAP inhibitors as potential therapeutics. However, the data already point to XIAP as an interesting target for therapy.

The strategy of inhibiting protein–protein interactions with a small molecule has also been applied to the design of antiviral and antibacterial compounds. White et al. [100] reported a small-molecule inhibitor of papilloma virus E1–E2 dimerization. The inandione inhibitor **14** (Fig. 3.14) binds to the hydrophobic pocket of the E2 protein as shown by the cocrystal structure of the complex (Fig. 3.15) [101]. A second weakly bound inandione molecule was also observed in the crystal structure, suggesting the presence of additional binding region on the E2 protein for exploiting

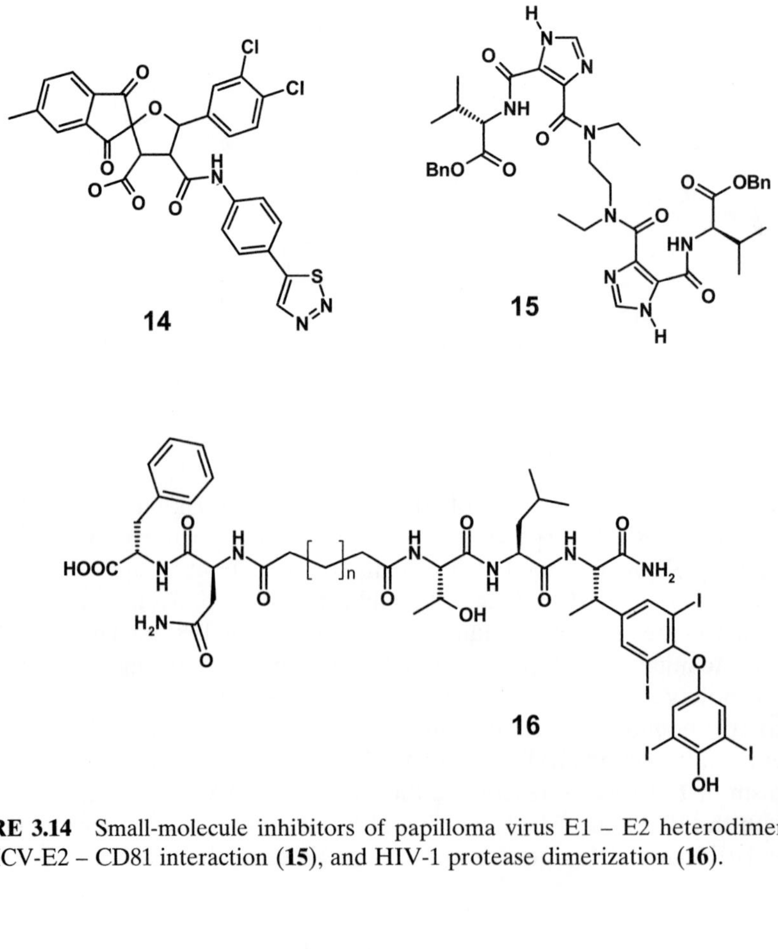

FIGURE 3.14 Small-molecule inhibitors of papilloma virus E1 – E2 heterodimerization (**14**), HCV-E2 – CD81 interaction (**15**), and HIV-1 protease dimerization (**16**).

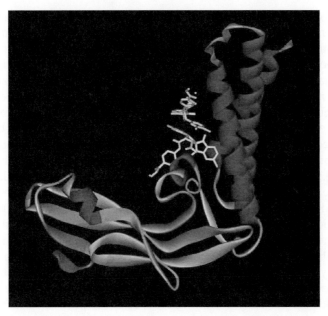

FIGURE 3.15   The structure of a small-molecule inhibitor, an inandione bound to papilloma virus E2 protein (PDB accession code 1R6N [101]). The inhibitor binding to E2 prevents E1–E2 heterodimerization and disrupts viral replication. A second weakly bound inhibitor (top) suggests that additional functional groups could be added to the side chains of the inhibitor to gain binding affinity.

inhibitor design. Todd and colleagues [41] developed molecules like **15** (Fig. 3.14), with a novel bis-imidazole scaffold, as mimics of helix D of CD81 that reversibly inhibited binding of HCV-E2 to CD81 receptor protein.

Inhibition of HIV-1 protease dimerization is a promising strategy for anti-HIV drug design as opposed to the active-site directed inhibitors. In this regard, Chmielewski and co-workers [102] discovered a nanomolar inhibitor (**16**, K_i = 71 nM, Fig. 3.14) of HIV-1 protease dimerization using a focused library approach. More importantly, the potent molecules of this class were equally active against wild-type and a mutant form of the enzyme. The mutant enzyme was resistant to active-site directed inhibitors, suggesting the importance of alternative drug design strategy.

3.4.3   Molecules Containing Porphyrin or Peptidocalixarene Scaffolds

Protein surface recognition by molecular architectures such as porphyrin and calixarene scaffolds has also been utilized in several instances. Hamilton and co-workers [103, 104] have used tetraphenylporphyrin derivatives to recognize the surface of cytochrome-*c* and identified subnanomolar binders. These molecules consist of peripheral anionic groups that bind positively charged Arg and Lys residues present on the cytochrome-*c* surface. The binding of phenylporphyrins induces unfolding of the protein, leading to disruption of tertiary and secondary structure. This denaturation of the protein facilitates proteolytic degradation. Another group used similar porphyrin-based derivates for blocking potassium channels. Trauner and colleagues [105] used porphyrins to match the fourfold symmetry of the homotetrameric human $K_v1.3$ potassium channel. Using competitive binding assays, the authors showed that tetraphenylporphyrin derivatives with peripheral cationic groups strongly interact with potassium channel, thereby reducing the current through the channel.

Several synthetic receptors containing calixarene scaffolds have been designed to bind protein surfaces to block protein–protein interactions or the entry of small molecules into the active site of certain enzymes [106–109]. For example, calix[8]arene receptors decorated with basic amino acids competitively inhibit recombinant lung tryptase by binding to the acidic residues at the central junction of the tetrameric protein [107]. These molecules, most likely, bind at the entrance of the active site and block the approach of the substrate. Similarly, peptidocalix[4]arenes have been shown to bind the surface of transglutaminase, inhibiting its acitivity [108]. However, the competition assays suggest that these molecules bind to the surface of protein other than the enzyme active site, causing a conformational change in the protein or sterically blocking the approach of the substrate. Aachmann et al. [109] have designed β-cyclodextrin that binds to a specific site on the insulin surface via its solvent-exposed aromatic side chain. These studies suggest that porphyrin and calixarene scaffolds are certainly promising candidates for protein surface recognition and further work in this area may lead to novel therapeutic agents.

3.5 CONCLUSION

Over the past decade, protein complexes have become prime targets for therapeutic intervention. This has opened immense opportunities in the treatment of hitherto incurable diseases such as cancer. A large number of protein pairs have been identified as drug targets with reported successful inhibitors, suggesting the possibility of fighting disease in near future. However, with the identification of hundreds of possible drug targets in the "class" of protein–protein interaction complexes, picking targets for inhibition by peptides, peptide mimetics, or small molecules is going to be critical. Many protein pairs have interfaces where a small, linear region of one protein binds into a hydrophobic cleft of the other. Inhibitors for such interfaces have been discovered, using several approaches ranging from screening to structure-based design, that display sufficient potency and cellular activity. Unfortunately, a potent, specifically binding molecule does not necessarily make a good drug. The true potential of these molecules as therapeutics will only be realized following successful clinical trials.

REFERENCES

1. Fregeau Gallagher NL, Sailer M, Niemczura WP, Nakashima TT, Stiles ME, Vederas JC. Three-dimensional structure of leucocin A in trifluoroethanol and dodecylphosphocholine micelles: spatial location of residues critical for biological activity in type IIa bacteriocins from lactic acid bacteria. *Biochemistry* 1997;36:15062–15072.
2. Ryan DP, Matthews JM. Protein–protein interactions in human disease. *Curr Opin Struct Biol* 2005;15:441–446.

3. Zhao L, Chmielewski J. Inhibiting protein–protein interactions using designed molecules. *Curr Opin Struct Biol* 2005;15:31–34.

4. Arkin M. Protein–protein interactions and cancer: small molecules going in for the kill. *Curr Opin Chem Biol* 2005;9:317–324.

5. Fletcher S, Hamilton AD. Protein surface recognition and proteomimetics: mimics of protein surface structure and function. *Curr Opin Chem Biol* 2005;9:632–638.

6. Sillerud LO, Larson RS. Design and structure of peptide and peptidomimetic antagonists of protein–protein interaction. *Curr Protein Pept Sci* 2005;6:151–169.

7. Pagliaro L, Felding J, Audouze K, Nielsen SJ, Terry RB, Krog-Jensen C, Butcher S. Emerging classes of protein–protein interaction inhibitors and new tools for their development. *Curr Opin Chem Biol* 2004;8:442–449.

8. Fry DC, Vassilev LT. Targeting protein–protein interactions for cancer therapy. *J Mol Med* 2005;83:955–963.

9. Bottger A, Bottger V, Garcia-Echeverria C, Chene P, Hochkeppel HK, Sampson W, Ang K, Howard SF, Picksley SM, Lane DP. Molecular characterization of the hdm2–p53 interaction. *J Mol Biol* 1997;269:744–756.

10. Kussie PH, Gorina S, Marechal V, Elenbaas B, Moreau J, Levine AJ, Pavletich NP. Structure of the MDM2 oncoprotein bound to the p53 tumor suppressor transactivation domain. *Science* 1996;274:948–953.

11. Fotouhi N, Graves B. Small molecule inhibitors of p53/MDM2 interaction. *Curr Top Med Chem* 2005;5:159–165.

12. Adams JM, Cory S. The Bcl-2 protein family: arbiters of cell survival. *Science* 1998;281:1322–1326.

13. Chao DT, Korsmeyer SJ. BCL-2 family: regulators of cell death. *Annu Rev Immunol* 1998;16:395–419.

14. Cory S, Huang DC, Adams JM. The Bcl-2 family: roles in cell survival and oncogenesis. *Oncogene* 2003;22:8590–8607.

15. O'Neill J, Manion M, Schwartz P, Hockenbery DM. Promises and challenges of targeting Bcl-2 anti-apoptotic proteins for cancer therapy. *Biochim Biophys Acta* 2004;1705:43–51.

16. Wang S, Yang D, Lippman ME. Targeting Bcl-2 and Bcl-XL with nonpeptidic small-molecule antagonists. *Semin Oncol* 2003;30:133–142.

17. Sattler M, Liang H, Nettesheim D, Meadows RP, Harlan JE, Eberstadt M, et al. Structure of Bcl-xL–Bak peptide complex: recognition between regulators of apoptosis. *Science* 1997;275:983–986.

18. Petros AM, Nettesheim DG, Wang Y, Olejniczak ET, Meadows RP, Mack J, et al. Rationale for Bcl-xL/Bad peptide complex formation from structure, mutagenesis, and biophysical studies. *Protein Sci* 2000;9:2528–2534.

19. Wang JL, Zhang ZJ, Choksi S, Shan S, Lu Z, Croce CM, Alnemri ES, Korngold R, Huang Z. Cell permeable Bcl-2 binding peptides: a chemical approach to apoptosis induction in tumor cells. *Cancer Res* 2000;60:1498–1502.

20. Petros AM, Medek A, Nettesheim DG, Kim DH, Yoon HS, Swift K, Matayoshi ED, Oltersdorf T, Fesik SW. Solution structure of the antiapoptotic protein bcl-2. *Proc Natl Acad Sci USA* 2001;98:3012–3017.

21. Muchmore SW, Sattler M, Liang H, Meadows RP, Harlan JE, Yoon HS, et al. X-ray and NMR structure of human Bcl-xL, an inhibitor of programmed cell death. *Nature* 1996;381:335–341.

22. Schimmer AD, Dalili S, Batey RA, Riedl SJ. Targeting XIAP for the treatment of malignancy. *Cell Death Differ* 2006;13:179–188.

23. Shiozaki EN, Chai J, Rigotti DJ, Riedl SJ, Li P, Srinivasula SM, Alnemri ES, Fairman R, Shi Y. Mechanism of XIAP-mediated inhibition of caspase-9. *Mol Cell* 2003;11: 519–527.

24. Web: Drugs used in the treatment of HIV infection. http://wwwfdagov/oashi/aids/viralshtml. 2000.

25. Liu Z, Sun C, Olejniczak ET, Meadows RP, Betz SF, Oost T, Herrmann J, Wu JC, Fesik SW. Structural basis for binding of Smac/DIABLO to the XIAP BIR3 domain. *Nature* 2000;408:1004–1008.

26. Jing N, Tweardy DJ. Targeting Stat3 in cancer therapy. *Anticancer Drugs* 2005;16: 601–607.

27. Becker S, Groner B, Muller CW. Three-dimensional structure of the Stat3beta homodimer bound to DNA. *Nature* 1998;394:145–151.

28. Sahai E, Marshall CJ. RHO-GTPases and cancer. *Nat Rev Cancer* 2002;2:133–142.

29. Worthylake DK, Rossman KL, Sondek J. Crystal structure of Rac1 in complex with the guanine nucleotide exchange region of Tiam1. *Nature* 2000;408:682–688.

30. Gao Y, Dickerson JB, Guo F, Zheng J, Zheng Y. Rational design and characterization of a Rac GTPase-specific small molecule inhibitor. *Proc Natl Acad Sci USA* 2004;101:7618–7623.

31. Tucker GC. Integrins: molecular targets in cancer therapy. *Curr Oncol Rep* 2006;8: 96–103.

32. Humphries MJ. The molecular basis and specificity of integrin–ligand interactions. *J Cell Sci* 1990;97:585–592.

33. D'Andrea LD, Del Gatto A, Pedone C, Benedetti E. Peptide-based molecules in angiogenesis. *Chem Biol Drug Des* 2006;67:115–126.

34. Dechantsreiter MA, Planker E, Matha B, Lohof E, Holzemann G, Jonczyk A, Goodman SL, Kessler H. N-methylated cyclic RGD peptides as highly active and selective alpha(V)beta(3) integrin antagonists. *J Med Chem* 1999;42:3033–3040.

35. Dimitrov DS. Virus entry: molecular mechanisms and biomedical applications. *Nat Rev Microbiol* 2004;2:109–122.

36. zur Hausen H. Papillomaviruses and cancer: from basic studies to clinical application. *Nat Rev Cancer* 2002;2:342–350.

37. Baseman JG, Koutsky LA. The epidemiology of human papillomavirus infections. *J Clin Virol* 2005;32:S16–S24.

38. Abbate EA, Berger JM, Botchan MR. The X-ray structure of the papillomavirus helicase in complex with its molecular matchmaker E2. *Genes Dev* 2004;18:1981–1996.

39. Bartosch B, Vitelli A, Granier C, Goujon C, Dubuisson J, Pascale S, Scarselli E, Cortese R, Nicosia A, Cosset FL. Cell entry of hepatitis C virus requires a set of co-receptors that include the CD81 tetraspanin and the SR-B1 scavenger receptor. *J Biol Chem* 2003;278:41624–41630.

40. Cormier EG, Tsamis F, Kajumo F, Durso RJ, Gardner JP, Dragic T. CD81 is an entry coreceptor for hepatitis C virus. *Proc Natl Acad Sci USA* 2004;101:7270–7274.

41. VanCompernolle SE, Wiznycia AV, Rush JR, Dhanasekaran M, Baures PW, Todd SC. Small molecule inhibition of hepatitis C virus E2 binding to CD81. *Virology* 2003;314:371–380.

42. Wagner CE, Mohler ML, Kang GS, Miller DD, Geisert EE, Chang YA, Fleischer EB, Shea KJ. Synthesis of 1-boraadamantaneamine derivatives with selective astrocyte vs C6 glioma antiproliferative activity. A novel class of anti-hepatitis C agents with potential to bind CD81. *J Med Chem* 2003;46:2823–2833.

43. Peiris JS, Guan Y, Yuen KY. Severe acute respiratory syndrome. *Nat Med* 2004; 10:S88–S97.

44. Li W, Moore MJ, Vasilieva N, Sui J, Wong SK, Berne MA, et al. Angiotensin-converting enzyme 2 is a functional receptor for the SARS coronavirus. *Nature* 2003;426:450–454.

45. Xiao X, Chakraborti S, Dimitrov AS, Gramatikoff K, Dimitrov DS. The SARS-CoV S glycoprotein: expression and functional characterization. *Biochem Biophys Res Commun* 2003;312:1159–1164.

46. Wong SK, Li W, Moore MJ, Choe H, Farzan M. A 193-amino acid fragment of the SARS coronavirus S protein efficiently binds angiotensin-converting enzyme 2. *J Biol Chem* 2004;279:3197–3201.

47. Li F, Li W, Farzan M, Harrison SC. Structure of SARS coronavirus spike receptor-binding domain complexed with receptor. *Science* 2005;309:1864–1868.

48. Schwarz-Linek U, Werner JM, Pickford AR, Gurusiddappa S, Kim JH, Pilka ES, et al. Pathogenic bacteria attach to human fibronectin through a tandem beta-zipper. *Nature* 2003;423:177–181.

49. Pilka ES, Werner JM, Schwarz-Linek U, Pickford AR, Meenan NA, Campbell ID, Potts JR. Structural insight into binding of *Staphylococcus aureus* to human fibronectin. *FEBS Lett* 2006;580:273–277.

50. Schwarz-Linek U, Pilka ES, Pickford AR, Kim JH, Hook M, Campbell ID, Potts JR. High affinity streptococcal binding to human fibronectin requires specific recognition of sequential F1 modules. *J Biol Chem* 2004;279:39017–39025.

51. Raibaud S, Schwarz-Linek U, Kim JH, Jenkins HT, Baines ER, Gurusiddappa S, Hook M, Potts JR. *Borrelia burgdorferi* binds fibronectin through a tandem beta-zipper, a common mechanism of fibronectin binding in staphylococci, streptococci, and spirochetes. *J Biol Chem* 2005;280:18803–18809.

52. Deane JE, Ryan DP, Sunde M, Maher MJ, Guss JM, Visvader JE, Matthews JM. Tandem LIM domains provide synergistic binding in the LMO4:Ldb1 complex. *EMBO J* 2004;23:3589–3598.

53. Ryan DP, Sunde M, Kwan AH, Marianayagam NJ, Nancarrow AL, Vanden Hoven RN, et al. Identification of the key LMO2-binding determinants on Ldb1. *J Mol Biol* 2006;359:66–75.

54. Matthews JM, Visvader JE. LIM-domain-binding protein 1: a multifunctional cofactor that interacts with diverse proteins. *EMBO Rep* 2003;4:1132–1137.

55. Hammond SM, Crable SC, Anderson KP. Negative regulatory elements are present in the human LMO2 oncogene and may contribute to its expression in leukemia. *Leuk Res* 2005;29:89–97.

56. Gadek TR. Strategies and methods in the identification of antagonists of protein–protein interactions. *Biotechniques Suppl* 2003;21–24.

57. Arkin MR, Wells JA. Small-molecule inhibitors of protein–protein interactions: progressing towards the dream. *Nat Rev Drug Discov* 2004;3:301–317.

58. Vassilev LT, Vu BT, Graves B, Carvajal D, Podlaski F, Filipovic Z, et al. *In vivo* activation of the p53 pathway by small-molecule antagonists of MDM2. *Science* 2004;303:844–848. Epub 2004 Jan 2002.

59. Benhar I. Biotechnological applications of phage and cell display. *Biotechnol Adv* 2001;19:1–33.

60. Clackson T, Hoogenboom HR, Griffiths AD, Winter G. Making antibody fragments using phage display libraries. *Nature* 1991;352:624–628.

61. Griffiths AD, Duncan AR. Strategies for selection of antibodies by phage display. *Curr Opin Biotechnol* 1998;9:102–108.

62. Hoogenboom HR, de Bruine AP, Hufton SE, Hoet RM, Arends JW, Roovers RC. Antibody phage display technology and its applications. *Immunotechnology* 1998;4:1–20.

63. Fields S, Song O. A novel genetic system to detect protein–protein interactions. *Nature* 1989;340:245–246.

64. Graessmann A, Graessmann M, Mueller C. Microinjection of early SV40 DNA fragments and T antigen. *Methods Enzymol* 1980;65:816–825.

65. Morgan DO, Roth RA. Analysis of intracellular protein function by antibody injection. *Immunol Today* 1988;9:84–88.

66. Valle G, Jones EA, Colman A. Anti-ovalbumin monoclonal antibodies interact with their antigen in internal membranes of *Xenopus* oocytes. *Nature* 1982;300:71–74.

67. Burke B, Warren G. Microinjection of mRNA coding for an anti-Golgi antibody inhibits intracellular transport of a viral membrane protein. *Cell* 1984;36:847–856.

68. Lobato MN, Rabbitts TH. Intracellular antibodies as specific reagents for functional ablation: future therapeutic molecules. *Curr Mol Med* 2004;4:519–528.

69. Tanaka T, Lobato MN, Rabbitts TH. Single domain intracellular antibodies: a minimal fragment for direct *in vivo* selection of antigen-specific intrabodies. *J Mol Biol* 2003;331:1109–1120.

70. Das D, Suresh MR. Producing bispecific and bifunctional antibodies. *Methods Mol Med* 2005;109:329–346.

71. Boder ET, Wittrup KD. Yeast surface display for screening combinatorial polypeptide libraries. *Nat Biotechnol* 1997;15:553–557.

72. Lipovsek D, Pluckthun A. *In-vitro* protein evolution by ribosome display and mRNA display. *J Immunol Methods* 2004;290:51–67.

73. Tse E, Lobato MN, Forster A, Tanaka T, Chung GT, Rabbitts TH. Intracellular antibody capture technology: application to selection of intracellular antibodies recognising the BCR-ABL oncogenic protein. *J Mol Biol* 2002;317:85–94.

74. Visintin M, Settanni G, Maritan A, Graziosi S, Marks JD, Cattaneo A. The intracellular antibody capture technology (IACT): towards a consensus sequence for intracellular antibodies. *J Mol Biol* 2002;317:73–83.

75. Lobato MN, Rabbitts TH. Intracellular antibodies and challenges facing their use as therapeutic agents. *Trends Mol Med* 2003;9:390–396.

76. Hudson PJ, Souriau C. Engineered antibodies. *Nat Med* 2003;9:129–134.

77. Hinoda Y, Sasaki S, Ishida T, Imai K. Monoclonal antibodies as effective therapeutic agents for solid tumors. *Cancer Sci* 2004;95:621–625.

78. Kritzer JA, Lear JD, Hodsdon ME, Schepartz A. Helical beta-peptide inhibitors of the p53–hDM2 interaction. *J Am Chem Soc* 2004;126:9468–9469.

79. Yin H, Lee GI, Park HS, Payne GA, Rodriguez JM, Sebti SM, Hamilton AD. Terphenyl-based helical mimetics that disrupt the p53/HDM2 interaction. *Angew Chem Int Ed Engl* 2005;44:2704–2707.

80. Yin H, Lee GI, Sedey KA, Rodriguez JM, Wang HG, Sebti SM, Hamilton AD. Terephthalamide derivatives as mimetics of helical peptides: disruption of the Bcl-x(L)/Bak interaction. *J Am Chem Soc* 2005;127:5463–5468.

81. Yin H, Lee GI, Sedey KA, Kutzki O, Park HS, Orner BP, Ernst JT, Wang HG, Sebti SM, Hamilton AD. Terphenyl-based Bak BH3 alpha-helical proteomimetics as low-molecular-weight antagonists of Bcl-xL. *J Am Chem Soc* 2005;127:10191–10196.

82. Walensky LD, Kung AL, Escher I, Malia TJ, Barbuto S, Wright RD, Wagner G, Verdine GL, Korsmeyer SJ. Activation of apoptosis *in vivo* by a hydrocarbon-stapled BH3 helix. *Science* 2004;305:1466–1470.

83. Sadowsky JD, Schmitt MA, Lee HS, Umezawa N, Wang S, Tomita Y, Gellman SH. Chimeric (alpha/beta + alpha)-peptide ligands for the BH3-recognition cleft of Bcl-XL: critical role of the molecular scaffold in protein surface recognition. *J Am Chem Soc* 2005;127:11966–11968.

84. Xiong JP, Stehle T, Zhang R, Joachimiak A, Frech M, Goodman SL, Arnaout MA. Crystal structure of the extracellular segment of integrin alpha Vbeta3 in complex with an Arg-Gly-Asp ligand. *Science* 2002;296:151–155. Epub 2002 Mar 2007.

85. Altmeyer R. Virus attachment and entry offer numerous targets for antiviral therapy. *Curr Pharm Des* 2004;10:3701–3712.

86. Moore JP, Doms RW. The entry of entry inhibitors: a fusion of science and medicine. *Proc Natl Acad Sci USA* 2003;100:10598–10602.

87. Web: Drugs used in the treatment of HIV infection. http://wwwfdagov/oashi/aids/viralshtml. Accessed 9 August 2006.

88. Ernst JT, Kutzki O, Debnath AK, Jiang S, Lu H, Hamilton AD. Design of a protein surface antagonist based on alpha-helix mimicry: inhibition of gp41 assembly and viral fusion. *Angew Chem Int Ed Engl* 2002;41:278–281.

89. Nozaki A, Ikeda M, Naganuma A, Nakamura T, Inudoh M, Tanaka K, Kato N. Identification of a lactoferrin-derived peptide possessing binding activity to hepatitis C virus E2 envelope protein. *J Biol Chem* 2003;278:10162–10173.

90. English EP, Chumanov RS, Gellman SH, Compton T. Rational development of beta-peptide inhibitors of human cytomegalovirus entry. *J Biol Chem* 2006;281:2661–2667.

91. Petros AM, Olejniczak ET, Fesik SW. Structural biology of the Bcl-2 family of proteins. *Biochim Biophys Acta* 2004;1644:83–94.

92. Wang JL, Liu D, Zhang ZJ, Shan S, Han X, Srinivasula SM, Croce CM, Alnemri ES, Huang Z. Structure-based discovery of an organic compound that binds Bcl-2 protein and induces apoptosis of tumor cells. *Proc Natl Acad Sci USA* 2000;97:7124–7129.

93. Qian J, Voorbach MJ, Huth JR, Coen ML, Zhang H, Ng SC, et al. Discovery of novel inhibitors of Bcl-xL using multiple high-throughput screening platforms. *Anal Biochem* 2004;328:131–138.

94. Tzung SP, Kim KM, Basanez G, Giedt CD, Simon J, Zimmerberg J, Zhang KY, Hockenbery DM. Antimycin A mimics a cell-death-inducing Bcl-2 homology domain 3. *Nat Cell Biol* 2001;3:183–191.

95. Sun H, Nikolovska-Coleska Z, Yang CY, Xu L, Liu M, Tomita Y, et al. Structure-based design of potent, conformationally constrained Smac mimetics. *J Am Chem Soc* 2004;126:16686–16687.

96. Sun H, Nikolovska-Coleska Z, Yang CY, Xu L, Tomita Y, Krajewski K, Roller PP, Wang S. Structure-based design, synthesis, and evaluation of conformationally constrained mimetics of the second mitochondria-derived activator of caspase that target the X-linked inhibitor of apoptosis protein/caspase-9 interaction site. *J Med Chem* 2004;47:4147–4150.

97. Sun H, Nikolovska-Coleska Z, Chen J, Yang CY, Tomita Y, Pan H, Yoshioka Y, Krajewski K, Roller PP, Wang S. Structure-based design, synthesis and biochemical testing of novel and potent Smac peptido-mimetics. *Bioorg Med Chem Lett* 2005;15:793–797.

 98. Li L, Thomas RM, Suzuki H, De Brabander JK, Wang X, Harran PG. A small molecule Smac mimic potentiates TRAIL- and TNFalpha-mediated cell death. *Science* 2004;305:1471–1474.

 99. Schimmer AD, Welsh K, Pinilla C, Wang Z, Krajewska M, Bonneau MJ, et al. Small-molecule antagonists of apoptosis suppressor XIAP exhibit broad antitumor activity. *Cancer Cell* 2004;5:25–35.

100. White PW, Titolo S, Brault K, Thauvette L, Pelletier A, Welchner E, et al. Inhibition of human papillomavirus DNA replication by small molecule antagonists of the E1–E2 protein interaction. *J Biol Chem* 2003;278:26765–26772.

101. Wang Y, Coulombe R, Cameron DR, Thauvette L, Massariol MJ, Amon LM, et al. Crystal structure of the E2 transactivation domain of human papillomavirus type 11 bound to a protein interaction inhibitor. *J Biol Chem* 2004;279:6976–6985.

102. Shultz MD, Ham YW, Lee SG, Davis DA, Brown C, Chmielewski J. Small-molecule dimerization inhibitors of wild-type and mutant HIV protease: a focused library approach. *J Am Chem Soc* 2004;126:9886–9887.

103. Aya T, Hamilton AD. Tetrabiphenylporphyrin-based receptors for protein surfaces show sub-nanomolar affinity and enhance unfolding. *Bioorg Med Chem Lett* 2003;13: 2651–2654.

104. Groves K, Wilson AJ, Hamilton AD. Catalytic unfolding and proteolysis of cytochrome C induced by synthetic binding agents. *J Am Chem Soc* 2004;126:12833–12842.

105. Gradl SN, Felix JP, Isacoff EY, Garcia ML, Trauner D. Protein surface recognition by rational design: nanomolar ligands for potassium channels. *J Am Chem Soc* 2003;125: 12668–12669.

106. Park HS, Lin Q, Hamilton AD. Modulation of protein–protein interactions by synthetic receptors: design of molecules that disrupt serine protease–proteinaceous inhibitor interaction. *Proc Natl Acad Sci USA* 2002;99:5105–5109.

107. Mecca T, Consoli GM, Geraci C, Cunsolo F. Designed calix[8]arene-based ligands for selective tryptase surface recognition. *Bioorg Med Chem* 2004;12:5057–5062.

108. Francese S, Cozzolino A, Caputo I, Esposito C, Martino M, Gaeta C, Troisi F, Neri P. Transglutaminase surface recognition by peptidocalix[4]arene diversomers. *Tetrahedron Lett* 2005;46:1611–1615.

109. Aachmann FL, Otzen DE, Larsen KL, Wimmer R. Structural background of cyclodextrin–protein interactions. *Protein Eng* 2003;16:905–912.

4

METHOD DEVELOPMENT FOR PRECLINICAL BIOANALYTICAL SUPPORT

MASOOD KHAN[1] AND NAIDONG WENG[2]

[1]*Covance Laboratories Inc., Chantilly, Virginia*
[2]*Johnson & Johnson Pharmaceutical Research & Development, Raritan, New Jersey*

Contents

Preclinical Development Handbook: ADME and Biopharmaceutical Properties,
edited by Shayne Cox Gad
Copyright © 2008 John Wiley & Sons, Inc.

4.1   PRECLINICAL BIOANALYTICAL SUPPORT USING LIQUID CHROMATOGRAPHY WITH TANDEM MASS SPECTROMETERS (LC-MS/MS)

4.1.1   Introduction

Preclinical development represents a critical stage in the progression from discovery to marketed pharmaceutical drug candidates that have passed initial discovery screening and are identified to possess some drug-like properties. Serious resources and financial commitments are now being made to vigorously test the drug candidates before they enter clinical trials. From a regulatory point of view, it is also essential to ensure the welfare of the volunteers and patients participating in the clinical trials by vigorously testing the safety using appropriate animal models. A series of questions concerning the toxicity, pharmacokinetic (PK) parameters, safety assessment, formulation optimization, and so on need to be answered.

Bioanalytical support plays a pivotal role in answering these questions. Timely bioanalytical support is essential to improve the success rate of drug candidates moving along the preclinical development pipeline and allows decisions to be made early to modify/improve the drug candidates or terminate the program. By definition, the goal of preclinical development support is attrition of the drug candidates with less favorable drug-like properties. The financial benefit of eliminating candidates from the drug development pipeline has been highlighted by Lee and Kerns [1].

Bioanalytical support at the preclinical development phase presents some unique challenges. The first unique challenge is the *Good Laboratory Practice* (GLP) *requirement.* Unlike discovery support, where bioanalytical support does not typically run under GLP compliance and oftentimes generic fast gradient methods are used to rank the drug candidates, preclinical bioanalytical support is under strict GLP regulations, where the data generated undergo rigorous regulatory scrutiny. The mindset is certainly shifted from the more creative discovery bioanalytical support to more compliance-oriented development bioanalytical support. Cutting-edge technology is only used at preclinical bioanalytical support with caution and only after these technologies meet the challenge of vigorous validations for staying in compliance will they be widely accepted as one of the primary tools for preclinical bioanalytical support.

The second unique challenge is to have good *metabolic selectivity coverage.* Usually at the early stages of preclinical studies, information on metabolites may not be well characterized and a definitive human absorption, distribution, metabolism, and excretion (ADME) study is usually not run until clinical studies. New microdosing paradigms are evolving, which, over time, may garner human metabolism information earlier. Yet, from the bioanalytical point of view, the limited information on metabolites normally available presents a challenge. It is often uncertain how many metabolites should be included in the assay. Insufficient coverage of metabolite measurement would leave inadequate coverage of the safety margin in clinical trials should a minor metabolite in an animal species become a significant one in humans. On the other hand, methods measuring too many metabolites could result in high failure rates, a highly undesirable feature that is not only costly but also leads to regulatory question regarding the validity of the entire method.

The third unique characteristic of the preclinical bioanalytical support is the very quick turnaround time for *method development, validation, and sample analysis* for multiple animal species (mouse, rat, dog, rabbit, monkey, etc.) and oftentimes for multiple matrices (plasma, urine, tissue, liver, brain, etc.). The requirements for the skill set and infrastructure of a bioanalytical laboratory supporting preclinical work could be different from those supporting clinical bioanalytical works. For clinical bioanalytical support, it is not unusual to have a group of scientists dedicated to method development and validation and then the methods are transferred to other chemists to run large sets of routine sample analysis that could last for several months to several years. For preclinical bioanalytical support, such a transition is also possible but requires a more vigorous method ruggedness test and more frequent communication between the method developer and chemists running the samples. Also, there is a need for a very quick turnaround as well as a heavy load on method development/validation instead of routine sample analysis. It is still desirable to free method developers from routine sample analysis so that they can focus on quality method development. In general, the ratio of method developers to sample analysts should be higher for supporting preclinical LC-MS/MS than for clinical LC-MS/MS.

The fourth unique characteristic is that at this stage one needs to think about a strategy of *streamlining the process at various stages of bioanalytical support*. Table 4.1 summarizes the major characteristics for the discovery, preclinical development, and clinical bioanalytical support. These three stages should not be viewed as three separate and consecutive ones, since each can extend well into the next stage. Streamlining the sample analysis process during the preclinical stage presents unique challenges in comparison with discovery or clinical bioanalytical supports, even though great effort has been made by many scientists in the pharmaceutical industry. In the discovery stage, a few generic methods are applied to many candidates, which make it easier to adopt a universal strategy to streamline and automate the process with the ultimate goal of generating data as quickly as possible to enable eliminating poor candidates. Data review by a quality assurance unit is not needed and reporting is usually kept quite simple. When the projects get transferred to the preclinical stage, an individual unique method needs to be developed and validated for each candidate to ensure the method meets the specific requirements specified in standard operating procedures (SOPs) as well as in regulatory guidance. The method will then be used for analyzing samples. Depending on the nature of the program, the sample numbers can vary quite significantly. The scientist needs to make sure that automation is applicable for real sample analysis [2, 3]. At the preclinical stage, emphasis is usually on method reproducibility and method specificity to ensure the highest quality data. However, one should not overlook the benefit of using automation when appropriate. Automation does reduce human errors and improve method reproducibility. Once the drug candidate moves into the clinical stage, automation and other means of improving sample processing become more important. The cost

TABLE 4.1   Bioanalytical Support for Discovery, Preclinical, and Clinical Studies

	Discovery	Preclinical	Clinical
Regulatory requirement	Non-GLP	GLP	Although GLPs only apply to preclinical studies, clinical falls under the guidance and by practice the same standards as the GLPs
LC-MS/MS method	Generic	Tuned to compound; requires extensive method development	Tuned to compound; extensive method development but could leverage preclinical methods
Validation	Minimal	Extensive validation to multiple matrices in multiple species	Extensive validation but limited to human samples; specificity tests to coadministered compounds
Validation strategy	Abbreviated method validation; minimal stability test	Full validation for one species and partial validation for other species including incurred sample reproducibility; has large curve range that may be problematic due to carry-over or ionization saturation	Full validation including incurred sample analysis; very sensitive method may be needed for high potency candidate
Sample analysis	Small sets of samples per compound but hundreds or thousands of compounds	Moderate numbers of samples for dozens of compounds	Large numbers of samples for very few compounds
Sample analysis strategy	Streamline process from sample collection to data generation; use of generic methods also allows easier set up for automation	Due to relatively small sets of samples and various methods tuned for each compound, automation is feasible but may not be feasible for some methods due to limited sample volumes	Quick turnaround time for sample analysis (automated sample preparation, multiplexing, UPLC) to allow data to be released

of automating clinical bioanalytical methods can easily be justified. The same clinical bioanalytical method can be used by multiple bioanalytical chemists within or even among different organizations to meet the demand of analyzing large sets of samples within a short period of time. The nature of clinical samples also makes automation more amenable for routine sample analysis. Sample volumes are typically several-fold higher than those in preclinical studies and are more suitable for automation. Like discovery bioanalytical support, sample analysis speed is likely to be the rate-limiting step for clinical bioanalytical support. Approaches for expediting sample analysis, such as multiplexing two high-performance liquid chromatography (HPLC) units into one mass spectrometer or ultra-pressure liquid chromatography (UPLC) using sub 2 μm columns, are frequently used.

The literature on general bioanalytical method development, validation, and sample analysis has been extensively reviewed [4–14], but a strategy focused on preclinical bioanalytical support would certainly be useful. In this chapter, we share our practical experience on preclinical bioanalytical support.

4.1.2 Regulatory Requirement

A distinguishing feature of preclinical bioanalytical support is the regulatory compliance. Standard operating procedures (SOPs) are used to address many aspects of the regulatory requirements, ranging from instrument qualification, maintenance, and calibration, to bioanalytical method validation, sample analysis, data management, and sample archiving. The goal of these SOPs is to ensure the highest data integrity that can pass regulatory scrutiny. These SOPs are usually drafted based on specific regulations and guidance from the U.S. Food and Drug Administration (FDA) and international regulatory agencies, based on various federal/state requirements and based on specific policies at each institution. The single most important regulatory guidance is the FDA guidance on bioanalytical method validation [15], which provides a general guideline on establishing important parameters, including method specificity/selectivity, sensitivity, linearity, accuracy, precision, stability, matrix effects, recovery, carry-over, and contamination. The method should also demonstrate reproducibility and accuracy of measurements for incurred samples and be suitable for its intended use. However, it is up to each institution to formulate its own SOPs based on this general guidance. It is well recognized that there is a gap between the spiked quality control (QC) samples and incurred samples [16, 17]. It is generally accepted industry-wide and by the regulatory agencies that the method should meet criteria such as selectivity, sensitivity, linearity, accuracy, precision, and stability using quality control samples that are prepared by spiking known amounts of analytes to the control matrix. However, QC samples may not entirely reflect the nature of the incurred samples and this fact is often neglected by the bioanalytical chemists, resulting in over- or underestimation of analytes due to various factors. Therefore, efforts should be made to address this gap to satisfy the regulatory compliance needs.

4.1.3 Batch Failure Rate

Batch failure rate has been particularly useful to assess the method ruggedness or reliability. High failure rates usually indicate inherent shortcomings of a given method and could be used by the FDA to reject the submitted data. Excluding execution errors, good bioanalytical methods should achieve at least 80% passing rate. All failed batches should also be documented and reported in both validation and sample analysis reports. Under no circumstances should the failed batches be omitted from the report. If the method has failed to demonstrate the acceptable batch passing rates during sample analysis, analysis should be placed on-hold and an investigation for the root cause should be initiated. Based on the conclusions of the root-cause analysis, the method may need to be modified and revalidated. A decision on analyzing samples in the failed batches should be judicious and the reanalysis should be authorized after an investigation. Testing into compliance by repeatedly reinjecting the failed batch until it passes acceptance criteria is definitely a red flag for regulatory authorities. Excessive manual peak reintegration, especially for standards and quality control samples, is also an indication of inherent problems in method ruggedness or data integrity and this practice should be avoided. One should be aware that, with multiple analytes (drug candidates with multiple metabolites), the overall batch failure rates can be significantly worse even if each single analyte has an acceptable 80% passing rate. Therefore, including too many metabolites in a method could potentially introduce bias to otherwise useful data from the parent compound and its most important metabolites. One approach is to have a separate non-GLP method for those metabolites whose significance to humans in not yet fully understood [18]. For the drug and significant metabolites, bioanalytical methods intended for GLP studies should be vigorously tested and validated to have a thorough assessment of the method reproducibility and ruggedness. It is costly and time consuming to troubleshoot the methods in the middle of sample analysis, especially for preclinical studies where quick turnaround is required.

4.1.4   Narrowing the Gap for Incurred Sample Analysis

Due to potential differences such as protein binding and metabolite conversion, quality control samples, which are prepared by spiking analytes of interest into the control blank matrix, cannot totally mimic incurred samples. This difference may lead to a significant bias for the quantitative bioanalysis and must be carefully evaluated. The importance of assessing method accuracy and reproducibility using incurred samples has been emphasized at the 3rd AAPS/FDA Bioanalytical Method Validation Workshop (commonly referred to as the Crystal City III meeting) [19]. It was suggested that evaluation of assay reproducibility and accuracy for the incurred samples needs to be performed on each species used for GLP toxicology studies. Method reproducibility could be assessed by repeat analysis of individual or pooled incurred samples. Analyzing individual incurred samples will generate a second set of data. A clear written policy should be established for how to handle this second set of data. One approach that avoids generating a second set of data is to use pooled samples. Pooled samples provide the same type of data as individual incurred samples, but they are not reportable as study data. Nevertheless, the argument against this pooling is that bias from individual samples could be averaged out. For example, dosing vehicle that can cause significant ion suppression and therefore biased quantitation is more predominant in the early time points and pooling with later time points may diminish such an effect. One approach to solve this issue is to pool samples from similar time points. Assessment of method accuracy for the incurred samples presents a major challenge. It would be extremely difficult to ascertain the method accuracy for the incurred samples since the true value is unknown. The feasible approaches to ascertain some level of method accuracy for incurred samples might be the addition of analytes to the incurred samples (standard addition) or comparison of results from two orthogonal methods. Even with these assessments, situations causing bias for the quantitation of incurred samples could still exist. One such possibility is the instability of the incurred samples during the sample collection procedure and sample storage. This may be even more pronounced for the large molecule therapeutics. Neither the standard addition approach nor the orthogonal method approach would detect such a problem. Therefore, as a bioanalytical scientist, one must be judicious when developing methods and make sure any issues that can cause potential method bias or poor reproducibility are resolved prior to the method validation. One common mistake when developing separate assays for parent compound and metabolite is the failure to investigate selectivity and stability toward the potential influence of the drug and other metabolites on each other. Each individual method may only contain the analytes to be measured in that method which does not typically reflect the entire content of incurred samples. Potential conversion between known analytes or between known and unknown metabolites may occur during the sample collection, storage, preparation, or postextraction, leading to quantitation bias. The extent of the bias depends on the conversion rate and the concentration ratio among these interconverting compounds. Typically, concentrations for the calibration standards and QCs are prepared in such a way that both concentrations increase or decrease proportionally. This approach allows the use of one common stock solution to prepare standards or QCs at lower concentrations. In most cases, this approach would be fine since for most of the drug candidates such a proportioned concentration change is indeed observed (Fig. 4.1a). However, for drug candidates such as prodrugs, the concentration ratio of prodrug versus active drug could be lopsided, as shown in Fig. 4.1b. At early time points, the prodrug concentration can be significantly higher than the drug concentration. Because of the labile nature of the prodrug, the drug concentration may be overestimated because of the conversion of prodrug to drug during storage, extraction, postextraction, and in the LC-MS/MS source. One approach to investigating this problem is to prepare additional quality control samples at nonequivalent concentrations.

4.1.5   Control Animal Samples

One important aspect of bioanalytical preclinical support is to analyze samples from the control animal groups, which are not given a dose of the drug candidate. Any positive finding in these control animal samples indicates potential contamination in the dosing, collection, storage, sample preparation, or analysis process and usually warrants a thorough investigation. In order to minimize potential contamination during the sample preparation and analysis, these control animal samples may be analyzed in a separate batch from the samples from dosed animals. Multiple matrix blank samples are also analyzed along with these control animal samples to assist the investigation into the source of contamination, should it occur. Determining whether the measured concentrations in the control animals follow any pharmacokinetic (PK) profile or the parent/metabolite ratio is consistent with *in vivo* observations

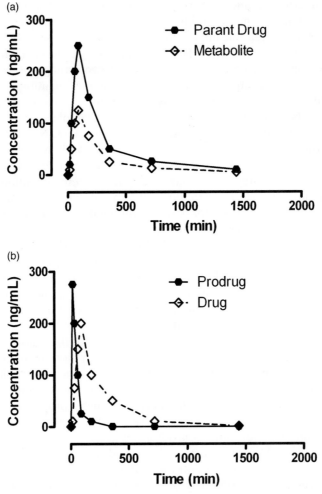

FIGURE 4.1 Typical PK profiles for parent drug/metabolite and prodrug/drug. Note the parallel concentration profile between parent drug and metabolite in (a) and the lopsided concentration profile between prodrug and drug in (b).

also provides good insight into the source of contamination. It might be necessary to have a dedicated laboratory and instruments to analyze the control animal samples if a drug candidate is highly potent and is dosed in very small amount.

4.1.6 Metabolic Selectivity Coverage During Drug Development

An industry report on drug metabolites in safety testing (commonly referred to as MIST) was published in 2002 [20]. After deliberation between industry and the FDA, a draft FDA *Guidance for Industry: Safety Testing of Drug Metabolites* was issued in 2005 [21]. Extensive characterization of the pharmacokinetics of unique and/or major human metabolites would be very useful to correlate metabolites and toxicological observations. At the Crystal City III meeting, it was agreed that a "tiered" method validation approach could be used for measuring unique and/or major metabolites in early drug development. A tiered validation approach would allow information to be gathered on human and animal metabolites with scientifically valid methods while deferring more labor-intensive GLP validations to later stages in the drug development when significant metabolites are identified. In order to identify which metabolites to measure, metabolites formed in several animal species and human liver microsomes *in vitro* are identified and their concentrations are measured. Yet, there is no guarantee that there is a direct correlation between the metabolites thus observed and the human metabolites observed *in vivo*. If unique human metabolites are found or major metabolites were observed at concentrations without safety margin from toxicology studies, it could present some unique challenges to bioanalytical scientists. It would be beneficial if human metabolites could be identified early during the drug development. With the advancement and availability of the highly sensitive accelerated mass spectrometry (AMS), one can perform exploratory human ADME by using the microdosing scheme suggested in the guidance for exploratory studies or by combining exploratory human ADME with single ascending dosing (SAD) [22].

In order to obtain meaningful results from the study, one also needs to pay attention to the metabolite stability *ex vivo*. Metabolite stability in plasma could be affected by enzymes, pH, anticoagulants, storage conditions, and freeze/thaw cycles. It is well known that acylglucuronides can degrade back to the original drug under neutral or basic pH [23]. Adjusting the pH to 3–5 would stabilize the acylglucuronides. Candidates can also be subject to hydrolysis due to esterases. An enzymatic inhibitor (sometimes more than one) is sometimes needed to stabilize both the parent compound and its metabolite(s). One should be aware that commercially purchased plasma may not have the same enzymatic activity as the plasma harvested from freshly drawn blood. It is advisable to confirm the metabolic stability using fresh matrix.

Another consideration related to metabolic specificity is the in-source fragmentation occurring at the LC-MS/MS interface. Under high temperature (300–600 °C) and high voltage (2–5 kV), phase II glucuronide metabolites may lose the glucuronide to form the original compound, which will show up in the aglycone analyte channel. If there is no chromatographic separation between them, overestimation of the aglycone compound may occur.

4.1.7 Method Development Strategy

Vigorous method development and optimization is essential in order to narrow the gap between spiked QC and incurred samples. The spiked QC samples only contain the added analytes while the incurred samples may contain additional known and unknown metabolites. In the early stages of preclinical bioanalytical support, information related to metabolite characteristics and stability may not be fully developed. As mentioned previously, metabolic specificity of the method needs to be carefully evaluated. Another unique feature of preclinical bioanalytical support is the dosing vehicle effect on the quantitation, especially when limited or minimal sample preparation and fast gradients are used.

With attaining high quality data as the ultimate goal, bioanalytical scientists strive to develop methods with good selectivity, high sensitivity, and faster throughput.

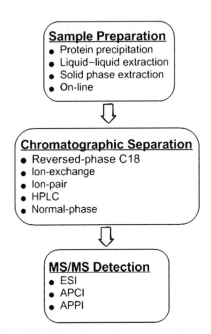

FIGURE 4.2 Three distinguished but interrelated stages (sample preparation, chromatographic separation, and MS/MS detection) of analysis of biological samples using LC-MS/MS.

Bioanalytical methods (chromatographic) typically consist of three important but interrelated parts: sample preparation, chromatography, and MS detection (Fig. 4.2). Many techniques can be employed for each of these parts. When developing a robust method, one needs to consider all three parts as an integrated system. Sometimes trade-offs need to be balanced. For example, if a simple sample preparation procedure, such as protein precipitation, is used, one may need to compensate for the potential ion suppression or in-source conversion of glucuronide metabolites to parent compound by using a more extensive chromatographic separation. Ideally, the mechanism for sample extraction and chromatography should be orthogonal to provide better method selectivity. A combination of reversed-phase solid-phase extraction (SPE) and reversed-phase LC may not provide sufficient separation power of metabolites or interferences. Of course, one will always need to keep in mind the analyte integrity during sample extraction, postextraction, and chromatography. Although liquid chromatography with ultraviolet or fluorescence detection (LC-UV/FLU) or gas chromatography with mass spectrometer detection (GC-MS) methods are still widely used and sometimes offer better methods than LC-MS/MS [24], the use of LC-MS/MS, owing to its intrinsic advantages, has nevertheless grown exponentially in the last decade and is used extensively for the preclinical bioanalytical support for small molecule therapeutics. The principle of MS is the production of ions from analyzed compounds that are separated or filtered based on their mass to charge ratio (m/z). Most applications for quantitative bioanalysis use tandem mass spectrometers (MS/MS) that employ two mass analyzers: one for the precursor ion in the first quadrupole and the other for the product ion in the third quadrupole after the collision–activated dissociation of the precursor ion in a collision cell (second quadrupole). Between the high pressure LC and the MS operated under a high-vacuum environment, interface connections that operate at atmospheric pressure, such as electrospray ionization (ESI), atmospheric-pressure chemical ionization (APCI), and atmospheric-pressure photoionization (APPI), have matured into highly reliable systems necessary for quantitative LC-MS/MS bioanalysis. On the chromatographic side, reversed-phase columns are extensively used but separation based on other retention mechanisms can also be used complementarily (e.g., normal-phase chromatography for chiral separations).

Sample Preparation   Protein precipitation (PPT), liquid/liquid extraction (LLE), and SPE are frequently used sample preparation techniques in the format of either individual tubes/cartridges or 96-well plates. Analytes of interest are released from protein when a protein precipitation reagent, such as organic solvents (e.g., acetonitrile, methanol), acids, or salt (e.g., ammonium sulfate), is added to the biological samples to denature the protein. These analytes stay in the supernatant after centrifugation and can be analyzed as is or can go through evaporation/reconstitution steps to make the injection compatible with the chromatographic condition. For highly protein-bound compounds, it is frequently necessary to release them from the proteins by adjusting the sample pH; otherwise, the analyte could be trapped in the precipitates. In principle, solid-phase extraction (SPE) is analogous to liquid/liquid extraction (LLE). As a liquid sample passes through the SPE, compounds are adsorbed onto the support or sorbent material. Interferences can then be selectively removed using washing solvents. Finally, the desired analytes may be selectively recovered by an elution solvent, resulting in a purified extract. The eluent can either be injected directly onto LC-MS/MS or go through the evaporation/reconstitution steps for further concentration enhancement and for compatibility with chromatographic conditions. Unlike protein precipitation, where universal extraction and recovery is usually achieved regardless of the chemical structures of the analytes, success using LLE and SPE to extract analytes largely depends on the chemistry of the molecules and the experience of the analyst. Although LLE and SPE usually give cleaner samples than protein precipitation and thus less matrix effects due to ion suppression and enhancement, their selectivity can result in differential recovery among parent compound and metabolites as well as the internal standards. This could place a limit on their use for simultaneous analysis of multiple analytes. Use of stable isotope-labeled (SIL) internal standards could compensate for this deficiency to some extent since the SIL internal standards usually have the same recovery and chromatographic characteristics as the unlabeled analytes.

Chromatography   With the initial sample clean-up using SPE, LLE, or PPT, unwanted compounds can still be present in higher concentrations than the analytes of interest. A second stage of cleanup, typically involving LC separation, further separates analytes of interest from the unwanted compounds. Without this further separation, those unwanted and present compounds in the MS/MS are not typically observed but present significant challenges. In the LC-MS interface, these compounds compete with analytes for ionization and cause inconsistent matrix effects that are detrimental to quantitative LC-MS/MS.

Reversed-phase LC has traditionally been used for quantitative LC-MS/MS. There are numerous types of reversed-phase columns, with the C18 column being the most predominant. With increasing organic solvent concentrations in the mobile phase, the analyte retention decreases. However, one should be aware of the potential bimodal retention on the reversed-phase column due to the residual silanol group [25]. This bimodel retention may cause retention shifts during the run or irreproducibility of the method. Of particular interest is the use of monolithic columns (available in C18 format) operated at a high flow rate. Compared to a particulate column, the monolithic column has a reduced pressure drop but still maintains high separation efficiency at high mobile phase flow rates. This is due to its unique bimodal pore structure, which consists of macropores (2 μm) and mesopores (13 nm) [26]. The mesopores provide the surface area for achieving adequate capacity while the macropores allow high flow rates because of higher porosity, resulting in reduced flow resistance. Monolithic columns have become increasingly popular for use in ultrafast bioanalysis of drug candidates using tandem mass spectrometric detection [27–29]. Another recent development in column technology is the fused-core column, specially designed for hyperfast chromatography under the tradename Halo. Due to the small and uniform 2.7 μm particle size and fused-core technology, the analytes travel in the column with reduced diffusion, resulting in improved column efficiency and reduced column backpressure. Sub 2 μm particle columns used for UPLC has also drawn lots of attention. Special LC units, designed to operate under a backpressure as high as 15,000 psi, allow fast chromatography. Hydrophilic interaction chromatography (HILIC) became a popular choice in the last several years. HILIC is similar to normal-phase LC in that the elution is promoted by the use of polar mobile phase. However, unlike classic normal-phase LC, where the water to the mobile phase has to be kept to minimal but constant levels, water is present in a significant amount (>5%). HILIC also uses water-miscible polar organic solvents such as acetonitrile instead of water-immiscible solvents like hexane and chloroform. LC-MS/MS using HILIC on silica columns has been extensively studied and reviewed [30, 31].

On-Line Extraction and Chromatography   On-line extraction is another frequently used technology. With the improvement in instrumentation and column technology [32], on-line sample extraction that is coupled into LC-MS/MS has developed as an important tool in the past few years. In general, this technique employs turbulent flow chromatography, in which extraction columns are packed with retaining particles of large size (e.g., 50 μm) on a commercially available device or on a regular homemade column switch device. Biological samples are injected directly onto the extraction column, usually after dilution with an aqueous buffer. The analytes are then washed either forward or backward onto the analytical column for further chromatographic separation prior to the MS/MS detection. Common on-line extraction systems use typical reversed-phase columns for both the extraction and analysis. In our laboratory, we have successfully employed a weak-cation extraction (WCX) column and HILIC analytical column to analyze an extremely polar quaternary amine compound. This compound has no retention at all on a reversed-phase column but has excellent retention and peak shape on a HILIC column. The analyte in plasma was loaded onto a WCX column with an aqueous mobile phase and the WCX column was then washed with acetonitrile to remove endogenous compounds. The analyte was then eluted off the WCX column, using acidified acetonitrile, onto the HILIC analytical column for a gradient elution.

Analyte Adsorption Issue   Loss of analytes during the collection of incurred samples, preparation of quality controls, storage, and analysis due to adsorption to the container should also be considered. Compound adsorption to storage containers often happens in sensitive LC-MS/MS assays, which causes nonlinear response and loss of sensitivity. The use of a zwitterionic detergent such as 3-[3-cholamidopropyl)-dimethylammonio]-1-propanesulfonate (CHAPS) as an additive in urine can prevent some analytes from adhering to surfaces during sample collection, storage, and preparation [33]. Protein binding of the drug candidate could also be significantly different for the quality control samples and incurred samples. If the analyte was not released from the protein prior to the extraction, quantitation bias could occur, depending on the extraction method. Xue et al. [34] observed the same issue with a liquid/liquid extraction method. For the plasma extraction method, two incubation steps were required after the addition of 5 mM ammonium acetate and the internal standard (stable isotope labeled) in acetonitrile to release the analyte bound to proteins prior to LLE with toluene.

4.1.8   Method Automation Strategy: From Preclinical to Clinical

As the candidates progress well, method development and validation for supporting human clinical trials will start well before the drugs enter the clinic. A well-established automated process, wherever possible, should be used to replace manual tasks early on in the preclinical stage. Automation results in greater performance consistency over time and in more reliable methods.

Standardization in sample collection can significantly enhance bioanalytical productivity. Preclinical samples could be collected in 96-well format [35] or transferred to 96-well format from a pierceable capped tube fitted with a nonleaking resealable polymer septum [36]. Automated 96-well plate technology for sample preparation is well established and accepted and has been shown to effectively replace manual tasks. The 96-well instruments can execute automated off-line extraction and sample cleanups. Automated SPE [37–40], LLE [41–46], and PPT [47, 48] can be performed in 96-well format. Both packed cartridges and disks in 96-well SPE formats have been successfully used. Further efficiency improvements were made when the organic extracts from SPE [49, 50] or LLE [51, 52] were injected directly onto the silica column with low aqueous–high organic mobile phases. While the commonly used SPE or LLE solvents are stronger elution solvents (not compatible) than a mobile phase on typical reversed-phase chromatography, they are weaker elution solvents (compatible) on the silica column with low aqueous–high organic mobile phases operated under HILIC. In this approach, the time-consuming and error-prone solvent evaporation and reconstitution steps are eliminated.

4.1.9   Matrix Effects and Recovery

The influence of matrix effects on quantitative bioanalytical LC-MS/MS has been well recognized [53, 54]. The U.S. Food and Drug Administration's (FDA) *Guidance for Industry on Bioanalytical Method Validation* requires the assessment of matrix effects during method validation for quantitative bioanalytical LC-MS/MS methods [55]. In a broad sense, matrix effects represent the impact of the matrix on the analysis of the analytes, including ion suppression/enhancement, differentiated recovery, and altered stability, and is certainly not just limited to quantitative bioanalytical LC-MS/MS. However, it has been generally accepted and proposed in the industry guidance that matrix effects for small molecule bioanalytical analysis is defined as the analyte ionization suppression or enhancement in the presence of matrix components that could originate from endogenous compounds such as phospholipids [56], metabolites, coadministered drugs, internal standards [57], dosing vehicles [58–60], mobile phase additives [61], and plastic tubes [62]. These effects are more pronounced with ESI than with APCI [63, 64]. There are several commonly used ways of measuring matrix effects. One approach is to compare the MS response of the analyte spiked postextraction with that in a neat solution [65–67]. Since there is no extraction involved, any signal loss or enhancement in the postextraction spiked sample will be assumed due to matrix effects. Another useful approach of assessing matrix effect is postcolumn infusion of an analyte into the MS detector. The extracted blank matrix is injected by an autosampler onto the analytical column [68–70]. The purpose of postcolumn infusion with the analyte is to raise the background level so that the matrix-induced suppression will show as negative peaks. An approach for assessing the lack of inconsistent matrix effect among individual samples is to measure the consistency for the results obtained from these types of experiments with samples from individual matrix lots (typically $n > 6$) [71–76].

Constanzer et al. [77] measured both absolute matrix effects by comparing the responses from postextraction spiked samples with those from neat solutions and relative matrix effects by measuring the consistency of the response factors from spiked matrix lots. Results from LC-MS/MS methods were compared to a validated non-MS method, such as LC-UV [78, 79], LC with fluorescence detector [80], enzyme-linked immunosorbent assay (ELISA) [81, 82], and fluorescence polarization assay [83], or to a different separation method such as GC [84]. Comparable results indicate lack of matrix effects or inconsistent matrix effects since this approach does not positively identify the magnitude of the matrix effects. Huang et al. [85] used LC-UV to detect the down-field matrix peaks that caused ion suppression for the analyte of interest and modified the chromatographic condition [85]. Recovery is determined by comparing the MS response of extracted samples with those spiked (postextraction) into a blank matrix. Because both samples have the matrix constituents present, the matrix effects can be considered the same for extracted samples and postextraction spiked samples. Any differences in responses can be considered as caused by extraction recovery.

4.1.10 Effect of Dosing Vehicles

In preclinical studies, dosing vehicles typically are used at high concentrations to dissolve the test compounds. These dosing vehicles, especially polymeric vehicles such as PEG 400 and Tween 80, can cause significant signal suppression for certain analytes when minimal sample cleanup is used. Table 4.2 shows a real-world example of the adverse effects of dosing vehicles. The results obtained using a fast gradient LC-MS/MS method with minimal retention are significantly lower than those

TABLE 4.2 Comparison of Results Obtained from the Same Set of IV Plasma Samples Containing PEG 400 When Two Different Gradient LC-MS/MS Methods Are Used

Time Postdose (h)	Results from the Extended Gradient Method (ng/mL)	Results from the Fast Gradient Method (ng/mL)
0.067	753	261
0.133	712	219
0.2	761	239
0.333	523	176
0.5	394	104
0.75	279	72.0
1	116	28.0
1.5	35.0	7.00
2	6.00	2.00

obtained from an extended gradient LC-MS/MS method. When these two sets of data were fitted into a noncompartment model, values for C_{max}, area under the curve (AUC), and clearance (Cl) were more than 300% different [59].

Effective means of minimizing this type of effect include better chromatographic separations, better sample cleanup, and alternative ionization methods. An easy way to check dosing vehicle effects is to fortify some quality control samples with the vehicle [86]. Significant differences in the measured values between fortified quality control samples and regular quality control samples indicate potential dosing vehicle effects.

4.1.11 Carry-over and Contamination

Carry-over should be differentiated from contamination. Carry-over is usually caused by liquid handlers for the sample preparation or autosamplers for the injection. Carry-over can be estimated and to some extent managed by prearranging the samples so that the consecutive samples are not impacted by the carry-over [87]. Nevertheless, carry-over should be evaluated during method development and validation and if possible reduced. Contamination could be systematic (such as contamination of a reagent with the analyte) or could be random (such as spillover of extraction solvents of two adjacent wells in a 96-well plate). Contamination is undesirable and is usually unmanageable. Care must be taken to minimize carry-over and contamination so that they will not negatively impact the assay results.

4.1.12 Misconception About Stable Isotope-Labeled Internal Standard

Use of stable isotope-labeled analyte as the internal standard has played a significant role in advancing quantitative bioanalytical LC-MS/MS methodology. Due to the high similarity of the physical and chemical characteristics of labeled and unlabeled analytes, almost identical sample extraction recovery and matrix effects could be expected. Potential loss of analyte during the sample preparation and signal suppression/enhancement due to matrix components can be effectively compensated for. However, the stable isotope-labeled internal standard will not compensate for analyte loss due to instability or adsorption to either container or proteins. Occasionally, stable isotope-labeled internal standards have been chromatographically separated from the analyte and have experienced different matrix effects [88].

Yang et al. [89] presented an interesting case study for diagnosis and trouble-shooting of problems associated with strong analyte–protein binding. The method was validated using a stable isotope-labeled internal standard with a LLE method using hexane as the extraction solvent. However, upon repeat analysis of the same samples, the concentration values increased fivefold from the original value. The concentration increased with each additional freeze/thaw cycle. It was found that this drug candidate has a strong protein binding and hexane is not sufficient to release the drug candidate from the protein. Freeze/thaw cycles gradually denatured the protein and weakened the binding, resulting in increases in the free and extract-able drug candidate concentration. A protein precipitation (PP) method was then used to inhibit the protein binding and to release the analyte. Consistent results were then obtained.

4.1.13   Troubleshooting Strategy

Successful method troubleshooting requires full understanding of all aspects of the bioanalytical method. For example, poor dynamic range can potentially be caused by many factors. A systematic investigation of the root cause would help resolve the issues. Table 4.3 provides a general investigational guide for the troubleshooting of poor linearity. Similar systematic investigations could be made to other important parameters for quantitative bioanalytical methods. One important parameter to

TABLE 4.3   Troubleshooting for Poor Linearity

Observation	Potential Root Cause
Response factors decrease at high end	Poor solubility?
	Correct reconstitution solvent and volume: analyte soluble in matrix?
	Saturation due to large curve range—at LC-MS/MS interface? At detector?
Response factors decrease at low end	Adsorption of analytes to container?
	Adsorption of analytes to 96-well plate?
	Loss of analytes in evaporation/reconstitution step?
	Adsorption of analyte to injector/tubing/column/source?
Abnormal high response at low end of the curve	Contamination?
	Carry-over?
Internal standard (ISTD) response increases with increased analyte concentration	Isotope effects or impurities from analyte?
	Adsorption of analytes and ISTD to the container?
ISTD response decreases with increased analyte concentration	Suppression from analyte to ISTD?
ISTD not tracking analyte	LC-MS matrix effect?
	Extraction recovery problem?
	Instability of analyte or ISTD in extract?
	Inadequate equilibrium for protein binding of ISTD?

review when performing troubleshooting, especially when troubleshooting a mismatch of calibration standards and quality controls, is the response factor. The response factor is the response ratio of the analyte versus internal standard normalized against the concentrations. Response factors should be consistent throughout the entire calibration range. Table 4.4 shows a troubleshooting example. At first glance, the accuracy results indicate that the two low levels of quality control samples (0.25 ng/mL and 0.75 ng/mL) are biased high based on the calculated accuracy results. However, a further review of the response factors shows that these two

TABLE 4.4   Troubleshooting for Poor Accuracy of Quality Control (QC) Samples[a]

Sample Name	Calculated Concentration (ng/mL)	Response Factor	Accuracy (%)	Sample Name	Calculated Concentration (ng/mL)	Response Factor	Accuracy (%)
CAL-200	205	0.0163	102.6	QC-0.25	0.298	0.01607	119.2
CAL-100	109	0.0173	109.3	QC-0.25	0.298	0.01611	119.4
CAL-50	47.7	0.0151	95.32	QC-0.25	0.296	0.01597	118.5
CAL-20	20	0.0158	100.1	QC-0.25	0.299	0.01617	119.8
CAL-10	10.3	0.0162	102.6	QC-0.25	0.297	0.01601	118.8
CAL-5	4.92	0.0155	98.35	QC-0.25	0.297	0.01601	118.8
CAL-2	2.03	0.0157	101.3	QC-0.75	0.883	0.01774	117.8
CAL-0.5	0.54	0.0157	107.9	QC-0.75	0.902	0.01813	120.3
CAL-0.25	0.241	0.0125	96.49	QC-0.75	0.86	0.01724	114.6
CAL-0.25	0.246	0.0128	98.54	QC-0.75	0.865	0.01734	115.3
CAL-0.5	0.518	0.0150	103.6	QC-0.75	0.878	0.01762	117
CAL-2	1.9	0.0147	95.15	QC-0.75	0.874	0.01754	116.5
CAL-5	4.72	0.0148	94.33	QC-160	166	0.01641	103.5
CAL-10	9.8	0.0155	98.01	QC-160	174	0.01724	108.7
CAL-20	19.8	0.0157	99.13	QC-160	166	0.01650	104
CAL-50	48.8	0.0155	97.64	QC-160	168	0.01666	105.1
CAL-100	97.9	0.0155	97.85	QC-160	167	0.01657	104.5
CAL-200	203	0.0161	101.7	QC-160	170	0.01680	106
Mean		0.01532	100	QC-75	80.6	0.01704	107.5
SD		0.001147	4.13	QC-75	78.7	0.01664	104.9
CV%		7.49	4.13	QC-75	81.1	0.01715	108.2
				QC-75	78.8	0.01665	105
				QC-75	79.2	0.01674	105.6
				QC-8	8.91	0.01757	111.3
				QC-8	8.67	0.01710	108.3
				QC-8	8.7	0.01717	108.8
				QC-8	8.44	0.01665	105.5
				QC-8	8.73	0.01723	109.2
				QC-8	8.8	0.01736	110
				Mean		0.016878	111.3
				SD		0.000576	5.93
				CV%		3.42	5.33

[a]Pay special attention to the lower response factors but good accuracy for CAL-0.25. QC samples have consistent response factors over the entire concentration range but poor accuracy caused by the lower response factor of CAL-0.25. Because this is $1/x^2$ weighted linear regression, the lowest standard (CAL-0.25) has the most significant weighting for the calculation of QC concentrations.

levels of quality control samples have the same response factors as the other levels of quality controls. It also reveals that the response factors dropped for the calibration standards at lower concentrations even though the calculated accuracy for these standards is excellent. Further investigation revealed that the compound in the spiking solution used to prepare calibration standards was impacted by adsorption onto the container. This simple example clearly demonstrates the importance of reviewing the response factors rather than only relying on the calculated accuracy for the troubleshooting.

4.1.14   Conclusion

Bioanalytical support for preclinical studies is complicated. Hence, bioanalytical scientists need to fully understand both the underlying sciences and regulatory requirements. They should always be aware of the potential pitfalls that could occur at any stage of the study. There are a number of parameters requiring evaluation during method development and validation. The method validation strategy should be tailored for the intended use.

4.2   PRECLINICAL BIOANALYTICAL SUPPORT USING LIGAND-BINDING ASSAY

4.2.1   Introduction

Much of the information discussed in Section 4.1 for the bioanalysis of small molecules may also apply to the bioanalysis of large molecule therapeutics as well. However, there are some unique challenges associated with quantification of large molecule therapeutics. These are due mainly to the nature of the molecules and limitations of the technology (e.g., ligand-binding assay (LBA)), used for bioanalysis.

Recombinant proteins and humanized monoclonal antibodies comprise an ever increasing larger proportion of protein therapeutics and, as a result, have posed new challenges and special needs. These molecules may not survive the typical sample handling conditions of the chromatographic assays. Moreover, these drugs are highly potent. Consequently, their blood concentration levels tend to be very low. Hence, the method of quantification for these entities must be very gentle, specific, and highly sensitive. Ligand-binding assays such as radioimmunoassay (RIA) and enzyme-linked immunosorbent assay (ELISA) are the techniques of choice for quantification of large molecule drugs in biological samples [90, 91].

In addition, due to their high molecular weight, there is always the possibility that large molecule therapeutics may elicit an immune response directed against the drug [92]. A small change in protein structure, even though it may comprise a very small proportion of the total protein, can induce a large immunogenic response. Therefore, regulatory agencies require immunogenicity evaluation for large molecule therapeutics even in the preclinical stage [93]. Consequently, there is an increasing need to develop novel assays that can detect and characterize the anti-drug antibodies (ADA) or immunogenicity of large molecule therapeutics. To accomplish this, the laboratory has to rely on several bioanalytical techniques and technologies to measure these changes including LBA.

Like any other bioanalytical method, the intended use of the LBA helps to determine the course of development and validation of the assay. Ligand-binding assays are used for (1) the quantitation of therapeutic entities to support the toxicokinetic / pharmacokinetic studies [91, 94] and (2) monitoring the level of surrogate biomarkers to support pharmacodynamic evaluation [95]. On the other hand, qualitative or quasiquantitative assays are generally used for the determination of anti-drug antibodies [92, 96]. The LBA developed for the bioanalytical support should not only be robust, reliable, and reproducible but should also be GLP compliant from a regulatory perspective. It can then be used for production, toxicology, and Phase I though IV testing. In view of the small sample volumes available in typical preclinical studies, it is even more compelling to design and develop a robust assay to reduce sample reanalysis.

In this section we provide a brief account of the ligand-binding assay technology, specific challenges associated with the GLP-compliant method development and validation of quantitative assays, and current industry and regulatory perspectives. Method development and validation for detection of anti-drug antibodies [92, 96] or quantification of biomarkers [95] may require slightly different strategies.

4.2.2   Ligand-Binding Assay Technology

A typical ligand-binding assay utilizes an analyte-specific binder (e.g., antibody, binding protein, drug, or receptor) to capture the analyte of interest. The captured analyte is detected by the "detector molecule," which is generally an antibody labeled with a radioisotope (e.g., ^{125}I), an enzyme (e.g., horseradish peroxidase, alkaline phosphatase), or another label (e.g., biotin, avidin). ELISA, the most commonly used ligand-binding assay, generally uses a detector molecule that is labeled with an enzyme. The extent of bound enzyme activity is measured by the changes in color intensity of the substrate solution. The color intensity is directly proportional to the concentration of analyte captured on the microtiter plate (see Fig. 4.3). A detailed description of the ligand-binding assay technology is beyond the scope of this chapter. Several books that provide in-depth information on ligand-binding assays, including ELISA, are included in the references [97, 98].

4.2.3   Using Ligand-Binding Assay in a GLP Environment

To support preclinical studies, an analyte-specific ligand-binding assay must be validated to conform to GLP regulations. In a GLP environment, like any other bioanalytical method, an LBA has a three-phase life cycle: (1) method development, (2) prestudy validation, and (3) in-study validation. Table 4.5 summarizes the assay assessment parameters that are addressed at various stages of the method life cycle. During method development, emphasis is focused on designing a robust and analyte-specific method for the intended use. This requires advanced planning and a careful consideration of (1) assay design and format, (2) critical reagent selection, (3) critical reagent stability evaluation, (4) matrix selection, (5) sample collection conditions, and (6) optimization of assay condition to achieve desired performance characteristics. Once a robust method has been developed, the prestudy validation becomes uncomplicated. The assay characteristics, including precision and accuracy, limits of quantification, and analyte stability, are formally confirmed during the

TABLE 4.5   Summary of Method Validation Assessment Parameters Over the Method Life Cycle

Performance Parameters	Development	Prestudy Validation	*In-Study Validation*
Critical reagents	Identify and procure	Apply	Apply
Assay format / batch size	Establish	Apply	Apply
Matrix of calibrators and controls	Establish	Confirm	Apply
Minimal required dilution	Establish	Confirm	Apply
Analyte stability	Initiate	Establish	Ongoing assessment
Specificity	Establish	Apply	Apply
Selectivity	Evaluate	Confirm	Apply
Calibration curve fitting algorithm	Establish	Confirm	Apply
LLOQ and ULOQ	Evaluate	Establish	Apply
Precision and accuracy	Evaluate (CV and RE)	Establish (CV and RE)	Apply (TE)
Run acceptance QC (low, medium, high)	Evaluate	Establish	Apply
Dilutional linearity	Establish	Confirm	Apply—confirm if extended
Batch size	Evaluate	Establish	Apply—confirm if extended
Robustness/ ruggedness	Evaluate	Establish	Monitor
Parallelism	Evaluate where possible	Evaluate where possible	Establish with incurred samples
Run acceptance criteria	N/A	Runs accepted based on calibration curve acceptance criteria	Runs accepted based on acceptable calibration curve and QC samples following 4-6-X rule

prestudy validation phase. These characteristics are monitored during the in-study validation phase in which study samples are analyzed [91, 94].

4.2.4 Ligand-Binding Assay Specific Challenges

The distinguishing characteristics of ligand-binding assays that separate them from chromatographic (e.g., LC-MS/MS) assays are summarized as follows.

1. The design of a sandwich ligand-binding assay takes advantage of the ability of an antibody to specifically bind to the analyte (drug). The amount of analyte

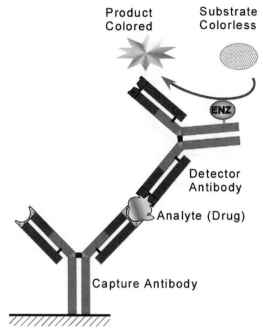

FIGURE 4.3 A sandwich enzyme linked immunosorbent assay (ELISA) with colorimetric endpoint.

is measured indirectly by the binding of a detector antibody conjugated to an enzyme or any other labeling molecule (Fig. 4.3). In a chromatographic assay the analyte is physically separated into distinct peaks. The area under the peak is precisely measured and is directly proportional to the analyte concentration. Due to the indirect measurements in LBA, the results are somewhat less precise, as reflected by coefficient of variation ($CV \leq 20\%$), than in chromatographic assays ($CV \leq 10\%$).

2. The biological samples are generally analyzed without pretreatment in a LBA, as opposed to the process of extracting analyte from samples prior to the chromatographic assay. Consequently, numerous matrix components including binding proteins, drugs, degrading enzymes, heterophilic antibodies, and anti-animal antibodies may have negative or positive interference in the assay performance.

3. Due to the limited analyte-binding capacity of the binder molecule (e.g., capture antibody), the typical calibration curves in these assays are nonlinear, as opposed to the linear curves in chromatographic assays. Consequently, the working range of quantification in an LBA is narrower than in the linear curves of chromatographic assays (Fig. 4.4). In preclinical studies, relatively high doses of drugs are administered. The resulting high concentration of drug in the study samples may require sample dilutions that could be several thousandfold.

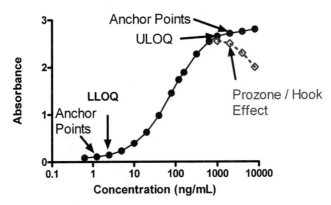

FIGURE 4.4 Prozone or Hook effect Illustration. A typical sigmoid calibration curve for a sandwich ELISA is shown with "anchor points" at both ends of the curve bracketing the calibrators at the LLOQ and ULOQ levels. A high dose Prozone or Hook effect is illustrated by suppression of signal (absorbance) with analyte at concentrations far above the ULOQ level.

4.2.5   Responding to the Challenge of Ligand-Binding Assay

For all assays, the key factor is the accuracy of the reported results [15]. In view of the above characteristics, besides method reproducibility considerations, one must pay special attention to establishing the method **(1)** specificity, **(2)** selectivity, **(3)** minimal required dilution, **(4)** dilutional linearity, and **(5)** analyte (drug) stability in the biological matrix [94]. Evaluation and validation of the method repeatability, precision, and accuracy for the LBA is described in detail elsewhere [91, 94].

Method Specificity   Demonstration of method specificity for the LBA could be a challenging task. The LBA is generally developed during the discovery phase when specific antibodies are raised against the drug molecule and are characterized. These antibodies are used to develop the initial ELISA method. Later, the assay is used to support preclinical and clinical studies. The specificity of the method is based mainly on the ability of these antibodies to specifically interact with the drug molecule as opposed to interacting with nondrug (i.e., cross-reactant) molecules.

Antibody specificity is generally evaluated by determining the cross-reactivity of the antibody with nondrug molecules, including coadministered drugs, drug metabolites, or molecules that are structurally related to the drug. To evaluate the antibody specificity, dose–response curves are generated using drugs of interest and potential cross-reactive compounds at significantly higher concentrations than the drug itself [97, 98]. The extent of acceptable cross-reactivity may depend on the relative concentration of the potential cross-reactant present in the study sample. An antibody with low cross-reactivity (e.g., <1%) with a potential cross-reactant may not be suitable if the concentration of the cross-reactant in the sample is at a very high concentration relative to the analyte (e.g., 1000-fold). In such cases, a sample cleanup method may be required to remove the cross-reactants prior to sample analysis. Similarly, an antibody with 20% cross-reactivity with a potential contaminant may be acceptable for use if the analyte itself is expected to be in great excess.

Method Selectivity   In a typical LBA, the samples are analyzed without pretreatment. Numerous matrix components that are present in the sample may affect the assay performance. The ability of the method to selectively quantify the analyte of interest in the presence of a variety of matrix components defines the method selectivity [15, 91, 94]. Method selectivity evaluation and validation is one of the most crucial and demanding tasks in establishing the LBA. During method development, at least 10 individual matrix samples from 10 normal animals or subjects (from normal or patient population) are assayed unspiked and spiked with the drug at a concentration near the lower end of the calibration curve. Acceptable recovery of drug (usually within 20% of the nominal concentration) in at least 80% of the samples is considered an indication that the method is selective. At this stage of assay development (where blank matrix is not available), the calibration curve may be prepared in the assay diluent. The results of the initial selectivity screening of matrix samples may be used to identify matrix samples that can be pooled to form a blank matrix pool. This pool can then be used for preparing the calibrators and the validation or QC samples [91, 94]. Method selectivity is confirmed during the prestudy validation, where both calibrators and control samples are spiked in the pooled biological matrix. In these experiments the selectivity is evaluated by assaying at least 10 individual matrix samples unspiked and spiked with the analyte near the lower limit of quantification (LLOQ).

Minimal Required Dilution of Sample   In assays where a strong matrix effect is observed, it may be necessary to determine the "minimal required dilution" (MRD) of the sample, that is, the dilution at which matrix interference is minimized to an acceptable level. Since the reportable concentration of analyte is the product of the measured concentration multiplied by the dilution factor, the practical limit of quantification will be greatly affected by the MRD of sample [94]. Hence, the target should be to develop a relatively more sensitive (with lower LLOQ) method where the MRD is higher. A method with smallest MRD that has acceptable interference and sensitivity for the intended use would be ideal.

Dilutional Linearity   Due to the narrow range of quantification in ligand-binding assays and the possible high concentration of analyte of interest in the sample (especially in preclinical studies), a number of samples may require dilution prior to analysis. Therefore, to avoid running highly concentrated "dilution controls" with each assay during sample analysis, dilutional linearity of sample at a wide range of dilutions is demonstrated during prestudy method validation. It should be noted that the final content of biological matrix should be identical to that in the calibration curve and/or QC samples. Therefore, dilutional linearity should be established subsequent to "method selectivity" evaluation, MRD establishment, and preparation of a blank matrix pool.

In some cases, it is observed that high concentration of analyte may suppress the signal, resulting in underestimation of analyte [99]. This phenomenon is known as the "Prozone" or "Hook" effect. A typical illustration of the effect is depicted in Fig. 4.4. Dilutional linearity evaluation may help in identifying this effect, especially for assays used to support preclinical studies. If this effect goes undetected, it may result in a gross underestimation of drug concentration in the samples where high concentrations of analyte are expected. A typical example is illustrated in Table 4.6

TABLE 4.6   Demonstration of Hook Effect and Dilutional Linearity[a]

Dilution (Fold)	Measured Concentration (pg/mL)[b]	Computed Concentration (pg/mL)	
Neat	231	231	Hook or
2	365	729	Prozone
4	674	2,698	effect
80	>ULOQ	Not computed	
160	>ULOQ	Not computed	
200	>ULOQ	Not computed	
400	755	302,078	
800	369	294,798	
1,600	178	285,226	Dilutional
3,200	93	297,229	linearity[c]
6,400	50	322,447	
12,800	26	335,578	
25,600	<LLOQ	Not computed	

[a]Data from this table is visually depicted in Fig. 4.5.
[b]Method ULOQ = 25 pg/mL; ULOQ = 1000 pg/mL.
[c]Average concentration (pg/mL) = 306,226 with 6.2% CV.

and Fig. 4.5. A sample from an escalating dose study, where high concentration of drug is expected, may be assayed "neat" (without dilution), giving a low measured concentration. This anomalous observation may call for an investigation. In trouble-shooting experiments, the sample may be re-assayed at a wide range of dilutions. In the illustration, it is observed that with increasing dilutions the measured concentration increased, reaching the ULOQ of the assay. Moreover, subsequent dilutions from 400-fold to 128,000-fold showed dilutional linearity. Computed concentrations, measured in the dilutional linearity range, provided a realistic estimate of the concentration of drug in samples. This scenario clearly illustrates the importance of Prozone or Hook effect evaluation and establishment of the dilutional linearity in an LBA.

Parallelism is another assay parameter that is conceptually similar to the dilutional linearity. It is evaluated when incurred samples become available. Plotting the responses generated by the diluted incurred samples versus the calibration curve gives a visual impression of parallelism. Various approaches to parallelism data have been described in the literature [95, 100]. A test of parallelism demonstrates that the analyte present in the sample is structurally similar to that used for generation of the calibration curve.

Analyte Stability in Biological Matrix   Biological matrices may vary from each other with respect to their chemical constituents including proteins and enzymes. Proteolytic enzyme composition may have a distinct effect on the stability of a drug in a biological matrix. Rat or mouse serum or plasma samples should be treated with special care. It has been our experience that an analyte that may be stable in rabbit or monkey serum may very well be highly unstable in rat or mouse serum. Therefore, in such cases, it may be necessary to collect the study samples in the

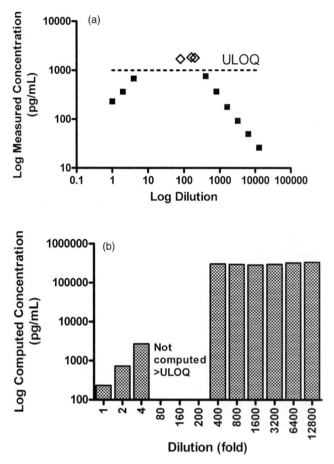

FIGURE 4.5 Illustration of the significance of dilutional linearity evaluation, especially in an assay where Prozone or Hook effect is present. (a) Initially with increasing dilutions the measured concentration in a sample increased, reaching or exceeding the ULOQ of the assay, demonstrating the suppression of response with high concentration of analyte. Subsequently, six dilutions showed a linear decrease in measured concentration with increasing dilutions of the sample. (b) The computed concentrations corrected for the dilution factor from 400-fold to 128,000-fold demonstrated dilutional linearity by showing that computed concentration is independent of the dilution factor in this range.

presence of a cocktail of proteolytic enzyme inhibitors and/or keep the samples on ice during analysis.

4.2.6   Using Commercial Kit Based Assays

Often commercial kits are used for quantification of drugs that are homologs of endogenous compounds or for the measurement of biomarkers in biological samples. Kits are generally designed for use in clinical or research lab environments. In order to adopt commercial kits for GLP-compliant bioanalytical work, one must redesign the composition and format of the control samples that are used to monitor the assay performance and to make assay acceptance decisions. It is of the utmost importance that a quality control strategy is designed in advance to evaluate and monitor the lot-to-lot variability of kits. Several multiplexed assay kits are also available commercially. Adaptation and validation of these kits for quantification of analytes of interest in biological matrices could be challenging and therefore should be thoroughly explored prior to sample analysis.

4.2.7 Industry and Regulatory Perspective

Historically, the focus of regulatory agencies has been on the chromatographic techniques for the quantification of small molecular weight drug entities that constituted the major proportion of drug development portfolios in the pharmaceutical industry. The first conference on bioanalytical method validation (commonly known as the Crystal City I conference), that was held in Crystal City, Virginia in 1990, addressed in depth the validation of chromatographic assays but paid little attention to nonchromatographic methods including immunoassays [101]. The search for LBA-specific guidance was started soon after the 1990 Crystal City conference. In 1998, one of the authors of this chapter (MK) organized a roundtable at the AAPS annual meeting in San Francisco. This was, perhaps, the first time that LBA-specific challenges were discussed on a public platform. This led to the publication of a white paper giving a comprehensive account of the pharmaceutical industry perspective on the validation of immunoassays for bioanalysis [91]. Soon after this publication in 2000, a historic workshop on bioanalytical method validation for macromolecules was sponsored by the AAPS and the FDA (1–3 March 2000). This workshop, for the first time, addressed the validation of a variety of methodologies for assays of large molecule therapeutics [102]. However, the scope of the workshop was too broad to reach a consensus. In May 2001, the FDA *Guidance for Industry: Bioanalytical Methods Validation* was issued [15]. It was thought that a focused approach was needed to address the special challenges associated with LBAs for large molecule therapeutics. Consequently, a subcommittee of the then newly formed Ligand Binding Assay Bioanalytical Focus Group (LBABFG) at the American Association of Pharmaceutical Scientists (AAPS) was set out to critically review the workshop summary report, evaluate exceptions to criteria in the guidance, and produce a consensus document. The LBABFG white paper was published in 2003 [94]. Around the same time, the AAPS sponsored a workshop (12–13 May 2003) mainly to address the "how to" of the validation of methods used for PK analysis of macromolecules [103]. Over the last four years, LBABFG white paper has provided valuable direction to LBA scientists working in regulatory compliant environments. In May 2006, the 3rd AAPS/FDA Bioanalytical Method Validation Workshop was held. With some changes, this workshop essentially endorsed the LBA method performance acceptance criteria proposed in the LBABFG white paper (Table 4.7). In the workshop, the recommended run acceptance rule of "4-6-30" (i.e., a minimum of 4 out of 6 QC samples are within 30% of their nominal values) has been changed to a "4-6-20" rule as stipulated in the conference report [19].

4.2.8 Conclusions

Ligand-binding assays are the technique of choice for bioanalytical support for preclinical and clinical studies for large molecule therapeutics. In view of the small sample volumes and high drug concentrations that are typically available in preclinical studies, one should design and develop a robust assay where reliable and repro-

TABLE 4.7   Comparison of LBA Specific Acceptance Criteria as Recommended by the LBABFG White Paper and AAPS/FDA 3rd Conference Report

Performance Characteristic	LBABFG White Paper	AAPS/FDA 3rd Conference Report	Recommended Changes in Conference Report
Validation Sample %RE	±20% ±25% at the LLOQ	±20% ±25% at the LLOQ and ULOQ	±25% RE extended to ULOQ level as well
Validation Sample %CV	±20% ±25% at the LLOQ	±20% ±25% at the LLOQ and ULOQ	±25% CV extended to ULOQ level as well
Validation Sample %TE	±30% ±40 at the LLOQ	±30% ±40% at the LLOQ and ULOQ	±40% TE extended to ULOQ level as well
In-study standards (excluding anchor points)	≥75% of standard points are ±20% RE (±25% RE at the LLOQ); at least six valid standard points must remain within limits	≥75% of standard points are ±20% RE (±25% RE at the LLOQ and ULOQ)	±25% RE extended to standard points at ULOQ level as well; number of acceptable points in a standard curve not specified
In-study quality controls	4-6-30[a] rule; at least 50% of QCs are valid at each level	4-6-20[a] rule; at least 50% of QCs are valid at each level; three levels analyzed in duplicate (six results)	Major changes: (1) QC acceptance limit is reduced from 30% RE to 20% RE; (2) three levels of QC samples in duplicate specified

[a]Exceptions allowed with justification.

ducible results are obtained and sample reanalysis is minimized. Moreover, the method specificity, selectivity, dilutional linearity, and reproducibility must be established and validated upfront to avoid potential problems that may be encountered during sample analysis. Method validation performance acceptance criteria for precision of measurements for LBA assays are much wider compared to that of chromatographic assays. Current white papers and workshop reports provide adequate recommendations for development, pre-study and in-study validation, and implementation of these assays to support regulatory compliant studies.

This chapter provides an overview of the current advance and trends in the bioanalytical area to support preclinical studies. It covers both conventional small molecule drugs and macromolecular BIOTEC therapeutic entities.

REFERENCES

1. Lee MS, Kerns ED. LC/MS applications in drug development. *Mass Spectrom. Rev* 1999;18:187–279.
*2. Dong H, Ouyang Z, Liu J, Jemal M. The use of a dual dye photometric calibration method to identify possible sample dilution from an automated multichannel liquid-handling system. *Clin Lab Med* 2007;27:113–122.

3. Gu H, Unger S, Deng Y. Automated Tecan programming for bioanalytical sample preparation with EZTecan. *Assay Drug Dev Technol* 2006;4:721–733.

4. Brewer E, Henion J. Atmospheric pressure ionization LC/MS/MS techniques for drug disposition studies. *J Pharm Sci* 1998;87:395–402.

5. Jemal M, Xia Y-Q. LC-MS development strategies for quantitative bioanalysis. *Curr Drug Metab* 2006;7:491–502.

6. Jemal M. High-throughput quantitative bioanalysis by LC/MS/MS. *Biomed Chromatogr* 2000;14:422–429.

7. Oliveira EJ, Watson DG. Liquid chromatography–mass spectrometry in the study of the metabolism of drugs and other xenobiotics. *Biomed Chromatogr* 2000;14:351–372.

8. Law B, Temesi D. Factors to consider in the development of generic bioanalytical high-performance liquid chromatographic–mass spectrometric methods to support drug discovery. *J Chromatogr B* 2000;748:21–30.

9. Plumb R, Dear GJ, Mallett DN, Higton DM, Pleasance S, Biddlecombe RA. Quantitative analysis of pharmaceuticals in biological fluids using high-performance liquid chromatography coupled to mass spectrometry: a review. *Xenobiotica* 2001;31:599–617.

10. Kyranos JN, Cai H, Wei D, Goetzinger WK. High-throughput high-performance liquid chromatography/mass spectrometry for modern drug discovery. *Curr Opin Biotechnol* 2001;12:105–111.

11. Triolo A, Altamura M, Cardinali F, Sisto A, Maggi CA. Mass spectrometry and combinatorial chemistry: a short outline. *J Mass Spectrom* 2001;36:1249–1259.

12. O'Connor D. Automated sample preparation and LC-MS for high-throughput ADME quantification. *Curr Opin Drug Discov Dev* 2002;5:52–58.

13. Ackermann BL, Berna MJ, Murphy AT. Recent advances in use of LC/MS/MS for quantitative high-throughput bioanalytical support of drug discovery. *Curr Top Med Chem* 2002;2:53–66.

14. Hopfgartner G, Bourgogne E. Quantitative high-throughput analysis of drugs in biological matrices by mass spectrometry. *Mass Spectrom Rev* 2003;22:195–214.

15. FDA. *Guidance for Industry: Bioanalytical Methods Validation.* US Department of Health and Human Services, Center for Drug Evaluation and Research, and Center for Veterinary Medicine, May 2001. Available at http://www.fda/cder/guidance/index.htm.

16. Jemal M, Schuster A, Whigan DB. Liquid chromatography/tandem mass spectrometry methods for quantitation of mevalonic acid in human plasma and urine: method validation, demonstration of using a surrogate analyte, and demonstration of unacceptable matrix effect in spite of use of a stable isotope analog internal standard. *Rapid Commun Mass Spectrom* 2003;17:1723–1734.

17. Jemal M, Ouyang Z, Powell ML. A strategy for a post-method-validation use of incurred biological samples for establishing the acceptability of a liquid chromatography/tandem mass-spectrometric method for quantitation of drugs in biological samples. *Rapid Commun Mass Spectrom* 2002;16:1538–1547.

18. Humphreys WG, Unger SE. Safety assessment of drug metabolites: characterization of chemically stable metabolites. *Chem Res Toxicol* 2006;19:1564–1569.

19. Viswanathan CT, Bansal S, Booth B, DeStefano AJ, Rose MJ, Sailstad J, Shah VP, Skelly JP, Swann PG, Weiner R. Workshop/conference report—Quantitative Bioanalytical methods validation and implementation: best practices for chromatographic and ligand binding assays, *AAPS* 2007;9(1): Article 4. Available at http://www.aapsj.org.

20. Baillie TA, Cayen MN, Fouda H, Gerson RJ, Green JD, Grossman SJ, Klunk LJ, LeBlanc B, Perkins DG, Shipley LA. Drug metabolites in safety testing. *Toxicol Appl Pharmacol* 2002;182:188–196.

21. US Food and Drug Administration. *Draft Guidance for Industry: Safety Testing of Drug Metabolites.* Available at www.fda.gov/cder/guidance.

22. Brown K, Tompkins EM, White INH. Applications of accelerator mass spectrometry for pharmacological and toxicological research. *Mass Spectrom Rev* 2006;25:127–145.

23. Bailey MJ, Dickinson RG. Acyl glucuronide reactivity in perspective: biological consequences. *Chem-Biol Interact* 2003;145:117–137.

24. Miles DR, Mesfin M, Mody TD, Stiles M, Lee J, Fiene J, Denis B, Boswell GW. Validation and use of three complementary analytical methods (LC-FLS, LC-MS/MS and ICP-MS) to evaluate the pharmacokinetics, biodistribution and stability of motexafin gadolinium in plasma and tissues. *Anal Bioanal Chem* 2006;385:345–356.

25. Chen Y-L, Felder L, Jiang X, Naidong W. Determination of ketoconazole in human plasma by high-performance liquid chromatography–tandem mass spectrometry. *J Chromatogr B* 2002;774:67–78.

26. Leinweber FC, Lubda D, Cabrera K, Tallarek U. Characterization of silica-based monoliths with bimodal pore size distribution. *Anal Chem* 2002;74:2470–2477.

27. Wu JT, Zeng H, Deng Y, Unger SE. High-speed liquid chromatography/tandem mass spectrometry using a monolithic column for high-throughput bioanalysis. *Rapid Commun Mass Spectrom* 2001;15:1113–1119.

28. Hsieh Y, Wang G, Wang Y, Chackalamannil S, Brisson, J-M, Ng K, Korfmacher WA. Simultaneous determination of a drug candidate and its metabolite in rat plasma samples using ultrafast monolithic column high-performance liquid chromatography/tandem mass spectrometry. *Rapid Commun Mass Spectrom* 2002;16:944–950.

29. Deng Y, Wu JT, Lloyd TL, Chi CL, Olah TV, Unger SE. High-speed gradient parallel liquid chromatography/tandem mass spectrometry with fully automated sample preparation for bioanalysis: 30 seconds per sample from plasma. *Rapid Commun Mass Spectrom* 2002;16:1116–1123.

30. Naidong W, Shou WZ, Chen, Y-L, Jiang X. Novel liquid chromatographic–tandem mass spectrometric methods using silica columns and aqueous-organic mobile phases for quantitative analysis of polar ionic analytes in biological fluids. *J Chromatogr B* 2001;754:387–399.

31. Naidong W. Bioanalytical liquid chromatography tandem mass spectrometry methods on underivatized silica columns with aqueous/organic mobile phases. *J Chromatogr B* 2003;796:209–224.

32. Herman JL. Generic method for on-line extraction of drug substances in the presence of biological matrices using turbulent flow chromatography. *Rapid Commun Mass Spectrom* 2002;16:421–426.

33. Tang YQ, Tollefson JA, Beato BD, Weng N. 2003 AAPS Annual Meeting, Salt Lake City, Utah, 26–30 October 2003.

34. Xue YJ, Pursley J, Arnold M. Liquid–liquid extraction of strongly protein bound BMS-299897 from human plasma and cerebrospinal fluid, followed by high-performance liquid chromatography/tandem mass spectrometry. *J Pharm Biomed Anal* 2007;43:1728–1736.

35. Zhang N, Rogers K, Gajda K, Kagel JR, Rossi DT. Integrated sample collection and handling for drug discovery bioanalysis. *J Pharm Biomed Anal* 2000;23:551–560.

36. Teitz DS, Khan S, Powell ML, Jemal M. An automated method of sample preparation of biofluids using pierceable caps to eliminate the uncapping of the sample tubes during sample transfer. *J Biochem Biophys Methods* 2000;45:193–204.

37. Allanson JP, Biddlecombe RA, Jones AE, Pleasance S. The use of automated solid phase extraction in the "96 well" format for high throughput bioanalysis using liquid

chromatography coupled to tandem mass spectrometry. *Rapid Commun Mass Spectrom* 1996;10:811–816.

38. Janiszewski J, Schneider R, Hoffmaster K, Swyden M, Wells D, Fouda H. Automated sample preparation using membrane microtiter extraction for bioanalytical mass spectrometry. *Rapid Commun Mass Spectrom* 1997;11:1033–1037.

39. Simpson H, Berthemy A, Burhrman D, Burton R, Newton J, Kealy M, Wells D, Wu D. High throughput liquid chromatography/mass spectrometry bioanalysis using 96-well disk solid phase extraction plate for the sample preparation. *Rapid Commun Mass Spectrom* 1998;12:75–82.

40. Eerkes A, Addison T, Naidong W. Simultaneous assay of sildenafil and desmethylsildenafil in human plasma using liquid chromatography–tandem mass spectrometry on silica column with aqueous-organic mobile phase. *J Chromatogr B* 2002;768:277–284.

41. Steinborner S, Henion J. Liquid–liquid extraction In the 96-well plate format with SRM LC/MS quantitative determination of methotrexate and its major metabolite in human plasma. *Anal Chem* 1999;71:2340–2345.

42. Jemal M, Teitz D, Ouyang Z, Khan S. Comparison of plasma sample purification by manual liquid–liquid extraction, automated 96-well liquid–liquid extraction and automated 96-well solid-phase extraction for analysis by high-performance liquid chromatography with tandem mass spectrometry. *J Chromatogr B* 1999;732:501–508.

43. Bolden RD, Hoke SH II, Eichold TH, McCauley-Myers DL, Wehmeyer KR. Semi-automated liquid–liquid back-extraction in a 96-well format to decrease sample preparation time for the determination of dextromethorphan and dextrorphan in human plasma. *J Chromatogr B* 2002;772:1–10.

44. Ramos L, Bakhtiar R, Tse FLS. Liquid–liquid extraction using 96-well plate format in conjunction with liquid chromatography/tandem mass spectrometry for quantitative determination of methylphenidate (Ritalin) in human plasma. *Rapid Commun Mass Spectrom* 2000;14:740–745.

45. Shen Z, Wang S, Bakhtiar R. Enantiomeric separation and quantification of fluoxetine (Prozac) in human plasma by liquid chromatography/tandem mass spectrometry using liquid–liquid extraction in 96-well plate format. *Rapid Commun Mass Spectrom* 2002;16:332–338.

46. Eerkes A, Shou WZ, Naidong W. Liquid/liquid extraction using 96-well plate format in conjunction with hydrophilic interaction liquid chromatography–tandem mass spectrometry method for the analysis of fluconazole in human plasma. *J Pharm Biomed Anal* 2003;31:917–928.

47. Watt AP, Morrison D, Locker KL, Evans DG. Higher throughput bioanalysis by automation of a protein precipitation assay using a 96-well format with detection by LC-MS/MS. *Anal Chem* 2000;72:979–984.

48. Shou WZ, Bu H-Z, Addison T, Jiang X, Naidong W. Development and validation of a liquid chromatography/tandem mass spectrometry (LC/MS/MS) method for the determination of ribavirin in human plasma and serum. *J Pharm Biomed Anal* 2002; 29:83–94.

49. Naidong W, Shou WZ, Addison T, Maleki S, Jiang X. Liquid chromatography/tandem mass spectrometric bioanalysis using normal-phase columns with aqueous/organic mobile phases—a novel approach of eliminating evaporation and reconstitution steps in 96-well SPE. *Rapid Commun Mass Spectrom* 2002;16:1965–1975.

50. Li AC, Junga H, Shou WZ, Bryant MS, Jiang X, Naidong W. Direct injection of solid-phase extraction eluents onto silica columns for the analysis of polar compounds isoniazid and cetirizine in plasma using hydrophilic interaction chromatography with tandem mass spectrometry. *Rapid Commun Mass Spectrom* 2004;18:2343–2350.

51. Song Q, Naidong W. Analysis of omeprazole and 5-OH omeprazole in human plasma using hydrophilic interaction chromatography with tandem mass spectrometry (HILIC-MS/MS)—eliminating evaporation and reconstitution steps in 96-well liquid/liquid extraction. *J Chromatogr B* 2006;830:135–142.

52. Naidong W, Zhou W, Song Q, Zhou S. Direct injection of 96-well organic extracts onto a hydrophilic interaction chromatography/tandem mass spectrometry system using a silica stationary phase and an aqueous/organic mobile phase. *Rapid Commun Mass Spectrom* 2004;18:2963–2968.

53. Matuszewski BK. Standard line slopes as a measure of a relative matrix effect in quantitative HPLC-MS bioanalysis. *J Chromatogr B* 2006;830:293–300.

54. Matuszewski BK, Constanzer ML, Chavez-Eng CM. Strategies for the assessment of matrix effect in quantitative bioanalytical methods based on HPLC-MS/MS. *Anal Chem* 2003;75:3019–3030.

55. FDA. *Guidance for Industry: Bioanalytical Methods Validation*. US Department of Health and Human Services, Center for Drug Evaluation and Research, and Center for Veterinary Medicine, May 2001. Available at http://www.fda/cder/guidance/index.htm.

56. Little JL, Wempe MF, Buchanan CM. Liquid chromatography–mass spectrometry/mass spectrometry method development for drug metabolism studies: examining lipid matrix ionization effects in plasma. *J Chromatogr B* 2006;833:219–230.

57. Sojo LE, Lum G, Chee P. Internal standard signal suppression by co-eluting analyte in isotope dilution LC-ESI-MS. *Analyst* 2003;128:51–55.

58. Tong XS, Wang J, Zheng S, Pivnichny JV, Griffin PR, Shen X, Donnelly M, Vakerich K, Nunes C, Fenyk-Melody J. Effect of signal interference from dosing excipients on pharmacokinetic screening of drug candidates by liquid chromatography/mass spectrometry. *Anal Chem* 2002;74:6305–6313.

59. Shou WZ, Naidong W. Post-column infusion study of the "dosing vehicle effect" in the liquid chromatography/tandem mass spectrometric analysis of discovery pharmacokinetic samples. *Rapid Commun Mass Spectrom* 2003;17:589–597.

60. Schuhmacher J, Zimmer D, Tesche F, Pickard V. Matrix effects during analysis of plasma samples by electrospray and atmospheric pressure chemical ionization mass spectrometry: practical approaches to their elimination. *Rapid Commun Mass Spectrom* 2003;17:1950–1957.

61. Mallet CR, Lu Z, Mazzeo JR. A study of ion suppression effects in electrospray ionization from mobile phase additives and solid-phase extracts. *Rapid Commun Mass Spectrom* 2004;18:49–58.

62. Mei H, Hsieh Y, Nardo C, Xu X, Wang S, Ng K, Korfmacher WA. Investigation of matrix effects in bioanalytical high-performance liquid chromatography/tandem mass spectrometric assays: application to drug discovery. *Rapid Commun Mass Spectrom* 2003;17:97–103.

63. Pommier F, Frigola R. Quantitative determination of rivastigmine and its major metabolite in human plasma by liquid chromatography with atmospheric pressure chemical ionization tandem mass spectrometry. *J Chromatogr B* 2003;784:301–313.

64. Dams R, Huestis MA, Lambert WE, Murphy CM. Matrix effect in bio-analysis of illicit drugs with LC-MS/MS: influence of ionization type, sample preparation, and biofluid. *J Am Soc Mass Spectrom* 2003;14:1290–1294.

65. Choi BK, Hercules DM, Gusev AI. Effect of liquid chromatography separation of complex matrices on liquid chromatography–tandem mass spectrometry signal suppression. *J Chromatogr A* 2001;907:337–342.

66. Lin ZJ, Desai-Krieger D, Shum L. Simultaneous determination of glipizide and rosiglitazone unbound drug concentrations in plasma by equilibrium dialysis and liquid chromatography–tandem mass spectrometry. *J Chromatogr B* 2004;801:265–272.

67. Arnold RD, Slack JE, Straubinger RM. Quantification of doxorubicin and metabolites in rat plasma and small volume tissue samples by liquid chromatography/electrospray tandem mass spectroscopy. *J Chromatogr B* 2004;808:141–152.

68. Bonfiglio R, King RC, Olah TV, Merkle K. The effects of sample preparation methods on the variability of the electrospray ionization response for model drug compounds. *J Chromatogr B* 1999;13:1175–1185.

69. Borges V, Yang E, Dunn J, Henion J. High-throughput liquid chromatography–tandem mass spectrometry determination of bupropion and its metabolites in human, mouse and rat plasma using a monolithic column. *J Chromatogr B* 2004;804:277–287.

70. Wang Y, Hochhaus G. Simultaneous quantification of beclomethasone dipropionate and its metabolite, beclomethasone 17-monopropionate in rat and human plasma and different rat tissues by liquid chromatography–positive electrospray ionization tandem mass spectrometry. *J Chromatogr B* 2004;805:203–210.

71. Jemal M, Huang M, Mao Y, Whigan D, Powell MD. Increased throughput in quantitative bioanalysis using parallel-column liquid chromatography with mass spectrometric detection. *Rapid Commun Mass Spectrom* 2001;15:994–999.

72. Zeng W, Wang AQ, Fisher AL, Musson DG. A direct injection high-throughput liquid chromatography tandem mass spectrometry method for the determination of a new orally active alphavbeta3 antagonist in human urine and dialysate. *Rapid Commun Mass Spectrom* 2003;17:2475–2482.

73. Chavez-Eng CM, Constanzer ML, Matuszewski BK. Determination of rofecoxib (MK-0966), a cyclooxygenase-2 inhibitor, in human plasma by high-performance liquid chromatography with tandem mass spectrometric detection. *J Chromatogr B* 2000;748:31–39.

74. Needham SR, Ye B, Smith R, Korte WD. Development and validation of a liquid chromatography–tandem mass spectrometry method for the determination of pyridostigmine bromide from guinea pig plasma. *J Chromatogr B* 2003;796:347–354.

75. Jemal M, Rao S, Gatz M, Whigan D. Liquid chromatography–tandem mass spectrometric quantitative determination of the HIV protease inhibitor atazanavir (BMS-232632) in human peripheral blood mononuclear cells (PBMC): practical approaches to PBMC preparation and PBMC assay design for high-throughput analysis. *J Chromatogr B* 2003;795:273–289.

76. Verhaeghe T, Diels L, de Vries R, de MeulDer M, de Jong J. Development and validation of a liquid chromatographic–tandem mass spectrometric method for the determination of galantamine in human heparinised plasma. *J Chromatogr B* 2003;789:337–346.

77. Constanzer ML, Chavez-Eng CM, Dru J, Kline KF, Matuszewski BK. Determination of a novel substance P inhibitor in human plasma by high-performance liquid chromatography with atmospheric pressure chemical ionization mass spectrometric detection using single and triple quadrupole detectors. *J Chromatogr B* 2004;806:243–250.

78. Zhou L, Glickman RD, Chen N, Sponsel WE, Graybill JR, Lam K-W. Determination of voriconazole in aqueous humor by liquid chromatography–electrospray ionization–mass spectrometry. *J Chromatogr B* 2002;776:213–220.

79. Lakso H, Norström A. Determination of dextropropoxyphene and nordextropropoxyphene in urine by liquid chromatography–electrospray ionization mass spectrometry. *J Chromatogr B* 2003;794:57–65.

80. Yang JZ, Bastian KC, Moore RD, Stobaugh JF, Borchardt RT. Quantitative analysis of a model opioid peptide and its cyclic prodrugs in rat plasma using high-performance

liquid chromatography with fluorescence and tandem mass spectrometric detection. *J Chromatogr B* 2002;779:269–281.

81. Inoue K, Wada M, Higuchi T, Oshio S, Umeda T, Yoshimura Y, Nakazawa H. Application of liquid chromatography–mass spectrometry to the quantification of bisphenol A in human semen. *J Chromatogr B* 2002;773:97–102.

82. Eriksson K, Östin A, Levin J-O. Quantification of melatonin in human saliva by liquid chromatography–tandem mass spectrometry using stable isotope dilution. *J Chromatogr B* 2003;794:115–123.

83. Keevil BG, Lockhart SJ, Cooper DP. Determination of tobramycin in serum using liquid chromatography–tandem mass spectrometry and comparison with a fluorescence polarisation assay. *J Chromatogr B* 2003;794:329–335.

84. Stokes P, O'Connor G. Development of a liquid chromatography–mass spectrometry method for the high-accuracy determination of creatinine in serum. *J Chromatogr B* 2003;794:125–136.

85. Huang Y, Zurlinden E, Lin E, Li X, Tokumoto J, Golden J, Murr A, Engstrom J, Conte J Jr. Liquid chromatographic–tandem mass spectrometric assay for the simultaneous determination of didanosine and stavudine in human plasma, bronchoalveolar lavage fluid, alveolar cells, peripheral blood mononuclear cells, seminal plasma, cerebrospinal fluid and tonsil tissue. *J Chromatogr B* 2004;799:51–61.

86. Leahy M, Felder L, Goytowski K, Shou W, Weng N. 52nd ASMS Conference on Mass Spectrometry and Allied Topics, Nashville, Tennessee, 23–27 May 2004.

87. Zeng W, Musson DG, Fisher AL, Wang AQ. A new approach for evaluating carry-over and its influence on quantitation in high-performance liquid chromatography and tandem mass spectrometry assay. *Rapid Commun Mass Spectrom* 2006;20:635–640.

88. Wang S, Cyronak M, Yang E. Does a stable isotopically labeled internal standard always correct analyte response? A matrix effect study on a LC/MS/MS method for the determination of carvedilol enantiomers in human plasma. *J Pharm Biomed Anal* 2007; 43:701–707.

89. Yang L, Wu N, Clement RP, Rudewicz PJ. Validation and application of a liquid chromatography–tandem mass spectrometric method for the determination of SCH 211803 in rat and monkey plasma using automated 96-well protein precipitation. *J Chromatogr B* 2004;799:271–280.

90. Khan MN. Immunoassay in drug development arena: an old player with new status. *J Clin Ligand Assay* 1999;22:242–253.

91. Findlay JWA, Smith WC, Lee JW, Nordblom GD, Das I, DeSilva BS, Khan MN, Bowsher RR. Validation of immunoassay for bioanalysis: a pharmaceutical industry perspective. *J Pharm Biomed Anal* 2000;21:1249–1273.

92. Wadhwa M, Bird C, Dilger P, Gaines-Das R, Thorpe R. Strategies for selection, measurements and characterization of unwanted antibodies induced by therapeutic biologicals. *J Immunol Methods* 2003;278:1–17.

93. Shankar G, Shores E, Wagner C, Mire-Sluis A. Scientific and regulatory considerations on the immunogenicity of biologics. *Trends Biotechnol* 2006;24:274–280.

94. DeSilva B, Smith W, Weiner R, Kelly M, Smolec J, Lee B, Khan M, Tacey R, Hill H, Celniker A. Recommendations for the bioanalytical method validation of ligand-binding assay to support pharmacokinetics assessment of macromolecules. *Pharm Res* 2003;20: 1885–1900.

95. Lee JW, Dewanarayan V, Barrett YC, Weiner R, Allison J, Fountain S, Keller S, Weinryb I, Green M, Duann L, Rogers JA, Millham R, O'Brian PJ, Sailstad J, Khan M, Ray C, Wagner JA. Fit-for-purpose method development and validation for successful biomarker measurements. *Pharm Res* 2006;32:312–328.

96. Mire-Sluis AR, Barett Y, Devanarayan V, Koren E, Liu H, Maia M, Parish T, Scott G, Shankar G, Shores E, Swanson SJ, Taniguchi G, Wierda D, Zuckerman LA. Recommendations for the design and optimization of immunoassays used in the detection of host antibodies against biotechnology products. *J Immunol Methods* 2004;289:1–16.

97. Crowther JR. *The ELISA Guidebook*, Methods in Molecular Biology, Vol 149. Totowa, NJ: Humana Press; 2001.

98. Wild D. *The Immunoassay Handbook*, 2nd ed. New York: Nature Publishing Group; 2001.

99. Rodbard D, Feldman Y, Jaffe ML, Miles Le EM. Kinetics of two-site immunoradiometeric (sandwich) assay II. *Immunochemistry* 1978;15:77–82.

100. Plikaytis BD, Holder PF, Pais LB, Maslanka SE, Gheesling LL, Carlone GM. Determination of parallism and nonparallelism in bioassay dilution curves. *J Clin Microbiol* 1994;32:2441–2447.

101. Shah VP, Midha KK, Dighe SV, McGiveray JJ, Skelly JO, Yacobi A, Laylogg T, Viswanathan CT, Cook CE, McDowall RD, Putman KA, Spector S. Analytical method validation: bioavailability, bioequivalence, and PK studies. *J Pharm Sci* 1992;81: 309–312.

102. Miller KJ, Bowsher RR, Celniker A, Gibbons J, Gupta S, Lee JW, Swanson J, Smith WC, Weiner RS. Workshop on bioanalytical method validation for macromolecules: summary report. *Pharm Res* 2001;18:1373–1383.

103. Smolec J, DeSilva B, Smith W, Weiner R, Kelly M, Lee B, Khan M, Tacey R, Hill H, Cekniker A. Bioanalytical method validation for macromolecules in support of pharmacokinetic studies. *Pharm Res* 2005;22:1425–1431.

5

ANALYTICAL CHEMISTRY METHODS: DEVELOPMENTS AND VALIDATION

IZET M. KAPETANOVIC[1] AND ALEXANDER V. LYUBIMOV[2]

[1]*NIH NCI Division of Cancer Prevention, Chemoprevention Agent Development Research Group, Bethesda, Maryland*
[2]*University of Illinois at Chicago, Chicago, Illinois*

Contents

Preclinical Development Handbook: ADME and Biopharmaceutical Properties,
edited by Shayne Cox Gad
Copyright © 2008 John Wiley & Sons, Inc.

5.1   INTRODUCTION

5.1.1   Background

Analytical methodology plays an integral part of drug development from the initial synthesis and manufacture through clinical trials and postmarketing monitoring. In new drug applications (NDAs), abbreviated new drug applications (ANDAs), biologics license applications (BLAs), or product license applications (PLAs), data must be submitted to establish that the analytical procedures used in testing meet proper FDA and ICH guidelines of accuracy and reliability. At the time of submission, the NDA, ANDA, BLA, or PLA should contain method validation information to support the adequacy of the analytical procedures. All analytical methods should be validated (to demonstrate that the analytical procedures are suitable for their intended use) prior to their use. The suitability of a compendial analytical procedure must be verified under the actual condition of use, but full validation is not required. As in all other preclinical pharmacology/toxicology studies, analytical assays should be conducted according to the FDA's Good Laboratory Practices (GLPs) (21 CFR part 58). Selective and sensitive validated analytical methods for the quantitative evaluation of drugs are critical for the successful conduct of preclinical safety and efficacy studies.

5.1.2   Purpose

Analytical methods are required for determination of the following:

- Active pharmaceutical ingredient (API)—manufacturing control, stability testing, shelf-life forecast.
- Synthetic contaminants, degradation products—manufacturing control, stability testing, shelf-life forecast.
- Pharmaceutical excipients (binders, disintegrants, lubricants, antioxidants and preservatives, suspending and dispersing agents, natural or artificial flavorings and colorings, coatings, etc.)—manufacturing control, stability testing. The *United States Pharmacopeia and the National Formulary* (USP-NF) contains information on the identity, strength, quality, and purity for more than 250 excipients including official test methods in analytical testing.
- Drug and metabolites in biological fluids and tissues—bioavailability, pharmacokinetics.

It is important to have validated analytical methods from the start and throughout the drug development process. The generic approach to method development involves three basic steps: sample preparation (clean up), separation, and detection. A schematic flow diagram depicting the most commonly used options is shown in Fig. 5.1. While general approaches to method development are similar, complexity and requirements of time and resources vary. For example, the *United States Pharmacopeia-National Formulary* (USP-NF) provides standard methods for pharmaceutical excipients, obviating a need for analytical method development, and will not be specifically addressed here. On the other hand, analysis in biological fluids and tissues is the most time and labor intensive due to complexity and variability

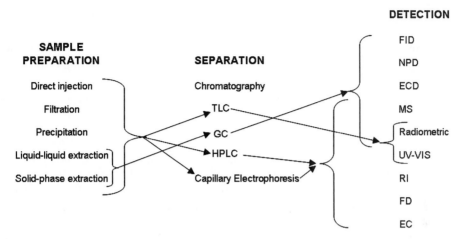

FIGURE 5.1   General scheme for developing an analytical method based on separation techniques. Most commonly used approaches are depicted.

of the biological matrices and the relatively low levels of analytes. Selection of appropriate sample preparation, separation, and detection approaches depends on the nature of the sample, the nature of the sample matrix, the concentration of analyte(s) in the matrix, the laboratory levels of skill and available resources, and so on.

5.2   ANALYTICAL METHOD DEVELOPMENT

5.2.1   Sampling and Handling

The proper sampling and handling of samples is one of the most important factors in a high quality analysis. The reader is referred to an excellent resource, Chapter 7 in *Quality Assurance Principles for Analytical Laboratories* [1], for details of sampling and handling. The main principles are described below.

There are three basic activities involved in solving an analytical problem: (1) collection and handling of the appropriate sample, (2) preparation of sample for analysis, and (3) analysis using an appropriate method.

These activities are independent of each other, but one significantly influences the others. Failure to observe standard procedures for sample collection, handling, and documentation often impairs the intended purpose of the analysis itself. In many cases, the collection of samples falls outside a laboratory's control. However, the laboratory must do all it can to receive appropriate, applicable, and defensible samples.

Key points for sampling are the following:

• The laboratory shall have a sampling plan and procedures for sampling when it carries out sampling of substances, materials, or products for subsequent testing or calibration.

- Sampling plans shall, whenever reasonable, be based on appropriate statistical methods.
- Sampling procedures shall describe the selection, sampling plan, withdrawal, and preparation of a sample or samples from a substance, material, or product to yield the required information.
- The laboratory shall have procedures for recording relevant data and operations relating to sampling.

It is extremely important to perform accurate subsampling (taking the appropriate test portion for analysis) in the laboratory. The number of samples to be analyzed in a given situation is limited by the resources available for the collection of the samples or for their analysis. Analyses of multiple samples always are preferred over single samples since single samples give no information on the homogeneity of the lot that was sampled. In addition, for single samples, the sampling error is also confounded with the analytical error. It is a common practice to collect several samples for test substance and dosage formulation analyses to assess homogeneity. For example, at least three samples from the top, middle, and bottom portions of the dietary admixture or dosage formulation should be collected and usually each portion is analyzed in triplicate to assess homogeneity. However, for a bioanalytical analysis, a single sample is usually analyzed because of limited volume of sample and high cost of each analysis. Each sample should be prepared in a way that it achieves homogeneity and should be handled in a manner that prevents alteration from the original composition. Even seemingly homogeneous materials such as liquids may be subject to sedimentation or stratification.

Shipment or delivery of the sample should be done under appropriate conditions (e.g., temperature) in a proper container package and with a proper label and should be accompanied by meaningful documentation, including Material Safety Data Sheet (MSDS) and instructions for sample storage upon delivery. The documentation consists of a chain-of-custody or similarly named document that accompanies the sample as it moves to and through the laboratory. A dependable record of sample handling is important. The sample shall be accepted by a designated person (a custodian in laboratories of appreciable size) who documents the action by completing a sample accountability record. This document will contain the sample number, the name of the product, and the date received; will indicate who received it; will describe the method of shipment or delivery, the packages received, and their condition; and will provide space for recording various storage locations before and after analysis. Deliveries of the sample, or parts of the sample, to the analyst, and its return, shall also be recorded on this form, as shall the signed statement concerning the final disposition of the reserve sample. A two-part form can be used for this purpose. One copy remains with the custodian and the other moves with the sample through the laboratory and is used by the supervisor for sample management purposes. Some laboratories use a Sample Receiving Log book for sample control. The information entered in the Log book is essentially the same as described for the two-part form.

For proper handling of the test samples and calibration items, the laboratory shall have written procedures for their transportation, receipt, handling, protection, storage, retention, and/or disposal. The laboratory shall have a system for identifying test and/or calibration items. The laboratory shall also have documented procedures and appropriate facilities to avoid deterioration, damage, loss, or cross-contamination of any test item or sample during storage and handling. All necessary environmental conditions, including special security arrangements for sample integrity as needed for some samples, shall be established, maintained, monitored, and recorded.

5.2.2   Sample Preparation

Sample preparation is a very important first and often critical step in the analytical method, especially when biological samples are involved. Typically, it is the most difficult and time-consuming step. The purpose of sample preparation is to isolate analytes of interest from interfering sample components, concentrate the analytes, and dissolve them in a suitable solvent for subsequent separation and detection. Sample preparation significantly impacts on the recovery, selectivity, sensitivity, reproducibility, and ruggedness of the analytical method. Sample cleanliness or, more often, a lack thereof may have a direct effect (e.g., full or partial chromatographic peak overlap) on detection and quantification of analytes of interest, but also an indirect effect (e.g., contamination of analytical column or mass spectrometry (MS) ion source, ionization suppression in MS). Not only can some of the interferences lead to a loss in sensitivity (e.g., ionization suppression in MS) [2], but this effect may be variable depending on individual samples [3]. However, in some instances, the coextracted materials may be helpful. For example, coextractants can neutralize active sites on glassware, injector, or column and thereby minimize adsorptive effects. Therefore, coextractants may have a positive or negative effect and should be considered during analytical method development. Consequently, it is strongly advisable that all comparisons of extracted biological samples be made to similar extracts of spiked blank biological matrix instead of neat solutions.

Commonly encountered sample problems include (1) lack of compatibility with chromatographic system (e.g., tendency to clog or degrade the analytical column), (2) being too dirty (presence of coextracted materials that interfere with separation or detection of analytes), and (3) being too dilute (sensitivity issue). More common approaches to sample preparation will be discussed later, while the less common ones (turbulent flow chromatography, monolithic chromatography, immunoaffinity, etc.) will not be included here.

Comparison of most commonly employed sample preparation techniques is presented in Table 5.1. In general, simpler, faster methods tend to generate dirtier samples, which tend to limit the number of injections that can be made on a column or into a chromatographic system before chromatographic or system conditions start to deteriorate.

Direct Injection   Direct injection approaches have been developed to facilitate and expedite analysis of biological samples and are more suitable for liquid as opposed to gas phase separation methods. They include direct injection with or without prior dilution, column switching, and restricted access medium (RAM) or internal surface reversed-phase (ISRP) column methods.

A simple dilution and injection approach is not commonly used because it requires high analyte concentration and/or high detector response to an analyte.

TABLE 5.1   Relative Comparison of Commonly Used Sample Preparation Methods

Factor	Direct Injection	Filtration	Precipitation	LLE	SPE
Simplicity	++++	+++++	+++++	+++	+++
Speed	+++	++++	++++	+	+++
Resultant sample cleanliness	++	+	+	+++++	+++++
Resultant analyte concentration	+	+	+	+	+++
Selectivity	+	+	+	+++	++++
Solvent consumption	++	+	+++	+++++	++
Possible injections per column	++	++	++	+++++	+++++

This straightforward approach may be suitable for analysis of simple matrices (e.g., API or formulated pharmaceutical product) but generally is not useful for the analysis of biological samples due to low analyte concentration and numerous complex interferences.

Column switching for separation and enrichment of analytes of interest has been in use for a long time [4]. Hagestam and Pinkerton [5] introduced an online cleaning method for HPLC analysis with a RAM/ISRP column [6–8]. RAM columns operate via both size exclusion and phase partitioning modes. Prefiltered samples are injected onto a RAM column, which retains small molecules in the inner hydrophobic pores while larger ones go to waste unretained. Subsequently, small molecules are eluted from the RAM column onto an analytical reversed-phase column, where they are concentrated prior to elution with an appropriate strength mobile phase. A number of manufacturers offer RAM columns with similar basic principles but some variations on the theme (e.g., http://www.registech.com/ram/#SPS). The advantages of this method include speed, simplicity, automation, potential increased safety for analysts due to lesser exposure, and applicability to varied biological, botanical, and environmental matrices. However, the online sample cleaning methods are, in general, subject to carry-over and injector clogging problems. Another drawback of the RAM method is a relatively low sensitivity. However, recent improvements in HPLC column technology and evolution of LC-MS and LC-MS/MS instrumentation have provided additional selectivity and sensitivity [8–10]. Hogendoorn et al. [11] demonstrated suitability of RAM columns for LC-MS/MS analysis of analytes with a wide range of polarities in human serum. Other similar techniques include size exclusion chromatography and turbulent flow chromatography (narrow bore columns packed with large particles) but will not be further discussed here.

The column switching approach utilizes switching valves to redirect the flow of a mobile phase between two columns—a cleanup column and an analytical separation column. Limitations include a requirement of mobile phase compatibility between the two columns. An example of column switching includes online solid phase extraction (SPE, to be discussed later). Good sensitivity and precision were reported in a comparison of online and offline SPE methods for measurement of six isoflavones and lignans in urine [12]. However, the online method was found to be more sensitive, precise, reproducible, and cost effective. Another variation involves a ternary-column system [13], which utilizes dual extraction columns in a parallel configuration. This allows use of one column for extraction while the other is being equilibrated and thereby decreasing the injection cycle time and increasing the sample throughput.

Filtration   Various filtration methods serve similar purposes and have similar advantages and disadvantages to those of protein precipitation (see next section). There are basically two types of filters: depth and screen. Depth filters are randomly oriented fibers that retain particles throughout the matrix rather than just on the surface. They have a higher load capacity than screen filters [14]. Screen filters are polymeric membranes that have a uniform distribution of pore sizes. They are relatively thin so that there is a minimal amount of liquid retention. Screen filters clog more rapidly than depth filters.

In developing a method that requires filtration, adsorption of the analyte onto the filter must be taken into account. For dilute solutions of adriamycin, more than 95% is adsorbed to cellulose ester membranes and about 40% to polytetrafluoro-ethylene membranes [15]. For more concentrated solutions, as would be encountered in bulk formulation testing, filter adsorption is not as important a concern. Nevertheless, the common practice is to discard the first several milliliters of the filtrate. For protein-based products, there is significant nonspecific binding to nylon-based microporous membranes and minimal binding to hydrophilic polyvinylidene fluoride membranes [16]. Ultrafiltration removes protein and protein-bound drug, which makes it suitable for plasma-free drug concentration measurements. Dialysis, on the other hand, is primarily useful for protein binding studies.

Precipitation   Protein precipitation or deproteinization (commonly acetonitrile, perchloric acid, or methanol) is also a relatively simple method of sample preparation and minimally eliminates interferences from large molecules. However, interferences from small molecules remain and this approach is more suited for analytical methods that offer additional selectivity such as LC-MS and LC-MS/MS. Precipitation with acetonitrile or methanol may be combined with subsequent extraction and may be used for HPLC or LC-MS/MS analytical methods, which employ these solvents as mobile phases. In addition, matrix-based interferences can create indirect problems in MS detection due to interference with the ionization process. Furthermore, sensitivity may also be an issue as this method does not include a preconcentration step. Matrix interferences place additional strain on the analytical system. Occasionally, sample dilution prior to precipitation may be needed to avoid trapping analytes within precipitated matrix. One significant advantage of protein precipitation is that it extracts all analytes regardless of their polarity. This overcomes limitations of other extraction methods (e.g., LLE, SPE), which may not effectively extract analytes with a wide range of polarities [17]. The precipitation approach is amenable to automation.

Liquid–Liquid Extraction (LLE)   LLE is one of the oldest and widely used methods for sample preparation. It is based on analyte (solute) partitioning between immiscible solvents according to relative analytes' solubilities in the solvents. In order to optimize separation in terms of recovery, selectivity, and sample cleanliness, several extractions with the same or different solvent combinations may be necessary. For example, acidic analytes can be extracted from acidified aqueous solution into organic solvent (e.g., methyl-*t*-butyl ether), followed by their extraction from methyl-*t*-butyl ether into a basic aqueous solution (e.g., ammonium hydroxide), which is neutralized, and analytes are back-extracted into methyl-*t*-butyl ether. Commonly used extraction solvents include hexane, methyl-*t*-butyl ether, ethyl acetate, chloroform, methylene chloride, and dilute acid or base. Modifiers such as a small percentage of isopropanol can also be added. Fine tuning in LLE can be carried out by judicious selection of solvents, solvent modifiers, solvent volumes, pH, and so on. Not all extractions need to involve aqueous and organic phases. There are some organic solvent combinations that are immiscible and can be used in LLE. For example, the acetonitrile : hexane combination is immiscible and can be used to clean somewhat polar analytes from lipophilic components in a biological matrix. LLE is labor intensive, slow, and not easily amenable to automation. Liquid handling stations are making automation more feasible. LLE generally requires large solvent consumption and solvent evaporation, which have environmental, safety, and health concerns. Finding a suitable solvent system and conditions may be difficult for simultaneous extraction of analytes with different polarities. There is also a tendency for emulsion formation, which introduces further complications. Adsorptive losses may result during evaporation and it may be necessary to pacify the active surface by sylation. Some solvents have a tendency for peroxide formation (e.g., diethyl ether, ethyl acetate) that can lead to analyte stability problems. Methyl-*t*-butyl ether has roughly similar polarity but a lesser propensity for peroxide formation and can often be substituted for those solvents.

Solid-Phase Extraction (SPE)   SPE is analogous to offline gradient liquid chromatography and has overtaken LLE in popularity as it lacks a number of the drawbacks associated with LLE. It is relatively easy to automate, requires small solvent volumes, can concentrate samples without evaporation, and yields cleaner extracts and higher recoveries for polar analytes. However, as mentioned earlier, there are cases where SPE may not be suitable for analytes with a broad range of polarities [17]. Earlier manufacturing problems in batch-to-batch reproducibility of the column materials have mostly been resolved. Cartridge columns with a wide variety of bonded phase packing materials (phases or sorbents) are commercially available (or custom prepared, if desired). Cartridge columns are obtainable in different sizes (e.g., 1 mL, 3 mL, 6 mL, 12 mL) with different amounts of packing material (e.g., 30 mg, 50 mg, 60 mg, 100 mg, 150 mg, 200 mg, 500 mg) to accommodate different sample sizes and not to mass or volume overload SPE columns. As a rough guide, nonionic silica-based sorbents can retain a mass of solute approximately equivalent to 1–5% of sorbent mass or 1–5 mg of solute per 100 mg of sorbent. Polymeric sorbents have a larger surface area and can accommodate solute up to 15% of sorbent mass. However, keep in mind that solute represents analytes plus coextracted material. As a rule of thumb, solvent volumes between 4 and 8 times the bed volume are needed to ensure appropriate conditioning, washing, and elution. Silica-based SPE columns have approximately 150 μL bed volume per 100 mg of sorbent, and polymeric sorbents about 250 μL per 100 mg of sorbent. Most commonly used sorbents comprise siloxane-bonded materials with different functional groups to provide normal-phase, reversed-phase, ion exchange, or mixed-mode chromatographic separation. General characteristics of different phases are summarized in Table 5.2. Some of the phases can operate in different modes. For

TABLE 5.2   Characteristics of Common Silica-Based SPE Phases

	Normal	Reversed	Ion Exchange
Sorbent functional group	Silica Cyano Diol Amino	Octadecyl (C18) Octyl (C8) Methyl (C1) Ethyl (C2) Phenyl	Strong cation exchange (SCX; pK_a 2.0–3.0): benzene sulfonylpropyl Strong anion exchange (SAX; pK_a 11.0–12.0): quarternary amine Amine (pK_a 9.5–10.5)
Analytes	Polar	Nonpolar	Ionized
Elution factor(s)	Solvent strength	Solvent strength	Ionic interaction (pH, ionic strength, counterion strength)
Increasing elution strength	Hexane Toluene Chloroform Methylene chloride Tetrahydrofuran Ethyl acetate Acetone Acetonitrile Isopropanol Methanol Water	Water Methanol Isopropanol Acetonitrile Acetone Ethyl acetate Tetrahydrofuran Methylene chloride Chloroform Toluene Hexane	Cations: Li^+ Na^+ NH^+ K^+, Mg^{2+} Ca^{2+} Anions: Hydroxide, fluoride, propionate Acetate, formate Phosphate, carbonate Sulfate Nitrate Citrate

example, cyano phase can be used either in normal-phase or reversed-phase mode and amino phase can be used in normal phase or anion exchange phase. Undesirable secondary interactions can occur with free silanol moieties and can be minimized by end-capping.

SPE cartridges require prior conditioning to remove any impurities from them and make the sorbent compatible with the sample solvent and allow sample retention. Two conditioning washes are commonly used (each 1–2 mL per 100 mg of sorbent): the first to clean the column and the second (similar to or weaker than the sample solvent) to make the column conducive to sample retention. Sample application and elution should not be performed too rapidly as sufficient residence time must be allowed for effective analyte–sorbent interaction. In order to avoid channeling, it is also important not to allow sorbent to dry between conditionings and prior to sample application. After cartridge conditioning, liquid sample (in the weakest strength solvent possible) is applied and allowed to pass through the column via gravity, pressure, or vacuum. Sample retained on the column should be washed with a stronger solvent than the one used in sample loading but weaker than solvent that would cause its elution. Elution of analytes should be performed with solvent strong enough to allow elution in a relatively small volume. This may avoid or minimize a need for a concentration step (e.g., evaporation) prior to sample analysis. Solvent combination may sometimes be necessary for elution (e.g., methanol:water) in order to minimize the elution volume and/or coelution of undesirable substances. Ion exchange phases require additional considerations. For effective analyte retention, sample pH should be at least 2 pH units lower or 2 pH units greater than the pK_a of the corresponding cation or anion so approximately 99% of analyte remains ionized. In addition, low ionic and high solvent strength promote retention and elution, respectively. The SPE phase and the solvent system can be selected depending on specific goals: analyte elution (interference retention), interference elution (analyte retention with subsequent elution; most common), or analyte concentration. While evaporation may not be necessary when using small elution volumes, it may be advantageous in order to further increase assay sensitivity and improve chromatographic behavior (e.g., peak shapes) by dissolving the extracted sample in the mobile phase or a weaker solvent. Chromatographic artifacts can be encountered when injecting samples, especially larger sample volumes, in a solvent significantly different from the mobile phase.

More recently, miniaturized SPE formats (SPE disks and pipette tips) have been developed. These allow use of smaller sample and elution volumes, provide large flow area, and avoid channeling. SPE disks can easily be adapted to an online 96-well approach.

Comparison of plasma sample purification by LLE, automated LLE (96-well collection plate with robotic liquid handling system), and automated SPE (96-well collection plate with robotic liquid handling system) [18] found total time for automated SPE to be slightly less than that for automated LLE, and both were three times faster than manual LLE. Total time for the automated SPE could be reduced further by a factor of 2 if the evaporation step was omitted. Analyst time was lower by a factor of 25 for the two automated methods as compared to the manual LLE. Overall results in terms of accuracy and precision were comparable for the three methods.

Advantage of SPE over simpler methods like precipitation is shown in Fig. 5.2. More effective cleanup yielded a cleaner chromatogram, decreased ionization suppression by coeluting matrix components, and thereby improved signal to noise by more than tenfold.

Solid-phase microextraction (SPME) represents another recent variation on the SPE method [19]. This method of preparation does not use solvent and the separation takes place on a fused-silica fiber, which is coated with a suitable stationary phase. The fiber is inserted into the sample and allowed to extract analytes via absorption and/or adsorption. Analytes are then eluted either thermally or via mobile phase. This technique can be used in conjunction with GC, CE, or HPLC and is nicely suited for MS.

Derivatization   Derivatization may sometimes be required in order to improve volatility, stability, chromatographic behavior, sensitivity, and selectivity. Ideally, derivatization reactions should be rapid, simple, and mild and should yield a single

Protein Precipitation

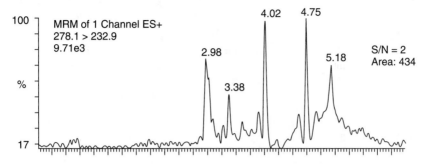

Oasis® MCX µElution Plate

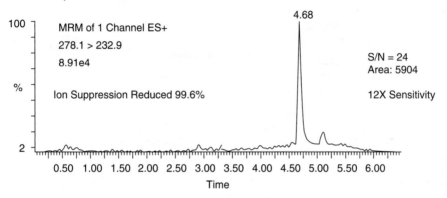

Amitriptyline 0.1 ng/mL in Human Plasma

FIGURE 5.2   Effect of sample cleanup on sensitivity in LC-MS. Upper chromatogram depicts sample after precipitation cleanup, while the lower tracing is for analogous sample following a SPE cleanup. (Used with permission from Waters Corp.)

product. Choice of derivatizing moiety depends on the need (e.g., stability, sensitivity, chirality), available derivatizable groups on the analyte (e.g., carboxyl, amine, hydroxyl, thiol), separation method (e.g., GC, HPLC), and detection method (e.g., electrochemical, ultraviolet, fluorescent). Tables 5.3 and 5.4 contain examples of commonly used derivatizing agents for GC and HPLC, respectively. In addition, derivatization can also improve ionization efficiency in atmospheric pressure ionization mass spectrometry (API-MS) and thereby improve sensitivity, which may be compromised by coextracted substances [20]. Derivatization can also help identify and characterize metabolites. For example, *N*-methyl-*N*-(*tert*-butyldimethylsilyl) derivatives tend to yield stable molecular (or quasimolecular) ions in mass spectrometry and thereby allow determination of molecular weight. Ions and fragments can be identified easier by using a mixture of deuterated and nondeuterated (or other stable labeled derivatizing agent) agents. A number of reviews have been published on various derivatizing techniques for the most common separation techniques including GC [21–24], HPLC [25–32], and capillary electrophoresis (CE) [26–28, 33, 34]. Other derivatization approaches have also been reported (e.g., combining sample preparation and derivatization) [35]. While derivatization offers pos-

TABLE 5.3 **Examples of Commonly Used GC Derivatizing Agents**

Functional Moiety	Derivatizing Agent	Enhanced Detector Response
Alcohols	Heptafluorobutyric anhydride	ECD
	Pentafluorobenzyl chloride	ECD
	Bis(trimethylsilyl)trifluoroacetamide (BSTFA)	
	N-Methyl-N-(t-butyldimethylsilyl)trifluoroacetamide (MTBSTFA)	
Amines (primary)	Chloroacetic anhydride	ECD
	Pentafluorobenzoyl chloride	ECD
	Pentafluorobenzaldehyde	ECD
	Bis(trimethylsilyl)trifluoroacetamide (BSTFA)	
	N-Methyl-N-(t-butyldimethylsilyl)trifluoroacetamide (MTBSTFA)	
Amines	Heptafluorobutyric anhydride	ECD
	Pentafluorobenzyl chloride	ECD
	Bis(trimethylsilyl)trifluoroacetamide (BSTFA)	
	N-Methyl-N-(t-butyldimethylsilyl)trifluoroacetamide (MTBSTFA)	
Amino acids	Acetic acid	
	Heptafluorobutyric anhydride	ECD
	Bis(trimethylsilyl)trifluoroacetamide (BSTFA)	
	N-Methyl-N-(t-butyldimethylsilyl)trifluoroacetamide (MTBSTFA)	
Carboxylic acids	Pentafluorobenzyl chloride	ECD
	Pentafluorobenzyl alcohol	ECD
	Diazomethane	
	Hydrochloric acid + methanol	
	Bis(trimethylsilyl)trifluoroacetamide (BSTFA)	
	N-Methyl-N-(t-butyldimethylsilyl)trifluoroacetamide (MTBSTFA)	
Phenols	Heptafluorobutylimidazole	ECD
	Pentafluorobenzyl chloride	ECD
	Bis(trimethylsilyl)trifluoroacetamide (BSTFA)	
	N-Methyl-N-(t-butyldimethylsilyl)trifluoroacetamide (MTBSTFA)	

sibilities for significant analytical improvements, appropriate caution needs to be exercised in order to avoid potential pitfalls, such as various artifacts with trimethylsilylation [36].

5.2.3 Analytical Techniques for Method Development

Nonseparation Methods

Absorption and Emission Spectroscopy

ULTRAVIOLET (UV)–VISIBLE (VIS) Spectrophotometry is a technique of detecting and measuring absorption of electromagnetic radiation by molecules with π or unshared electrons. The UV-VIS spectrum is divided into 200–380 nm (UV) and 380–800 nm (VIS) regions. The Beer–Lambert law is used for measurement of ana-

TABLE 5.4 Examples of Commonly Used HPLC Derivatizing Agents

Functional Moiety	Derivatizing Agent	Enhanced Detector Response
Alcohols	Benzoyl chloride	
	4-Dimethylamino-1-naphthoyl nitrile	FD
	3,5-Dinitrobenzyl chloride	
	p-Nitrobenzoyl chloride (4-NBCl)	
	p-Nitrophenyl chloroformate	
	p-Iodobenzensulfonyl chloride	
Amines (primary)	Benzoyl chloride	
	4-Chloro-7-nitrobenzo-2-oxa-1,3-diazole (NBD-Cl)	FD
	Dansyl chloride (DnS-Cl)	FD
	Flourescamine	FD
Amines	Benzoyl chloride	
	4-Chloro-7-nitrobenzo-2-oxa-1,3-diazole (NBD-Cl)	FD
	Dansyl chloride (DnS-Cl)	
	3,5-Dinitrobenzyl chloride	
	p-Nitrobenzoyl chloride (4-NBCl)	FD
	o-Phthaldialdehyde (OPT)	FD
Amino acids	Dansyl chloride (DnS-Cl)	FD
	Flourescamine	FD
	Pyridoxal	FD
	o-Phthaldialdehyde (OPT)	FD
Carboxylic acids	Benzyl bromide	
	p-Bromophenacyl bromide	
	4-bromomethyl-7-methoxycoumarin (Br-Mmc)	FD
	9,10-Diaminophenanthrene	FD
	Phenacyl bromide	
Ketones/aldehydes	p-Nitrobenzylhydroxylamine hydrochloride	
	2-Diphenylacetyl-1,3-indandione	FD
	2,4-Dinitrophenyl hydrazine	
Phenols	4-Chloro-7-nitrobenzo-2-oxa-1,3-diazole (NBD-Cl)	FD
	Dansyl chloride (DnS-Cl)	FD
	3,5-Dinitrobenzyl chloride	
Thiols	4-Chloro-7-nitrobenzo-2-oxa-1,3-diazole (NBD-Cl)	FD
	N-(9-Acridinyl)maleimide	FD

lytes. While UV-VIS detectors are commonly used for HPLC analysis, UV-VIS spectrophotometry without prior chromatographic separation is not well suited for complex biological samples. It is frequently used for analysis of API or other substances in the manufacturing process and in USP methods [37]. Further improvements in UV-VIS spectrophotometry are being made, for example, UV derivative spectrophotometry [38].

INFRARED (IR)   IR is a technique of detecting absorption of energy resulting from transitions between vibrational and rotational energy levels of molecules. It is in the

0.5–200 μm (20,000–50 cm^{-1}) region of the electromagnetic spectrum. IR is commonly used for characterization of API and in the manufacturing process [39, 40].

ATOMIC ABSORPTION SPECTROMETRY (AAS)   Primary applications of AAS in the pharmaceutical area involve quantification of metal ions, metal-containing organic compounds, and inorganic molecules (e.g., arsenic trioxide, different platinum analogues, silver, mercury, copper, palladium) [41–48] in drug formulations, tissues, and biological liquids. It is also used for trace element control in natural plant products and in synthesized drug substances [49–52]. AAS is also used for indirect measurements of organic substances based on formation of ion-paired complexes with the drugs [53–56].

AAS detects absorption or emission of light in thermally vaporized and extensively atomized molecules. Atomization is achieved via either flame aspiration or electrothermal atomization (graphite furnace). The former also allows emission analysis while the latter ashes components and diminishes matrix effects. Graphite-furnace atomic absorption spectrometry (GF AAS) is well suited for analysis of biological samples as it only requires very small sample size (20 μL) and provides increased sensitivity due to a longer residence time. More details on HGAAS (hydride generation atomic absorption spectrometry) can be found in Dědina and Tsalev [57]. All aspects of the theory, instrumentation, and practical usefulness of electrothermal atomization for analytical atomic spectrometry can be found in Jackson [58]. There are also some general guides on the theory and practice of AAS [59–62]. Recently, a fully validated GF AAS method has been described for the cancer chemotherapeutic oxaliplatin [48].

Ligand-Binding Assays   A ligand-binding assay (LBA) is a technique that uses specific antigen or antibody, capable of binding to the analyte, to identify and quantify substances. The antibody can be linked to a radioisotope (radioimmunoassay, RIA), to an enzyme that catalyzes an easily monitored reaction (enzyme-linked immunosorbent assay, ELISA), or to a highly fluorescent compound by which the location of an antigen can be visualized (immunofluorescence).

Because LBAs are indirect assays dependent on binding interactions, factors such as lipemic and hemolyzed samples, binding proteins, and anticoagulants that interfere with this process will destabilize the assay.

ELISA is a useful and powerful method in estimating ng/mL to pg/mL of test articles and metabolites in the solution, such as serum, urine, and culture supernatant. It is a relatively easy task to develop ELISA if "suitable" antibodies against materials of interest such as proteins, peptides, and drugs are readily available. ELISAs combine the specificity of antibodies with the sensitivity of simple enzyme assays by using antibodies or antigens coupled to an easily assayed enzyme. ELISAs can provide a useful measurement of antigen or antibody concentration. There are two main variations on this method: ELISA can be used to detect the presence of antigens that are recognized by an antibody or it can be used to test for antibodies that recognize an antigen. An ELISA is a five-step procedure: (1) coat the microtiter plate wells with antigen; (2) block all unbound sites to prevent false-positive results; (3) add antibody to the wells; (4) add IgG conjugated to an enzyme; and (5) react the substrate with the enzyme to produce a measurable colored product, thus indicating a positive reaction.

One of the most common types of ELISA is the "sandwich ELISA." The sandwich ELISA measures the amount of antigen between two layers of antibodies. The antigens to be measured must contain at least two antigenic sites, capable of binding to antibody, since at least two antibodies act in the sandwich. So sandwich assays are restricted to the quantitation of multivalent antigens such as proteins or polysaccharides. Sandwich ELISAs for quantitation of antigens are especially valuable when the concentration of antigens is low and/or they are contained in high concentrations of contaminating protein. When two "matched pair" antibodies are not available for the target, another option is the competitive ELISA. An advantage to the competitive ELISA is that nonpurified primary antibodies may be used. In order to utilize a competitive ELISA, one reagent must be conjugated to a detection enzyme, such as horseradish peroxidase. The enzyme may be linked to either the immunogen or the primary antibody. There are several different configurations for competitive ELISAs. The example below uses a labeled immunogen as the competitor. Briefly, an unlabeled purified primary antibody is coated onto the wells of a 96-well microtiter plate. This primary antibody is then incubated with unlabeled standards and unknowns. After this reaction is allowed to go to equilibrium, conjugated immunogen is added. This conjugate will bind to the primary antibody wherever its binding sites are not already occupied by unlabeled immunogen. Thus, the more immunogen in the sample or standard, the lower the amount of conjugated immunogen bound. The plate is then developed with substrate and color change is measured.

Ligand-binding assays, including immunoassays/antibody assays, are required to meet the established requirements for chemical assays. However, due to the nature of the ligand-binding assays, certain additional elements such as specificity must be more explicitly established and other elements such as accuracy and precision may meet a lesser standard, or be evaluated on a sample-to-sample basis. The principal elements of a method validation are discussed in ICH Q2A and Q2B and in the U.S. FDA guidance on bioanalytical method validation. The exceptions or additional elements as they apply to validation of ligand-binding assay are described [63]. The criteria for acceptance of method validation, prestudy validation, and in-study validation are described in great detail in this document. In contrast to other analytical methods, LBA are inherently nonlinear. Because four- and five-parameter logistic curves are used to create calibration curves, a large number of calibrators should be used to most accurately describe the curve. The LBA should additionally be validated for cross-reactivity to metabolites and comedications. This evaluation should be performed at high levels and in combination to thoroughly demonstrate selectivity or to determine specific cross-reactivity for each competing analyte.

Greater latitude in precision is allowed for these types of assays. The precision and accuracy should be evaluated during the method validation by analyzing 4 sets of QC samples at LLOQ, low, medium, and high levels in duplicate in 6 different batches. For assays not capable of meeting the nominal acceptance criteria, greater criteria can be set but the precision should be evaluated for each sample analyzed by preparing and analyzing multiple aliquots of each sample. For accuracy in each batch, 4 out of 6 QC samples must be within ±15% of nominal concentration but the two failed QC samples may not be at the same level (4-6-15 rule). When separation (or cleanup) is used for samples but not for calibrators, the recovery of this separation or cleanup step must be determined and used to correct reported sample concentrations. Possible approaches to assess recovery are the use of a radiolabeled tracer analyte or an internal standard not recognized by the antibody and measured using another technique. Assessment of analyte stability should be performed in whole matrix, not treated, stripped, or prepared matrix. Matrix effects are particularly troublesome in immunoassay methods. The effect of matrix and nonspecific binding must be evaluated and documented in a number of different ways during the method validation: (1) serial dilution of reference analyte with matrix and then the evaluation of response to known concentration; (2) the calibration curve in matrix versus buffer; (3) parallelism between diluted samples and reference analyte; and (4) non specific binding. For the in-study validation, acceptance criteria should follow the 4-6-30 rule (4 out of 6 samples should be within ±30% of nominal concentration).

More recently, recommendations for the development and implementation of bioanalytical method validation for macromolecules in support of pharmacokinetic and toxicokinetic assessments were published in detail [64]. Briefly, values of ±20% (25% at the lower limit of quantification (LLOQ)) are recommended as default acceptance criteria for accuracy (% relative error (RE), mean bias) and interbatch precision (% coefficient of variation (CV)). In addition, as the secondary criterion for method acceptance, it was proposed that the sum of the interbatch precision (%CV) and the absolute value of the mean bias (%RE) be less than or equal to 30%. This added criterion is recommended to help ensure that in-study runs of test samples will meet the proposed run acceptance criteria of 4-6-30. Exceptions to the proposed process and acceptance criteria are appropriate when accompanied by a sound scientific rationale.

Usually, if possible, the LBA should be cross-validated with a chemical method such as LC/MS [65–67]. LBAs are widely used for macromolecular measurements in blood, urine, and other biological liquids [68–72], monitoring of drug–protein interactions [73], and small molecular measurements in different biological fluids [65, 74–76].

Isotope Assays

RADIOISOTOPE ANALYSIS Isotopes of elements contain nuclei with the same number of protons, but different numbers of neutrons. In general, atoms where the number of protons does not equal the number of neutrons tend to be unstable. Some isotopes are stable and some are not. Both stable and unstable isotopes are used in analytical methods. An unstable isotope has an excess of neutrons in its nucleus. To eliminate the surplus, the nucleus decays to a different nucleus by emitting particles and energy. Radioactive nuclides are also known as radioisotopes.

Radioisotopes have proved to be an indispensable tool in biomedical research and have played a pivotal role in the investigation of absorption, distribution, metabolism, and excretion (ADME) properties of new chemical entities over the past several decades [77–79]. The main advantage of using radioisotopes in studying the disposition of new drug candidates is the ease of detection and the achievement of high sensitivity, especially when compounds with high specific activity are used. There are two main types of radiochemical analysis: (1) isotope dilution assay and (2) neutron activation analysis.

Isotope Dilution Assay (IDA)   The IDA is a method of quantitative analysis based on the measurement of the isotopic abundance of a nuclide after dilution by mixing with one or more of its isotopes [80]. The activity ratio or isotopic ratio of the mixture defines the concentration of the analyte, which is a tremendous advantage for measurement since quantitative separation of the analyte from nonradioactive components is not required.

Reverse dilution analysis involves addition of nonradioactive (cold) drug or metabolite to a sample containing low levels (per weight basis) of radiolabeled drug in order to isolate a radioactive substance. Subsequent purification (usually via crystallization and recrystallizations) to constant specific activity demonstrates the original presence of the compound added.

The principal limitation to IDA is the availability of a suitable spike substance or tracer [81]. The half-life and type of radiation emitted by a radiotracer are very important, as is the purity. The half-life must be long enough so that sufficient activity is available during the analysis for good counting statistics. However, too long half-lives can be a problem because of low specific activities and storage and disposal problems. The IDA can be used as the analytical technique to quantify the absolute abundances of the isotopes excreted in the experiment.

An injection of a radioisotopically labeled drug can be used to determine blood, plasma, or urine levels and their temporal profile by liquid scintillation or gamma counting and measurement of activities in serially derived samples. Liquid scintillation counters can be used to measure total sample radioactivity. In addition, radioactivity of individual components can be determined after chromatographic separation by using an online radiometric chromatographic detector or by collecting chromatographic fractions and using a liquid scintillation detector.

More recently, accelerator mass spectrometry (AMS) has also been introduced into the field of pharmacology and toxicology [82–84]. The sensitivity is due to the fact that this technique measures radioactive atoms directly instead of merely their decay, and thus AMS is approximately one million times more sensitive than liquid scintillation. The main advantage of this technique is its exquisite sensitivity in the attamole range. High sensitivity allows for microdosing studies and human Phase 0 studies.

Positron Isotopes   Among beta-emitters, at least 95% of all samples used in metabolism and toxicology studies are labeled with either tritium (^3H) or carbon-14 (^{14}C). Perhaps 1–3% of samples contain phosphorus-32 (^{32}P) and less than 1% include all other beta-emitters combined. Of these samples, probably 99% contain one isotope by itself with 1% or less being a mixture of two isotopes, almost always $^3H + {}^{14}C$. Other commonly used positron isotopes are ^{11}C, ^{13}N, ^{15}O, and ^{18}F.

When beta-emitters such as ^3H and ^{14}C decay, they release into their surroundings an electron (beta particle), which may have different kinetic energy.

Carbon-14 is a weak β-ray emitter (155 keV). A maximum specific activity of 62.4 mCi per milliatom of carbon or 4460 mCi/g is more than sufficient for most PK studies, where typical doses of carbon-14-labeled drugs are approximately 10–20 μCi. Long physical half-life (5.7×10^3 yr) is an advantage that allows calculating specific activity without having to consider losses due to spontaneous decay. Biological half-life for a bound compound is 12 days and 40 days for an unbound isotope. Many carbon-14-labeled drugs can be prepared in the analyst's laboratory.

Tritium (^{3}H) is a weak β-ray emitter (i.e., maximum = 18.6 keV) with significantly lower energy than ^{14}C. Tritium-labeled drugs of higher specific activity than those labeled with carbon-14 must be used to achieve equivalent sensitivities in detection. Tritium (^{3}H) has a long physical half-life of 12.3 yr and usually a biological half-life of 10–12 days, which depends on the nature of the labeled molecule.

Sulfur-35 is an artificially produced β-emitting isotope. The β particles' energy of ^{35}S exceeds that of ^{14}C. This has prompted the use of ^{35}S-labeled drugs in pharmaceutical analysis. The short physical half-life (87.9 days) and low number of drugs containing sulfur limits the overall utility of ^{35}S in the analysis of drugs and metabolites in biologic fluids.

Phosphorus-32 is another artificially produced β-emitting isotope. The β particles' energy of ^{32}P exceeds that of ^{14}C. Because of a short physical half-life (14.3 days), it requires calculation of loss of radioactivity due to spontaneous decay. Phosphorus occurs in an extremely small number of drugs and therefore is of low importance in biopharmaceutical analysis.

Gamma Isotopes   The most commonly used gamma isotopes are ^{125}I, and ^{99m}Tc. Other commonly used gamma isotopes are ^{111}In, ^{123}I, and ^{153}Sm.

Gamma-emitters, upon their decay, give off discrete packets of energy (gamma rays) in the form of photons rather than particles. Gamma emission is monoenergetic as contrasted to the broad energy distribution of beta-emitters. Thus, for a radioisotope such as iodine-125 (^{125}I), all of the gamma emissions have the identical energy of 35 keV. Iodine-125 has been most useful in the development of radiolabeled antibodies for certain radioimmunoassays. It is also used in labeling proteins and hormones. Since a small number of therapeutic agents have iodine atoms as a part of their molecular structure, ^{125}I labeling is of little direct benefit in preparing radiolabeled small molecule drugs.

Technetium-99m is used primarily in imaging analysis. A short biological half-life (6 hours) and sufficient physical half-life (1 day) make it ideal for gamma imaging resolution.

Positron emitters are more appropriate for the direct labeling of drug molecules since the gamma-emitting radionuclides are rarely an integral part of the drug molecule structure. The positron (β-emitting) radionuclides are used for *in vitro* and *in vivo* experiments. The gamma-emitting radionuclides are useful for *in vivo* imaging.

The following are the most frequently used radiolabeling techniques: isotope exchange reactions, introduction of a foreign label, labeling with bifunctional chelating agents, biosynthesis, recoil labeling, and excitation labeling. Details and recommendations for radiolabeling can be found in Saha [85].

High chemical and radioactive purity of the labeled drugs is very important for successful ADME and PK studies. The loss of efficacy of a labeled compound over a period of time may result from radiolysis and depends on the physical half-life of the radionuclide, the solvent, any additive, the labeled molecule, the nature of emitted radiations, and the nature of the chemical bond between the radionuclide and the molecule. Radiolysis is decomposition by radiation of labeled compounds emitted by the radionuclides present in them. Radiolysis introduces a number of radiochemical impurities in the sample of labeled material and one should be cautious about these unwanted products. Autoradiolysis occurs when the chemical bond breaks down by radiation from its own molecule. Indirect radiolysis is caused by the decomposition of the solvent by the radiation, producing free radicals that can break down the chemical bond of the labeled compounds. To help prevent indirect radiolysis, the pH of the solvent should be neutral because more reactions of this nature can occur at alkaline or acidic pH. Higher specific activity results in greater effect of radiolysis. The longer the half-life of the radionuclide, the more extensive the radiolysis will be. Usually a period of three physical half-lives or a maximum of 6 months is suggested for shelf life.

Detection   Different detection means are employed for beta and gamma measurement but after the initial detection both employ essentially the same electronics to count the number of events detected as well as the same software to process the recorded results.

For beta detection, because the beta particles that are most often used have such low penetrating power, in the process known as "liquid scintillation counting," a discrete sample or a column eluate is usually mixed with special energy transfer solvents and chemicals ("scintillators"), which produce light when a radioactive decay takes place. Alternatively, a column eluate, but never a discrete sample, is allowed to flow over particulate solid ("solid scintillator") matter, which emits light when a radioactive decay occurs on the surface or in close proximity to it.

Because gamma radiation is pure energy and has no mass, it is much more penetrating than beta-particle emission of the same energy. Therefore, the preferred detector for gamma-rays is a cylindrical block of specially activated sodium iodide, one face of which is optically coupled to a photomultiplier with the sides and other face, and the photomultiplier as well, enclosed in a thin aluminum shell. Gamma radiation penetrates the shell, is stopped by the very dense sodium iodide producing light, which is then measured by the photomultiplier. Light production by this means is approximately five times that of a comparable energy beta-particle with liquid scintillator.

Whole-body autoradiography (WBA) is a routine and traditional method of detection on X-ray film. It is successfully used for tissue distribution studies [86, 87]. Whole-body radioluminography is a new method of radiation detection based on a phosphorus imaging technique, offering particular benefits of being much more sensitive and having much wider linear measurement range than traditional X-ray film techniques. This method is successfully and extensively used for tissue distribution studies [78, 88] and is especially attractive in combination with different chromatographic methods on extracts of tissues for studying the metabolic fate of the radiolabel [86].

Neutron Activation Analysis (NAA)   NAA is one of the most sensitive techniques used for qualitative and quantitative elemental analysis of multiple major, minor, and trace elements in various samples [89, 90]. For many elements, NAA offers sensitivities that are superior to those possible by any other technique. Moreover, the accuracy and precision of the technique are such that NAA is still one of the primary analytical methods used by the National Institute of Standards and Technology (NIST) to certify the concentration of elements in Standard Reference Materials (SRMs) [91]. In typical NAA, stable nuclides (^AZ, the target nucleus) in the sample undergo neutron capture reactions in a flux of (incident) neutrons. The radioactive nuclides (^{A+1}Z, the compound nucleus) produced in this activation process will, in most cases, decay through the emission of a beta particle (β–) and gamma-ray(s) with a unique half-life. A high-resolution gamma-ray spectrometer is used to detect these "delayed" gamma-rays from the artificially induced radioactivity in the sample for both qualitative and quantitative analysis. One of the principal advantages of NAA is that biological samples in the liquid or solid state can be irradiated and little or no cleanup is necessary. Samples are typically collected, irradiated, and analyzed directly in plastic holders. Care must be taken to avoid contact with metal equipment or other contaminants containing trace levels of metals. NAA is nearly free of any matrix interference effects as the vast majority of samples are completely transparent to both the probe (the neutron) and the analytical signal (the gamma-ray). Moreover, because NAA can most often be applied instrumentally (no need for sample digestion or dissolution), there is little if any opportunity for reagent or laboratory contamination. However, interferences can occur when different elements in the sample produce gamma-rays of nearly the same energy. Usually this problem can be circumvented by choosing alternate gamma-rays for these elements or by waiting for the shorter-lived nuclide to decay prior to counting. Other interferences can occur if another type of nuclear reaction concurrently produces the radionuclide of interest. The accuracy of NAA is generally high, although precision values in the range of ± 5–10% (RSDs) have been quoted for this technique.

The instrumentation used to measure gamma-rays from radioactive samples generally consists of a semiconductor detector, associated electronics, and a computer-based, multichannel analyzer (MCA/computer). Most NAA labs operate one or more hyperpure or intrinsic germanium (HPGe) detectors.

Over the last several years there has been a growing interest in the use of *in situ* radiotracers to test new pharmaceuticals and dosage forms being developed for commercial distribution [92–94]. These methodologies offer significant advantages in the evaluation of encapsulations, time release, clearance, and the distribution of the pharmaceutical in animal and human models [95]. Recent work [96] evaluated the sensitivity, accuracy, and precision of NAA to measure serum iohexol (contrast agent) at concentrations necessary for estimating GFR. NAA is also used for elemental analysis of some herbal plants [97].

Readers are referred to *Fundamentals of Nuclear Pharmacy* by G. B. Saha [85] for details on theory and practice of radioisotope methods. This is a comprehensive book describing radiopharmaceuticals currently in use, covering radioactivity, radiation detectors, production of radionuclides, generators, radiopharmaceuticals, and practical recommendations on radiolabeling.

Properties of some radioactive isotopes useful in biology are presented in Table 5.5.

Safety Radioactivity users must follow the institutional Radiation Safety Office instructions, complete special training, and work in a licensed laboratory. The Radiation Safety Office conducts periodical inspections in the user's lab. As with all laboratories, no eating or drinking is allowed in labs used for radioactive work.

When radiation passes through matter, it forms ions by knocking electrons loose from their atoms. This separation of electrons from their atoms is called ionization. Ionization makes X-rays and gamma-rays different from other electromagnetic

TABLE 5.5   Properties of Some Radioactive Isotopes Useful in Biology

Element	Half-life	Beta Energy[a]	Gamma Energy[a]
Barium (^{137}Ba)	2.6 min	None	0.662
Calcium (^{45}Ca)	165 days	0.258	0.0125
Carbon (^{14}C)	5730 years	0.156	None
Cesium (^{137}Cs)	30 years	0.511, 1.176	0.661
Chlorine (^{36}Cl)	3.1×10^5 years	0.714	None
Cobalt (^{60}Co)	5.26 years	0.315, 0.663, 1.49	1.17, 1.33, 2.16
Hydrogen (^{3}H)	12.26 years	0.01861	None
Iodine (^{131}I)	8.07 days	Several (600 keV)	Several (364 keV)
Iodine (^{125}I)	60 days	None	35 keV
Iron (^{59}Fe)	45 days	1.573, 0.475, 0.273	Several (1292 keV)
Lead (^{210}Pb)	21 years	0.015	0.0465
Phosphorus (^{32}P)	14.3 days	1.710	None
Phosphorus (^{33}P)	25 days	0.249	None
Potassium (^{42}K)	12.4 hours	3.52, 1.97	Several
Sulfur (^{35}S)	88 days	0.167 (similar to ^{14}C)	None
Zinc (^{65}Zn)	243.6 days	Positron = 0.325	0.34, 0.77, 1.12

[a]Maximum energies in million (mega) electron volts. Where the term "several" is listed, individual values can be obtained from the *Handbook of Chemistry and Physics* [188]. Specific activity is the rate of disintegration per unit quantity of the isotope and is frequently expressed as Ci/mole, mCi/mmole, or dpm/mole

radiation such as light rays or radio waves. Ionization changes the nature of biological molecules. As the amount of energy released (as the radioisotope naturally decays) increases, ionization effects increase, as well as the amount of required protection. For instance, ^{3}H is a very low-energy radioisotope (18 keV) and paper can be used as a shield. ^{32}P is a relatively low-energy radioisotope (1.71 MeV) and requires Plexiglas shields. ^{125}I also is a low-energy isotope (35 keV), but because it also emits gamma-rays, lead shields are required for protection.

Radiation can cause somatic and genetic effects in biological organisms. All radioisotopes are hazardous when they get inside the body. Gamma- or high-energy beta-emitters are external hazards.

STABLE ISOTOPE ANALYSIS   Stable isotopes are nonradioactive chemical tracers. Stable isotope ratios are measured by mass spectrometric analyses of either bulk phases or specific compounds. Jasper [98, 99] discussed ten major points regarding the properties and uses of stable isotopes in pharmaceuticals, including the suggestion of "isotope product authenticity" of APIs and drug products.

Stable isotopes are also very useful in pharmacokinetic studies. Stable labeled and nonlabeled drug can be simultaneously administered by different routes in order to determine absolute bioavailability. Stable labeled drug can also be administered while the subject is at steady state to determine the steady-state pharmacokinetic profile without requiring drug withdrawal [100]. Stable isotope tagging methods are also being used in proteomic research [101].

The isotope dilution assay using a stable isotope is suitable for pharmacokinetic and pharmacodynamic studies of proteins and polypeptides. This method involves the use of target protein analogues labeled with stable isotopes (such as deuterium or ^{15}N). These nonradioactive analogues have different molecular masses and act as internal standards. In a typical experiment, a known amount of the analogue is added to the biological sample to be analyzed prior to any sample handling. After appropriate extraction and purification processes, the final mass spectrometric analysis allows the direct identification of the target compound and its analogue by virtue of their respective molecular masses. In addition, it enables a precise quantification on the basis of the relative intensities of the observed signals (principle of isotope dilution).

The IDA completely avoids the use of radioactive material and is not susceptible to errors arising from immunological cross-reactivity with closely related compounds (e.g., precursors, analogues, maturation or degradation fragments). The measured molecular masses further allow the unambiguous identification of the target compound at a sub-pM level with a clear distinction between its endogenous and injected forms, thus allowing for simultaneous *in vivo* quantitative investigations of both native endogenous and injected compounds [102, 103].

Separation Methods   Relative comparison of different aspects of most commonly employed separation techniques is presented in Table 5.6 and characteristics of each will be discussed next.

Chromatography   Chromatography is an analytical technique used to separate components of a mixture based on their partitioning between a flowing mobile (gaseous or liquid) phase and a stationary phase. *LC/GC* journal (http://www.lcgcmag.com/lcgc/) is a good practical source of articles about chromatographic issues and applications and periodically distributes a very helpful wallchart guide to LC (or GC) troubleshooting.

Quantification of chromatographically separated peaks is accomplished by measurements of peak areas or peak heights. For well behaved peaks, areas tend to be more precise than heights, but heights tend to be less dependent on flow rate than areas. Band broadening by neighboring peaks and noisy baselines may also affect accuracy of area measurements. Column degradation and method of integration (peak deconvolution algorithm used to identify start and stop integration markers and connection between them) may also affect accuracy.

Internal standard or external standard methods can be used for calibration and quantification. In the internal standard method, a known amount of one or more compounds with similar physicochemical properties to the analyte(s) is added

TABLE 5.6   Relative Comparison of Most Commonly Used Separation Methods

Factor	TLC	GC	HPLC	CE
Resolution	+	++++	+++	++++
Clean sample requirement	+	++++	++	++
Potential sensitivity	+	++++	++++	+++
Need for derivatization	+	++++	+	+
Different separation mode options	+	+++	++++	++++
Available sensitive/selective detectors	+	++++	++++	++++
Automation	+	++++	++++	+++
System cost	+	++++	++++	+++

(spiked) along with known amounts of analyte(s) to calibration samples prior to sample processing. Calibration is based on peak height or area response ratio of analyte to the internal standard. When using mass spectrometric detection, stable labeled (nonradioactive) compounds make ideal standards due to their physico-chemical similarity to the analytes. External standard calibration is based on samples only spiked with known amounts of analytes and therefore this approach requires reproducible recovery, dilutions, injections, and constant instrument behavior.

Carry-over is not an uncommon problem in automated chromatographic methods [104]. It can have a significant negative impact on all aspects of method development and validation. Causes for carry-over vary, for example, hardware problems (presence of dead volume in chromatographic plumbing), the nature of the solvent, or analyte solubility. The latter can often be eliminated by appropriate modification of the solvent, its pH, the ionic strength, or the addition of an organic modifier. In some cases, a wash step may be required to minimize any carry-over. While neither ICH nor FDA guidelines specifically address carry-over, chromatographers consider less than 20% of the lowest level of quantitation (LLOQ) as the general acceptance criterion.

Another potential problem during analytical procedures concerns analyte stability, including analyte interconversion [105, 106]. For example, retinoids may undergo stereoisomerization and some statins may undergo interconversion between lactone and open hydroxy carboxylic acid forms. In order to avoid analytical artifacts, appropriate analytical measures and QC samples need to be employed [105, 106].

THIN LAYER CHROMATOGRAPHY (TLC)   TLC is a simple, quick, and inexpensive procedure that gives a rapid answer as to how many components are in a mixture. TLC is also used to support the identity of a compound in a mixture when the R_f (R_f = distance of migration of the sample zone/distance of the mobile phase front) of a compound is compared with the R_f of a known compound (preferably both run on the same TLC plate). Pharmaceutical applications of TLC include analysis of starting raw materials, intermediates, pharmaceutical raw materials, formulated products, and drugs and their metabolites in biological media [107, 108].

In conventional TLC, the stationary phase is a powdered adsorbent that is fixed to an aluminum, glass, or plastic plate. The mixture to be analyzed is loaded near the bottom of the plate. The plate is placed in a reservoir of solvent so that only the bottom of the plate is submerged. This solvent is the mobile phase; it moves up the plate by capillary action, causing the components of the mixture to distribute between the adsorbent on the plate and the moving solvent, thus separating the components of the mixture so that the components are separated into separate "spots" appearing from the bottom to the top of the plate. The stationary phase (the adsorbent: silica gel or alumina) is polar, and the polarities of both the component of the mixture and the solvent used as the mobile phase are the determining factors in how fast the compound travels.

When the solvent has reached the top of the plate, the plate is removed from the developing chamber and dried, and the separated components of the mixture are visualized. Automation of locating spots is possible with commercially available spotters and plate readers.

Zone identification is confirmed by offline or online coupling of TLC with visible/ultraviolet (UV), Fourier transform infrared (FTIR), Raman, and mass spectrometry (MS). The most common method for detection is the use of a densitometer, which measures diffusely reflected light from the sample spot in the UV-VIS range. Video-densitometric quantitation is also used [109]. Instrumental development methods, such as overpressure layer chromatography (OPLC) or automated multiple development (AMD), can provide separations with increased resolution.

Additional information about the sample is gained by using two-dimensional TLC with two different mobile phases. After the first separation and evaporation of the mobile phase, the plate is turned by 90 degrees and a second TLC run is performed using a different type of mobile phase. A further development is the use of high performance thin layer chromatography (HPTLC). Reduction of layer thickness (down to 100 μm) and particle size (down to 5 μm) of the stationary phase leads to an improved separation within a shorter time. An HPTLC procedure takes approximately 10 min (conventional TLC up to 15–20 min). A major disadvantage is the smaller sample capacity. The very small layer thickness of approximately 10 μm and the absence of any kind of binder in combination with the framework of this stationary phase lead to new and improved properties of this ultrathin layer chromatographic (UTLC) silica-gel plate [110].

TLC elution patterns usually extrapolate to column chromatography elution patterns. Since TLC is a much faster procedure than column chromatography, TLC is used to determine the best solvent system for column chromatography. As you increase the polarity of the solvent system, all mixture components move faster (and vice versa with lowering the polarity). The ideal solvent system is simply the system that separates the components. For instance, in determining the solvent system for a flash chromatography procedure, the ideal system is the one that moves the desired component of the mixture to a TLC R_f of 0.25–0.35 and that will separate this component from its nearest neighbor by the difference in TLC R_f values of at least 0.20. Therefore, a mixture is analyzed by TLC to determine the ideal solvent(s) for a flash chromatography procedure.

Comparative studies have often found that HPTLC is comparative in accuracy and precision but superior to HPLC in terms of total cost and time required for pharmaceutical analyses [107, 108]. Recently, several HPTLC methods were developed and completely validated for different classes of pharmaceuticals in herbal extracts [108, 111, 112], bulk drugs and dosage forms [113–117], and plasma [118, 119].

Some advantages of the offline arrangement (HPTLC) as compared to an online process, such as column high performance liquid chromatography (HPLC), have been outlined [107, 117] and include the following:

1. There is the availability of a great range of stationary phases with unique selectivities for mixture components.
2. Ability to choose solvents for the mobile phase is not restricted by low UV transparency or the need for ultrahigh purity.
3. Repetition of densitometric evaluation can be achieved under different conditions without repeating the chromatography in order to optimize quantification since all sample fractions are stored on the plate.
4. High sample throughput can be achieved since many samples can be chromatographed simultaneously.

5. The cost of solvent purchase and disposal is minimal since the required amount of mobile phase per sample is small.

6. Accuracy and precision of quantification is high because samples and standards are chromatographed and measured under the same conditions on a single TLC plate.

7. Sensitivity limits of analysis are typically at nanogram (ng) to picogram (pg) levels.

Despite these advantages, HPLC is the preferred method of the majority of analytical laboratories for routine drug measurements because of its higher resolution, better automation, and superior quantitative detection. More detailed information on the principles, theory, practice, instrumentation, and applications of TLC and HPTLC can be found in the literature [107, 120]. A lot of practical tips are described by Elke Hahn-Deinstrop [121].

GAS CHROMATOGRAPHY (GC)   Gas chromatography separates volatile mixture components by partitioning between the inert gas mobile phase and the liquid stationary phase on a solid support. Older glass or steel packed columns (2–$6\,m \times 2$–$4\,mm$ i.d.) have for the most part been superseded by thin fused-silica capillary columns (10–$30\,m \times 0.05$–$0.53\,mm$ i.d.). Capillary columns provide much greater separation efficiency (resolution) but are susceptible to sample overloading (as evidenced by long tailing peaks). Wide-bore capillary columns ($0.53\,mm$ i.d.) can be used to minimize overloading problems. Suitable choice of capillary injector (split, splitless, on-column) depends on the nature of the mixture to be analyzed (sample cleanliness, analyte concentration, analyte stability, etc.). Split injection is the most common. Only about 1% or less of the sample goes on the column. The splitless injection technique allows application of the entire sample onto a column and is useful for relatively clean samples containing very small amounts of analytes. On-column injection is made directly onto the column at a low temperature and also allows the sample to condense in a narrow band. It is useful for thermally labile analytes that may decompose in the injection port.

Resolution and run times can be optimized by appropriate column temperature programming. Some commonly observed GC problems include tailing, fronting and ghost peaks, and column bleed. Tailing peaks are usually indicative of undesirable secondary interaction of analyte(s) with the system, for example, active or contaminated surfaces (injector inlet liner, septum, transfer lines), poor column cut, or cold spots. Active or contaminated surfaces need to be pacified and/or cleaned. Column overload usually causes fronting peaks (gradual rise and abrupt peak fall). It can be avoided by decreasing the analyte amount and/or increasing the thickness of the stationary phase, internal diameter of the column, or the column temperature. Ghost peaks commonly arise from a contaminated system, most commonly the injector, and may be resolved by appropriate cleaning. Column bleed is always present to some degree but is increased by excessive column temperature, system (mainly injector and column) contamination, or system leaks allowing column exposure to oxygen. Column conditioning or correction of those problems may be needed.

TABLE 5.7   Relative Comparison of Most Commonly Used GC Detectors

Factor	FID	NPD	ECD	MS
Sensitivity	100 pg	10 pg	100 fg	10 pg
Selectivity	+	++	+++	++++
Dynamic range	++++	++	+	+++
Compound sensitivity	General	Nitrogen, phosphorus	Halogens, nitrates	General
Structural information	+	+	+	++++

GC techniques generally offer better resolution and sensitivity than other chromatographic techniques, including HPLC. However, requirements for volatile and thermally stable analytes introduce a limitation for GC analysis of some compounds. This drawback can be overcome with prior derivatization to impart volatility and/or stability.

Detection   The most common detection methods are flame ionization, nitrogen phosphorus, electron capture, and mass spectrometry. Comparison of commonly used GC detectors is presented in Table 5.7.

1. *Flame Ionization Detector (FID).* FID detects most organic compounds by ionizing the column eluate in a hydrogen-air flame. It is the most commonly used GC detector and exhibits good sensitivity and wide dynamic range.

2. *Nitrogen Phosphorus Detector (NPD).* NPD, also known as a thermionic detector, responds almost exclusively and in a very sensitive manner to compounds containing nitrogen or phosphorus. It differs from FID by having a rubidium or cesium silicate bead, which when heated emits electrons. Nitrogen or phosphorus compounds affect the resultant thermionic emission, generating a signal. The bead is consumable and requires periodic replacement.

3. *Electron Capture Detector (ECD).* ECD utilizes a nickel-63 beta (electron) emitting source, which ionizes a carrier gas. Electronegative compounds (e.g., halogens, nitrates) interact with the generated ions, leading to detection of these compounds. ECD is extremely sensitive to electronegative compounds but has a somewhat limited dynamic range. It requires a general radioactive license and periodic wipe testing.

4. *Mass Spectrometer (MS).* MS will be discussed in the HPLC section below.

HIGH PERFORMANCE LIQUID CHROMATOGRAPHY (HPLC)   HPLC separates the dissolved components of a mixture by their equilibration between the liquid mobile phase and a stationary phase. Separation may occur via adsorption, partitioning, ion exchange, or size exclusion. The principles described earlier for SPE sorbent phases are generally applicable to HPLC column packings. Table 5.8 describes the physical properties of commonly employed HPLC solvents. Commonly used mobile phases are described in Table 5.9.

Reversed-phase (partition) and normal-phase (adsorption) separations are most commonly employed in HPLC analyses. Silica gel and alumina adsorption chromatography has been mostly superseded by the emergence of bonded (derivatized) silicas. Bonded phases contain a constant amount of liquid phase coated on an inert solid support. This technological improvement was instrumental in resolving prior reproducibility problems. Present normal-phase technology utilizes cyano, amine, or diol moieties bonded to the stationary phase via siloxane bridges. Normal-phase

TABLE 5.8   Physical Properties of Solvents Commonly Used in HPLC

Solvent	BP (°C)	Viscosity (mPa·s) (20°C)	Polarity Index (P')	Density (g/mL)	UV Cutoff (nm)
Acetic acid	118	1.31	6.2	1.049	255
Acetonitrile	82	0.34	5.8	0.78	190
Chloroform	61	0.57	4.1	1.49	245
Ethyl acetate	77	0.46	4.3	0.90	255
n-Hexane	69	0.31	0.06	0.66	192
Methanol	65	0.55	5.1	0.79	206
Methyl-*t*-butyl ether	55	0.28	2.5	0.76	210
Methylene chloride	40	0.41	3.4	1.33	233
Potassium phosphate					215
1-Propanol	97	2.26	4.0	0.80	210
2-Propanol	82	2.86	4.3	0.79	205
Tetrahydrofuran	66	0.55	4.2	0.88	212
Triethylamine		0.38			
Trifluoroacetic acid	72			1.54	210
Water	100	1.00	10.2	1.00	180

TABLE 5.9   Commonly Used HPLC Mobile Phases

Compound	Reversed Phase	Normal Phase	Ion Exchange	Size Exclusion
Primary solvents (adjust mobile phase strength)	Methanol Acetonitrile Tetrahydrofuran (Propanol)	Methylene chloride Acetonitrile Methanol Methyl-*t*-butyl ether Ethyl acetate	Water	Water
Secondary solvents (diluents)	Water	Hexane	Buffers: Phosphates Acetate Citrate Trifluoroacetate	Buffer
Modifiers	Buffers: Phosphate Acetate Triethylamine EDTA (Ion pairing: Octyl sulfonate, Tertiary butyl ammonium) TFA			

HPLC employs a nonpolar mobile phase and a polar stationary phase. The mobile phase consists of organic solvents and more lipophilic compounds elute first. Some of the drawbacks of normal-phase HPLC include irreversible adsorption, poor reproducibility (sensitive to water content; deactivation), slow equilibration, and peak tailing.

Reversed-phase column packings employ different length alkyl chains (e.g., C_1, C_2, C_4, C_8, C_{18}, C_{30}), phenyl, or cyano moieties bonded to the stationary phase via siloxane bridges. Reversed-phase HPLC employs a polar mobile phase and a nonpolar stationary phase. Elution order, at least in a first approximation, follows hydrophobicity, where polar compounds elute first. The main mode of separation is via partitioning, but there is also the possibility of secondary interactions due to residual silanol groups. These weakly acidic residual silanols can interact with analytes via ion-exchange, hydrogen bonding, or dipole–dipole mechanisms and can cause peak tailing and long retention times. Using end-capped columns (smaller groups bonded to residual silanols) or a basic modifier like triethylamine can minimize unwanted secondary interactions. Modifiers can also be used to minimize undesirable interactions with stationary phase or control analyte ionization. Ion pairing can be used to neutralize ionic or partially ionized species. Alkyl (methane, heptane) sulfonic acids or tetra alkyl (methyl, butyl) ammonium salts are commonly used as ion-pairing reagents (5–10 mM) for bases and acids, respectively. Tetra alkyl ammonium salts can also be used to block residual silanols. Addition of EDTA to the mobile phase can eliminate problems due to minor metal cation impurities.

Advantages of reversed-phase over normal-phase HPLC include the option to use optically transparent solvents (e.g., methanol, acetonitrile), greater compatibility with biological samples and electrochemical detection, relatively rapid equilibration, possibility of gradient elution, and control of secondary equilibria (equilibrium of solute in the mobile phase or stationary phase, i.e., ionization, ion pairing). The most commonly used solvents in reversed-phase HPLC are methanol and acetonitrile. Acetonitrile offers certain advantages over methanol, for example, lower UV cutoff, lower viscosity and thus lower backpressures, lesser tendency for out-gassing (bubble formation), and higher elution strength. On the other hand, buffer salts and ion-pairing agents are more soluble in methanol. The most commonly used buffers are phosphate and acetate. Phosphate buffers have a larger pH buffering range and greater transparency in UV, but lower solubility in organic solvents and lesser volatility. Gradient elution (stepwise or continuous) in reversed-phase HPLC offers a possibility of improved resolution and sensitivity, reduced run time, and better peak shapes. However, gradient chromatography can lead to baseline drifts. Reversed-phase HPLC is a workhorse for biomedical applications.

Ion-exchange chromatography is based on a reversible exchange of ions between stationary and mobile phases. Column packing uses polystyrene resins cross-linked with divinylbenzene, sulfonated to form strong cation exchanger (SCX), or quarternized amine to form strong anion exchanger (SAX). Similar principles apply to ion-exchange HPLC as already discussed for the SPE sorbent phases and will not be further discussed here.

Size exclusion (gel filtration) chromatography uses an aqueous mobile phase for separation of large organic molecules (proteins, polyptides) based on analyte molecular weight. Retention is mostly determined by size of the pores in the stationary phase. Larger molecules elute first because they tend to be excluded from the pores. Columns are selected such that pore size is consistent with the molecular weight composition of the sample.

Some of the more common HPLC problems include high, low, or cycling pressure; leaks; retention time shifting; and peak shape problems. High pressure is commonly caused by blockage in the system (e.g., inline filter or a frit on the guard column or analytical column). This may be due to coextracted material or buffer salt precipitation. Cleaning or replacement of a filter or frits may resolve these problems. Low pressure may be caused by bubbles in the pump or a leak. Bubbles may be due to improperly degassed mobile phases or leaky check valves, which may need to be cleaned or replaced. Cycling pressure is usually caused by bubbles in a pump head or dirty check valves and may be resolved by degassing the mobile phase and purging the pump or cleaning or replacing a check valve. Retention problems may also be due to leaks, bubbles, and check valve problems. Changes in chemistry (e.g., mobile phase composition or flow) would also cause similar symptoms. Unidirectional, time-related changes in retention times are most likely due to column aging and may require column cleaning with stronger solvents or its replacement. Column aging may also cause peak shape problems and may also require column cleaning or replacement. Peak shape problems may also be due to the mobile phase (e.g., improperly prepared), lack of modifier to minimize undesirable secondary column interactions, or use of a strong injection solvent. Leaks may be due to improperly cut or tightened fittings, excessive system pressure, or worn pump or injector rotor seals.

There are several considerations to be made in selecting a suitable HPLC system, including solubility of analytes, nature of the sample matrix, nature of the functional groups on the analyte(s), required sensitivity and selectivity, and nature of the inherent detectability or ability to impart selective detectability. A good reference book on HPLC method development is by Snyder et al. [122].

Detection   The most common HPLC detection methods are ultraviolet/visible, fluorescent, mass spectrometric, and infrared. Comparison of the most commonly used HPLC detectors is presented in Table 5.10. Desirable detector characteristics include high sensitivity, low drift, low noise, low dead volume, fast response, wide dynamic range, reliability, simplicity, and relative insensitivity to operational conditions (temperature, mobile phase composition, flow rate, etc.).

Sensitivity and specificity may be enhanced by appropriate derivatization. Post column derivatization allows separation to be independent of the derivatizing

TABLE 5.10   Relative Comparison of Most Commonly Used HPLC Detectors

Factor	UV/VIS	FD	EC	RID	MS
Sensitivity	1 ng	1 pg	5 pg	100 ng	5 pg
Selectivity	++	+++	+++	+	++++
Dynamic range	+++	++	+	+	++++
Compound sensitivity	General	Aromatics with conjugated pi electrons	Phenols, catechols, nitrosamines	General	General
Structural information	+++	++	++	+	++++
Environmental sensitivity	+	+++	++++	++++	++

moiety, which could minimize separation and also avoid on-column stability issues (e.g., *o*-phthalaldehyde).

1. *Ultraviolet/Visible (UV/VIS) and Photodiode-Array (PDA) Detector.* UV/VIS detectors are analyte property (as opposed to bulk property) detectors. They can be based on single (filter), variable (monochromator), or multiple wavelengths (multiple diodes). A fixed wavelength detector (discrete source, mostly 254 nm) is generally more sensitive than a variable one.

A variable wavelength detector (continuum source with monochromator), on the other hand, allows selection of a wavelength of maximum sensitivity and/or specificity.

A PDA (rapid scanning) provides the most information as it allows quantification at wavelength(s) of maximum sensitivity and/or selectivity, spectral resolution of chromatographically overlapping components, and collection of absorption spectra for peak identification. It collects the entire UV spectrum (all wavelengths simultaneously) several times during the elution of a chromatographic peak and provides three-dimensional data information: time, wavelength, and absorbance unit response. The PDA is commonly used for peak purity determination (Fig. 5.3).

2. *Fluorescence Detector (FD).* Fluorescent molecules absorb light energy and emit it at a lower frequency as electrons return to the ground state from the excited singlet state. An FD is several orders of magnitude more sensitive for compounds with appropriate functional groups (e.g., rigid aromatic compounds with conjugated pi electrons) than the UV detector. It also provides enhanced selectivity, as less than 15% of organic compounds fluoresce. Additional selectivity can be achieved with variable excitation and emission (two monochromators). Further fine-tuning can be accomplished by judicious selection of excitation and emission wavelengths. While an FD offers greater selectivity and sensitivity for fluorescent compounds, it is also more sensitive to environmental factors (e.g., temperature, pressure).

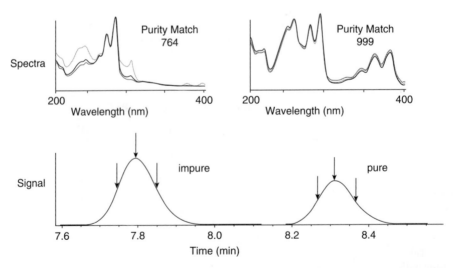

FIGURE 5.3   Use of a PDA for peak purity determination. A PDA (top traces) can detect impurities even when they are not evident from the UV chromatographic signal (bottom traces). (Used with permission from C. Huber, LabCompliance.)

3. *Electrochemical (EC) Detector.* Detection with EC is based on oxidation/reduction reactions at a suitable detector. EC provides enhanced sensitivity and selectivity for analytes with appropriate functional groups (e.g., phenols, catecholamines, nitrosamines). For example, EC detection can be employed in *in vitro* drug metabolism studies where a small amount of phenolic metabolite is being formed in the presence of huge excess of substrate—the latter being transparent in this detector [123]. An EC detector can be operated in either the oxidative or reductive mode, but the former is more commonly employed and is not subject to interferences by oxygen. Electrodes require frequent cleaning, depending on the nature of the samples and mobile phase. In the most prevalent mode, amperometric, a fixed potential applied to the electrode (most commonly glassy carbon) oxidizes (or reduces) the analyte with only a small fraction of analyte (~10%) being involved in electron transfer. In coulometric mode, 100% of the analyte is involved in electron transfer and thus is independent of mobile phase flow. While it offers absolute quantitation by Faraday's law, the coulometric mode requires a large-area electrode, which is more susceptible to contamination. Resultant noise offsets 100% analyte conversion without improvement in signal-to-noise (S/N) ratio.

4. *Refractive Index Detector (RID).* While being a universal detector, this bulk property detector has several inherent limitations: it is very temperature sensitive, it requires the same mobile phase composition throughout the run, the baseline is often difficult to stabilize, and it has relatively poor sensitivity.

5. *Radiometric Detector.* A radiometric detector is primarily used for detection of beta-emitters (^3H, ^{14}C, ^{32}P), soft gamma-emitters, or positron-emitters. Radioactive label imparts specificity and allows detection and quantification in biological matrices without concern about nonradioactive interferences. It is especially useful for metabolite detection and pharmacokinetic studies.

6. *Mass Spectrometer Detector.* Mass spectrometric detection adds another dimension to selectivity based on mass/charge (m/z) ratio. In addition to quantification, it also allows identification and characterization of analytes and metabolites [124]. Increased sensitivity and selectivity for quantification can be obtained with selected ion monitoring (SIM) in which only a few selected characteristic ions are monitored. Several ionization modes are possible and are selected to best fit the analyte and sample. Electron impact (EI) is the oldest ionization mode and provides extensive fragmentation and yields important and reproducible structural information. Positive chemical ionization (PCI) provides soft ionization (little excess energy in the molecule), causing lesser fragmentation than EI, and yields information on protonated molecular ions or adducts and molecular weight. It can provide additional sensitivity and specificity over EI. Negative chemical ionization (NCI)—electron capture—provides extreme sensitivity for suitable molecules (containing halogens or nitro groups) or molecules that can be appropriately derivatized (e.g., pentafluorobenzyl) to make them amenable to NCI. Atmospheric pressure ionization (API-MS) techniques, electrospray ionization (ESI), and atmospheric pressure chemical ionization (APCI) are popular because they combine solvent elimination and ionization in a single step, but some compounds do not ionize using this approach. ESI is a softer ionization than APCI and can be useful for ionization of polar and less volatile components. APCI, on the other hand, is more robust and less susceptible to ion suppression by coeluting substances. Both

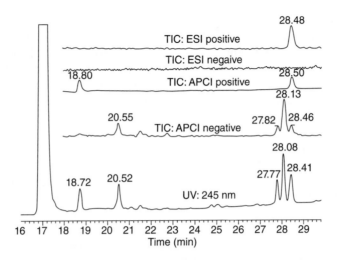

FIGURE 5.4   Effect of different modes of API-MS on detection. The bottom UV trace (245 nm) indicates presence of three impurity components eluting between 27 and 29 min. The top four traces represent corresponding total ion current (TIC) response in different modes of API-MS. (Used with permission from the publisher [190].)

ESI and APCI can operate in either positive or negative mode. Sometimes significant improvements in the sensitivity of API-MS methods can be achieved by derivatization (introduction of permanently charged or readily ionized moieties in ESI or high proton or electron affinities in APCI) or mobile phase modification to facilitate adduct formation [20]. It is also important to keep in mind that response in any ionization mode is compound specific as illustrated in Fig. 5.4. As shown for three unknown compounds eluting between 27 and 29 minutes, response varied markedly using different modes in API-MS. Additional structural information or sensitivity/selectivity is achievable using tandem mass spectrometry or MS/MS techniques (see later discussion).

Several mass spectrometric analyzers are used for drug analyses. The most prevalent is a quadrupole. It has a mass range up to 4000 amu (atomic mass units) and represents a reasonable mixture of mass resolution, linear range, ease of use, and cost. It is also available in a triple quad configuration, TQMS (tandem mass spectrometry), where the middle quadrupole serves as a collision cell to allow for collision-induced dissociation (CID) and operation in MS/MS mode. Parent ions from the first quadrupole undergo further fragmentation in the collision cell to yield daughter ions detectable in the third quadrupole. The process is also known as selected reaction monitoring (SRM) and provides increased selectivity and sensitivity and helps overcome background interferences. MS/MS mode is also useful in peak purity assessment, as shown in Fig. 5.5. HPLC UV and MS monitoring showed a single chromatographic peak. Two largely abundant ions were coeluting in the MS tracings. Further fragmentation in the MS/MS mode of the larger mass ion did not generate the other coeluting smaller mass ion, suggesting that the latter was not spontaneously generated from the former and that it belongs to another species (i.e., the chromatographic peak was impure).

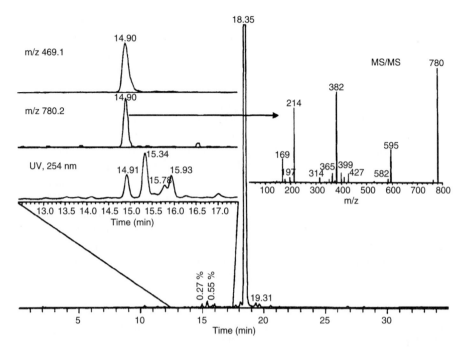

FIGURE 5.5 Detection of coeluting impurity using MS/MS. Left panel shows a UV trace and expanded/enlarged UV and MS (two coeluting ions) traces. Right panel depicts MS/MS spectrum of the larger mass ion that lacks the lower mass ion. (Used with permission from the publisher [190].)

An ion trap represents another quadrupole configuration. Advantages of the ion trap include compact size and ability to trap and accumulate ions and thereby increase signal-to-noise ratio. Trapped ions can be further fragmented and ion trap instruments provide an economical alternative to tandem mass spectrometers. Serial trapping and fragmentation theoretically allow MS^n. Time-of-flight (TOF) analyzers offer several advantages, including high mass resolution, very high mass range, and high mass accuracy. Enhanced mass resolution with TOF instruments provides improved selectivity. A TOF analyzer [124] can also be used in MS/MS mode by combining it with another TOF, a quadrupole, or an ion trap analyzer. Use of LC/MS in the pharmaceutical arena has been reviewed in the literature [8, 125].

As already discussed, matrix effects (presence of coeluting substances) leading to ionization suppression can cause serious problems in mass spectrometric analyses, especially the EIS [2, 3].

While LC-MS offers sensitivity and selectivity and is presently a very popular technique, it is not suitable for all analytical applications [126] and is not a substitute for expertise in chemistry and chromatography.

Capillary Electrophoresis (CE)   CE comprises a family of techniques capable of separating a variety of compounds. A recent review [127] describes this separation technique and includes several application examples. The unifying principle in CE is electrical field-driven separation, with migration rate based on analyte size and charge in the presence of an applied voltage. An electric field is applied across a fused silica capillary with the front end of the capillary immersed in the sample. There are a number of different modes of performing CE separation, including capillary zone electrophoresis (CZE), micellar kinetic electrochromatography (MKEC), and capillary electrochromatography (CEC). CZE is most widely used due to its simplicity and versatility and is applicable to separation of any charged species, including positively and negatively charged species in the same run, but not neutral species. MKEC incorporates pseudopartitioning and thereby also allows separation of neutral species. CEC is a hybrid of CZE and HPLC. CE detectors include UV, fluorescence, electrochemical, and mass spectrometers. In general, some advantages of CE include high resolution, speed, high throughput, small sample size requirement, small reagent consumption, ability to separate most molecules (small and large, even whole organisms), feasible miniaturization, and chiral analysis. It is applicable to both small [128] and large molecules [129]. The major deficiency of CE relative to HPLC has been the higher limit of quantification resulting from small sample volumes and short path length. However, sensitivity improvements (online derivatization, preconcentration, electrokinetic injection, etc.) have been and are being made [128].

Development of various multichannel microfluid devices is under way in order to increase speed and throughput and reduce sample size requirements [130–132] in CE. These include multiplexed CE [131] and microchip electrophoresis [130].

Chiral Methods   The common occurrence of chirality (e.g., sugars, amino acids, enzymes) in nature has been known for several centuries, and more recently the stereoselective nature (three-dimensional drug–receptor interaction) of drugs has also become more appreciated and addressed. Recent advances in synthetic [133] and analytical methods (see later discussion) are making development of enantiomeric drugs more technically feasible. The FDA (http://www.fda.gov/cder/guidance/stereo.htm) and other regulatory agencies worldwide are recommending that enantiomers with the best drug characteristics be developed instead of racemates. Enantiomers have identical physical and chemical properties but may behave very differently in an asymmetric milieu. Stereoisomers are frequently distinguished by biological systems and may have different qualitative and quantitative pharmacokinetic and pharmacodynamic (pharmacological and/or toxicological) properties [134]. Therefore, efficacy and safety issues may exist with enantiomers [135]. For example, only the *d*-enantiomer of methylphenidate is active for treatment of the attention deficit hyperactivity disorder and is also significantly more bioavailable. Racemic terodiline has two enantiomers with similar activity for treatment of urinary incontinence. However, cardiotoxicity due to its *R*-isomer led to its withdrawal from the market. In addition, enantiomers may also have a very different metabolic profile and may affect each other's metabolism [136]. There is a growing consensus that new chiral drugs should be developed as single enantiomers (eutomers) and older racemic drugs should be reevaluated and used as pure active enantiomers if supported by clinical data [137]. During drug development, analysis of the formulated racemate should include stereochemical composition. Phase 1 or 2 pharmacokinetic data should address potential interconversion between enantiomers. Conventional analytical methods cannot separate enantiomers without introduction of an asymmetric environment. Direct (chiral chromatography or addition of chiral modifier to the mobile phase) and indirect (chromatography following chiral derivatization) analytical approaches can be employed for analyses of chiral compounds and have recently been reviewed [138–141]. Different separation methods (including TLC, GC, CE, and HPLC) have been employed for chiral analysis [141]. Currently, EC and HPLC are most commonly employed for chiral analysis and their application has been the subject of a number of recent reviews [140, 142–149]. Different chiral derivatization approaches have also been used [22, 24, 29, 31]. Miniaturization efforts are under way to improve throughput and speed and reduce sample volume size and include microchip EC [130] and nanotechnology [150].

5.3   ANALYTICAL METHOD VALIDATION

5.3.1   Installation, Operation, Performance Qualification, and Maintenance of Instrumentation

Current regulations do not provide clear and authoritative guidance for validation/qualification of analytical instruments. Therefore, the American Association of Pharmaceutical Scientists, the International Pharmaceutical Federation (FIP), and the International Society for Pharmaceutical Engineering (ISPE) cosponsored a workshop entitled "A Scientific Approach to Analytical Instrument Validation," held in Arlington, Virginia, on 3–5 March 2003. The report describing conclusions of this workshop is published in [151].

The various parties at this workshop agreed that processes are "validated" and instruments are "qualified." Therefore, the phrase "analytical instrument qualification (AIQ)" will be used in lieu of "analytical instrument validation" [151]. Analytical instrument qualification (AIQ) is documented evidence that an instrument performs suitably for its intended purpose and that it is properly maintained and calibrated. AIQ is often broken down into four main phases (Fig. 5.6):

- Design qualification (DQ) for setting functional and performance specifications (operational specifications).
- Installation qualification (IQ) for performing and documenting the installation in the selected user environment.
- Operational qualification (OQ) for testing the equipment in the selected user environment to ensure that it meets the previously defined functional and performance specifications.
- Performance qualification (PQ) for testing that the system consistently performs as intended for the selected application.

The *design qualification* **(DQ)** activity is most suitably performed by the instrument developer/manufacturer. Since the instrument design is already in place for commercial (off-the-shelf) systems, the user does not need to repeat all aspects of

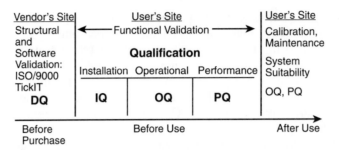

FIGURE 5.6 The validation timeline. Activities under each phase are usually performed in each phase indicated in the figure. In some cases, it may be more appropriate to combine a given activity or perform it with another phase. If performed under the other phase, it is not necessary to repeat the activity under the phase where the activity is listed.

DQ. However, users should ensure that instruments have all the necessary functions and performance criteria that will enable them to be successfully implemented for the intended application and that the manufacturer has adopted a quality system for developing, manufacturing, and testing. Users should also establish that manufacturers and vendors adequately support installation, service, and training. As part of the design qualification process, the vendor should be qualified. This may be done by review of established and documented quality systems (e.g., ISO 9001) at the supplier or by a direct audit.

Installation qualification **(IQ)** is a documented collection of activities needed to install an instrument in the user's environment. The IQ process can be divided into two steps—*preinstallation* and *physical installation*. During preinstallation, all the information pertinent to the proper installation, operation, and maintenance of the instrument is reviewed. Site requirements and the receipt of all of the parts, pieces, and manuals necessary to perform the installation are confirmed. During physical installation, serial numbers are recorded, and all of the fluidic, electrical, and communication connections are made for components in the system. Documentation describing how the instrument was installed, who performed the installation, and other miscellaneous details should be archived. Only after a successful IQ is the instrument ready for OQ testing.

Operational qualification **(OQ)** is the process of demonstrating that an instrument will function according to its operational specification in the user's environment. OQ ensures that the specific modules of the system (or entire system) are operating according to the defined specifications for accuracy, linearity, and precision. This process may be as simple as verifying the module self-diagnostic routines, or may be performed in more depth by running specific tests to verify, for example, detector wavelength accuracy, flow rate, or injector precision. OQ tests can be modular or holistic. Modular testing of individual components of a system may facilitate interchange of such components without requalification and should be done whenever possible. Holistic tests, which involve the entire system, are acceptable in lieu of modular testing [152]. Having successfully completed OQ testing, the instrument is qualified for use in regulated samples testing.

The sample type of tests possible during OQ, which apply to a high performance liquid chromatography (HPLC) unit, can be applied: pump flow rate, gradient linearity, detector wavelength accuracy, detector linearity, column oven temperature, peak area precision, and peak retention time precision. A more intensive list of tests for HPLC is proposed by Grizanti and Zachowski [153]. Bansal et al. [151] consider that OQ tests may not be required to be repeated at a regular interval. Rather, when the instrument undergoes major repairs or modifications, relevant OQ tests should be repeated to verify whether the instrument continues to operate satisfactorily.

Performance qualification **(PQ)** is the process of demonstrating that an instrument consistently performs according to a specification appropriate for its routine use. PQ testing is conducted under actual running conditions across the anticipated working range. In practice, however, OQ and PQ frequently blend together, particularly for linearity and precision (repeatability) tests, which can be conducted more easily at the system level [153]. For HPLC, the PQ test should use a method with a well-characterized analyte mixture, column, and mobile phase. It should incorporate the essence of the System Suitability section of the general chromatography chapter ⟨621⟩ in the USP. Again, proper documentation should be archived to support the PQ process. PQ tests are performed routinely, for example, each time the instrument is used. PQ tests should be performed independent of the routine analytical testing performed on the instrument [151]. In practice, PQ can mean system suitability testing, where critical key system performance characteristics are measured and compared with documented, preset limits. For example, a well characterized standard can be injected five or six times and the standard deviation of amounts are then compared with a predefined value. The analysis of quality control (QC) samples with construction of quality control charts has been suggested as another way of performing PQ. Control samples with known amounts are interspersed among actual samples at intervals determined by the total number of samples, the stability of the system, and the specified precision. The advantage of this procedure is that the system performance is measured more or less continuously under conditions that are very close to the actual application [154].

Documented procedures should exist that instruct the operators on what to do if the system does not meet the criteria. When PQ test(s) fail to meet specifications, the instrument requires maintenance or repair. For many instruments a periodic preventive maintenance (PM) may also be recommended. Relevant PQ test(s) should be repeated after the needed maintenance or repair to ensure that the instrument remains qualified.

Suggested PM and PQ procedures and their recommended frequency for several analytical instruments are contained in Appendix A of *Quality Assurance Principles for Analytical Laboratories* [1] and in *Analytical Method Validation and Instrument Performance Verification* [155].

On completion of equipment qualification, documentation should be available that consists of:

- Design qualification document
- Vendor qualification checklist

- Installation qualification document (includes description of hardware and software)
- Procedures for testing
- Qualification test reports with signatures and dates
- Entries on instrument ID in the laboratory's instrument database
- PQ test procedures and representative results

Software used for analytical work can be classified into the following categories:

- Firmware
- Instrument control, data acquisition, and processing software
- Stand-alone software

1. *Firmware.* The computerized analytical instruments contain integrated chips with low-level software (firmware). Such instruments will not function without properly operating firmware, and users usually cannot alter the firmware's design or function. Firmware is thus considered a component of the instrument itself. Indeed, qualification of the hardware is not possible without operating it via its firmware. So when the hardware (i.e., analytical instrument) is qualified at the user's site, it essentially qualifies the integrated firmware. No separate on-site qualification of the firmware is needed. Any changes made to firmware versions should be tracked through change control of the instrument.

2. *Instrument Control, Data Acquisition, and Processing Software.* Software for instrument control, data acquisition, and processing for many of today's computerized instruments is loaded on a computer connected to the instrument. Operation of the instrument is then controlled via the software, leaving fewer operating controls on the instrument. Also, the software is needed for data acquisition and post-acquisition calculations. Thus, both hardware and software are critical to providing analytical results.

The manufacturer should perform the DQ, validate this software, and provide users with a summary of validation. At the user's site, holistic qualification, which involves the entire instrument and software system, is more efficient than modular validation of the software alone. Thus, the user qualifies the instrument control, data acquisition, and processing software by qualifying the instrument according to the AIQ process defined earlier.

3. *Stand-Alone Software.* An authoritative guide for validating stand-alone software, such as Laboratory Information Management System (LIMS), is available [156]. The validation process is administered by the software developer, who also specifies the development model appropriate for the software. It takes place in a series of activities planned and executed through various stages of the development cycle. The user-site testing is an essential part of the software development cycle. However, the user-site testing, though essential, is only part of the validation process for stand-alone software and does not constitute complete validation. Refer to this guide for activities needed to be performed at the user's site for testing stand-alone software used in analytical work.

Instrument Categories   Based on the level of qualification needed, it is convenient to categorize instruments into three groups—A, B, and C, as defined below [151]. Each group is illustrated by some example instruments. The list of instruments provided as illustration is not meant to be exhaustive, nor can it provide the exact category for an instrument at a user's site. The exact category of an instrument should be determined by the user for the specific instrument or application.

1. *Group A Instruments.* Conformance of Group A instruments to user requirements is determined by visual observation. No independent qualification process is required. Example instruments in this group include light microscopes, magnetic stirrers, mortars and pestles, nitrogen evaporators, ovens, spatulas, and vortex mixers.

2. *Group B Instruments.* Conformance of Group B instruments to user requirements is performed according to the instruments' standard operating procedures. Their conformity assessments are generally unambiguous. Installation of Group B instruments is relatively simple and causes of their failure are readily discernible by simple observations. Example instruments in this group include balances, incubators, infrared spectrometers, melting point apparatus, muffle furnaces, pH meters, pipettes, refractometers, refrigerator-freezers, thermocouples, thermometers, titrators, vacuum ovens, and viscometers.

3. *Group C Instruments.* Conformance of Group C instruments to user requirements is highly method specific, and the conformity bounds are determined by their application. Installing these instruments can be a complicated undertaking and may require the assistance of specialists. A full-qualification process, as outlined in this document, should apply to these instruments. Example instruments in this group include atomic absorption spectrometers, differential scanning calorimeters, densitometers, diode-array detectors, electron microscopes, elemental analyzers, flame absorption spectrometers, gas chromatographs, high-pressure liquid chromatographs, inductively coupled argon plasma emission spectrometers, mass spectrometers, microplate readers, near-infrared spectrometers, Raman spectrometers, thermal gravimetric analyzers, UV/VIS spectrometers, and X-ray fluorescence spectrometers.

5.3.2 Validation Parameters and Definition

Validation is a constant, evolving process starting before an instrument is placed online, and continuing long after method development and transfer. A well defined and documented validation process provides regulatory agencies with evidence that the system and method are suitable for their intended use.

The purpose of method validation [157] is to demonstrate that an analytical method is acceptable for its intended use in terms of the criteria below. Assay qualification differs from assay validation in that its intent is to demonstrate that an accepted method (e.g., compendial method from the USP) is suitable for the intended analysis under actual conditions of use. USP provides regulatory guidance for compendial method validation (USP 25-NF 20). When using USP or NF methods, it is not required to demonstrate their accuracy and reliability. Criteria to be used in

TABLE 5.11   ICH Validation Characteristics

Procedure (ICH Q2A) Product Specification	ID Test Present/ Absent	Quantitative Limit Test ≤20%	Qualitative Limit Test ≤5%	Content Purity ≥80%	Content Range 40–60%
Accuracy	No	Yes	No	Yes	Yes
Repeatability	No	Yes	No	Yes	Yes
Specificity	Yes	Yes	Yes	Yes	Yes
Linearity	No	Yes	No	Yes	Yes
Range	No	Yes	No	Yes	Yes
LOD	No	No	Yes	No	No
LOQ	No	Yes	No	No	No

method validation are described in ICH (International Conference on Harmonisation) guidelines Q2A (http://www.fda.gov/cder/guidance/ichq2a.pdf) [158] and Q2B (http://www.fda.gov/cder/guidance/1320fnl.pdf) [159]. Their brief descriptions are included below and details, including tolerances and acceptance criteria, can be found in those guidelines. In addition, FDA Draft Guidance 2396 (http://www.fda.gov/cder/guidance/2396dft.pdf) [160] provides additional information on analytical procedures and methods validation in CMC (chemistry, manufacturing, and controls) documentation and FDA Guidance 4252 provides information on bioanalytical method validation (http://www.fda.gov/cder/guidance/4252fnl.pdf) [161]. Systematic approaches to the acceptance/rejection decision for chromatographic methods and hypothesis testing have been reviewed [162]. ICH validation characteristics for different tests are summarized in Table 5.11.

Specificity   Specificity (some guidances use the term *selectivity*) is the ability to assess unequivocally the analyte in the presence of components that may be expected to be present (e.g., impurities, degradants, matrix).

Accuracy and Precision   The accuracy represents an agreement between measured and theoretical values. Precision refers to variability in the data from replicate determinations. Precision and accuracy are depicted schematically in Fig. 5.7. Five samples per concentration should be used to validate a bioanalytical method in terms of accuracy and precision. The mean value should be within 15% of the theoretical value with a coefficient of variation (CV) of 15%, except for LLOQ, where these should be within 20%. QC samples should represent low, middle, and high concentrations of experimental values.

Limit of Detection (LOD) and Limit of Quantification (LOQ)   LOD refers to the lowest amount of analyte that can be detected (distinguishable from background) but not adequately accurate or precise to be quantified. It is commonly based on 3:1 signal-to-noise ratio (SNR) or as 3 times the standard deviation of the response divided by the slope of the calibration curve.

LOQ refers to the lowest and the highest concentrations that can be quantified with adequate accuracy and precision. It is commonly based on 10:1 SNR or as 10 times the standard deviation of the response divided by the slope of the calibration curve.

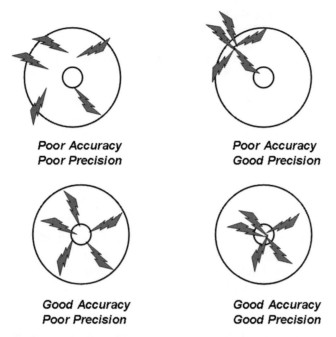

Poor Accuracy
Poor Precision

Poor Accuracy
Good Precision

Good Accuracy
Poor Precision

Good Accuracy
Good Precision

FIGURE 5.7 Schematic depiction of accuracy and precision.

Linearity and Range Linearity refers to direct proportionality between measurement values (response) and analyte concentrations. Commonly 5 to 8 concentrations are used to generate the standard curve. Mathematical transformations to allow linearity may be applied if shown scientifically appropriate.

Range refers to concentrations between the low and high limit of quantification and should bracket the concentration in experimental samples.

Stability Potential degradation of samples, standards, controls, and critical reagents during storage (including freeze–thaw cycles when relevant) should be evaluated and attention paid to expiration dates. Stress studies can be performed by exposing analytes to acid, base, heat, UV light, oxidizers, and so on in order to assess their stability.

Ruggedness Ruggedness refers to reproducibility under normal but variable conditions (e.g., different instruments, operators, laboratories, reagent lots, analytical column lots).

Robustness Robustness refers to the analytical method's ability to remain unaffected by small changes in operational parameters (e.g., temperature, mobile phase composition or flow rate, injection volume) and is used to define acceptable tolerances.

Transferability and Revalidation After a method has been validated, it is ready to be transferred to other laboratories that will be using the method. Documentation of the method should include a detailed written procedure, a method validation

TABLE 5.12   System Suitability Parameters and Recommendations[a]

Parameter	Recommendation
Capacity factor (k')	The peak should be well resolved from other peaks and the void volume; generally, $k' > 2.0$
Repeatability	RSD $\leq 1\%$ for $N \geq 5$ is desirable
Relative retention	Not essential as long as the resolution is stated.
Resolution (R_s)	$R^s > 2$ between the peak of interest and the closest eluting potential interferent (impurity, excipient, degradation product, internal standard, etc.).
Tailing factor (T)	$T \leq 2$
Theoretical plates (N)	In general, should be >2000

[a]Details of determination of these parameters are presented in Ref. 189.

report, system suitability criteria, and a plan for the method's implementation. General acceptance criteria for the method's intended purpose should also be included. The new user should plan on spending time verifying method performance prior to the method being implemented.

At some time during the lifetime of a method, for one reason or another, it may become necessary to revalidate the method. Revalidation can be carried out in a reactive or proactive manner. Reactive revalidation may be performed in response to changes in incoming raw material, manufacturing batch changes, formulation changes, or any other changes (dilutions, sample preparation) in the method. A total revalidation from scratch is usually not necessary in these instances, but enough revalidation should be performed to address the issues at hand as dictated by the needs and use of the method. Proactive revalidation may be undertaken to take advantage of new technology, or perhaps to automate a previously complex, labor-intensive, and/or time-consuming manual procedure. In such cases, revalidation may be more comprehensive, depending on the undertaking. System suitability tests are based on the concept that the equipment, electronics, analytical operations, and samples constitute an integral system that can be evaluated as a whole.

System Suitability   System suitability is determined by checking a system to ensure system performance before or during the analysis of unknowns. For example, for HPLC, parameters such as plate count, tailing factors, resolution, and reproducibility (%RSD retention time and area for six repetitions) are determined and compared against the specifications set for the method. These parameters are measured during the analysis of a system suitability "sample" that is a mixture of main components and expected by-products. Table 5.12 lists the terms to be measured and their recommended limits obtained from the analysis of the system suitability sample for the HPLC analytical method.

5.3.3   Guidelines: ICH, FDA, AOAC, USP, ISO 9000, and ISO 17025

When the ICH was first established, one of the objectives was to organize an International Conference on Harmonization, hence the name given to the initiative. The name of ICH has now, perhaps, become more associated with the process of harmonization, than the actual conferences, although these have been extremely important for ensuring that the process of harmonization was carried out in a transparent manner and that there was an open forum in which to present and discuss ICH recommendations. ICH is a joint initiative involving both regulators and industry as equal partners in the scientific and technical discussions of the testing procedures that are required to ensure and assess the safety, quality, and efficacy of medicines.

The focus of the ICH has been on the technical requirements for medicinal products containing new drugs. The vast majority of those new drugs and medicines are developed in Western Europe, Japan, and the United States of America and therefore, when the ICH was established, it was agreed that its scope would be confined to registration in those three regions.

The ICH Topics are divided into four major categories and ICH Topic Codes are assigned according to these categories: *Quality Topics*, that is, those relating to chemical and pharmaceutical Quality Assurance, which are relevant to this chapter, are divided into the following subcategories: Q1 Stability Testing, Q2 Validation, Q3 Impurity Testing, Q4 Pharmacopoeias (not implemented yet), Q5 Quality of Biotechnological Products, and Q9 Risk Management.

Q1A (R2): Stability Testing of New Drug Substances and Products (Second Revision)   This guideline [163] has been revised a second time in order to accommodate for the consequences of Q1F and reached Step 4 of the ICH process on 6 February 2003. This guideline provides recommendations on stability testing protocols including temperature, humidity, and trial duration. Furthermore, the revised document takes into account the requirements for stability testing in Climatic Zones III and IV in order to minimize the different storage conditions for submission of a global dossier.

Q1B: Photostability Testing of New Drug Substances and Products   The tripartite harmonized ICH guideline [164] was finalized (Step 4) in November 1996. This forms an annex to the main stability guideline and gives guidance on the basic testing protocol required to evaluate the light sensitivity and stability of new drugs and products.

Q1C: Stability Testing for New Dosage Forms   The tripartite harmonized ICH guideline [165] was finalized (Step 4) in November 1996. It extends the main stability guideline for new formulations of already approved medicines and defines the circumstances under which reduced stability data can be accepted.

Q1D: Bracketing and Matrixing Designs for Stability Testing of Drug Substances and Drug Products   The tripartite harmonized ICH guideline [166] was finalized (Step 4) in February 2002. This document describes general principles for reduced stability testing and provides examples of bracketing and matrixing designs.

Q1E: Evaluation of Stability Data   The tripartite harmonized ICH guideline [167] was finalized (Step 4) in February 2003. This document extends the main guideline by explaining possible situations where extrapolation of retest periods/ shelf-lives beyond the real-time data may be appropriate. Furthermore, it provides examples of statistical approaches to stability data analysis.

Q1F: Stability Data Package for Registration Applications in Climatic Zones III and IV   The tripartite harmonized ICH guideline [168] was finalized (Step 4) in February 2003. This document provides guidance on specific stability testing requirements for Climatic Zones III and IV. Besides proposing acceptable storage conditions for long-term and accelerated studies, it gives guidance on data to cover situations of elevated temperature and/or extremes of humidity. The referenced literature provides information on the classification of countries according to climatic zones.

The most important for this chapter are Q2A and Q2B ICH guidelines already mentioned.

Q2A: Text on Validation of Analytical Procedures   The tripartite harmonized ICH text [158] was finalized (Step 4) in October 1994. This identifies the validation parameters needed for a variety of analytical methods. It also discusses the characteristics that must be considered during the validation of the analytical procedures, which are included as part of registration applications.

Q2B: Validation of Analytical Procedures—Methodology   The tripartite harmonized ICH text [159] was finalized (Step 4) in November 1996. It extends the guideline Q2A to include the actual experimental data required, along with the statistical interpretation, for the validation of analytical procedures.

Q3A(R): Impurities in New Drug Substances (Revised Guideline)   First recommended for adoption at Step 4 of the ICH process on 30 March 1995, the guideline [169] was revised under Step 2 of the ICH process on 7 October 1999 and recommended for adoption under Step 4 on 7 February 2002 by the ICH Steering Committee.

The guideline addresses the chemistry and safety aspects of impurities, including the listing of impurities in specifications, and defines the thresholds for reporting, identification, and qualification. Revision of the guideline has allowed clarification of some inconsistencies, revision of the decision tree, harmonizing with Q3B, and addressing some editorial issues.

Q3B(R): Impurities in New Drug Products (Revised Guideline)   This guideline [170] was revised and finalized under Step 4 in February 2003. It complements the guideline on impurities in new drug substances and provides advice in regard to impurities in products containing new, chemically synthesized drug substances. The guideline specifically deals with those impurities that might arise as degradation products of the drug substance or from interactions between drug substance and excipients or components of primary packaging materials. The guideline sets out a rationale for the reporting, identification, and qualification of such impurities based on a scientific appraisal of likely and actual impurities observed, and of the safety implications, following the principles elaborated in the parent guideline. Threshold values for reporting and control of impurities are proposed, based on the maximum daily dose of the drug substance administered in the product.

Q3C: Impurities—Guideline for Residual Solvents   The tripartite harmonized ICH guideline [171] was finalized (Step 4) in July 1997. This recommends the use of less toxic solvents in the manufacture of drug substances and dosage forms, and sets pharmaceutical limits for residual solvents (organic volatile impurities) in drug products.

Q5C: Quality of Biotechnological Products—Stability Testing of Biotechnological/Biological Products The tripartite harmonized ICH guideline [172] was finalized (Step 4) in November 1995. This document augments the stability guideline (Q1A above) and deals with the particular aspects of stability test procedures needed to take account of the special characteristics of products in which the active components are typically proteins and/or polypeptides.

Q9: Quality Risk Management The tripartite harmonized ICH guideline [173] was finalized (Step 4) in November 2005. This guideline provides principles and examples of tools of quality risk management that can be applied to all aspects of pharmaceutical quality including development, manufacturing, distribution, and the inspection and submission/review processes throughout the lifecycle of drug substances and drug (medicinal) products, biological and biotechnological products, including the use of raw materials, solvents, excipients, packaging and labeling materials.

Two FDA guidelines—FDA Draft Guidance 2396, *Analytical Procedures and Methods Validation, Chemistry, Manufacturing and Controls Documentation* [160], and FDA Guidance 4252, *Bioanalytical Method Validation* [161]—are important documents regulating analytical methods validation in addition to ICH guidelines.

United States Pharmacopoeia 26, National Formulary 21, Chapter 1225 describes validation of compendial methods [174]. In 2005 the USP proposed revisions to the method validation guidelines published in Chapter 1225 [175]. For the most part, the revisions were made to continue to harmonize with ICH terminology, for example, using the word "procedures" instead of "methods" [176]. The term "pharmaceutical products" is replaced by the term "pharmaceutical articles" to indicate that the guidelines apply to both drug substances and drug products. Another major change is the use of the term "intermediate precision" and the deletion of the section and use of the term "ruggedness." Use of the term ruggedness has been falling out of favor ever since implementation of the original ICH guideline on terminology [158].

Also in 2005, the USP published a proposed new chapter, Chapter 1226, entitled "Verification of Compendial Procedures" [177]. The purpose of this new general information chapter is to provide guidelines for verifying the suitability of a compendial procedure under conditions of actual use. This new chapter summarizes what is necessary to confirm that the compendial procedure works for a particular drug substance, excipients, or dosage form by *verifying* a subset of validation characteristics rather than completing a full validation. The intent is to provide guidance on how to verify that a compendial procedure that is being used for the first time will yield acceptable results utilizing the laboratory's personnel, equipment, and reagents. Verification consists of assessing selected "analytical performance characteristics," described in Chapter 1225, to generate appropriate relevant data as opposed to repeating the entire validation process.

The ISO 9000 family [178–180] was published on 15 December 2000 by the International Organization for Standardization (ISO). These revised standards are identified by the "2000" in their designation. ISO 9001:2000 [179] specifies requirements for a quality management system for any organization that needs to demonstrate its ability to consistently provide product that meets customer and applicable regulatory requirements and aims to enhance customer satisfaction. ISO 9001:2000 has been organized in a user-friendly format with terms that are easily recognized by all business sectors. The standard is used for certification/registration and contractual purposes by organizations seeking recognition of their quality management system. ISO 9001:2000 specifies requirements for a quality management system where an organization (1) needs to demonstrate its ability to consistently provide product that meets customer and applicable regulatory requirements, and (2) aims to enhance customer satisfaction through the effective application of the system, including processes for continual improvement of the system and the assurance of conformity to customer and applicable regulatory requirements.

All requirements of this international standard are generic and are intended to be applicable to all organizations, regardless of type, size, and product provided. Recently, the ISO has published a new edition of the standard in the ISO 9000 family that defines the vocabulary and describes the fundamentals of quality management systems. ISO 9000:2005, *Quality Management Systems—Fundamentals and Vocabulary* [181], introduces no changes to the descriptions of the fundamentals of quality management systems (QMSS), as presented in the previous edition published in 2000. However, some definitions have been added and explanatory notes expanded or added.

ISO/IEC 90003:2004 [182] provides guidance for organizations in the application of ISO 9001:2000 to the acquisition, supply, development, operation, and maintenance of computer software and related support services. It replaces the old ISO 9000-3 1997 software standard. The American Society for Quality (ASQ) published ANSI/ISO/ASQ Q9000-2000 Series—*Quality Management Standards* [183], which are American National Standards on quality management and quality assurance that are internationally recognized as being identical to the ISO 9000:2000 quality standards.

The ISO/IEC Guide 25, *General Requirements for the Competence of Calibration and Testing Laboratories* [184], has been the internationally recognized basic document for accreditation of laboratories including chemical analysis. The attainment of accreditation is mandatory for some regulatory work areas and frequently is the basis of contracts for analytical work. In 2000 the draft was replaced by ISO/IEC DIS 17025, *General Requirements for the Competence of Testing and Calibration Laboratories* [185]. A new version of ISO/IEC 17025 was issued on 15 May 2005 (ISO/IEC 17025:2005) [186]. The American Association for Laboratory Accreditation (A2LA) provides accreditation and certification in accordance with ISO/IEC 17025:2005.

The ISO 17025 standard states that if testing and calibration laboratories comply with ISO 17025, they also operate in accordance with ISO 9001 or ISO 9002. However, calibration against ISO 9001 and 9002 does not itself demonstrate the competence of the laboratory to produce technically valid data and results. While ISO/IEC Guide 25 was mainly focused on technical controls, the new guide includes more management and administrative controls from the ISO 9001 and ISO 9002 quality standards. ISO/IEC 17025 is the most specific document for quality systems for laboratories. The U.S. FDA is implementing it in their labs and all regulated laboratories may look at ISO/IEC 17025 as a basis for their operation as many elements will also be subject to FDA audits.

The impact of ISO/IEC 17025 on analytical instrumentation and test methods is similar to the impact GLP and GMP regulations have. Instrument hardware should be calibrated, tested, and verified for performance, and it should be maintained to assure a continuous performance. The performance of hardware should be periodically reverified according to a well documented schedule. Software should be validated by the user or vendor firm and verified by the end-user for proper performance. Analytical methods must be validated if nonstandard methods are used.

Specific to some extent to ISO 9000 and ISO/IEC 17025 is the requirement to trace calibration devices such as reference standards or reference test devices back to national or international standards. All tools used for calibration and performance verification of instruments should be well maintained and calibrated. Training records should be kept for all individuals who perform the calibration and verification.

5.3.4   Good Laboratory Practice (GLP)

Analytical laboratories should follow GLPs for all preclinical drug development studies.

The basic GLP requirements for analytical laboratories include the following:

- Established, controlled, *standard operating procedures* (SOPs) for sample handling, instrument operation, test methods, data handling, and analyst training.
- Use of *labeled, traceable reagents* properly stored and used within expiration dates.
- Use of *traceable reference standards* as testing controls.
- Maintenance of *controlled, complete laboratory notebooks*, including raw data archiving and retrieval systems.
- Having *calibrated, regularly maintained equipment* for every step in sample storage, handling, and testing.
- *Documentation* of all activities performed in operations related to GLP samples, including personnel qualifications and training records.

Attention to five steps of data acquisition for product analysis can help to focus on the goals of compliance activities: analyses should be planned, performed, monitored, recorded, and reported. Viewing these as distinct activities can greatly enhance a facility's ability to follow GLPs.

1. *Planning.* Designate a study protocol and a study director. The protocol should include descriptions of the nature and purpose of the study, sample information, dates, test methods used, justifications, and references. Any modifications to the protocol must be signed and dated. The study director is the party responsible for adhering to compliance activities. Contract laboratories should designate a study director to coordinate efforts with the client's in-house preclinical study director.

2. *Performing.* Facilities where the analytical work is done should be of suitable size, design, and construction for analyses. SOPs should describe all aspects of sample handling (such as receipt, identification, labeling, and storage) and instrument use (such as maintenance, calibration, and monitoring—including refrigerators, freezers, water baths, incubators, etc.). Equipment should be of adequate capacity and suitably located. Personnel should be experienced in the methods they perform and have documented training.

3. *Monitoring.* Analysis systems need to be examined by a quality assurance unit, who will review database information, data analysis, and the final report. A statement should be attached to the final report documenting review by this unit.

4. *Recording.* This includes documentation, data generation and analysis, and data storage and retrieval. It includes everything from the study protocol, procedures, final reports, and audits, to personnel qualifications, equipment records, and sample records.

5. *Reporting.* A final study report should be delivered to the client, describing the nature and purpose of the study, the protocols used, the samples tested, the results, references to raw data (including computer files), and any applicable literature references. All data should be signed and dated, with corrections in the protocol or report included as amendments.

5.3.5   Method Validation Protocol

A validation plan is a written plan stating how validation will be conducted, including test parameters, product characteristics, production equipment, and decision points on what constitutes acceptable results. USP Chapter 1225 [174] on validation of analytical methods specifically addresses terms and definitions, but leaves protocol and methodology open for interpretation. The ICH guidelines on method validation methodology, ICH Q2A and ICH Q2B [158, 159], and the U.S. FDA *Guidance for Industry: Bioanalytical Method Validation* [161] fill this gap. Full or partial validation may be required. Full validation (usually on three different days) is performed when developing and implementing a method for the first time, when a new drug entity is used, and when metabolites are added to an existing assay for quantification. Partial validation (may be performed in 1–2 days) is used for modification of already validated methods. Partial validation can range from as little as one intraassay accuracy and precision determination to nearly full validation. Before outlining an experimental design or protocol, however, it is necessary to make some basic assumptions. These assumptions include:

1. Selectivity has been previously demonstrated or is measured and documented during the course of the validation protocol.
2. The method has been developed and optimized to the point where it makes sense investing time and effort in validating the method. Indeed, robustness should be the first parameter investigated.
3. Once data are generated, statistically valid approaches are used to evaluate it and make decisions, thus removing some of the subjectivity of method validation.

Given that the above three steps are addressed in one way or another, the following stepwise protocol can be proposed for method validation (each specific protocol depends on the nature of the method).

Step 1. On day 1, a linearity test (except for LBAs) over five levels for both the drug substance and dosage form is performed. Comparison of the results between the drug substance and dosage form fulfills the accuracy requirement.

Step 2. At the end of day 1, six repetitions are performed at 100% of the drug substance for repeatability.

Step 3. Steps 1 and 2 are repeated over two additional days for intermediate precision.

Step 4. LLOQ is evaluated (as needed) by analyzing the drug substance over five levels, plus six repetitions for precision.

Step 5. Baseline noise is evaluated over six repetitions of blank injections for the determination of LLOD (if required).

In this manner, a logical stepwise approach to method validation using ICH methodology can be performed. As stated previously, the use of the appropriate statistical tests (Students-t, Cochran, Dixon, and Fisher tests) allows for less subjective decisions to be made regarding the data, reducing method validation to a much more objective undertaking. For example, the Grubbs Procedure described in Ref. [187] may be used to exclude outliers. A rigorous use of statistics may in turn lend itself to some degree of automation in the future.

5.4 CONCLUSION

Analytical technologies continue to evolve, leading to further improvements in sensitivity and selectivity. There are many analytical tools (instrumentations, techniques, computations) presently available to analysts. Selection of tools to be used should be based on the nature of the analyte(s), analytical goals (sensitivity, selectivity, etc.), sample matrix, and sample stability. Tools should not be used blindly but with an analyst's understanding of theory, techniques, instrumentation, and their inherent limitations. While high throughput is desirable, analyses should not become only a matter of inputting samples into analytical machines and merely accepting numerical machine output. Analytical methods need to be subject to appropriate method validation (based on requirements of the most recent guidelines), including periodic instrument testing and calibration, and should incorporate appropriate quality control measures. In addition, stability of analyte(s) needs to be considered from the time of sample collection through final analytical measurement.

REFERENCES

1. Garfield FM, Klesta E, Hirsch J, Eds. *Quality Assurance Principles for Analytical Laboratories*, 3rd ed. Gaithersburg: AOAC International; 2000.

2. Taylor PJ. Matrix effects: the Achilles heel of quantitative high-performance liquid chromatography-electrospray-tandem mass spectrometry. *Clin Biochem* 2005;38(4):328–334.

3. Jemal M, Schuster A, Whigan DB. Liquid chromatography/tandem mass spectrometry methods for quantitation of mevalonic acid in human plasma and urine: method validation, demonstration of using a surrogate analyte, and demonstration of unacceptable matrix effect in spite of use of a stable isotope analog internal standard. *Rapid Commun Mass Spectrom* 2003;17(15):1723–1734.

4. Roth W, Beschke K, Jauch R, Zimmer A, Koss FW. Fully automated high-performance liquid chromatography. A new chromatograph for pharmacokinetic drug monitoring by direct injection of body fluids. *J Chromatogr* 1981;222(1):13–22.

5. Hagestam IH, Pinkerton TC. Internal surface reversed-phase silica supports for liquid chromatography. *Anal Chem* 1985;57:1757–1763.

6. Haque A, Stewart JT. Direct injection HPLC analysis of some non-steroidal anti-inflammatory drugs on restricted access media columns. *Biomed Chromatogr* 1999;13(1):51–56.

7. Rbeida O, Chiap P, Lubda D, Boos KS, Crommen J, Hubert P. Development and validation of a fully automated LC method for the determination of cloxacillin in human plasma using anion exchange restricted access material for sample clean-up. *J Pharm Biomed Anal* 2005;36(5):961–968.

8. Hopfgartner G, Bourgogne E. Quantitative high-throughput analysis of drugs in biological matrices by mass spectrometry. *Mass Spectrom Rev* 2003;22(3):195–214.

9. Veuthey JL, Souverain S, Rudaz S. Column-switching procedures for the fast analysis of drugs in biologic samples. *Ther Drug Monit* 2004;26(2):161–166.

10. Heinig K, Bucheli F. Application of column-switching liquid chromatography–tandem mass spectrometry for the determination of pharmaceutical compounds in tissue samples. *J Chromatogr B Analyt Technol Biomed Life Sci* 2002;769(1):9–26.

11. Hogendoorn EA, van Zoonen P, Polettini A, Marrubini Bouland G, Montagna M. The potential of restricted access media columns as applied in coupled-column LC/LC-TSP/MS/MS for the high-speed determination of target compounds in serum. Application to the direct trace analysis of salbutamol and clenbuterol. *Anal Chem* 1998;70(7):1362–1368.

12. Kuklenyik Z, Ye X, Reich JA, Needham LL, Calafat AM. Automated online and off-line solid-phase extraction methods for measuring isoflavones and lignans in urine. *J Chromatogr Sci* 2004;42(9):495–500.

13. Xia YQ, Whigan DB, Powell ML, Jemal M. Ternary-column system for high-throughput direct-injection bioanalysis by liquid chromatography/tandem mass spectrometry. *Rapid Commun Mass Spectrom* 2000;14(2):105–111.

14. Adamovics JA, Ed. *Chromatographic Analysis of Pharmaceuticals*, 2nd ed. New York: Marcel Dekker; 1997.

15. Bosanquet AG. Stability of solutions of antineoplastic agents during preparation and storage. *Cancer Chemother Pharmacol* 1986;17:1.

16. Pitt AM. The nonspecific protein binding of polymeric microporous membranes. *J Parenteral Sci Technol* 1987;41(2):110.

17. Catz P, Shinn W, Kapetanovic IM, Kim H, Kim M, Jacobson EL. Simultaneous determination of myristyl nicotinate, nicotinic acid, and nicotinamide in rabbit plasma by liquid chromatography–tandem mass spectrometry using methyl ethyl ketone as a deproteinization solvent. *J Chromatogr B* 2005;829(1–2):123–135.

18. Jemal M, Teitz D, Ouyang Z, Khan S. Comparison of plasma sample purification by manual liquid–liquid extraction, automated 96-well liquid–liquid extraction and automated 96-well solid-phase extraction for analysis by high-performance liquid chromatography with tandem mass spectrometry. *J Chromatogr B Biomed Sci Appl* 1999; 732(2):501–508.

19. Vas G, Vekey K. Solid-phase microextraction: a powerful sample preparation tool prior to mass spectrometric analysis. *J Mass Spectrom* 2004;39(3):233–254.

20. Gao S, Zhang ZP, Karnes HT. Sensitivity enhancement in liquid chromatography/atmospheric pressure ionization mass spectrometry using derivatization and mobile phase additives. *J Chromatogr B Analyt Technol Biomed Life Sci* 2005;825(2):98–110.

21. Ahuja S. Derivatization in gas chromatography. *J Pharm Sci* 1976;65(2):163–182.

22. Schurig V. Practice and theory of enantioselective complexation gas chromatography. *J Chromatogr A* 2002;965(1–2):315–356.

23. Halket JM, Zaikin VV. Derivatization in mass spectrometry-3. Alkylation (arylation). *Eur J Mass Spectrom (Chichester)* 2004;10(1):1–19.

24. Srinivas NR, Shyu WC, Barbhaiya RH. Gas chromatographic determination of enantiomers as diastereomers following pre-column derivatization and applications to pharmacokinetic studies: a review. *Biomed Chromatogr* 1995;9(1):1–9.

25. Danielson ND, Targove MA, Miller BE. Pre- and postcolumn derivatization chemistry in conjunction with HPLC for pharmaceutical analysis. *J Chromatogr Sci* 1988;26(8): 362–371.

26. Fukushima T, Usui N, Santa T, Imai K. Recent progress in derivatization methods for LC and CE analysis. *J Pharm Biomed Anal* 2003;30(6):1655–1687.

27. Krull IS, Deyl Z, Lingeman H. General strategies and selection of derivatization reactions for liquid chromatography and capillary electrophoresis. *J Chromatogr B Biomed Appl* 1994;659(1–2):1–17.

28. Li F, Zhang C, Guo X, Feng W. Chemiluminescence detection in HPLC and CE for pharmaceutical and biomedical analysis. *Biomed Chromatogr* 2002;17(2–3):96–105.

29. Toyo'oka T. Resolution of chiral drugs by liquid chromatography based upon diastereomer formation with chiral derivatization reagents. *J Biochem Biophys Methods* 2002; 54(1–3):25–56.

30. Ohkura Y, Kai M, Nohta H. Fluorogenic reactions for biomedical chromatography. *J Chromatogr B Biomed Appl* 1994;659(1–2):85–107.

31. Sun XX, Sun LZ, Aboul-Enein HY. Chiral derivatization reagents for drug enantioseparation by high-performance liquid chromatography based upon pre-column derivatization and formation of diastereomers: enantioselectivity and related structure. *Biomed Chromatogr* 2001;15(2):116–132.

32. Imai K. Derivatization in liquid chromatography. *Adv Chromatogr* 1987;27:215–245.

33. Bardelmeijer HA, Lingeman H, de Ruiter C, Underberg WJ. Derivatization in capillary electrophoresis. *J Chromatogr A* 1998;807(1):3–26.

34. Bardelmeijer HA, Waterval JC, Lingeman H, van't Hof R, Bult A, Underberg WJ. Pre-, on- and post-column derivatization in capillary electrophoresis. *Electrophoresis* 1997;18(12–13):2214–2227.

35. Rosenfeld JM. Solid-phase analytical derivatization: enhancement of sensitivity and selectivity of analysis. *J Chromatogr A* 1999;843(1–2):19–27.

36. Little JL. Artifacts in trimethylsilyl derivatization reactions and ways to avoid them. *J Chromatogr A* 1999;844(1–2):1–22.

37. Salgado HR, Oliveira CL. Development and validation of an UV spectrophotometric method for determination of gatifloxacin in tablets. *Pharmazie* 2005;60(4):263–264.

38. Lastra OC, Lemus IG, Sanchez HJ, Perez RF. Development and validation of an UV derivative spectrophotometric determination of losartan potassium in tablets. *J Pharm Biomed Anal* 2003;33(2):175–180.

39. Forbes RA, Persinger ML, Smith DR. Development and validation of analytical methodology for near-infrared conformance testing of pharmaceutical intermediates. *J Pharm Biomed Anal* 1996;15(3):315–327.

40. Fountain W, Dumstorf K, Lowell AE, Lodder RA, Mumper RJ. Near-infrared spectroscopy for the determination of testosterone in thin-film composites. *J Pharm Biomed Anal* 2003;33(2):181–189.

41. Kumana CR, Au WY, Lee NS, Kou M, Mak RW, Lam CW, Kwong YL. Systemic availability of arsenic from oral arsenic-trioxide used to treat patients with hematological malignancies. *Eur J Clin Pharmacol* 2002;58(8):521–526.

42. Jacobs SS, Fox E, Dennie C, Morgan LB, McCully CL, Balis FM. Plasma and cerebrospinal fluid pharmacokinetics of intravenous oxaliplatin, cisplatin, and carboplatin in nonhuman primates. *Clin Cancer Res* 2005;11(4):1669–1674.

43. Goodisman J, Hagrman D, Tacka KA, Souid AK. Analysis of cytotoxicities of platinum compounds. *Cancer Chemother Pharmacol* 2005;19:1–11.

44. Lansdown AB, Williams A, Chandler S, Benfield S. Silver absorption and antibacterial efficacy of silver dressings. *J Wound Care* 2005;14(4):155–160.

45. Al-Saleh I, Shinwari N, El-Doush I, Billedo G, Al-Amodi M, Khogali F. Comparison of mercury levels in various tissues of albino and pigmented mice treated with two different brands of mercury skin-lightening creams. *Biometals* 2004;17(2):167–175.

46. Gorter RW, Butorac M, Cobian EP. Examination of the cutaneous absorption of copper after the use of copper-containing ointments. *Am J Ther* 2004;11(6):453–458.

47. Brun PH, DeGroot JL, Dickson EF, Farahani M, Pottier RH. Determination of the *in vivo* pharmacokinetics of palladium-bacteriopheophorbide (WST09) in EMT6 tumour-bearing Balb/c mice using graphite furnace atomic absorption spectroscopy. *Photochem Photobiol Sci* 2004;3(11–12):1006–1010.

48. Brouwers EE, Tibben MM, Joerger M, van Tellingen O, Rosing H, Schellens JH. Determination of oxaliplatin in human plasma and plasma ultrafiltrate by graphite-furnace atomic-absorption spectrometry. *Anal Bioanal Chem* 2005;382(7):1484–1490.

49. Liu Y. Determination of ten trace elements in Chinese traditional medicines by atomic absorption spectrometry. *Guang Pu Xue Yu Guang Pu Fen Xi* 2000;20(3):373–375.

50. Gomez MR, Soledad C, Olsina RA, Silva MF, Martinez LD. Metal content monitoring in *Hypericum perforatum* pharmaceutical derivatives by atomic absorption and emission spectrometry. *J Pharm Biomed Anal* 2004;34(3):569–576.

51. Arce S, Cerutti S, Olsina R, Gomez MR, Martinez LD. Determination of metal content in valerian root phytopharmaceutical derivatives by atomic spectrometry. *J AOAC Int* 2005;88(1):221–225.

52. Niemela M, Kola H, Eilola K, Peramaki P. Development of analytical methods for the determination of sub-ppm concentrations of palladium and iron in methotrexate. *J Pharm Biomed Anal* 2004;35(3):433–439.

53. Abdel-Ghani NT, Youssef AF, Awady MA. Cinchocaine hydrochloride determination by atomic spectrometry and spectrophotometry. *Farmaco* 2005;60(5):419–424.

54. Khalil S, Borham N. Indirect atomic absorption spectrometric determination of pindolol, propanolol and levamisole hydrochlorides based on formation of ion-associates with

ammonium reineckate and sodium cobaltinitrite. *J Pharm Biomed Anal* 2000;22(2): 235–240.

55. Avad MM, Shalaby AA, Abdellatef HE, Hosny MM. Spectrophotometric and AAS determination of ramipril and enalapril through ternary complex formation. *J Pharm Biomed Anal* 2002;15(2):311–321.

56. Salem H, Askal H. Colourimetric and AAS determination of cephalosporins using Reineck's salt. *J Pharm Biomed Anal* 2002;29(1–2):347–354.

57. Dědina J, Tsalev DL. *Hydride Generation Atomic Absorption Spectrometry*. Hoboken, NJ: Wiley; 1995.

58. Jackson KW, Ed. *Electrothermal Atomization for Analytical Atomic Spectroscopy*. Hoboken, NJ: Wiley; 1999.

59. Butcher DJ, Sneddon J. *A Practical Guide to Graphite Furnace Atomic Absorption Spectrometry*. Hoboken, NJ: Wiley; 1998.

60. Haswell SJ, Ed. *Atomic Absorption Spectrometry: Theory Design and Applications*. St Louis, MO: Elsevier; 1991.

61. Ebdon L, Evans EH, Fisher AS, Hill SJ. *An Introduction to Analytical Atomic Spectrometry*. Hoboken, NJ: Wiley; 1998.

62. Welz B, Sperling M. *Atomic Absorption Spectrometry*, 3rd ed. Hoboken, NJ: Wiley; 1999.

63. DeSilva B, Smith W, Weiner R, Kelley M, Smolec J, Lee B. Recommendations for the bioanalytical method validation of ligand-binding assays to support pharmacokinetic assessments of macromolecules. *Pharm Res* 2003;20(11):1885–1900.

64. Smolec JM, DeSilva B, Smith W, Weiner R, Kelly M, Lee B, Khan M, Tacey R, Hill H, Celniker A, Shah V, Bowsher R, Mire-Sluis A, Findlay, JWA, Saltarelli M, Quarmby V, Lansky D, Dillard R, Ullmann M, Keller S, Karnes HT. Bioanalytical method validation for macromolecules in support of pharmacokinetic studies. *Pharm Research* 2005;22(9): 1425–1431.

65. Lyubimov AV, Garry VF, Carlson RE, Barr DB, Baker SE. Simplified urinary immunoassay for 2,4-D: validation and exposure assessment. *J Lab Clin Med* 2000;136:116–124.

66. Laloup M, Tilman G, Maes V, De Boeck G, Wallemacq P, Ramaekers J, Samyn N. Validation of an ELISA-based screening assay for the detection of amphetamine, MDMA and MDA in blood and oral fluid. *Forensic Sci Int* 2005;153(1):29–37.

67. Allen KR, Azad R, Field HP, Blake DK. Replacement of immunoassay by LC tandem mass spectrometry for the routine measurement of drugs of abuse in oral fluid. *Ann Clin Biochem* 2005;42(Pt 4):277–284.

68. Rothen-Weinhold A, Besseghir K, De Zelicourt Y, Gurny R. Development and evaluation *in vivo* of a long-term delivery system for vapreotide, a somatostatin analogue. *J Control Release* 1998;52(1–2):205–213.

69. Brown-Augsburger P, Yue XM, Lockridge JA, McSwiggen JA, Kamboj D, Hillgren KM. Development and validation of a sensitive, specific, and rapid hybridization–ELISA assay for determination of concentrations of a ribozyme in biological matrices. *J Pharm Biomed Anal* 2004;34(1):129–139.

70. Xie H, Audette C, Hoffee M, Lambert JM, Blattler WA. Pharmacokinetics and biodistribution of the antitumor immunoconjugate, cantuzumab mertansine (huC242-DM1), and its two components in mice. *Pharmacol Exp Ther* 2004;308(3):1073–1082.

71. Zhang Q, Wang GJ, Sun JG. Pharmacokinetics of recombinant human basic fibroblast growth factor in mice using a radioiodination method combined with SDS-PAGE and a sandwich enzyme-linked immunosorbent assay. *Eur J Drug Metab Pharmacokinet* 2004;29(3):163–168.

72. Ito Y, Tosh B, Togashi Y, Amagase K, Kishida T, Kishida T, Sugioka N, Shibata N, Takada K. Absorption of interferon alpha from patches in rats. *J Drug Target* 2005;13(6); 383–390.

73. Yang XX, Hu ZP, Chan SY, Zhou SF. Monitoring drug–protein interaction. *Clin Chim Acta* 2006;365(1–2):9–29.

74. Mealey KL, Peck KE, Bennett BS, Sellon RK, Swinney GR, Melzer K, Gokhale SA, Krone TM. Systemic absorption of amitriptyline and buspirone after oral and transdermal administration to healthy cats. *J Vet Intern Med* 2004;18(1):43–46.

75. Saita T, Fujito H, Mori M. A specific and sensitive assay for gefitinib using the enzyme-linked immunosorbent assay in human serum. *Biol Pharm Bull* 2005;28(10):1833–1873.

76. Higashi Y, Ikeda Y, Yamamoto R, Yamashiro M, Fujii Y. Pharmacokinetic interaction with digoxin and glucocorticoids in rats detected by radio-immunoassay using a novel specific antiserum. *Life Sci* 2005;77(9):1055–1067.

77. Dalvie D. Recent advances in the applications of radioisotopes in drug metabolism, toxicology and pharmacokinetics. *Curr Pharm Des* 2002;6(10):1009–1028.

78. McCarthy KE. Recent advances in the design and synthesis of carbon-14 labelled pharmaceuticals from small molecule precursors. *Curr Pharm Des* 2000;6:1057–1083.

79. Mao J, Xu Y, Wu D, Almassain B. Pharmacokinetics, mass balance and tissue distribution of a novel DNA alkylating agent, VNP40101M, in rats. *AAPS PharmSci* 2002;4(4) *article 24*:1–7.

80. Van Grieken R, de Bruin M. Nomenclature for Radioanalytical Chemistry: IUPAC Recommendation 1994. *Pure & Appl Chem* 1994;66:2513.

81. Fassett JD. Isotopic and nuclear analytical techniques in biological systems: a critical study. Part X. Elemental isotope dilution analysis with radioactive and stable isotopes. *Pure & Appl Chem* 1995;67(11):1943–1949.

82. White INH, Brown K. Techniques: the application of accelerator mass spectrometry to pharmacology and toxicology. *Trends Pharmacol Sci* 2004;25(8):442–447.

83. Choi MH, Skipper PL, Wishnok JS, Tannenbaum SR. Characterization of testosterone 11ß-hydroxylation by human liver microsomal cytochromes P450. *Drug Metab Dispos* 2005;33(6):714–718.

84. Sarapa N, Hsyu PH, Lappin G, Garner RC. The application of accelerator mass spectrometry to absolute bioavailability studies in humans: simultaneous administration of an intravenous microdose of ^{14}C-nelfinavir mesylate solution and oral nelfinavir to healthy volunteers. *J Clin Pharmacol* 2005;45(10):1198–1205.

85. Saha GB. *Fundamentals of Nuclear Pharmacy*, 5th ed. New York: Springer-Verlag; 2004, p 383.

86. d'Argy R, Sundwall A. Quantitative whole-body radioluminography—future strategy for balance and tissue distribution studies. *Regul Toxicol Pharmacol* 2000;31:S57–S62.

87. Solon EG, Balani SK, Lee FW. Whole-body autoradiography in drug discovery. *Curr Drug Metab* 2002;3(5):451–462.

88. Steinke W, Archimbaud Y, Becka M, Binder R, Busch U, Dupont P, Maas J. Quantitative distribution studies in animals: cross-validation of radioluminography versus liquid-scintillation measurement. *Regul Toxicol Pharmacol* 2001;31:S33–S43.

89. Ehmann WD, Vance DE. *Radiochemistry and Nuclear Methods of Analysis*. Hoboken, NJ: Wiley; 1991.

90. Alfassi ZB. *Chemical Analysis by Nuclear Methods*. Hoboken, NJ: Wiley; 1994.

91. Robouch P, Eguskiza M, Maguregui MI, Pomme S, Pauwels J. k0-NAA, a valuable tool for reference-material producers. *Fresenius J Anal Chem* 2001;370(2–3):255–258.

92. Digenis GA, Sandefer EP, Beihn RM, Parr AF. Dual-isotope imaging of neutron-activated erbium-171 and samarium-153 and the *in vivo* evaluation of a dual-labeled bilayer tablet by gamma scintigraphy. *Pharm Res* 1991;8(10):1335–1340.

93. Awang MB, Hardy JG, Davis SS, Wilding IR, Parry SJ. Radiolabeling of pharmaceutical dosage forms by neutron activation of samarium-152. *J Labelled Compounds Radiopharmaceuticals* 1993;33(10):941–948.

94. Awang MB, Hardy JG, Davis SS, Pimm MV, Parry SJ, Wilding IR. Evaluation of [153]Sm-diethylenetriaminepentaacetic acid for radiolabelling of pharmaceutical dosage forms by neutron activation. *Nucl Med Biol* 1994;21(7):905–909.

95. Ohta A, Siraishi F, Nagahara T, Tomura K. Neutron activation analysis of biological samples. *Nippon Rinsho* 1996;54(1):207–214.

96. Albert DA, Cohen AJ, Mandelbrot DA, Reinhardt CP, Dickson EW. Neutron-activation analysis: a novel method for the assay of iohexol. *J Lab Clin Med* 2003;141(2): 106–109.

97. Rajurkar NS, Pardeshi BM. Analysis of some herbal plants from India used in the control of diabetes mellitus by NAA and AAS techniques. *Appl Radiat Isot* 1997; 48(8):1059–1062.

98. Jasper JP. The increasing use of stable isotopes in the pharmaceutical industry. *Pharm Tech* 1999;23(10):106–114.

99. Jasper JP. Quantitative estimates of precision for molecular isotopic measurements. *Rapid Commun Mass Spectrom* 2001;15:1554–1557.

100. Kapetanovic IM, Kupferberg HJ. Stable isotope methodology and gas chromatography mass spectrometry in a pharmacokinetic study of phenobarbitol. *Biomed Mass Spectrom* 1980;7:47–52.

101. Schneider LV, Hall MP. Stable isotope methods for high-precision proteomics. *Drug Discov Today* 2005;10(5):353–363.

102. Stöcklin R, Arrighi J-F, Hoang-Van K, Vu L, Cerini F, Gilles N, Genet R, Markussen J, Offord RE, Rose K. Positive and negative labelling of human proinsulin, insulin and C-peptide with stable isotopes: new tools for metabolic and pharmacokinetic studies. In Chapman J, Ed. *Protein and Peptide Analysis: Advances in the Use of Mass Spectrometry,* Methods in Molecular Biology. Totowa, NJ: Humana Press; 2000, Vol 146, pp 293–315.

103. Kippen AD, Cerini F, Vadas L, Stöcklin R, Vu L, Offord RE, Rose K. Development of an isotope dilution assay for precise determination of insulin, C-peptide and proinsulin levels in non-diabetic and type II diabetic individuals with comparison to immunoassay. *J Biol Chem* 1997;272:12513–12522.

104. Vallano PT, Shugarts SB, Woolf EJ, Matuszewski BK. Elimination of autosampler carryover in a bioanalytical HPLC-MS/MS method: a case study. *J Pharm Biomed Anal* 2005;36(5):1073–1078.

105. Jemal M, Xia YQ. Bioanalytical method validation design for the simultaneous quantitation of analytes that may undergo interconversion during analysis. *J Pharm Biomed Anal* 2000;22(5):813–827.

106. Wang CJ, Pao LH, Hsiong CH, Wu CY, Whang-Peng JJ, Hu OY. Novel inhibition of cis/trans retinoic acid interconversion in biological fluids—an accurate method for determination of trans and 13-cis retinoic acid in biological fluids. *J Chromatogr B Analyt Technol Biomed Life Sci* 2003;796(2):283–291.

107. Sherma J. Chromatographic methods of analysis—thin layer chromatography. In *Encyclopedia of Pharmaceutical Technology*, 2nd ed. New York: Dekker Encyclopedias Taylor and Francis Group LLC; 2002, pp 426–439.

108. Coran SA, Giannellini V, Bambagiotti-Alberti M. High-performance thin-layer chromatographic-densitometric determination of secoisolariciresinol diglucoside in flaxseed. *J Chromatogr A* 2004;1045(1–2):217–222.

109. Petrovic M, Kastelan-Macan M, Ivankovic D, Matecic S. Video-densitometric quantitation of fluorescence quenching on totally irradiated thin-layer chromatographic plates. *J AOAC Int* 2000;83(6):1457–1462.

110. Hauck HE, Schultz M. Ultrathin-layer chromatography. *J Chromatogr Sci* 2002;40(10): 550–552.

111. Agrawal H, Kaul N, Paradkar AR, Mahadik KR. HPTLC method for guggulsterone I. Quantitative determination of E- and Z-guggulsterone in herbal extract and pharmaceutical dosage form. *J Pharm Biomed Anal* 2004;36:33–41.

112. Babu SK, Kumar KV, Subbaraju GV. Estimation of *trans*-resveratrol in herbal extracts and dosage forms by high-performance thin-layer chromatography. *Chem Pharm Bull* 2005;53(6):691–693.

113. Mahadik KR, Paradkar AR, Agrawal H, Kaul N. Stability-indicating HPTLC determination of tizanidine hydrochloride in bulk drug and pharmaceutical formulations. *J Pharm Biomed Anal* 2003;33(4):545–552.

114. Makhija SN, Vavia PR. Stability indicating HPTLC method for the simultaneous determination of pseudoephedrine and cetirizine in pharmaceutical formulations. *J Pharm Biomed Anal* 2001;25(3–4):663–667.

115. Campbell AN, Sherma J. Development and validation of a high-performance thin-layer chromatographic method with densitometric detection for determination of bisacodyl in pharmaceutical tablets. *ACTA Chromatogr* 2003;13:109–116.

116. Agrawal H, Mahadik KR, Paradkar AH, Kaul N. Stability indicating HPTLC determination of linezolid as bulk drug and in pharmaceutical dosage form. *Drug Dev Ind Pharm* 2003;29(10):1119–1126.

117. Kaul N, Agrawal H, Patil B, Kakad A, Dhaneshwar SR. Application of stability-indicating HPTLC method for quantitative determination of metadoxine in pharmaceutical dosage form. *Il Farmaco* 2005;60:351–360.

118. Pandya KK, Mody VD, Satia MC, Modi IA, Chakravarthy BK, Gandhi TP. High-performance thin-layer chromatographic method for the detection and determination of lansoprazole in human plasma and its use in pharmacokinetic studies. *J Chromatogr B Biomed Sci Appl* 1997;693(1):199–204.

119. Savale HS, Pandya KK, Gandhi TP, Modi IA, Modi RI, Satia MC. Plasma analysis of celiprolol by HPTLC: a useful technique for pharmacokinetic studies. *J AOAC Int* 2001;84(4):1252–1257.

120. Adamovics JA, ed. *Chromatographic Analysis of Pharmaceuticals*. New York: Marcel Dekker; 1997.

121. Hahn-Deinstrop E. *Applied Thin-Layer Chromatography. Best Practices and Avoidance of Mistakes*. Weinheim, Germany: Wiley-VCH; 2000.

122. Snyder LR, Kirkland JJ, Glajch JL. *Practical HPLC Method Development*, 2nd ed. Hoboken, NJ: Wiley-Interscience; 1997.

123. Clarke NJ, Rindgen D, Korfmacher WA, Cox KA. Systematic LC/MS metabolite identification in drug discovery. *Anal Chem* 2001;73(15):430A–439A.

124. Volmer DA, Sleno L. Mass analyzers: an overview of several designs and their applications, Part I. *Spectroscopy* 2005;20(11):20–26.

125. Ackermann BL, Berna MJ, Murphy AT. Recent advances in use of LC/MS/MS for quantitative high-throughput bioanalytical support of drug discovery. *Curr Top Med Chem* 2002;2(1):53–66.

126. Vallano PT, Shugarts SB, Kline WF, Woolf EJ, Matuszewski BK. Determination of risedronate in human urine by column-switching ion-pair high-performance liquid chromatography with ultraviolet detection. *J Chromatogr B Analyt Technol Biomed Life Sci* 2003;794(1):23–33.

127. Watzig H, Gunter S. Capillary electrophoresis—a high performance analytical separation technique. *Clin Chem Lab Med* 2003;41(6):724–738.

128. Altria KD, Elder D. Overview of the status and applications of capillary electrophoresis to the analysis of small molecules. *J Chromatogr A* 2004;1023(1):1–14, 720–723.

129. Hempel G. Biomedical applications of capillary electrophoresis. *Clin Chem Lab Med* 2003;41(6):720–723.

130. Belder D, Ludwig M. Microchip electrophoresis for chiral separations. *Electrophoresis* 2003;24(15):2422–2430.

131. Pang HM, Kenseth J, Coldiron S. High-throughput multiplexed capillary electrophoresis in drug discovery. *Drug Discov Today* 2004;9(24):1072–1080.

132. Koh HL, Yau WP, Ong PS, Hegde A. Current trends in modern pharmaceutical analysis for drug discovery. *Drug Discov Today* 2003;8(19):889–897.

133. Federsel HJ. Asymmetry on large scale: the roadmap to stereoselective processes. *Nat Rev Drug Discov* 2005;4(8):685–697.

134. Islam MR, Mahdi JG, Bowen ID. Pharmacological importance of stereochemical resolution of enantiomeric drugs. *Drug Safety* 1997;17(3):149–165.

135. Srinivas NR, Barbhaiya RH, Midha KK. Enantiomeric drug development: issues, considerations, and regulatory requirements. *J Pharm Sci* 2001;90(9):1205–1215.

136. Torchin CD, McNeilly PJ, Kapetanovic IM, Strong JM, Kupferberg HJ. Stereoselective metabolism of a new anticonvulsant drug candidate, losigamone, by human liver microsomes. *Drug Metab Dispos* 1996;24(9):1002–1008.

137. Waldeck B. Three-dimensional pharmacology, a subject ranging from ignorance to overstatements. *Pharmacol Toxicol* 2003;93(5):203–210.

138. Srinivas NR. Simultaneous chiral analyses of multiple analytes: case studies, implications and method development considerations. *Biomed Chromatogr* 2004; 18(10):759–784.

139. Srinivas NR. Evaluation of experimental strategies for the development of chiral chromatographic methods based on diastereomer formation. *Biomed Chromatogr* 2004; 18(4):207–233.

140. Haginaka J. Pharmaceutical and biomedical applications of enantioseparations using liquid chromatographic techniques. *J Pharm Biomed Anal* 2002;27(3–4):357–372.

141. Ward TJ. Chiral separations. *Anal Chem* 2002;74(12):2863–2872.

142. Amini A. Recent developments in chiral capillary electrophoresis and applications of this technique to pharmaceutical and biomedical analysis. *Electrophoresis* 2001;22(15): 3107–3130.

143. Andersson S, Allenmark SG. Preparative chiral chromatographic resolution of enantiomers in drug discovery. *J Biochem Biophys Methods* 2002;54(1–3):11–23.

144. Bonato PS. Recent advances in the determination of enantiomeric drugs and their metabolites in biological fluids by capillary electrophoresis-mediated microanalysis. *Electrophoresis* 2003;24(22–23):4078–4094.

145. Millot MC. Separation of drug enantiomers by liquid chromatography and capillary electrophoresis, using immobilized proteins as chiral selectors. *J Chromatogr B Analyt Technol Biomed Life Sci* 2003;797(1–2):131–159.

146. Rizzi A. Fundamental aspects of chiral separations by capillary electrophoresis. *Electrophoresis* 2001;22(15):3079–3106.

147. Scriba GK. Selected fundamental aspects of chiral electromigration techniques and their application to pharmaceutical and biomedical analysis. *J Pharm Biomed Anal* 2002; 27(3–4):373–399.

148. Scriba GK. Pharmaceutical and biomedical applications of chiral capillary electrophoresis and capillary electrochromatography: an update. *Electrophoresis* 2003;24(15): 2409–2421.

149. Misl'anova C, Hutta M. Role of biological matrices during the analysis of chiral drugs by liquid chromatography. *J Chromatogr B Analyt Technol Biomed Life Sci* 2003; 797(1–2):91–109.

150. Martin CR, Kohli P. The emerging field of nanotube biotechnology. *Nat Rev Drug Discov* 2003;2(1):29–37.

151. Bansal SK, Layloff T, Bush ED, Hamilton M, Hankinson EA, Landy JS. Qualification of analytical instruments for use in the pharmaceutical industry: a scientific approach. *AAPS PharmSciTech* 2004;5(1):E22.

152. Furman WB, Layloff TP, Tetzlaff J. Validation of computerized liquid chromatographic Systems. *J AOAC* 1994;77:1314–1318.

153. Grisanti V, Zachowski EJ. Operational and performance qualification. *LCGC North America* 2002;20 (4):356–362.

154. Huber L. *Validation and Qualification in Analytical Laboratories*. Boca Raton, FL: CRC Press; 1999.

155. Chan CC, Herman Lam H, Lee YC, Xue-Ming Zhang XM, Eds. *Analytical Method Validation and Instrument Performance Verification*. Hoboken, NJ: Wiley; 2004.

156. US Food and Drug Administration. *General Principles of Software Validation. Final Guidance for Industry and FDA Staff*. Rockville, MD: US Department of Health and Human Services, Food and Drug Administration; Jan 2002.

157. Shah VP, Midha KK, Findlay JW, Hill HM, Hulse JD, McGilveray IJ. Bioanalytical method validation—a revisit with a decade of progress. *Pharm Res* 2000;17(12): 1551–1557.

158. ICH Q2A: Text on Validation of Analytical Procedures. Fed Reg 1995;60 FR11260. http://www.fda.gov/cder/guidance/ichq2a.pdf.

159. ICH Q2B: Validation of Analytical Procedures: Methodology. Fed Reg 1997; 62 FR 27463. http://www.fda.gov/cder/guidance/1320fnl.pdf.

160. *Guidance for Industry: Analytical Procedures and Methods Validation, Chemistry, Manufacturing and Controls Documentation*. Rockville, MD: US Deptartment of Health and Human Services, Food and Drug Administration; 2000. http://www.fda.gov/cder/guidance/2396dft.pdf.

161. *Guidance for Industry: Bioanalytical Method Validation*. Rockville, MD: US Deptartment of Health and Human Services, Food and Drug Administration; 2001.

162. Hartmann C, Smeyers-Verbeke J, Massart DL, McDowall RD. Validation of bioanalytical chromatographic methods. *J Pharm Biomed Anal* 1998;17(2):193–218.

163. ICH Q1A(R2): Stability Testing of New Drug Substances and Products (Second Revision). *Fed Reg* 2003;68(225). http://www.ich.org/MediaServer.jser?@_ID=419&@_MODE=GLB.

164. ICH Q1B: Photostability Testing of New Drug Substances and Products. *Fed Reg* 1997;62(95):27115–27122.   http://www.ich.org/MediaServer.jser?@_ID=412&@_ MODE=GLB.

165. ICH Q1C: Stability Testing for New Dosage Forms. *Fed Reg* 1997;62(90)25634–25635. http://www.ich.org/MediaServer.jser?@_ID=413&@_MODE=GLB.

166. ICH Q1D: Bracketing and Matrixing Designs for Stability Testing of Drug Substances and Drug Products. *Fed Reg* 2003;68(11):2339–2340. http://www.ich.org/MediaServer. jser?@_ID=414&@_MODE=GLB.

167. ICH Q1E: Evaluation of Stability Data. *Fed Reg* 2004;69(110):32010–32011. http://www. ich.org/MediaServer.jser?@_ID=415&@_MODE=GLB.

168. ICH Q1F: Stability Data Package for Registration Applications in Climatic Zones III and IV. *Fed Reg* 2003;68(225):65717–65718. http://www.ich.org/MediaServer.jser?@_ ID=416&@_MODE=GLB.

169. ICH Q3A(R): Impurities in New Drug Substances (Revised Guideline). *Fed Reg* 2003;68(68):6924–6925. http://www.ich.org/MediaServer.jser?@_ID=422&@_ MODE=GLB.

170. ICH Q3B(R): Impurities in New Drug Products (Revised Guideline). *Fed Reg* 2003;68(220):64628–64629. http://www.ich.org/MediaServer.jser?@_ID=421&@_ MODE=GLB.

171. ICH Q3C: Impurities: Guideline for Residual Solvents. *Fed Reg* 1997;62(247):67377. http://www.ich.org/MediaServer.jser?@_ID=423&@_MODE=GLB.

172. ICH Q5C: Quality of Biotechnological Products: Stability Testing of Biotechnological/ Biological Products. *Fed Reg* 1996;61:36466. http://www.ich.org/MediaServer. jser?@_ID=427&@_MODE=GLB.

173. Q9: Quality Risk Management. *Fed Reg* 2005;70(151):45722–45723. http://www.ich.org/ LOB/media/MEDIA1957.pdf.

174. United States Pharmacopoeial Convention. *United States Pharmacopoeia 26, National Formulary 21, ⟨1225⟩ Validation of Compendial Methods*. Rockville, MD: United States Pharmacopoeial Convention; 2003.

175. *Pharmacopeial Forum* 2005;31(2):549.

176. Swartz ME, Kull IS. Validation, qualification, or verification. *LCGC North America* 2005;23(10):47.

177. *Pharmacopeial Forum* 2005;31(2):555.

178. ISO 9000:2000 *Quality Management Systems—Fundamentals and Vocabulary*. Geneva, Switzerland: International Organization for Standardization; 2000.

179. ISO 9001:2000 *Quality Management System—Requirements*. Geneva, Switzerland: International Organization for Standardization; 2000.

180. ISO 9002:2000 *Production and Installation QMS Only*. Geneva, Switzerland: International Organization for Standardization; 2000.

181. ISO 9000:2005 *Quality Management Systems—Fundamentals and Vocabulary*. Geneva, Switzerland: International Organization for Standardization; 2005.

182. ISO/IEC 90003:2004 Software *Engineerin—Guidelines for the Application of ISO 9001:2000 to Computer Software*. Geneva, Switzerland: International Organization for Standardization; 2004.

183. ANSI/ISO/ASQ Q9000-2000 *Series—Quality Management Standards*. Milwaukee: ASQ Quality Press; 2001.

184. ISO/IEC Guide 25: *General Requirements for the Competence of Calibration and Testing Laboratories*, 3rd edition. Geneva, Switzerland: International Organization for Standardization; 1990.

185. ISO/IEC DIS 17025: *General Requirements for the Competence of Testing and Calibration Laboratories*. Geneva, Switzerland: International Organization for Standardization; 1998.

186. ISO/IEC 17025:2005 *General Requirements for the Competence of Testing and Calibration Laboratories*. Geneva, Switzerland: International Organization for Standardization; 2005.

187. Taylor JK. *Quality Assurance of Chemical Measurements*. Chelsea, MI: Lewis Publishers; 1987, p 36.

188. Lide D. *Handbook of Chemistry and Physics*, 86th ed. Boca Raton, FL: CRC Press; 2005.

189. Reviewer Guidance: Validation of Chromatographic Methods. Rockville, MD: US Department of Health and Human Services, Food and Drug Administration, Center for Drug Evaluation and Research (CDER); 1994. http://www.fdagov/cder/guidance/cmc3.pdf.

190. Ermer J, Vogel M. Applications of hyphenated LC-MS techniques in pharmaceutical analysis. *Biomed Chromatogr* 2000;14(6):373–383.

6

CHEMICAL AND PHYSICAL CHARACTERIZATIONS OF POTENTIAL NEW CHEMICAL ENTITY

ADEGOKE ADENIJI AND ADEBOYE ADEJARE*

Philadelphia College of Pharmacy, University of the Sciences in Philadelphia, Philadelphia, Pennsylvania

Contents

6.1   INTRODUCTION

A new chemical entity (NCE) is a compound that has not been approved as a pharmaceutical agent for a particular indication. In the United States, the approving body is the Food and Drug Administration (FDA) and most countries have a similar agency [1]. The compound may be an already approved drug being evaluated for a

---

*Corresponding author.

Preclinical Development Handbook: ADME and Biopharmaceutical Properties,
edited by Shayne Cox Gad
Copyright © 2008 John Wiley & Sons, Inc.

new indication or a novel compound. New regulations, the ever increasing demand for drugs worldwide, and an unprecedented need to drive drug prices lower challenge the pharmaceutical companies and point to the need to put more lead compounds into the development pipeline [2]. While these chemical entities are constantly being synthesized or isolated from natural sources in various academic and industrial laboratories throughout the world, very few compounds make it to the market as drugs. It is estimated that only one out of every 5000 synthesized compounds ends up on the market as a therapeutically useful drug [3].

Elucidation of the chemical and physical properties of a potential NCE is critical to drug discovery efforts as part of "pharmaceutical profiling." Knowledge of these properties could give insight into how the compound acts or binds to the target receptor to elicit desired or undesired effects and also help with formulation studies [4, 5]. Based on these properties, some compounds could be dismissed as possible drug candidates. For instance, a compound being proposed for intravenous administration that has very poor aqueous solubility might not be favorably considered because of envisaged problems with formulation and bioavailability. Indeed, the fate of many NCEs are decided immediately after the chemical and physical properties of the compounds are determined. These properties often serve as indices by which a compound will be judged for its "drugability" and likelihood of eliciting the desired response. Thus, the journey to the market for a compound that becomes a drug begins with determination of its basic chemical and physical properties such as the mass, structure, solubility, and stability. Further physicochemical characterizations, for example, if the compound has different polymorphs, may follow should the compound exhibit a desired biological profile. However, those may not be warranted if a "cut" decision is made at an earlier stage. A stage-appropriate characterization is therefore critical for every potential NCE for maximization of resources. The most common chemical and physical characterization methods for a novel potential NCE and two examples will be described. If the potential NCE is already approved for an indication, then many pertinent chemical and physical properties would have been determined and are likely to be in literature. This brief chapter focuses on small molecules although many of the methods described have been adapted to characterize therapeutic proteins and other macromolecules.

6.2   DETERMINATION OF MASS

Most drugs are small molecules with mass in the range 100–1000 amu. There are, however, notable exceptions such as lithium salts at the lower end, while peptides, proteins, and antibodies being used in therapy could have masses much greater than 1000 amu. The mass of a compound is the sum of the atomic masses of its constituent elements. It is generally expected that a non-ionic compound with low molecular mass will be absorbed more readily than one with high mass under similar conditions, such as being in the same chemical class and dosage form. This is particularly true for orally administered drugs. Lipinski's rule of five [6, 7] indicates that a molecular mass less than or equal to 500 is essential for passive absorption of an orally administered drug. There are several methods used to determine the molecular mass of a compound. These methods include vapor density, vapor pressure osmometry, cryoscopy, elemental analysis, and undoubtedly the most popular and important, mass spectrometry [8–11]. Mass spectrometry (MS) and elemental analysis are the two major techniques used in mass determination. MS is a very versatile tool that is applicable in several fields of science and new applications are being found. It involves a high energy bombardment of the molecule of interest to generate charged fragments, which are detected based on the mass/charge ratio. The mass of the compound is established by the mass of the molecular ion or those of its fragments. The molecular formula and the structure of the compound can also be obtained by studying the fragmentation pattern of the compound [9, 10]. MS has also been widely used in determining the structures of proteins and other macromolecules. Quite often, the molecular masses of such peptides and proteins can be inferred from fragment ions.

Elemental analysis, on the other hand, determines the composition of a sample by giving the amount (usually percentage weight) of each element that is present in the sample. It is often based on oxidation of an organic compound at elevated temperatures to produce gaseous molecules of the elements of interest, which are then separated and analyzed [11]. It is very useful as it gives values from which the empirical formula of the compound can be calculated. The molecular formula can then be determined from the empirical formula and molecular weight. By determining the proportion of the constituent elements of a compound, the purity of the compound can also be established.

6.3   STRUCTURE ELUCIDATION

Most drugs are weakly acidic or basic organic compounds [12]. The determination of structure helps to identify the functional groups on the compound, validate the synthetic or isolation pathway, and initiate structure–activity relationship studies that are very important in drug discovery [13]. It also helps to determine physicochemical parameters. The process of structure elucidation involves determining the elements present and their bonding arrangements in the compound and establishes the identity of the chemical entity. Several methods are used for structure elucidation, most of which are spectroscopic. Of these, nuclear magnetic resonance (NMR) is the most versatile and is thus a key tool in determining structures of molecules. NMR exploits the ability of certain nuclei to align themselves either with or against the field when placed in a magnetic field. Since the effective magnetic field experienced by these nuclei is influenced by the electronic environment in their proximity (e.g., the presence of a neighboring strongly electronegative atom), information about atom connectivity can be deduced from spectra analysis [14]. Both ^{1}H- and ^{13}C-NMR are widely used but several other nuclei such as ^{19}F and ^{31}P are also utilized [14–16].

Ultraviolet/Visible (UV/Vis) spectroscopy and particularly infrared (IR) spectroscopy are also widely used. UV/Vis spectroscopy gives information about the presence of chromophores (i.e., conjugated double bonds), which are responsible for selective absorption of radiation in a given wavelength range [14]. IR spectroscopy gives information about functional groups in the molecule. Both methods are based on the ability of compounds to absorb a fraction of incident radiation. In IR spectroscopy, the absorption frequency confirms the presence of particular functional groups (e.g., carbonyl, hydroxyl, and aryl) since these values are consistent and only slightly influenced by adjacent groups in the molecule. There are charts and tables in the literature that list the absorption frequencies of common organic functional groups and they can be used as reference. The electronic collection of spectra and the availability of spectra simulating software have increased the usefulness of these and other spectroscopic techniques.

Polarimetry measures the ability of a sample to rotate plane polarized light. It is critical for the characterization of optically active or chiral compounds. The specific rotation of a chemical compound. $[\alpha]_D^T$ is defined as the observed angle of rotation α, when light of 589 nm wavelength (the sodium D line) is passed through a sample with a pathlength of 0.1 m and a sample concentration of 1 g/ml at temperature T. It is usually measured at 20 °C. It is applicable for both qualitative and quantitative purposes since the extent of light rotation is dependent on the molecular structure and the concentration of the sample. Thus, it can be used to determine enantiomeric purity of a sample.

X-ray crystallography gives vital information about the crystal structure of a compound using diffraction techniques. It allows for measurement of atomic connectivity, bond lengths, bond angles, and torsion angles, thereby giving very detailed information about the structure of a compound [14]. The compounds, however, need to be crystallizable, which is sometimes very difficult, especially for large macromolecules such as protein and DNA complexes. For small molecules, it can be used to determine absolute configurations at chiral centers. This can become very important in discovery efforts as it can help explain compound reactivity and binding to receptors (proteins), which contain many chiral centers.

6.4 PURITY

The presence of impurities in an NCE can not only affect the physicochemical properties but could also preclude correct assessment of the bioactivity and toxicity profiles of the target compound. It is generally desirable that the compound be available in a very pure form before incorporation into any dosage form for *in vitro* or *in vivo* studies. Several methods including some that have been discussed earlier can be used to assess the purity of a compound. These methods include NMR, mass spectrometry, chromatography, UV spectroscopy, IR spectroscopy, and polarimetry. However, in many cases, the very first test to determine the purity is melting point (mp) for solids and boiling point (bp) for liquids. A broad range of values for either parameter is usually indicative of impurity [17]. The mp and bp as well as the refractive index and density are defining characteristics of a compound. Refractive index measures the ratio of the velocity of light in air to that in the sample at a particular wavelength, temperature, and pressure.

Chromatography separates mixtures based on the different rates of movement of the components along an adsorbent medium. Ever since its invention by the Russian botanist Mikhail Tswett in the early twentieth century [18], its application has increased tremendously to earn it a place of pride in analytical science. From the relatively simple thin layer chromatography (TLC) to the more technical gas chromatography (GC) and high performance liquid chromatography (HPLC), chromatographic techniques allow for separation of the components of a sample based on the ease of mobility through a stationary phase. The presence of a single band in TLC or a single peak in HPLC or GC suggests high purity of the new compound. Various detectors can be used, from UV to fluorescence to MS. Chromatographic techniques are used not only to determine purity but also in purification [19]. The high sensitivity shown by the low limit of detection of these techniques has been employed in quantitative compound determination in plasma and other matrices, where they have been used to detect nanogram/milliliter concentrations of drugs [20, 21]. A major advantage of chromatographic techniques is that they can be adapted for quantitative determinations and/or joined with other techniques to give hyphenated methods (e.g., LC-MS). HPLC has also been used in determining purity of enantiomers [22, 23]. In such cases, a chiral column or derivatization technique to give diastereomers is employed.

6.5 SOLUBILITY AND LIPOPHILICITY

Solubility of a sample in a solvent refers to the amount of the sample that will dissolve in the given solvent at a particular temperature. It is generally desirable for a drug molecule to have some level of water solubility. Poor water solubility can present many problems from reliability and reproducibility of several *in vitro* tests to significant formulation issues [7, 24]. Solubility is typically measured using the shake flask method. The shake flask method involves adding an excess amount of a solid sample to a flask containing a specified amount of buffer; the saturated solution is then agitated until it attains equilibrium, after which the undissolved sample is separated from the solution and the concentration of the sample is determined usually by UV spectroscopy or another applicable technique [25].

Since most drugs are weak acids or bases [11], the pK_a is an important parameter used to study and predict the behavior of an NCE in a physiological environment. The pK_a or *dissociation constant* is a measure of the acid strength of a compound. It allows for determination of the predominant state of an ionizable compound at any given pH and therefore affects solubility of the compound. In general, aqueous solubility increases with ionization. The pK_a can be determined using several methods such as capillary electrophoresis, liquid chromatography, and potentiometry.

The relevant equations are

$$pK_a = -\log K_a \tag{6.1}$$

Acids: $HA \rightleftharpoons H^+ + A^-$

$$K_a = [H^+][A^-]/[HA], \quad \text{where } [\,] = \text{molar concentration} \tag{6.2}$$

Bases: $HB^+ \rightleftharpoons H^+ + B$

$$K_a = [H^+][B]/[HB^+] \tag{6.3}$$

Lipophilicity refers to the tendency of a compound to partition into nonpolar (organic) versus aqueous environments [26]. Log P refers to the logarithm of the partition coefficient and it is the most common measure of lipophilicity of a compound. The partition coefficient is a constant that defines the ratio of a compound in aqueous medium to the compound in an immiscible solvent at equilibrium. The most commonly used organic solvent for biological purposes is 2-octanol. The partition coefficient is probably one of the most important physicochemical properties that infer the crossing of a drug across biological membranes, binding to proteins, and, consequently, the activity and the ease of excretion from the body. The partition coefficient has been shown to correlate with the activity of many classes of drugs [27, 28]. A compound with log $P > 5$ is usually not considered a good candidate in drug development [6, 7] because it is considered to be too lipophilic.

$$\log P = \log_{10}(\text{Partition coefficient}) \qquad (6.4)$$

where Partition coefficient, $P = [\text{Organic}]/[\text{Aqueous}]$.

It is generally desirable for an NCE to possess enough water solubility so that it can dissolve in body fluids while also possessing sufficient lipophilicity to cross biological membranes. Log P describes the partitioning for a neutral and un-ionizable molecule, which is often not the case. For ionizable compounds, log P is expected to change with pH. The relationship between log P and pH is described by the log distribution coefficient (log D), also called the apparent partition coefficient. Log D, unlike log P, changes with pH as it depends on the acidic or basic nature of the compound. The log D at pH 7.4 is often used as an index of the behavior of a sample in plasma.

$$\text{Distribution coefficient, } D = [\text{Un-ionized}]_{(o)}/[\text{Un-ionized}]_{(aq)} + [\text{Ionized}]_{(aq)} \qquad (6.5)$$

$$\log D = \log_{10}(\text{Distribution coefficient}) \qquad (6.6)$$

$$\log D_{(pH)} = \log P - \log(1 + 10^{(pH - pK_a)}) \quad \text{for acids} \qquad (6.7)$$

$$\log D_{(pH)} = \log P - \log(1 + 10^{(pK_a - pH)}) \quad \text{for bases} \qquad (6.8)$$

6.6   STABILITY

Physical and chemical stability considerations become essential to estimate how long the NCE can be stored without significant decomposition. Stability is usually determined by monitoring particular properties of the compound over a period of time, usually days or weeks and sometimes months, under specified storage conditions, which are often designed to be more unfavorable (stress testing) than the envisioned storage conditions [29, 30]. The stability of the compound is assessed in the presence of elevated temperature, light, high relative humidity (75% or higher), varying pH range, and an oxidative environment.

6.7   PROTEINS AND PEPTIDES

Peptides usually exhibit poor *in vivo* stability, pharmacokinetics, and bioavailability. These often pose a major challenge to drug discovery and development efforts. Therefore, most drugs are small molecules or peptidomimetics [31]. With advances in drug delivery and more sophisticated equipment, an increasing number of peptides and proteins are being used in therapy [32, 33].

6.8   MISCELLANEOUS TECHNIQUES

There are many other techniques used to decipher other chemical and/or physical properties of an NCE. Examples include circular dichroism (CD), Raman spectroscopy, and differential scanning calorimetry (DSC). CD is a type of absorption spectroscopy often used to determine optical properties and secondary structures of molecules. While it can be used for any optically active molecule, it is more critical in cases of biomolecules such as sugars, amino acids, peptides, and proteins when embarking on structural determination. It measures the difference in the absorption of right- and left-circularly polarized light as a function of wavelength. It is used extensively to study secondary protein structures: how the secondary structure of a molecule changes as a function of temperature or the concentration of denaturing agents, thus making it a vital tool in assessing the physical and chemical stability of peptides and proteins. Raman spectroscopy is a technique that is used to study the vibrational, rotational, and low frequency modes in a system. Its use derives from the Raman effect, which is the inelastic scatter of photons following light incidence. Its principal use is to identify a compound based on a fingerprint that is unique to the compound, since vibrational information is very specific for chemical bonds in molecules. The fingerprint region of organic molecules is in the range of 500–2000 cm^{-1}. More uses are being discovered for MS. High resolution MS is being accepted as a substitute for elemental analysis by several journals. Purity of amines is sometimes difficult to determine using chromatographic techniques. An MS-based technique that can help identify amine impurities using hydrogen/deuterium exchange has been developed [34].

DSC is a thermoanalytical method that measures the difference in heat absorbed by a chemical compound and a reference as a function of temperature when the two are subjected to the same regulated temperature conditions. It measures the changes in heat flow as the sample and reference undergo any physical transformation, such as phase transition. It is related to several parameters of a compound and is thus used mainly to establish identity and purity of chemical compounds among other uses such as polymorph characterization [35, 36].

6.9   CASE STUDIES

For illustration, we now examine the chemical and physical characterizations of two new potential NCEs.

Example A.   4-Fluoro-*N*-(adamantan-2-yl)-benzenesulfonamide (Fig. 6.1) is a novel compound that was designed and synthesized as a gamma secretase inhibitor [37, 38]. Gamma secretase is an enzyme involved in amyloid precursor protein processing to give amyloid peptides, which are the building blocks of the plaques found in the brains of patients with Alzheimer's disease (AD). It has been hypothesized that gamma secretase inhibitors can halt the onset and/or progression of AD. After synthesis, the melting point for the target compound was determined to be 150–152 °C. The narrow range suggested good purity for the sample. Elucidation of the structure was carried out using IR spectroscopy and NMR, the results of which

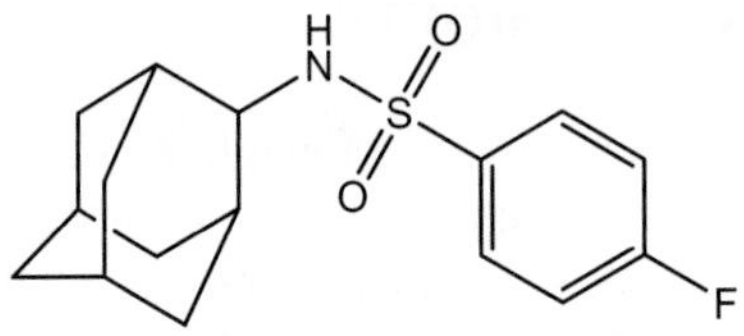

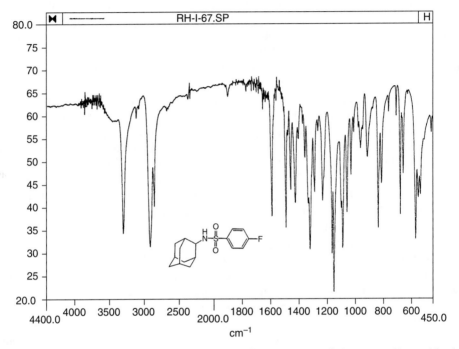

FIGURE 6.1   Structure of 4-fluoro-*N*-(adamantan-2-yl)-benzenesulfonamide.

FIGURE 6.2   FT-IR spectrum of 4-fluoro-*N*-(adamantan-2-yl)-benzenesulfonamide in KBr.

confirmed the presence of the expected functional groups. IR (KBr) cm^{-1}: 3300 (NH); 1322, 1166 (O=S=O); 1234 (Ar—F) (Fig. 6.2). The ^{1}H-, ^{13}C-, and ^{19}F-NMR results further confirmed the presence of the expected functional groups; the results are shown in Fig. 6.3. The molecular mass determination using mass spectrometry and elemental analysis, the results of which are shown below, also support the proposed structure of the compound.

MS ESI (*m/z*, species, %): 308.3, [M—H]$^{-}$, 100% as shown in Fig. 6.4.

The elemental analysis of the compound showed the proportion of the constituent elements to be the following. Calculation for $C_{16}H_{20}FNO_2S$: C, 62.11; H, 6.52; F, 6.14; N, 4.53. Found: C, 62.06; H, 6.49; F, 6.43; N, 4.37. The "found" is within ±0.4 of the calculated values and thus consistent with the proposed structure.

^{1}H-NMR (CDCl$_3$) δ: 7.9 (s, 2H, 2 × Ar—CH), 7.4–7.1 (d, 2H, 2 × Ar—H), 4.9 (s, 1H, 1 × NH), 3.4 (s, 1H, 1 × CH), 1.8–1.5 (m, 15H, 5 × CH$_2$, 5 × CH).

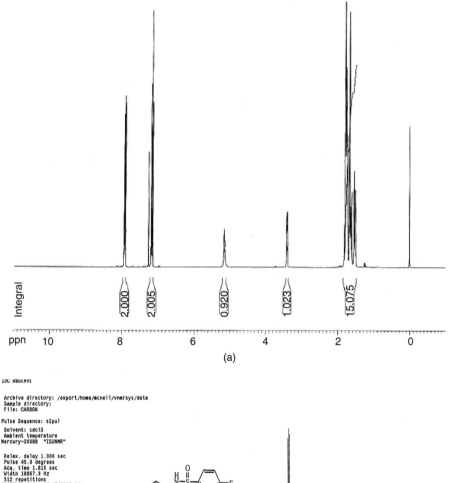

13C OBSERVE

Archive directory: /export/home/mcneil/vnmrsys/data
Sample directory:
File: CARBON

Pulse Sequence: s2pul

Solvent: cdcl3
Ambient temperature
Mercury-300BB "ISUNMR"

Relax. delay 1.000 sec
Pulse 45.0 degrees
Acq. time 1.815 sec
Width 18867.9 Hz
512 repetitions
OBSERVE C13, 75.4549300 MHz
DECOUPLE H1, 300.0805374 MHz
Power 40 dB
continuously on
WALTZ-16 modulated
DATA PROCESSING
Line broadening 1.0 Hz
FT size 131072
Total time 24 min, 51 sec

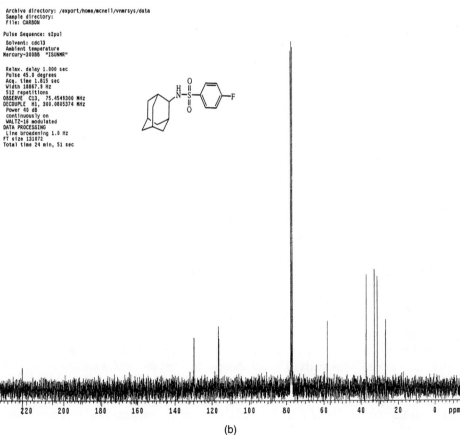

FIGURE 6.3 (a) H-NMR, (b) ^{13}C-NMR, and (c) ^{19}F-NMR of 4-fluoro-*N*-(adamantan-2-yl)-benzenesulfonamide in CDCl$_3$.

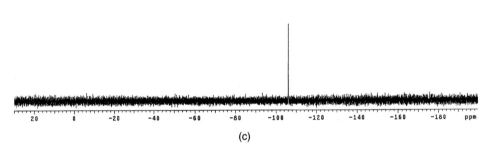

Archive directory: /export/home/pharmacy/vnmrsys/data
Sample directory: RW-I-67f_22May2003
File: FLUORINE

Pulse Sequence: s2pul

Solvent: CDCl3
Ambient temperature
Mercury-300BB "ISUNMR"

Relax. delay 1.500 sec
Pulse 30.0 degrees
Acq. time 0.300 sec
Width 64935.1 Hz
16 repetitions
OBSERVE F19, 282.3565651 MHz
DATA PROCESSING
Line broadening 0.3 Hz
FT size 65536
Total time 0 min, 31 sec

(c)

FIGURE 6.3 *Continued*

^{13}C-NMR (CDCl$_3$) δ: 130 (s, 2C, 1 × Ar—CF, 1 × Ar—CSO$_2$), 116 (s, 4C, 4 × Ar—CH), 58 (s, 1C, 1 × CHN), 37 (s, 2C, 2 × CH), 33 (s, 2C, 2 × CH), 31 (s, 4C, 4 × CH$_2$), 27 (s, 1C, 1 × CH$_2$).

The equilibrium solubility of this compound in water and phosphate buffers (pH 7.4 and 11.50) were determined at 23.0 ± 1.0 °C by dissolving the compound in 2 mL of the appropriate solvent, shaking, and then centrifuging at 220 rpm for 48 h. The concentration of the drug was measured by UV spectrophotometry.

Determination of the pK_a was conducted using the shake flask method, while the log P(octanol/water) was determined using both the shake flask method and HPLC with UV detection. It was also calculated using commercially available software, ChemDraw Ultra®. The agreement of the values gives some confidence in terms of getting a good handle on the lipophilicity of the compound. The results of the solubility, pK_a, and log P determination are given in Table 6.1.

In summary, the compound possesses adequate water solubility to dissolve in intestinal fluid and the partition coefficient of 3.4 suggests that the compound possesses acceptable lipophilicity. The compound also has molecular weight of 309.4. It has only one hydrogen bond (HB) donor group (less than the maximum of 5) and less than 10 hydrogen bond acceptor groups, with a generous count reflecting 4. Based on Lipinski's rule of five (Fig. 6.5), one could conclude that this compound

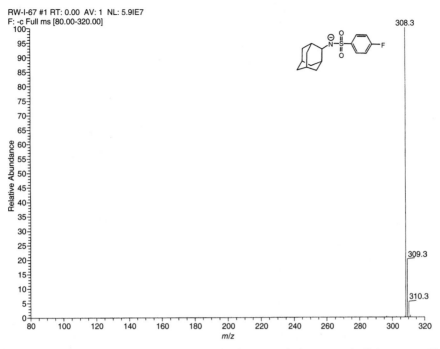

RW-I-67 #1 RT: 0.00 AV: 1 NL: 5.9lE7
F: -c Full ms [80.00-320.00]

FIGURE 6.4 Electrospray mass spectrum of 4-fluoro-*N*-(adamantan-2-yl)-benzenesulfon-amide *m/z* 308.3, in MeOH.

TABLE 6.1   Solubility, log *P*, and p*K*ₐ of 4-Fluoro-*N*-(adamantan-2-yl)-benzenesulfonamide

Solubility (23.0 ± 1.0 °C) (μg/mL)	
Water	120 ± 50
Phosphate buffer (pH 7.4)	200 ± 30
Phosphate buffer (pH 11.50)	270 ± 60
Log partition coefficients	
Calculated	3.44
Shake flask method	3.36 ± 0.16
HPLC	3.31 ± 0.01
pK_a	10.36 ± 0.11

falls "inside the box" and thus has the appropriate physicochemical properties necessary for absorption in an oral formulation.

Example B   (2*R*)-3-(4-fluoro-1-naphthyloxy)-1-(*tert*-butyl-amino) 2-propanol (Fig. 6.6) was synthesized to determine the effect of fluorine substitution on the aromatic ring on adrenergic receptor activities [23, 39]. Similar compounds are potent beta-adrenergic receptor antagonists and are used in the control of blood pressure. Upon completion of synthesis, the melting point of the free base was found to be 56–57 °C, while that of the hydrochloride salt was 165–166 °C. The sharp melting points were indicative of good purity. The structure of the compound was determined using data

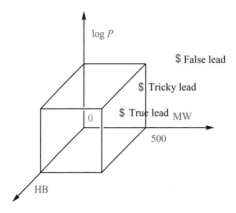

FIGURE 6.5   Optimal properties for orally active compounds are found within the "log *P*-HB-MW" box.

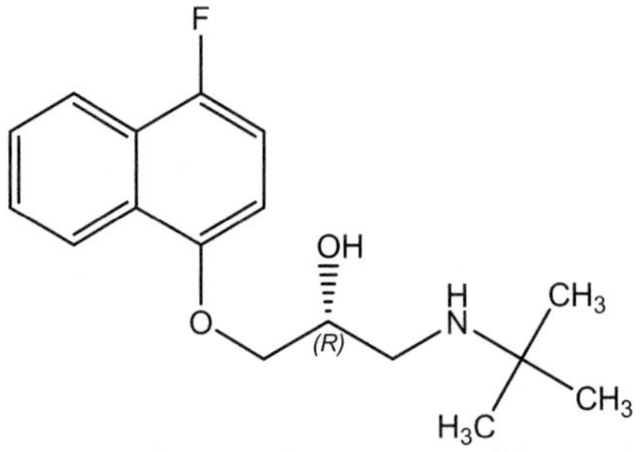

FIGURE   6.6 Structure   of   (2*R*)-3-(4-fluoro-1-naphthyloxy)-1-(*tert*-butyl-amino) 2-propanol.

from the proton NMR analysis of the sample: ^{1}H-NMR (CDCl$_3$) δ: 8.27–7.40 (m, 4H, aryl H), 7.0–7.10 (t, 1H aryl H), 6.75–6.65 (dd, 1H aryl H), 4.10 (s 2H, **CH$_2$**CHOH), 2.95–2.40 (m, 3H, **CHOHCH$_2$N**), 1.11 (s, 9H, C(**CH$_3$**)$_3$). This was supported by the molecular mass determination using mass spectrometry. The base peak was at 292 (M + 1) with the next major peak being 236 (M + 1 – 56), which is due to the cleavage of the *t*-butyl group. The elemental analysis of the hydrochloride salt gave C$_{17}$H$_{23}$NFO$_2$Cl, which further supported the structure proposed. The optical rotation values of the free base and hydrochloride salt were determined to be $[\alpha]_D^{25} = +3.71°$ (c = 1.96, EtOH) and $[\alpha]_D^{25} = +13.2°$ (c = 0.81, EtOH), respectively. Enantiomeric purity of the compound was evaluated by HPLC with UV detection. There was a major peak at 3.7 minutes for the *R*-enantiomer (98%) and a very minor peak at 3.15 minutes for the *S*-enantiomer.

6.10   CONCLUSION

As the cost of drug discovery and development continues to rise, the need to make important "cut" decisions as early in the process as possible is more pertinent now than ever. Along with potency and efficacy of the compound to elicit the desired biological effects, the importance of determining appropriate chemical and physical properties cannot be overemphasized, as they could play a key role in the "cut" decisions. Advances in technology have produced several methods, many of which have been highlighted in this chapter and are at the disposal of the medicinal chemist to characterize a potential new chemical entity.

REFERENCES

1. http://www.fda.gov/cder/about/smallbiz/exclusivity.htm.
2. Bradley D. High (throughput) mass. *Modern Drug Discov* 2003;6(4):43–45.
3. Tufts Centre for the Study of Drug Development. Backgrounder: how new drugs move through the development and approval process, 2001. http://csdd.tufts.edu/NewsEvents/RecentNews.asp?newsid=4.
4. Martin A. *Physical pharmacy*, 4th ed. Philadelphia: Lea & Febiger; 1993, Ch 4, pp 77–78.
5. Dewitte RS, Kolovanov E. *Pharmaceutical Profiling in Drug Discovery for Lead Selection.* Arlington, VA: AAPS Press; PUBX; 2004, Vol 1, Ch 2, pp 27–28.
6. Lipinski CA, Lombardo F, Dominy BW, Feeney PJ. Experimental and computational approaches to estimate solubility and permeability in drug discovery and development settings. *Adv Drug Deliv Rev* 1997;23:4–25.
7. Lipinski CA. Drug like properties and the cause of poor solubility and poor permeability. *J Pharmacol Toxicol Methods* 2000;44:235–249.
8. Gupta PK. Solutions and phase equilibra. In *Remington: The Science and Practice of Pharmacy*, 21st ed. Baltimore: Lippincott Williams &Wilkins; 2005, Ch 16, pp 224–228.
9. Skoog DA, Holler FJ, Nieman TA. *Principles of Instrumental Analysis*, 5th ed. Belmont, CA: Brooks/Cole and Thomson Learning; 1998, Ch 33, pp 524–528.
10. Chaudhry AK, Singh GS, Stephenson GA, Ackermann BL. Instrumental methods of analysis. In *Remington: The Science and Practice of Pharmacy*, 21st ed. Baltimore: Lippincott Williams & Wilkins; 2005, Ch 34, pp 633–636.
11. Skoog DA, Holler FJ, Nieman TA. *Principles of Instrumental Analysis*, 5th ed. Belmont, CA: Brooks/Cole and Thomson Learning; 1998, Ch 33, pp 844–845.
12. Zimmerman JJ, Feldman S. Physical–chemical properties and biological activity. In *William Foye's Principles of Medicinal Chemistry*, 2nd ed. Philadelphia: Lea & Febiger; 1981, Ch 2, pp 39–40.
13. Verkman AS. Drug discovery in academia. *Am J Physiol Cell Physiol* 2004;286:C465–C474.
14. Chaudhry AK, Singh GS, Stephenson GA, Ackermann BL. Instrumental methods of analysis. In *Remington: The Science and Practice of Pharmacy*, 21st ed. Baltimore: Lippincott Williams & Wilkins; 2005, Ch 34, pp 635–640.
15. Dalvit C, Fagerness PE, Hadden DTA, Sarver RW, Stockman BJ. Fluorine-NMR experiments for high-throughput screening: theoretical aspects, practical considerations, and range of applicability. *J Am Chem Soc* 2003;125(25):7696–7703.
16. Morgan KR, MacLachian DJ. ^{31}P solid state NMR studies of the structure of amine-intercalated a-zirconium phosphate. 2. Titration of a-zirconium phosphate with *n*-propylamine and *n*-butylamine. *J Phys Chem* 1992;96:3458–3464.
17. Eaton DC. *Laboratory Investigations in Organic Chemistry*. New York: McGraw-Hill; 1989, Experiment 2, pp 65–67.

18. Skoog DA, Holler FJ, Nieman TA. *Principles of Instrumental Analysis*, 5th ed. Belmont, CA: Brooks/Cole and Thomson Learning; 1998, Ch 26, pp 674–677.

19. Nopper B, Kohen F, Wilchek M. A thiophilic adsorbent for the one-step high performance liquid chromatography purification of monoclonal antibodies. *Anal Biochem* 1989;180(1):66–71.

20. Permuleter JS, Loftin S, Carl JL, Karimi. M. Modified high-performance liquid chromatography with electrochemical detection method for plasma measurement of levodopa, 3-*O*-methyldopa, dopamine, carbidopa and 3,4-dihydroxyphenylacetic acid. *J Chromatogr B* 2006;836:120–123.

21. Axe BP. Trace level detection and quantification of ethyl-diazoacetate by reverse phase high performance liquid chromatography and UV detection. *J Pharm Biomed Anal* 2006;41:804–810.

22. Saito M, Morris S, Yomota C, Iwaya K, Kudo K. Determination of enantiomeric purity of hyoscyamine from scopolia extract using HPLC-CD without chiral separation. *Enantiomer* 2000;5(3–4):369–375.

23. Adejare A, Deal SA, Day MS. Syntheses and β-adrenergic binding affinities of (*R*)- and (*S*)-fluoronaphthyloxypropanolamines. *Chirality* 1999;11:144–148.

24. Lipinski CA. Avoiding investment in doomed drugs. *Curr Drug Discov* 2001;Apr:17–19.

25. Comer JEA. High throughput measurement of log *D* and pK_a in drug bioavailability: estimation of solubility, permeability, absorption and bioavailability. In *Methods and Principles in Medicinal Chemistry, Volume 18*. Weinheim: Wiley-VCH; 2003, Ch 2, pp 21–45.

26. Di. L, Kerns EH. Pharmaceutical profiling in drug discovery. *Drug Discov Today* 2003;8(7):316–323.

27. Chui, W-K, Tsun-Hon Wong P, Thenmozhiyal JC. Anticonvulsant activity of phenylmethylenehydantoins: a structure–activity relationship study. *J Med Chem* 2004; 47:1527–1535.

28. Kurz H, Hofstetter A, Teschemacher H, Herz A, The importance of lipid-solubility for the central action of cholinolytic drugs. *Neuropharmacology* 1965;4(4):207–218.

29. Xu XH, Song JZ, Qaio CF, Tai J, Cheung S, Han QB. Stability and cytotoxicity of gambogic acid and its derivative gambogoic acid. *Biol Pharm Bull* 2005;28(12):2335–2337.

30. Trissel LA, Zhang Y, Xu Q. Physical and chemical stability of gemcitabine hydrochloride solutions. *J Am Pharm Assoc* 1999;39(4):509–513.

31. Lipinski C, Hopkins A. Navigating chemical space for biology and medicine. *Nature* 2004;432:855–861.

32. Kirkpatrick P, Lebbos J, LaBonte J. Fresh from the pipeline: enfuvirtide. *Nat Rev Drug Discov* 2003;2:345–346.

33. Gefter ML, Wallner BP. Peptide treatment for allergic diseases. *Clin Immunol Immunopathol* 1996;80(2):105–109.

34. Adejare A, Brown PW. Hydrogen/deuterium exchange to differentiate fragments ions from pseudomolecular ions by electrospray tandem mass spectrometry. *Anal Chem* 1997;69(8):1525–1529.

35. Skoog DA, Holler FJ, Nieman TA. *Principles of Instrumental Analysis*, 5th ed. Belmont, CA: Brooks/Cole and Thomson Learning; 1998, Ch 31, pp 805–808.

36. Martin A. *Physical Pharmacy*, 4th ed. Philadelphia: Lea & Febiger; 1993, Ch 2, pp 46–48.

37. Wells RM. *Design and synthesis of non-peptide rigid sulfonamide gamma secretase inhibitors*. MS thesis, Idaho State University, 2003.

38. Adejare A, El-Gendy AM. Membrane permeability related physicochemical properties of a novel γ-secretase inhibitor. *Int J Pharm* 2004;280:45–55.

39. Adejare A, Sciberras SS. Syntheses and β-adrenergic activities of (*R*)-fluoronaphthyloxy-propanolomaine. *Pharm Res* 1997;14(4):533–536.

7

PERMEABILITY ASSESSMENT

Srinivas Ganta, Puneet Sharma, and Sanjay Garg
University of Auckland, Auckland, New Zealand

Contents

7.1 INTRODUCTION

Drug discovery is a lengthy and costly process with a very low probability of success. Approximately 50% of the investigational new drugs (INDs) fail in preclinical and

Preclinical Development Handbook: ADME and Biopharmaceutical Properties,
edited by Shayne Cox Gad
Copyright © 2008 John Wiley & Sons, Inc.

clinical phases of the drug development process. The major reasons for such a high proportion of failures are poor biopharmaceutical properties, including low aqueous solubility, inadequate intestinal permeability, chemical instability, intestinal or hepatic metabolism, and systemic clearance. The advent of combinatorial chemistry and high throughput screening (HTS) has allowed the synthesis of thousands of compounds a day, leading to the rapid identification of therapeutically active compounds (i.e., hits and leads). Despite this dramatic increase in the speed of synthesis and screening, the number of drugs reaching the market has not increased in similar proportions.

However, the success rate is beginning to rise with the increase in availability of many *in vitro* screening techniques, which can be used for early prediction of new chemical entity (NCE) permeability through biological barriers and other physico-chemical properties. It helps medicinal chemists to design compounds that exhibit the right pharmaceutical characteristics and avoid wasting valuable resources on developing molecules that are not likely to become successful drugs.

Drug permeability is considered an important parameter in drug discovery and lead optimisation; it is essential to have reliable methods of predicting the *in vivo* permeability by thoughtful use of *in vitro* permeability models.

7.2   NATURE AND PERMEABILITY OF SOME PHYSIOLOGICAL BARRIERS

The main physiological permeation barriers to be crossed by drugs are epithelia and endothelia. Epithelia cover the surface of the body and line various cavities. Endothelia line the blood capillaries so as to regulate the distribution of compounds between the blood and the interstitial fluids. Despite their extensive biochemical differences, they serve as highly selective permeability barriers, separating internal and external environments. Oral bioavailability is a highly desirable property for molecules under investigation in drug discovery, because approximately 90% of all marketed drugs are administered orally. The principal physiological barrier that drugs have to cross to enter the systemic circulation is the gastrointestinal mucosa. Alternatively, drugs can also be absorbed through the skin, cornea, and buccal, sublingual, nasal, vaginal, or rectal mucosa. Some of these routes have been explored as alternative paths for the delivery of drugs that are inactivated by first-pass metabolism. Another important physiological barrier is the blood–brain barrier (BBB), which separates the blood from the central nervous system. Due the difference in anatomical structure of the epithelia throughout the body, different drug application routes are impeded by different barriers.

7.3   DRUG TRANSFER PROCESS THROUGH A PHYSIOLOGICAL MEMBRANE

According to the *fluid mosaic model*, the structure of the cellular membrane is described as an interrupted phospholipid bilayer capable of both hydrophilic and hydrophobic interactions [1]. The membrane model for the understanding of relevant drug transport processes across the biological membranes is shown in Fig. 7.1.

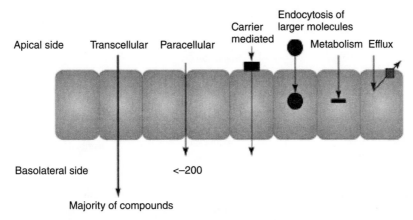

FIGURE 7.1 Different routes of drug entry from the intestine into the bloodstream. (From Ref. 52, with permission from Elsevier.)

1. The majority of the lipophilic drugs are absorbed via passive diffusion across the cellular membrane—transcellular transport [2].
2. Transcellular passage is the main route for both intestinal epithelium and BBB.
3. The hydrophilic molecules (molecular weight or MW < 200) passes through the water-filled tight junctions formed by fusion of adjacent cells—paracellular transport [3].
4. The MW cutoff for paracellular transport may be 400–500 [4]. However, paracellular permeation is negligible in brain endothelium.
5. Drug molecules transported against concentration gradient by active energy consuming transporter proteins, P-glycoprotein (P-gp)—carrier mediated transport [5].
6. Some carriers can permeate in the direction of the concentration gradient without consumption of energy—facilitated transport.
7. The high MW compounds (e.g., peptides and proteins) usually take another transcellular route—endocytosis or transcytosis [6].

7.4 PHYSICOCHEMICAL PROPERTIES DETERMINING MEMBRANE PERMEATION

The tenets of molecular properties influence drug permeability through various physiological membranes. The relevant physicochemical descriptors for membrane permeability, and their interrelationships, are presented in Fig. 7.2 [7].

7.4.1 Lipophilicity

Because of the lipid nature of cell membranes, a molecule's lipophilicity has long been considered an important factor in drug design. The most common expression of lipophilicity is the logarithm of the partition coefficient ($\log P$). Since the

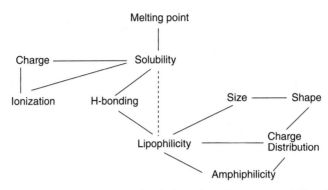

FIGURE 7.2 Physicochemical properties influencing drug permeability. (From van de Waterbeemd H. *Eur J Pharm Sci* 1993; 7, with permission from Elsevier.)

membranes are primarily lipophilic in nature and with the lipid domain playing an important role in their barrier function, the relationship between log P and permeability is nonlinear, with a decrease in permeability at both low and high log P values. These nonlinearities are theorized to be due to the limited diffusion of poorly lipophilic molecules into the lipophilic cell membrane, or the preferential partitioning of highly lipophilic molecules into the phospholipid cell membrane, preventing passage through the aqueous portion of the membrane [8, 9].

7.4.2 Molecular Size

Molecular size is believed to play a distinct role in permeation processes and can be a further limiting factor in oral drug absorption. The paracellular transport highly depends on the molecular size due to the *sieving effect*, the molecular weight limit for the paracellular permeation being approximately 400–500 [4]. The bigger the molecule is, the harder it is to diffuse. Diffusion coefficients across biological membranes have been shown to be highly dependent on molecular mass. It has been concluded that the permeation of drugs with MW < 300 Da is not significantly influenced by the physicochemical properties of the drug, which will mostly permeate through aqueous channels of the membrane. By contrast, the rate of permeation is highly sensitive to molecular size for compounds with MW > 300 Da. The Lipinski rule of five proposes an upper MW limit of 500 as being the limit for orally absorbed compounds [10].

7.4.3 Hydrogen Bonding Property

The hydrogen bonding ability (an estimate of hydrophilicity) of a molecule is an important property for cellular membrane permeability [11]. Conradi et al. [3] believe that the relative contributions of both lipophilicity and hydrogen bonding must be considered, as opposed to hydrophobicity alone. Lipids within membranes contain hydrophilic parts that have hydrogen bonding acceptor groups. These groups bond to the hydrogen bond donating solutes, preventing the solutes from penetrating the membranes and slowing down the diffusion process [12].

7.4.4   pH Partition (pK_a)

The majority of drugs in use are either weak acids or bases and, depending on the pH, exist in an ionized or un-ionized form. Membranes are more permeable to un-ionized forms of drugs than to ionized species due to the greater lipid solubility of the un-ionized forms and the highly charged nature of the cell membranes. However, Palm et al. [13] reported that the molecules with an un-ionized fraction of <10%, a common state for many drugs in the intestinal pH range, were permeable across Caco-2 cell membranes. As discussed by these authors, a variety of examples exist where ionized molecules are permeable, deviating from classical pH partition theory.

7.4.5   Solubility

Solubility is a major factor in determining drug absorption through physiological membranes. Poor aqueous solubility is likely to result in poor absorption, since the drug diffusing through intestinal membrane is proportional to its concentration gradient between the lumen of the intestine and blood. Therefore, even drugs with high permeation rate show a low absorption. Conversely, the highly aqueous soluble drugs are well absorbed despite low or moderate permeation.

7.5   BIOPHARMACEUTICS CLASSIFICATION SYSTEM (BCS) IN DRUG PRODUCT OPTIMIZATION

The biopharmaceutics characteristics like solubility and permeability are vital in drug discovery and lead optimization due to the dependence of drug absorption on these two properties. The BCS is derived based on these two main properties [14–17]. By knowing a drug solubility and intestinal permeability, the BCS classifies drugs into one of the four categories (Fig. 7.3).

Class I drugs are highly soluble and highly permeable. Drug discovery programs are targeted to achieve Class I drugs, which are ideal candidates for oral delivery. Class II drugs are highly permeable across the gut by virtue of their high lipophilic-

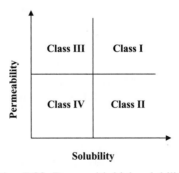

FIGURE 7.3   Model depicting BCS. Drugs with high solubility and high permeability are grouped into Class I; low solubility and high permeability into Class II; high solubility and low permeability into Class III; and low solubility and low permeability into Class IV.

ity. The bioavailability of products containing these compounds is likely to be dissolution rate limited due to low solubility. However, as drug dissolution is the rate-limiting step, the *in vitro* permeability data obtained from different experimental models may not accurately predict the *in vivo* absorption. Class III drugs are highly soluble but have less intrinsic permeability due to their physicochemical properties. For this reason dissolution is very rapid but absorption is permeability rate limited. Class IV drugs exhibit low solubility and low permeability. Low and variable oral bioavailability for these drugs is anticipated because of the combined limitation of solubility and permeability. Strategies to improve both solubility and permeability should be established for these molecules.

The BCS is considered by the U.S. Food and Drug Administration (FDA) as a fundamental principle to define the rate and extent of absorption of a drug product. It has published several guidance based on the BCS covering scale-up and postapproval changes [18] and has allowed waiver of *in vivo* bioequivalence studies [19]. However, accurate use of permeability methods to measure the drug permeability is a critical component for this classification. The scientific aspects of the BCS have been extensively discussed and have been the subject of numerous studies [20, 21].

7.6   EXPERIMENTAL MODELS FOR THE EVALUATION OF DRUG PERMEATION

The need to screen drugs for their absorption characteristics has increased significantly in recent years due to use of techniques like combinatorial chemistry. An ideal screening tool should be fast and easy to use, require small amounts of the compound, be relatively inexpensive, and give reliable predictions. In practice, such ideal testing methods are not easy to develop. While evaluating the usefulness of these different methods in drug discovery, it is important to know exactly what each technique measures and how this can help identify potentially successful or unsuccessful compounds. In the following section, we look at key techniques for evaluating and predicting the drug permeability and critically assess their advantages and limitations in drug discovery and development.

7.6.1   Predicting Drug Permeability from Physicochemical Parameters

During drug development, laboratories might use computational approaches to predict the absorption potential of new chemical entities. These computational methods are based on lipophilicity, hydrogen bonding, and molecular size. It has long been recognized that these physicochemical descriptors are related to membrane permeability [22], although this relationship is often obscured when structurally different compounds are studied [23].

Lipophilicity: log **P** *and log* **D**   Drug lipophilicity is commonly used as a predictor of membrane permeability because transcellular permeation is dependent on the lipophilicity of the compound. The molecule requires a certain affinity for the phospholipid structure in order to enter the cell membrane [24]. Fick's first law of diffusion describes the passive transport of the drug across the membrane as being

TABLE 7.1   Computer Programs for Log P Calculations

Computer Program	Software Package/Vendor
PrologP and Prolog P	PALLAS/CompuDrug Chemistry Ltd.
ACD/logP and logD	Version 3.0/Advanced Chemistry Development Inc.
ALOGP	Tsar 3.1/Oxford Molecular Group
CLIP/logP	University of Lausanne
CLOGP	Pcmodels/Daylight CIS, CLOGP/Biobyte
HINT/logP	Edusoft
KLOGP	Multicase Inc.
LISP	O. Raevsky
LOGKOW	Syracuse Research Corp.
SCILOGP	SCILOGP/Scivision
TLOGP	TLOGP 1.0/Upstream Solutions
XLOGP	XLOGP V 2.0/Institute of Physical Chemistry, Peking University
ALOGPS	ALOGPS 2.1/Virtual Computational Chemistry Laboratory
MLOGP	DRAGON 3.0

proportional to the membrane–water partition coefficient. These coefficients are conventionally expressed as the n-octanol–water partition coefficient (log P), which is the concentration ratio of the compound between n-octanol and aqueous phase at equilibrium. The distribution coefficient D (log D) is pH dependent in the case of ionizable compounds.

The log P and log D are traditionally determined by the shake flask method using an n-octanol–water biphasic system. This has been one of the most suitable models of the lipidic biological membranes, due to the resemblance of n-octanol to lipids—with its long alkyl chain and the polar hydroxyl group. However, the log P and log D values for a single compound can vary as a result of different experimental conditions [25]. Both log P and log D are used for prediction of drug absorption, which can subsequently be measured by more sophisticated and standardized techniques like potentiometer titration of the compound in the biphasic system [26].

In the drug development program, an early estimate of log P and log D values can be determined by computational approaches. Many computational approaches have been developed to estimate log P [27, 28], including the popular C log P [29] and A log P [30] algorithms (Table 7.1). These approaches can calculate log P values using software programs and are based on data for either atomic contributions or molecular fragments, or on molecular properties such as the molecular lipophilicity potential (MLP) [31], molar volume, and hydrogen bonding.

Liposomal Partitioning   Liposomes are lipid bilayer vesicles that can be used as membrane models in partition studies [32] with the potentiometric titration method [33]. The phosphatidylcholine liposomes seem to provide a more accurate partition system for absorption prediction than the n-octanol–buffer system. Beigi et al. [34] demonstrated a chromatographic technique for partition studies in liposomal systems. Liposomes of different lipid composition were immobilized in small agarose–dextran gel beads and packed into chromatography columns. The capacity factor of 12 compounds related well to their fraction absorbed in humans.

Chromatographic Methods   The elution times in chromatography represent the partitioning behavior of the compound between stationary and mobile phases. Chong et al. [35] introduced immobilized artificial membrane (IAM) columns containing phosphatidylcholine or similar lipid-like ligands covalently bonded to silica particles. This lipid monolayer is similar to the lipid membrane in partition studies. This high performance liquid chromatography (HPLC) technique can be used to study the partition of a solute. In spite of the end capping, the solutes also interact with uncapped silanol groups, in addition to the lipid ligands. Once this problem is solved, IAM columns are likely to provide a good tool for absorption prediction.

Hydrogen Bonding   Hydrogen bonding can be measured experimentally by allowing a compound to distribute between two solvents, of which only one can form hydrogen bonds. This is expressed as $\Delta \log P$, which is the difference between the *n*-octanol–water $\log P$ and an alkane–water $\log P$ [36], where *n*-octanol is the solvent that permits hydrogen bonding. $\Delta \log P$ has shown good correlation with membrane permeability in numerous studies. El Tayar et al. [37] found correlation of $\Delta \log P$ with skin absorption. $\Delta \log P$ was also compared with brain permeability. Optimal permeability was predicted for $\log D$ between 0 and 3 and $\Delta \log P < 2$ [38]. The main shortcoming of the $\Delta \log P$ method is that it requires two experimental determinations for each compound, since *n*-octanol is miscible with alkane and it is not possible to measure $\Delta \log P$ directly.

For reasonable prediction of membrane permeability, the hydrogen bonding capacity is calculated by counting the number of hydrogen bond donor atoms (hydrogens) attached to oxygen and nitrogen and hydrogen bond acceptor atoms (oxygens and nitrogens) [10], or counting the number of lone pair electrons [39]. Recently, more accurate methods of calculating hydrogen bonding capacity have been introduced. These include MolSurf [40], which calculates hydrogen bonding properties based on quantum mechanics, and Hybot [41], which is based on experimental results for the formation of complexes between hydrogen bond donors and acceptors.

Molecular Size   As a molecular size descriptor, often the molecular weight is used in predicting the drug permeability. The paracellular permeability of drug compounds was successfully modeled based on MW as discussed earlier. Molecular size is not only a component of lipophilicity, but also of the diffusion coefficient ($\log D$) in physiological membranes. A rather strong dependence on molecular size has been observed for transcellular diffusion in physiological membranes. Camenisch et al. [42] reported that the physiological membrane permeability of high MW compounds is overestimated when using $\log D$ as a predictor. This effect is important for compounds with MW > 500. For compounds that have similar $\log D$ values, Caco-2 permeabilities were lower for high MW compounds as compared with compounds of lower MW. Camenisch et al. [2] reviewed suggestions for the correction of partition coefficients with MW functions that were made by several authors. In the case of BBB penetration, a correlation between logarithm of the BBB permeation and logarithm of MW also existed [43].

Polar Surface Area (PSA)   The polar surface area (PSA) is the molecular surface area associated with hydrogen bonding acceptor atoms (i.e., oxygen and nitrogen)

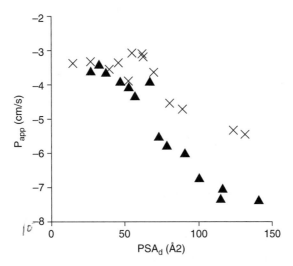

FIGURE 7.4 Relationship between dynamic polar surface area and drug permeability in perfused human jejunum (×) and in Caco-2 cell monolayers (▲). (From Ref. 46, with permission from Elsevier.)

plus the area of the hydrogen atoms attached to these heteroatoms—which are known as hydrogen donors. This model has been introduced to account for the neglected intramolecular hydrogen bond formation [44]. The dynamic polar surface area (PSAd) is the statistical average of the PSA of the low energy conformations of a molecule. The areas were calculated for an aqueous environment using atomic van der Waals radii. The smaller the PSAd of a compound, the better it permeates the biological barrier. Good inverse linear correlation was observed between the permeability across a Caco-2 model and the water-accessible PSA of six β-blockers and their ester prodrugs. Figure 7.4 shows the PSAd correlated to permeability in the human jejunum for 13 structurally different drugs investigated by Winiwarter et al. [45]. A comparison is also seen from the Caco-2 cell monolayer permeabilities for 14 model compounds presented by Stenberg et al. [46].

The long calculation time for the low energy conformations of large and flexible molecules is a limitation with this model. Stenberg et al. [46] noted that the relationship may break if the data for drugs that undergo intestinal metabolism or active transport, or have solubility problems, is included in the calculations. Therefore, integration of all these events into a computational model is vital.

Lipinski's Rule of Five Approach   In a common computational approach for absorption and permeability, Lipinski et al. [10] introduced the simple "rule of five" approach for the quick evaluation of new chemical entities. This model states that absorption or permeation of a compound is more likely to be poor when the calculated MW > 500, log P > 5, hydrogen bond donors > 5, and hydrogen bond acceptors > 10. The numbers of hydrogen bond donors and acceptors are simply calculated by the counting method described. If any two of these criteria are met, poor absorption or permeability is to be anticipated. This rule is based on a variety of calculated properties among several thousand drugs belonging to different therapeutic categories; therefore, certain drugs falling outside the rule, for example, orally active drugs like antibiotics, antifungals, vitamins, and cardiac glycosides, violate the rule of five. These drugs have structural similarities that allow them to act as substrates for biological transporters; therefore, they are outside the rule of five approach.

7.6.2   Cell Culture Based Models for Permeability Study

Caco-2 Cell Model   The Caco-2 cell model is a well characterized and widely used *in vitro* model in the field of drug permeability studies [6, 47]. It has been considered the gold standard technique and has been used to standardize other absorption assessment methods [48, 49]. Caco-2 cells are grown on a filter support in a multiple well format and permeability is measured by the movement of molecules from one side of the cell monolayer to the other (Fig. 7.5).

Caco-2 cells derived from a human colon adenocarcinoma exhibit many *in vivo* intestinal cell characteristics by having tight intercellular junctions and microvilli and expressing intestinal enzymes and transporters (e.g., P-gp). Due to these similarities, the permeation characteristics of drugs across Caco-2 cell lines correlate with their human intestinal permeation characteristics; therefore, it has been recommended that the Caco-2 model can be used to predict the absorption of drugs in humans. An essential component of studies using Caco-2 cells is the culture of intact monolayer on permeable supports and the assessment of their integrity or cell damage either by measuring transepithelial electrical resistance or by using a paracellular flux marker such as mannitol [49]. Since this model is quicker to use, more convenient, and produces more reproducible data than animal studies, its use in the early stages of drug development can lead to savings in time and money and avoid the unnecessary use of experimental animals. Moreover, Caco-2 assays are relatively accessible and easier for higher throughput than the excised tissue assays.

Many drugs are absorbed by passive diffusion; therefore, physiochemical descriptors of the drugs are expected to play a vital role in this process. Caco-2 cell permeability data have frequently been plotted against log P or log D, molecular weight, or some descriptor for H bonding [44]. The sigmoidal relationship has been identified between the hydrogen bonding properties of the solutes and permeability coefficients through Caco-2 cell monolayers [50].

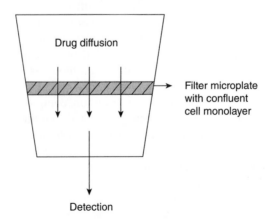

FIGURE 7.5   Caco-2 cell line model.

Although, Caco-2 cells can give evidence that a compound will be well absorbed, it is difficult to predict the compounds showing low or modest permeability. Other complications with Caco-2 cells include (1) variable expression of P-gp, metabolizing enzymes, and active transport systems [35, 51]; (2) interexperimental and interlaboratory variability, such as genetic change and sensitivity to differing culture conditions and protocols [49]; and (3) Caco-2 culture is laborious and costly—around 3–21 days are required to generate a confluent layer of cells [52].

Madin–Darby Canine Kidney (MDCK) Cell Model   Apart from Caco-2 cells, the other models that are most frequently used for permeability studies are MDCK and LLC-PK1 cells. When the MDCK cells are cultured under standard conditions, they differentiate into polarized columnar epithelial cells and form tight cellular junctions. The main advantage of MDCK cells is shorter culture times, which can be equal to 24 hours. A good correlation was reported between permeation of passively absorbed drugs in Caco-2 and MDCK cells [53]. The permeability coefficients of hydrophilic compounds are usually lower in Caco-2 cells than in MDCK cells. Whereas Caco-2 cells originate from human colon adenocarcinoma cells, MDCK cells are from dog kidney cells, and thus the expression levels of intestinal transporters would be different in these two cell lines [54]. Hence, the MDCK model has to be extensively characterized to confirm the correlation of transport mediated drug permeability to human absorption.

Lewis Lung Carcinoma–Porcine Kidney (LLC-PK1) Cell Model   LLC-PK1 cells are derived from normal pig kidneys. When cultured, these cells rapidly develop into a well formed monolayer with bush boarders and microvilli on their apical cell surface [55]. Several investigators have reported the use of these cells in passive cellular diffusion [56, 57]. As with MDCK cells, these cells also possess different transporters on their surface. A study has shown that uracil was transported by sodium-dependent and -independent pathways in LLC-PK1 cells; on the other hand, in Caco-2 cells uracil was transported independently of sodium pathway [18]. These differences in the transport mechanism can be attributed to differences in the origin of the cells types and the transporters that are expressed on these cells. Thus, further studies are warranted to determine the correlation between the LLC-PK1 cells and *in vivo* human absorption.

HT29 Cell Model   The role of mucus on drug permeability is largely ignored, since Caco-2 cells are a widely used model in permeability studies and they are devoid of this property. Certain clones of HT29 cells produce mucus. The wild-type HT29 cells grown on media containing galactose lead to the selection of a subclone of HT29 cells that form polarized cell monolayers and secrete mucus. A study has shown that the presence of the mucus layer in HT29-H resulted in lower permeability coefficients than Caco-2 monolayers in a testosterone permeability study. This indicates that the mucus layer accounts for most of the permeability resistance to testosterone. An attempt has been made to coculture the Caco-2 cells with HT29-MTX or HT29-H cells [58] in order to provide representative characteristics of intestinal mucosa.

The major application of the cell culture based model is screening of chemical libraries for compounds that have favorable permeability characteristics. Caco-2

TABLE 7.2   Cell Culture Models Used for Permeability Assessment

Cells	Origin	Special Characteristics
Caco-2	Human colon adenocarcinoma	Well characterized and widely used Express some relevant efflux transporters; expression of influx transporters is variable
MDCK	Dog kidney epithelial cells	Polarized cells with low expression of ABC transporters, ideal for transfection
LLC-PK1	Pig kidney epithelial cells	Polarized cells with low intrinsic transport expression, ideal for transfection
HT-29	Human colon	Contains mucus-producing goblet cells
TC-7	Caco-2 subclone	Similar to Caco-2
IEC-18	Rat small intestine cells	Provides a size selective barrier for paracellularly transported compounds

cells grow very slowly in 3–21 days; this time is too long for the drug discovery industry. Other cell models (MDCK and LLC-PK1) can grow much faster and be available for studies in 5–7 days. However, recent improvements in culture media like the addition of 10% fetal bovine serum, manipulation of the seeding density, and use of BIOCOT® transwell plates can reduce the time required for cell growth. Various cell culture models used for permeability assessment are described in Table 7.2.

Data Analysis from the Cell Cultured Models   The permeability coefficients (P_{eff}) through the cell monolayers are calculated from the following equation [48, 59]:

$$P_{eff} = \frac{V_A}{A(C_D - C_A)} \times \frac{dC_A}{dt} \tag{7.1}$$

where

- dC_A/dt (mg/s·mL) is the increase of drug concentration in the receiver chamber over the time period considered.
- A (cm^2) is the membrane surface area exposed to the compound.
- V_A (mL) is the solvent volume in the acceptor chamber.
- C_A and C_D (mg/mL) are the initial drug concentrations in the receiver and donor chambers, respectively.

Permeability rate (dC_A/dt) is calculated by plotting the amounts of drug measured over the linear diffusion range and determining the slope of the plot. P_{eff} from the equation is only valid under the experimental conditions, where a constant concentration gradient exists, so that backdiffusion is avoided. Under that condition, C_D is almost constant and C_A is negligible compared to C_D. In several findings, experimental conditions are usually accepted as sufficiently accurate for P_{eff} calculation, if the concentration difference between the donor and acceptor compartments does not diverge by more than 10% in the time interval studied [55].

7.6.3 Parallel Artificial Membrane Permeability Assay (PAMPA)

An alternative to the cell cultured models is the parallel artificial membrane permeability assay (PAMPA), which is a method for predicting passive permeability [60]. Recently, it has been suggested that artificial membrane methods such as PAMPA could soon replace high throughput screening Caco-2 assays [61], because PAMPA is an excellent biomimetic model, in terms of high throughput, reproducibility, and especially cost.

PAMPA is performed in a 96 micotiter well plate containing two parts. All the wells at the bottom part are filled with buffer solution. The top part contains a series of filter-immobilized artificial membranes composed of lipids, which match with the wells in the lower part. One-half of the filters on the top part are treated with an organic solvent, which supposedly acts as the cell membrane, and the other half are wetted with methanol/buffer. The test compound under investigation is applied to the top filters and the rate of appearance of the compound in the bottom wells should reflect the diffusion across the lipid layer. In a recent study by Lipinski et al. [62], a good correlation was found between diffusion in the PAMPA system and percentage absorption in humans for a selected series of compounds.

The filter immobilized artificial membranes are prepared by dispersing a phospholipid with the help of an organic solvent on a filter [60]. The various PAMPA models reported in the literature are presented in Table 7.3.

The problem of precipitation with low solubility compounds—when working at clinically relevant doses in cellular assays—is prevented in recent PAMPA models [63]. The limitations of the system include the lack of influx and efflux transporters, enzymes, and paracellular pathways.

7.6.4 Tissue Based Models for Permeability Study

Excised intestinal segments have been used to study intestinal drug absorption. The compound under investigation in a solution is applied to one side (mucosa or serosa) of the mucosa and the rate of drug absorption is determined by estimating

TABLE 7.3 Membrane Compositions of PAMPA Models

Assay	Model	Phospholipid Constituents[a]	Organic Solvent
Egg-PAMPA	Lecithin	10% Egg lecithin, cholesterol	n-Dodecane
BM-PAMPA	Biomimetic	0.8% PC, 0.8% PE, 0.2% PS, 0.2% PI, 1% cholesterol	1,7-Octadiene
HDM-PAMPA	Hexadecane	100% n-Hexadecane	n-hexadecane
DOPC-PAMPA	Synthetic phospholipid	2% Dioleylphosphatidyl choline	n-Dodecane
BBB-PAMPA	Blood–brain barrier	2% Porcine brain lipid extract (PC, PE, PS, PI, PA, cerebrosides)	n-Dodecane
DS-PAMPA	Double sink	20% Phospholipid mixture (PC, PE, PI, PA, triglycerides)	n-Dodecane

[a]PC, phosphatidyl choline; PE, phosphatidyl ethanolamine; PS, phosphatidyl serine; PI, phosphatidylinositol; PA, phosphatidic acid.

either the disappearance of drug from the drug solution or appearance of drug on the serosal side. These models preserve the characteristics of the biological membranes and also help in determining absorption across different gastrointestinal segments. Limited viability and versatility are the limitations with this type of preparation.

Everted Intestinal Segments   Isolated intestinal segment is a simple technique used to measure the intestinal transport of a drug. In this model, the permeability assessment is carried out through a segment of the intestine, with the musculature intact. Commonly, rat intestine is used, although absorption in other animal models, such as monkey, also correlate well with human absorption [64]. To prepare the rings, a selected segment of the intestine is isolated immediately after euthanizing the animal, washed in ice-cold buffer to remove debris and digestive products, and tied at one end with a piece of suture. The closed end is carefully pushed through the intestine using a glass rod, resulting in eversion of the intestine, which is then cut into small rings, typically 2–4 mm wide [65]. Next, the rings are incubated in buffer at 37 °C containing the compound under investigation, and shaken well in a water bath. After a set time, the drug uptake is suppressed by rinsing the rings with ice-cold saline or buffer. The rings are then blotted dry, weighed, and then dissolved or processed for assay. Any segment of the intestine can be used to prepare a large number of rings. This model can be used to study both active and passive transport pathways especially that of amino acids and peptides [66]. A major disadvantage associated with this model is the lack of maintenance of viability in the isolated rings, due to absence of blood supply and nerves. Some other factors like drug metabolism and accumulation in the mucosa could lead to an overestimation of true drug absorption. For example, one such early study found that, for several beta-lactam antibiotics, absorption based on luminal disappearance was roughly twice the true amount transported across the tissue [67].

Everted Intestinal Sacs   In this method, a 2–4 cm section of the intestine is tied off at one end and everted similar to the intestinal ring method. The sac is filled with buffer, tied off at the other end, and placed in a flask with oxygenated (95% O_2/5% CO_2) buffer solution as a test compound. Drug absorption is measured by sampling the solution inside and outside the sac. Unlike the *in vivo* situation, everted intestinal sacs only include the mucosa plus underlying muscle layers, which could lead to biased absorption values. Although this method is relatively simple and allows several experiments to be performed using tissue from just one intestine, it differs from the *in vivo* situation and drug accumulation in the muscle layer can lead to poor recovery of the drug.

Diffusion Cells   Diffusion cells have been used to determine the transport of compound in living tissues, one of the first approaches being the so-called Ussing chamber. In this method, the long intestinal mucosal sheets are cut into mucosal strips of adequate size (~2 cm) and are clamped between two glass chambers filled with buffer. The compound under study is added to the donor compartment, and the accumulation of the compound at the other side of the membrane (acceptor side) is measured as a function of time. The permeability of the compound is calculated from the following equation:

$$P_{eff} = \frac{dc}{dt} \times \frac{V}{A \times C} \tag{7.2}$$

where dc/dt is the change in concentration in the receptor compartment per unit time, V is the receptor volume, and A is the area available for diffusion. P_{eff} is usually expressed in centimeters per second (cm/s). This method has been used to evaluate *in vitro* permeability with varying degrees of success. For example, intestinal mucosa of rat mounted in an Ussing chamber was useful in describing the regional variability in GIT absorption of a mixed series of compounds [68].

7.6.5 *In Situ* Model of Intestinal Drug Permeability

Single-Pass Perfusion Model Several different models of the single-pass perfusion system have been used [69–71]. In these *in situ* models the viability of the tissue is maintained, as the whole animal is used and the blood vessels and lymphatics are intact. This technique has been widely used to study both active and passive transport pathways [69, 71, 72]. In addition, the effect of various factors such as drug concentration, intestinal region, and flow rate can be studied. In the closed loop model, a solution containing the diluted drug is added to a segment of the intestine, and the intestine is closed. After a set time the intestine is excised and the drug content is analyzed [73]. Conversely, in the open loop model, the proximal and the distal end of a segment of the intestine are canulated with a glass tube. The drug is then pumped through the intestine and the ratio of drug in and out is measured.

The steady-state effective intestinal permeability coefficient (P_{eff}) is calculated according to the parallel-tube model [74]:

$$P_{eff} = \frac{-Q_{in} In(C_{out}/C_{in})}{2\pi r L} \tag{7.3}$$

where Q_{in} is the perfusion flow rate through the intestine segment (mL/s), and C_{in} and C_{out} correspond to the inlet and outlet concentrations (μg/mL), respectively. r is the radius of the intestinal loop (cm) and L is the length of the loop (cm). From the equation, it can be seen that by varying the length of the intestinal segment, the effect of transit time on drug absorption can also be studied [55, 66]. Even with these advantages, use of the single-pass perfusion model is limited because in this model the disappearance of the drug from the intestine is used to predict permeability. However, the rate of decrease in drug concentration does not always equal the rate of drug absorption; for example, drugs can interact with the lipid membrane [75]. Furthermore, the proximal and distal content of the lumen can enter the test segment of the intestine, making it difficult to control conditions such as flow rate [76].

Prediction of oral absorption in human beings is important in the early stage of the drug discovery process. *In vitro* assays in Caco-2 and MDCK models are frequently used for that purpose. However, an *in situ* technique might be more accurate in estimation of absorption. One such study [77] found that effective permeability coefficients determined in rats by single-pass intestinal perfusion for 14 compounds were correlated to the values obtained from humans.

Single-Pass Perfusion of the Dog Intestine (Loc-I-Gut)   The Loc-I-Gut is a very effective model for investigating regional jejunum permeability. It is a perfusion instrument consisting of six channels and two inflatable latex balloons, which are set 10 cm apart [78]. The purpose of the balloons is to isolate the segment of the intestine that is being studied and to prevent the leakage of the proximal and distal luminal content into the selected area. It has been reported that less than 2% of the luminal content leaked into the jejunum when the balloons were inflated [76]. The tube is inserted into the proximal jejunum by using fluoroscopic techniques. Air is then pumped into the balloons, inflating them and creating a 10 cm separated jejunal segment. Insertion and setting up of the tube usually takes about an hour and the infusion rate is about 2–3 mL/min. A nonabsorbable marker such as ^{14}C-PEG 4000 is used in the perfusion solution to check the integrity of the balloons during the experiment [79]. In the dog model the drug permeability was calculated using the well-stirred model because it is assumed that the hydrodynamics are similar to the corresponding model in the human intestine. The P_{eff} can be calculated as [76]

$$P_{eff} = \frac{Q_{in}(C_{in} - C_{out})/C_{out}}{2\pi r L} \qquad (7.4)$$

where Q_{in} is the perfusion flow rate, r is the radius of the tube, L is the length of the tube, C_{in} is the infused drug concentration entering the tube, and C_{out} is the diffusate concentration leaving the tube. The Loc-I-Gut model is also used for perfusion of suspended drug particles in human jejunum. In this model, the *in vivo* dissolution of the drug can be directly estimated by measuring the concentration of drug either in dissolved or in solid-state form [80]. The major limitation to this model is that it is invasive. Intubation may affect the normal physiology and function of the GI tract. Furthermore, the fluid that is used to flush out the drug from the tube may affect the absorption of the drug [81].

7.6.6   Whole Animal Models

InteliSite Capsule   The InteliSite® capsule (Innovative Devices LLC, Raleight, NC) is a rapid and noninvasive technique for measuring site-specific permeability of a drug [82]. The permeability is assessed through measurement of the drug in the systematic circulation. When the capsule reaches the target site it is activated. Activation is accomplished by placing the magnetic field generator next to the subject's abdomen. This magnetic field is sensed by a receiver and is converted to heat. The heat will cause the shape memory alloys to straighten. This in turn results in the rotation of the interior sleeve in relation to the outer sleeve and the drug is released. Gamma scintigraphy and pharmacokinetics analysis are used to evaluate and measure drug absorption [81]. Pithavala et al. [81] evaluated the pharmacokinetic properties of ranitidine in eight volunteer subjects using the InteliSite capsule [81]. The result of the study correlated well with data available in the literature. Thus, it can be concluded that these capsules are a valuable tool for studying regional drug absorption.

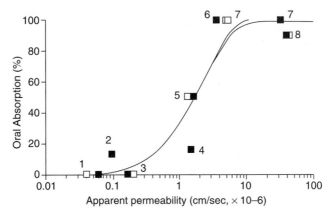

FIGURE 7.6 Correlation between the permeability coefficient (in cell culture) and fraction absorbed in human (From Ref. 83, with permission from Elsevier.)

7.7 *IN VITRO* AND *IN VIVO* CORRELATION (IVIV)

In order to use any experimental model for human permeability prediction, the drug permeability from the model has to correlate well with human absorption. To validate a permeability model, compounds with known absorption in humans are used and P_{eff} is calculated. Figure 7.6 [83] shows the general shape of the curve of fraction absorbed in human versus the *in vitro* P_{eff}. Any small change (such as the pH of the buffer or the intubation time) in the way that the techniques are carried out can effect the P_{eff} of the drug, and the curve may shift to left or right or alter its steepness. Therefore, well designed and validated techniques are to be used within laboratories to correlate the data collected.

Furthermore, in the case of animal models, there needs to be a correlation between the animal's P_{eff} and the fraction absorbed in human. It has been shown that rat and human jejunum P_{eff} of passively absorbed drugs correlate well [84]. Once the correlation is demonstrated for a series of compounds, then the experimental results can be used to make intelligent decisions about those compounds that can be further studied in animals.

7.8 CONCLUSION

Identifying appropriate models for permeation study of a new molecule is a very challenging task, but there are several options available to the pharmaceutical scientist. Careful review and selection of appropriate methods is crucial to a successful drug development program. The key feature that governs the process is *in vitro* and *in vivo* correlation in permeability studies. There is a potential to develop models that can provide good correlation.

REFERENCES

1. Singer SJ, Nicolson GL. The fluid mosaic model of the structure of cell membranes. *Science* 1972;175:720–731.

2. Camenisch G, Folkers G, van de Waterbeemd H. Review of theoretical passive drug absorption models: historical background, recent development and limitations. *Pharm Acta Helv* 1996;71:309–327.

3. Conradi RA, Burton PS, Borchardt RT. Physico-chemical and biological factors that influence a drug's cellular permeability by passive diffusion. *Methods Principles Med Chem* 1996;4:233–252.

4. Artursson P, Ungell A-L, Lofroth J-E. Selective paracellular permeability in two models of intestinal absorption: cultured monolayers of human intestinal epithelial cells and rat intestinal segments. *Pharm Res* 1993;10:1123–1129.

5. Hunter J, Hirst BH, Simmons NL. Drug absorption limited by *p*-glycoprotein-mediated secretory drug transport in human intestinal epithelial Caco-2 cell layers. *Pharm Res* 1993;10:743–749.

6. Artursson P, Palm K, Luthman K. Caco-2 monolayers in experimental and theoretical predictions of drug transport. *Adv Drug Deliv Rev* 1996;22:67–84.

7. van de Waterbeemd H. The fundamental variables of the biopharmaceutics classification system (BCS): a commentary. *Eur J Pharm Sci* 1998;7:1–3.

8. Hansch C, Clayton JM. Lipophilic character and biological activity of drugs. II. Parabolic case. *J Pharm Sci* 1973;1–21.

9. Kararli TT. Gastrointestinal absoption of drugs. *Crit Rev Ther Drug Carrier Syst* 1989;6:39–86.

10. Lipinski CA, Lombardo F, Dominyl BW, Feeney PJ. Experimental and computational approaches to estimate solubility and permeability in drug discovery and development settings. *Adv Drug Deliv Rev* 1997;23:3–26.

11. Diamond JM, Wright EM. Molecular forces governing non-electrolyte permeation through cell membranes. *Proc R Soc B Biol Sci* 1969;172:273–316.

12. Urtti ALS. Minimizing systemic absorption of topically administered ophthalmic drugs. *Surv Ophthalmol* 1993;37:435–456.

13. Palm K, Luthman K, Ros J, Grasjo J, Artursson P. Effect of molecular charge on intestinal epithelial drug transport: pH-dependent transport of cationic drugs. *J Pharmacol Exp Ther* 1999;291:435–443.

14. Dressman JB, Amidon GL, Fleisher D. Absorption potential: estimating the fraction absorbed for orally administered compounds. *J Pharm Sci* 1985;74:588–589.

15. Gordon LA, Hans L, Vinod PS, John RC. A theoretical basis for a biopharmaceutic drug classification: the correlation of *in vitro* drug product dissolution and *in vivo* bioavailability. *Pharm Res* 1995;12:413–420.

16. Sinko PJ, Leesman GD, Amidon GL. Predicting fraction dose absorbed in human using a macroscopic mass balance approach. *Pharm Res* 1991;8:979–988.

17. Symillides PEMMY. Toward a quantitative approach for the prediction of the fraction of dose absorbed using the absoption potential concept. *Biopharm Drug Dispos* 1989;10:43–53.

18. CDER/FDA. *Guidance for Industry*. Immediate release solid oral dosage forms: scale-up and post-approval changes. Washington DC: FDA;1995.

19. CDER/FDA. *Guidance for Industry*. Waiver of *in vivo* bioavailability and bioequivalence studies for immediate release solid oral dosage forms based on a biopharmaceutics classification system. Washington DC: FDA;2000.

20. Yu LX, Amidon GL, Polli JE, Zhao H, Mehta MU, Conner DP, Shah VP, Lesko LJ, Chen ML, Lee VHL, Hussain AS. Biopharmaceutics classification system: the scientific basis for biowaiver extensions. *Pharm Res* 2002;19.

21. Blume HH, Schug BS. The biopharmaceutics classification system (BCS): Class III drugs—better candidates for BA/BE waiver? *Eur J Pharm Sci* 1999;9:117–121.

22. Hans C, Steward AR, Iwasa J. The correlation of localization rates of benzeneboronic acids in brain and tumor tissue with substituent constants. *Mol Pharmacol* 1965;1:87–92.

23. Artursson P, Karlsson J. Correlation between oral drug absorption in humans and apparent drug permeability coefficients in human intestinal epithelial (Caco-2) cells. *Biochem Biophys Res Commun* 1991;175:880–885.

24. Kramer SD. Absorption prediction from physicochemical parameters. *Pharm Sci Technol Today* 1999;2:373–380.

25. Hansch C, Leo A. *Substituent Constants for Correlation Analysis in Chemistry and Biology.* Hoboken, NJ: Wiley-Interscience;1979.

26. Avdeef A. pH-metric log *P*. II: Refinement of partition coefficients and ionization constants of multiprotic substances. *J Pharm Sci* 1993;82:183–190.

27. Carrupt P, Testa B, Gaillard P. *Computational Approaches to Lipophilicity: Methods and Applications.* Hoboken, NJ: Wiley-VCH;1997.

28. Mannhold R, Cruciani G, Dross K, Rekker R. Multivariate analysis of experimental and computational descriptors of molecular lipophilicity. *J Comput Aided Mol Des* 1998;12:573–581.

29. Leo AJ, Hoekman D. Calculating *P*(oct) with no missing fragments; the problem of estimating new interaction parameters. *Perspect Drug Discov Des* 2000;18:19–38.

30. Ghose AK, Viswanadhan VN, Wenoloski JJ. Prediction of hydrophobic (lipophilic) properties of small organic molecules using fragmental methods: an analysis of ALOGP and CLOGP methods. *J Phys Chem A* 1998;102:3762–3772.

31. Testa B, Carrupt PA, Gaillard P, Billois F, Weber P. Lipophilicity in molecular modelling. *Pharm Res* 1996;13:335–343.

32. Balon K, Riebesehl BU, Muller BW. Drug liposome partitioning as a tool for the prediction of human passive intestinal absorption. *Pharm Res* 1999;16:882–888.

33. Avdeef A, Box KJ, Comer JEA, Hibbert C, Tam KY. pH-Metric log *P* 10. Determination of liposomal membrane–water partition coefficients of ionizable drugs. *Pharm Res* 1998;15:209–215.

34. Beigi F, Gottschalk I, Lagerquist Hagglund C, Haneskog L, Brekkan E, Zhang Y, Osterberg T, Lundahl P. Immobilized liposome and biomembrane partitioning chromatography of drugs for prediction of drug transport. *Int J Pharm* 1998;164:129–137.

35. Chong S, Dando SA, Soucek KM, Morrison RA. *In vitro* permeability through Caco-2 cells is not quantitatively predictive of *in vivo* absorption for peptide-like drugs absorbed via the dipeptide transporter system. *Pharm Res* 1996;13:120–123.

36. Seiler P. Interconversion of lipophilicities from hydrocarbon/water systems into octanol/water system. *Eur J Med Chem* 1974;9:473–479.

37. el Tayar NTR, Testa B, Carrupt PA, Hansch C, Leo A. Percutaneous penetration of drugs: a quantitative structure–permeability relationship study. *J Pharm Sci* 1991;80:744–749.

38. ter Laak AM, Tsai RS, Donne-Op den Kelder GM, Carrupt PA, Testa B, Timmerman H. Lipophilicity and hydrogen-bonding capacity of H1-antihistaminic agents in relation to their central sedative side-effects. *Eur J Pharm Sci* 1994;2:373–384.

39. Ren S, Das A, Lien EL. QSAR analysis of membrane permeability to organic compounds. *J Drug Target* 1996;4:103–107.

40. Norinder U, Svensson P. Descriptors for amino acids using MolSurf parametrization. *J Comput Chem* 1998;19:51–59.

41. Raevsky OA, Grigor'ev VY, Kireev DB, Zefirov NS. Complete thermodynamic description of H-bonding in the framework of multiplicative approach. *Quantitative Structure–Activity Relationships* 1992;11:49–63.

42. Camenisch G, Alsenz J, van de Waterbeemd H, Folkers G. Estimation of permeability by passive diffusion through Caco-2 cell monolayers using the drugs' lipophilicity and molecular weight. *Eur J Pharm Sci* 1998;6:313–319.

43. Hansch C, Bjorkroth JP, Leo A. Hydrophobicity and central nervous system agents: on the principle of minimal hydrophobicity in drug design. *J Pharm Sci* 1987;76:663–687.

44. Palm K, Luthman K, Ungell A-L, Strandlund G, Artursson P. Correlation of drug absorption with molecular surface properties. *J Pharm Sci* 1996;85:32–39.

45. Winiwarter S, Bonham NM, Ax F, Hallberg A, Lennernas H, Karlen A. Correlation of human jejunal permeability (*in vivo*) of drugs with experimentally and theoretically derived parameters. A multivariate data analysis approach. *J Med Chem* 1998;41:4939–4949.

46. Stenberg P, Luthman K, Artursson P. Virtual screening of intestinal drug permeability. *J Control Release* 2000;65:231–243.

47. Yee S. *In vitro* permeability across Caco-2 cells (colonic) can predict *in vivo* (small intestinal) absorption in man—fact or myth. *Pharm Res* 1997;14:763–766.

48. Camenisch G, Folkers G, van de Waterbeemd H. Comparison of passive drug transport through Caco-2 cells and artificial membranes. *Int J Pharm* 1997;147:61–70.

49. Hidalgo IJ. Assessing the absorption of new pharmaceuticals. *Curr Top Med Chem* 2001;1:385–401.

50. Palm K, Stenberg P, Luthman K, Artursson P. Polar molecular surface properties predict the intestinal absorption of drugs in humans. *Pharm Res* 1997;14:568–571.

51. van de Waterbeemd H. Property based design: optimization of drug absorption and pharmacokinetics. *J Med Chem* 2001;44:1313–1333.

52. Hamalainen MD, Frostell-Karlsson A. Predicting the intestinal absorption potential of hits and leads. *Drug Discov Today Technol* 2004;4:397–405.

53. Ribadeneira MD, Aungst BJ, Eyermann CJ, Huang S-M. Effects of structural modifications on the intestinal permeability of angiotensin II receptor antagonists and the correlation of *in vitro*, *in situ*, and *in vivo* absorption. *Pharm Res* 1996;13:227–233.

54. Balimane PV, Chong S. Cell culture-based models for intestinal permeability: a critique. *Drug Discov Today* 2005;10:335–343.

55. Anderberg EK, Nystrom C, Artursson P. Epithelial transport of drugs in cell culture. VII: Effects of pharmaceutical surfactant excipients and bile acids on transepithelial permeability in monolayers of human intestinal epithelial (Caco-2) cells. *J Pharm Sci* 1991;81:879–887.

56. Terada T, Saito H, Mukai M, Inui KI. Recognition of beta-lactam antibiotics by rat peptide transporters, PEPT1 and PEPT2, in LLC-PK1 cells. *Am J Physiol Renal Physiol* 1997;273:706–711.

57. Thwaites DT, Hirst BH, Simmons NL. Passive transepithelial absorption of thyrotropin-releasing hormone (TRH) via a paracellular route in cultured intestinal and renal epithelial cell lines. *Pharm Res* 1993;10:674–681.

58. Hilgendorf C, Spahn-Langguth H, Regardh CG, Lipka E, Amidon GL, Langguth P. Caco-2 versus Caco-2/HT29-MTX co-cultured cell lines: permeability via diffusion, inside- and outside-directed carrier-mediated transport. *J Pharm Sci* 2000;89:63–75.

59. Hilgers AR, Conradi RA, Burton PS. Caco-2 cell monolayers as a model for drug transport across the intestinal mucosa. *Pharm Res* 1990;7:902–910.

60. Kansy M, Senner F, Gubernator K. Physicochemical high throughput screening: parallel artificial membrane permeation assay in the description of passive absorption processes. *J Med Chem* 1998;41:1007–1010.

61. Lipinski CA. Observation on current ADMET technology: no uniformity exists. Paper presented at the *Proceedings of the Annual Meeting of the Society of Biomolecular Screening*, The Hauge, The Netherlands.

62. Lipinski CALF, Dominy BW, Feeney PJ. Experimental and computational approaches to estimate solubility and permeability in drug discovery and development. *Adv Drug Deliv Rev* 1997;23:3–25.

63. Kansy M, Avdeef A, Fischer H. Advances in screening for membrane permeability: high-resolution PAMPA for medicinal chemists. *Drug Discov Today Technol* 2004;1:349–355.

64. Chiou WL, Buehler PW. Comparison of oral absorption and bioavailability of drugs between monkey and human. *Pharm Res* 2002;19:868–874.

65. Mummaneni V, Dressman JB. Intestine uptake of cimetidine and ranitidine in rats. *Pharm Res* 1994;11:1599–1604.

66. Stewart BH, Chan OH, Lu RH, Reyner EL, Schmid HL, Hamilton HW, Steinbaugh BA, Taylor MD. Comparison of intestinal permeabilities determined in multiple *in vitro* and *in situ* models: relationship to absorption in humans. *Pharm Res* 1995;12:693–699.

67. Sugawara M, Saitoh H, Iseki K, Miyazaki K, Arita T. Contribution of passive transport mechanisms to the intestinal absorption of beta-lactam antibiotics. *J Pharm Pharmacol* 1990;42:314–318.

68. Ungell A-L, Nylander S, Bergstrand S, Sjoberg A, Lennernas H. Membrane transport of drugs in different regions of the intestinal tract of the rat. *J Pharm Sci* 1998;87:360–366.

69. Kirn D-C, Burton PS, Borchardt RT. A correlation between the permeability characteristics of a series of peptides using an *in vitro* cell culture model (Caco-2) and those using an *in situ* perfused rat ileum model of the intestinal mucosa. *Pharm Res* 1993;10:1710–1714.

70. Lowther N, Fox R, Faller B, Nick H, Jin Y, Sergejew T, Hirschberg Y, Oberle R, Donnelly H. *In vitro* and *in situ* permeability of a "second generation" hydroxypyridinone oral iron chelator: correlation with physico-chemical properties and oral activity. *Pharm Res* 1999;16:434–440.

71. Fagerholm U, Nilsson D, Knutson L, Lennernas H. Jejunal permeability in humans *in vivo* and rats *in situ*: investigation of molecular size selectivity and solvent drag. *Acta Physiol Scand* 1999;165:315–324.

72. Piyapolrungroj N, Zhou, YS, Li C, Liu G, Zimmermann E, Fleisher D. Cimetidine absorption and elimination in rat small intestine. *Drug Metab Dispos* 2000;28:65–72.

73. Aulton M. *Pharmaceutics: The Science of Dosage Form Design*, 2nd ed. Edinburgh; New York: Churchill Livingstone; 2002.

74. Komiya I, Park JY, Kamani A, Ho NFH, Higuchi WI. Quantitative mechanistic studies in simultaneous fluid flow and intestinal absorption using steroids as model solutes. *Int J Pharm* 1980;4:249–262

75. Balimane PV, Chong S, Morrison, RA. Current methodologies used for evaluation of intestinal permeability and absorption. *J Pharmacol Toxicol Methods* 2000;44:301–312.

76. Lennernas H, Ahrenstedt O, Hallgren R, Knutson L, Ryde M, Paalzow LK. Regional jejunal perfusion, a new *in vivo* approach to study oral drug absorption in man. *Pharm Res* 1992;9:1243–1251.

77. Salphati L, Childers K, Pan L, Tsutsui K, Takahashi L. Evaluation of a single-pass intestinal-perfusion method in rat for the prediction of absorption in man. *J Pharm Pharmacol* 2001;53:1007–1013.

78. Petri N, Tannergren C, Holst B, Mellon FA, Bao Y, Plumb GW, Bacon J, O'Leary KA, Kroon PA, Knutson L, Forsell P, Eriksson T, Lennernas H, Williamson G. Absorption/metabolism of sulforaphane and quercetin, and regulation Of phase II enzymes, In human jejunum *in vivo*. *Drug Metab Dispos* 2003;31:805–813.

79. Takamatsu N, Kim O-N, Welage LS, Idkaidek NM, Hayashi Y, Barnett J, Yamamoto R, Lipka E, Lennernås H, Hussain A, Lesko L, Amidon GL. Human jejunal permeability of two polar drugs: cimetidine and ranitidine. *Pharm Res* 2001;18:742–744.

80. Bonlokke L, Hovgaard L, Kristensen HG, Knutson L, Lennernas H. Direct estimation of the *in vivo* dissolution of spironolactone, in two particle size ranges, using the single-pass perfusion technique (Loc-I-Gut(R)) in humans. *Eur J Pharm Sci* 2001;12:239–250.

81. Pithavala YK, Heizer WD, Parr AF, O'Connor-Semmes RL, Brouwer KLR. Use of the InteliSite® capsule to study ranitidine absorption from various sites within the human intestinal tract. *Pharm Res* 1998;15:1869–1875.

82. InteliSite data sheet, www.innovativedevices.com.

83. Bailey CA, Bryla P, Malick AW. The use of the intestinal epithelial cell culture model, Caco-2, in pharmaceutical development. *Adv Drug Deliv Rev* 1996;22:85–103.

84. Fagerholm U, Johansson M, Lennernås H. Comparison between permeability coefficients in rat and human jejunum. *Pharm Res* 1996;13:1336–1342.

8

HOW AND WHERE ARE DRUGS ABSORBED?

MARIVAL BERMEJO AND ISABEL GONZALEZ-ALVAREZ

University of Valencia, Valencia, Spain

Contents

8.1 INTRODUCTION

A drug or a xenobiotic, in order to exert its pharmacological or toxic effects, must interact with its receptors at their action sites or therapeutic target. The essential step is therefore the absorption of the substance, that is, its entry from outside the body, unless the administration is done directly into the bloodstream. In this chapter, we review the biological barriers that the drug must cross in order to enter the body, which mechanisms are implicated in this process, and how the physiological characteristics of the administration route affect the absorption rate and extent.

Preclinical Development Handbook: ADME and Biopharmaceutical Properties,
edited by Shayne Cox Gad
Copyright © 2008 John Wiley & Sons, Inc.

8.2   ABSORPTION IMPACT ON DRUG BIOAVAILABILITY

The terms absorption and bioavailability are often used interchangeably when there is actually a conceptual difference between them. *Bioavailability* is a measurement of the rate and extent of therapeutically active drug that reaches the systemic circulation and is available at the site of action [1, 2]. *Absorption* is the movement of drug molecules across biological barriers from the site of administration. In some cases absorption has been defined as the movement from the administration site into the systemic circulation, but this definition could be misleading if in the pathway to the blood circulation the drug crosses a metabolic organ or tissue. The systemic availability F_{sys} is the result of absorption and all possible losses before arriving at the systemic circulation:

$$F_{sys} = F_a \cdot F_m$$

where F_a is the fraction absorbed and F_m is the fraction escaping first-pass extraction. From the equation, it is easy to conclude that F_a, the fraction absorbed, represents the upper limit for systemic availability in the absence of any presystemic losses of the drug on its way to the systemic circulation. It is therefore clear, that the absorption process is relevant to the availability of the drug at the action sites.

On the other hand, it is necessary to be aware of the terminology classically applied to some administration routes: if the drug does not reach the systemic circulation, then it is considered that no absorption occurs, and therefore the administration is considered to be topical. This is the case, for instance, for ophthalmic administration or for the topical administration of drugs on the skin. The entry of drug into those tissues is called *penetration* or *permeation* but not absorption, because the drug is not intended to reach the systemic circulation. This nomenclature then leads to the conclusion that the drug is bioavailable (as it reaches its action sites) but not absorbed into the bloodstream (or does not present systemic absorption).

Throughout the chapter, the difference between absorption and bioavailability for those administration routes that involve a first pass through a metabolic organ (mainly liver) or tissue (i.e., intestinal tissue) is stressed, and the drug is considered absorbed once it is inside the body.

The next step is to analyze the factors affecting F_a by the different routes of drug administration. As described in this chapter, absorption is a transport phenomenon that can be described mechanistically, in order to identify the limiting steps. The complexity of the barriers—subcellular, cellular, or multicellular—are also addressed.

8.3   HOW: ABSORPTION MECHANISMS

The complexity and number of barriers that the drug has to cross before reaching the bloodstream differs from one route of administration to other, but in all the cases the barriers are integrated by semipermeable cell membranes. They are composed of a bimolecular lipid matrix, containing mostly cholesterol and phospholipids. The lipids provide stability to the membrane and determine its permeability characteristics. Globular proteins, of various sizes and composition, embedded in the matrix are involved in transport and function as receptors for cellular regulation. Drugs may cross a biologic barrier by passive diffusion, facilitated passive diffusion, active transport, or endocytosis.

8.3.1 Passive Diffusion

Passive diffusion involves the movement of drug molecules down a concentration or electrochemical gradient without the expenditure of energy. Passive diffusion does not involve a carrier, is not saturable, and shows a low structural specificity [3]. Passive absorption of drug can be done by two pathways: paracellular and transcellular.

A paracellular pathway consists of the diffusion of xenobiotics across the intercellular spaces or tight junctions, aqueous pores, or fenestrae [4–6]. These junctions are more or less leaky, depending on the tissue, and allow the diffusion of water and small solutes. In general, the main restriction for using this route is the molecular size followed by the electric repulsion between the ionized groups of the molecules and the ionized groups in the constituents of the aqueous pathways [7–9].

From a mathematical point of view, paracellular diffusion follows the same diffusion law that is applied to transcellular diffusion. The passive movement of molecules down a concentration gradient is described by Fick's law. The process is depicted in Fig. 8.1.

$$J = \frac{1}{A} \cdot \frac{dM}{dt} = P \cdot \Delta C = \frac{D \cdot (K_1 \cdot C_{\text{aq-outside}} - K_2 \cdot C_{\text{aq-inside}})}{h}$$

where J represents the net flux, that is, the net rate of diffusion through the membrane surface (g/(cm^2·s)); P is the permeability coefficient (cm/s); D is the diffusion coefficient of the solute in the membrane (cm^2/s); ΔC is the concentration gradient across the membrane (g/cm^3); and K_1 and K_2 are the partition coefficients of the solute in the membrane (at both sides).

As can be seen from this equation, there are several factors that affect the diffusion of the molecules, such as lipophilicity, pH/pK_a, size, and area of the absorptive

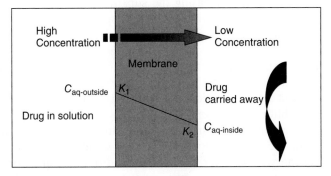

FIGURE 8.1 Scheme of the process of passive diffusion across biological membranes. The driving force for diffusion is the concentration gradient. The partition coefficient of the xenobiotic in the lipid bilayer is one of the main determinants of resistance to transport.

surface. Diffusion coefficients of drugs in the membrane increase with drug lipophilicity and decrease with molecular weight. On the other hand, it is the nonionized fraction of the molecules that mostly contributes to the overall transport, as the nonionized fraction has the highest partition coefficient.

The Henderson-Hasselbalch equation can be used to calculate the relative proportions of the ionized and nonionized forms of the drug [10]:

$$\text{For acids:} \quad \% \text{ ionized} = \frac{100}{1 + 10^{(pK_a - pH)}}$$

$$\text{For bases:} \quad \% \text{ ionized} = \frac{100}{1 + 10^{(pH - pK_a)}}$$

In other words, mass diffusion per unit area of a weakly acid drug will be higher from a more acid medium while mass diffusion per unit area of a weakly basic drug will be favored from a more alkaline medium.

A second consequence of the solute ionization in biological fluids is *ion trapping* phenomenon. When the pH of the fluids is different on both sides of the membrane, the solute will be trapped on the side favoring its ionization. A similar phenomenon is produced by the binding to macromolecules, for instance, proteins, as only the free drug is able to diffuse across the membrane.

8.3.2   Carrier Mediated

In addition to the passive diffusional processes over lipid membranes or between cells, substances can be transferred through the lipid phase of biological membranes through specialized systems, that is, active transport and facilitated diffusion [11].

Facilitated Diffusion   Facilitated diffusion involves the participation of a carrier molecule, so this mechanism also shows selectivity and saturation, but the transport occurs always from a higher concentration to a lower concentration area and thus it does not require any energy source [12].

One theory is that a carrier component combines reversibly with the substrate molecule at the cell membrane exterior, and the carrier–substrate complex diffuses rapidly across the membrane, releasing the substrate at the interior surface. The carrier transports only substrates with a relatively specific molecular configuration, and the process is limited by the availability of carriers.

Active Transport   Active transport of a xenobiotic is an energy requiring process that is saturable (i.e., is limited by the number of protein transporters present) and could proceed against a concentration gradient. Active transport can be affected by the presence of inhibitors [12]. There are two kinds of active transporters: primary active transporters use energy coming from the hydrolysis of ATP; while secondary active transporters use the energy coming from some electrochemical gradient generated by a primary transporter, for instance, a difference in H^+ or Na^+ ion concentration. Symporters transport the drug and the cotransported molecule or ion in the same direction, while antiporters transport the drug and the ion in opposite directions.

The active transport process can be described in mathematical terms using the Michaelis–Menten equation, as the binding of the solute to the carrier molecule and its translocation to the other side of the membrane have several similarities to the sustrate–enzyme interaction:

$$J_{active} = \frac{dM}{A \cdot dt} = \frac{V_{max} \cdot C}{K_m + C}$$

where V_{max} is the maximal transport velocity (mass/(area·time)), C is the drug concentration, and K_m is the drug concentration at which velocity of transport is $\frac{1}{2}V_{max}$.

When $C \gg K_m$,

$$J \simeq \frac{V_{max} \cdot C}{C} \simeq V_{max}$$

and the rate of the transport process becomes independent of the concentration. But when the drug concentration is much lower than K_m (i.e., $K_m \gg C$), then

$$J \simeq \frac{V_{max}}{K_m} \cdot C$$

and the transport process follows an apparent first order kinetic.

When a drug is able to be absorbed by passive diffusion and active transport, the total flux is the sum of the passive and active fluxes, as can be seen in Fig. 8.2.

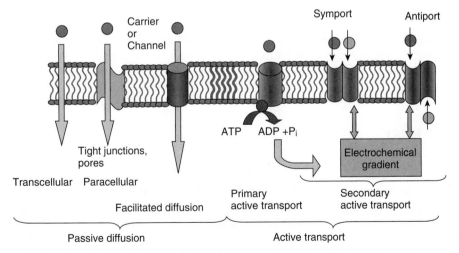

FIGURE 8.2 Transport flux as a function of drug concentration for a substance transported by passive diffusion, active transport, or a combination of both processes.

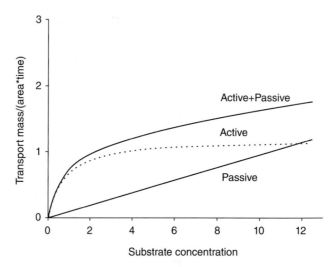

FIGURE 8.3 Summary of the transport mechanisms that xenobiotics use for crossing biological membranes (with the exception of endocytosis).

8.3.3 Endocytosis

Endocytosis is also called vesicle mediated transport. The molecules or particles are engulfed by a cell. The cell membrane invaginates, encloses the fluid or particles, then fuses again, forming a vesicle that later transports them across the membrane to the inside of the cell. This mechanism also requires energy expenditure. This diffusion is dependent on the size of the pore and the molecular weight of the chemical. Phagocytosis is the type of endocytosis where an entire cell is engulfed. Pinocytosis is when the external fluid is engulfed. Receptor-mediated endocytosis occurs when the material to be transported binds to certain specific molecules in the membrane. Examples include the transport of insulin and cholesterol into animal cells. Endocytosis probably plays a minor role in drug absorption, except for protein drugs.

In summary, chemicals can be introduced into the body by various mechanisms that are represented in Fig. 8.3. Once the drug is in the systemic circulation it has access to its target tissue or receptors by using some of the aforementioned mechanisms.

8.4 WHERE

8.4.1 Absorption Routes: Enteral Versus Parenteral

A tablet inside our stomach is, technically, outside the body. This image helps to define the two main groups of administration routes. Anything that is administered in the intestinal tract is using the enteral route (from *enteron* = intestine). By exclusion, all the other administration routes are defined as parenteral (*par* = outside). Enteral routes include buccal and sublingual, rectal, and oral. Among the parenteral routes we can distinguish those that require a needle to introduce the drug to the depot site (e.g., subcutaneous or intramuscular routes) and those using other mucosal surfaces or epithelial barriers (e.g., nasal, ophthalmic, or transpulmonary).

Selection of the route of administration involves the evaluation of many different factors, from the physicochemical characteristics of the drug, which determine its ability to cross the barriers, to the pharmacological action, which could require a fast absorption rate to assure a quick onset of response. Chronic therapies require ease of use and patient friendly routes. Lastly, the existence of the appropriate technology could limit the use of an administration route if a suitable dosage form is not in place.

8.4.2 Routes of Drug Administration and Physiological Variables Affecting Xenobiotic Absorption

A prerequisite to absorption by any administration route is drug dissolution. Any solid drug products (e.g., tablets) have to disintegrate and deaggregate in order to release the drug particles and to allow drug dissolution. The solubility of the drug in biological fluids at the administration site determines the gradient for diffusion, while permeability in the membrane establishes the resistance to the transport. For most administration routes these two factors—drug solubility and drug membrane permeability—are the main factors governing drug absorption.

Enteral Routes   Enteral absorption routes comprise all those involving any part of the gastrointestinal tract, that is, buccal and sublingual, rectal, and the so-called oral route that requires swallowing the substance, and its access to the intestine.

Oral   The oral route of administration is the most used and convenient for patients. The gastrointestinal tract is a complex environment from the standpoint of drug absorption; therefore, a deep understanding of gastrointestinal physiology is essential to determine how and where drugs and xenobiotics are absorbed from the oral route [13, 14]. The main physiological factors that must be considered to understand nutrients and drug absorption are summarized in Table 8.1 and are discussed in this section.

The gastrointestinal system includes the gastrointestinal tract and all the organs that secrete substances into it. The main functions are digestion, secretion, absorption, and motility [15]. The gastrointestinal tract begins in the mouth and continues

TABLE 8.1 Physiological Factors Affecting Drug Absorption from the Gastrointestinal Tract [17]

Membrane permeability
Luminal pH
Intestinal secretions presence of food
Surface area
Transit time
Disease state
Water fluxes
Mucus and unstirred water layer (UWL)

with the esophagus, which is the pathway to the stomach. The stomach is a sac-like organ with a quite acidic environment (pH ranging from 2 in fasted state to 5 or 6 in fed state) thanks to the secretion of hydrochloric acid by parietal cells. This acidic environment constitutes the first line of immune protection of the gastrointestinal tract and, on the other hand, is the first barrier against absorption, as many substances are not stable in this environment.

Digestion's final stages and most absorption occur in the next section: the small intestine. The small intestine is divided into three segments. The initial short one, the duodenum, receives the secretions of the pancreas and liver through a common duct. The pH of this segment ranges from 5 near the stomach to 7 at the final portion. The jejunum has a thicker and more vascular wall and along with the duodenum is the site where most digestion and absorption occur, so actually the small intestine has a big functional reserve. The last portion, the ileum, is the longest segment, a little narrower in diameter and with a pH rather constant at 6.5–7. Only a small portion of water, salts, and undigested material reach the large intestine. The large intestine has three parts: cecum, colon, and rectum. Between the small and large intestines there is a valve that prevents the material from going back. The large intestine has some enzymes, which are able to metabolize some drugs, along with a big population of bacteria that contribute to the fermentation of undigested residues. The large intestine is responsible for absorbing water and electrolytes and for the formation, storage, and evacuation of feces [13].

There is extensive folding on the intestinal surface. There are folds extending from the surface of the geometrical cylinder. In the surface of the folds, there are finger-like projections called villi. Villi contain absorptive cells and goblet cells. The absorptive cells are characterized by the small projections of their apical membranes that are called brush border or microvilli. The apical membrane is highly specialized and contains enzymes, binding sites, and transporters. Other important features are the tight junctions, which play a major role in regulating paracellular permeability of water and solutes. Permeability of junctional complexes is higher in the upper intestine than in the ileum.

Figure 8.4 shows how the combination of folds, villi, and microvilli increases the surface available for absorption about 600 times [15]. Each villus is occupied by a blind-ended lymphatic vessel (called a lacteal) and by a capillary network, whose drainage leads to the hepatic portal vein. That means that any substance absorbed in the intestinal epithelium must cross the liver before arriving in the systemic circulation. During this first passage through the liver, the nutrients, xenobiotics, and drugs can be metabolized, reducing the fraction of substance that finally arrives in the systemic circulation. This is the *first-pass effect* whose effect on bioavailability is analyzed later. On the other hand, during the passage through the liver the drug or xenobiotic could be excreted into the bile and again reach the small intestine, where it is again absorbed. This process is called enterohepatic circulation and could affect the disposition of the compound.

The large intestine has folds but no villi. The smaller surface area available for absorption and the smaller amount of fluid present in the large intestine are reflected, in general, in a lower permeability for xenobiotics; but, on the other hand, the longer residence time in this area may compensate for the lower permeability and makes the large intestine a suitable target area for prolonged release drug formulations [16, 17].

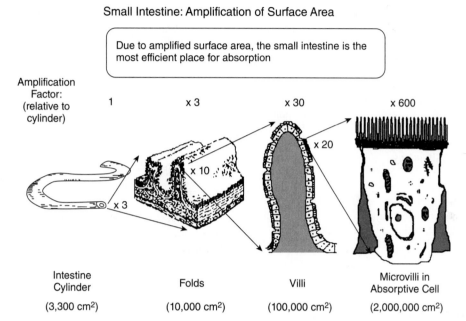

Small Intestine: Amplification of Surface Area

Due to amplified surface area, the small intestine is the most efficient place for absorption

Amplification
Factor:
(relative to
cylinder)

1   x 3   x 30   x 600

x 20

x 10

x 3

Intestine Cylinder	Folds	Villi	Microvilli in Absorptive Cell
(3,300 cm²)	(10,000 cm²)	(100,000 cm²)	(2,000,000 cm²)

FIGURE 8.4   Anatomical modifications of the intestinal system that increase the available surface for absorption. (From Ref. 15, with permission from Modern Biopharmaceutics™.)

Gastrointestinal secretions contribute to the digestion and absorption of nutrients. The main gastrointestinal secretions, their main components, and the substances they contribute to digestion are summarized in Table 8.2 [14].

Carbohydrates are digested into monosaccharides, proteins are hydrolized into amino acids or small peptides, and fat droplets are transformed into free fatty acids and monoglycerides. The resulting compounds from digestion as well as fat-soluble and water-soluble vitamins are absorbed by some of the absorption mechanisms explained in the previous section. All essential nutrients including proteins, carbohydrates, fats, vitamins, and minerals are substrates of some active or facilitated carrier system. There are excellent reviews about the nature and diversity of intestinal transporters [12, 18–21].

Another process of particular relevance for fat absorption that may also influence drug absorption is emulsification. Emulsification of fat droplets, thanks to mechanical disruption and the presence of emulsifying agents (bile salts and phospholipids), increase the surface available for lipase action, thus increasing the rate of lipid digestion. The digestion products are incorporated into the core of aggregates known as micelles. Micelles consist of bile salts, fatty acids, monoglycerides, and phospholipids, all clustered together with the polar ends of each molecule oriented toward the surface. The micelles release their contents near the lipid bilayer and, in consequence, the released molecules can diffuse easily across the intestinal lining. Fat-soluble vitamins follow the pathway for fat absorption, and any other highly lipophilic molecule could also be incorporated in the micellar phase. Thus, for instance, any interference with the secretion of bile decreases the absorption of fat-soluble vitamins.

TABLE 8.2   Main Gastrointestinal Secretions, Their Components, and the Nutrients They Contribute to Digestion [14]

Secretion	Main Components	Digestion
Saliva 1–1.5 liters/day pH ~ 8 at secretion rate	Water Electrolytes Mucus Lysozyme α-Amylase	Disaccharides
Gastric fluid 1.5–2 liters/day	Mucus Hydrochloric acid Pepsinogen (pepsin precursor) Intrinsic factor	All Proteins Essential for vitamin B_{12} absorption
Pancreatic secretions 1–1.5 liters/day	Bicarbonate Trypsin, chymotrypsin, carboxypeptidases α-Amylase Pancreatic lipase	Neutralizes acid from stomach Protein Disaccharides Fatty acids
Bile 0.5–1 liter/day	Bile salts Cholesterol Phospholipids Bile pigments Proteins Bicarbonate, electrolytes	Fat digestion
Intestinal fluid 2 liters/day	Electrolytes Water Mucus	

Water is the most abundant substance in chyme. Around 9 liters of ingested and secreted fluids enter the small intestine each day, but only 1.5 liters passes onto the large intestine, since 80% of the fluid is absorbed in the small intestine. Finally, only 150 grams of feces, consisting about 100 mL water and 50 g of solid material, is normally eliminated each day [14, 15]. The amount of water present in the gastrointestinal system is relevant for ensuring the complete dissolution of the administered dose. Some drugs present a dose-limited absorption when there is not enough water in the luminal fluids to allow the complete dissolution during transit time.

ABSORPTION OF DRUGS AND XENOBIOTICS   The two main factors affecting rate and extent of absorption are drug permeability and solubility in intestinal fluids. Solubility of the drug determines the highest gradient for drug diffusion across the membrane. This concept is represented in Fig. 8.5.

Chemical stability or phenomena such as aggregation and complexation with luminal components may reduce the drug concentration in the lumen. Solubility and drug concentration in the luminal fluids are functions of the molecule pK_a for weak acids and bases and the pH of the luminal fluids. The presence of different intestinal secretions and the change in secretion rate because of the presence of food changes luminal pH, as summarized in Fig. 8.6.

"First Law of Drug Absorption"

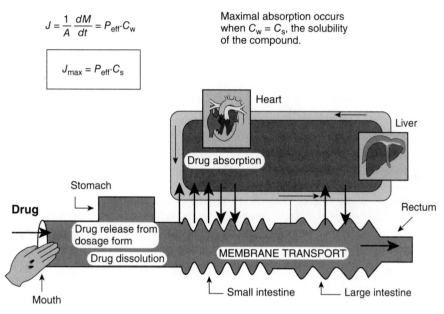

$$J = \frac{1}{A}\frac{dM}{dt} = P_{\text{eff}} \cdot C_{\text{w}}$$

$$J_{\max} = P_{\text{eff}} \cdot C_{\text{s}}$$

Maximal absorption occurs when $C_{\text{w}} = C_{\text{s}}$, the solubility of the compound.

Heart

Liver

Drug absorption

Stomach

Drug

Rectum

Drug release from dosage form

Drug dissolution

MEMBRANE TRANSPORT

Mouth

Small intestine

Large intestine

FIGURE 8.5   Factors determining rate and extent of absorption in the gastrointestinal tract.

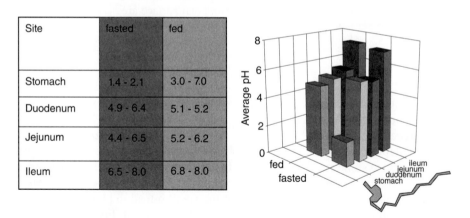

Site	fasted	fed
Stomach	1.4 - 2.1	3.0 - 7.0
Duodenum	4.9 - 6.4	5.1 - 5.2
Jejunum	4.4 - 6.5	5.2 - 6.2
Ileum	6.5 - 8.0	6.8 - 8.0

FIGURE 8.6   Average intestinal pH values in the gastrointestinal tract in the fasted and fed states. Data from Dressman et al. [85].

Finally, if the drug is administered in a solid form, any factor affecting its dissolution rate will have an impact on the rate and extent of absorption, so particle size may be relevant, in particular, for those substances of low solubility.

Permeability of the drug, as well as its permeation mechanism, depends on several molecular properties. Some of them are summarized in Table 8.3 [22]. Drugs administered by the oral route may cross the intestinal membrane by all the

TABLE 8.3 Molecular Descriptors Related to Drug Permeability in the Intestinal Epithelium

---

Lipophilicity As drug partitioning into the cell membrane is one of the steps in membrane transport, lipophilicity is widely used as a predictor of drug permeability. Lipophilicity has two principal components, molecular size and hydrogen bonding potential [25, 87–90].

Molecular Weight (MW) This is a component of lipophilicity as well as diffusion coefficient in biological membranes and fluids. A rather strong dependence between transcellular diffusion and molecular size has been observed. Compounds with MW < 200 are able to pass through the intestinal membrane by the paracellular pathway along with diffusion through the transcellular route. Compounds with MW > 250 use the transcellular route but further increases of the molecular weight (MW > 500) consequently lead to a decrease in membrane diffusion [91].

Hydrogen Bonding The absorption ability of a molecule depends on the number and the strength of the hydrogen bonds that the molecule is able to form with water molecules, because the first step to enter into the membrane is the desolvation of the molecule. Hydrogen bonding capacity is detrimental for transport into the nonpolar environment of the cell membrane. Thus, these properties along with lipophilicity are good descriptors of drug permeation [92].

Polar Surface Area (*PSA*) The PSA of a molecule is defined as the area of its van der Waals surface that arises from oxygen or nitrogen atoms plus the area of the hydrogen atoms attached to these heteroatoms. As such, PSA is clearly related to the capacity to form hydrogen bonds. Drugs with PSAd < 60 Å^2 would be completely absorbed (fraction absorbed, FA > 90%). Drugs with PSAd > 140 Å^2 would be absorbed less than 10%.

Nonpolar Surface Area Nonpolar substituents facilitate membrane transport and hydrophobic compounds generally have higher permeabilities than hydrophilic ones (with similar hydrogen bonding properties). Nonpolar surface area can also correlate with membrane permeability. In general, this parameter is included in correlations along with PSA [88, 93–95].

Source: Adapted from Ref. 22.

previously mentioned mechanisms: passive diffusion, facilitated passive diffusion, active transport, or pinocytosis.

The paracellular pathway, between the epithelial cells, is both size (MW, volume) and charge dependent [6, 23, 24]; cations seem to penetrate the negatively charged tight junctional system much more easily than anions [23]. On the other hand, the available surface area for paracellular intestinal absorption has been estimated to be about 0.01% of the total surface area of the small intestine [4, 6].

Due to the lipidic nature of the intestinal membrane, the ability of the molecules to diffuse across it is dependent on their lipophilicity [25, 26]. In particular, one of the main factors affecting drug permeability is the distribution coefficient, which depends on the pH of the luminal fluids. As has been described, the pH of the luminal contents changes along the gastrointestinal tract and it is different in the fasted versus the fed state. That affects the solubility of ionizable compounds and their distribution coefficient; so, in general, permeability also varies along the gastrointestinal tract for a given solute [27].

The unstirred water layer (UWL) adjacent to the intestinal lining was considered to be the rate-limiting step for intestinal permeability of high permeability compounds [28]. However, several *in vivo* studies have clearly reported that the thickness of this UWL is significantly thinner than was previously assumed, thanks to the motility of the gastrointestinal tract [29, 30].

There is now enough evidence about the involvement of intestinal transporters in the absorption of drugs [31]. Targeting intestinal transporters by means of development of prodrugs has been a successful strategy for improving oral absorption. For example, the intestinal peptide transporter is utilized in order to increase the bioavailability of several classes of peptidomimetic drugs, especially ACE inhibitors and beta-lactam antibiotics [19]. The bioavailability of poorly absorbed drugs can be improved by utilization of the transporters responsible for the intestinal absorption of various solutes and/or by inhibiting the transporter involved in the efflux system [32–35].

The last relevant physiological factor that determines drug absorption is intestinal motility, as this function limits the intestinal transit time of any solute. Since the small intestine is the main site for drug absorption, gastric emptying is the first limiting step for the access of the drug to the intestine. The average gastric emptying time is around 30 minutes, transit time in the small intestine is around 3 hours, and transit time in the large intestine is much more variable but an average of 3 days has been reported [15, 36]. Some factors affecting the gastric emptying rates of liquids are described in Table 8.4.

Solid emptying is slower than liquid emptying; also, emptying depends on the caloric content of the meal (as for liquids), and particles of size bigger than 2 mm remain in the stomach until the next "housekeeping wave" that completely empties the stomach [15].

Intestinal peristalsis is stimulated by voluminous meals and hypertonic contents. Anticholinergic drugs slow intestinal movements while cholinergic drugs stimulate transit, so simultaneous administration of these drugs with food may affect absorption.

To complete the description of this route of absorption, it is necessary to remember again the difference between absorption and oral bioavailability. Win L. Chiou [1] defined absorption as the movement of drug across the outer mucosal membranes of the gastrointestinal tract; while, in general, the systemic availability (F_{sys}) is defined as the fraction of the amount (dose) of the xenobiotic (drug) that reaches the systemic circulation. As described previously, during first passage through the liver and also during passage through the intestinal cells, the drug could be biotransformed by the intestinal or hepatic enzymes. In mathematical terms, this process is expressed as follows:

$$F_{sys} = F_a \cdot (1 - E_g) \cdot (1 - E_h) \tag{8.1}$$

TABLE 8.4   Factors Affecting Gastric Emptying Rates of Liquids [15]

Gastric Emptying	Comment
Volume	Larger volume, faster emptying rate
Osmotic pressure	Iso-osmotic content empties faster than hyper- or hypotonic solutions
pH	
Caloric content	Higher caloric content slows emptying
Viscosity	Higher viscosity delays emptying

where F_a is the fraction absorbed, E_g is the gut extraction ratio, and E_h is the hepatic extraction ratio. $(1 - E_g)$ is the fraction escaping intestinal metabolism and $(1 - E_h)$ represents the fraction escaping liver metabolism. In the absence of any presystemic losses, systemic bioavailability equals the fraction absorbed.

Buccal and Sublingual   Administration of drugs using the oral cavity is an option well accepted by patients. Oral mucosa is relatively permeable with a rich blood supply [37–39]. A second advantage is the avoidance of first-pass effect and presystemic elimination in the GI tract. These factors make the oral mucosal cavity a potential alternative for systemic drug delivery [40].

Within the oral cavity, delivery of drugs can be made through the sublingual mucosa or by placing the dosage form in the mucosa lining the internal face of the cheeks, which is called the buccal route.

Oral mucosa is a stratified epithelium with a turnover time around 5–6 days [41]. It is estimated that the permeability of the buccal mucosa is 4–4000 times greater than that of the skin [42]. The buccal area has 40–50 cell layers, whereas the sublingual zone is slightly thinner. Oral mucosa is keratinized and relatively impermeable in all the areas that suffer mechanical stress, but the sublingual and buccal areas are not keratinized, rendering them more permeable [41, 43, 44]. In general, the permeabilities of the oral mucosa decrease in the order of sublingual > buccal > palatal [41].

For significant drug absorption, the drug must have a prolonged exposure to the mucosal surface so the drug taste must be acceptable to the patient [45].

The absorption potential of the buccal mucosa is influenced by the lipid solubility and therefore the permeability of the solution (osmosis), the ionization (pH), and the molecular weight of the substances. Because the pH of saliva is usually 6.5–6.9, absorption is favored for drugs with a high pK_a [41, 46].

The basic drug transport mechanism for buccal epithelium is passive diffusion, as for other epithelia in the body. There are two major routes involved: transcellular (intracellular) and paracellular (intercellular) [47]. The intercellular spaces are the major barrier to permeation of lipophilic compounds and the cell membrane acts as the major transport barrier for hydrophilic compounds. The route that predominates, however, is generally the one that provides the least amount of hindrance to passage [40]. Some authors have suggested the presence of a specialized transport system for cephadroxyl in the human buccal membrane [48].

One of the major disadvantages associated with buccal drug delivery is the low flux, which results in low drug bioavailability and the lack of dosage form retention at the site of absorption. Consequently, bioadhesive polymers have extensively been employed in buccal drug delivery systems.

To sum up, the buccal mucosa offers several advantages for controlled drug delivery for extended periods of time and is a promising area for systemic delivery of orally inefficient drugs (such as potent peptide and protein drug molecules). However, the need for safe and effective buccal permeation/absorption enhancers is a crucial component for a prospective future in the area of buccal drug delivery.

Sublingual literally means "under the tongue." Sublingual mucosa is more permeable than buccal mucosa. Because of the high permeability and the rich blood supply, the sublingual route is capable of producing a rapid onset of action, but the area is continuously washed by a high amount of saliva, making the buccal area more suitable for placement of retentive dosage forms. In clinical practice, sublingual drug administration is applied in the field of cardiovascular drugs, steroids, some barbiturates, and enzymes and it has been explored as an alternative for vitamins and minerals, which are found to be readily absorbed by this method. It could be especially useful for those who experience difficulty in swallowing tablets.

Rectal   Absorption through the rectal mucosa is, in general, irregular and not complete so it can not be considered a first delivery option. The acceptance of the rectal route varies among countries but rectal delivery could be a convenient, alternative route when other routes are not available. The following situations represent opportunities for rectal administration:

- Patients having difficulty swallowing, nausea, vomiting, or gastric pain.
- Uncooperative or nonconscious patients.
- When access to the intravenous route is difficult.
- For drugs unstable in the gastrointestinal tract.
- For drugs with high first-pass effect.
- When a slow and prolonged input could have therapeutic interest.

For instance, rectal administration is used for anticonvulsants [49], nonnarcotic and narcotic analgesics, theophylline, antiemetics, and antibacterial agents and for inducing anesthesia in children [50, 51].

Its principal advantage is that it is independent of gastrointestinal tract motility and rate of gastric emptying [52].

However, this route should be avoided in the following situations:

- Painful anal conditions (fissures or inflamed hemorrhoids).
- Immunosuppressed patients in whom even minimal trauma could lead to formation of an abscess [53].
- Elderly patients with diarrhea.
- Patients physically unable to place the suppository.

The rectal route also has other disadvantages. There may be a great deal of variation among individuals regarding the necessary dose. Moreover, the rectal dose generally must be higher than the dose administered intravenously or orally, as absorption is slower and incomplete.

In humans, the rectum comprises the last 12–19 cm of the large intestine and the rectal epithelium is formed by a single layer of columnar or cuboidal cells and goblet cells; its surface area is about 200–400 cm^2. The absorbing surface area of the rectum is considerably smaller than that of the small intestine, as the former lacks villi and microvilli. However, the epithelia in the rectum and the upper intestinal tract are histologically similar, giving them comparable abilities to absorb drugs. The rectal mucosa is richly vascularized.

Drugs absorbed via the inferior and middle rectal veins can in part avoid first-pass metabolism because the blood flow from these veins bypasses the portal system and empties into the vena cava. First-pass effects are not completely avoided, however, as there are anastomoses among inferior and middle veins with the superior one. The drugs absorbed via the superior rectal veins are transported to the liver via the portal system [54–56].

For a number of drugs the extent of rectal absorption has been reported to exceed oral values, which may reflect partial avoidance of hepatic first-pass metabolism after rectal delivery. This phenomenon has been reported for morphine, metoclopramide, ergotamine, lidocaine (lignocaine), and propranolol [54, 57].

Passive diffusion is the predominant mechanism of absorption and it is mainly dependent on the molecular weight, liposolubility, and degree of ionization of molecules. The contribution of other mechanisms, such as carrier mediated transport or pinocytosis, can be considered negligible. Paracellular diffusion is more restricted than in the upper zone of the gastrointestinal tract due to the lower permeability of the tight junctions in this area. The rate of rectal transmucosal absorption is affected by different factors: for example, the surface area available for absorption is small, particularly for drugs in solid dosage forms, which provide less extensibility than liquid forms. The volume present in the rectal cavity is also variable among patients but generally the volume is small and the viscosity is high. Diluent volume is also an important determinant of rectal drug uptake, as demonstrated with methohexital administered rectally for preprocedure sedation [58].

Lipophilic drugs are better absorbed than hydrophilic ones. Rectal pH may also influence drug uptake by altering the amount of drug that is ionised [59]. The pH of the rectal vault in children ranges from 7.2 to 12.2 [60]. This pH range favors absorption of barbiturates that will remain in a nonionized state because their pK_a is near the physiologic range (~7.6). The greater lipid solubility of nonionized drugs enhances their movement across the membrane. Finally, in a similar way to the small intestine where transit time limits absorption, rectal retention of the drug determines the absorption. Retention time, in many cases, is affected by the nature of the drug excipients. Hydrophilic excipients are more irritating for the rectal mucosa and increase peristaltic movements, reducing retention time.

Parenteral Routes (Noninjectables)

Transpulmonary   The respiratory system consists of two main areas—the conducting and the respiratory regions. The first one is responsible for filtering and humidifying the air entering the respiratory region, where gas interchange takes place. The conducting region is formed by the nasal cavity, nasopharynx, bronchi, and bronchioles. Airways distal to the bronchioles and the alveoli constitute the respiratory region.

The transpulmonary route has classically been used for drugs intended to exert a local action in the lungs and more recently for systemic administration. In the first case, it allows the delivery of high drug concentration directly to the action site. In this way, the same therapeutic effect can be obtained with a fraction of the dose administered by any other systemic route, and simultaneously systemic and adverse effects are minimized. In general, a rapid onset of action can be achieved. For systemic action, the transpulmonary route offers the advantages of being a friendly needle-free option, with a huge absorptive surface area ($100\,m^2$) of a highly permeable membrane in the alveolar region (0.2–0.7 μm). Compared to the gastrointestinal tract, the possibility of enzymatic degradation is reduced, and large molecules can be absorbed in part thanks to a prolonged residence time, as the mucociliary clearance is less marked in the lung periphery.

Nevertheless, there are also barriers against absorption through this route. The respiratory system is designed to prevent the entry of particles. The airway geometry, the humidification mechanisms, and the mucociliary clearance contribute to this process and then constitute barriers for transpulmonary absorption. Once in the lower parts of the respiratory tract, the drug has to deal with the lung surfactant, surface lining fluid, the epithelium and basement membranes, and the capillary endothelium before arriving at the blood flow.

The main factors affecting the amount of drug that is finally deposited in the deep lung are the particle size and density. The combination of both factors defines the aerodynamic diameter, which is actually the factor governing the deposition site. The relation between particle diameter and aerodynamic diameter of a spherical particle is defined by the following equation:

$$d_a = \sqrt{\frac{\rho}{\rho_a}} \cdot d$$

where d_a is the aerodynamic diameter, d is the particle diameter, ρ is the particle density, and $\rho_a = 1\,g/cm^3$.

Particles of mean aerodynamic diameter of 1–3 μm deposit minimally in the mouth and throat and maximally in the lung's parenchymal (i.e., alveolar or "deep lung") region. Tracheobronchial deposition is maximal for particles with aerodynamic diameters between 8 and 10 μm. Particles possessing an aerodynamic diameter smaller than 1 μm (although greater than several hundred nanometers) are mostly exhaled, and particles larger than 10 μm have little chance of making it beyond the mouth.

Once deposited in the lungs, inhaled drugs are (1) cleared from the lungs, (2) absorbed into the systemic or lymphatic circulation, or (3) degraded via drug metabolism.

Mucociliary Clearance. Mucus is secreted by goblet cells and submucosal glands forming a double sol-gel layer covering the ciliated epithelium. Mucociliary clearance can be impaired in some pathological conditions either by impairment or ciliary movement or by the production of thicker mucus.

Absorption. Lipophilic molecules pass easily through the airway epithelium via passive transport. Hydrophilic molecules cross via paracellular pathways, such as tight junctions, or by active transport via endocytosis and exocytosis. The rate of protein absorption from the alveoli is size dependent. Effros and Mason [61] demonstrated an inverse relationship between alveolar permeability and molecular weight.

Metabolism. The lung is the only organ through which the entire cardiac output passes. The liver first-pass effect is thus avoided through this route, but metabolism during the passage through the epithelium can still happen even if the relevance of metabolic clearance in the lung for systemic availability of inhaled drug is not well understood. All metabolizing enzymes found in the liver are found to a lesser extent in the lung: phase 1 cytochrome P450 (CYP450) enzymes, flavin-containing monooxygenases (FMOs), monoamine oxidase (MAO), aldehyde dehyrogenase, NADPH-CYP450 reductase, esterases, and proteases are all present in the lung. The monooxygenase system metabolizes fatty acids, steroids, and lipophilic xenobiotics. Esterase presents in high concentrations in alveolar macrophages, and to a lesser degree in alveolar type I and II cells. Proteins and peptides are subject to hydrolysis by proteases. However, for most proteins degradation in the alveoli is not a major clearance mechanism, with >95% of proteins, including insulin, being absorbed intact from the lung periphery.

Nasal   The nasal mucosa is a promising site for the delivery of many drugs, including proteins and other large biomolecules that do not have good absorption through other routes. The nasal cavity is easily accessible and extensively vascularized, and compounds administered via this route avoid the hepatic first-pass effect. In this respect, it should be an ideal route for noninvasive delivery. In addition, absorption of drug at the olfactory region of the nose provides a potential pathway for a pharmaceutical compound to be available to the central nervous system. The nasal delivery of vaccines is another very attractive application in terms of efficacy and patient acceptance. However, there are a number of factors that limit its utility. The physiology of the nasal cavity presents the most significant barrier to drug absorption. Limiting factors include rapid mucociliary clearance, enzymatic degradation in the mucus layer, and low permeability of the nasal epithelium [62–66].

The nasal vestibule and atrium are the less permeable areas in the nasal cavity, whereas the respiratory region (turbinate) is the most permeable thanks to the increased surface area and the rich vasculature. This latter area has a large surface area ~150–160 cm^2 because of the presence of microvilli. The pH of the zone varies between 5.5 and 6.5 in adults and between 5.0 and 7.0 in children.

The mechanisms for drug absorption in this area include passive diffusion (para- and transcellular), carrier mediated transport, and transcytosis. Lipophilic drugs are well absorbed with bioavailabilities reaching 100%; but permeability is low for polar molecules (including low molecular weight drugs and large peptides and proteins). In general, absorption is restricted for drugs with molecular weights higher than 1000 daltons.

Deposition of the formulation in the anterior portion of the nose provides a longer nasal residence time but permeability is lower in this area; whereas deposition in the posterior zone, where the permeability is higher, provides shorter residence times. This shorter residence time is due to the mucociliary clearance, which must be maintained for normal physiological functions, such as the removal of dust, allergens, and bacteria. A prolonged residence time in the nasal cavity may also be achieved by using bioadhesive polymers, microspheres, and chitosan or by increasing the viscosity of the formulation. Nasal mucociliary clearance can also be stimulated or inhibited by drugs, excipients, preservatives, and/or absorption enhancers and thus affect drug delivery to the absorption site.

Several proteases and amino peptidases present in the nasal mucosa might affect the stability of proteins and peptides; nevertheless, the level of proteolytic activity is much lower than that in the gastrointestinal tract. Peptides may also form complexes with immunoglobulins (Igs) in the nasal cavity, leading to an increase in the molecular weight and a reduction of permeability.

A linear inverse correlation has been reported between the absorption of drugs and molecular weight up to 300 daltons. Absorption decreases significantly if the molecular weight is greater than 1000 daltons, except with the use of absorption enhancers.

These enhancers work by a variety of mechanisms, such as by modifying the phospholipid bilayer, leaching out protein from the membrane, or even stripping off the outer layer of the mucosa. Some of these enhancers also have an effect on the tight junctions and/or work as enzymatic inhibitors. The main problem associated with enhancers is that most of them cause significant mucosal damage at the concentrations required to enhance nasal absorption. Some of the enhancers that have been investigated include bile salts, dihydrofusidates, surfactants, and fatty acid derivatives.

Chitosan, a bioadhesive polymer, has been shown to improve the absorption by increasing the contact time between the drug and the nasal membrane and, hence, its retention on the nasal mucosa. It also had an effect on paracellular transport. Other bioadhesive materials are carbopol, cellulose agents, starch, and dextran. The use of cyclodextrins as a means of enhancing solubility and/or absorption also looks promising [67, 68].

Ophthalmic Systemic absorption of drugs from the ocular route is considered, in general, a nondesired effect. The main objective of the application of a drug on the front of the eye is to exert some effect in the eye and the annex structures. There are five potential targets for ophthalmic drugs: the precorneal structures (conjunctiva and eyelids), the cornea, the posterior and anterior chambers, the vitreous cavity, and the retina (Fig. 8.7). Preocular structures, cornea, and the anterior and

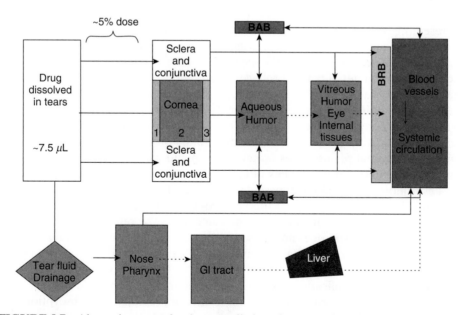

FIGURE 8.7 Absorption route for drugs applied on the eye surface. BAB, blood aqueous barrier; BRB, blood retinal barrier; 1, epithelium; 2, stroma; 3, endothelium. (Adapted from Ref. 86.)

posterior chambers can be accessed by topical application but the posterior side of the eye is difficult to reach from the eye surface, and, in general, systemic administration by another route or intraocular injection is used to deliver drugs to the vitreous cavity. The main pathway for drugs to enter the anterior chamber is via the cornea. Some large and hydrophilic drugs prefer the conjunctival and scleral route, and then diffuse into the ciliary's body [69], while small lipophilic compounds permeate through the corneal pathway.

On the other hand, reaching the anterior part of the eye from the systemic circulation is difficult due to the existence of the blood–ocular (blood–aqueous and blood–retinal) barrier, similar to the hematoencephalic barrier. The tight junctions of the capillary endothelial cells restrict the entry of substances from the blood into the aqueos humor and/or into the retina [70].

Once the drug is dissolved in the tear fluid, its residence time in the conjunctival sac is short (between 2 and 5 minutes) because of the drainage of the instillation fluid with tears and the tear turnover. Drainage rates decrease with increased viscosity of the instilled fluid but increase with increased volume of the instilled fluid because the eye tends to maintain the normal tear volume around 7.5 μL. If the drug is irritating to the eye or the conjunctiva, it will induce lacrimation and decrease residence time. The drug from the lacrimal duct arrives at the nose and then pharynx and can be swallowed and reach the gastrointestinal tract. From all these routes the drug can be absorbed, and potentially it could cause adverse effects. The drug in the tears is either absorbed by the conjunctiva, sclera, or cornea. The conjunctiva is a richly irrigated mucosa covering the inside of the eyelids and sclera. Its surface is higher than the corneal surface as well as its permeability, so this absorption pathway competes with the corneal route, reducing intraocular bioavailability.

The corneal barrier is formed by a series of three layers without blood supply: epithelium, stroma, and endothelium. The outer layer is a multistratified epithelium representing 10% of the total thickness. Between the epithelium and the stroma lies Bowman's membrane, containing strong collagen fibers, which help the cornea maintain its shape. Ninety percent of the thickness corresponds to the stroma, which is constituted by a net of parallel collagen fibrils and high water content. The endothelium pumps water from the cornea, keeping it clear. Epithelium and endothelium are lipophilic, while the stroma is a barrier for hydrophobic compounds. Lipophilicity, molecular weight, and ionization degree are the main factors affecting corneal permeability as well as the degree of binding to the protein content of the lacrimal fluid [71]. Lacrimal pH oscillates around 7.0–7.4 and has a low buffering capacity; thus, the pH and buffering capacity of the instillation solution could affect ophthalmic absorption. The optimum apparent partition coefficient (octanol/pH 7.4 buffer) for corneal absorption is in the range of 100–1000. It was shown that increasing molecular size of the permeating substance decreases the rate of paracellular permeation, as the pore size does not allow permeation of big molecules. Nevertheless, transcellular diffusion is the main pathway for most drugs used in the clinic [69].

Transdermal   The application of drug substances over the skin could have two different purposes: acting locally over the skin surface or providing drug absorption into the systemic circulation. Cutaneous administration refers, in general, to the first purpose while transdermal absorption defines the incorporation of a drug inside the body, crossing the skin in order to reach the blood vessels and exert systemic effects.

The advantage of the transdermal route over other routes is its large accessible surface area (average surface $1.8\,m^2$) and the avoidance of drug degradation in the gastrointestinal tract. Nevertheless, the skin by itself has homeostatic and protective functions, and it is a formidable barrier membrane, thanks mainly to the contribution of the stratum corneum (SC).

SKIN PHYSIOLOGY   There are two important layers to human skin: the epidermis, and the dermis, which contains blood vessels. The skin contains annex structures that include sweat and sebaceous glands and hair follicles. These structures cross the skin from the dermis and open on the epidermis surface.

The stratum corneum (or horny layer) is the top layer of the skin and varies in thickness from 10 to 20μm depending on the region of the body. It is composed of 15–20 layers of dead, flat, and keratinized epidermal cells (keratinocytes) surrounded by a lipid matrix, which renders this structure as the most significant barrier to diffusion and drug transport. The viable epidermis lies below the stratum corneum. Its cells have a greater degree of hydration, so diffusion is faster through this area. Viable epidermis contains melanocytes, which provide skin with pigmentation and Langerhans cells (antigen-presenting cells to the immune system). Finally, the dermis is the layer containing the blood vessels, sensory neurons, and a lymphatic network. The thickness of the dermis (1 mm) is approximately 100 times the thickness of the stratum corneum.

DRUG PERMEATION   Generally, drug absorption into the skin occurs by passive diffusion according to Fick's law. The transport rate is directly proportional to the surface area of the skin and inversely proportional to the thickness of the stratum corneum. Regarding the physicochemical characteristics of the compound, drug hydrosolubility, lipophilicity, and molecular weight, as well as charge, are the main factors affecting permeation, as in other routes where passive diffusion is the main mechanism. There is in most cases a parabolic relationship between the drug lipophilicity (expressed as octanol–water partition coefficient) and the permeation rate [72, 73]. This kind of correlation appears because compounds with low partition coefficient ($\log P$) present little partitioning into the skin and therefore low permeability, while compounds with high partition coefficient also give low permeability due their inability to partition out of the stratum corneum. The generally accepted range of $\log P$ for maximum permeation is between 1 and 3 [74]. For hydrophilic or charged molecules, resistance to transport is higher due to the lipid-rich nature of the stratum corneum and its low water content. Transport of lipophilic drug molecules is facilitated by their dissolution into intercellular lipids around the cells of the stratum corneum.

There are two main pathways by which drugs can cross the skin and reach the systemic circulation (see Fig. 8.8): the transfollicular and transepidermal pathways.

The *transfollicular route* is through the hair follicles and sebaceous glands. Hair follicles and sebaceous glands penetrate through the stratum corneum, allowing more direct access to the dermal microcirculation. Some hydrophilic substances can diffuse through this pathway. However, due to the low relative surface area (around 1%), very little drug actually crosses the skin via this route.

The *transepidermal pathway* consists of two paths. The *transcellular* represents the shortest path. However, the drug must cross environments of hydrophilic

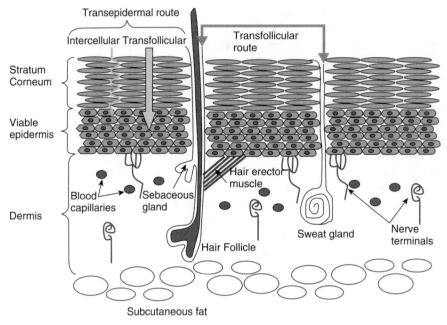

FIGURE 8.8   Skin structure and main pathways for transdermal absorption.

TABLE 8.5   Physiological Factors Relevant for Drug Penetration Through the Skin

Age	Neonates, elderly People: higher permeability [96]
Ethnicity	Controversial results in the literature: skin more permeable in Caucasians and Asians versus blacks, or no difference detected [97–99]
Body areas	Most permeable areas: mucous membranes, scrotal skin, eyelids Intermediate permeability: face, chest/back, buttocks, abdomen, upper arms/legs Less permeable zones: palms, feet soles, nails
Skin condition	Hydration degree: hydrated skin is more permeable [100] Irritation: if stratum corneum is broken, permeability is increased [100] Temperature: warmer skin is more permeable Eczema: increased permeability Psoriasis: thicker skin but disrupted barrier function; reported increase in permeability for low molecular drugs and for some high molecular entities [101]

(keratinocytes) and liphophilic nature (extracellular lipids) and that means that the substance needs a balanced hydrophilic–liphophilic nature to be able to follow this route and in general most substances find high resistance to permeation. The *intercellular* pathway is the more common pathway. Nevertheless, even if the thickness of the SC is very small, the tortuosity of the diffusion pathway around the cells increases the resistance to drug penetration.

Some physiological factors affecting drug penetration across the skin are summarized in Table 8.5.

Examples of drugs that are administered via the transdermal route include clonidine, estradiol, fentanyl, nicotine, nitroglycerin, scopolamine, testosterone, oxybutynin, and the combination products norelgestromin/ethinyl estradiol and estradiol/norethindrone acetate. The common characteristics is that they are all molecules of low molecular weight but with enough potency to be active at low blood concentrations (few ng/mL or less) [75].

Vaginal

VAGINAL PHYSIOLOGY   The human vagina is a slightly S-shaped tube that communicates the cervix of the uterus with the external body surface. The tube is collapsed with the anterior and posterior walls in contact with each other. The average length of the vagina is 8–12 cm [76].

The vaginal wall is comprised of an epithelial layer, a muscular layer, and the tunica adventitia. During the menstrual cycle, the thickness of the vaginal epithelial cell layer changes by approximately 200–300 μm. The surface of the vagina is composed of numerous folds or rugae. The rugae provide distensibility, support, and an increased surface area for the vaginal wall [76].

The primary venous drainage occurs via the pudendal veins. The vaginal, uterine, vesical, and rectosigmoid veins from the middle and upper vagina lead the blood flow to the inferior vena cava, thus bypassing the hepatic portal system.

Age, hormone status, and pregnancy cause changes in vaginal physiology as well as the pH changes due to several factors including semen, menstruation, estrogen status, and bacterial colonization. Reproductive hormones control the thickness of the vaginal epithelium, with estradiol 17-β (E2) thickening the epithelium and hypoestrogenism resulting in atrophy [77]. The vaginal fluid ranges mostly a transudate from vaginal and cervical cells but also contains vulvar secretions, cervical mucus, endometrial and oviductal fluids, and microorganisms and their metabolic products.

The normal average vaginal pH in healthy women of reproductive age ranges from 3.8 to 4.2. This acidic environment is maintained by the production of lactic acid by the vaginal microflora and it constitutes part of the defensive mechanism of the vaginal mucosa. The amount and composition of the vaginal fluid also changes throughout the menstrual cycle. Women of reproductive age produce fluid at a rate of 3–4 g/4 h, while this amount decreases by 50% in postmenopausal women. The human vaginal fluid may contain enzymes, enzyme inhibitors, proteins, carbohydrates, amino acids, alcohols, hydroxylketones, and aromatic compounds.

VAGINAL ABSORPTION   Vaginal delivery is a potential option for both local and systemic delivery. Vaginal mucosa possess several advantages when other routes of administration fail, such as avoidance of first-pass metabolism. On the other hand, this route of administration could be used for particular purposes, such as providing prolonged absorption from sustained release formulations or achieving local therapeutic effects while avoiding systemic administration and potential adverse effects of the drug. In general, the vaginal route provides good systemic absorption mostly for low molecular weight drugs [78].

Enzymatic activity of vaginal epithelium and vaginal fluids are two physiological factors that have shown to have influence on vaginal absorption. The external cell layers and the basal cell layers of the vagina retain most of the enzyme activity. Among the enzymes present, proteases are likely to be the prominent barrier for the absorption of intact peptide and protein drugs into the systemic circulation [79]. The absorption of a drug that is poorly water soluble may be increased when the fluid volume is higher. However, the presence of overly viscous cervical mucus may present a barrier to drug absorption and increased fluid volume may remove the drug from the vaginal cavity and subsequently reduce absorption [80].

Since many drugs are weak electrolytes, the pH may change their degree of ionization and affect the absorption of drug. As in other membranes, the ionization decreases the permeability of the drug as the un-ionized form has the higher permeability [80].

Physicochemical properties such as molecular weight, lipophilicity, ionization, and surface charge can influence vaginal drug absorption [79]. Lipophilicity, in general, increases drug permeability but low molecular weight lipophilic drugs are likely to be absorbed more than large molecular weight lipophilic or hydrophilic drugs. On the other hand, the molecular weight cutoff above which compounds are not absorbed may be higher for the vagina than other mucosal surfaces, such as the small intestine or colon [81]. Drugs with molecular weight >300 Da have shown a higher permeability in *in vitro* models of vaginal mucosa compared to small intestine and colon [81].

In conclusion, knowledge about the relationship between physicochemical properties and human vaginal permeability is still very limited; much work needs to be done in this area.

Parenteral Routes (Injectables)   Parenteral drug administration comprises all the nonenteral routes. Some of the parenteral routes require a needle for placing the drug at the absorption site. The most used extravascular parenteral routes are intradermal, subcutaneous, and intramuscular, which are represented in Fig. 8.9. Drug has to cross different barriers to be absorbed from the depot compartment.

Intradermal   The dermis is a layer underneath the epidermis, which contains the blood capillaries and nerve terminations. In general, the body area used to administer intradermal injections is the upper part of the arm and/or the back. It is used mainly for diagnostic agents, vaccines, or desensitization agents (a method to reduce or eliminate an organism's negative reaction to a substance or stimulus). The maximum volume to be administered by this route is 0.1 mL. Intradermal drugs diffuse slowly from the injection site into local capillaries, and the process is a little faster with drugs administered subcutaneously.

Subcutaneous   This route of administration can be used in either short-length or chronic therapies. The drug is injected, or the delivery system is placed in the interstitial tissue beneath the dermis. The most used zones for subcutaneous injection are the upper arm, the upper thigh, the lower part of the abdomen, or the upper part of the back. Maximal volume is around 2 mL. The blood supply to the subcutaneous tissue is less than the blood supply to the underlying muscular tissue; thus, subcutaneous absorption can be slower than intramuscular absorption. Nevertheless, compared to the oral route, subcutaneous absorption can be more rapid and predictable. The following factors can alter the absorption rate through this route:

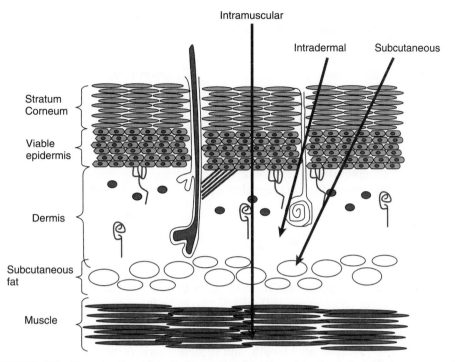

FIGURE 8.9 Parenteral routes of drug administration: intradermal, subcutaneous, and intramuscular. The injection depth determines where the drug depot is formed.

heating or massaging the injection zone (to increase absorption), coadministering vasodilators or hyaluronidase (to increase diffusion rate), or administering epinephrine to cause vasoconstriction (and thus decrease absorption rate).

Intramuscular This route is easier and less risky to use than the intravenous one, but it is more painful and the action onset is slower as it requires an absorption step. The injection is done in the muscular layer right under the subcutaneous tissue, avoiding blood vessels and nerves. The main sites of absorption are: deltoid muscle (up to 2 mL), gluteus muscle (5 mL), vastus lateralis muscle (upper thigh 15 mL). The absorption rate through this route depends on physiological factors, such as blood flow, exercise, and injection depth. The physicochemical characteristics of the drugs can also affect absorption rate (see Table 8.6) and in some cases the drug precipitates in the intramuscular depot further delaying the absorption.

Absorption Routes Once the drug is injected, a depot is formed in contact with the surrounding tissue. From the depot the drug can reach blood capillaries or lymphatic capillaries. Absorption proceeds through the blood or lymph, depending mainly on the drug molecular weight. Drugs with molecular weight higher than 2000 daltons preferentially use lymphatic vessels, while drugs with lower molecular weight are absorbed in the blood vessels. Blood capillaries have a thin wall formed by endothelial cells constituting a lipid barrier with aqueous pores and intercellular spaces called fenestrations. Pores and fenestrations represent only 0.1–0.2% of the capillaries' surface but the flow of water and soluble substances through them can

TABLE 8.6   Factors Affecting Parenteral Absorption by the Intradermal, Subcutaneous, and Intramuscular Routes

Physiological Factors	Physicochemical Factors
Blood flow	Lipophilicity
Muscular activity	Solubility
Vasoconstriction degree	Dissolution rate
Medium viscosity	pK_a

be very fast. Parenteral drug absorption occurs by passive diffusion through the lipid barrier or convective diffusion through the pores and fenestrations. Both processes can be described using Fick's diffusion law:

$$\frac{dQ_a}{dt} = \left(\frac{D \cdot P \cdot S}{L \cdot V_a} + \frac{D' \cdot S'}{\eta \cdot L' \cdot V_a} \right) \cdot Q_a$$

where dQ_a/dt is absorption rate from the depot compartment; Q_a, the amount of drug in the depot compartment; D, diffusion coefficient in the lipid membrane; P, partition coefficient; S, membrane surface; L, membrane thickness; V_a, volume of parenteral deposit; D', aqueous diffusion coefficient; S', aqueous pores and fenestration surface; L', average pore length; and η, medium viscosity.

Considering all the terms inside the parentheses as constants, the process is described as first order kinetics. In consequence, the absorption rate is directly proportional to the diffusion coefficient, available surface, and partition coefficient and inversely proportional to the membrane thickness, pore length, and medium viscosity. Absorption rate can be increased by including vasodilators or diffusion agents (hyaluronidase) in the drug formulation or decreased by using vasoconstrictors and thickening agents.

The drug's properties that exhibit more influence on drug absorption rate are those affecting dissolution rate and lipophilicity. Dissolution rate is conditioned by the particle size, crystalline structure, and polymorphs. Lipophilicity influences the drug's partitioning into the membrane and this factor depends on the drug's pK_a and the pH of the fluid, as the un-ionized form is more lipophilic. All these factors are summarized in Table 8.6.

In the last decades new needle-free technologies have been developed for injectable delivery. Needle-free injectors are devices that do not use a needle to place the drug in its depot site. The mechanism involves high pressure to push the drug formulation through the skin to the desired site. Pressure is produced by using either a gas (carbon dioxide or nitrogen) or a spring device. The pressure forces the medication through a small opening in the device while it is held against the skin. This creates a fine stream of the medication that penetrates the skin [82, 83].

Other Parenteral Routes   Intraspinal (epidural and intrathecal) delivery of drugs is an alternative route used mainly for anesthesia and pain-killer medications, in particular, when patients experience intolerable side effects from systemic drugs. Intraspinal delivery can be given into the epidural space or into the intrathecal space [84].

Drugs delivered epidurally also circulate systemically. By contrast, drugs delivered intrathecally circulate only in the cerebropsinal fluid (CSF). In both cases, the drugs administered by the intraspinal route bypass the blood–brain barrier. However, epidurally administered drugs must first cross the dura (the protective outer layer of the spinal cord) before entering the CSF. Therefore, when the epidural route of delivery is used, more time and higher doses are required for the drugs to exert the same effect compared with intrathecal delivery.

REFERENCES

1. Chiou WL. The rate and extent of oral bioavailability versus the rate and extent of oral absorption: clarification and recommendation of terminology. *J Pharmacokinet Pharmacodyn* 2001;28(1):3–6.

2. Shargel L, Yu ABC. *Applied Biopharmaceutics & Pharmacokinetics*, 4th ed. Stamford, CT: Appleton & Lange; 1999.

3. Mayerson M. *Principles of Drug Absorption. Modern Pharmaceutics edition.* New York: Marcel Dekker; 1995.

4. Artursson P. Epithelial transport of drugs in cell culture. I: A model for studying the passive diffusion of drugs over intestinal absorptive (Caco-2) cells. *J Pharm Sci* 1990;79(6):476–482.

5. Artursson P, Magnusson C. Epithelial transport of drugs in cell culture. II: Effect of extracellular calcium concentration on the paracellular transport of drugs of different lipophilicities across monolayers of intestinal epithelial (Caco-2) cells. *J Pharm Sci* 1990;79(7):595–600.

6. Artursson P, Ungell AL, Lofroth JE. Selective paracellular permeability in two models of intestinal absorption: cultured monolayers of human intestinal epithelial cells and rat intestinal segments. *Pharm Res* 1993;10(8):1123–1129.

7. Fagerholm U, Borgstrom L, Ahrenstedt O, Lennernas H. The lack of effect of induced net fluid absorption on the *in vivo* permeability of terbutaline in the human jejunum. *J Drug Target* 1995;3(3):191–200.

8. Fagerholm U, Nilsson D, Knutson L, Lennernas H. Jejunal permeability in humans *in vivo* and rats *in situ*: investigation of molecular size selectivity and solvent drag. *Acta Physiol Scand* 1999;165(3):315–324.

9. Lennernas H, Ahrenstedt O, Ungell AL. Intestinal drug absorption during induced net water absorption in man; a mechanistic study using antipyrine, atenolol and enalaprilat. *Br J Clin Pharmacol* 1994;37(6):589–596.

10. Hasselbalch K. Die Berechnung der Wasserstoffzahl des Blutes aus der freien und gebundenen Kohlensäure desselben und die Sauerstoffbindungen des Blutes als Funktion der Wasserstoffzahl. *Biochemistry* 1916;78:112.

11. Adibi SA. The oligopeptide transporter (Pept-1) in human intestine: biology and function. *Gastroenterology* 1997;113(1):332–340.

12. Sadee W, Drubbisch V, Amidon GL. Biology of membrane transport proteins. *Pharm Res* 1995;12(12):1823–1837.

13. Martinez MN, Amidon GL. A mechanistic approach to understanding the factors affecting drug absorption: a review of fundamentals. *J Clin Pharmacol* 2002;42(6):620–643.

14. DeSesso JM, Jacobson CF. Anatomical and physiological parameters affecting gastrointestinal absorption in humans and rats. *Food Chem Toxicol* 2001;39(3):209–228.

15. *Modern Biopharmaceutics*. [computer program]. Version 6.03; Amidon GL, Bermejo M. TSRL, Inc; 2003.

16. Kararli TT. Comparison of the gastrointestinal anatomy, physiology, and biochemistry of humans and commonly used laboratory animals. *Biopharm Drug Dispos* 1995;16(5): 351–380.

17. Dressman JB, Bass P, Ritschel WA, Friend DR, Rubinstein A, Ziv E. Gastrointestinal parameters that influence oral medications. *J Pharm Sci* 1993;82(9):857–872.

18. Oh DM, Amidon GL. Overview of membrane transport. *Pharm Biotechnol* 1999;12:1–27.

19. Oh DM, Han HK, Amidon GL. Drug transport and targeting. Intestinal transport. *Pharm Biotechnol* 1999;12:59–88.

20. Kunta JR, Sinko PJ. Intestinal drug transporters: *in vivo* function and clinical importance. *Curr Drug Metab* 2004;5(1):109–124.

21. Shin HC, Landowski CD, Amidon GL. Transporters in the GI tract. In Waterbeemd V-d, Lennernäs H, Pirtursson P, Eds. *Drug Bioavailability/Estimation of Solubility, Permeability and Absorption*. Weinheim, Germany: Wiley-VCH; 2003.

22. Bermejo M, Ruiz-Garcia A. Oral permeability predictions—-from *in silico* to *in vivo* models. *Business Briefing Pharma Tech* 2002;175–180.

23. Karlsson J, Ungell A, Grasjo J, Artursson P. Paracellular drug transport across intestinal epithelia: influence of charge and induced water flux. *Eur J Pharm Sci* 1999;9(1): 47–56.

24. Pade V, Stavchansky S. Estimation of the relative contribution of the transcellular and paracellular pathway to the transport of passively absorbed drugs in the Caco-2 cell culture model. *Pharm Res* 1997;14(9):1210–1215.

25. Bermejo M, Merino V, Garrigues TM, et al. Validation of a biophysical drug absorption model by the PATQSAR system. *J Pharm Sci* 1999;88(4):398–405.

26. Taylor DC, Pownall R, Burke W. The absorption of beta-adrenoceptor antagonists in rat *in-situ* small intestine; the effect of lipophilicity. *J Pharm Pharmacol* 1985; 37(4):280–283.

27. Hendriksen BA, Felix MV, Bolger MB. The composite solubility versus pH profile and its role in intestinal absorption prediction. *AAPS PharmSci* 2003;5(1):E4.

28. Lennernas H. Does fluid flow across the intestinal mucosa affect quantitative oral drug absorption? Is it time for a reevaluation? *Pharm Res* 1995;12(11):1573–1582.

29. Anderson BW, Levine AS, Levitt DG, Kneip JM, Levitt MD. Physiological measurement of luminal stirring in perfused rat jejunum. *Am J Physiol* 1988;254(6 Pt 1):G843–G848.

30. Levitt MD, Furne JK, Strocchi A, Anderson BW, Levitt DG. Physiological measurements of luminal stirring in the dog and human small bowel. *J Clin Invest* 1990;86(5): 1540–1547.

31. Tsuji A, Tamai I. Carrier-mediated intestinal transport of drugs. *Pharm Res* 1996;13(7): 963–977.

32. Benet LZ, Cummins CL, Wu CY. Unmasking the dynamic interplay between efflux transporters and metabolic enzymes. *Int J Pharm* 2004;277(1–2):3–9.

33. Fischer V, Einolf HJ, Cohen D. Efflux transporters and their clinical relevance. *Mini Rev Med Chem* 2005;5(2):183–195.

34. Wagner D, Spahn-Langguth H, Hanafy A, Koggel A, Langguth P. Intestinal drug efflux: formulation and food effects. *Adv Drug Deliv Rev* 2001;50(Suppl 1):S13–S31.

35. Suzuki H, Sugiyama Y. Role of metabolic enzymes and efflux transporters in the absorption of drugs from the small intestine. *Eur J Pharm Sci* 2000;12(1):3–12.

36. Kimura T, Higaki K. Gastrointestinal transit and drug absorption. *Biol Pharm Bull* 2002;25(2):149–164.

37. de Vries ME, Bodde HE, Verhoef JC, Junginger HE. Developments in buccal drug delivery. *Crit Rev Ther Drug Carrier Syst* 1991;8(3):271–303.

38. Squier CA. The permeability of oral mucosa. *Crit Rev Oral Biol Med* 1991;2(1):13–32.

39. de Vries ME, Bodde HE, Busscher HJ, Junginger HE. Hydrogels for buccal drug delivery: properties relevant for muco-adhesion. *J Biomed Mater Res* 1988;22(11):1023–1032.

40. Shojaei AH. Buccal mucosa as a route for systemic drug delivery: a review. *J Pharm Pharm Sci* 1998;1(1):15–30.

41. Harris D, Robinson JR. Drug delivery via the mucous membranes of the oral cavity. *J Pharm Sci* 1992;81(1):1–10.

42. Galey WR, Lonsdale HK, Nacht S. The *in vitro* permeability of skin and buccal mucosa to selected drugs and tritiated water. *J Invest Dermatol* 1976;67(6):713–717.

43. Wertz PW, Squier CA. Cellular and molecular basis of barrier function in oral epithelium. *Crit Rev Ther Drug Carrier Syst* 1991;8(3):237–269.

44. Squier CA, Cox P, Wertz PW. Lipid content and water permeability of skin and oral mucosa. *J Invest Dermatol* 1991;96(1):123–126.

45. Chan KK, Gibaldi M. Effects of first-pass metabolism on metabolite mean residence time determination after oral administration of parent drug. *Pharm Res* 1990;7(1):59–63.

46. Streisand JB, Zhang J, Niu S, McJames S, Natte R, Pace NL. Buccal absorption of fentanyl is pH-dependent in dogs. *Anesthesiology* 1995;82(3):759–764.

47. Narawane LVHL. *Absorption Barriers. Harwood Academic*, Switzerland: AG de Boer; 1994.

48. Kurosaki YNH, Terao K, Nakayama T, Kimura T. Existence of specialized absorption mechanism for cephadroxyl, an aminocephalosporin antibiotic, in the human oral cavity. *Int J Pharm* 1992;82:165–169.

49. Graves NM, Kriel RL. Rectal administration of antiepileptic drugs in children. *Pediatr Neurol* 1987;3(6):321–326.

50. Roelofse JA, van der Bijl P, Stegmann DH, Hartshorne JE. Preanesthetic medication with rectal midazolam in children undergoing dental extractions. *J Oral Maxillofac Surg* 1990;48(8):791–797; discussion 797.

51. Malinovsky JM, Lejus C, Servin F, et al. Plasma concentrations of midazolam after i.v., nasal or rectal administration in children. *Br J Anaesth* 1993;70(6):617–620.

52. Hanning CD. The rectal absorption of opioids. In Benedetti C, Chapman CR, Giron G, Eds. *Advances in Pain Research and Therapy*. Philadelphia: Lippincott-Raven; 1990; 14:259–268.

53. Alternative routes of drug administration—advantages and disadvantages (subject review). American Academy of Pediatrics. Committee on Drugs. *Pediatrics* 1997;100(1):143–152.

54. van Hoogdalem EJ, de Boer AG, Breimer DD. Pharmacokinetics of rectal drug administration. Part II. Clinical applications of peripherally acting drugs, and conclusions. *Clin Pharmacokinet* 1991;21(2):110–128.

55. Choonara IA. Giving drugs per rectum for systemic effect. *Arch Dis Child* 1987; 62(8):771–772.

56. Khalil SN, Florence FB, Van den Nieuwenhuyzen MC, Wu AH, Stanley TH. Rectal methohexital: concentration and length of the rectal catheters. *Anesth Analg* 1990; 70(6):645–649.

57. van Hoogdalem E, de Boer AG, Breimer DD. Pharmacokinetics of rectal drug administration. Part I. General considerations and clinical applications of centrally acting drugs. *Clin Pharmacokinet* 1991;21(1):11–26.

58. Forbes RB, Vandewalker GE. Comparison of two and ten percent rectal methohexitone for induction of anaesthesia in children. *Can J Anaesth* 1988;35(4):345–349.

59. Jantzen JP, Erdmann K, Witton PK, Klein AM. The effect of rectal pH values on the absorption of methohexital. *Anaesthesist* 1986;35(8):496–499.

60. Jantzen JP, Tzanova I, Witton PK, Klein AM. Rectal pH In children. *Can J Anaesth* 1989;36(6):665–667.

61. Effros RM, Mason GR. Measurements of pulmonary epithelial permeability *in vivo. Am Rev Respir Dis* 1983;127(5 Pt 2):S59–S65.

62. Arora P, Sharma S, Garg S. Permeability issues in nasal drug delivery. *Drug Discov Today* 2002;7(18):967–975.

63. Turker S, Onur E, Ozer Y. Nasal route and drug delivery systems. *Pharm World Sci* 2004;26(3):137–142.

64. Illum L. Nasal drug delivery: new developments and strategies. *Drug Discov Today* 2002;7(23):1184–1189.

65. Illum L. Nasal drug delivery—possibilities, problems and solutions. *J Control Release* 2003;87(1–3):187–198.

66. Illum L, Jabbal-Gill I, Hinchcliffe M, Fisher AN, Davis SS. Chitosan as a novel nasal delivery system for vaccines. *Adv Drug Deliv Rev* 2001;51(1–3):81–96.

67. Chavanpatil MD, Vavia PR. The influence of absorption enhancers on nasal absorption of acyclovir. *Eur J Pharm Biopharm* 2004;57(3):483–487.

68. Davis SS, Illum L. Absorption enhancers for nasal drug delivery. *Clin Pharmacokinet* 2003;42(13):1107–1128.

69. Hornof M, Toropainen E, Urtti A. Cell culture models of the ocular barriers. *Eur J Pharm Biopharm* 2005;60(2):207–225.

70. Hosoya K, Tomi M. Advances in the cell biology of transport via the inner blood–retinal barrier: establishment of cell lines and transport functions. *Biol Pharm Bull* 2005;28(1):1–8.

71. Reichl S, Dohring S, Bednarz J, Muller-Goymann CC. Human cornea construct HCC— an alternative for *in vitro* permeation studies? A comparison with human donor corneas. *Eur J Pharm Biopharm* 2005;60(2):305–308.

72. Kim MK, Lee CH, Kim DD. Skin permeation of testosterone and its ester derivatives in rats. *J Pharm Pharmacol* 2000;52(4):369–375.

73. Lopez A, Llinares F, Cortell C, Herraez M. Comparative enhancer effects of Span20 with Tween20 and Azone on the *in vitro* percutaneous penetration of compounds with different lipophilicities. *Int J Pharm* 2000;202(1–2):133–140.

74. Thomas BJ, Finnin BC. The transdermal revolution. *Drug Discov Today* 2004;9(16): 697–703.

75. Kalia YN, Merino V, Guy RH. Transdermal drug delivery. Clinical aspects. *Dermatol Clin* 1998;16(2):289–299.

76. Dezarnaulds G, Fraser IS. Vaginal ring delivery of hormone replacement therapy—a review. *Expert Opin Pharmacother* 2003;4(2):201–212.

77. Buchanan DL, Kurita T, Taylor JA, Lubahn DB, Cunha GR, Cooke PS. Role of stromal and epithelial estrogen receptors in vaginal epithelial proliferation, stratification, and cornification. *Endocrinology* 1998;139(10):4345–4352.

78. Woolfson AD, Malcolm RK, Gallagher R. Drug delivery by the intravaginal route. *Crit Rev Ther Drug Carrier Syst* 2000;17(5):509–555.

79. Alexander NJ, Baker E, Kaptein M, Karck U, Miller L, Zampaglione E. Why consider vaginal drug administration? *Fertil Steril* 2004;82(1):1–12.

80. Hussain A, Ahsan F. The vagina as a route for systemic drug delivery. *J Control Release* 2005;103(2):301–313.

81. van der Bijl P, Van Eyk AD. Comparative *in vitro* permeability of human vaginal, small intestinal and colonic mucosa. *Int J Pharm* 2003;261(1–2):147–152.

82. Furness G. Needle-Free and Auto Injectors—Management Forum Conference. An update on technology and application. 23–24 Feb 2004, London, UK. *IDrugs* 2004;7(4):329–330.

83. Ajmani D. Going from needles to needle-free injectables. *Drug Deliv Technol* 2004; http://www.drugdeliverytech.com/cgi-bin/articles.cgi?idArticle=318

84. Paice JA, Magolan JM. Intraspinal drug therapy. *Nurs Clin North Am* 1991;26(2): 477–498.

85. Dressman JB, Amidon GL, Reppas C, Shah VP. Dissolution testing as a prognostic tool for oral drug absorption: immediate release dosage forms. *Pharm Res* 1998;15(1): 11–22.

86. Loftssona T, Jarvinen T. Cyclodextrins in ophthalmic drug delivery. *Adv Drug Deliv Rev* 1999;36(1):59–79.

87. Kamm W, Hauptmann J, Behrens I, et al. Transport of peptidomimetic thrombin inhibitors with a 3-amidino-phenylalanine structure: permeability and efflux mechanism in monolayers of a human intestinal cell line (Caco-2). *Pharm Res* 2001;18(8):1110–1118.

88. Stenberg P, Luthman K, Ellens H, et al. Prediction of the intestinal absorption of endothelin receptor antagonists using three theoretical methods of increasing complexity. *Pharm Res* 1999;16(10):1520–1526.

89. Casabo VG, Nunez-Benito E, Martinez-Coscolla A, Miralles-Loyola E, Martin-Villodre A, Pla-Delfina JM. Studies on the reliability of a bihyperbolic functional absorption model. II. Phenylalkylamines. *J Pharmacokinet Biopharm* 1987;15(6):633–643.

90. Dowty ME, Dietsch CR. Improved prediction of *in vivo* peroral absorption from *in vitro* intestinal permeability using an internal standard to control for intra- and inter-rat variability. *Pharm Res* 1997;14(12):1792–1797.

91. Camenisch G, Folkers G, van de Waterbeemd H. Shapes of membrane permeability–lipophilicity curves: extension of theoretical models with an aqueous pore pathway. *Eur J Pharm Sci* 1998;6(4):325–329.

92. Norinder U, Osterberg T, Artursson P. Theoretical calculation and prediction of intestinal absorption of drugs in humans using MolSurf parametrization and PLS statistics. *Eur J Pharm Sci* 1999;8(1):49–56.

93. Palm K, Luthman K, Ungell AL, Strandlund G, Artursson P. Correlation of drug absorption with molecular surface properties. *J Pharm Sci* 1996;85(1):32–39.

94. Clark DE. Rapid calculation of polar molecular surface area and its application to the prediction of transport phenomena. 2. Prediction of blood–brain barrier penetration. *J Pharm Sci* 1999;88(8):815–821.

95. Clark DE. Rapid calculation of polar molecular surface area and its application to the prediction of transport phenomena. 1. Prediction of intestinal absorption. *J Pharm Sci* 1999;88(8):807–814.

96. Roskos KV, Maibach HI. Percutaneous absorption and age. Implications for therapy. *Drugs Aging* 1992;2(5):432–449.

97. Lotte C, Wester RC, Rougier A, Maibach HI. Racial differences in the *in vivo* percutaneous absorption of some organic compounds: a comparison between black, Caucasian and Asian subjects. *Arch Dermatol Res* 1993;284(8):456–459.

98. Gean CJ, Tur E, Maibach HI, Guy RH. Cutaneous responses to topical methyl nicotinate in black, Oriental, and Caucasian subjects. *Arch Dermatol Res* 1989;281(2):95–98.

99. Kompaore F, Marty JP, Dupont C. *In vivo* evaluation of the stratum corneum barrier function in blacks, Caucasians and Asians with two noninvasive methods. *Skin Pharmacol* 1993;6(3):200–207.

100. Tsai JC, Sheu HM, Hung PL, Cheng CL. Effect of barrier disruption by acetone treatment on the permeability of compounds with various lipophilicities: implications for the permeability of compromised skin. *J Pharm Sci* 2001;90(9):1242–1254.

101. Gould AR, Sharp PJ, Smith DR, et al. Increased permeability of psoriatic skin to the protein, plasminogen activator inhibitor 2. *Arch Dermatol Res* 2003;295(6):249–254.

9

ABSORPTION OF DRUGS AFTER ORAL ADMINISTRATION

Luis Granero and Ana Polache

University of Valencia, Valencia, Spain

Contents

Preclinical Development Handbook: ADME and Biopharmaceutical Properties,
edited by Shayne Cox Gad
Copyright © 2008 John Wiley & Sons, Inc.

9.1   INTRODUCTION

Drugs are most commonly given orally and the oral route is the preferred one for the administration of new therapeutic agents. After oral administration, drugs must be absorbed through the gastrointestinal tract to achieve the systemic circulation and exert their pharmacological effects. The successful formulation of an optimized oral drug delivery system requires a detailed consideration and a good understanding of the intestinal absorption process, its possibilities and limitations. In fact, peroral delivery of new hydrophilic drugs, which include macromolecules frequently with null or scarce capacity of absorption through the intestinal barrier, is one of the greatest challenges in biopharmaceutical research.

Recent years have seen rapid developments in the field of intestinal absorption: more detailed insights into the structure and organization of intestinal mucosa (e.g., increased knowledge of tight junction physiology and regulation), new approaches to overcoming the problems associated with poor intestinal drug absorption (e.g., the use of paracellular enhancers), and novel methods for assessing the permeability of intestinal mucosa.

The goal of the present chapter is to give an overview and update on the concepts, possibilities, and limitations of drug absorption after oral administration. First, we introduce the anatomical and physiological aspects of the gastrointestinal tract, since they are decisive to understanding the absorption processes, and analyze the possible pathways of drug intestinal absorption. Second, the primary factors that influence oral drug absorption (e.g., physiological, physicochemical, and technological variables) are covered. Third, we analyze the use of permeation enhancers as a way to increase the rate and extent of drugs across the intestinal barrier. Fourth, we review the different methodologies (*in vitro, in situ*, and *in vivo*) that allow an investigator to establish the suitability of a drug candidate and to solve problems associated with drug intestinal absorption.

9.2   ANATOMY AND PHYSIOLOGY OF THE HUMAN GASTROINTESTINAL TRACT

The gastrointestinal tract (GIT) consists of a hollow muscular tube starting from the oral cavity, where food enters the mouth, continuing through the pharynx, esophagus, stomach, and intestines, to the rectum and anus, where food is expelled. There are various accessory organs that assist the tract by secreting enzymes to help break down food into its component nutrients. Thus, the salivary glands, liver, pancreas, and gallbladder have important functions in the digestive system. Food is propelled along the length of the GIT by peristaltic movements of the muscular walls.

The primary purpose of the GIT is to break down food into nutrients, which can be absorbed into the body to provide energy. First, food must be ingested into the mouth to be mechanically processed and moistened. Second, digestion occurs mainly in the stomach and small intestine, where proteins, fats, and carbohydrates are chemically broken down into their basic building blocks. Smaller molecules are then absorbed across the epithelium of the small intestine and subsequently enter the circulation. The large intestine plays a key role in reabsorbing excess water. Finally, undigested material and secreted waste products are excreted from the body via defecation (passing of feces).

9.2.1 Basic Structure

The GIT is a muscular tube lined by a special layer of cells, called epithelium. The contents of the tube are considered external to the body and are in continuity with the outside world at the mouth and the anus. Although each section of the tract has specialized functions, the entire tract has a similar basic structure with regional variations. The wall is divided into four layers as follows (beginning with the luminal surface): (1) mucosa, (2) submucosa, (3) muscularis externa, and (4) serosa (mesentery). The three outer layers are similar throughout most of the tract; however, the mucosa has distinctive structural and functional characteristics.

1. *Mucosa.* The innermost layer of the digestive tract has specialized epithelial cells supported by an underlying connective tissue layer called the lamina propria. The lamina propria contains blood vessels, nerves, lymphoid tissue, and glands that support the mucosa. Depending on its function, the epithelium may be simple (a single layer) or stratified (multiple layers). Areas such as the mouth and esophagus are covered by a stratified squamous (flat) epithelium so they can survive the wear and tear of passing food. Simple columnar (tall) or glandular epithelium lines the stomach and intestines to aid secretion and absorption. The inner lining is constantly shed and replaced, making it one of the most rapidly dividing areas of the body. Beneath the lamina propria is the muscularis mucosa. This comprises layers of smooth muscle, which can contract to change the shape of the lumen.

2. *Submucosa.* The submucosa surrounds the muscularis mucosa and consists of fat, fibrous connective tissue, and larger vessels and nerves. At its outer margin there is a specialized nerve plexus called the submucosal plexus or Meissner plexus. This supplies the mucosa and submucosa.

3. *Muscularis Externa.* This smooth muscle layer has inner circular and outer longitudinal layers of muscle fibers separated by the myenteric plexus or Auerbach plexus. Neural innervations control the contraction of these muscles and hence the mechanical breakdown and peristalsis of the food within the lumen.

4. *Serosa (Mesentery).* The outer layer of the GIT is formed by fat and another layer of epithelial cells called mesothelium.

9.2.2 Stomach

The stomach is a J-shaped expanded bag, located just left of the midline between the esophagus and small intestine. It is divided into four main regions and has two borders called the greater and lesser curvatures. The first section is the *cardia*, which surrounds the cardial orifice where the esophagus enters the stomach. The *fundus* is the superior, dilated portion of the stomach that has contact with the left dome of the diaphragm. The *body* is the largest section between the fundus and the curved portion of the J. This is where most gastric glands are located and where most mixing of the food occurs. Finally, the *pylorus* is the curved base of the stomach. Gastric contents are expelled into the proximal duodenum via the pyloric sphincter. The inner surface of the stomach is contracted into numerous longitudinal folds called *rugae*. These allow the stomach to stretch and expand when food enters. The stomach can hold up to 1.5 liters of material.

The functions of the stomach include (1) the short-term storage of ingested food, (2) mechanical breakdown of food by churning and mixing motions, (3) chemical digestion of proteins by acids and enzymes, and (4) killing bugs and germs by acidification. Most of these functions are achieved with the aid of the secretion of stomach juices by gastric glands in the body and fundus. Some cells are responsible for secreting acid and others secrete enzymes to break down proteins.

9.2.3   Small Intestine

The small intestine is composed of the duodenum, jejunum, and ileum. It averages approximately 6 m in length, extending from the pyloric sphincter of the stomach to the ileocecal valve separating the ileum from the cecum. The small intestine is compressed into numerous folds and occupies a large proportion of the abdominal cavity. The duodenum is the proximal C-shaped section that curves around the head of the pancreas. The duodenum serves a mixing function as it combines digestive secretions from the pancreas and liver with the contents expelled from the stomach. The start of the jejunum is marked by a sharp bend, the duodenojejunal flexure. It is in the jejunum where the majority of digestion and absorption occurs. The final portion, the ileum, is the longest segment and empties into the cecum at the ileocecal junction.

The small intestine performs the majority of digestion and absorption of nutrients. Partly digested food from the stomach is further broken down by enzymes from the pancreas and bile salts from the liver and gallbladder. These secretions enter the duodenum at the ampulla of Vater. After further digestion, food constituents such as proteins, fats, and carbohydrates are broken down to small building blocks and absorbed into the body.

The lining of the small intestine (Fig. 9.1) is made up of numerous permanent folds called plicae circulares or folds of Kerckring. Each plica has numerous villi (folds of mucosa) and each villus is covered by epithelium containing several specialized cells; some are responsible for absorption, the enterocytes, while others secrete digestive enzymes and mucus to protect the intestinal lining from digestive actions. Enterocytes in the small intestine are cells clearly specialized in absorption, having in their luminal pole the so-called microvilli (brush border). This anatomical structure is designed to increase the surface area for absorption by a factor of several hundred.

All the structure in the small intestine is conceived to increase effective surface for absorption (Fig. 9.2). The initial increase in surface area is due to the projection within the lumen of folds of mucosa. As indicated earlier, lining the entire epithelial surface are finger-like projections, the villi. These villi range in length from 0.5 to 1.5 m, and it has been estimated that there are about 10–40 villi/mm^2 of mucosal surface. Projecting from the villi surface are the microvilli, which represent the final large increase in the surface area of the small intestine. There are approximately 600 microvilli protruding from each enterocyte lining the villi. Relative to the initial

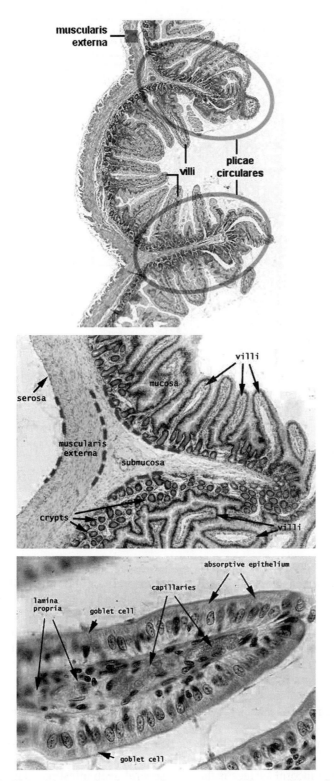

FIGURE 9.1 Photomicrographs showing the structure of the small intestine (jejunum). Magnification increases from the upper to the lower panel.

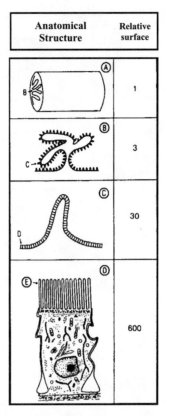

Anatomical Structure	Relative surface
Ⓐ B	1
Ⓑ C	3
Ⓒ D	30
Ⓓ Ⓔ	600

FIGURE 9.2   Schematic representation of the increase in the effective surface of the small intestine mucosa, relative to a simple cylinder, as a consequence of its particular structural features: Ⓐ simple cylinder, Ⓑ plicae circulares, Ⓒ villi, Ⓓ enterocyte, and Ⓔ microvilli.

surface of a smooth cylinder, the folds, villi, and microvilli increase the effective surface area by factors of 3, 30, and 600, respectively.

9.2.4   Large Intestine

The large intestine is horseshoe shaped and extends around the small intestine like a frame. It consists of the appendix, cecum, ascending, transverse, descending, and sigmoid colon, and the rectum. It has a length of approximately 1.5 m and a width of 7.5 cm. The cecum is the expanded pouch that receives material from the ileum and starts to compress food products into fecal material. Food then travels along the colon. The wall of the colon is made up of several pouches (haustra) that are held under tension by three thick bands of muscle (taenia coli). The rectum is the final 15 cm of the large intestine. It expands to hold fecal matter before it passes through the anorectal canal to the anus. Thick bands of muscle, known as sphincters, control the passage of feces.

   The mucosa of the large intestine lacks villi seen in the small intestine. Thus, the effective surface area for absorption is clearly lower than that existing in the small intestine. The mucosal surface is flat with several deep intestinal glands. Numerous goblet cells line the glands that secrete mucus to lubricate fecal matter as it solidifies.

The functions of the large intestine can be summarized as (1) the accumulation of unabsorbed material to form feces, (2) some digestion by bacteria the bacteria responsible for the formation of intestinal gas, and (3) reabsorption of water, salts, sugar, and vitamins.

9.2.5 Liver, Gallbladder, and Pancreas

The liver, gallbladder, and pancreas, although not part of the gut, have been included, since these organs secrete materials vital to the digestive and certain absorptive functions of the gut.

The liver is a large, reddish-brown organ situated in the right upper quadrant of the abdomen. It is surrounded by a strong capsule and divided into four lobes, namely, the right, left, caudate, and quadrate lobes. The liver has several important functions. It acts as a mechanical filter by filtering blood that travels from the intestinal system. It detoxifies several drugs and endogenous metabolites including the breakdown of bilirubin and estrogen. In addition, the liver has synthetic functions, producing albumin and blood clotting factors. However, its main roles in digestion are in the production of bile and metabolism of nutrients. All drugs and nutrients absorbed by the intestines pass through the liver and are processed before traveling to the rest of the body. The bile produced by cells of the liver enters the intestines at the duodenum. Here, bile salts break down lipids into smaller particles so there is a greater surface area for digestive enzymes to act.

The gallbladder is a hollow, pear-shaped organ that sits in a depression on the posterior surface of the liver's right lobe. It consists of a fundus, body, and neck. It empties via the cystic duct into the biliary duct system. The main functions of the gallbladder are storage and concentration of bile. Bile is a thick fluid that contains enzymes to help dissolve fat in the intestines. Bile is produced by the liver but stored in the gallbladder until it is needed. Bile is released from the gallbladder by contraction of its muscular walls in response to hormone signals from the duodenum in the presence of food.

Finally, the pancreas is a lobular, pinkish-grey organ that lies behind the stomach. Its head communicates with the duodenum and its tail extends to the spleen. The organ is approximately 15 cm in length with a long, slender body connecting the head and tail segments. The pancreas has both exocrine and endocrine functions. Endocrine refers to production of hormones, which occurs in the islets of Langerhans. The islets produce insulin, glucagon, and other substances and these are the areas damaged in diabetes mellitus.

The exocrine (secretory) portion makes up 80–85% of the pancreas and is the area relevant to the gastrointestinal tract. It is made up of numerous acini (small glands) that secrete contents into ducts, which eventually lead to the duodenum. The pancreas secretes fluid rich in carbohydrates and inactive enzymes. Secretion is triggered by the hormones released by the duodenum in the presence of food. Pancreatic enzymes include carbohydrases, lipases, nucleases, and proteolytic enzymes that can break down different drugs and components of food. These are secreted in an inactive form to prevent digestion of the pancreas itself. The enzymes become active once they reach the duodenum.

9.2.6   Structure and Composition of Intestinal Membrane

Drug absorption is ultimately the penetration of the drug across the intestinal membrane and its appearance unchanged in the blood draining the GIT. The term intestinal membrane is misleading since, as we commented earlier, this membrane is not a unicellular structure, but really a number of unicellular membranes parallel to one another and separated by aqueous fluid regions bounded by these membranes. Whatever the case, drug absorption implies a movement of drug molecules across biological membranes and, therefore, it could be useful to remember their basic structure and composition.

The biological membranes are bilipid layers. In a real cell the membrane phospholipids create a spherical three-dimensional lipid bilayer shell around the cell. The hydrophobic hydrocarbon chains of the phospholipids orient toward each other, creating a hydrophobic environment within the membrane. This leaves the charged phosphate groups facing out into the hydrophilic environment. The membrane is approximately 5 nm thick. This bilipid layer is semipermeable, meaning that some molecules are allowed to pass freely (diffuse) through the membrane. Molecules can diffuse through the membrane at differing rates depending on their ability to enter the hydrophobic interior of the membrane bilayer. The most accepted biological membrane model is referred to as the *fluid mosaic model* [1]. In this model lipid bilayers are fluid, and individual phospholipids diffuse rapidly throughout the two-dimensional surface of the membrane. These fluid bilayers include proteins, cholesterol, and other types of molecules besides phospholipids. Membrane proteins diffuse throughout the membrane in the same fashion, although at a slower pace because of their massive size (a phospholipid may be 650 daltons, and a medium sized protein can be 100,000 daltons). From time to time a given phospholipid will "flip-flop" through the membrane to the opposite side, but this is uncommon. To do so required the hydrophilic head of the phospholipid to pass fully through the highly hydrophobic interior of the membrane, and for the hydrophobic tails to be exposed to the aqueous environment.

There are also molecules of cholesterol embedded in the membrane. Cholesterol is a necessary component of biological membranes. Cholesterol breaks up the van der Waals interactions and close packing of the phospholipid tails. This disruption makes the membrane more fluid. Therefore, one way for a cell to control the fluidity of its membrane is by regulating its level of cholesterol in the cell membrane. Another way is to regulate the ratio of saturated to unsaturated hydrocarbon chains of the phospholipids. A group of phospholipids with saturated hydrocarbon chains can pack close together and form numerous van der Waals bonds that hold the phospholipids to each other. Phospholipids with unsaturated hydrocarbon side chains break up those van der Waals bonds and the tight packing by preventing the phospholipids from getting close together.

The cell membrane plays host to a large amount of protein, which is responsible for its various activities. The amount of protein differs between species and according to function; however, the typical amount in a cell membrane is 50%. These proteins are undoubtedly important to a cell. Three groups of membrane proteins can be identified:

1. *Integral Proteins.* They are located spanning the membrane and thus have a hydrophilic cytosolic domain that interacts with internal molecules, a hydrophobic membrane-spanning domain that anchors it within the cell membrane, and a hydro-

philic extracellular domain that interacts with external molecules. Examples of these integral proteins, also known as transmembrane proteins, are ion channels, proton pumps, transport proteins and efflux transporters, such as P-glycoprotein, and G protein-coupled receptors.

2. *Lipid Anchored Proteins.*   They are located covalently bound to single or multiple lipid molecules, which hydrophobically insert into the cell membrane and anchor the protein. The protein itself is not in contact with the membrane. Examples are G proteins.

3. *Peripheral Proteins.*   They are attached to integral proteins, or associated with the head groups of membrane lipids. As such, these proteins are not in contact with the hydrophobic membrane core and therefore associate only at the cytosolic and extracellular faces. They tend to have only temporary interactions with permanent membrane proteins, and once reacted, the molecule dissociates to carry on its work in the cytoplasm. Examples are some enzymes and some hormones.

It is also important to remember that the cell membrane, being exposed to the outside environment, is an important site of cell communication. As such, a large variety of protein receptors and identification proteins, such as antigens, are present on the surface of the membrane.

9.3   PATHWAYS OF DRUG ABSORPTION

For oral drugs to be therapeutically effective, they have to possess favorable characteristics to cross the biological membrane into the systemic circulation and reach the site of action: that is, they must be absorbed. Once a drug molecule is in solution, it has the possibility to be absorbed. At the intestinal epithelial cell surface, there are two pathways that are potentially available to molecules. Transepithelial transport of drugs can be achieved either across the cell (*transcellular* or *intracellular pathway*) or through the junctions that hold the cells together (*paracellular* or *intercellular pathway*) (Fig. 9.3). Historically, the transcellular pathway has received more

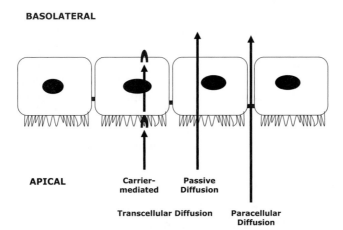

FIGURE 9.3   Schematic representation of the potential transcellular and paracellular pathways of drug intestinal absorption.

attention. However, the increasing understanding of tight junction physiology and regulation has shed light on the paracellular route.

9.3.1 Transcellular Pathway

In the transcellular or intracellular route, drugs are absorbed by passive diffusion, facilitated diffusion, or an active transport system (Fig. 9.3). Since these absorption mechanisms are discussed in Chapter 8, we will not dwell upon it in this chapter.

Passive diffusion (linear or first-order kinetics) is the predominant pathway taken by most oral drugs. Passive diffusion indicates that the transfer of a compound from an aqueous phase (intestinal lumen) through a membrane may be described by physicochemical laws and by the properties of the membrane. The driving force for diffusion across the membrane is the gradient concentration of the drug across the membrane. It is essential for a molecule to have characteristics with low molecular size and relatively high lipophilicity in order to pass across the intestinal membrane by this pathway. Factors influencing transcellular passive diffusion in the GIT are well studied and are reviewed here.

Facilitated diffusion is a process in which a molecule specifically and reversibly binds to its carrier protein in the enterocyte membrane. It crosses the membrane associated with the carrier and is then released to the cytoplasm of the cell. As with passive diffusion, facilitated diffusion can only occur down a gradient of chemical potential, since no energy source is required. The process follows the kinetic of enzymes, being saturable and subject to inhibition by competitive inhibitors. Actually, there are not many unequivocal examples of facilitated diffusion for drug molecules.

Active transport of drugs requires both membrane associated carrier proteins and an energy source, in order that the drug molecules could be transported up a gradient of concentration. Active transport satisfies the following criteria: (1) it is saturable, (2) metabolic inhibitors inhibit transport, and (3) substrate analogues compete with the drug for the active site on the carrier [2]. Absorption by specialized carrier mechanism from the small intestine has been shown to exist for several drugs having chemical structures that are very similar to essential nutrients for which the intestine has a specialized transport mechanism [3].

In direct contrast with specialized transport of a drug into epithelial cells is a process refered to as *efflux transport*, which implies the facilitated movement of a drug out of the cell. Today, it is well demonstrated that this mechanism exists in epithelial cells of the gastrointestinal tract. There is a cell surface glycoprotein (P-glycoprotein, P-gp) that is responsible for this mechanism. P-gp is believed to be responsible for poor intestinal uptake of several classes of compounds. The P-gp protein could be inhibited and the process may be saturated. The former is the basis for many drug–drug and drug–nutrients interactions, and the latter limits the efficacy of the transporter. Both situations may have repercussions in the intestinal absorption of drugs.

9.3.2 Paracellular Pathway

The paracellular route can be defined as the aqueous pathway along the intercellular space between adjacent cells, which is restricted by tight junctions (TJs) at the most apical part of the cells (Fig. 9.3). The aqueous nature of this route makes it favorable for the absorption (through passive diffusion) of small hydrophilic solutes (nutrients, ions, etc.). TJs are dynamic structures, which normally regulate the trafficking of nutrients, medium sized compounds ($\leq 15\,\text{Å}$), and relatively large amounts of fluids between the intestinal lumen and the submucosa [4]. Tight junction permeability differs according to the type of permeant involved, its size, and its charge. The molecular size cutoff for this route is approximately 500 Da [5].

Paracellular transport was belittled for much of the last century and was not considered an effective pathway until the 1960s, when it was discovered that molecules of different sizes can cross the epithelium via the paracellular route [6]. Today, it is well known that the flux across the TJs can be considerable, and that the permeability and selectivity of the junctions can be regulated [7]. Thus, in the last decades many efforts have been made to increase paracellular transport of less absorbable drugs—the use of enhancers being the most promising and studied strategy [8]. This topic is covered in Section 9.5, including an overview of the structure and function of this pathway.

9.4 FACTORS AFFECTING DRUG INTESTINAL ABSORPTION

Factors affecting gastrointestinal drug absorption have been classified into three broad categories. These have been summarized in Table 9.1. In the following, we analyze in a brief manner their influence on intestinal drug absorption.

9.4.1 Physicochemical Factors Affecting Gastrointestinal Drug Absorption

The primary physicochemical properties of a drug influencing absorption across gastrointestinal membrane are solubility, particle size, crystal form, lipophilicity, dissociation constant, and molecular weight.

Solubility Low aqueous solubility is a frequently encountered reason for poor oral absorption. Absorption requires that drug molecules be in solution at the absorption site. For that, drug molecules contained in the dosage forms must be delivered and then they must dissolve in the gastrointestinal fluids at the absorption site. Dissolution depends in part on the solubility of the drug. Together with solubility, the rate of dissolution is another variable to consider. In fact, there are cases of compounds with very low aqueous solubility, which have fully adequate oral bioavailability. This can occur because the rate of dissolution being a rapid phenomenon in spite of the overall solubility being low.

TABLE 9.1 Factor Affecting Gastrointestinal Drug Absorption

Physicochemical Factors	Physiological Factors	Technological Factors
Solubility	Gastric emptying and GIT motility	Pharmaceutical dosage form
Particle size		
Crystal form	Degradation and excretion processes in the GIT	Manufacturing processes
Lipophilicity		
Dissociation constant		

Polar solutes are more soluble in water than in organic media, whereas the opposite is true for nonpolar solutes. When the drug is ionizable, ionized species are more soluble in water than their un-ionized counterparts. On the other hand, solubility of weak acids or bases in aqueous medium is dependent on pH. For these compounds with acidic or basic functional groups, both solubility and rate of dissolution can be improved by suitable choice of salt forms.

The presence of charged groups can aid in solubility. However, charge, particularly high charge density, can have a negative impact on drug absorption since charged species do not readily penetrate the lipoidal membrane (*vide infra*). In such cases the reduction in charge by chemical modification can be a useful strategy. In other cases, charge also can have a negative impact on drug absorption by forming water-insoluble complexes or salts with the gastrointestinal contents.

Particle Size   Surface area of drug particles influences the rate of drug dissolution and, therefore, drug absorption. Particle size determines the surface area of the solid. Small particles have greater surface area than larger particles and, consequently, they dissolve more rapidly. One important exception is constituted by the hydrophobic drugs. In this case, some examples have shown that the dissolution rate can increase with increasing particle size. For example, the rate of dissolution of the hydrophobic drug phenacetin increases as particle size increases from 0.11–0.15 mm to 0.50–0.71 mm [9]. It is probable that decreasing particle size of a hydrophobic drug actually decreases its effective surface area (i.e., the portion of surface without adsorbed air and actually in contact with dissolving fluid). In these cases, the addition of a surface-active agent significantly increases the effective surface area, improving the rate of dissolution and therefore the rate and extent of absorption.

Particle size appears to have little influence on the absorption of high aqueous solubility drug molecules. However, absorption of drugs such as griseofulvin, a molecule with low solubility in water, is highly dependent on the particle size. In these cases, strategies that increase particle surface area will result in improvement of drug absorption. The effective surface-area may be increased by physically reducing the particle size or by adding surface-active agents to the dosage form.

Crystal Form   The physicochemical properties of crystal forms are influenced by the intermolecular forces present. Crystals with weak attractive forces between molecules exhibit greater solubility than those with strong attractive forces. In this sense, solubility could be dependent on the crystal form. There are a number of drugs with different crystal forms (polymorphs) and, in these cases, they can show differences in dissolution rates and, consequently, in absorption. For example, the rate of absorption of chloramphenicol appears to be directly related to the solubility of the different polymorphs of its palmitate ester [10].

Lipophilicity   Gastrointestinal membranes are lipoidal in nature; therefore, they are more permeable to lipid-soluble drug substances. Lipid solubility of the diffusing species will influence, in part, passive diffusion across biological membranes. Lipid solubility of a drug is determined by the presence of nonpolar groups in the structure of the drug molecule, as well as by the presence of ionizable groups that are affected by local pH. It is logical to suppose that when an ionizable group exists in the drug molecule, it is very important, in order to improve lipophilicity, that this group would be in the un-ionized state. High lipid solubility values must be accompanied, however, by adequate water solubility. When the water solubility is too low, a significant concentration of the drug molecule cannot be achieved at the membrane surface and absorption may be inefficient in spite of favorable lipid solubility.

The relative lipophilic to hydrophilic balance of the entire molecule can be described by the oil/water partition coefficient ($K_{o/w}$). In general, this parameter can be used as a predictor of the ability of a drug molecule to be absorbed by passive diffusion across lipoidal membranes. As $K_{o/w}$ increases, the rate of absorption increases. However, there are several exceptions to this general rule. Highly branched compounds are absorbed more slowly and small polar molecules more readily than would be expected based on their $K_{o/w}$ values.

The absorption of a hydrophilic drug may often be enhanced through appropriate structural modifications that increase $K_{o/w}$ of the compound (e.g., esterification). For example, esterification of one of the carboxylic groups of enalaprilat results in a significant increase in oral bioavailability [11].

Dissociation Constant   The presence of ionizable groups in the drug molecule can condition the absorption across biological membranes. The importance of ionization in drug absorption is based on the observation that the nonionized form of the drug has a greater $K_{o/w}$ than the ionized form; therefore, the nonionized form of the drug in solution penetrates lipoidal membranes of the gastrointestinal tract more rapidly than the ionized species. The rate of absorption of an ionizable drug is therefore dependent on the concentration of its nonionized species at the absorption site, which is, as predicted by the Henderson–Hasselbalch equation, a function of the pK_a of the compound and the pH of the medium.

$$\text{For acidic drugs:} \quad f = \frac{1}{1 + 10^{(\text{pH} - pK_a)}} \tag{9.1}$$

$$\text{For basic drugs:} \quad f = \frac{1}{1 + 10^{(pK_a - \text{pH})}} \tag{9.2}$$

where f is the nonionized fraction.

The pH of the gastrointestinal tract ranges from 1.2 to 3.5 in the stomach, 5.0 to 6.0 in the duodenum, and 6.5 to 8.0 in the jejunum and large intestine. For acidic drugs with pK_a values between 2.5 and 7.5, the un-ionized fraction f decreases with increases in pH. The same is true for bases with pK_a values between 5 and 11.

A number of studies have related and quantified the influence of pH and pK_a on drug absorption in the gastrointestinal tract. These studies resulted in the so-called pH-partition theory. Briefly, this theory states that only the nonionized form of an ionizable drug is able to penetrate biological membranes because only this form has an adequate $K_{o/w}$. As a result, acidic drugs should best be absorbed from media with pH $< pK_a$, whereas basic compounds would best be absorbed from media with pH $> pK_a$. This does not mean that acidic drugs are best absorbed in the stomach and basic drugs best absorbed in small intestine. Even though the pH-partition theory provides a useful guide in predicting general trends in passive drug absorption, some inconsistencies have been observed. The primary limitation of this theory derives from the assumption that only nonionized drug is absorbed, when in fact the ionized form of low to medium molecular weight drugs can be absorbed by passive diffusion through the pores (actually known as the paracellular route, *vide supra*), albeit at a slower rate. In fact, some models of intestinal drug absorption [12] propose that for ionized compounds, with low to medium molecular weight (below 250), diffusion through this route is the major contributor of absorption. For extremely low molecular weight, highly hydrophilic compounds, this route may be the only one. As the molecular weight and, consequently, the $K_{o/w}$ increase, passage through the transcellular route (i.e., through the lipoidal membrane) will predominate. For intermediate molecular weight drugs, diffusion using both routes will be possible.

9.4.2 Physiological Factors Affecting Gastrointestinal Drug Absorption

Once a drug molecule is in solution, it has the potential to be absorbed. However, there are a number of variables, other than the physicochemical ones, that can condition the absorption process. In the following sections we review the main physiological factors related to drug absorption.

Gastric Emptying and GIT Motility   When an oral dosage form is swallowed by a patient, it travels through the GIT, starting this travel in the stomach. At this point, the dosage form must break down into small granules and particles and release the drug in order to facilitate its dissolution in the gastrointestinal fluids. Because the stomach has a reduced membrane surface area relative to small intestine, very frequently, the rate of drug absorption in this area is very low. So the rate at which the drug gets to the small intestine can condition the rate of absorption. Gastric emptying is the normal physiological process that controls the progression of the gastric contents toward the duodenum. Knowledge of the factors controlling gastric emptying is important because this process can control the rate of absorption in the small intestine.

There is a general consensus that gastric emptying (measured from the remaining volumes in the stomach after ingestion) follows first-order kinetics [13] especially when liquid or small volumes of semisolids are ingested. The half-life of the process ranges from 10 to 60 min in the case of fluids or semisolids, whereas this time increases up to 4 hours when nondisintegrating solids are ingested. Since, for the majority of the drugs, absorption occurs in the small intestine, the start of the absorption process will be conditioned by gastric emptying. When the intrinsic absorbability of the drug is elevated, gastric emptying become a rate-determining step of drug absorption. For example, paracetamol has good absorbability in the small intestine. Clements et al. [14] showed that, when this drug is orally administered, the absorption rate constant is highly correlated with the rate of gastric emptying.

Gastric emptying rate can be modified by several factors. For example, light physical activity stimulates gastric emptying, whereas strenuous exercise delays it. The volume of the ingested meal is another important factor conditioning gastric emptying. So Hunt and Macdonald [15] found that the half-life of gastric emptying increased from 7 min for a 50 mL standard meal to 50 min for a 1250 mL ingestion. The viscosity of the meal also conditions the rate of gastric emptying. Liquids abandon the stomach faster than semisolids. Nondigestible solids with size ≥ 2 mm in diameter are handled by the stomach quite differently from liquids and will remain in the stomach for a long period (up to 12 hours). Concurrent drug therapy may also affect the rate of gastric emptying. Thus, cholinergic drugs increase the rate of emptying [16].

Delays in stomach emptying may decrease the rate of availability of a drug. The extent of availability, however, may be increased, decreased, or unaffected. For poorly water-soluble drugs, the extent of availability can be significantly reduced when the drug is ingested under fasting conditions. So Welling et al. [17] showed that erythromycin availability was reduced when 250 mg tablets were taken on a fasting stomach relative to that obtained when tablets were ingested after high fat, high protein, and high carbohydrate meals.

Concurrent drug therapy may increase or decrease intestinal motility. Such changes may increase, decrease, or have no effect on the extent of availability of the drug. So the concomitant use of metoclopramide, a drug that increases the gastrointestinal motility, can reduce the extent of availability of drugs with low values of rate of dissolution. For example, digoxin bioavailability is reduced in the presence of metoclopramide probably due to the increase in intestinal motility, so there is insufficient time for the release of digoxin from its dosage form and the subsequent dissolution in the gastrointestinal fluids before it abandons the GIT [18]. However, digoxin bioavailability increases in the presence of propantheline, a drug that slows gastrointestinal motility [18].

Degradation and Excretion Processes in the Gastrointestinal Tract   Several processes in the GIT can reduce the extent of availability of a drug administered by the oral route. The main processes that can reduce the extent of availability are given in Table 9.2.

Some drugs can interact with endogenous or exogenous substances present in the gastrointestinal fluids, forming insoluble complexes. For example, biliary salts can interact with drugs such as neomycin and kanamycin, forming insoluble and nonabsorbable complexes.

Chemical degradation, especially pH-dependent reactions, can occur in the gastrointestinal fluids. Several polypeptides, nucleotides, or fatty acids may be susceptible to enzymatic degradation by several enzymes present in the gastrointestinal fluids. The role of the gastrointestinal microflora on the metabolism of drugs has long been recognized. In humans less than 1000 organisms/mL are usually found in the gastric juice. Only if the pH is high (>4) are relatively large numbers of bacteria found. The bacterial flora in the proximal jejunum is sparse, with increasing number in the distal small intestine. The number of organisms increases markedly in the

TABLE 9.2   Factors Reducing the Extent of Drug Absorption

Factors Acting in the Lumen of the GIT (Before Membrane Penetration)	Factors Acting After Membrane Penetration
Adsorption and nonsoluble complex formation	Gut wall metabolism
Chemical degradation	Gut secretion by efflux transporters
Enzymatic degradation	
Bacterial degradation	

large intestine. Microorganisms are capable of carrying out a multitude of reactions, and some of these reactions may have toxicological significance. Most of the metabolic transformations mediated by the microflora fall into the category of hydrolytic reactions, reactions involving the removal of various groups (e.g., dehydroxylations, descarboxylations, dealkylations) and reductive reactions.

Many drugs and toxic compounds that enter the body via the GIT suffer metabolism in the mucosal cells. In fact, enterocytes in the upper segment of the small intestine express, at high concentrations, two forms of cytochrome P450 (CYP3A4 and CYP3A5) that can potentially limit the availability of drugs [19]. Oxidation reactions mediated by CYP and also conjugation reactions play an important role in the metabolism of drugs in the small intestine [20]. For example, drugs such as midazolam or felodipine are subjected to an intense first-pass effect at the intestinal membrane [21, 22]. However, although it would seem that drug metabolism within the mucosal cells would serve only to reduce its extent of availability, in some cases, this process may enhance bioavailability. For example, clindamycin palmitate is a more stable form than the clindamycin HCl solution. The palmitate ester is rapidly hydrolyzed into the parent drug and its use increases the availability of clindamycin after oral administration [23]. Molecules such as clindamycin palmitate are chemical derivatives of drugs usually made to enhance the pharmaceutical properties (e.g., lipophilicity) of the parent molecule. These derivatives are called prodrugs.

Another recently described process that reduces the extent of bioavailability is the excretion process by efflux transporters in the small intestine. In this process, the drug—once it penetrates the intestinal membrane and is in the cytoplasm of the enterocyte—is subjected to a secretion process mediated by a transporter and is translocated, again, into the intestinal lumen. This process is mediated by an ATP-binding transmembrane transporter called P-glycoprotein. P-glycoprotein is a protein that belongs to the ATP-binding cassette (ABC) family. P-glycoprotein functions as a transmembrane efflux pump that translocates its substrates from its intracellular domain to its extracellular domain. P-glycoprotein is assumed to be one of the most important ABC transporters for drug disposition in humans. It is now established that P-glycoprotein is expressed constitutively in small intestine and in other organs. As a result of its anatomical localization, P-glycoprotein limits drug entry into the body after oral drug administration as a result of its expression in the luminal (apical) membrane of enterocytes [24].

Recently, it has been shown that enterocytes simultaneously express the major drug-metabolizing enzymes CYP3A and the efflux transporter P-glycoprotein [19]. This leads to a drug efflux–metabolism alliance, which increases the access of drug to metabolism by CYP3A4 through repeated cycles of absorption and efflux, further reducing the possibility of the drug reaching the systemic circulation unaltered.

9.4.3 Technological Factors Affecting Gastrointestinal Drug Absorption

As well as the physicochemical and physiological factors affecting intestinal drug absorption, there are technological variables that could affect the rate and extent of drug absorption. We have classified these variables into two subcategories: factors depending on pharmaceutical dosage form and manufacturing factors.

Pharmaceutical Dosage Form   In considering, in a general manner, the availability of drugs from various classes of dosage forms, drugs administered in solution usually produce the most available drug product, assuming that the drug does not precipitate in the stomach and is not deactivated there. The second most available dosage form would be drug dispersed in a fine suspension, followed by micronized drug in a capsule, uncoated tablets, and finally by the coated tablets. In formulating and designing drug products, this ranking should be kept in mind.

The reason for this different availability is the difference in processes involved in drug release from the dosage form. Once the dosage form reaches the stomach, it must break down (if it is a solid dosage form) and release the therapeutic agent. Disintegration and dissolution are the key processes that precede the absorption process from a solid dosage form. As mentioned earlier, dissolution of the drug in the gastrointestinal fluid is the first step for drug absorption. The disintegration process increases the surface area of the dosage form and, in general, will increase the rate of dissolution. Disintegration is not a prerequisite when a pharmaceutical suspension or solution is employed.

Release of the therapeutic agent can be affected by the nonactive ingredients included in the dosage form. For example, for drugs formulated as tablets, diluents, disintegrants, binders, lubricants, surfactants, and even colorants can affect the release of the drug from the pharmaceutical dosage form as measured by the rate of dissolution in *in vitro* tests. Their proper choice becomes more critical when formulating water-insoluble drugs and when the total concentration of the drug in the dosage form is small.

Manufacturing Processes   In addition to the above-mentioned variables, the characteristics and processing of the dosage form could have great influence on drug availability. Variables such as process of granulation method or compressional force in production of tablets can significantly affect the bioavailability of the drug [25].

9.5 INTESTINAL PERMEABILITY ENHANCEMENT: POSSIBILITIES AND LIMITATIONS

In the last decade incredible advances have been made in the application of molecular biology and biotechnology, which have led to a revolution in the development of new therapeutic compounds. These new drugs must be properly delivered in the body to have the desired pharmacological effect. In this challenging task, it is essential to consider the biopharmaceutical and pharmacokinetic properties of the drug, particularly those concerning intestinal absorption and bioavailability (BA) after oral administration. The oral route is the preferred administration route, and it must be taken into account that the newer promising drugs, especially peptides and proteins, cannot be developed as oral products because of their null or scarce bioavailability. In general, these are hydrophilic compounds, of medium to high molecular weight, and sometimes containing strongly charged functional groups—implying that transport across the intestinal barrier occurs essentially via the paracellular pathway [26]. The contribution of this pathway to intestinal absorption is considered to be small, since this pathway occupies less than 0.1% of the total surface area of the intestinal epithelium [27], and the presence of tight junctions (TJs) between the epithelial cells limits drug absorption. Therefore, for the above-mentioned drugs, the main cause of low bioavailability is their poor intestinal permeability. Thus, considerable attention has been directed at finding ways to increase the paracellular transport of these compounds—the use of enhancers being the most promising and studied strategy [8, 28]. In recent years, knowledge of tight junction physiology and regulation has increased [29], which has facilitated the search for compounds capable of enhancing absorption via the paracellular pathway. To obtain maximum benefit from such enhancing compounds, it is necessary to confirm that reduced membrane permeability is the cause (or at least the main cause) of poor drug bioavailability. Moreover, the activity of an absorption enhancer should be inmediate and should coincide with the presence of the drug at the absorption site [8, 30]. In these cases, an increase in intestinal absorption would be achieved, leading to an enhancement in drug bioavailability, which in turn would allow oral administration of the drug and also a reduction in inter- and intrasubject variability in plasma concentrations and therefore in therapeutic effects.

In this section, we analyze the possibilities and limitations of the most promising intestinal paracellular enhancers. The basic anatomic and physiological properties of the paracellular route are first examined in order to better understand the absorption process, which could help in the selection of the appropriate enhancer. Interest has focused on medium chain fatty acids and chitosan and its derivatives, since these are the most studied and effective enhancers. In fact, the medium chain fatty acid sodium caprate is being used as an absorption enhancer in the clinical setting in Japan, Denmark, and Sweden. There have been no reports of serious side effects [31–33]. Additionally, the results obtained with the more recent paracellular enhancers are presented. Previous reviews are recommended for in-depth insight into this topic [4, 8, 28, 34].

9.5.1 Structure and Function of the Intestinal Paracellular Pathway

The junctional complex found in the apical portion of adjacent cells is composed of three distinct regions: tight junctions or zonula occludens, zonula adherens, and macula adherens or desmosome (Fig. 9.4). Paracellular permeability is primarily regulated by the TJs, because this is the rate-limiting barrier of the transport pathway. TJs have been described as gates (selectively allowing the passage of small hydrophilic compounds) and as fences (forming an intermembrane diffusion barrier maintaining enterocyte polarity and excluding potentially toxic molecules). These two functions are not separate unrelated phenomena [29]. It is becoming increasingly clear that TJs in themselves constitute the product of a global polarizing process; their role therefore does not seem to correspond to that of a simple fence [35].

In the last years some light has been shed on the architecture and regulation of TJs. Because a complete review of TJ structure, function, and molecular regulation is beyond the scope of this chapter, and has previously been done [35–38], only a brief summary of the more relevant aspects of the subject and its repercussions on paracellular permeability are presented here.

Under the transmission electron microscope, tight junctions appear as a series of focal contacts between the plasma membrane of two adjacent cells. In early freeze-fracture electron microscopy sections, the tight junctional complex appeared as a

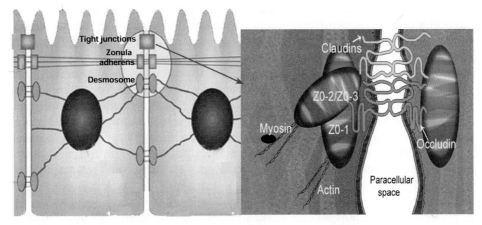

FIGURE 9.4 (Left) The functional complex located in the apical part of adjacent entero-cytes (tight junctions, zonula adherens, and desmosomes) is depicted. (Right) Schematic representation of the protein interactions at tight junctions. The interaction is only repre-sented in one part of the illustration. Other proteins have been localized to the cytoplasmic surface of tight junctions, although they are not represented. For more information see the text. (From Ref. 34, with permission.)

dense network of interdigitating strands or fibrils in the plane of the plasma mem-brane [39]. At some points the strands showed discontinuities, which might corre-spond to "pores" [40], and which would imply channel-like permeability (i.e., fluctuating aqueous pores embedded in the fibrils would account for diffusion through TJs). This early concept has progressed little and it is presently also postu-lated that fibrils on one cell interact with fibrils on an adjacent cell to seal the para-cellular space and define the permeability characteristics [36]. To date, the commonly held view is that increases in paracellular permeability under perturbed or patho-logical conditions result from the dilatation of existing tight junction pores [41]. In contrast, the composition of the fibrils is now well known. Fibrils are formed by at least two types of tetra-spanning transmembrane proteins: occludin and claudin (Fig. 9.4). Occludin is a 65 kDa phosphoprotein [42–44]. The findings reported to date are consistent with a functional role for occludin in defining the barrier [45, 46]. Claudins are a family of proteins, named from the Latin *claudere*, "to close." They appear to represent the major structural components of tight junction strands [47]. Recent studies have proposed that claudins are the pore-forming structures in TJs [48, 49]—thus strongly supporting the idea that claudins confer specific selectiv-ity to paracellular transport. Furthermore, a dense cytoplasmic network of proteins has been described at the TJs. These are referred to as tight junction associated proteins (TJAPs), and are designated ZO-1, ZO-2, and ZO-3. As can be seen in Fig. 9.4, these proteins interact among each other (ZO-1 and ZO-2 are bound to each other and to 130 kDa protein, ZO-3) and also serve as a link between occludin and the actin filaments of the cytoskeleton [28]. The association of TJs with the apical perijunctional actomyosin ring seems to regulate global TJ permeability [38]. It is also known that the barrier assembly and permeability characteristics of TJs are influenced by many cellular signaling mechanisms—although these remain largely undefined [50]. Therefore, despite rapid progress in knowledge of TJ structure and molecular physiology, their function in the context of paracellular permeability is still far from fully clear.

In summary, evidence now exists to suggest that the regulation of paracellular permeability by the TJ is a complex process, illustrated by the diversity in functional reactions of this structure. At present, apart from conventional permeability studies, several probes have become available for detecting changes in activation of intracellular proteins, such as the protein kinase C isotypes. Moreover, *in situ* imaging techniques are being used [37]. Studies in the field of diseases originated by paracellular permeability alterations (food allergies, malabsorption syndromes, and inflammatory bowel diseases such as Crohn's disease and ulcerative colitis) also contribute to our understanding of paracellular transport. In future, all such intense research can contribute to secure in-depth knowledge of the control mechanisms implicated in paracellular transport and its modulation, which may have great repercussions for drug delivery.

9.5.2 Intestinal Paracellular Enhancers

As already outlined, attempts to reduce the absorption barrier are mainly based on the use of paracellular permeation enhancers as auxiliary agents in oral drug delivery systems [8]. Before presenting the potential compounds that could be used as enhancers, several general aspects are considered.

General Considerations   According to Aungst [8] there are several critical issues to consider in the selection of a compound as a potential absorption enhancer for use in drug delivery: the degree of bioavailability enhancement achieved, the influence of formulation and physiological variables, the possible toxicity originated by the enhancing action, and the mechanism of permeation enhancement.

On the other hand, once the enhancer has been selected it should be highlighted that the efficacy of absorption enhancer, in terms of intensity and duration of its effect, depends on the concentration at its site of action. Therefore, it is necessary to have the means to control this concentration or at least to be able to regulate it within a certain effective concentration range. This, nevertheless, might be difficult to achieve in some cases, since many variables, as outlined before, influence the actual concentration of drug and/or enhancer at a specific site in the GIT. Alternatively, the application of controlled release dosage forms could be more effective in maintaining concentrations of enhancer in the effective range [51].

The vast majority of data published on the use of intestinal paracellular enhancers have been obtained using *in vitro* and *in situ* methodologies. The possibilities and limitations of these techniques are evaluated in the following section. The effectiveness of any compound for enhancing intestinal permeation must also be assessed by *in vivo* studies. The degree of bioavailability enhancement, as well as the effect on C_{max} and the area under the curve (AUC), are the indicators most commonly used in studies of this kind. The *in vivo* setting clearly constitutes a more complex and dynamic environment, which hampers assessment of the promoting effect. Furthermore, the formulation used to administer the drug and promoter (solution, capsules, microcapsules, enteric-coated capsules, suppositories) could influence the efficacy of an absorption enhancing excipient. Similarly, the route of administration used (peroral, intrajejunal, intracolonic, rectal) is directly related to the success of oral drug bioavailability enhancement. For more information on the factors influencing the *in vivo* performance of permeation enhancers, readers are referred to the reviews by Aungst [8] and Ward et al. [28].

Medium Chain Fatty Acids (MCFAs)   Based on research conducted in the last decade, it has become clear that several sodium salts of medium chain fatty acids (caprylate C8 (CH_3—$(CH_2)_6$—COOH), caprate C10 (CH_3—$(CH_2)_8$—COOH), and laurate C12 (CH_3—$(CH_2)_{10}$—COOH)) are able to enhance the paracellular permeability of hydrophilic compounds. Lindmark et al. [52] carried out a comparative study with these three fatty acids and sodium caproate (C6). They showed that C8, C10, and C12 (but not C6) exhibit dose-dependent enhancing effects on mannitol transport across cell monolayers—with C12 being the most effective enhancer. Interestingly, the lowest concentrations to enhance transport of the marker molecule were in the vicinity of their critical micellar concentration (CMC), which in turn differs considerably for each.

Among these MCFAs, sodium caprate is the most extensively studied and the only absorption-enhancing agent included in a marketed drug product. It is added in a suppository formulation intended for human use in Sweden and Japan [33]. Since this fatty acid has a low molecular weight, it could be absorbed from the intestine even more quickly than the drug itself [8]. The numerous studies conducted with C10 have addressed different aspects such as its enhancing effect on the permeability of compounds with different molecular weights (MWs), its concentration and time-dependent effects, and its toxicity and mechanism of action.

Most published data on *sodium caprate* as an absorption enhancer have been obtained using *in vitro* and *in situ* techniques. Collectively, the results obtained using these methodologies indicate that C10 can enhance intestinal permeability of low (MW 180–400) and high (MW 4000–19,000) molecular weight *marker molecules* [31, 52–56]. However, the authors point out that the effect would be significant only for substances of MW ≤ 1200 g/mol; that is, in the case of larger molecules, permeability enhancement would not result in a significant increase in the dose fraction absorbed [57]. Regarding the effects on *drug* permeability, sodium caprate enhances intestinal permeability of cefmetazole [58], ebitaride (a pentapeptide ACTH analogue) [57], peptide drugs [53, 59], and epirubicin, an anticancer drug [60]. Nevertheless, it is worth pointing out that Raiman et al. [61] have recently found that C10 (10 mM) does not affect the permeability of the bisphosphonate drug clodronate across Caco-2 cell monolayers.

In all of the studies just mentioned, the sodium caprate concentration used was in the vicinity of its CMC (i.e., 13 mM). Several research groups, using Caco-2 cells, have shown the C10 enhancement effect on membrane permeability to be concentration dependent [31, 52, 53]. We have also recently observed this *concentration-dependent effect in vitro* (Caco-2 cell) using acamprosate, an alcoholic antirelapse drug (unpublished data). However, when we performed the experiments *in situ* [62] and *in vivo* with rats, this effect disappeared. Our results agree with those obtained *in vivo* by Raoof et al. [63] in pigs. According to their data, the enhancing capacity of C10 is dose independent.

Regarding the *time-dependent effect* of C10 on intestinal permeability, studies carried out by Anderberg et al. [54], using Caco-2 cells, showed significant time-dependent effects at 13 mM and higher concentrations (16 mM). These experiments were performed after long incubations (approximately 1 h) with C10. Since the immediate effect of the enhancer is presumably more relevant than the long-term effect *in vivo*, Lindmark et al. [32], in Caco-2 cell monolayers, determined both the long- and short-term effects. According to their results, the time-dependent effect of sodium caprate 13 mM upon permeability can be separated into two phases: an initial phase (10–20 min) in which a rapid increase in permeability was observed, and a later phase characterized by a slow but more prolonged enhancement in permeability. Kamm et al. [59] have also shown C10 absorption enhancement to be markedly dependent on incubation time in Caco-2 cells.

The local *toxicity* of sodium caprate in the small intestine is one of the main concerns with use of this fatty acid in pharmaceutical products. The toxicity of C10 has been extensively studied *in vitro*. Considering that cytotoxicity depends on the concentration and duration of exposure, comparisons among results obtained in experiments using different protocols may not always be valid. Cell damage can be assessed by several methods (morphological observations, the release of biological markers, and the recovery of transepithelial electrical resistance (TEER))—a fact that further complicates the drawing of firm conclusions. A closer examination of the reported data suggests that C10 at effective concentrations (around 13 mM) does not affect epithelial viability [64] and does not cause serious cytotoxicity—its effects moreover being reversible [53, 55, 65, 66].

The studies performed *in vivo* with sodium caprate are not as numerous as those using *in vitro* and *in situ* techniques. The drugs involved in these investigations have been peptides, antibiotics, and polar, high MW *drugs* such as antisense oligonucleotides or glycyrrhizin. When the drug and enhancer are administered as a solution, the effective C10 doses in the reported studies are comparable. Closer examination shows that all these doses are in the range of 0.1–0.5 mmol/kg. Curiously, when these amounts are transformed into concentrations, the values obtained are in some cases quite different and clearly higher (25–1000 mM) than those tested in the *in vitro* models [34]. Most investigations have been performed in rats, although dogs, pigs, rabbits, and even humans have also been used [34]. As a whole, it can be concluded that this medium chain fatty acid is capable of improving oral drug bioavailability. However, it must be stressed that only two studies have been carried out to date in humans, and no effect was reported in one of them [67].

It is worth mentioning that two studies have compared the *in vivo* enhancing effect of several medium chain fatty acids [68, 69], concluding that the strength of this effect is in the following order: caprate > laurate > caprylate. Hence, sodium caprate seems to be the most potent promoter among the MCFAs tested.

In vivo studies analyzing the toxicity of C10 are scarce but in concordance. This fatty acid, at the doses tested, was well tolerated by the intestinal mucosa, and no membrane damage was observed [53, 63, 68].

In conclusion, sodium caprate can be considered a promising agent for use as an enhancing excipient in drug delivery. The C10 effect is dependent on its permeability in the tissue upon which it is required to act. Further studies are needed to confirm its null or low toxicity, and to evaluate its enhancing efficacy for each particular drug substance.

Chitosan and Its Derivatives   High MW polymers such as chitosan and its derivatives have gained considerable attention as permeation enhancers. Because of their high MW, these polymers are supposedly not absorbed from the gut, and systemic side effects are thus excluded. In addition, prolonged localization in the mucosa is ensured, which in turn would prolong the promoting effect. Chitosan and its derivatives are also of great interest as excipients and drug carriers in the pharmaceutical field, due to their biodegradability, biocompatibility, and recent FDA application [34].

Chitosan is a partially deacetylated form of chitin, which is present in crustacean shells, insects, and fungi, as well as in some microorganisms (Fig. 9.5). Chitosan is actually a denomination describing a series of polymers with different molecular weights (from 50 to 2000 kDa) and degrees of deacetylation. These two factors are very important for the physicochemical properties of chitosan and thus exert a major impact on its promoting effects (as discussed later).

The effect of chitosan on intestinal permeability across tight junctions was first reported by Artursson et al. [70]. These authors found chitosan glutamate to enhance ^{14}C-mannitol transport *in vitro* (Caco-2 cell monolayers). Posteriorly, it was

(a)

Chitin
- Natural structural component of crustacean shells
- Most common natural polymer apart from cellulose
- Biodegradable. Nontoxic

(b)

Chitosan
- High molecular weight
- Soluble in dilute acids pH<6.5
-Polyamine
- Biodegradable. Nontoxic

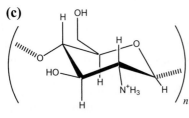

(c)

Chitosan-cationic
- High positive charge
-Strong film forming properties
- Compatible with cations
- Forms complexes with anions
- Biodegradable. Nontoxic

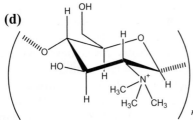

(d)

N-Trimethyl chitosan
- High positive charge
- Soluble in pH< 9
- Enhancing intestinal absorption properties
- Biodegradable. Nontoxic

FIGURE 9.5 Chemical structures and properties of chitosan and its derivatives. (From Ref. 34, with permission.)

confirmed that chitosan hydrochloride and chitosan glutamate, in a slightly acidic environment, increase the permeation of low molecular weight *markers* as well as of large hydrophilic compounds (PEG-4000 and fluorescein dextrans) in intestinal epithelial cells. It was also found that both salts are insoluble at pH 7.4 and prove to be ineffective as permeation enhancers [71, 72].

Regarding the effect of chitosan salts on *drug* intestinal permeability *in vitro*, there is general agreement that these polymers are potent absorption enhancers for poorly absorbed drugs such as atenolol and peptide drugs. Studies with buserelin, 9-deglycinamide 8-arginine vasopressin (DGAVP), and insulin have evidenced a strong increase in the transport of these drugs in the presence of chitosan glutamate and chitosan hydrochloride (acidic environment) [34].

Schipper et al. [73] reported that the molecular weight and degree of deacetylation of chitosans influence their effects on Caco-2 permeability and cytotoxicity. Accordingly, one chitosan with an intermediate degree of deacetylation and high molecular weight had good enhancing characteristics and low cytotoxicity. Chitosan toxicity has been further evaluated by other researchers based on trypan blue exclusion studies and confocal laser scanning microscopy [71]. No deleterious effects on the cells were demonstrated. Thus, the general opinion regarding chitosan salt toxicity *in vitro* appears to be that it offers a very safe toxicity profile.

In vivo studies of the enhancing effects of chitosan on intestinal absorption are scarce but concordant. Chitosan hydrochloride has been observed to increase drug (buserelin, octreotide acetate) bioavalibility in rats and pigs in an acidic environment [34]. Hence, the chitosan pH-dependent effect observed *in vitro* was also confirmed *in vivo*. The explanation for this phenomenon is based on the fact that chitosan, being a weak base, loses its positive charge in neutral and basic media—thus proving to be ineffective as an absorption enhancer [74].

To overcome the solubility limitations of chitosans at neutral and basic pH, *N-trimethyl chitosan chloride* (*TMC*) *derivatives* (Fig. 9.5d) are obtained. These derivatives display much greater aqueous solubility than chitosan at neutral and alkaline pH values [75]. Consequently, a great volume of data have been published on the intestinal enhancing properties of these polymers.

In vitro, TMC derivatives are especially effective in enhancing the transport of small hydrophilic compounds (e.g., mannitol), although they also improve the transport of large molecules (drugs) such as buserelin, insulin, DGAVP, and octreotide acetate [34]. Throughout the multiple studies performed *in vitro*, the researchers have abundantly shown the degree of quaternization to play an important role in the absorption-enhancing properties of these polymers, especially in neutral and basic environments. There is general agreement that the promoting effect of TMC derivatives increases with an increase in their degree of quaternization [34]. Discrepancies exist regarding the optimum degree of quaternization. Thus, maximum absorption enhancement of mannitol and buserelin was recorded with TMC 60 (degree of quaternization 60%) [31, 76]. However, it has recently been reported that the best and maximum permeation-enhancing results are achieved with TMC 49 (degree of quaternization 48.8%) [77, 78]. The few *in vivo* studies reported to date are relatively recent and have been conducted using TMC derivatives with a high degree of quaternization (TMC 40 and TMC 60), and involving the same *drugs* tested *in vitro*—that is, buserelin and octreotide acetate [31, 79]. All these data reveal increased drug bioavailability when the drug is administered intraduodenally in rats and pigs, with TMC 40 and TMC 60 at neutral pH values. Moreover, a concentration-dependent effect of these polymers was observed [79]. No toxicity studies have been presented to date.

TMC derivatives are only suitable for improving the intestinal absorption of macromolecular therapeutic agents with neutral or basic properties due to its positive charge. Hence, when chitosan salts and TMC were evaluated for their compatibility with low molecular weight heparin (LMWH), a highly anionic polysaccharide, strong aggregation was observed with subsequent fiber formation and precipitation. To overcome this problem, another chitosan derivative has been synthesized: *mono-N-carboxymethyl chitosan* (*MCC*) [80]. This polymer is perfectly soluble in aqueous environments at neutral and alkaline pH values and is compatible with anionic and neutral compounds. MCC was evaluated as a potential absorption enhancer of LMWH *in vitro* (Caco-2 cell monolayers) and *in vivo* (rats) [80]. Both the *in vitro* and *in vivo* results indicated that MCC derivatives are capable of significantly increasing the intestinal absorption of LMWH. Moreover, these polymers were seen to present nontoxic characteristics. The authors concluded that carboxymethyl modifications of chitosan may be suitable absorption enhancers for the peroral delivery of anionic macromolecules.

In summary, it can be concluded that chitosan and its derivatives are promising excipients for use as enhancers in the peroral delivery of poorly absorbed drugs.

Zonula Occludens Toxin (Zot)   The great interest in the peroral administration of poorly absorbing therapeutic agents has led to the development of innovative strategies. This is the case, for instance, of *zonula occludens toxin* (Zot), a 45 kDa protein elaborated by *Vibrio cholerae* that is able to reversibly regulate tight junction permeability [81]. This toxin interacts with a specific intestinal epithelial surface receptor, with subsequent activation of a complex cascade of intracellular events that lead to a protein kinase C-dependent polymerization of actin microfilaments strategically localized to regulate the paracellular pathway, and consequently leading to opening of the TJs at a toxin concentration as low as $1.1 \times 10^{-13} M$ [82, 83]. The potential of Zot to enhance the paracellular transport of marker compounds and drugs was first investigated by Fasano et al. [84]. These authors showed that Zot reversibly enhances rabbit intestinal permeability to insulin *in vitro* in the jejunum and ileum, although no substantial changes were detected in the colon. Posteriorly, Cox et al. [85] demonstrated that Zot enhances transport across Caco-2 cell monolayers of low and *high molecular weight markers*. It was also shown that the *in vitro* permeabilities of drugs with low oral bioavailability such as paclitaxel, acyclovir, and cyclosporine and enamione anticonvulsants were increased with Zot. Furthermore, the enhancing properties of Zot were found to be reversible and nontoxic [81–85]. Recent studies have identified a smaller 12 kDa fragment of Zot, referred to as ΔG [86]—this fragment being responsible for the intrinsic tight junction modulation activity. In 2003, Salama et al. [87] reported that this biologically active fragment (ΔG) is able to increase mannitol permeability across Caco-2 cell monolayers. ΔG was found to be noncytotoxic at the concentration tested. These authors also examined the *in vivo* effect of ΔG using the rat as animal model. When mannitol was administered intraduodenally with ΔG only, no significant differences were observed in terms of the pharmacokinetic parameters. However, when the active fragment was used in the presence of protease inhibitors (PIs), significant increases were obtained for C_{max} and AUC of mannitol. Thus, protease inhibitors are necessary to minimize ΔG enzymatic degradation secondary to proteases/peptidases. Furthermore, ΔG was also able to increase the AUC and C_{max} for macromolecules [82]. Recently, it has been reported that ΔG significantly increased the *in vivo* oral absorption of some low bioavailable *drugs* (cyclosporin A, ritonavir, saquinavir, and acyclovir) in the presence of protease inhibitors [88]. In the opinion of the authors, these studies illustrate the potential usefulness of ΔG in enhancing oral drug delivery.

Thiolated Polymers   An alternative class of permeation enhancers is represented by *thiolated polymers*—also called thiomers. These are polymers in which the thiol groups are covalently bound. It has been shown that polycarbophyl polymers (PCP) display permeation-enhancing effects [89]. This property, however, could be significantly improved as a result of the covalent attachment of cysteine (Cys) to this polymer (*PCP-Cys*) (Fig 9.6a), as has recently been shown by Clausen and Bernkop-

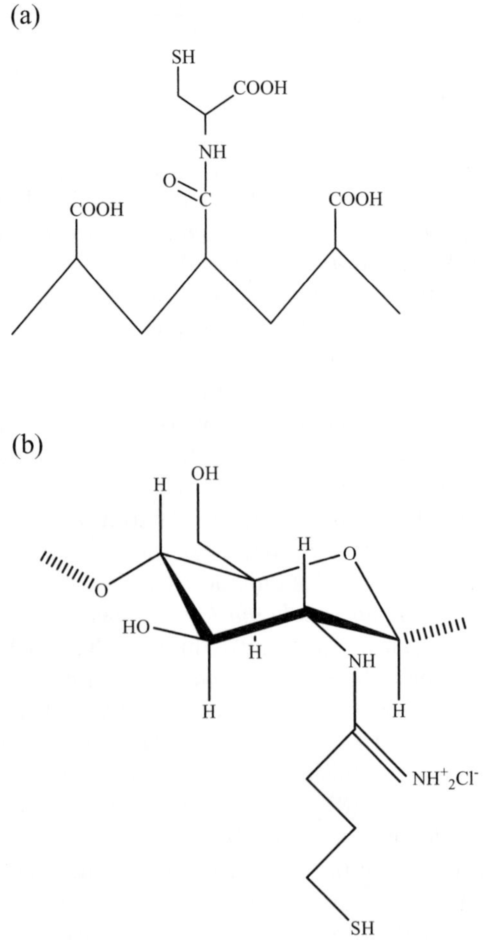

FIGURE 9.6   Chemical structure of (a) polycarbophyl-cysteine conjugate and (b) chitosan-4-thio-butylamidine. (From Ref. 34, with permission.)

Schnürch [90]. Accordingly, this thiolated polymer (PCP-Cys) is able to significantly increase the transport of *marker compounds* (sodium fluorescein) and *peptide drugs* (bacitracin-fluorescein isothiocyanate and insulin-fluorescein isothiocyanate) across the intestinal mucosa of guinea pigs (*in vitro* studies). The thiol groups, covalently attached to the polymer, seem to be responsible for the improved permeation-enhancing properties of these conjugates. Furthermore, the improved mucoadhesive properties of these polymers provide a somewhat prolonged residence time, which in some cases can lead to additional improvement in drug bioavailability. They are not absorbed from the GIT due to the high molecular mass. Based on all these features, the authors concluded that the thiolated polymers could constitute a promising excipient for the development of peptide drug delivery systems. Posteriorly, this same research group explored the mechanism of action of thiolated PCP-Cys in depth [91], showing that these compounds exert their permeation-enhancing effects via glutathione. It seems that PCP-Cys can transform oxidized glutathione (GSSG) into reduced glutathione (GSH), prolonging GSH concentration at the apical membrane. GSH is reportedly capable of inhibiting protein tyrosine phosphatase (PTP) activity by almost 100%, which results in a higher extent of phosphorylated tyrosine groups on the extracellular loops of the membrane protein occludin, leading to the opennig of the TJs [92].

Other thiolated polymers such as sodium carboxymethylcellulose-cysteine, chitosan-cysteine and chitosan-4-thio-butylamidine (chitosan-TBA) (Fig. 9.6b) [34] have also displayed permeation-enhancing properties for hydrophilic compounds and drugs when evaluated using *in vitro* techniques. The addition of the permeation mediator GSH improves this effect. This association is referred to as a *thiomer/GSH system* [93]. Different thiomer/glutathione systems have been used depending on the hydrophilic macromolecular drugs tested. Hence, for salmon calcitonin, a peptide drug of net cationic charge, chitosan-TBA was used. In contrast, insulin and low molecular weight heparin are anionic drugs—thus being incompatible with chitosan. In these cases, an anionic thiolated polymer—poly(acrylic acid)—cysteine conjugate—was used. When *in vivo* experiments were performed, a significantly improved pharmacological efficacy/bioavailability was achieved by using these systems. These results are in good agreement with those obtained *in vitro*. The authors concluded that due to their high efficacy and minimal toxicological risks, the thiomer/GSH systems represent a promising new generation of oral permeation-enhancing delivery systems for hydrophilic macromolecules [93]. Recently, the same research group has shown that the combination of thiomer/GSH system with bromelain, a proteolytic enzyme, represents a promising strategy in order to raise the *in vivo* efficacy of orally administered hydrophilic macromolecular drugs [92].

Nitric Oxide (NO) Donors   In 1995, Salzman et al. [94] showed that sodium nitroprusside (SNP), an NO donor, induced a concentration-dependent increase in fluorescein sulfonic acid transport in Caco-2 cell monolayers. Similarly, Utoguchi et al. [95] reported that *S*-nitroso-*N*-acetyl-penicillamine (SNAP), another NO donor, was able to greatly enhance the rectal absorption of insulin—this effect being concentration dependent. Posteriorly, Yamamoto et al. [96] also observed this absorption-enhancing effect on 5(6)-carboxyfluorescein transport with other NO donors such as NO5 (3-(2-hydroxy-1-methylethyl)-2-nitrosohydrazino)-1-propanamine) and NO12 (*N*-ethyl-2-(1-ethyl-hydroxy-2-nitrosohydrazino)-ethanamine), using an *in vitro*

Ussing chamber method and the rat jejunum and colon. Regional differences in the promoting effect of NO12 were found (colon > jejunum). Their findings also demonstrated NO12 action to be mediated by nitric oxide, with partial inclusion of dilatation of tight junctions in the epithelium. As these agents exhibit low toxicity, the authors suggested that NO donors may be useful for enhancing the intestinal absorption of poorly absorbing drugs.

9.5.3 Technologies in Development

Gastrointestinal Permeation Enhancement Technology™ (GIPET™) is a proprietary solid-dose/microemulsion-based medium-chain fatty acid technology by Merrion Pharmaceuticals. In the first format of GIPET (GIPET I), enteric-coated tablets, comprising a pH-sensitive coating and a drug, were synthesized. The second variation of the technology (GIPET II) consisted of microemulsions of mono- and diglyceride mixtures of C8 and C10 entrapped with the drug in an enteric-coated soft gel capsule. GIPET I and II have been tested orally in rats, dogs, and humans, primarily to establish safety profiles but also to demonstrate efficay. Afterwards, these formulations have shown efficacy in human Phase I oral delivery studies of drugs comprising both single- and repeat-dosing regimes. Oral bioavailability of alendronate, desmopressin, and low molecular weight heparin in humans was increased using GIPET formulations compared with unformulated controls. Importantly, Phase I trials revealed no toxicity of concern and this was also observed in subjects receiving multiples doses of GIPET. The absorption-promoting effects of GIPET are transient and complete in less than 1 hour as shown in additional human studies [97]. According to the researchers involved in these studies, GIPET formulations have genuine potential as platform technology for safe and effective oral drug delivery of a wide range of poorly permeable drugs.

9.5.4 Limitations of Intestinal Promotion of Drugs

In 1995, Amidon et al. [98] reported the biopharmaceutical classification system (BCS) for oral delivery of inmediate release products [98], which was adopted by the FDA in 2000. The major outcome of this classification was to group major drug classes according to whether they had oral delivery issues related to solubility or permeability issues, neither of these issues, or both. So drugs that are soluble but poorly absorbed, including most peptides and newer drugs (Class III), are amenable to epithelial permeation enhancement. As outlined earlier, over the past fifteen years many attempts to promote oral absorption of poorly absorbed drugs (Class III) have been carried out but, unfortunately, some of them have failed. It must be highlighted that achieving a sucessful oral formulation with enhancers for a poorly absorbed drug implies that there is access to the appropiate intestinal region for a sufficient amount of time, release of intact soluble drug and enhancer, and an acceptable but reversible degree of epithelial cell permeability enhacement. Bearing this in mind, the limitations for paracellular permeation enhancement by oral formulation include the inability to deliver therapeutic levels over a sustained period, the requirement for massive amounts of material, and safety aspects regarding the long-term integrity of the intestinal epithelium. Additional limitations include the inability to follow through with practical and reproducible solid dose formulations in scale-up manufacturing. Once the targeted pharmacokinetic and pharmacodynamic profile is achieved in humans, the formulation must have a safety profile to allow it to be given to patients on a repeated basis.

9.6 METHODOLOGIES FOR STUDYING INTESTINAL ABSORPTION

Assessments of rate, extent, site, and mechanism of intestinal absorption have been performed by a variety of experimental techniques in humans and animals with *in vitro*, *in situ*, and *in vivo* preparations. Details of the most common methodologies currently in use in experimental animals are given next, along with a discussion of the utility and limitations of each. It is the judicious use of these techniques that can help identify drug candidates that will be absorbed in humans. It is well recognized that human intestinal permeability cannot be accurately predicted based on a single methodology (*in vitro*, *in situ*, or *in vivo*) [99, 100] since each kind of method covers only some of the factors involved in the intestinal absorption and does not take into account other factors that may be important. Moreover, it must be highlighted that although animals provide the opportunity to gain much valuable information through screening, investigators must remain aware that the results cannot be extrapolated directly and exactly to humans.

9.6.1 *In Vitro* Techniques

Different *in vitro* methods utilizing tissues from rodents and other species have been developed to screen compounds for oral absorption and elucidate the mechanism involved in the intestinal transport, which could be decisive in obtaining maximum bioavailability. Cell cultures have also been shown to constitute a highly valuable tool in the decision making process to select candidates for *in vivo* clinical studies at early stage drug discovery and development [101].

Two *in vitro* biological methods are discussed. These are diffusion chambers equipped with intestinal tissues from animal origin and cultured cells.

Diffusion Cells Using Tissues   At the end of the 1960s Schultz et al. [102] developed a method for the direct measurement of unidirectional influx of amino acids from the mucosal bathing solution into the intestinal epithelium. This method was a modification of the so-called Ussing chamber widely used to evaluate drug absorption. Posteriorly, the Shultz method was slightly modified by B.G. Munck, who performed a lot of experiments in order to study the intestinal absorption of amino acids from a mechanistic point of view [103, 104]. Other researchers adopted this technique to gain insight into the absorption mechanism of some drugs (e.g., acamprosate) [105] and trace elements such as Zn [106].

In this method, a chosen segment of the intestine of the animal (rat, rabbit, or guinea pig) is excised, opened along the mesenteric attachment, and rinsed in ice-cold buffer. Each segment is mounted on a Lucite plate with the mucosal surface facing upward and a Lucite block is clamped on top of the plate. The Lucite plate is depicted in Fig. 9.7. In this way, four mucosal areas, each of approximately $0.35\,cm^2$, can be exposed at the bottom of the wells, where the solution is oxygenated and stirred with high rates of O_2 flow. The use of two blocks allows eight measurements

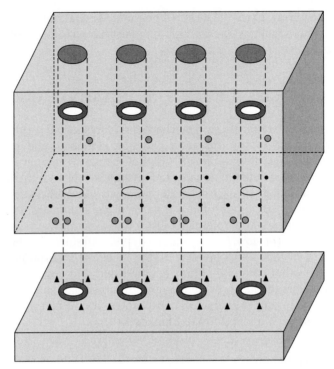

FIGURE 9.7   Schematic representation of a Lucite plate, where the segment of the intestine is mounted, and the Lucite block that is clamped on top of the plate.

from each rat. With guinea pigs and rabbits, 4 blocks can be used, allowing 16 measurements from each animal. The serosal surface of the tissue rests on moistened filter paper and is not exposed to the mucosal solution. After mounting, the tissues are preincubated at 37 °C, in a properly designed chamber (Fig. 9.8). The tissues are incubated for 15 min with a drug-free solution containing 5 mM glucose, which was then withdrawn. The well and mucosal surface are gently wiped with soft paper to remove the adhered incubation fluid before the test solution (containing the radiolabeled drug to test and radiolabeled PEG-4000) is injected. The 0.5 min incubation period is terminated by aspiration of the incubation fluid and flushing of the well with an ice-cold 300 mM mannitol solution. The mannitol wash serves to terminate the exposure both by diluting the remaining test solution and by suddenly cooling the tissues. The exposed tissues are then punched out, briefly rinsed in ice-cold mannitol solution, blotted on hard filter paper, and extracted for 18 h in 0.1 M HNO$_3$. Aliquots of tissue extract and test solution are assayed for drug content. Usually radiolabeled drugs are used since, as outlined before, the exposition time is very short so the amount of transported compound is really low. So the extract and tissue solution are analyzed by liquid scintillation spectrometry. The amount of radiolabeled PEG-4000 was used to correct for extracellular contamination; thus corrected, the radiolabeled drug activity is used to calculate the rate of influx across the brush border membrane. The unidirectional drug influx, J, is expressed in concentration/cm^2·h.

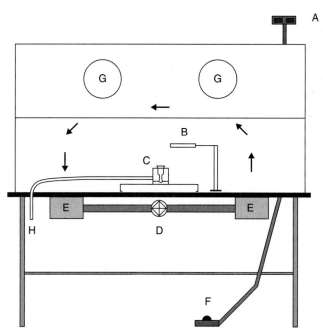

FIGURE 9.8   Schematic representation of the chamber used to incubate and oxygenate the tissue mounted in the Lucite plate: A, digital time and temperature controller; B, thermic sound; C, Lucite plate; D, air turbine; E, air inlet and outlet; F, chronometer pulsator; G, access to chamber inside; H, oxygen inlet.

This technique is simple and rapid, and a reduced number of animals, are used in comparison with the *in situ* and *in vivo* methods. Conditions of temperature, oxygenation, and availability of nutrients and energy sources can be controlled more closely for mechanistic studies than is possible *in situ* or *in vivo*. Moreover, researchers can study differences in regional absorption of drugs, which is not possible in cell cultures. The limitations include the problems associated with the use of radiolabeled compounds and the lack of mesenteric circulation, which is not a physiological condition. Another drawback of any *in vitro* system is the intrinsic variability that can be seen in the permeation data.

Intestinal Cell Cultures   Within the past decades the use of monolayers of human intestinal epithelial cells for evaluating drug absorption has become possible. Actually, it was impossible to culture normal, mature enterocytes so colon adenocarcinoma cell lines (Caco-2 cells, HT29, T84) are used. Although isolated from a colon tumor, these cells all show an enterocyte-like differentiation; however, the degree of differentiation is variable (Table 9.3). These cells are relatively well defined while there is also no interference by feedback and/or other mechanism, which are present in intact organs or animals.

The most used cell line from human origin is the Caco-2 cell line. Even though these cells display colon-like properties regarding transepithelial electrical resistance (TEER) and passive permeability to drugs, their morphology, expression of brush border enzymes, and carriers for nutrients resemble more closely small

TABLE 9.3   Degree of Differentation of Epithelial Cell Lines Originating from Human Colon Carcinoma

	Differentiation		
Cell Line	Tight Junctions	Apical Brush Border (Microvilli + Enzyme)	Mucus Secretion
Caco-2 cells	+	+	0
HT29	+	+/−	+/−
T84	+	0	0

Source: Adapted from Ref. 120.

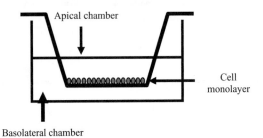

FIGURE 9.9   Schematic setup for transport studies in culture cell lines. Sampling can be carried out from the apical and/or basolateral chamber.

intestinal enterocytes [107]. Several studies have demonstrated the usefulness of these cells as a model for intestinal drug transport. According to published results, the properties of this cell line are the same as normal intestinal epithelium in *in vivo* model systems and are useful for studying transport of hydrophilic as well as lipophilic compounds. A vast amount of work has been done in characterizing the Caco-2 cell line. Several carrier and receptor systems have been identified. Moreover, in some studies, a correlation between human intestinal drug absorption after oral administration and permeability in Caco-2 cells was established [108].

Figure 9.9 illustrates the culturing system whereby the Caco-2 cells are seeded, usually onto polycarbonate filter support on which a polarized cell monolayer is formed within a few days and differentiates into absorptive intestinal cells. The microporous support allows access to drug to both the apical and basolateral sides of the epithelium, which means that drug transport could be studied in both the apical to basolateral and the basolateral to apical. The result of transport experiments can be expressed as the permeability, P_{app}, in cm/s.

The tight junctions in the Caco-2 cell monolayers resemble the junctions in the human colon, resulting in far higher TEER than typical for small intestine tissue. The higher TEER makes these cells a useful and widespread method for studying both pharmacological pretreatments and direct additives on cell integrity because the paracellular permeability of a typical nonpermeant such as PEG-4000 or mannitol can easily be monitored. The direct measurement of TEER is also used as a method to evaluate cell monolayer integrity. To measure TEER values, a four-electrode system, which measures the resistance of a cell monolayer on permeable support, could be used. The results of TEER measurements can be expressed as absolute values or as percentages of the initial values, which is preferable when TEER values are measured after various treatments since variability in the starting values between monolayers exists and different measurement setups might result in different absolute values.

One of the major advantages of the use of intestinal cell cultures lies in its possible application to high throughput screening (HTS) strategies. This model has a high potential for HTS because the cells are rather simple to culture in high quantities and in a reproducible manner. Keep in mind that to time and cost-effectively develop a new drug application, the selection of candidates for clinical studies has to be made during an early-decision process made with *in vitro* data. So *in vitro* permeability and solubility screening has become a routine measurement in drug discovery and development. In some cases, the fraction of drug absorbed in humans could be predicted by *in vitro* Caco-2 cell permeability. In addition, *in vitro* permeability and solubility data can be used to classify compounds according to the BCS system and, subsequently, to direct formulation optimization strategies [101]. Another important advantage is that, as analyzed in the previous section, Caco-2 cells are also a valuable tool to investigate absorption-enhancement of poorly absorbable drugs. Furthermore, the mechanism of action of absorption-enhancing compounds may be elucidated and if combined with microscopical techniques, the paracellular enhancement could be visualized [108].

Apart from these advantages, Caco-2 cells also have striking disadvantages. First, these are cells with tighter tight junctions than those present in the small intestine. This might give rise to underpredictions of the permeabilities of hydrophilic compounds with a low *in vivo* uptake. Second, transporter substrates usually demonstrate lower permeability than their actual permeability *in vivo*, due to the low transporter expression levels in Caco-2 cells [101]. Third, between laboratories, or even batch-to-batch, variability can occur. These limitations should be taken into consideration when assessing the "developability" of a drug and during the decision making process for selecting candidates, before processing a drug to clinical studies.

9.6.2   *In Situ* Techniques

The isolation of segments of the gastrointestinal tract *in situ* in anesthetized animals with intact mesenteric blood flow is widely used to gain valuable information as to the site and mechanism of drug absorption and permeability assessment [2]. Different *in situ* preparations (single-pass perfusion, recirculating perfusion, oscillating perfusion, and static perfusion) have been used. One of the most employed techniques is the *in situ* rat gut preparation described by Doluisio et al. [109]. In short, after anesthetizing the rats, the abdomen is opened through a middle incision and a selected segment of intestine is cannulated at either end. After rinsing with physiological saline to eliminate fecal residue and debris, an isotonic drug solution properly buffered is perfused at 37 °C. At selected times (usually every 5 min for a total of 30 min), the solution is forced out of alternate ends of the segment and sampled. Drug concentration in the samples is quantified and used for calculations. The corresponding kinetic parameters (first-order absorption rate constant, k_a, or V_{max} and K_m) can be estimated. In some cases, it is necessary to correct for water reabsorption in order to obtain the actual concentration. A nonabsorbable water marker, such as phenol red, or radiolabeled PEG-4000 could be used. Since our previous experience with these markers was not entirely satisfactory, an alternative method based on the direct measurement, at fixed times, of the remaining volumes of the test solutions perfused independently in selected animals was developed [110]. This technique has proved to be very useful in studying the correlation between gastrointestinal absorption and partition constants for homologous series of xenobiotics [110, 111], the influence of synthetic and natural bile acid surfactants on passive diffusion of xenobiotics [112, 113], and the mechanism of drug absorption. For example, intestinal transport of baclofen, cefadroxil, and cefuroxime axetil through carrier-mediated transport has been evidenced [114–116]. More recently, we have reported, by using this technique, that acamprosate, an anti-craving drug, is absorbed in the small intestine of the rat by passive diffusion [100]. All these investigations have helped to solve problems related with the low bioavailability of the drugs studied. The influence of the potential inhibitors and/or enhancers as well as the participation of the P-gp in the absorption of drugs could also be evaluated [100, 117, 118].

With the use of any of the *in situ* techniques, intact circulation is maintained in such a way that absorbed drugs are taken away from the basement membrane in a more normal physiological manner than in the *in vitro* techniques discussed above. Particularly, with the *in situ* rat gut preparation, absorption rates that are near to *in vivo* values are obtained [12], which allow one to fit absorption models more easily to experimental data. Recently, the *in situ* single-pass perfusion model has proved to be a robust means of assessing permeability for BCS classification [119]. The drawbacks inherent in these techniques are the effects of anesthesia and the short time that the preparations are viable.

9.6.3   *In Vivo* Techniques

The *in vivo* studies in laboratory animals are needed to validate the results obtained *in vitro* or *in situ* in order to avoid the risk of inaccurate predictions. Furthermore, it should be borne in mind that *in vivo* studies are also required during formulation development.

Usually, animals were placed under anesthesia and subjected to surgical cannulation of a vein (e.g., jugular vein) to facilitate blood sampling. Oral administration of the drug is performed usually by gastric intubation. If it is requiered, the animals can be housed in metabolic cages in order to collect urine and feces. Once the sampling period is over, the samples are properly processed to obtain plasma and urine concentrations, which are used for kinetic calculations (C_{max}, AUC, bioavailability). Whole animal studies are also useful for investigating specific parts of the absorption process. For example, chronic portal vein cannulae may be inserted surgically and maintained patent for sampling portal venous blood after oral administration. A portal-vein cannula also allows drug infusions to simulate presentation of drug to the liver by controlled-release devices.

One of the main disadvantages of *in vivo* animal studies is that they are impractical for the screening of a large number of compounds due to the intensive work, slow speed, high cost, and lack of automation. Additionally, *in vivo* oral bioavailability studies in animals are not always predictive of bioavailability in humans. Nevertheless, in spite of these limitations, *in vivo* studies provide some initial estimates of how well a compound is absorbed, the variables that affect absorption (including enhancers), and the probability that the compound undergoes first-pass metabolism.

REFERENCES

1. Singer SJ, Nicolson GL. The fluid mosaic model of the structure of cell membranes. *Science*. 1972;175:720–731.

2. Loper AE, Gardner CR. Gastrointestinal absorption of drugs. In Swarbrick J, Boylan JC, Eds. *Encyclopedia of Pharmaceutical Technology*, Volume 6. New York: Marcel Dekker; 1988, pp 385–413.

3. Tsuji A, Tamai I. Carrier-mediated intestinal transport of drugs. *Pharm Res* 1996;13(7): 963–977.

4. Salama NN, Eddington ND, Fasano A. Tight junction modulation and its relationship to drug delivery. *Adv Drug Deliv Rev* 2006;58:15–28.

5. He Y-L, Murby S, Warhurst G, Gifford L, Walker D, Ayrton J, Eastmond R, Rowland M. Species differences in size discrimination in the paracellular pathway reflected by oral bioavailability of poly(ethylene glycol) and D-peptides. *J Pharm Sci* 1998;87:626–633.

6. Lindeman P, Solomon AK. Permeability of luminal surface of intestinal mucosal cells. *J Gen Physiol* 1962;45:801–810.

7. Cerejido M. *Tight Junctions*. Boca Raton, FL: CRC Press; 1992.

8. Aungst BJ. Intestinal permeation enhancers. *J Pharm Sci* 2000;89(4):429–442.

9. Finholt P. Influence of formulation on dissolution rate. *Acad Pharm Sci* 1974;106–146.

10. Aguiar AJ, Krc J Jr, Kinkel AW, Samyn JC. Effect of polymorphism on the absorption of chloramphenicol from chloramphenicol palmitate. *J Pharm Sci* 1967;56:847–853.

11. Ulm EH, Hichens M, Gomez HJ, Till AE, Hand E, Vassil TC, Biollaz J, Brunner HR, Schelling JL. Enalapril maleate and a lysine analogue (MK-521): disposition in man. *Br J Clin Pharm* 1982;14:357–362.

12. Pla-Delfina JM, Moreno J. Intestinal absorption–partition relationships: a tentative functional nonlinear model. *J Pharmacokinet Biopharm* 1981;9:191–215.

13. Hunt JN. Gastric emptying and secretion in man. *Physiol Rev* 1959;39:491–533.

14. Clements JA, Heading RC, Nimmo WS, Prescott LF. Kinetics of acetaminophen absorption and gastric emptying in man. *Clin Pharmacol Ther* 1978;24:420–431.

15. Hunt JN, Macdonald I. The influence of volume on gastric emptying. *J Physiol* 1954;126:459–474.

16. Nimmo J, Heading RC, Tothill P, Prescott LF. Pharmacological modification of gastric emptying: effects of propantheline and metoclopromide on paracetamol absorption. *Br Med J* 1973;1(5853):587–589.

17. Welling PG, Huang H, Hewitt PF, Lyons LL. Bioavailability of erythromycin stearate: influence of food and fluid volume. *J Pharma Sci* 1978;67:764–766.

18. Manninen V, Apajalahti A, Melin J, Karesoja M. Altered absorption of digoxin in patients given propantheline and metoclopramide. *Lancet* 1973;24(7800):398–400.

19. Suzuki H, Sugiyama Y. Role of metabolic enzymes and efflux transporters in the absorption of drugs from the small intestine. *Eur J Pharm Sci* 2000;12:3–12.

20. Lin JH, Chiba M, Baillie TA. Is the role of the small intestine in first-pass metabolism overemphasized? *Pharm Rev* 1999;51:135–158.

21. Regardh CG, Edgar B, Olsson R, Kendall M, Collste P, Shansky C. Pharmacokinetics of felodipine in patients with liver disease. *Eur J Clin Pharmacol* 1989;36:473–479.

22. Paine MF, Shen DD, Kunze KL, Perkins JD, Marsh CL, McVicar JP, Barr DM, Gillies BS, Thummel KE. First-pass metabolism of midazolam by the human intestine. *Clin Pharmacol Ther* 1996;60:14–24.

23. Barr WH, Riegelman S. Intestinal drug absorption and metabolism. I. Comparison of methods and models to study physiological factors of *in vitro* and *in vivo* intestinal absorption. *J Pharm Sci* 1970;59:154–163.

24. Fromm MF. Importance of P-glycoprotein at blood–tissue barriers. *Trends Pharmacol Sci* 2004;25:423–429.

25. McGinity JW, Stavchansky SA, Martin A. *Bioavailability in Tablet Technology*. New York: Marcel Dekker; 1981;269–449.

26. Hayashi M, Sakai T, Hasegawa Y, Nishikawahara T, Tomioka H, Iida A, Shimizu N, Tomita M, Awazu S. Physiological mechanism for enhancement of paracellular drug transport. *J Control Release* 1999;62:141–148.

27. Pappenheimer JR. Physiological regulation of transepithelial impedance in the intestinal mucosa of rats and hamsters. *J Membr Biol* 1987;100:137–148.

28. Ward PD, Tippin TK, Thakker DR. Enhancing paracellular permeability by modulating epithelial tight junctions. *Pharm Sci Technol* 2000;3(10):346–358.

29. Madara JL. Regulation of the movement of solutes across tight junctions. *Annu Rev Physiol* 1998;60:143–159.

30. Thanou MM, Florea BI, Langemeÿer MW, Verhoef JC, Junginger HE. N-trimethylated chitosan chloride (TMC) improves the intestinal permeation of the peptide drug buserelin *in vitro* (Caco-2 cells) and *in vivo* (rats). *Pharm Res* 2000;17:27–31.

31. Sakai M, Imai T, Ohtake H, Azuma H, Otagiri M. Effects of absorption enhancers on the transport of model compounds in Caco-2 cell monolayers: assessment by confocal laser scanning microscopy. *J Pharm Sci* 1997;86(7):779–785.

32. Lindmark T, Kimura Y, Artursson P. Absorption enhancement through intracellular regulation of tight junction permeability by medium chain fatty acids in Caco-2 cells. *J Pharmacol Exp Ther* 1998;284:362–369.

33. Takahashi K, Murakami T, Yumoto R, Hattori T, Higashi Y, Yata N. Decanoic acid induced enhancement of rectal absorption of hydrophilic compounds in rats. *Pharm Res* 1994;11(10):1401–1404.

34. Cano-Cebrián MJ, Zornoza T, Granero L, Polache A. Intestinal absorption enhancement via the paracellular route by fatty acids, chitosans and others: a target of drug delivery. *Curr Drug Deliv* 2005;2:9–22.

35. Cereijido L, Shoshani L, Contreras RG. Molecular physiology and pathophysiology of tight junctions. I. Biogenesis of tight junctions and epithelial polarity. *Am J Physiol Gastrointestinal Liver Physiol* 2000;279:G477–G482.

36. Mitic LL, Van Itallie CM, Anderson JM. Molecular physiology and pathophysiology of tight junctions I. Tight junction structure and function: lessons from mutant animals and proteins. *Am J Physiol Gastrointestinal Liver Physiol* 2000;279:G250–G254.

37. Karczewski J, Groot J. Molecular physiology and pathophysiology of tight junctions III. Tight junction regulation by intracellular messengers: differences in response within and between epithelia. *Am J Physiol Gastrointestinal Liver Physiol* 2000;279:G660–G665.

38. Nusrat A, Turner JR, Madara JL. Molecular physiology and pathophysiology of tight junctions. IV. Regulation of tight junctions by extracellular stimuli: nutrients, cytokines, and immune cells. *Am J Physiol Gastrointestinal Liver Physiol* 2000;279:G851–G857.

39. Gumbiner B. Structure, biochemistry, and assembly of epithelial tight junctions. *Am J Physiol* 1987;253:C749–C758.

40. Claude P. Morphological factors influencing transepithelial permeability: a model for the resistance of the zonula occludens. *J Membr Biol* 1978;39:219–332.

41. Watson CJ, Rowland M, Warhurst G. Functional modeling of tight junctions in intestinal cell monolayers using polyethylene glycol oligomers. *Am J Physiol Cell Physiol* 2001;281:C388–C397.

42. Furuse M, Hirase T, Itoh M, Nagafuchi A, Yonemura S, Tsukita S. Occludin: a novel integral membrane protein localizing at tight junctions. *J Cell Biol* 1993;123:1777–1788.

43. Ando-Akatsuka Y, Saitou M, Hirase T, Kishi M, Sakakibara A, Itoh M, Yonemura S, Furuse M, Tsukita S. Interspecies diversity of the occludin sequence: cDNA cloning of human, mouse, dog, and rat-kangaroo homologues. *J Cell Biol* 1996;133:43–47.

44. Saitou M, Ando-Akatsuka Y, Itoh M, Furuse M, Inazawa J, Fujimoto K, Tsukita S. Mammalian occludin in epithelial cells: its expression and subcellular distribution. *Eur J Cell Biol* 1997;73:222–231.

45. Tsukita S, Furuse M. Occludin and claudins in tight-junction strands: leading or supporting players? *Trends Cell Biol* 1999;9:268–273.

46. Van Itallie CM, Anderson JM. Occludin confers adhesiveness when expressed in fibroblasts. *J Cell Sci* 1997;110:1113–1121.

47. Furuse M, Sasaki H, Fujimoto K, Tsukita S. Single gene product, claudin-1 or -2, reconstitutes tight junction strands and recruits occludin in fibroblasts. *J Cell Biol* 1998;143; 391–401.

48. Simon DB, Lu Y, Choate KA, Velazquez H, Al-Sabban E, Praga M, Casari G, Bettinelli A, Colussi G, Rodríguez SJ, McCredie D, Milford D, Sanjad S, Lifton RP. Paracellin-1, a renal tight junction protein required for paracellular Mg^{2+} resorption. *Science* 1999;285; 103–106.

49. Tsukita S, Furuse M. Pores in the wall: claudins constitute tight junction strands containing aqueous pores. *J Cell Biol* 2000;149:13–16.

50. Anderson JM, Van Itallie CM. Tight junctions and the molecular basis for regulation of paracellular permeability. *Am J Physiol* 1995;269:G467–G475.

51. De Boer A, Breimer D. GI-tract absorption enhancement: general introduction and simulation of time–concentration-effect profiles of absorption enhancers. In de Boer AG, Ed. *Drug Absorption Enhancement.* Chur, Switzerland: Harwood Academic Publishers; 1994, Vol 3, pp 155–176.

52. Lindmark T, Nikkila T, Artursson P. Mechanisms of absorption enhancement by medium chain fatty acids in intestinal epithelial Caco-2 cell monolayers. *J Pharmacol Exp Ther* 1995;275(2):958–964.

53. Chao AC, Nguyen JV, Broughall M, Griffin A, Fix JA, Daddona PE. *In vitro* and *in vivo* evaluation of effects of sodium caprate on enteral peptide absorption and on mucosal morphology. *Int J Pharm* 1999;191(1):15–24.

54. Anderberg EK, Lindmark T, Artursson P. Sodium caprate elicits dilatations in human intestinal tight junctions and enhances drug absorption by the paracellular route. *Pharm Res* 1993;10(6):857–864.

55. Quan YS, Hattori K, Lundborg E, Fujita T, Murakami M, Muranishi S, Yamamoto A. Effectiveness and toxicity screening of various absorption enhancers using Caco-2 cell monolayers. *Biol Pharm Bull* 1998;21(6):615–620.

56. Lindmark T, Schipper N, Lazarova L, de Boer AG, Artursson P. Absorption enhancement in intestinal epithelial Caco-2 monolayers by sodium caprate: assessment of molecular weight dependence and demonstration of transport routes. *J Drug Target* 1998;5(3):215–223.

57. Artursson P, Karlsson J. Correlation between oral drug absorption in humans and apparent drug permeability coefficients in human intestinal epithelial (Caco-2) cells. *Biochem Biophys Res Commun* 1991;175:880–885.

58. Tomita M, Sawada T, Ogawa T, Ouchi H, Hayashi M, Awazu S. Differences in the enhancing effects of sodium caprate on colonic and jejunal drug absorption. *Pharm Res* 1992;9(5):648–653.

59. Kamm W, Jonczyk A, Jung T, Luckenbach G, Raddatz P, Kissel T. Evaluation of absorption enhancement for a potent cyclopeptidic alpha(nu)beta(3)-antagonist in a human intestinal cell line (Caco-2). *Eur J Pharm Sci* 2000;10:205–214.

60. Lo YL, Huang JD. Effects of sodium deoxycholate and sodium caprate on the transport of epirubicin in human intestinal epithelial Caco-2 cell layers and everted gut sacs of rats. *Biochem Pharmacol* 2000;59(6):665–672.

61. Raiman J, Törmälehto S, Yritys K, Junginger H, Mönkkönen J. Effects of various absorption enhancers on transport of clodronate through Caco-2 cells. *Int J Pharm* 2003;261: 129–136.

62. Zornoza T, Cano MJ, Polache A, Granero L. Pharmacology of acamprosate: an overview. *CNS Drug Rev* 2003;9(4):359–374.

63. Raoof AA, Ramtoola Z, McKenna B, Yu RZ, Hardee G, Geary RS. Effect of sodium caprate on the intestinal absorption of two modified antisense oligonucleotides in pigs. *Eur J Pharm Sci* 2002;17:131–138.

64. Söderholm JD, Oman H, Blomquist L, Veen J, Lindmark T, Olaison G. Reversible increase in tight junction permeability to macromolecules in rat ileal mucosa *in vitro* by sodium caprate, a constituent of milk fat. *Dig Dis Sci* 1998;43(7):1547–1552.

65. Uchiyama T, Sugiyama T, Quan YS, Kotani A, Okada N, Fujita T, Muranishi S, Yamamoto A. Enhanced permeability of insulin across the rat intestinal membrane by various absorption enhancers: their intestinal mucosal toxicity and absorption-enhancing mechanism of *N*-lauryl-beta-D-maltopyranoside. *J Pharm Pharmacol* 1999;51(11):1241–1250.

66. Yamamoto A, Okagawa T, Kotani A, Uchiyama T, Shimura T, Tabata S, Kondo S, Muranishi S. Effects of different absortion enhancers on the permeation of ebirbatide, an ACTH analogue, across intestinal membranes. *J Pharm Pharmacol* 1997;49(11): 1057–1061.

67. Lennernäs H, Gjellan R, Hällgren R, Graffner J. The influence of caprate on rectal absorption of phenoxymethylpenicillin: experience from an *in-vivo* perfusion in humans. *J Pharm Pharmacol* 2002;54:499–508.

68. Ishizawa T, Hayashi M, Awazu S. Enhancement of jejunal and colonic absorption of fosfomycin by promoters in the rat. *J Pharm Pharmacol* 1987;39:892–895.

69. Sasaki K, Yonebayashi S, Yoshida M, Shimizu K, Aotsuka T, Takayama K. Improvement in the bioavailability of poorly absorbed glycyrrhizin via various non-vascular administration routes in rats. *Int J Pharm* 2003;265:95–102.

70. Artursson P, Lindmark T, Davis SS, Illum L. Effect of chitosan on the permeability of monolayers of intestinal epithelial cells (Caco-2). *Pharm Res* 1994;11:1358–1361.

71. Kotzé AF, Lueßen HL, de Leeuw BJ, de Boer AG, Verhoef JC, Junginger HE. Comparison of the effect of different chitosan salts and *N*-trimethyl chitosan chloride on the permeability of intestinal epithelial cells (Caco-2). *J Control Release* 1998;51:35–46.

72. Kotzé AF, Lueßen HL, de Boer AG, Verhoef JC, Junginger HE. Chitosan for enhanced intestinal permeability: prospects for derivatives soluble in neutral and basic environments. *J Pharm Sci* 1998;7:145–151.

73. Schipper NGM, Vårum KM, Artursson P. Chitosans as absorption enhancers for poorly absorbable drugs. 1: Influence of molecular weight and degree of acetylation on drug

transport across human intestinal epithelial (Caco-2) cells. *Pharm Res* 1996;13(11):1686–1692.

74. Van der Lubben IM, Verhoef C, Borchard G, Junginger HE. Chitosan and its derivatives in mucosal drug and vaccine delivery. *Eur J Pharm Sci* 2001;14:201–207.

75. Kotzé AF, Lueßen HL, de Leeuw BJ, Verhoef JE, Brussee J, Junginger HE. *N*-trimethyl chitosan chloride as a potential absorption enhancer across mucosal surfaces: *in vitro* evaluation in intestinal epithelial cells (Caco-2). *Pharm Res* 1997;14:1197–1202.

76. Thanou MM, Kotzé AF, Scharringhausen T, Lueßen HL, de Boer AG, Verhoef JC, Junginger HE. Effect of degree of quaternization of *N*-trimethyl chitosan chloride for enhanced transport of hydrophilic compounds across intestinal caco-2 cell monolayers. *J Control Release* 2000;64:15–25.

77. Jonker C, Hamman JH, Kotzé AF. Intestinal paracellular permeation enhancement with quaternised chitosan: *in situ* and *in vitro* evaluation. *Int J Pharm* 2002;238:205–213.

78. Hamman JH, Schultz CM, Kotzé AF. *N*-trimethyl chitosan chloride: optimum degree of quaternization for drug absorption enhancement across epithelial cells. *Drug Dev Ind Pharm* 2003;29:161–172.

79. Thanou MM, Verhoef JC, Marbach P, Junginger HE. Intestinal absorption of octreotide: *N*-trimethyl chitosan chloride (TMC) ameliorates the permeability and absorption properties of the somatostatin analogue *in vitro* and *in vivo*. *J Pharm Sci* 2000;89:951–957.

80. Thanou MM, Nihot MT, Jansen M, Verhoef JC, Junginger HEJ. Mono-*N*-carboxymethyl chitosan (MCC), a polyampholytic chitosan derivative, enhances the intestinal absorption of low molecular weight heparin across intestinal epithelia *in vitro* and *in vivo*. *J Pharm Sci* 2001;90:38–46.

81. Fasano A, Bernadette B, Pumplin D, Wasserman SS, Tall BD, Ketley JM, Kaper JB. *Vibrio cholerae* produces a second enterotoxin, which affects intestinal tight junctions. *Proc Natl Acad Sci USA* 1991;88:5242–5246.

82. Salama NN, Fasano A, Thakar M, et al. The effect of ΔG on the transport and oral absorption of macromolecules. *J Pharm Sci* 2004;93(5):1310–1319.

83. Wang W, Uzzau S, Goldblum E, Fasano A. Human zonulin, a potential modulator of intestinal tight junctions. *J Cell Sci* 2000;113:4435–4440.

84. Fasano A, Uzzau S. Modulation of intestinal tight junctions by zonula occludens toxin permits enteral administration of insulin and other macromolecules in an animal model. *J Clin Invest* 1997;99(6):1158–1164.

85. Cox D, Raje S, Gao H, Salama NN, Eddington ND. Enhanced permeability of molecular weight markers and poorly bioavailable compounds across Caco-2 cell monolayers using the absorption enhancer, zonula occludens toxin. *Pharm Res* 2002;19:1680–1688.

86. Di Pierro M, Lu R, Uzzau S, Wang W, Margaretten K, Pazzani C, Maimone F, Fasano A. Zonula occludens toxin structure–function analysis. Identification of the fragment biologically active on tight junctions and of the zonulin receptor binding domain. *J Biol Chem* 2001;276:19160–19165.

87. Salama NN, Fasano A, Ruliang L, Eddington ND. Effect of the biologically active fragment of zonula occludens toxin, delta G, on the intestinal paracellular transport and oral absorption of mannitol. *Int J Pharm* 2003;251:113–121.

88. Salama NN, Fasano A, Thakar M, Eddington ND. The impact of ΔG on the oral bioavailability of low bioavailable therapeutic agents. *J Pharmacol Exp Ther* 2005;312:199–205.

89. Lueßen HL, Rentel CO, Kotzé AF, Lehr CM, de Boer AG, Verhoef JC, Junginger HE. Mucoadhesive polymers in peroral peptide drug delivery. IV. Polycarbophil and chitosan

are potent enhancers of peptide transport across intestinal mucosae in vitro. *J Control Release* 1997;45(1):15–23.

90. Clausen AE, Bernkop-Schnürch A. *In vitro* evaluation of the permeation-enhancing effect of thiolated polycarbophil. *J Pharm Sci* 2000;89:1253–1261.

91. Clausen AE, Kast CE, Bernkop-Schnürch A. The role of glutathione in the permeation enhancing effect of thiolated polymers. *Pharm Res* 2002;19(5):602–608.

92. Guggi D, Bernkop-Schnürch A. Improved paracellular uptake by the combination of different types of permeation enhancers. *Int J Pharm* 2005;288:141–150.

93. Bernkop-Schnürch A, Kast CE, Guggi D. Permeation enhancing polymers in oral delivery of hydrophilic macromolecules: thiomer/GSH systems. *J Control Release* 2003;93: 95–103.

94. Salzman AL, Menconi MJ, Unno N, Ezzel RM, Casey DM, Gonzalez PK, Fink MP. Nitric oxide dilates tight junctions and depletes ATP in cultured Caco-2BBe intestinal epithelial monolayers. *Am J Physiol* 1995;268:6361–6373.

95. Utoguchi N, Watanabe Y, Shida T, Matsumoto M. Nitric oxide donors enhance rectal absorption of macromolecules in rabbits. *Pharm Res* 1998;15:870–876.

96. Yamamoto A, Tatsumi H, Maruyama M, Uchiyama T, Okada N, Fujita T. Modulation of intestinal permeability by nitric oxide donors: implications in intestinal delivery of poorly absorbable drugs. *J Pharm Exp Ther* 2001;296:84–90.

97. Leonard TW, Lynch J, McKenna MJ, Brayden DJ. Promoting absorption of drugs in humans using medium-chain fatty acid-based solid dosage forms: GIPET. *Expert Opin Drug Deliv* 2006;3(5):685–692.

98. Amidon GL, Lennernas H, Shah VP, Crison JR. A theoretical basis for a biopharmaceutic drug classification: the correlation of *in vitro* drug product dissolution and *in vivo* bioavailability. *Pharm Res* 1995;12(3):413–420.

99. Balimane PV, Chong S, Morrison RA. Current methodologies used for evaluation of intestinal permeability and absorption. *J Pharmacol Toxicol Methods* 2000;44(1):301–312.

100. Zornoza T, Cano-Cebrian MJ, Nalda-Molina R, Guerri C, Granero L, Polache A. Assessment and modulation of acamprosate intestinal absorption: comparative studies using *in situ, in vitro* (CACO-2 cell monolayers) and *in vivo* models. *Eur J Pharm Sci* 2004;22(5):347–356.

101. Sun D, Yu L, Hussain MA, Wall DA, Smith RL, Amidon GL. *In vitro* testing of drug absorption for drug "developability" assessment: forming an interface between *in vitro* preclinical data and clinical outcome. *Curr Opin Drug Discov Dev* 2004;7(1):75–85.

102. Schultz SG, Curran PF, Chez RA, Fuisz RE. Alanine and sodium fluxes across mucosal border of rabbit ileum. *J Gen Physiol* 1967;50:1241–1260.

103. Munck BG. Transport of imino acids and non-α–amino acids across the brush-border membrane of the rabbit ileum. *J Membr Biol* 1985;83:15–24.

104. Munck LK, Munck BG. Chloride-dependence of amino acid transport in rabbit ileum. *Biochim Biophys Acta* 1990;1027:17–20.

105. Más-Serrano P, Granero L, Martín-Algarra RV, Guerri C, Polache A. Kinetic study of acamprosate absorption in rat small intestine. *Alcohol Alcohol* 2000;35(4):324–330.

106. Condomina J, Zornoza-Sabina T, Granero L, Polache A. Kinetics of zinc transport *in vitro* in rat small intestine and colon: interaction with copper. *Eur J Pharm Sci* 2002;16:289–295.

107. Wilson G, Hassan IF, Dix CJ, Wlliamsson I, Shah R, Mackay R, Artursson P. Transport and permeability properties of human Caco-2 cells: an *in vitro* model of the intestinal epithelial cell barrier. *J Control Release* 1990;11:25–40.

108. Noach A, Hurni M, De Boer A, Breimer D. The paracellular approach: drug transport and its enhancement via the paracellular pathway. In de Boer A, Ed. *Drug Absorption Enhancement*. Chur, Switzerland: Harwood Academic Publishers; 1994, Vol 3, pp 291–324.

109. Doluisio JT, Billups NF, Dittert LW, Sugita ET, Swintosky JV. Drug absorption. I. An *in situ* rat gut technique yielding realistic absorption rates. *J Pharm Sci* 1969;58:1196–1200.

110. Martín-Villodre A, Plá-Delfina JM, Moreno J, Pérez-Buendía D, Miralles J, Collado E, Sánchez-Moyano E, Del Pozo A. Studies on the reliability of a bihyperbolic functional absorption model. I. Ring-substituted anilinas. *J Pharmacokinet Biopharm* 1986;14(6): 615–633.

111. Casabó VG, Núñez-Benito E, Martínez-Coscollá A, Miralles-Loyola E, Martín-Villodre A, Plá-Delfina JM. Studies on the reliability of a bihyperbolic functional absorption model. II. Phenylalkylamines. *J Pharmacokinet Biopharm* 1987;15(6):633–643.

112. Bermejo MV, Pérez-Varona AT, Segura-Bono MJ, Martín-Villodre A, Plá-Delfina JM, Garrigues TM. Compared effects of synthetic and natural bile acid surfactants on xenobiotic absorption I. Studies with polysorbate and taurocholate in rat colon. *Int J Pharma* 1991;69:221–231.

113. Garrigues TM, Collado EF, Fabra-Campos S, Pérz-Buendía MD, Martín-Villodre A, Plá-Delfina JM. Absorption–partition relationships for true homologous series of xenobiotics as a possible approach to study mechanisms of surfactants in absorption. III. Aromatic amines and cationic surfactants. *Int J Pharm* 1989;57:189–196.

114. Merino M, Peris-Ribera JE, Torres-Molina F, Sánchez-Picó A, García-Carbonell MC, Casabó VG, Martín-Villodre A, Plá-Delfina JM. Evidence of a specialized transport mechanism for the intestinal absorption of baclofen. *Biopharm Drug Dispos* 1989;10: 279–297.

115. Sánchez-Pico A, Peris-Ribera JE, Toledano C, Torres-Molina F, Casabo VG, Martin-Villodre A, Pla-Delfina JM. Nonlinear intestinal absorption kinetics of cefradoxil in the rat. *J Pharm Pharmacol* 1989;41:179–185.

116. Ruiz-Carretero P, Merino-Sanjuan M, Nacher A, Casabo VG. Pharmacokinetic models for the saturable absorption of cefuroxime axetil and saturable elimination of cefuroxime. *Eur J Pharm Sci* 2004;21(2–3):217–223.

117. Polache A, Plá-Delfina JM, Merino M. Partially competitive inhibition of intestinal baclofen absorption by beta-alanine, a nonessential dietary amino acid. *Biopharm Drug Dispos* 1991;12:647–660.

118. Rodriguez-Ibanez M, Nalda-Molina R, Montalar-Montero M, Bermejo MV, Merino V, Garrigues TM. Transintestinal secretion of ciprofloxacin, grepafloxacin and sparfloxacin: *in vitro* and *in situ* inhibition studies. *Eur J Pharmacokinet Biopharm* 2003;55(2):241–246.

119. Kim JS, Mitchell S, Kijek P, Tsume Y, Hilfinger J, Amidon GL. The suitability of an *in situ* perfusion model for permeability determinations: utility for BCS class I biowaiver requests. *Mol Pharm* 2006;3(6):686–694.

120. Anderberg EK, Artursson P. Cell cultures to access drug absorption enhancement. In de Boer A, Ed. *Drug Absorption Enhancement*. Chur, Switzerland: Harwood Academic Publishers; 1994, pp 101–118.

10

DISTRIBUTION: MOVEMENT OF DRUGS THROUGH THE BODY

JAYANTH PANYAM[1] AND YOGESH PATIL[2]

[1]*University of Minnesota, Minneapolis, Minnesota*
[2]*Wayne State University, Detroit, Michigan*

Contents

10.1 INTRODUCTION

10.1.1 Drug Distribution

Drug distribution refers to the reversible movement of drug from blood to various tissues of the body [1]. Following entry into the systemic circulation, a drug

Preclinical Development Handbook: ADME and Biopharmaceutical Properties,
edited by Shayne Cox Gad
Copyright © 2008 John Wiley & Sons, Inc.

distributes into different tissues, the rate and extent of which is dependent on the drug's physicochemical properties and the blood flow to the tissues. The rate and extent of distribution to different tissues, in turn, affects the duration and magnitude of therapeutic effect and toxicity [2]. This chapter explores the various factors that affect drug distribution and the different approaches available to modify drug distribution.

10.1.2 Effect of Distribution on Drug Action

The intensity and duration of therapeutic effects derived from drugs other than those exerting an immediate, irreversible action depend, theoretically, on maintaining adequate concentrations of the active form of the drug at receptor sites [3]. For the purpose of this chapter, receptor sites are considered to be target sites located anywhere in the body that combine with a drug or its active metabolite to produce a pharmacological effect. To elicit a therapeutic effect, a drug has to distribute from the systemic circulation to its site of action [4]. Therefore, it is important to consider the effect of distribution in selecting an appropriate dose, dosage form, dosage interval, and route of administration; appropriate modification of these parameters permits attainment of effective concentrations of the active form of a drug at receptor sites [5].

For blood levels of a drug to correlate with pharmacological effect, the concentration of the drug in blood must be in equilibrium with the concentration of drug at the receptor site through which it produces its effect [6]. Furthermore, the pharmacological response being investigated must bear a direct relationship to the drug's concentration at the receptor site [5, 6]. Certain drugs, such as monoamine oxidase and cholinesterase inhibitors, must accumulate at receptor sites to a certain concentration before pharmacological effects will ensue [7]. During this initial period of drug accumulation at receptor sites, no direct relationship between the drug level in blood and pharmacological effects may be seen. Thus, the distribution process could make a graded response (response proportional to drug concentration), giving the impression of a quantal response (response does not have a linear relationship with drug concentration) [8].

10.2 DRUG DISTRIBUTION INTO DIFFERENT COMPARTMENTS

10.2.1 Distribution Among Plasma/Blood, Tissues, Organs, and Body Fluids

After absorption into the bloodstream, drugs tend to distribute into all body water. The total body water can be divided into intravascular, extracellular, and intracellular water [9]. For a 70 kg person, the total body water is about 42 L. The intravascular water accounts for about 3 L of the total body water while the extracellular and intracellular waters account for 16 L and 23 L, respectively [2]. Drugs that permeate freely through cell membranes become distributed, in time, throughout the body water. Drugs that pass readily through or between capillary endothelial cells, but do not penetrate other cell membranes, are distributed into the extracellular fluid space [10]. Occasionally, the drug molecule may be so polar, large, or highly

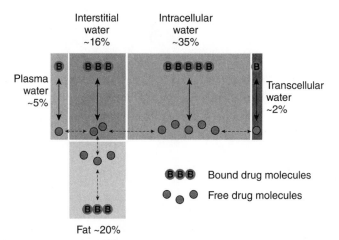

FIGURE 10.1 The main body fluid compartments, expressed as a percentage of body weight. Drug molecules exist in bound or free form in each compartment, but only the free drug is able to move between the compartments. (From Ref. 11, with permission.)

bound to plasma proteins that it remains in the intravascular space after IV administration [2].

In all these body fluid compartments, drug molecules are present in either protein-bound or unbound form (Fig. 10.1), with the equilibrium existing between the unbound form of the drug in different tissues [11]. Furthermore, drugs that are weak acids or bases will exist as an equilibrium mixture of ionized or un-ionized forms, the position of the equilibrium depending on the pH of the compartment. Un-ionized and lipophilic drug molecules can generally diffuse from interstitial space across the cell membrane into the cytoplasm of a cell, while ionized and highly polar drugs cannot readily diffuse across the cell membrane [12].

The effect of pH on diffusion of drugs across a cell membrane could be understood from the gastric pouch experiments [13]. It was shown that drugs cross the gastric epithelium in their nonionized form, and that the ionized form penetrates very slowly, if at all. In the experiments, various acidic and basic drugs were administered intravenously to dogs with gastric pouches, and the concentrations of drug in gastric juice and plasma were measured. At steady state, basic drugs appeared in gastric juice in concentrations ranging from 1 to 40 times that of plasma. In contrast, acidic drugs appeared in gastric juice in low concentrations, which ranged from 0 to 0.6 that of plasma. The results were explained in terms of a model system in which gastric juice is separated from plasma by a barrier permeable only to the nonionized form of a weak electrolyte (Fig. 10.2) [7]. At steady state, the concentrations of nonionized drug in plasma and gastric juice are the same (correcting for the degree of plasma binding), but the concentrations of the ionized form are unequal because of the difference in the pH of the two fluids. Accordingly, the total concentration of drug (ionized plus nonionized) on both sides of the gastric mucosa is a function of the pH of the two fluids and the dissociation constant of the drug. From this relationship, it can readily be calculated that a basic drug will be more concentrated in tissues with acidic pH than in plasma, and an acidic drug will be more concentrated in plasma than in tissues with acidic pH [7].

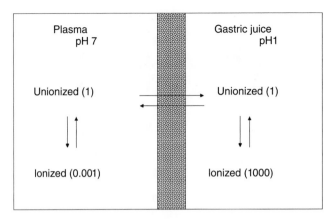

FIGURE 10.2   The theoretical distribution of an organic base, pK_a 4, between plasma and gastric juice, assuming that the fluids are separated by a boundary permeable only to the unionized drug molecule. (From Ref. 7, with permission.)

Drugs may also undergo redistribution in the body after initial high levels are achieved in tissues that have a rich vascular supply. As the plasma concentration falls, drug readily diffuses back from a tissue with initial high concentration into the circulation to be quickly redistributed to other tissues with high blood-flow rates, such as the muscles. Then, over time, the drug also becomes deposited in tissues with poor blood supply, such as the fat depots [14]. Some drug molecules are distributed to eliminating organs like liver and kidney. Many drugs are not distributed equally throughout the body but tend to accumulate in certain specific tissues or fluids [15, 16]. For example, chloroquine mainly accumulates in liver, tetracycline in bone and teeth, and iodine in thyroid glands.

10.2.2   Volume of Distribution (V_D)

Anatomically, the total volume of body water available for a drug to distribute into is about 42 L [2]. If all drugs were to distribute into all of body water equally, then the initial plasma concentration of all drugs for a given intravenous bolus dose of the drug would be similar. However, this is rarely the case. The plasma concentration of the drug appears to be as if the total body water was less than or greater than 42 L. The reason for the discrepancy is twofold. First, most drugs do not distribute evenly in all body water. Second, only the drug concentration in the intravascular compartment is measurable. Two extreme cases of distribution should be considered for a better understanding. Some molecules like Evan's blue are strictly localized within the intravascular compartment. When the concentration of Evan's blue in the plasma is measured, it appears as if the total volume in which the molecule is distributed is small. For example, following a 100 mg IV bolus dose, the initial plasma concentration measured would be about 100 mg/3 L = 33 mg/L. Now, if the dose (100 mg) and initial concentration (33 mg/L) were used to estimate the volume, this would be about 3 L. For the other extreme, consider a drug molecule like quinine, which accumulates extensively in intracellular water. When the concentration of such a drug molecule in the plasma is measured, it appears as if the total volume in which the drug is distributed is large. For example, consider a drug molecule that shows 90% partitioning out of the intravascular water. Thus, following a 100 mg dose, 10 mg will stay in the intravascular water while 90 mg will be distributed into extravascular water. The initial concentration measured for this drug after an IV bolus dose would theoretically be about 10 mg/3 L = 3.3 mg/L. If the dose and initial concentration were used to estimate the volume, this would be about 33 L.

In order to account for these differences, the term *apparent volume of distribution* is used. Apparent volume of distribution (V_D) is the volume that must be considered in estimating the amount of drug in the body from the concentration of drug found in the sampling compartment [1]. Volume of distribution relates the concentration of the drug in plasma (C_P) and the amount of drug in the body (A), as in the following equation:

$$V_D = \frac{A}{C_P}$$

Some drugs have V_D as small as 5 L while others have a V_D of 50,000 L. Since V_D is not a true anatomic/physiologic space, it is called *apparent* volume of distribution. Volume of distribution is a measure of the tendency of a drug to move out of blood/plasma to other tissue sites. Thus, the larger the volume of distribution, the more extensively is the drug distributed outside the vasculature. Volume of distribution is useful in the determination of plasma drug concentration when a known amount of drug is in the body or conversely in the determination of dose required to achieve a particular plasma concentration. Examples of drugs with small and large volumes of distribution are shown in Table 10.1 [11]. It is important to note that volume of distribution is dependent on a patient's body weight and is often quoted with the units of L/kg [11].

10.3   FACTORS AFFECTING DRUG DISTRIBUTION

There are several factors that affect the rate and extent of drug distribution. Blood perfusion to a tissue and permeability of the drug across cell membrane play an important role in determining the rate of distribution. Extent of distribution is mainly affected by molecular weight, lipid solubility, pK_a, and protein binding of the drug. Presence of drug efflux transporters and genetic differences in transporter activity in different patient populations also significantly affect drug distribution.

10.3.1   Rate of Distribution

Distribution of drugs from blood to different tissues is a two-step process [11]. The first step involves the transport of drug by blood to different tissues. The second step is the transport of the drug from blood into the tissue across the cell membrane. For lipophilic, small molecular weight drugs that can cross cell membranes efficiently, transport to the tissue is the rate-limiting step, while for hydrophilic and large molecular weight drugs, transport across the cell membrane is the rate-limiting step. Thus, depending on the drug's characteristics, drug distribution could be either permeability limited or perfusion limited.

TABLE 10.1   Distribution Volumes for Some Drugs Compared with Volume of Body Fluid Compartments

Volume (L/kg body weight)	Compartment	Volume of Distribution (V_D; L/kg body weight)	
0.05	Plasma	0.05–0.1	Heparin
			Insulin
		0.1–0.2	Warfarin
			Sulfamethoxazole
			Glibenclamide
			Atenolol
0.2	Extracellular fluid	0.2–0.4	Tubocurarine
		0.4–0.7	Theophylline
0.55	Total body water		Ethanol
			Neostigmine
			Phenytoin
		1–2	Methotrexate
			Indomethacin
			Paracetamol
			Diazepam
			Lidocaine
		2–5	Glyceryl trinitrate
			Morphine
			Propranolol
			Digoxin
			Chlorpromazine
		>10	Nortriptyline

Permeability-Limited Distribution   The cell membrane separates extra- and intracellular compartments. The cell membrane allows a bidirectional, dynamic, and selective exchange of organic molecules, ions, and gas molecules between the two compartments. Small, noncharged lipid molecules pass through the membrane freely. Small polar molecules (carbon dioxide, water) can also pass cell membranes easily following their concentration gradient. Most hydrophilic molecules and macromolecules cannot cross the cell membrane effectively [17].

Thus, cell permeability is the limiting factor in the tissue distribution of polar and high molecular weight drugs. For such drugs, equilibrium is reached faster in tissues without permeability constraints, even though these tissues may have a lower perfusion rate. For example, brain has a perfusion rate of 0.5 mL/min/mL while muscle has a perfusion rate of 0.025 mL/min/mL. However, the cell junctions in the brain capillary endothelium are tighter than those found in the muscle capillary endothelium. Lipophilic drugs that can cross the cell membrane efficiently reach equilibrium faster in brain than in muscle while polar molecules reach equilibrium faster in muscles [18].

Cell permeability varies in characteristics depending on the tissue [19]. The endothelial cells of the brain capillaries, which are more tightly joined to one another than those found in other capillaries, contribute to the slower diffusion of water-soluble drugs into brain. Another barrier to water-soluble drugs is the glial connective tissue cells (astrocytes), which form an astrocytic sheath close to the basement membrane of the brain capillary endothelium [14]. The tight junctions between brain vascular endothelial cells lead to high endothelial electrical resistance, in the range of 1500–$2000\,\Omega\cdot\text{cm}^2$ (pial vessels), as compared to 3–$33\,\Omega\cdot\text{cm}^2$ in other tissues [20, 21]. Thus, polar compounds cannot enter the brain effectively but can enter the interstitial fluids of most other tissues [22].

Even within a tissue, the distribution of a drug may vary between the different regions of the tissue. For example, drugs penetrate into the brain cortex more rapidly than into white matter, probably because of the greater delivery rate of drug via the bloodstream to the tissue [23]. The consequences of the diverse rates of entry of different drugs into the CNS include the following: (1) water-soluble or ionized drugs will not enter the CNS very well; (2) low ionization, low plasma–protein binding, and a fairly high lipid–water partition coefficient confer ready penetration; and (3) direct injections into the CSF often produce unexpected effects [24, 25].

Perfusion-Limited Distribution For most lipophilic drugs with small molecular weight, cell membranes do not create any barrier to their distribution [26]. For such drugs, distribution to different tissues is mainly governed by the blood perfusion rate to that tissue. Perfusion rate is often expressed as milliliter of blood per minute per unit volume of tissue. Perfusion rate could be as much as $10\,\text{mL/min/mL}$ for lungs to only $0.025\,\text{mL/min/mL}$ for resting muscle (Table 10.2) [1].

TABLE 10.2 Blood Flow, Perfusion Rate, and Relative Size of Different Organs and Tissues Under Basal Conditions in a Standard 70 kg Human[a]

Organ[b]	Percent of Body Volume	Blood Flow (mL/min)	Percent of Cardiac Output	Perfusion Rate (mL/min/mL of Tissue)
Adrenal glands	0.03	25	0.2	1.2
Blood	7	$(5000)^b$	(100)	—
Bone	16	250	5	0.02
Brain	2	700	14	0.5
Fat	20[c]	200	4	0.03
Heart	0.4	200	4	0.6
Kidneys	0.5	1100	22	4
Liver	2.3	1350	27	0.8
Portal	1.7 (gut)	(1050)	(21)	—
Arterial	—	(300)	(6)	—
Lungs	1.6	(5000)	(100)	10
Muscle (inactive)	43	750	15	0.025
Skin (cool weather)	11	300	6	0.04
Spleen	0.3	77	1.5	0.4
Thyroid gland	0.03	50	1	2.4
Total Body	*100*	*5000*	*100*	*0.071*

[a]Compiled and adapted from data in Guyton AC. *Texbook of Medical Physiology*, 7th ed. Philadelphia: Saunders; 1986, p 230; Lentner C, Ed. *Geigy Scientific Tables, Volume 1*. Edison, NJ: Ciba-Geigy; 1981; and Davies B, Morris T. Physiological parameters in laboratory animals and humans. *Pharm Res* 1993;10:1093–1095.

[b]Some organs (e.g., stomach, intestines, and pancreas) are not included.

[c]Includes fat within organs.

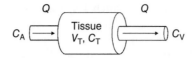

FIGURE 10.3   Perfusion-limited tissue distribution: Q = rate of blood flow; C_A = arterial concentration; C_V = venous concentration; V_T = tissue volume; and C_T = tissue concentration.

All other factors (membrane permeability, protein binding, pH, etc.) remaining equal, well-perfused tissues take up more drug than poorly perfused tissues. There is a direct correlation between tissue perfusion rate and time to distribute to a tissue. This can be explained as follows.

Consider a tissue T whose volume is V_T and the concentration of the drug in the tissue is C_T (Fig. 10.3). The rate of blood flow to the tissue is Q. If C_A is concentration of the drug in arterial blood and C_V is the concentration of the drug in venous blood, then the rate of presentation of the drug to the tissue is given by $Q \cdot C_A$, while the rate of leaving of drug from the tissue is given by $Q \cdot C_V$. The net rate of drug uptake by the tissue is $Q \cdot (C_A - C_V)$.

The amount of the drug in the tissue is obtained using the volume of the tissue and the concentration of the drug in the tissue: amount of drug in tissue = $V_T \cdot C_T$. The relative affinity of the drug for the tissue can be defined in terms of a partition coefficient K_P, where $K_P = C_T/C_V$. Rearranging this relationship, and substituting for C_T in the above equation, we get

$$\text{Amount of drug in tissue} = V_T \cdot K_P \cdot C_V$$

The exit of the drug from the tissue can be defined by the fractional rate of exit, which is given by

$$\text{Fractional rate of exit} = k_T = \text{Rate of exit/Amount in tissue}$$

Substituting for rate of exit and the amount of the drug in the tissue, we get

$$k_T = (Q \cdot C_V)/(V_T \cdot K_P \cdot C_V) = (Q/V_T)/K_P$$

where Q/V_T is perfusion rate of tissue and K_P is the partition coefficient of the drug for the tissue. The time to distribute into a tissue is given by tissue distribution half-life (time for 50% distribution):

$$\text{Tissue distribution half-life} = 0.693/k_T = 0.693 K_P/(Q/V_T)$$

If each organ has the same ability to store the drug (K_P is equal), then the distribution half-life is governed by the blood flow Q and the volume (size) V_T of the organ. A large blood flow to the organ decreases the distribution time; whereas a large organ size increases the distribution time because a longer time is needed to fill a large organ volume with drug. Also, it is important to note that if a tissue has a long distribution half-life, a long time is needed for the drug to leave the tissue when blood level decreases. If arterial concentration is maintained constant, tissue concentration goes up but rate of uptake decreases with time. Tissue concentration (C_T) at any time t is given by the following relationship:

$$C_T = K_P C_A (1 - e^{-k_T t})$$

Equilibrium in tissue concentration and the loss of drug from tissue take longer the poorer the perfusion and the greater the partitioning of drug into the tissue.

10.3.2 Extent of Distribution

Factors like molecular weight, lipid solubility, pH–pK_a, and protein binding play an important role in determining the extent of drug distribution. It is important to note that all the above factors also affect the rate of drug distribution into the tissue.

Molecular Weight The diffusion of a molecule across a cell membrane depends mainly on its molecular size, the diffusion coefficient for small molecules being inversely proportional to the square root of molecular weight. Consequently, while large molecules diffuse at a slower rate than small ones, the effect of molecular weight for most drug molecules is modest. Most drugs fall within the molecular weight range 200–1000, and variations in aqueous diffusion rate have only a small effect on their overall pharmacokinetic behavior. However, beyond this molecular weight range, diffusion of molecules across cell membranes is considerably limited. For compounds with molecular diameter above 100 Å, transfer across membranes is significantly slow [11].

Lipid Solubility Distribution of drugs is significantly influenced by lipid solubility. Lipid solubility affects the ability of the drug to bind to plasma proteins and to cross lipid membrane barriers [27]. A drug needs to be lipid soluble to penetrate membranes, unless there is an active transport system for the drug or the drug is so small that it can pass through the aqueous channels in the membrane. For weakly acidic and weakly basic drugs, ionization, and therefore lipid solubility, is pH dependent (see pH–pK_a discussion). As discussed earlier, very high lipid solubility can result in a drug initially partitioning preferentially into highly vascularized lipid-rich areas. Subsequently, these drugs slowly redistribute into body fat, where they may remain for long periods of time.

pH–pK_a Most drugs are weak acids or bases and therefore exist in both un-ionized and ionized forms, the ratio of the two forms varying with pH. For a weak base, the ionization reaction is

$$BH^+ \xrightarrow{\ K_a\ } B + H^+$$

The negative logarithm of the acid dissociation constant is designated by the symbol pK_a and is given by the Henderson–Hasselbalch equation:

$$pK_a = pH + \log_{10}([BH^+]/[B])$$

For a weak acid,

$$AH \xleftrightarrow{K_a} A^- + H^+$$

$$pK_a = pH + \log_{10}([AH]/[A^-])$$

Drug accumulates on the side of a membrane where pH favors greater ionization of drug. This is known as the pH-partition hypothesis [28]. Only un-ionized nonpolar drug can permeate through the lipid membrane, and at equilibrium, the concentration of the un-ionized species is the same on both sides, but there will be more total drug on the side on which the degree of ionization is greater. Basic drugs tend to accumulate in tissues with pH values lower than the pK_a of the drug; conversely, acidic drugs concentrate in regions of higher pH, provided that the free drug is sufficiently lipid soluble to be able to penetrate the membranes that separate the compartments. Even small differences in pH across membranes, such as those that exist between CSF (pH 7.3) and plasma (pH 7.4), milk (pH 6.5–6.8) and plasma, renal tubular fluid (pH 5.0–8.0) and plasma, and inflamed tissue (pH 6.0–7.0) and healthy tissue (pH 7.0–7.4), can lead to unequal distribution of drugs [11].

Figure 10.4 shows how a weak acid (e.g., aspirin, pK_a 3.5) and a weak base (e.g., pethidine, pK_a 8.6) would be distributed at equilibrium between three body compartments, namely, plasma (pH 7.4), alkaline urine (pH 8), and gastric juice (pH 3). Within each compartment, the ratio of ionized to un-ionized drug is governed by the pK_a of the drug and the pH of that compartment [11]. It is assumed that the un-ionized species can cross the membrane and therefore reaches an equal concentration in each compartment. The ionized species is assumed not to cross at all. The result is that, at equilibrium, the total (ionized + un-ionized) concentration of the drug will be different in the different compartments, with an acidic drug being concentrated in the compartment with high pH ("ion trapping"), and vice versa [29]. The concentration gradients produced by ion trapping can theoretically be very large, if there is a large pH difference between compartments. Thus, aspirin would be concentrated more than fourfold with respect to plasma in alkaline renal tubule, and about 6000-fold in plasma with respect to the acidic gastric contents. Such large gradients, however, are unlikely to be achieved in reality for two main reasons. First, the attribution of total impermeability to the charged species is not realistic, and even a small permeability will considerably attenuate the concentration difference that can be reached. Second, body compartments rarely approach equilibrium. Neither the gastric contents nor the renal tubular fluid stands still, and the resulting flux of drug molecules reduces the concentration gradients well below the theoretical equilibrium conditions. The pH-partition mechanism nonetheless correctly explains some of the qualitative effects of pH changes in different body compartments on the pharmacokinetics of weakly acidic or basic drugs, particularly in relation to penetration of the blood–organ barriers. Values of pK_a for some common drugs are shown in Fig. 10.5 [1].

Protein Binding Binding to proteins in tissue, dissolution in adipose tissue, formation of nondiffusible complexes in tissues such as bone, incorporation into specific storage granules, or binding to selective sites in tissues all impede movement of drugs in the body and account for differences in the cellular and organ distribution

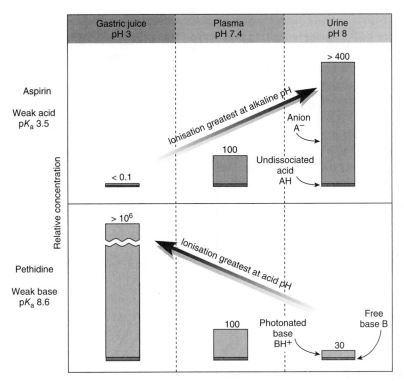

FIGURE 10.4 Theoretical partition of a weak acid (aspirin) and a weak base (pethidine) between aqueous compartments (urine, plasma, and gastric juice) according to the pH difference between them. Numbers represent relative concentrations (total plasma concentration = 100). It is assumed that the uncharged species in each case can permeate the cellular barrier separating the compartments and therefore reaches the same concentration in all three. Variations in the fractional ionization as a function of pH give rise to the large total concentration differences with respect to plasma. (From Ref. 11, with permission.)

of particular drugs [30, 31]. Extensive plasma–protein binding will cause more of the drug to stay in the central blood compartment, because only the unbound or free fraction of a drug can diffuse out of capillaries into tissues. Therefore, drugs that bind strongly to plasma proteins tend to have lower volumes of distribution. Similarly, drugs that bind extensively to tissue proteins (proteins outside the vascular compartment) tend to have large volumes of distribution [32].

The most important binding of drugs in circulation is to plasma albumin, which comprises about 50% of the total plasma proteins and binds the widest range of drugs [33]. Acidic drugs commonly bind to albumin, while basic drugs often bind to α_1-acid glycoproteins and lipoproteins (Table 10.3) [34]. Many endogenous substances, steroids, vitamins, and metal ions are bound to globulins. A drug may become bound to plasma proteins to a greater or lesser degree, depending on a number of factors, for example, plasma pH, concentration of plasma proteins, concentration of the drug, the presence of another agent with a greater affinity for the limited number of binding sites, and the presence of acute-phase proteins during active inflammatory conditions [9]. The degree of plasma–protein binding and the

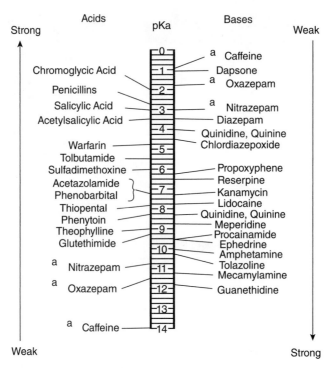

FIGURE 10.5 The pK_a values of acidic and basic drugs vary widely. Some of drugs are amphoteric (a): that is, they have both acidic and basic functional groups. (From Ref. 1, with permission.)

TABLE 10.3   Potential Binding Sites of Proteins for Various Drugs

Binding Sites	Drugs
For Acidic Agents:	
Albumins	Bilirubin, bile acids, fatty acids, vitamin C, salicylates, sulfonamides, barbiturates, phenylbutazone, penicillins, tetracyclines, probenecid
For Basic Agents:	
Globulins, α_1, α_2, β_1, β_2, γ	Adenosine, quinacrine, quinine, streptomycin, chloramphenicol, digoxin, ouabain, coumarin

affinity of a drug for the nonspecific protein-binding sites are of great clinical significance in some instances and much less so in others [35]. For example, a potentially toxic compound (such as dicumarol) may be 98% bound, but if for any reason it becomes only 96% bound, then the concentration of the free active drug that becomes available in the plasma is doubled, with potentially harmful consequences. The concentration of a drug administered in overdose may exceed the binding capacity of the plasma protein and lead to an excess of free drug, which can distribute into various target tissues and produce exaggerated effects. Of equal importance is the readiness with which drugs dissociate from plasma proteins. Those that are more tightly bound tend to have much longer elimination half-lives, because they are released gradually from the plasma protein reservoir. The long-acting sulfonamides are good examples of this phenomenon.

10.3.3   Role of Transporters

Drug transporters, proteins that transport drugs across the cell membrane, either from or to the intravascular compartment, play an important role in determining drug disposition. Transporters have been shown to be important in the disposition of endogenous compounds, drugs, and other xenobiotics in many organs such as the intestine, liver, kidney, and brain [36–39]. This section focuses on the role of primary transport proteins like ATP-binding cassette transporters and secondary and tertiary transporters like organic cation and anion transporters in the distribution of drugs.

Primary Transporters (ATP-Binding Cassette Transporters)   It is now well recognized that membrane efflux transporters, especially P-glycoprotein (P-gp), play an important role in determining the absorption, distribution, metabolism, excretion, and toxicology (ADMET) behaviors of many drugs and molecules in development. Many of the important mammalian efflux transporters are members of the adenosine triphosphate (ATP)-binding cassette (ABC) superfamily, where transport is driven by hydrolysis of ATP. The first member of this family to be discovered was P-gp. P-gp is a 170 kDa, integral membrane protein found in most organisms from bacteria to humans. It was originally identified as a key reason for the development of multidrug resistance in certain cancers [40]; however, constitutive expression of P-gp in many normal tissues such as intestinal epithelia, hepatocytes, kidney proximal tubules, blood–brain barrier endothelia, and placental trophoblast demonstrates its protective roles in limiting drug absorption and distribution, contributing to pharmacokinetics, and potentially impacting pharmacodynamics and toxicity [41, 42]. A list of P-gp substrates is shown in Table 10.4. The tissue localization and probable role of transport proteins in drug absorption, distribution, and excretion are depicted in Fig. 10.6.

P-gp is only one of 48 known transporters belonging to seven subfamilies (A–G) [43]. So the potential for other transporters to affect drug disposition is high. As the importance of transport proteins in drug disposition emerges, it is also clear that these transport proteins are saturable, inducible, can be inhibited, and display some degree of polymorphism—factors that need to be considered with respect to variability in drug disposition and response [44–47].

As discussed earlier, the extent of membrane permeability is largely governed by the physicochemical properties of drugs, and lipophilicity is generally considered a key determinant in extent of drug absorption, hepatic transport, and brain penetration. However, increased lipophilicity alone is not predictive of increased permeability when the transport proteins contribute to drug transport across the membrane. While determining the kinetics of drug movement across a barrier, contributions of both passive diffusion and active transport have to be considered. The flux of a drug across a membrane is linearly related to drug concentration, if only passive diffusion is present. Active transport (forward transport or efflux) is usually saturable at high concentrations. If both passive diffusion and active transport are present, net flux will depend on the relative contribution of the two processes and the concentration

TABLE 10.4   List of P-Glycoprotein Substrates

Anthracyclines (doxorubicin, daunomycin, epirubicin)
Acridines (m-AMSA)
Azatoxins (azatoxin)
Benzxoheptalene compounds (colchicine)
Benzothiazepines (diltiazem)
Dihydropyridines (azidopine, nicardipine)
Epipodophyllotoxins (etoposide)
Isoquinolines (cepharantine)
Macrolides (FK506)
Organometallic cations (99mTc-sestamibi)
Peptides (actinomycin D, bleomycin, cyclosporin A, valinomycin)
Phenothiazines (chlorpromazine)
Phenylalkylamines (verapamil, tiapamil)
Pyrroloindoles (mitomycin C)
Quinolines (chloroquine, quinidine)
Rhodamines (rhodamine 123)
Steroids (aldosterone, corticosterone, cortisol, dexamethasone, testosterone)
Taxanes (paclitaxel, docetaxel)
Vinca alkaloids (vincristine, vinblastine)
Other (digoxin, Hoechst 33342)

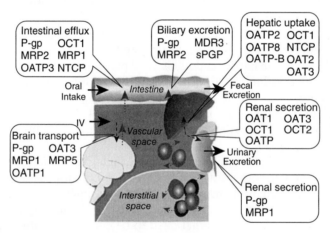

FIGURE 10.6   Tissue localization and role of transport proteins in drug disposition. (From Ref. 19, with permission.)

of drug. At very high concentrations, the contribution of active transport to the kinetics of drug flux across the membrane is minimized.

Secondary and Tertiary Transporters (Driven by an Exchange or Cotransport of Intracellular and/or Extracellular Ions)   Besides the ATP family of transporters, other transporters, such as the organic anion transporters (OATs) and the organic cation transporters (OCTs) are present in the human body and significantly influence drug distribution [48].

Organic anion transporters (OATs) play an essential role in the disposition of clinically important anionic drugs, including antiviral drugs, antitumor drugs, antibiotics, antihypertensives, and anti-inflammatory agents. The activities of OATs are directly linked to drug toxicity and drug–drug interactions. So far, four members of the OAT family have been identified: OAT1, OAT2, OAT3, and OAT4 [49]. These transporters share several common structural features including 12 transmembrane domains, multiple glycosylation sites localized in the first extracellular loop between transmembrane domains 1 and 2, and multiple phosphorylation sites present in the intracellular loop between transmembrane domains 6 and 7 and in the carboxyl terminus. The impact of these structural features on the function of these transporters has just begun to be explored. OAT1 and OAT3 are predominantly expressed in the kidney and brain. OAT2 is predominantly expressed in liver. OAT4 is present mainly in placenta and kidney. These transporters are multispecific with a wide range of substrate recognition [49].

OAT1 has been shown to interact with a wide range of organic anion drugs such as nonsteroidal anti-inflammatory drugs (NSAIDs), β-lactam antibiotics, antiviral drugs, diuretics, antitumor drugs, and angiotensin-converting enzyme inhibitors. The prototype substrate for OAT1 is para-aminohippuric acid (PAH) [50]. OAT2 interacts with organic anion drugs, such as NSAIDs, and antibiotics. Unlike for OAT1, PAH is a low affinity substrate for OAT2. For OAT3, the prototype substrates are sulfate- and glucuronide-conjugated steroids. OAT3 also interacts with various drugs and endogenous substances such as NSAIDs, antitumor drugs, H2-receptor antagonists, prostaglandins, diuretics, angiotensin-converting enzyme inhibitors, β-lactam antibiotics, and various neurotransmitter metabolites. PAH is a low affinity substrate for OAT3. OAT4 interacts with sulfate-conjugated steroids, antibiotics, and ochratoxin A and shows very little transport of PAH. Compared with OAT1 and OAT3, OAT4 has much narrower substrate specificity [51].

Organic cation transporters (OCTs) are critical in drug absorption, targeting, and disposition. It has become increasingly clear that multiple mechanisms are involved in organic cation transport in the key tissues responsible for drug absorption and disposition: kidney, liver, and intestine. Drugs from a wide array of clinical classes—including antihistamines, skeletal muscle relaxants, antiarrhythmics, and adrenoceptor blocking agents—are organic cations. In addition, several endogenous bioactive amines—such as dopamine, choline, and N1-methylnicotinamide (NMN)—are organic cations. Since many of these molecules (pK_a 8–12) are polar and positively charged at physiologic pH, OCTs generally are involved in the absorption, distribution, and elimination of these compounds [52].

10.3.4 Pharmacogenetic Factors

Pharmacogenetics deals with inherited differences in response to drugs. It is well recognized that most medications exhibit wide interpatient variability in their efficacy and toxicity. For many drugs, these interindividual differences are due, in part, to polymorphisms in genes encoding drug-metabolizing enzymes, drug transporters, and/or drug targets (e.g., receptors, enzymes). Pharmacogenomics is aimed at elucidating the genetic basis for differences in drug efficacy and toxicity, and it uses genome-wide approaches to identify the network of genes that govern an individual's response to drug therapy.

Polymorphism   The best recognized examples are genetic polymorphisms of drug-metabolizing enzymes, which affect about 30% of all drugs [53]. Loss of function of thiopurine *S*-methyltransferase (TPMT) results in severe and life-threatening hematopoietic toxicity if patients receive standard doses of mercaptopurine and azathioprine. Gene duplication of cytochrome P4502D6 (CYP2D6), which metabolizes many antidepressants, has been identified as a mechanism of poor response in the treatment of depression. There is also a growing list of genetic polymorphisms in drug targets that have been shown to influence drug response. In this section, we discuss genetic polymorphisms in drug transporters that are involved in drug distribution.

As previously described, many drugs are substrates of active transporters, membrane proteins that maintain cellular homeostasis by importing and exporting endogenous compounds. Because of their localization in intestinal, hepatic, and renal epithelial cells, these transporters are important in the absorption, distribution, bioavailability, and elimination of many drugs. Moreover, they can be important in targeting drugs to organs because they are localized in blood–organ barriers.

Genetic polymorphisms affecting a transporter's expression or affinity for substrates can alter drug concentrations at the site of action despite similar blood concentrations. MDR1, MRPs, OATPs, OCTs, OATs, and nucleoside transporters are of particular interest because they transport exogenous substrates, including drugs, as well as endogenous compounds. P-gp, the product of *ABCB1* gene, has received much attention because its substrates include many important drugs. Systemic screening initially revealed 15 genetic variants of human *ABCB1*. A total of 28 SNPs have now been identified; those in exons 21 (G2677T) and 26 (C3435T) are of particular interest because they affect expression or function [47, 55]. Although several studies have addressed the association of these variants with disposition and effects of P-gp substrates, controversy remains about the influence of different variants on pharmacokinetics and pharmacodynamics. Tissues studied so far have shown an average eight- to tenfold difference in P-gp expression. The 3435CC and 3435TT genotypes show a two- to threefold difference in P-gp expression in duodenum, kidney, peripheral leukocytes, and placenta, with substantial overlap between genotypes. This modest difference suggests a moderate impact of the *ABCB1* genotypes on the disposition and effects of P-gp substrates; nongenetic factors probably play an important role in modifying P-gp expression. Differences of ~25–35% in the bioavailability and renal clearance of digoxin in relation to the exon 21 or exon 26 SNP have been reported [56–59]. Several studies [60, 61] have addressed the relevance of *ABCB1* polymorphism to dose requirements, blood concentrations, chronic rejection, and chronic nephrotoxicity in renal transplant patients receiving the calcineurin inhibitors cyclosporin A and tacrolimus.

P-gp expressed on the luminal side of endothelial cells of the brain capillaries significantly limits the transfer of many drugs from blood to brain, as evidenced by a huge increase in brain-to-blood concentration in the P-gp knockout mouse [54]. Because many CNS-active drugs are P-gp substrates, differences in *ABCB1* expression at the blood–brain barrier could help explain why patients with identical plasma drug concentrations respond differently and have different side effects. The consequences of genetic polymorphism have been assessed *in vivo* for another transporter of relevance for drug therapy, OATP-C (SCP1B1), which facilitates the uptake of drug substrates from the blood into the hepatocyte. The relatively common

TABLE 10.5 Genetic Polymorphisms of Human Transporters

BSEP	Conjugates	Not yet elucidated
MDR-1	Natural product anticancer drugs, CYP3A4 substrates, digoxin	Not yet elucidated
MRPs	Glutathione, glucuronide, and sulfate conjugates, nucleoside antivirals	Not yet elucidated

variant OATP-C*5 is associated with markedly reduced transporter function [62]. Carriers of the *5 allele have high plasma concentrations of the OATP-C substrate pravastatin [63–65], suggesting impaired uptake of pravastatin by hepatocytes. Indeed, pravastatin concentrations in hepatocytes are low, which results in less inhibition of cholesterol synthesis as assessed by decreased lathosterol concentration and lathosterol/cholesterol ratio [65]. Whether cholesterol-lowering efficacy is impaired in carriers of these variants during long-term treatment is yet unknown. A profound impact of OATP-C polymorphism was recently demonstrated for the antidiabetic drug repaglinide, for which AUC values were approximately three times higher in carriers of the variant *5 allele than in wild-type subjects. This effect was associated with a more pronounced reduction of blood glucose levels [65].

Table 10.5 provides a list of human drug transporters that exhibit functional genetic polymorphisms and their substrates [66].

10.4 MODIFYING DRUG DISTRIBUTION

A number of drugs often exhibit undesirable pharmacokinetic properties. Some of these include unfavorable distribution profiles such as lack of penetration into target tissues or binding to specific tissues that could result in toxicity. A number of approaches are available to modify the distribution profile of a drug. These include alterations in the chemical structure of the drug, use of another drug that alters the pharmacokinetics of the drug under investigation, and encapsulation of the drug in a delivery system.

10.4.1 Alterations in Chemical Structure: Prodrug Design

Prodrug design strategies have been employed to improve the efficacy of drugs with undesirable pharmacokinetic properties such as chemical instability and lack of specificity. Targeted prodrug design represents a strategy for site-directed and efficient drug delivery. Targeting of drugs to transporters and receptors to aid in site-specific carrier-mediated absorption is emerging as a novel and clinically significant approach. Various prodrugs have been successful in achieving the goals of enhanced availability and are therefore considered to be an important tool in biopharmaceutics.

Strategies in targeted prodrug design include antibody-directed enzyme prodrug therapy, gene-directed enzyme prodrug therapy, and peptide transporter-associated prodrug therapy. The term *prodrug* or *proagent* was first introduced to signify pharmacologically inactive chemical derivatives that could be used to alter the physicochemical properties of drugs, in a temporary manner, to increase their usefulness and/or to decrease associated toxicity [67]. Often, use of the term prodrug implies a covalent link between a drug and a chemical moiety, although some authors also use it to characterize some forms of salts of the active drug molecule. Although there is no universal definition for a prodrug itself, and the definition may vary, generally prodrugs can be defined as pharmacologically inert chemical derivatives that can be converted *in vivo* to active drug molecules, enzymatically or nonenzymatically, to exert a therapeutic effect. Ideally, the prodrug should be converted to the original drug at the target site of action, followed by subsequent rapid elimination of the released derivatizing group [68, 69].

Prodrugs can be designed to target specific enzymes or carriers by considering enzyme–substrate specificity or carrier–substrate specificity in order to overcome various undesirable drug properties. This type of "targeted-prodrug" design requires considerable knowledge of particular enzymes or carrier systems, including their molecular and functional characteristics. Targeted prodrug designs are classified into two categories: (1) targeting specific enzymes and (2) targeting specific membrane transporters.

Prodrug Design Targeting Enzymes   In prodrug design, enzymes can be recognized as presystemic metabolic sites or prodrug–drug *in vivo* reconversion sites. Usually, targeting enzymes to reduce the presystemic metabolism is more successfully achieved by irreversible chemical modification rather than by a prodrug approach. Therefore, our discussion focuses on the enzymes as *in vivo* reconversion targets for prodrugs. The enzyme-targeted prodrug approach can be used to improve oral drug absorption, as well as site-specific drug delivery. In the case of improving oral drug absorption, gastrointestinal enzymes may be the main targets for prodrug design, and the use of a nutrient moiety as a derivatizing group permits more specific targeting for gastrointestinal enzymes to improve oral drug absorption [70]. These prodrugs have the additional advantage of producing nontoxic nutrient by-products when they regenerate the active drugs *in vivo*.

Site-specific drug delivery can be obtained from tissue-specific activation of a prodrug, which is the result of metabolism by an enzyme that is either unique for the tissue or is present at a higher concentration (compared with other tissues); thus, it activates the prodrug more efficiently. This type of site-specific drug delivery has been of particular interest in cancer chemotherapy. Appropriately designed prodrugs have been found to be effective in the treatment of animal tumors possessing high levels of an activating enzyme [71, 72]. However, clinical results were disappointing when it was found that human tumors containing appropriately high levels of the activating enzymes were rare and that the high levels of activating enzymes were not associated with any particular type of tumor [73]. Recently, new therapies have been proposed to overcome this limitation of prodrug therapy. These new approaches are referred to as ADEPT (antibody-directed enzyme prodrug therapy) and GDEPT (gene-directed enzyme prodrug therapy), which attempt the localization of prodrug activation enzymes into specific cancer cells prior to prodrug administration.

Prodrug Design Targeting the Membrane Transporters   Although the classical approach to improve membrane permeability of polar drugs uses lipophilic derivatives to increase passive membrane penetration, the targeted prodrug approach uses transporters designed for facilitating membrane transport of polar nutrients such as amino acids and peptides. There is direct and indirect evidence for the participation of carrier-mediated membrane transport mechanisms, where several hydrophilic compounds seem to be absorbed efficiently via specific transporters [74]. Therefore, targeting specific membrane transporters is particularly important when prodrugs are polar or charged. Prodrugs can be designed to structurally resemble endogenous compounds and to be transported by specific carrier proteins. In this case, prodrugs may have the additional advantage of producing nontoxic by-products when prodrugs are converted to the parent drug molecules. The brain uptake of the potent glycine-NMDA receptor antagonists, such as 7-chlorokynurenic acid and 5,7-dichlorokynurenic acid, was significantly improved by their respective prodrugs, L-4-chlorokynurenine and L-4,6-dichlorokynurenine, which are amino acid derivatives [70]. L-4-chlorokynurenine was shown to be rapidly delivered into the brain by the large neutral amino acid transporter of the blood–brain barrier and to be converted intracellularly to its parent drug, 7-chlorokynurenic acid [70]. Furthermore, there have been some reports on prodrug design targeting peptide transporters, including peptidyl derivatives of methyldopa and alafosfalin and tripeptidyl prodrugs of foscarnet [75–77]. Developing prodrugs targeting specific membrane carriers requires considerable knowledge of the carrier proteins, including their distribution and substrate specificity.

10.4.2 Pegylation

Pegylation refers to the modification of a therapeutic agent by the attachment of poly(ethylene glycol) (PEG) molecules through covalent conjugation to the therapeutic agent. Pegylation may be an effective method of delivering therapeutic proteins and modifying their pharmacokinetic properties, in turn modifying pharmacodynamics, via a mechanism dependent on altered binding properties of the native protein [78]. PEG moieties are inert, long-chain amphiphilic molecules produced by linking repeating units of ethylene oxide [79]. A large number of potential PEG molecules are available, and they can be produced in different configurations, including linear or branched structures, and in different molecular weights (Fig. 10.7). Using pegylation to increase the size and molecular weight of a therapeutic protein

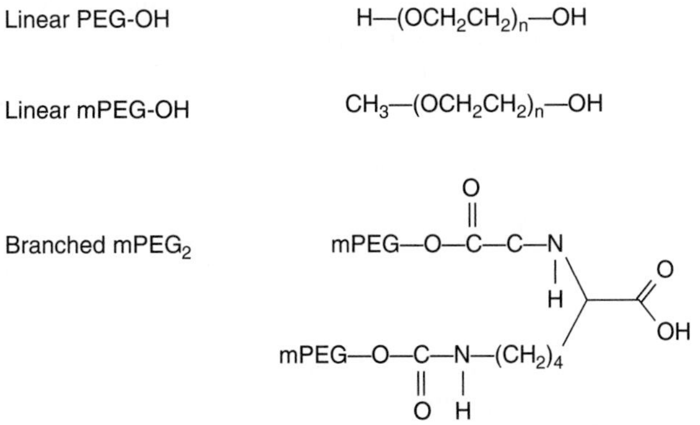

FIGURE 10.7 Structural formulas of poly(ethylene glycol) (PEG) molecules. mPEG = monomethoxypoly(ethylene glycol). (From Ref. 80, with permission.)

alters the immunological, pharmacokinetic, and pharmacodynamic properties of the protein in ways that can extend its potential uses [80, 81]. Goals for chemically coupling PEG to peptide and protein drugs include decreased renal clearance and, for some products, more sustained absorption after subcutaneous administration as well as restricted distribution [82]. These pharmacokinetic changes may result in more constant and sustained plasma concentrations, which can lead to increases in clinical effectiveness when the desired effects are concentration dependent. Maintaining drug concentrations at or near a target concentration for an extended period of time is often clinically advantageous and is particularly useful in antiviral therapy, since constant antiviral pressure should prevent replication and may thereby suppress the emergence of resistant variants [83]. Additionally, PEG modification may decrease adverse effects caused by the large variations in peak-to-trough plasma drug concentrations associated with frequent administration and by the immunogenicity of unmodified proteins. Pegylated proteins may have reduced immunogenicity because PEG-induced steric hindrance can prevent immune recognition [84]. Furthermore, pegylation can enhance targeting of peptides and proteins to tumor tissue through enhanced permeation and retention (EPR) effect [78]. Tumor tissues have a very porous vasculature, and large molecular weight compounds (like pegylated drugs) have enhanced permeation into tumor tissue. Once permeated into the tumor, they are retained in the tumor for a prolonged period of time due to poor drainage from tumor. This EPR effect associated with pegylation has also been used to improve the therapeutic effectiveness of a number of drug molecules like doxorubicin [85, 86]. Pegylation has also been used to improve the circulation times of nanometer-size delivery systems such as liposomes and nanoparticles [87]. Table 10.6 lists the potential types of PEG conjugates.

TABLE 10.6   Types of PEG Conjugates

Conjugate Type	Properties and Applications[a]
Small molecule drugs	Improved solubility, controlled permeability through biological barriers, longevity in bloodstream, controlled release
Affinity ligands and cofactors	Used in aqueous two-phase partitioning systems for purification and analysis of biological macromolecules and cells; enzymatic reactors
Peptides	Improved solubility, conformational analysis, biologically active conjugates
Proteins	Resistance to proteolysis, reduced immunogenicity and antigenicity, longevity in bloodstream, tolerance induction; uses include therapeutics, organic-soluble reagents, bioreactors
Saccharides	New biomaterials, drug carriers
Oligonucleotides	Improved solubility, resistance to nucleases, cell membrane permeability
Lipids	Used for preparation of PEG-grafted liposomes
Liposomes and particulates	Longevity in bloodstream, RES evasion
Biomaterials	Reduced thrombogenicity, reduced protein and cell adherence

[a]PEG, poly(ethylene glycol); RES, reticuloendothelial system.

10.4.3   Use of Another Drug to Modify Distribution

A drug molecule that affects the pharmacokinetics of a second drug can be used clinically to modify the disposition, and therefore the pharmacodynamics, of the second drug. This phenomenon has been used previously to modify the absorption and elimination of a number of drugs. Classic examples include the use of probenecid to decrease the urinary excretion of penicillin [88] and the use of vasoconstrictors to decrease the rate of absorption of local anesthetics from subcutaneous injection site [89]. Use of hyperosmotic mannitol to transiently open up the tight junctions of the blood–brain barrier represents one of the earliest attempts to use one agent to modify the distribution of another drug [90]. With increasing knowledge of the effects of transporters on drug distribution and pharmacokinetics, a number of attempts have been made to use the inhibitors of these transporters to improve the distribution profile of drugs. Because the use of inhibitors of P-gp have been the most studied, this is discussed further.

As discussed earlier, P-gp is overexpressed in many normal tissues such as the capillary endothelium of the blood–brain barrier (BBB), the intestinal epithelium, and also in tumor tissues. Overexpression of P-gp in the blood–brain barrier results in the reduced transport of P-gp substrates into the brain. The significance of this problem is highlighted by the estimations that up to 98% of the newly developed small molecules will not cross the BBB [91]. This limits the number of drugs available for treating diseases like epilepsy [92], stroke and brain injury [93], brain cancer [94], HIV infection of the brain [95], and amyotrophic lateral sclerosis [96]. Numerous preclinical studies and a few clinical studies have indicated the potential of P-gp inhibitors to enhance brain delivery of P-gp substrates [91, 94, 97–99]. P-gp inhibition was evaluated as a means of increasing the brain delivery of the peripherally acting opioid loperamide [100]. Healthy volunteers received a single oral dose of loperamide with or without the P-gp inhibitor quinidine. The central effect of loperamide (change in ventilatory response in response to carbon dioxide) was only observed in volunteers receiving both loperamide and quinidine, indicating the ability of the P-gp inhibitor to enhance the brain delivery of P-gp substrates. Other case studies have demonstrated the use of the P-gp inhibitor verapamil to enhance the brain delivery of anticonvulsant drugs in refractory epilepsy [101, 102].

Many important anticancer agents like doxorubicin and paclitaxel are substrates of P-gp. Overexpression of P-gp in tumor cells results in the development of drug resistance. Initial clinical trials with P-gp inhibitors to treat resistant tumors were performed with "first generation" P-gp inhibitors such as cyclosporin, which were already in use for other indications [103]. Absence of confirmation of P-gp expression in the tumors and P-gp inhibitor toxicity at doses administered to achieve serum concentrations comparable to those that were effective in animal models resulted in the failure of these drugs in clinical trials [104]. Second generation inhibitors (e.g., PSC 833) were developed solely for the purpose of overcoming drug resistance [105]. These agents were tested in clinical trials in various malignancies for which there was evidence that P-gp is expressed or associated with a poorer therapeutic outcome [106]. One major limitation of these trials, however, was the reduction in anticancer drug doses that was required with concurrent administration of inhibitor [107]. P-gp inhibitors increased the serum levels of the coadministered chemotherapeutic agent. A number of studies found that reduction in the dose led to a number of patients being undertreated, which could have contributed to the failure of these combination treatments [107]. Pharmacokinetic interactions between the P-gp inhibitor and the drug could also result from the inhibitor's ability to inhibit other proteins involved in drug metabolism such as cytochrome P450 [108] P-gp inhibitors with fewer pharmacokinetic interactions are being developed [109], and functional assays to verify the role of P-gp in drug resistance, such as sestamibi imaging, are proving helpful in assessing the development of the newer inhibitors [110]. A number of other approaches to overcome P-gp that are currently in development include the use of monoclonal antibodies against P-gp [111, 112], antisense oligonucleotides [113], pH-sensitive polymeric micelles [114], Pluronic[(r)] copolymers [115], peptide-based transmembrane inhibitors [116], and inhibitors of signal transduction [117].

10.4.4 Encapsulation in Delivery Systems

A delivery system is often used to encapsulate a drug, because of the following advantages: (1) prolonged drug availability in the body because of sustained release of the drug from the delivery system; (2) enhanced availability of the drug at the target site—by choosing appropriate formulation parameters, a favorable tissue distribution profile could be obtained; and (3) enhanced stability of the drug due to protection from drug-metabolizing enzymes. Sustained (or continuous) release of a drug from a delivery system involves slow diffusion of the drug out of a polymeric matrix and/or slow degradation of the polymer over time. Pulsatile release is sometimes the preferred method of drug delivery, as it closely mimics the way in which the body naturally produces hormones such as insulin. It is achieved by using drug-carrying polymers that respond to specific stimuli (e.g., exposure to light, changes in pH or temperature) [118].

Choice of the delivery system often depends on the route of administration, nature of the drug, and nature of the disease. Applications involving intravenous administration require the use of nanometer-size delivery systems. This is necessary to reach distant target sites perfused by fine capillaries (diameter $\approx 1\,\mu m$) and to prevent embolism. Colloidal drug carrier systems such as micelles, vesicle and liquid crystal dispersions, as well as nanoparticle dispersions consisting of small particles of 10–400 nm diameter have been found useful as intravenous drug delivery systems. Figure 10.8 demonstrates different types of drug carriers. When developing these formulations, the goal is to obtain systems with optimized drug loading and release properties, long shelf-life, and low toxicity [119].

Micelles formed by self-assembly of amphiphilic block copolymers (5–50 nm) in aqueous solutions are of great interest for drug delivery applications [120]. Drugs can be physically entrapped in the core of block copolymer micelles and transported at concentrations that can exceed their intrinsic water solubility. Moreover, the hydrophilic blocks can form hydrogen bonds with the aqueous surroundings and form a tight shell around the micellar core. As a result, the contents of the hydrophobic core are effectively protected against hydrolysis and enzymatic degradation. In addition, the corona may prevent recognition by the reticuloendothelial system and therefore preliminary elimination of the micelles from the bloodstream.

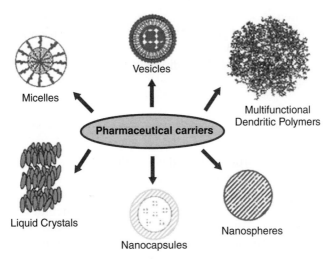

FIGURE 10.8 Schematic of various pharmaceutical carriers. (From Ref. 120, with permission.)

Functionalization of block copolymers with crosslinkable groups can increase the stability of the corresponding micelles and improve their temporal control. Substitution of block copolymer micelles with specific ligands is a very promising strategy to achieve targeted drug delivery.

Liposomes are a form of vesicles that consist either of many, a few, or just one phospholipid bilayer [121]. The polar character of the liposomal core enables polar drug molecules to be encapsulated. Amphiphilic and lipophilic molecules are solubilized within the phospholipid bilayer according to their affinity toward the phospholipids. Channel proteins can be incorporated without loss of their activity within the hydrophobic domain of vesicle membranes, acting as a size-selective filter, only allowing passive diffusion of small solutes such as ions, nutrients, and antibiotics. Thus, drugs that are encapsulated in a nanocage functionalized with channel proteins are effectively protected from premature degradation by proteolytic enzymes. The drug molecule, however, is able to diffuse through the channel, driven by the concentration difference between the interior and the exterior of the nanocage.

Dendrimers are nanometer-sized, highly branched, and monodisperse macromolecules with symmetrical architecture [122]. They consist of a central core, branching units, and terminal functional groups. The core, together with the internal units, determines the environment of the nanocavities and consequently their solubilizing properties, whereas the external groups determine the solubility and chemical behavior of these polymers. Targeting effectiveness is affected by attaching targeting ligands at the external surface of dendrimers, while their stability and protection from the phagocytosis is achieved by functionalization of the dendrimers with PEG chains.

Nanocapsules are vesicular systems in which the drug is confined to a cavity surrounded by a polymer membrane, while nanospheres are matrix systems in which the drug is physically and uniformly dispersed [123]. Biodegradable polymeric nanoparticles have many applications in the controlled release of drugs, in targeting particular organs/tissues, as carriers of DNA in gene therapy, and in their ability to deliver proteins, peptides, and genes to the target tissue. Like for other nanocarriers, pharmacokinetics and the biodistribution profile of nanoparticles may be altered by varying the surface properties (e.g., addition of PEG chains) and attaching specific tissue-targeting ligands on the surface.

10.5 CONCLUSION

Distribution plays an important role in determining the magnitude and duration of a drug's therapeutic effect. Drug distribution is influenced by physical properties of the drug as well as physiologic factors such as blood perfusion, protein binding, and transporter activity. A number of physical and chemical methods are available to alter the distribution of the drug. These allow the therapeutic use of drug molecules that would otherwise have unfavorable distribution in the body.

REFERENCES

1. Tozer TN. *Clinical Pharmacokinetics Concepts and Applications*, 3rd ed. Baltimore: Lippincott Williams & Wilkins; 1995, pp 137–140.

2. Shargel L. *Applied Biopharmaceutics and Pharmacokinetics*, 4th ed. New York: McGraw-Hill; 1999, pp 281–291.

3. Dvorchik BH, Vesell ES. Pharmacokinetic interpretation of data gathered during therapeutic drug monitoring. *Clin Chem* 1976;22:868–878.

4. MacKichan JJ. Pharmacokinetic consequences of drug displacement from blood and tissue proteins. *Clin Pharmacokinet* 1984;9(Suppl 1):32–41.

5. Lin JH, Lu AY. Role of pharmacokinetics and metabolism in drug discovery and development. *Pharmacol Rev* 1997;49:403–449.

6. Aarons LJ, Rowland M. Kinetics of drug displacement interactions. *J Pharmacokinet Biopharm* 1981;9:181–190.

7. Vesell ES. Clinical pharmacology: a personal perspective. *Clin Pharmacol Ther* 1985;38: 603–612.

8. Aarons L, Salisbury R, Alam-Siddiqi M, Taylor L, Grennan DM. Plasma and synovial fluid kinetics of flurbiprofen in rheumatoid arthritis. *Br J Clin Pharmacol* 1986;21: 155–163.

9. Schuhmann G, Fichtl B, Kurz H. Prediction of drug distribution *in vivo* on the basis of *in vitro* binding data. *Biopharm Drug Dispos* 1987;8:73–86.

10. Lloyd JB. Lysosome membrane permeability: implications for drug delivery. *Adv Drug Deliv Rev* 2000;41:189–200.

11. Rang HP, Ritter JM, Moore PK, Lamb P. *Pharmacology*, 4th ed. Edinburgh: Churchill Livingstone; 2001, pp 91–105.

12. Hogben CA, Tocco DJ, Brodie BB, Schanker LS. On the mechanism of intestinal absorption of drugs. *J Pharmacol Exp Ther* 1959;125:275–282.

13. Shore ML. Biological applications of kinetic analysis of a two-compartment open system. *J Appl Physiol* 1961;16:771–782.

14. Schanker LS. Passage of drugs across body membranes. *Pharmacol Rev* 1962;14: 501–530.

15. Olanoff LS, Anderson JM. Controlled release of tetracycline–III: A physiological pharmacokinetic model of the pregnant rat. *J Pharmacokinet Biopharm* 1980;8:599–620.

16. Ingbar SH, Freinkel N. The influence of ACTH, cortisone, and hydrocortisone on the distribution and peripheral metabolism of thyroxine. *J Clin Invest* 1955;34:1375–1379.

17. Artursson P, Karlsson J. Correlation between oral drug absorption in humans and apparent drug permeability coefficients in human intestinal epithelial (Caco-2) cells. *Biochem Biophys Res Commun* 1991;175:880–885.

18. Taylor DC, Pownall R, Burke W. The absorption of beta-adrenoceptor antagonists in rat *in-situ* small intestine; the effect of lipophilicity. *J Pharm Pharmacol* 1985;37:280–283.

19. Simons K, Vaz WL. Model systems, lipid rafts, and cell membranes. *Annu Rev Biophys Biomol Struct* 2004;33:269–295.

20. Crone C, Christensen O. Electrical resistance of a capillary endothelium. *J Gen Physiol* 1981;77:349–371.

21. Butt AM, Jones HC, Abbott NJ. Electrical resistance across the blood–brain barrier in anaesthetized rats: a developmental study. *J Physiol* 1990;429:47–62.

22. Tamai I, Tsuji A. Transporter-mediated permeation of drugs across the blood–brain barrier. *J Pharm Sci* 2000;89:1371–1388.

23. Tsuji A. Small molecular drug transfer across the blood–brain barrier via carrier-mediated transport systems. *NeuroRx* 2005;2:54–62.

24. Ecker GF, Noe CR. *In silico* prediction models for blood–brain barrier permeation. *Curr Med Chem* 2004;11:1617–1628.

25. Suzuki H, Sugiyama Y. [Kinetic analysis of the disposition of hydrophilic drugs in the central nervous system (CNS): prediction of the CNS disposition from the transport properties in the blood–brain and blood–cerebrospinal fluid barriers]. *Yakugaku Zasshi* 1994;114:950–971.

26. Upton RN, Doolette DJ. Kinetic aspects of drug disposition in the lungs. *Clin Exp Pharmacol Physiol* 1999;26:381–391.

27. Avdeef A. Physicochemical profiling (solubility, permeability and charge state). *Curr Top Med Chem* 2001;1:277–351.

28. Obata K, Sugano K, Saitoh R, Higashida A, Nabuchi Y, Machida M, Aso Y. Prediction of oral drug absorption in humans by theoretical passive absorption model. *Int J Pharm* 2005;293:183–192.

29. Sue YJ, Shannon M. Pharmacokinetics of drugs in overdose. *Clin Pharmacokinet* 1992;23:93–105.

30. Levy G. Effects of plasma protein binding of drugs on duration and intensity of pharmacological activity. *J Pharm Sci* 1976;65:1264–1265.

31. Tocco DJ, deLuna FA, Duncan AE, Hsieh JH, Lin JH. Interspecies differences in stereoselective protein binding and clearance of MK-571. *Drug Metab Dispos* 1990;18:388–392.

32. Lin JH, deLuna FA, Ulm EH, Tocco DJ. Species-dependent enantioselective plasma protein binding of MK-571, a potent leukotriene D4 antagonist. *Drug Metab Dispos* 1990;18:484–487.

33. Eap CB, Cuendet C, Baumann P. Binding of *d*-methadone, *l*-methadone, and *dl*-methadone to proteins in plasma of healthy volunteers: role of the variants of alpha 1-acid glycoprotein. *Clin Pharmacol Ther* 1990;47:338–346.

34. Ruiz-Cabello F, Erill S. Abnormal serum protein binding of acidic drugs in diabetes mellitus. *Clin Pharmacol Ther* 1984;36:691–695.

35. Ryan DP, Matthews JM. Protein-protein interactions in human disease. *Curr Opin Struct Biol* 2005;15:441–446.

36. Kim RB. Transporters and drug discovery: why, when, and how. *Mol Pharm* 2006;3:26–32.

37. Zhang L, Strong JM, Qiu W, Lesko LJ, Huang SM. Scientific perspectives on drug transporters and their role in drug interactionst. *Mol Pharm* 2006;3:62–69.

38. Loo TW, Clarke DM. Recent progress in understanding the mechanism of P-glycoprotein-mediated drug efflux. *J Membr Biol* 2005;206:173–185.

39. Choo EF, Leake B, Wandel C, Imamura H, Wood AJ, Wilkinson GR, Kim RB. Pharmacological inhibition of P-glycoprotein transport enhances the distribution of HIV-1 protease inhibitors into brain and testes. *Drug Metab Dispos* 2000;28:655–660.

40. Gottesman MM, Ling V. The molecular basis of multidrug resistance in cancer: the early years of P-glycoprotein research. *FEBS Lett* 2006;580:998–1009.

41. Calcagno AM, Ludwig JA, Fostel JM, Gottesman MM, Ambudkar SV. Comparison of drug transporter levels in normal colon, colon cancer, and Caco-2 cells: impact on drug disposition and discovery. *Mol Pharm* 2006;3:87–93.

42. Schinkel AH, Jonker JW. Mammalian drug efflux transporters of the ATP binding cassette (ABC) family: an overview. *Adv Drug Deliv Rev* 2003;55:3–29.

43. Dean M, Hamon Y, Chimini G. The human ATP-binding cassette (ABC) transporter superfamily. *J Lipid Res* 2001;42:1007–1017.

44. Sugiyama Y, Ito K. Future prospects for toxicokinetics: prediction of drug disposition and adverse effects in humans from *in vitro* measurements of drug metabolism, transport and binding. *J Toxicol Sci* 1998;23(Suppl 4):647–652.

45. Greiner B, Eichelbaum M, Fritz P, Kreichgauer HP, von Richter O, Zundler J, Kroemer HK. The role of intestinal P-glycoprotein in the interaction of digoxin and rifampin. *J Clin Invest* 1999;104:147–153.

46. Edwards DJ, Fitzsimmons ME, Schuetz EG, Yasuda K, Ducharme MP, Warbasse LH, Woster PM, Schuetz JD, Watkins P. 6 ,7 -Dihydroxybergamottin in grapefruit juice and Seville orange juice: effects on cyclosporine disposition, enterocyte CYP3A4, and P-glycoprotein. *Clin Pharmacol Ther* 1999;65:237–244.

47. Kerb R, Hoffmeyer S, Brinkmann U. ABC drug transporters: hereditary polymorphisms and pharmacological impact in MDR1, MRP1 and MRP2. *Pharmacogenomics* 2001;2: 51–64.

48. Inui KI, Masuda S, Saito H, Cellular and molecular aspects of drug transport in the kidney. *Kidney Int* 2000;58:944–958.

49. You G. Towards an understanding of organic anion transporters: structure–function relationships. *Med Res Rev* 2004;24:762–774.

50. Masuda S, Inui K. [Molecular mechanisms on drug transporters in the drug absorption and disposition]. *Nippon Rinsho* 2002;60:65–73.

51. Sekine T, Cha SH, Endou H. The multispecific organic anion transporter (OAT) family. *Pflugers Arch* 2000;440:337–350.

52. Thomas MC, Tikellis C, Kantharidis P, Burns WC, Cooper ME, Forbes JM. The role of advanced glycation in reduced organic cation transport associated with experimental diabetes. *J Pharmacol Exp Ther* 2004;311:456–466.

53. Meyer UA. The molecular basis of genetic polymorphisms of drug metabolism. *J Pharm Pharmacol* 1994;46(Suppl 1):409–415.

54. Schinkel AH. Pharmacological insights from P-glycoprotein knockout mice. *Int J Clin Pharmacol Ther* 1998;36:9–13.

55. Schwab M, Eichelbaum M, Fromm MF. Genetic polymorphisms of the human MDR1 drug transporter. *Annu Rev Pharmacol Toxicol* 2003;43:285–307.

56. Sakaeda T, Nakamura T, Okumura K. Pharmacogenetics of MDR1 and its impact on the pharmacokinetics and pharmacodynamics of drugs. *Pharmacogenomics* 2003;4:397–410.

57. Kurata Y, Ieiri I, Kimura M, Morita T, Irie S, Urae A, Ohdo S, Ohtani H, Sawada Y, Higuchi S, Otsubo K. Role of human MDR1 gene polymorphism in bioavailability and interaction of digoxin, a substrate of P-glycoprotein. *Clin Pharmacol Ther* 2002;72:209–219.

58. Gerloff T, Schaefer M, Johne A, Oselin K, Meisel C, Cascorbi I, Roots I. MDR1 geno-types do not influence the absorption of a single oral dose of 1 mg digoxin in healthy white males. *Br J Clin Pharmacol* 2002;54:610–616.

59. Verstuyft C, Schwab M, Schaeffeler E, Kerb R, Brinkmann U, Jaillon P, Funck-Brentano C, Becquemont L. Digoxin pharmacokinetics and MDR1 genetic polymorphisms. *Eur J Clin Pharmacol* 2003;58:809–812.

60. Haufroid V, Mourad M, Van Kerckhove V, Wawrzyniak J, De Meyer M, Eddour DC, Malaise J, Lison D, Squifflet JP, Wallemacq P. The effect of CYP3A5 and MDR1 (ABCB1) polymorphisms on cyclosporine and tacrolimus dose requirements and trough blood levels in stable renal transplant patients. *Pharmacogenetics* 2004;14:147–154.

61. Krijt J, Vackova M, Kozich V. Measurement of homocysteine and other aminothiols in plasma: advantages of using tris(2-carboxyethyl)phosphine as reductant compared with tri-*N*-butylphosphine. *Clin Chem* 2001;47:1821–1828.

62. Tirona RG, Kim RB. Pharmacogenomics of organic anion-transporting polypeptides (OATP). *Adv Drug Deliv Rev* 2002;54:1343–1352.

63. Ieiri I, Suzuki H, Kimura M, Takane H, Nishizato Y, Irie S, Urae A, Kawabata K, Higuchi S, Otsubo K, Sugiyama Y. Influence of common variants in the pharmacokinetic genes (OATP-C, UGT1A1, and MRP2) on serum bilirubin levels in healthy subjects. *Hepatol Res* 2004;30:91–95.

64. Mwinyi J, Johne A, Bauer S, Roots I, Gerloff T. Evidence for inverse effects of OATP-C (SLC21A6) 5 and 1b haplotypes on pravastatin kinetics. *Clin Pharmacol Ther* 2004;75:415–421.

65. Niemi M, Schaeffeler E, Lang T, Fromm MF, Neuvonen M, Kyrklund C, Backman JT, Kerb R, Schwab M, Neuvonen PJ, Eichelbaum M, Kivisto KT. High plasma pravastatin concentrations are associated with single nucleotide polymorphisms and haplotypes of organic anion transporting polypeptide-C (OATP-C, SLCO1B1). *Pharmacogenetics* 2004;14:429–440.

66. Evans WE, Johnson JA. Pharmacogenomics: the inherited basis for interindividual differences in drug response. *Annu Rev Genomics Hum Genet* 2001;2:9–39.

67. Albert A. Chemical aspects of selective toxicity. *Nature* 1958;182:421–422.

68. Stella VJ, Charman WN, Naringrekar VH. Prodrugs. Do they have advantages in clinical practice? *Drugs* 1985;29:455–473.

69. Banerjee PK, Amidon GL. Physicochemical property modification strategies based on enzyme substrate specificities I: rationale, synthesis, and pharmaceutical properties of aspirin derivatives. *J Pharm Sci* 1981;70:1299–1303.

70. Han HK, Amidon GL. Targeted prodrug design to optimize drug delivery. *AAPS Pharm Sci* 2000;2:E6.

71. Cobb LM, Hacker T, Nolan J. NAD(P)H nitroblue tetrazolium reductase levels in apparently normoxic tissues: a histochemical study correlating enzyme activity with binding of radiolabelled misonidazole. *Br J Cancer* 1990;61:524–529.

72. Knox RJ, Connors TA. Prodrugs in cancer chemotherapy. *Pathol Oncol Res* 1997;3: 309–324.

73. Bagshawe KD. Antibody-directed enzyme prodrug therapy for cancer: its theoretical basis and application. *Mol Med Today* 1995;1:424–431.

74. Mizuma T, Ohta K, Hayashi M, Awazu S. Comparative study of active absorption by the intestine and disposition of anomers of sugar-conjugated compounds. *Biochem Pharmacol* 1993;45:1520–1523.

75. Swaan PW, Tukker JJ. Carrier-mediated transport mechanism of foscarnet (trisodium phosphonoformate hexahydrate) in rat intestinal tissue. *J Pharmacol Exp Ther* 1995;272:242–247.

76. Grappel SF, Giovenella AJ, Nisbet LJ. Activity of a peptidyl prodrug, alafosfalin, against anaerobic bacteria. *Antimicrob Agents Chemother* 1985;27:961–963.

77. Oh DM, Han HK, Amidon GL. Drug transport and targeting. Intestinal transport. *Pharm Biotechnol* 1999;12:59–88.

78. Caliceti P, Veronese FM. Pharmacokinetic and biodistribution properties of poly(ethylene glycol)–protein conjugates. *Adv Drug Deliv Rev* 2003;55:1261–1277.

79. Veronese FM, Pasut G. PEGylation, successful approach to drug delivery. *Drug Discov Today* 2005;10:1451–1458.

80. Harris JM, Martin NE, Modi M. Pegylation: a novel process for modifying pharmacokinetics. *Clin Pharmacokinet* 2001;40:539–551.

81. Francis GE, Delgado C, Fisher D, Malik F, Agrawal AK. Polyethylene glycol modification: relevance of improved methodology to tumour targeting. *J Drug Target* 1996;3: 321–340.

82. Mukai Y, Yoshioka Y, Tsutsumi Y, Phage display and PEGylation of therapeutic proteins. *Comb Chem High Throughput Screen* 2005;8:145–152.

83. Florence AT, Jani PU. Novel oral drug formulations. Their potential in modulating adverse effects. *Drug Saf* 1994;10:233–266.

84. Delgado C, Francis GE, Fisher D. The uses and properties of PEG-linked proteins. *Crit Rev Ther Drug Carrier Syst* 1992;9:249–304.

85. Crawford J. Clinical uses of pegylated pharmaceuticals in oncology. *Cancer Treat Rev* 2002;28(Suppl A):7–11.

86. Crawford J. Clinical benefits of pegylated proteins in oncology. *Cancer Treat Rev* 2002;28(Suppl A):1–2.

87. Bhadra D, Bhadra S, Jain P, Jain NK. Pegnology: a review of PEG-ylated systems. *Pharmazie* 2002;57:5–29.

88. Bergholz H, Erttmann RR, Damm KH. Effects of probenecid on plasma/tissue distribution of ^{14}C-benzylpenicillin in rats. *Experientia* 1980;36:333–334.

89. Adriani J, Naraghi M. The pharmacologic principles of regional pain relief. *Annu Rev Pharmacol Toxicol* 1977;17:223–242.

90. Black KL, Ningaraj NS. Modulation of brain tumor capillaries for enhanced drug delivery selectively to brain tumor. *Cancer Control* 2004;11:165–173.

91. Pardridge WM. Blood–brain barrier drug targeting: the future of brain drug development. *Mol Interv* 2003;3:90–105, 51.

92. Volk HA, Loscher W. Multidrug resistance in epilepsy: rats with drug-resistant seizures exhibit enhanced brain expression of P-glycoprotein compared with rats with drug-responsive seizures. *Brain* 2005;128:1358–1368.

93. Liu XD, Pan GY, Xie L, Hou YY, Lan W, Su Q, Liu GQ. Cyclosporin A enhanced protection of nimodipine against brain damage induced by hypoxia-ischemia in mice and rats. *Acta Pharmacol Sin* 2002;23:225–229.

94. Fellner S, Bauer B, Miller DS, Schaffrik M, Fankhanel M, Spruss T, Bernhardt G, Graeff C, Farber L, Gschaidmeier H, Buschauer A, Fricker G. Transport of paclitaxel (Taxol) across the blood–brain barrier *in vitro* and *in vivo*. *J Clin Invest* 2002;110:1309–1318.

95. Kim RB, Fromm MF, Wandel C, Leake B, Wood AJ, Roden DM, Wilkinson GR. The drug transporter P-glycoprotein limits oral absorption and brain entry of HIV-1 protease inhibitors. *J Clin Invest* 1998;101:289–294.

96. Kirkinezos IG, Hernandez D, Bradley WG, Moraes CT. An ALS mouse model with a permeable blood–brain barrier benefits from systemic cyclosporine A treatment. *J Neurochem* 2004;88:821–826.

97. Bauer B, Hartz AM, Fricker G, Miller DS. Modulation of P-glycoprotein transport function at the blood–brain barrier. *Exp Biol Med (Maywood)* 2005;230:118–127.

98. Boyle FM, Eller SL, Grossman SA. Penetration of intra-arterially administered vincristine in experimental brain tumor. *Neuro-oncol* 2004;6:300–305.

99. Kemper EM, Boogerd W, Thuis I, Beijnen JH, van Tellingen O. Modulation of the blood–brain barrier in oncology: therapeutic opportunities for the treatment of brain tumours? *Cancer Treat Rev* 2004;30:415–423.

100. Sadeque AJ, Wandel C, He H, Shah S, Wood AJ. Increased drug delivery to the brain by P-glycoprotein inhibition. *Clin Pharmacol Ther* 2000;68:231–237.

101. Iannetti P, Spalice A, Parisi P. Calcium-channel blocker verapamil administration in prolonged and refractory status epilepticus. *Epilepsia* 2005;46:967–969.

102. Summers MA, Moore JL, McAuley JW. Use of verapamil as a potential P-glycoprotein inhibitor in a patient with refractory epilepsy. *Ann Pharmacother* 2004;38:1631–1634.

103. Ferry DR, Traunecker H, Kerr DJ. Clinical trials of P-glycoprotein reversal in solid tumours. *Eur J Cancer* 1996;32A:1070–1081.

104. Shabbits JA, Krishna R, Mayer LD. Molecular and pharmacological strategies to overcome multidrug resistance. *Expert Rev Anticancer Ther* 2001;1:585–594.

105. Twentyman PR, Bleehen NM. Resistance modification by PSC-833, a novel non-immunosuppressive cyclosporin [corrected]. *Eur J Cancer* 1991;27:1639–1642.

106. Oza AM. Clinical development of P glycoprotein modulators in oncology. *Novartis Found Symp* 2002;243:103–115; discussion 115–118, 180–185.

107. Fracasso PM, Brady MF, Moore DH, Walker JL, Rose PG, Letvak L, Grogan TM, McGuire WP. Phase II study of paclitaxel and valspodar (PSC 833) in refractory ovarian carcinoma: a gynecologic oncology group study. *J Clin Oncol* 2001;19:2975–2982.

108. Ma MK, McLeod HL, Westervelt P, Fracasso PM. Pharmacokinetic study of infusional valspodar. *J Clin Pharmacol* 2002;42:412–418.

109. Agrawal M, Abraham J, Balis FM, Edgerly M, Stein WD, Bates S, Fojo T, Chen CC. Increased 99mTc-sestamibi accumulation in normal liver and drug-resistant tumors after the administration of the glycoprotein inhibitor, XR9576. *Clin Cancer Res* 2003;9:650–656.

110. Bigott HM, Prior JL, Piwnica-Worms DR, Welch MJ. Imaging multidrug resistance P-glycoprotein transport function using microPET with technetium-94m-sestamibi. *Mol Imaging* 2005;4:30–39.

111. Haus-Cohen M, Assaraf YG, Binyamin L, Benhar I, Reiter Y. Disruption of P-glycoprotein anticancer drug efflux activity by a small recombinant single-chain Fv antibody fragment targeted to an extracellular epitope. *Int J Cancer* 2004;109:750–758.

112. Mechetner EB, Roninson IB. Efficient inhibition of P-glycoprotein-mediated multidrug resistance with a monoclonal antibody. *Proc Natl Acad Sci USA* 1992;89:5824–5828.

113. Kang H, Fisher MH, Xu D, Miyamoto YJ, Marchand A, Van Aerschot A, Herdewijn P, Juliano RL. Inhibition of MDR1 gene expression by chimeric HNA antisense oligonucleotides. *Nucleic Acids Res* 2004;32:4411–4419.

114. Lee ES, Na K, Bae YH. Doxorubicin loaded pH-sensitive polymeric micelles for reversal of resistant MCF-7 tumor. *J Control Release* 2005;103:405–418.

115. Batrakova EV, Li S, Elmquist WF, Miller DW, Alakhov VY, Kabanov AV. Mechanism of sensitization of MDR cancer cells by Pluronic block copolymers: selective energy depletion. *Br J Cancer* 2001;85:1987–1997.

116. Tarasova NI, Seth R, Tarasov SG, Kosakowska-Cholody T, Hrycyna CA, Gottesman MM, Michejda CJ. Transmembrane inhibitors of P-glycoprotein, an ABC transporter. *J Med Chem* 2005;48:3768–3775.

117. Xu D, Ye D, Fisher M, Juliano RL. Selective inhibition of P-glycoprotein expression in multidrug-resistant tumor cells by a designed transcriptional regulator. *J Pharmacol Exp Ther* 2002;302:963–971.

118. Langer R. Drug delivery and targeting. *Nature* 1998;392:5–10.

119. Kayser O, Lemke A, Hernandez-Trejo N. The impact of nanobiotechnology on the development of new drug delivery systems. *Curr Pharm Biotechnol* 2005;6:3–5.

120. Muller Goymann CC. Physicochemical characterization of colloidal drug delivery systems such as reverse micelles, vesicles, liquid crystals and nanoparticles for topical administration. *Eur J Pharm Biopharm* 2004;58:343–356.

121. Hart SL. Lipid carriers for gene therapy. *Curr Drug Deliv* 2005;2:423–428.

122. Iwamura M. [Dendritic systems for drug delivery applications]. *Nippon Rinsho* 2006;64:231–237.

123. Mayer C. Nanocapsules as drug delivery systems. *Int J Artif Organs* 2005;28:1163–1171.

11

THE BLOOD–BRAIN BARRIER AND ITS EFFECT ON ABSORPTION AND DISTRIBUTION

A. G. DE BOER[1] AND P. J. GAILLARD[2]

[1]University of Leiden, Leiden, The Netherlands
[2]to-BBB Technologies BV, Leiden, The Netherlands

Contents

11.1 INTRODUCTION

The central nervous system (CNS) is a sanctuary site and is protected by various barriers. These regulate brain homeostasis and the transport of endogenous and exogenous compounds by controlling their selective and specific uptake, efflux, and

Preclinical Development Handbook: ADME and Biopharmaceutical Properties,
edited by Shayne Cox Gad
Copyright © 2008 John Wiley & Sons, Inc.

metabolism in the brain. Unfortunately, potential drugs for the treatment of most brain diseases are therefore often not able to cross these barriers. As a result, various drug delivery and targeting strategies are currently being developed to enhance the absorption and distribution of drugs into the brain. This chapter discusses the biology and physiology of the blood–brain barrier (BBB) and the blood–cerebrospinal fluid barrier with respect to drug transport (absorption, distribution), the *in vitro* and *in vivo* methods to measure BBB transport, and the possibilities to deliver large molecular drugs, by viral and receptor-mediated nonviral drug delivery, to the (human) brain.

11.2 BARRIERS IN THE BRAIN

There are three barriers that limit drug transport to the brain parenchyma. These are the blood–brain barrier (BBB) localized in the capillaries in the brain, the blood–cerebrospinal fluid barrier (BCSFB) that is presented by the choroid plexus epithelium in the ventricles, and the ependyma that is an epithelial layer of cells covering the brain tissue in the ventricles and limits the transport of compounds from the CSF to the brain tissue.

11.2.1 Blood–Brain Barrier (BBB)

In 1885 Ehrlich [1] was the first to show evidence for the existence of a barrier between blood and brain. He injected vital dyes intravenously and found that, in contrast to other tissues, it did not stain the brain [1]. His successor, Goldman [2], injected these dyes into the cerebral spinal fluid, after which staining of the brain was observed, but not of the peripheral organs. Since this seminal discovery, much research has been performed on the (patho) physiology and pharmacology of the BBB (see also other reviews [3–9]).

The current knowledge is that the BBB is situated at the interface of blood and brain and its primary function is to maintain the homeostasis of the brain. Furthermore, the BBB is not uniform throughout the brain, since the capillaries in the circumventricular organs (CVOs) are fenestrated [10, 11]. Figure 11.1 gives a schematic representation of the barriers present in the CNS.

The human BBB has a total blood vessel length of approximately 600 km. In fact, every cubic centimeter of the cortex comprises the amazing sum of 1 km of blood vessels. It has an estimated surface area of approximately $20 m^2$, which is claimed to be similar to the BCSFB [12, 13]. However, the surface area of the BCSFB is facing the CSF and not the blood, which makes the BBB, based on total blood flow and its wide vascular bed, functionally the most important global influx barrier for solutes to reach the brain [10, 11].

The BBB is mainly formed by brain capillary endothelial cells (BCECs) [14], although other cell types such as pericytes, astrocytes, and neuronal cells also play an important role in the function of the BBB [15–19]. BCECs are different from peripheral endothelial cells, as can be seen schematically in Fig. 11.2 (in which the specific surroundings of the brain capillaries are shown). BCECs have specific characteristics, such as tight junctions, which prevent paracellular transport of small and large (water-soluble) compounds from blood to the brain [14, 20, 21]. Furthermore,

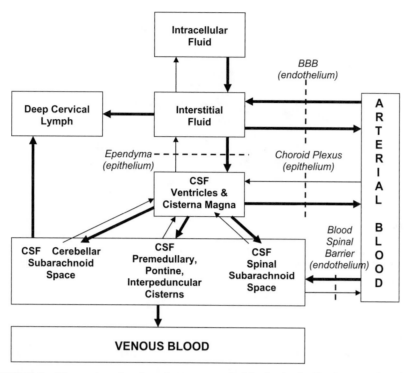

FIGURE 11.1 The various barriers that one can find in the brain (broken lines) representing the blood–brain barrier, the blood–cerebrospinal fluid (CSF) barrier, the brain–CSF barrier, and the blood–spinal barrier. The blood–brain barrier has the largest surface area and is therefore considered to be the most important influx barrier for solutes to reach the brain. In addition, paths are shown for fluid movement (solid arrows) between cerebral intracellular fluid (ICF), intrastitial fluid (ISF), cerebrospinal fluid (CSF), blood, and lymphatics. Thick arrows represent major paths of fluid movement under normal conditions. Thin arrows represent minor paths of fluid movement under normal conditions. (Adapted from Ref. 45.)

transcellular transport from blood to brain is limited as a result of low vesicular transport, high metabolic activity, and a lack of fenestrae [15]. It functions as a physical, a metabolic [22–24], and an immunological barrier [25]. In addition, receptors at the BBB may play a role in brain signaling (e.g., insulin receptor [26], LRP1,2 receptor [27]). These specific characteristics of the BBB are induced and maintained by the (endfeet of) astrocytes, surrounding the BCECs [15, 28], as well as by neuronal endings, which can directly innervate the BCECs [14, 29]. Pericytes also play a role at the BBB, as they share the continuous capillary basement membrane with the BCECs [30]. Their phagocytotic activity forms an additional BBB property [10]. Furthermore, pericytes regulate endothelial homeostasis by inducing the endothelial release of plasminogen-activator inhibitor-1 (PAI-1), thereby negatively regulating brain endothelial fibrinolysis [31].

Until now, many transport systems have been discovered that play an important role in maintaining BBB integrity and brain homeostasis but also influence drug transport to the brain. These comprise carrier-mediated transport (CMT) and receptor-mediated transport (RMT) systems including cationic and anionic influx

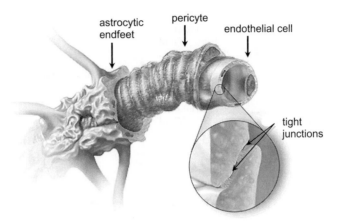

FIGURE 11.2   Schematic representation of surrounding pericytes (covering about 20–30% of the capillary surface) and astrocytic endfeet projecting on the endothelial cells of the cerebral capillaries that induce and maintain the blood–brain barrier. In contrast, endothelial cells of peripheral capillaries do not form a tight barrier because they lack the specific input of these brain cells. See text for details. (Reprinted with permission from G. Miller, *Science* 2002;297:1116–1118. Illustration: C Slayden. © 2002 AAAS.)

and efflux systems like P-glycoprotein [32, 33], multidrug resistance proteins [34, 35], nucleoside transporters, organic anion transporters (OATs), organic cation transporters (OCTs), large amino acid transporter, and the RMT systems like the transferrin-1 and -2 receptors, the melanotransferrin receptor [27], and the scavenger receptors SB-AI and SB-BI [36–38].

Because of the complex interactions between cell types and the transport of compounds to and from the brain, as well as the dynamic regulation of the BBB properties (e.g., receptor expression, formation of tight junctions), the "multitasking" BBB [39], or the "neurovascular unit" [5, 40], is considered to be an organ protecting the brain [36]. In addition, these properties are influenced by disease and drug effects, which will change the functionality of the BBB under such conditions and will influence drug delivery to the brain [6, 7, 41].

11.2.2   Blood–Cerebrospinal Fluid Barrier (BCSFB) and Ependyma

The BCSFB is a rather complicated system (see other reviews also [42–44]). It comprises mainly the choroidal and arachnoidal epithelium giving access to the ventricular and subarachnoidal CSF, respectively. Considering its location and the direction of the CSF flow, the choroidal epithelium at the choroid plexuses (CPs) can be considered to be the most important part of the BCSFB, which are located in the lateral ventricles and in the third and fourth ventricles. The CP functions as a physical, an enzymatic, and an immunological barrier and plays a role in drug metabolism, drug transport, repair, and signaling. It presents phase I–III enzymes [43]. Phase I enzymes are used for functionalization of drugs and include cytochrome P450 isoform (CYP2B1,2) and monoamine oxidase. Phase II enzymes are used for conjugation of drugs and include glutathione and glucuronosyl transferases. Phase III enzymes include transporters like Na-dicarboxylate cotransporter, the ascorbic acid transporter, the organic anion transporter (OAT), the organic anion transporter polypeptide 1 and 2 (OATP1,2), the organic cation transporter (OCT), equilibrating and concentrative nucleotide transporters (ENTs and CNTs), and multidrug transporters like P-gp and MRP1 [4, 33, 34, 36]. Furthermore, the CP seems to be involved in repair by secreting neuroprotective compounds and acting as a site of neurogenesis [43]. In addition, the CPs express many receptors and several of them are involved in signaling between the immune system and the brain ([46]) and pathology of the CP has been found in many CNS disease conditions [43].

In humans the total volume of the CSF is about 160 mL and the formation rate is about 0.35–0.40 mL/min. It is produced mainly by the CPs (60%) and the other part (40%) via ultrafiltration by brain capillaries [47]. It flows from the lateral to the third and fourth ventricles and subsequently into the cisterna magna and other large basal cisterns (see Fig. 11.1). From there the CSF flows posterior and downward into the subarachnoid space around the spinal cord and upward around the cerebral hemispheres. Via the arachnoidal villi in the subarachnoidal space the CSF flows outward into venous blood.

Since the endothelium in the blood capillaries in the CP is fenestrated, resistance to drug transport seems to be presented by (gap) junctions of the CP epithelium, which are more permeable than the tight junctions of the BBB endothelium [42]. Moreover, blood flow in the CP blood capillaries seems to be 5–10 times higher than the mean cerebral blood flow [43, 46, 48]. In addition, it has been calculated that the total surface area of all CPs is of the same order of magnitude as the entire BBB [13]. All these facts together allow for the possibility of substantial drug transport via the CPs into the CSF. However, as mentioned before, the surface area of the BCSFB is facing the CSF and not the blood, which makes drug transport to the CSF less effective. Moreover, from the point of view of drug transport to the brain parenchyma, the BCSFB has some disadvantages. Once a drug is in the CSF, an additional barrier for the transport of molecules is presented by the ependyma covering the ventricles. The ependyma is a single layer of epithelial cells connected by (gap) junctions and seems to be rather permeable, particularly to small molecular lipophilic compounds, while permeability for macromolecular drugs has been claimed (see also in Section 11.4.1, Direct Injection/Infusion of Macromolecular Drugs) [42].

11.3   METHODS TO MEASURE DRUG TRANSPORT TO THE BRAIN

11.3.1   *In Vitro* Methods

Research on drug transport across the BBB and BBB functionality has been very much enhanced by the availability of *in vitro* BBB (co)culture systems and many attempts have been made to develop such systems [49–60]. In addition, the use of such systems allows a detailed investigation of BBB related phenomena at the (sub)cellular level in the absence of feedback systems from the rest of the body. This makes it much easier to study *in vitro* BBB transport and BBB functionality by (pharmacological) intervention techniques like the application of receptor agonists and antagonists, blockers of transporters and enzymes, interference RNA and (anti)gene approaches, and the influence of disease.

BBB (co)culture systems comprise primary isolated cells (including their isolation procedures) or cell lines, the use of endothelial cells alone or cocultured with astrocytes (rat fetal or C_6-glioma), the application of epithelial cells as a BBB model, and the use and availability of human cell lines [61]. One of the most important issues is the variability and transference of data between laboratories [62] and the pitfalls in performing experiments and evaluating permeability data [63].

Primary Isolated Cells

Comparison of Isolation Procedures   Preparation of the *in vitro* BBB from primary isolated cells involves the isolation of capillaries and culture of BCECs alone or in combination with astrocytes or astrocyte conditioned medium. The first step in the culture of BCECs is the isolation of brain capillaries or brain capillary fragments. These can be isolated from human, bovine, porcine, and rat brain by various procedures, all starting with the grey matter of the brain [64]. Although human material would be most ideal from a scientific point of view, it is less easily available, and therefore most routinely applied procedures start from animal brains. Preferentially, bovine or porcine brains are used because of their larger mass and therefore the large amount of brain capillaries that can be isolated. The isolation procedures that have been used most frequently can be classified into nonenzymatic mechanical, combined mechanical–enzymatic, or enzymatic procedures [65–69]. The typical main steps in the various procedures are shown in Table 11.1.

The *enzymatic procedure* [65, 66] is rather time consuming (about 8 h). Following mincing of the brains into 1–2 mm cubes, two enzymatic and two separation steps are performed to isolate brain capillaries. First, an incubation step is performed with dispase followed by a dextran centrifugation/separation; and second, an incubation step with dispase/collagenase is followed by a Percoll gradient separation.

The *mechanical procedure* [55, 67] is fast and lasts 1–2 h for the isolation of capillaries from bovine brain. The brains are homogenized using two different potters. Subsequently, two filtration steps are applied: first, one isolating the material that stays behind on a 150 μm mesh, and second, one that collects the material, including capillaries that go through a 200 μm mesh.

The *combined mechanical–enzymatic procedure* [68, 69] lasts for about 4 h. It comprises the homogenization of brains by a Wheaton homogenizer followed by a filtration step through a 150 μm nylon mesh. The trapped material is subsequently treated with collagenase/DNAse and filtered through a 200 μm nylon mesh. The capillary fraction is collected by centrifugation and may be stored at −80 °C by freezing in a mix of fetal calf serum and 10% (v/v) DMSO.

Culture of BCECs   Brain capillaries may be plated and cultured in culture flasks. The BCECs, which have grown out of the capillaries, may be isolated by (micro)trypsinization and plated in culture flasks or on (polycarbonate) porous filters. Cecchelli's group [55, 67] claims that the mechanical procedure results in pure BCEC cultures: first, because of the isolation of brain capillaries (not arterioles and venules) that is provided by a selective adhesion at an extracellular matrix of corneal endothelial cells, and second, because of a microtrypsinization that avoids contamination by other cell types. In the other two methods, collagen (human placenta type IV) and human plasma fibronectin [69] or rat-tail collagen with fibronectin [65, 66]

TABLE 11.1 Overview of the Main Steps in the Various Brain Capillary and Brain Capillary Endothelial Cell (BCEC) Isolation Procedures

Mechanical [55, 67]	Mechanical–Enzymatic [68, 69]	Enzymatic [65, 66]
Bovine brain grey matter	Bovine brain grey matter	Bovine brain grey matter
Homogenization (with two different potters)	Homogenization (Wheaton homogenizer)	Minced to 1–2 mm cubes
Filtration step 1 (<150 μm mesh)	Filtration step 1 (<150 μm mesh)	Dispase incubation (2.5 h)
Filtration step 2 (>200 μm mesh)	Collagenase/DNAse incubation (1 h)	Dextran centrifugation
Selective adhesion of capillaries at CEC[a] matrix)	Filtration step 2 (>200 μm mesh)	Collagenase/dispase incubation (4 h)
Growing BCECs	Selective adhesion of capillaries at collagen type IV)[b] and fibronectin[c] matrix	Percoll gradient
Collection of BCECs by microtrypsinization	Growing BCECs	Selective adhesion of capillaries at rat-tail collagen and fibronectin matrix
Plating BCECs and astrocytes at bottom of well	Collection of BCECs by trypsinization	Growing BCECs
	Plating BCECs and astrocytes at the other side of the filter	Collection of BCECs by trypsinization Plating BCECs

[a]CEC, corneal endothelial cell.
[b]Human placenta type IV collagen.
[c]Human plasma fibronectin.
Source: From Ref. 362, with permission.

replace the selective isolation of capillaries by the corneal endothelial cell matrix. This avoids the periodical isolation of corneal endothelial cells. The selectivity of the latter two methods is further guaranteed/enhanced by the application of either a Percoll gradient [65] or the time for attachment (2–4 h) of the capillary fragments at the collagen/fibronectin coating [69]. In addition, the application of 50% ACM in the procedure of Gaillard et al. [69] enhances the selective outgrowth of BCECs. Subsequently, in one step BCECs can be selectively collected following a short trypsinization time (<1.5 min). By this procedure one can obtain enough BCECs to get about 1000 (24 wells) filters from one isolation. The method of Audus and Borchardt [65, 66] also results in the isolation of capillaries and subsequently in a large amount of endothelial cells. In addition, the procedure of Dehouck et al. [55, 67] results in a substantial amount of BCECs to cover filters (about 300), but BCECs have to be passed at least 4–7 times. Unfortunately, passing primary cultured cells will eventually lead to a loss of BBB properties. In this respect, the preservation of properties is in our opinion an important issue and it has been shown that several can be reinduced by astrocytes [70–72].

The mechanical isolation procedure reduces the risk of losing surface molecules, which can occur during enzymatic treatment, particularly when aspecific proteases are applied and when these are not reinduced. This risk is less following collagenase treatment since this is a more selective enzyme. Therefore, induction of surface molecules is particularly important for enzymatically isolated cells, since it helps to reinduce BBB properties/molecules. In addition, it may be worthwhile to know that endothelial cells have the special property to transdifferentiate from one phenotype to another by the influence of environmental factors [73].

Importance of Astrocytes in BBB Culture Systems   BCECs may be grown to confluency alone or in the presence of ACM or astrocytes. The use of astrocytes or ACM enhances the expression of various surface molecules and transporters and increases paracellular tightness [49–51, 68, 70–72].

Most frequently, astrocytes isolated from newborn rats and rat C_6-glioma cells have been used. Together with bovine or porcine BCECs, one obtains xenogenic coculture systems, which are very useful in studying drug transport and BBB functionality. In addition, preliminary data from our lab show that it is possible to construct an allogenic system of bovine BCECs with bovine astrocytes. However, these astrocytes were obtained from brains of 6–8 month old calves, which grow significantly slower than astrocytes of newborn rats and prolong culture time. A rat allogenic BBB coculture system has been established comprising rat BCECs and fetal rat astrocytes [74], and a mouse syngenic BBB coculture model has also been developed [75]. However, the disadvantage of these systems is that the amount of endothelial cells that can be obtained from mouse and rat brain is rather small in comparison to bovine and porcine brain and therefore these procedures are not yet suitable for large scale production of cocultures.

Astrocytes can be seeded at the bottom of (mostly polycarbonate) porous filters and at the bottom of the well. This may give rise to differences in endothelial functionality since factors released by the astrocytes influence BBB endothelial cells [67, 70–72]. Therefore, to study BBB functionality, particularly under acute stress conditions, endothelial cells and astrocytes should be in contact or in close approximation to each other for an optimal feedback. This is less necessary in studying only endothelial permeability of drugs. However, it may be argued that due to pharmacodynamic effects of drugs, increased or decreased endothelial permeability may be found caused by a less adequate feedback by astrocytes and astrocytic factors.

Other Cells in BBB Cultures   Other cells that may occur following isolation of BCECs are pericytes and fibroblasts. Pericytes are normally present at the BBB and are surrounded by a basement membrane and have been shown to induce separately specific enzymes in BCECs [76]. In addition, it has been argued that pericytes are necessary to establish an *in vivo*-like BBB cell culture model [31]. Fibroblasts are present in brain tissue, but not very much is known about their influence at the BBB. Other cells may also have an important action in BBB cell culture systems, such as neurons, microglia, and monocytes, and it may be argued that combinations of these cells should be present in a BBB cell culture system for optimal functionality. This has been described for an *in vitro* BBB model comprising human BCECs, human fetal astrocytes, human macrophages, and neuronal (human teratocarcinoma) cells [77]. Other systems have been developed comprising cultured monolayers of brain endothelial cell lines or selected epithelial cell lines, combined with astrocyte and neuron cultures that present a novel three-dimensional technique for the screening of neurotoxic compounds [78].

As mentioned before, human material is rather difficult to obtain regularly in large quantities. A good alternative is the use of human umbilical vein endothelial cells (HUVECs). These can be rather easily obtained and when cultured under proper conditions, such as with astrocytes, a human-like BBB system may be obtained [79]. Alternatively, human endothelial cells from skin capillaries can be used in combination with postnatal rat astrocytes [80]. Such systems are convenient for several purposes (such as transcellular lipophilic/hydrophilic transport and carrier/receptor-mediated transport) and are easy to obtain in large quantities. Still, it may be expected that the functionality of such cells is different from primary cultured BCECs (with respect to tightness, up/downregulation of transporters, etc.) although this has not been demonstrated until now.

Application of Barrier Enhancers   It has been shown that several compounds like cAMP, phosphodiesterase inhibitors, glucocorticoids, and interferon-α,β may be used to enhance the tightness of BBB endothelial monolayers [68, 69, 81, 82]. In addition, the application of basic fibroblast growth factor (bFGF; secreted by astrocytes [83, 84]) is important in growing/establishing functional and tight BBB cell culture systems [55] and in the induction of BBB properties [84].

Application of these enhancers has increased the ease of culture and the properties of the cell culture system. However, apart from the lack of functional influence of astrocytes, the question that still has to be answered is how these compounds influence other aspects of BBB functionality in addition to endothelial tightness.

Endothelial Cell Lines   Various immortalized brain capillary endothelial cell lines have been derived. These are made by transfection of these cells with an immortalizing gene. An overview of the most frequently used cell lines is given in Table 11.2. These cell lines have various properties that resemble *in vivo* BBB capillary endothelial cells. The advantage of cell lines is their ease in culture, their purity, and the fact that there is no need for a periodic isolation of capillaries from brains. Since these cell lines are obtained by immortalization, it may be expected that their functionality will be changed compared to primary cultured BCECs. This is illustrated by the fact that most of these cell lines are rather permeable (paracellular leakiness), which limits their use in studying BBB transport. The application of these cells is particularly useful for (immuno)histochemical identification of extra- and intracellular molecules, for studying morphological aspects of endothelial cells, and so on. In addition, barrier enhancers (see also previous paragraph) may be used to improve the tightness of these monolayers. Recently, a human brain immortalized endothelial cell line was established by transfection of the human telomerase or SV40 T antigen. This cell line (hCMEC/D3) represents a stable, well characterized, and well differentiated human brain endothelial cell line and offers opportunities for BBB research [61].

Tumor Cell Systems   The application of rat C_6-glioma cells makes the culture of astrocytes much easier. This provides the same advantages as with cell lines. Table 11.3 gives an overview of the various sources of astrocytes and their application in

TABLE 11.2   Overview of the Used Immortalized Brain Capillary Endothelial Cell Lines

Cell Line	Source	References
SV-BEC	Bovine	100
t-BBEC-117	Bovine	101
BBEC-SV	Bovine	102
RBEC1	Rat	103
TR-BBB	Rat	104
RBE4	Rat	105
CR3	Rat	106
RCE-T1	Rat	107
GPNT	Rat	108, 109
GP8.3	Rat	110
TM-BBB	Mouse	111
MBEC	Mouse	112
S5C	Mouse	113
PBMEC/C1-2	Porcine	114
SV-HEC	Human	115
BB19	Human	116
HBEC-51	Human	117

Source: From Ref. 363, with permission.

TABLE 11.3   Astrocytes Used in Coculture with Endothelial or Epithelial Cells of Various Sources

Astrocyte	Coculture with Endothelium[a]
Newborn rat astrocyte	BCECs (bovine) [55, 67, 69]
Newborn rat astrocyte cell line (A_7)	BCECs (bovine) [118]
C_6-rat glioma	BCECs (bovine) [119]
C_6-rat glioma	HUVECs (human) [79]
C_6-rat glioma	RBE4 (rat) [120]
C_6-rat glioma	Aortic (bovine) [121]
TR-AST (rat)[b] [122]	
Newborn mouse astrocytes	BCECs (mouse) [75]
Human fetal astrocytes	BCECs (human) [77]

Astrocyte	Coculture with Epithelium[a]
C_6-rat glioma	ECV304 (human) [81]
C_6-rat glioma	MDCK (dog) [80]
Human 1321N1 astrocyte cell line	ECV304 (human) [81]

[a]HUVECs, human umbilical vein endothelial cells; RBE4, rat brain immortalized capillary endothelial cell line; ECV, T24 human bladder epithelial carcinoma cell line; MDCK, dog kidney epithelial cell line; BCECs, brain capillary endothelial cells.
[b]Conditionally immortalized astrocyte type II.
Source: From Ref. 362, with permission.

BBB coculture systems. The application of tumor astrocytic cell lines introduces the consequence of a tumor phenotype in BBB cocultures. This may be very helpful if one is interested in the blood–tumor barrier in the brain because the homeostasis of the tumor–BBB endothelium may be different. Surface molecules and transporters may be up- or downregulated and may give leads for tumor targeting. These arguments make these BBB systems more suitable to study only passive hydrophilic or lipophilic drug transport. Since active transport processes may be differentially regulated under tumor conditions, the results of such transport studies are less relevant for those under "healthy" BBB conditions. Therefore, these tumor BBB coculture systems are not suitable to study active transport processes and functionality under other than tumor conditions. Apart from the tumor phenotype, these BBB coculture systems differ with respect to the source of the endothelial cells, while the ECV304 (recently characterized as a T24 bladder epithelial carcinoma cell, see [58]) and MDCK (dog kidney epithelial cell line) cell lines represent epithelium. It has recently been shown that the basal transendothelial electrical resistance (TEER) of ECV304 monolayers could be enhanced by human 1321N1 astrocytes and primary rat astrocytes and that relatively tight monolayers could be obtained [81]. However, the replacement of endothelial cells by epithelial cells may have some consequences. In the first place, endothelial cells are longitudinal cells with a thickness of 2–4 μm in contrast to MDCK cells that are columnar cells with a thickness of more than 20 μm. Second, (drug) metabolism by epithelial cells may be quite different from endothelial cells; and third, transporters may be up- or downregulated and absent or mutated.

Variability and Transference of Results Between BBB Culture Systems   BBB culture systems have been the subject of a Concerted Action within the EEC entitled *Drug Transport Across the BBB: New Experimental Strategies*, involving 21 research groups from 9 European countries [85]. The focus of this Concerted Action was on the optimization, harmonization, and validation of brain-microvessel-endothelial cell culture and microdialysis to develop and study new experimental strategies for drug transport to the brain. The various BBB culture systems have been described in the report of this Concerted Action including the sources of variability [62]. Furthermore, pitfalls in evaluating BBB data should be noted in order to avoid bias and misinterpretation of results [63]. Here we want to indicate and compare the various properties of the most frequently applied BBB (co)culture systems. In addition, others have indicated the need for validated BBB culture systems [86, 87]. It has been discussed elsewhere that the transference of data from various BBB culture systems and the evaluation of the results would be enhanced if these were obtained in a well validated context [62]. Presently, there is no laboratory-to-laboratory validation of BBB systems and only individual researchers characterize and validate their BBB systems by the expression of various surface molecules and enzymes, paracellular marker molecules (^{14}C-mannitol, ^{14}C-sucrose, fluorescein, and FITC-dextran MW 4000), and the measurement of the transendothelial electrical resistance (TEER) [82, 88]. In addition, since TEER values measured before the experiment do not guarantee BBB tightness during the experiment, this method is very helpful to estimate BBB performance during and after the experiment also. Efforts have been focused on the use and validation of *in vitro* BBB systems to estimate BBB transport of drugs and on the *in vitro/in vivo* correlation of BBB drug transport by the ECVAM (European Center for Validation of Alternative Methods) [89, 90].

Furthermore, the misinterpretation of results due to biased *in vitro* conditions may be a serious point [63]. Physiologically relevant *in vitro* conditions (pH, serum proteins, unstirred water layer, cellular retention, and use of artificial membranes) should be established as much as possible and recommendations have been made to optimize *in vitro* systems accordingly [63].

Application of BCEC Cocultures in Research   BBB (co)cultures are useful to study a whole variety of phenomena. These include transport processes like passive hydrophilic (paracellular) transport, passive lipophilic transport, carrier- or receptor-mediated (transcellular) transport, and fluid-phase and adsorptive-mediated transport. The discovery of efflux transporters like P-glycoprotein and MRPs (reviewed in [34–38, 91]) and influx transporters like the amino acid, the monocarboxylic acid, the cationic drug, the hexose, the nucleotide, and the peptide transport systems (reviewed by [92]) have contributed much to our understanding of BBB transport. In addition, drug metabolism [22–24], the effect of specific agents and conditions on the functionality of the BBB including disease state, the visualization of drug transport routes by confocal laser scanning microscopy (CFLM) [93], and the measurement of the transendothelial electrical resistance [80] can be studied.

Particularly, disease state is an important BBB condition to be studied, since it has been shown to change BBB functionality and therefore drug transport to the brain [80]. In addition, inflammatory conditions, which may occur in multiple sclerosis, Alzheimer disease, AIDS-related dementia, meningitis, and encephalitis, can be induced at the *in vitro* BBB by applying lipopolysaccharide (LPS), TNF-α, IL-1β, and NO [6, 7, 9, 75]. Under such disease conditions, BBB permeability, functionality, and drug transport can be studied together with (pharmacological) intervention. The application of functional genomics and the phage-display technique to BBB coculture systems is in this respect very interesting in order to identify transcribed genes and expressed surface molecules under various conditions including disease state.

Conclusions   The presently available *in vitro* BBB (co)culture systems have their specific properties and can be used for specific goals (see Table 11.4). These goals can be passive hydrophilic and lipophilic drug transport, the study of active transport processes, and BBB functionality. It may be clear that for the study of passive drug transport through the BBB, sophisticated BBB systems are not required. However, since monolayers may be leaky, a wrong interpretation may be obtained on the contribution of para- and transcellular transport to the total transport and corrections should be made [94]. BBB coculture systems that resemble as much as possible the *in vivo* BBB must be used when active transport processes and the study of BBB functionality are involved. Tumor (co)culture systems are more useful to study the tumor BBB, while other systems [67, 69] are more useful to study active BBB processes and BBB functionality under healthy and disease conditions.

The influence of BBB pathology and the influence of disease mediators like LPS, NO, and radical oxygen species/radical nitrogen species (ROS/RNS) on BBB permeability is well known, particularly with respect to paracellular permeability [6, 7, 9, 75]. In addition, disease may up- or downregulate active transcellular transport systems (transporters and transcytosis mechanisms). Less is known about the influences of the pharmacodynamic effects of drugs at the BBB, which may increase (e.g., glucocorticoids) [82, 95] or even decrease (doxorubicin, vinblastine given together

TABLE 11.4   Overview of the Various *In Vitro* BBB Coculture Systems Involving the Use of C$_6$-Rat Glioma Cells

E/A Coculture	Useful for Study of	Not Ideally Suited for Study of	References
Endothelium/astrocyte coculture			
HUVEC (human)/ C$_6$-glioma (rat)	L; H; CLSM	BBB-F; BBB-D; DT; DM; DE	79
BCEC (human)/ human fetal A	L; H; CLSM; DT; DM; DE "human"-BBB; BBB-F; BBB-D		77
BCEC (bovine)/ newborn (rat) A-cell line	L; H; CLSM	BBB-F; BBB-D; DT; DM; DE	118
BCEC (bovine)/ newborn rat A	L; H; CLSM; DT; DM; DE "normal"-BBB; BBB-F; BBB-D		67, 69
BCEC (mouse)/ newborn mouse A	L; H; CLSM; DT; DM; DE "normal"-BBB; BBB-F; BBB-D		75
BCEC (bovine)/ C$_6$-glioma (rat)	L; H; tumor-BBB; CLSM	BBB-F; BBB-D; DT; DM; DE	119
RBE4 (rat)/ C$_6$-glioma (rat)	L; H; tumor-BBB; CLSM	BBB-F; BBB-D; DT; DM; DE	120
Epithelium/astrocyte coculture			
MDCK (dog)/ C$_6$-glioma (rat)	L; H; CLSM	BBB-F; BBB-D; DT; DM; DE	123
ECV304 (human)/ C$_6$-glioma (rat)	L; H; CLSM	BBB-F; BBB-D DT; DM; DE	81
ECV304 (human)/ 1321N1 (human)	L; H; CLSM	BBB-F; BBB-D DT; DM; DE	81

Abbreviations: E/A, endothelial or epithelial coculture with astrocytes; A, astrocyte; L, passive lipophilic transport; H, passive hydrophilic (paracellular transport); BBB-F, BBB functionality; BBB-D, BBB diseases; DM, drug metabolism; DE, drug effects; DT, BBB drug influx and efflux transport systems; CLSM, confocal laser scanning microscopy.
Source: From Ref. 362, with permission.

with a P-gp inhibitor) paracellular tightness [72, 96, 97]. In addition, several diseases in the brain (multiple sclerosis, Alzheimer disease, AIDS-related dementia, meningitis, epilepsy, tumors, etc.) are the primary or secondary cause of BBB permeability. Therefore, it is important to consider the pharmacodynamic (therapeutical or toxicological) effects of drugs at the BBB also.

Variability [62] and physiologically relevant *in vitro* conditions [63] are probably the main obstacles to the transference of results between laboratories. An interesting example is the expression of P-glycoprotein in BCECs depending on cell culture conditions. Barrand et al. [98] have shown that mdr1a–P-gp in cultured rat BCECs was downregulated and changed into the expression of mdr1b–P-gp. In addition, it has been shown that P-gp expression in bovine BCECs could be upregulated again by rat astrocytes [72]. Similar data have been published by Zhang et al. [99], where the expression of MRPs (at mRNA level) in brain capillaries was qualitatively and quantitatively different from those in BCEC monolayers. Therefore, it may be stressed again, that the systems to be used are well characterized morphologically, biochemically, and functionally. Together with the use of validation markers [86] and physiologically relevant *in vitro* conditions, this will lead to an optimal transference of BBB data between laboratories [62, 63, 89, 90].

11.3.2 *In Vivo* Methods

Although the *in vitro* systems have evolved into sophisticated and functional models of the BBB, they may result in quantitative and qualitative differences in BBB transport due up- or downregulation of transporters and species differences. Therefore, it is necessary to verify and validate the obtained *in vitro* data *in vivo*. This requires the application of animal-based methods. There are several methods; however, their applicability depends on the sensitivity and selectivity to measure drug concentrations in the brain of fast and poor BBB/brain penetrating compounds, the estimation of local concentrations in the brain or whole brain distribution, and the measurement of single-time concentrations versus concentration time profiles. Therefore, it is essential to understand the possibilities and limitations of these methods for the estimation of BBB transport including the role of drug influx and efflux transporters at the BBB [36].

Here we briefly discuss the following methods in the context of their possibilities and limitations to estimate BBB transport: brain uptake index (BUI), multiple pass techniques, brain efflux index (BEI), *in situ* brain perfusion, CSF (cerebrospinal fluid) sampling (unit impulse response), positron emission tomography (PET), magnetic resonance techniques (imaging (MRI), spectroscopy (MRS)), quantitative autoradiography (QAR), and intracerebral microdialysis. Most of these methods are invasive in contrast to the noninvasive ones like PET and NMR.

Brain Uptake Index (BUI)   This is one of the oldest techniques (1970) to estimate the uptake (via the BBB and/or blood–CSF barrier) of drugs/compounds into the brain [124, 125]. The method is widely used, rapid, and relatively cheap and the surgery is easy. It is a single passage technique and comprises the intra-arterial administration (common carotid artery) of a solution containing a reference (mostly a ^{14}C-labeled compound) and a test compound (preferentially a ^{3}H-labeled compound) under anesthesia. The basic idea is that the reference compound can easily penetrate the brain and the test compound less. Following a short time (15 s) the animal is decapitated and brain concentrations of test and reference compounds are measured and related to the plasma concentration. This ratio is a measure for the brain uptake of the test compound that is expressed as a percentage of the penetration of the reference compound. This procedure is very suitable for compounds that are labile or fast metabolized. Its drawback is that the exposure to the brain is very short and results from BUI studies cannot easily be related to cerebrovascular permeability. These are dependent on blood flow, brain region, and time between injection and decapitation. Therefore, this procedure is not suitable for poorly penetrating compounds including peptides and proteins. Another limitation is that the total injected dose does not reach the whole brain since about 20% of the drug enters the internal carotid artery while 80% reaches the external carotid artery.

Brain Efflux Index (BEI) The BEI has recently (1996) been developed [126, 127]. It comprises the estimation of the efflux of compounds from the brain following microinjection (maximal 1 µL) at a specific site in the brain, compared to a reference compound (^{14}C-carboxy-inulin) that has a limited BBB permeability. Following decapitation at variable times, the brain and plasma concentration of compound and reference can be estimated. The BEI is expressed as the percentage of the ratio of drug effluxed from the brain and the drug injected into the brain. The apparent elimination rate constant can be calculated by plotting the log(BEI) versus time. Subsequently, the efflux clearance of compounds from the brain can be calculated. The technique is cheap and the surgery is moderately easy.

Multipassage Techniques These techniques have been developed to circumvent several of the drawbacks of the BUI method and were originally designed by Brodie et al. [128]. The exposure is much longer and thus measurable brain concentrations of poorly penetrating compounds can be obtained. Later on, mathematical models were developed to calculate the permeability surface area (PS) product after an intravenous bolus administration [129]. Generally, the concentration of the drug in the brain is divided by the integral of the plasma drug concentration and time (AUC). This results in the estimation of the clearance of drug from blood or plasma to brain and is expressed as the PS product for BBB and/or BCSFB transport. For an accurate estimation of the PS of slowly penetrating compounds, it is essential to correct for the amount of drug in the vascular bed of the brain. Furthermore, it has been speculated that the PS product was time dependent [130].

The multiple-passage/multiple-time-point techniques provide information about the time course of brain uptake [128, 131, 132]. Originally, these experiments were performed by maintaining plasma steady-state concentrations and following the time course of brain uptake by sacrificing groups of animals at different time points. BBB transport can be estimated when the concentration difference between brain or CSF and plasma relative to the plasma concentration is plotted versus time. Later on, this procedure was further developed to intravenous bolus administration [133]. Ultimately, the PS products can be calculated by the Renkin–Crone equation [134]. The interesting advantage of this equation is that the amount of drug penetrating the brain can also be estimated by positron emission tomography (PET) and computer tomography (CT) scans, which allow a noninvasive measurement of BBB permeability in humans [135]. An additional advantage is that the regional blood volume does not have to be estimated. However, since brain sampling can only be done after sacrificing the animal, it is not possible to study the time profile of BBB transport in a single animal. The technique is cheap and the surgery easy to perform.

In Situ Brain Perfusion Techniques These were developed (1984) to avoid (non-brain) metabolism of the test compound and to fully control the passage of the BBB and/or the BCSFB. These techniques do not require estimation of the regional blood volumes to correct brain concentrations. In this technique the common carotid artery is ligated and the (^{14}C-labeled) reference and (^{3}H-labeled) test compounds are perfused retrograde via the external into the internal carotid artery under anesthesia [136]. Following perfusion the animal is decapitated and the brain is collected and analyzed for reference and test compounds. The use of two test compounds (a highly diffusible one and the other an intravascular marker compound) allows an accurate estimation of the PS product [129]. The problem with this technique is that in rats the common carotid artery has branches between the neck region and the brain. Therefore, to ensure the delivery of compounds to the brain, these branches have to be ligated. Guinea pigs do not have these branches and are therefore more convenient animals to use in this respect [137]. The technique is cheap and surgery is easy.

Unit Impulse Response Procedure   This procedure together with numerical deconvolution [138–140] has been applied (1989) to estimate BBB and/or BCSFB transport based on serial CSF sampling in the *cisterna magna* [141]. This procedure allows the construction of a complete time–transport profile in a single anesthetized animal. It requires the estimation of a weighing function comprising the characterization of the disposition of a drug in the brain. This is achieved by injecting a compound in the lateral ventricle of the brain, followed by sampling of the CSF. Subsequently, the compound is given intravenously and plasma and CSF samples have to be collected. The BBB input profile can be obtained by a mathematical procedure called deconvolution [139, 140]. Principally, one can obtain information on passive and active transport processes in the brain. Essentially, the cumulative cleared plasma volume is plotted against time. When a straight line is obtained, its slope represents the uptake clearance. In the case of nonlinearity, the V_{max} and K_m can in principle be estimated. The method has been applied to lipophilic drugs like atenolol, acetaminophen, and antipyrine [141]. The advantage of this technique is that it avoids the occurrence of backdiffusion from brain to blood. The costs of the technique and the complexity of the surgery are moderate.

Positron Emission Tomography (PET)   Regional BBB and BCSFB permeability and drug transport can be investigated by PET [142]. This technique employs the intravenous administration (bolus or infusion) of positron emitting isotopes like ^{18}F, ^{13}N, ^{11}C, or ^{15}O. By this technique brain and plasma concentrations can be followed over a long time. Subsequently, one analyzes the data by pharmacokinetic models that describe the transport of tracers (uptake, distribution, and elimination). In 1955, this technique was developed by Davson [143]. The advantage of the technique is that the transport of tracers can be visualized and studied in whole brain over time. However, the technique is expensive and the preparation and stability of the tracers are matters of concern. Essentially, tracer concentrations are measured and no distinction can be made between parent compound, metabolite, and protein bound or unbound tracer. Nevertheless, this technique is sensitive and therefore very helpful in diagnostic purposes such as the localization of tumors in the brain and also in studying local differences in BBB permeability and BBB transport. P-gp functionality has been investigated with ^{11}C-verapamil in mdr1a (+/+) and (−/−) mice [142, 144]. The PET procedure underestimated the uptake of ^{11}C-verapamil in the brain. However, in patients, pretreatment with cyclosporin A increased ^{11}C-verapamil levels in GLC4/P-gp tumors (184%) and in brains (1280%). This pharmacokinetic effect was clearly visualized with PET [145].

Quantitative Autoradiography (QAR)   This method was initially applied in 1951 by Campbell [146] and later on used to visualize the distribution of radioactive tracers across the BBB and/or the BCSFB [131]. Typically, these are ^{3}H- of ^{14}C-labeled compounds that are given intravenously. Following administration, the animals are sacrificed after various times, brains collected, and slices prepared. Subsequently, autoradiographs are prepared that can be scanned by a computer driven densitometer. The technique is cheap and easy to perform. The spatial resolution of QAR is high; however, the time resolution is rather low since one animal has to be used for one time point. Other drawbacks are that no distinction can be made between parent compound and metabolites, and protein bound and unbound compounds.

Intracerebral Microdialysis   This method was developed in the late 1950s and measures particularly local concentrations of compounds in the extracellular fluid (ECF) of the brain or the CSF. It is an invasive method and longitudinal, I-shaped or semicircular probes can be used [147]. The time to perform experiments has to be evaluated carefully with respect to periprobe tissue reactions that may occur [148]. The method has been successfully applied in the estimation of BBB transport of various compounds [148–151]. The advantage of this method is that concentration–time profiles can be obtained of unbound compounds in the extracellular fluid in the brain. The spatial resolution of this technique is relatively high, and a highly sensitive and selective analytical technique is essential for estimation of concentrations of compounds in the ECF. Presently, HPLC combined with mass spectroscopy methods result in high selectivity and sensitivity. The surgery is moderately difficult and the costs are moderate.

An essential factor is the estimation of the *in vivo* recovery of the microdialysis probe. This describes the relation between the concentration of the compound in the fluid around the probe and that in the dialysate. *In vitro* recovery is mainly dependent on the perfusate composition and flow rate, the physicochemical characteristics of the compound, temperature, and probe characteristics. In addition, *in vivo* recovery is influenced by the para- and transcellular transport of compounds through brain tissue and the blood supply in terms of vascularization and blood flow [147]. *In vivo* recovery can be estimated by the "nonet flux" (measurement of recovery under serial steady-state conditions in one animal) [152] and the "dynamic nonet flux" (measurement of recovery under one but different steady-state conditions in different groups of animals) [153] methods and by the internal standard, the retrodialysis, and reverse dialysis methods (reviewed in Ref. 147).

Intracerebral microdialysis allows the estimation of the local BBB time transport profile of unbound compounds in the ECF of the brain and in the CSF. It can distinguish between parent compound and metabolite(s). The analytical technique to estimate the substances in the ECF or CSF must be very sensitive and selective. In addition, the conversion of dialysate concentrations to real extracellular concentrations in the brain is very much determined by the procedure to estimate *in vivo* recovery.

Magnetic Resonance Techniques   These comprise magnetic resonance imaging (MRI, initially applied in the late 1970s) and magnetic resonance spectroscopy (MRS, initially applied in the 1950s) and are noninvasive techniques. They do not require the use of ionizing radiation or the use of iodinated contrast compared to X-ray computed tomography (CT). They comprise the direct or indirect monitoring and recording of the spatiotemporal distribution of molecular or cellular processes for biochemical, biologic, diagnostic, or therapeutic applications [154]. The techniques employ ^{1}H-, ^{13}C-, and ^{31}P-labeled compounds that are injected intravenously. This allows evaluation of a variety of parameters in the brain related to anatomy, physiology, and metabolism, like macrophage infiltration, cytotoxic edema, cerebral blood flow and volume, and metabolic processes [155]. Depending on the technique used, slice-based as well as true 3D images can be obtained [156]. MRI techniques have been developed into functional MRI (fMRI) techniques, which measure regional blood volume and flow, regional diffusion of water (diffusion tensor imaging—DTI) [157, 158], and regional blood oxygenation level dependence (BOLD) [159, 160]. In addition, when combining a contrast enhancing principle (superparamagnetic iron oxide—SPIO; Mn^{2+}, Gd^{3+}) [160] with a target-specific carrier moiety (receptor ligand, antibody, cell), highly specific information on targeted molecular interactions can be obtained by molecular (brain) imaging [161]. This is very important from the diagnostic and therapeutic (e.g., disease progression) point of view. However, the problem is to deliver these agents through the BBB, and successful strategies have to be developed to accomplish this. Nevertheless, MRI has been used to investigate BBB permeability and leakage involved in brain diseases including neurodegenerative diseases [157, 162]; various brain tumors [163, 164], multiple sclerosis [165, 166], early infarcts, and inflammatory lesions can be studied [157] in addition to age related changes in brain tissue [158]. Moreover, since there are many disease models in small animals, MRI can be used to study these (brain) disease processes dynamically [156].

MRS has been used successfully to quantify phenylalanine (Phe) concentrations in the brain of patients with phenylketonuria and to estimate its BBB transport (PKU) [167]. In addition, it was shown that BBB transport parameters determined the clinical outcome in phenylketonuria [168]. In studies with multiple sclerosis (MS) patients, it was demonstrated that the earliest detectable event in the development of a new lesion was the increase in permeability of the BBB that was associated with inflammation [169]. It was shown that when the inflammation declined, edema resolved. With ^{1}H-MRS a correlation was shown between a decrease in N-acetylaspartate (NAA) concentrations (a marker of neuronal or axonal damage) and clinical disability [170].

With these techniques one can differentiate between parent compound and its metabolites as well as between free and unbound drug concentrations. The sensitivity and its spatial resolution are limited but resolutions ranging from 300 to 500 μm throughout the human brain and 50 to 100 μm through the rodent brain should be possible in reasonable scan times [159]. The latter are presently up to 2 hours while another disadvantage is that the technique is expensive [162]. Nevertheless, magnetic resonance techniques are very convenient to estimate BBB time transport profiles of poorly and fast brain-penetrating compounds.

Conclusions   Various methods have been developed to estimate drug transport to and from the brain. Table 11.5 shows an overview of the typical properties of the reviewed methods. Presently the brain perfusion method is one the most frequently used methods in animals. It allows the estimation of brain uptake of fast and poorly penetrating compounds at single times. In addition, when more animals are used a concentration–time profile can be obtained. The BEI method is applicable in the

TABLE 11.5 Applicability[a] of Various Methods to Estimate Drug Transport and Distribution in the Brain

Method	Fast Penetrating Compounds	Poor Penetrating Compounds	Single Concentration at Single Time	Concentration–Time Course in Single Animal	Brain Distribution[b]	Costs	Surgery
BUI	+	−	+	−	−	Cheap	Easy
Multipassage techniques	+	+	+	−	−	Cheap	Easy
BEI	+	+	+	−	−	Cheap	Moderately easy
Brain perfusion	+	+	++	−	−	Cheap	Easy
Impulse response method	+	+	++	+	− (CSF)	Cheap	Moderately difficult
PET	+	+	+	++ (human)	+ (WB)	Expensive	Easy
QAR	+	+	+	−	++ (WB)	Cheap	Easy
MRI/MRS	+	+		++ (human)	+ (WB)	Expensive	Easy
Intracerebral microdialysis	+	+		+	+ (local)	Moderate	Moderately difficult

[a]+, applicable; ++, very good applicability; −, not appplicable.
[b]WB, whole brain; CSF, only in cerebrospinal fluid.

same way and allows the measurement of brain efflux of compounds. The BUI, BEI, multipassage techniques, brain perfusion, and the impulse response method (only in CSF) do not give information on brain distribution. In contrast, PET, QAR, MRI/MRS, and intracerebral microdialysis provide information on the brain concentration–time course and brain distribution of compounds in one single animal. However, the resolution varies, with that of QAR and intracerebral microdialysis > PET and MRI/MRS. In addition, QAR gives information on whole brain distribution of compounds and intracerebral microdialysis only gives information about the unbound concentration in the brain area where the probe has been implanted. Both methods are suitable for routine use in animals while intracerebral microdialysis has been used to monitor patients with brain trauma [171]. In particular, PET and MRI/MRS can be applied in humans and can allow the estimation of the concentration–time course of compounds and their distribution in the whole brain. Moreover, the advantage of MRI/MRS is that a distinction can be made between metabolites and unbound and bound drug.

11.4   STRATEGIES FOR DRUG DELIVERY TO THE BRAIN

For many diseases of the brain, such as Alzheimer disease, Parkinson disease, stroke, depression, schizophrenia, epilepsy, and migraine headache, the drugs on the market are far from being ideal, let alone curative. A significant part of the problem is the poor BBB penetration of most of the drugs in development against neuronal targets for treatment of these disorders. This includes approximately 98% of the small molecules and nearly 100% of large molecules, such as recombinant proteins or gene-based medicines [12]. Therefore, much effort is put toward delivery and targeting of drugs to the brain [10, 12, 172]. Drug delivery to the brain can be achieved via several methods, including local invasive (direct injection/infusion) delivery, induction of enhanced permeability, and the application of global physiological targeting strategies. Apart from the delivery of small molecules (e.g., <500 Da) to the brain, the global delivery of large hydrophilic molecules, including enzymes, interference RNA (RNAi), and genes, present a serious problem.

11.4.1   Local Brain Delivery by Direct Injection/Infusion of Drugs into the Brain

Because of the lack of ability to target via the vascular route to the brain, invasive methods, like direct injection or infusion and convection enhanced delivery, have been applied to macromolecular drugs as well as to the delivery of viral vectors. These are reviewed in the following paragraphs.

Direct Injection/Infusion of Macromolecular Drugs   Intracerebral ventricular (ICV) or intrathecal drug infusion comprises direct injection/infusion of drug into the CSF. However, as mentioned before, CSF is completely drained into the venous circulation, and drugs still have to cross the ependymal brain–CSF barrier. This has shown to be feasible particularly for many small (mostly lipophilic [45, 172]) drugs following intraventricular administration. In addition, it was shown that compounds with MW < 5000 rapidly penetrate the ependyma but that penetration into the brain parenchyma was limited due to diffusion, tortuosity, transcapillary loss, cell uptake, and binding [173, 174]. As a result, the infused drug has minimal access to the paren-chyma by diffusion (Fig. 11.3C) [175]. In addition, it was shown that compounds with MW > 5000 very poorly penetrated the brain parenchyma even when they were administered intraventricularly. It was shown that following a 3–5 h infusion of ^{14}C-inulin in the lateral ventricle of dogs, only an appreciable uptake in tissues lining the ventricle was found [176] and intraventricular injection of ^{125}I-brain-derived neurotrophic growth factor [177] in rats resulted in a very poor uptake by the brain parenchyma. Very recently, it was elegantly demonstrated that the uptake of ^{125}I-insulin-like growth factor-1 (MW 7.7 kDa) following intraventricular infusion was very poor by brain parenchyma and was rapidly cleared from the cerebrospinal fluid compartment mainly into blood [178]. In addition, these authors stated that under healthy conditions the CSF flow direction will probably be different from that under disease conditions and that further investigations are required in this respect. Furthermore, experimental data in human parkinsonian patients indicate that intra-ventricular GDNF infusion by a Medtronic device was biologically active but did not improve parkinsonism symptoms, possibly because GDNF (dimer with MW 33–45 kDa) did not sufficiently reach the target tissues [179].

Direct infusion into the brain has also been applied. The delivery of GDNF by direct infusion into the putamen of parkinsonian patients in one study showed

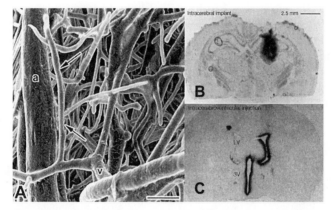

FIGURE 11.3   Drug delivery via the vascular route will enable widespread distribution of the drug to each single neuron within the brain (note that the bar in panel A indicates a length of 25 µm, which is about the size of a single neuron). (A) Scanning electron micrograph of a vascular cast of a mouse brain (a, artery; v, vein). (Reprinted from Satomi et al., Cerebral vascular abnormalities in a murine model of hereditary hemorrhagic telangiectasia. *Stroke* 2003;34(33):783–789. © 2003, with permission from Lippincott Williams & Wilkins.) (B) Minimal diffusion of [^{125}I]-nerve growth factor (NGF) after intracerebral implantation of a biodegradable polymer (note that the bar indicates a length of 2.5 mm, which was also the size of the implant). (Reprinted from Krewson et al., Distribution of nerve growth factor following direct delivery to brain interstitium. *Brain Res* 1995;680(1–2):196–206. © 1995, with permission from Elsevier.) (C) ICV injection of [^{125}I]-brain-derived neurotrophic factor (BDNF). (Reprinted from Yan et al., Distribution of intracerebral ventricularly administered neurotrophins in rat brain and its correlation with trk receptor expression. *Exp Neurol* 1994;127(1):23–36. © 1994, with permission from Elsevier.) Note that the neurotrophin does not distribute into the brain beyond the ipsilateral ependymal surface.

general improvement over time [180] while a Phase II clinical trial could only demonstrate "potential efficacy" [181]. Indeed, Amgen decided to confirm its previous decision to stop a Phase II clinical trial with GDNF infusions into the putamen of 48 patients because "scientific results indicated that allowing patients to continue treatment could potentially cause permanent harm, complicating an already devastating disease" [182].

A variant of this is *convection enhanced drug delivery*, where a positive pressure infusion in brain parenchyma has been applied to increase drug uptake [183–185]. In addition, uptake was significantly improved when the viscosity of the infusate was increased [183], which seems to be caused by a similar mechanism (osmotic opening) as has been applied by Kroll and Neuwelt [186]. Good results have been shown by large volume infusion of naked DNA in the tail vein or legs where temporarily blood flow was inhibited; however, this is not applicable to the brain [187, 188].

Furthermore, brain implants have been used for the local delivery of drugs to the brain (Fig. 11.3B). Indeed, it has been shown that polymeric implants (poly(ethylene-*co*-vinyl acetate)) containing ^{125}I-nerve-growth factor into rat brain were effective for local delivery, but unfortunately not for global delivery, of the drug [189].

In conclusion, because of the fenestrated capillaries in the CPs and their total surface area that is comparable to the BBB, drug transport into the CSF could be substantial. However, apart from the need of direct injection into brain parenchyma or infusion into the ventricles, for drugs that have to reach their target by passive diffusion, the direction of the CSF flow in the ventricles, the presence of the ependymal barrier (particularly for compounds with MW > 5000), and the direction of the flow of the interstitial fluid in the brain parenchyma are major obstacles for an effective global penetration into the brain.

Direct Injection/Infusion of Viral Vectors   Gene therapy [190–193] is meant to deliver genetic material with a therapeutic function encoding proteins (e.g., enzymes) or siRNA/shRNA to somatic cells [194]. In addition, gene therapy could provide a long-term effect following one single administration. However, genes are hydrophilic and charged and are large molecules that cannot pass cell membranes and tight cellular layers like the BBB. Therefore, means have to be found and developed to transport genes to the desired site of action.

Viruses have evolved over millions of years to obtain optimal mechanisms for gene delivery to host cells, which makes them applicable as a biological vector system to deliver genetic material to brain cells. There is a broad range of viral vectors available but the most commonly used are adeno-associated virus (AAV) vectors and lentivirus (LV) vectors. Important issues in viral gene delivery are stable transgene expression, limited immunogenicity, the induction of an inflammatory response, the (lack of) cell specific targeting efficiency, safety, toxicity, and the need for packaging cell lines [195].

Brain tropism (e.g., brain targeting) varies from virus to virus and has been shown not to be sufficient to pass the BBB following intravenous administration; therefore, the virus has to be injected directly into the brain. Moreover, various viral vectors have affinities for specific brain cells [190–196]. This could be improved if viral vectors could be produced with a homing/targeting device at their surface. Furthermore, the selectivity of gene transcription in the brain can be strongly enhanced by application of brain selective promoters like the myelin basic protein (MBP) promoter [197], the neuron-specific enolase (NSE) promoter [198–200], the platelet-derived growth factor-β (PDGB-β) promoter [201, 202], the glial fibrillary acid protein (GFAP) promoter [203], and synthetic promoters like the CMV plus human growth hormone first intron enhancer and the CMV-chicken β-actin promoter [204, 205]. Moreover, the addition of a posttranscriptional regulatory element of the woodchuck hepatitis virus (WPRE) has enhanced the expression of GFP [206, 207]. Similarly, application of the replication origin (oriP) and Epstein–Barr nuclear antigen (EBNA-1) elements [208] can enhance episomal transcription of plasmids [209]. However, it has been indicated that application of such elements could induce tumorgeneity, which makes them not readily applicable in humans [210].

The Tet and Cre-Lox systems are other regulatory systems that have been applied, particularly for viruses that integrate their genetic material into the genome [211]. The Tet system can upregulate the expression of GFP in rat brain in the absence of doxycycline [212] while the Cre-Lox system allows a conditional but irreversible gene modification [213].

The *adeno-associated virus* (AAV) is a human parvovirus and contains a ssDNA. There are approximately 35 known serotypes. Several of them have been engineered into recombinant viral vectors from which the rAAV1, rAAV2, and rAAV5 are most widely used to deliver genes to the brain [193, 214–217]. In particular, these serotypes are most effective in the transduction of neurons [215, 218]. The attractive feature of the virus is that its replication is dependent on coinfection with a lytic helper virus, which precludes the reversion into a replication competent virus [219].

rAAV vectors are capsid virions composed of a nucleic acid genome surrounded by a proteinaceous shell. The composition of the capsid determines which cells they bind to and may enter. They enter the cell following binding to heparin sulfate proteoglycan (HSPG) receptors. Two other coreceptors seem to be helpful in this and finally the dsDNA enters the nucleus through the pore [220, 221].

Once in the cell, the rAAV genome is maintained as an extrachromosomal element or episomal element [190, 222–224], which eliminates the risk of proto-oncogene activation or endogenous gene inactivation, which may occur following insertion into the host genome [223]. Nevertheless, random integration of rAAV material does irregularly occur [190, 223, 225]. The episome might replicate along with the endogenous cellular DNA but can also be maintained as a nonreplicating extrachromosomal element [190]. In nondividing cells, the episome can be maintained as a stable element, resulting in long-term transgene expression in cells [190, 222–224, 226]. In addition, a safe and long-term correction of genetic diseases in animal models following a single administration has been demonstrated [191]. These viruses can be produced under current Good Manufacturing Practices (cGMPs) as outlined in the Code of Federal Regulations (21CFR) in the United States [191]. This all guarantees that pure and high-quality rAAV vectors can be produced for human use.

Expression of rAAV2 delivered vectors in animals has been shown for brain-derived neurotrophic factor (BDNF) in atrophy of spinal neurons [227]; and glial cell line mediated neurotrophic factor (GDNF), tyrosine hydroxylase (TH), aromatic L-amino acid decarboxylase (AADC), and guanosine triphosphate cyclohydrolase (GCH) in Parkinson disease [228–234]. In addition, rAAV vectors are effective in the treatment of lysosomal storage diseases like mucopolysaccharidosis type I, II, and VII [235] and Niemann–Pick A [236]. In addition, it was demonstrated in mice that by targeting the deep cerebellar nuclei with AAV1 vectors capable of axonal transport, it was possible to get a widespread distribution throughout the cerebellum [236].

The major problem in delivering rAAV vectors to the brain is to get global brain transduction. This holds particularly for disorders caused by single-gene mutations such as lysosomal storage disorders and leukodystrophies, where a global brain transduction is desirable. Some vectors have been shown to have an enhanced neurotropism when expressing peptides that mimic binding domains for cytoplasmic dynein or NMDA receptors [237]. In addition, other viral vectors have been constructed that express capsid proteins that function as homing devices for targeted delivery of genes [238].

Another disadvantage is the occurrence of immune responses when animals have been treated with rAAV vectors, since this has resulted in killing of the transduced cells by cytotoxic T cells [190, 223, 225, 239, 240]. It was argued that this was caused by a slow uncoating of the rAAV in contrast to rapid uncoating [241, 242]. In addition, a humoral response can be elicited, which results in the production of antibodies. Moreover, memory cells are produced that will boost a strong humoral response when the same antigen is detected again. In this way, memory cells prevent the possibility of vector readministration [223].

Another feature is the packaging capacity of viruses. For rAAVs this is rather small (~4.5 kb) [190, 225, 243]. However, this may be increased up to 36 kb [244] by using (gutless) vectors, where as many viral genes as possible are deleted, only using those for the packaging sequence and sequences that define the beginning and end of the viral genome [190, 224, 240].

Lentivirus (LV) *vectors* are very promising vehicles to deliver therapeutic genes into the brain [190, 193, 194]. LV vectors are capsid virions surrounded by a lipid bilayer envelope [190]. LV vectors enter the cell following binding to HSPG; following membrane fusion, the virus moves along the microtubule by dynein-mediated transport. Finally, the dsDNA enters the nucleus through the pore [190]. LV vectors have a moderate packaging capacity with a maximum of 8 kb. LV vectors can be used to transduce a broad range of dividing as well as nondividing cells. In contrast to the rAAV vectors, they integrate into the host genome [196] and should therefore provide a longer and more stable transgene expression. However, they could also activate a proto-oncogene [190, 223, 224, 245] but since most CNS cells are terminally differentiated, the risk of tumorigenesis seems to be diminished [190, 225]. Nevertheless, the risk that vital genes are inactivated by random integration exists [190, 223, 245].

Furthermore, LV vectors seem to have a low immunogenicity. This seems to be caused by the fact that the genomes of these vectors do not encode any viral proteins. Indeed, low immunogenicity and prolonged transgene expression in the presence of preexisting lentiviral immunity was found, which should be encouraging for future use of these vectors in brain gene therapy [246].

Although viral delivery systems enter the cell by receptor-mediated endocytosis, this cell entry is not selective/specific since they can enter various cells, including brain cells, because of the lack of the expression of a selective/specific homing device. Therefore, rAAV and LV vectors can only effectively be delivered to the brain by direct local injection/infusion. However, the diffusion from the site of administration in the brain is minimal; therefore, the region of cells that is transduced is restricted to a few millimeters from this site [190, 224]. To compensate for poor brain diffusion, usually the vector is administered by injections at multiple sites to increase the area of vector delivery. However, injection is associated with injury at the injection site, which could evoke a damaging response.

LV vectors have already been applied for gene therapy of various (brain) diseases like lysosomal storage diseases, Sandhoff disease and mucopolysaccharidosis I [247, 248], Parkinson disease [249, 250], ALS [251], epilepsy [252], prion disease [253], brain tumors [254], and the delivery of growth factors [250, 255].

In summary, one can say that today viral gene delivery to the brain can be efficient. Many applications have been demonstrated for brain gene therapy by rAAV and LV vectors, showing an increasing interest in the use of LV vectors. Critical points in this respect are global versus local delivery including the ability to reach the desired site of action (targeting efficiency). This may be improved considerably when homing/targeting devices are expressed at the outer surface of the virus particle [238], which will allow the vascular and global delivery of these systems to the CNS, thereby avoiding damage caused by direct injection/infusion. The selectivity of delivery can be further enhanced when tissue-selective/specific promoters are included in the vectors. rAAV vectors stay mainly episomal, while LV vectors integrate into the genome with the possibility to activate proto-oncogenes. Furthermore, immunological reactions may occur, but these seem to be reduced following application of LV vectors. In addition, rAAV and LV vectors have a rather small to moderate packaging capacity and can safely be produced under well controlled conditions.

With respect to invasive brain drug delivery strategies, one may conclude that these can be effective for local delivery (e.g., tumors) but not for the administration of drugs against more widespread diseases, including diffuse tumors and metastases. Therefore, since every neuron has its own capillary, the only route for an effective global delivery of biopharmaceutical drugs to the brain is the vascular route by application of nonviral systems. This is discussed further in the next section.

11.4.2 Global Brain Delivery by Vascular Nonviral Drug Administration

The advantage of the vascular route is the widespread transport by blood of the infused drug across the whole brain [256]. As has been mentioned, approximately each neuron has its own brain capillary for oxygen supply as well as the supply of other nutrients (see also Fig. 11.3A). This means that the vascular route is a very promising one for drug targeting and delivery to the whole brain. However, the main problem for drug transport to the brain is BBB passage.

Drug Transport Across the BBB   There are various possibilities for drug transport across the BBB as shown in Fig. 11.4. Passive diffusion depends on lipophilicity and molecular weight [257]. Furthermore, the ability of a compound to form hydrogen bonds will limit its diffusion through the BBB [258]. In general, Lipinski's rule of five, as well as Abraham's equation, can be used to predict the passive transport of a drug molecule across the BBB [259–261]. Transport of hydrophilic compounds via the paracellular route is limited, while lipophilic drugs smaller than 400–600 Da may freely enter the brain via the transcellular route.

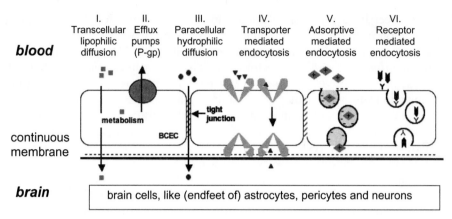

FIGURE 11.4   The various transport processes that may occur at the blood–brain barrier. (Adapted from Ref. 297.)

Active transport systems can be divided into absorptive-, carrier-, or receptor-mediated transcytosis. Absorptive-mediated transcytosis is initiated by the binding of polycationic substances (such as most cell-penetrating peptides) to negative charges on the plasma membrane [262, 263]. This process does not involve specific plasma membrane receptors. Upon binding of the cationic compound to the plasma membrane, endocytosis occurs, followed by the formation of endosomes. However, vesicular transport is actively downregulated in the BBB to protect the brain from nonspecific exposure to polycationic compounds. Therefore, forcing drugs to enter the brain by absorptive-mediated transcytosis goes against the neuroprotective barrier function, as demonstrated for anionic and cationic nanoparticles that disrupt the BBB [264].

Carrier-mediated transcytosis is used for the delivery of nutrients, such as glucose, amino acids, and purine bases, to the brain [265–267]. At least eight different nutrient transport systems have been identified, each transporting a group of nutrients of the same structure. Carrier-mediated transcytosis is substrate selective and the transport rate is dependent on the degree of occupation of the carrier [267, 268]. Therefore, only drugs that closely mimic the endogenous carrier substrates will be taken up and transported into the brain.

In contrast, receptor-mediated transcytosis enables larger molecules, such as peptides, proteins, and genes, to specifically enter the brain. Classical examples of receptors involved in receptor-mediated transcytosis are the insulin receptor [269], the transferrin receptor [270, 271], and the transporters for low density lipoprotein [272], leptin [273], and insulin-like growth factors [274].

Besides many influx mechanisms, several efflux mechanisms exist at the BBB as well. The best known is P-glycoprotein (P-gp) [33–37, 275, 276]. P-gp is a transmembrane protein, located at the apical membrane of the BCEC. It has a high affinity for a wide range of cationic and lipophilic compounds and therefore limits transport to the brain of many drugs including cytotoxic anticancer drugs, antibiotics, hormones, and HIV protease inhibitors [277]. Other multidrug resistance (MDR) efflux mechanisms at the BBB include the MDR related protein (MRP), such as MRP 1, 2, 5, and 6 [278]. In addition, as mentioned before (see Section 11.2.1), many other transporters are present at the BBB, like the organic anion transporter (influx and efflux), the organic cation transport system (influx), and the nucleoside transporter system (influx) [36, 37].

In conclusion, research over the years has shown that the BBB is a dynamic organ, which combines restricted diffusion to the brain for endogenous and exogenous compounds with specialized transport mechanisms for essential nutrients.

Global Brain Delivery by Enhanced Passive Vascular Drug Delivery Large molecules (e.g., drug conjugates) or drug delivery systems (nanosized carrier systems including polymers, emulsions, micelles, liposomes, and nanoparticles) may reach the brain by passive targeting similar to small molecules, meaning that their distribution is mainly determined by physicochemical and physiological conditions [279–281]. Mostly this results in a very poor distribution into the brain. However, enhanced distribution may be obtained when the permeability of blood vessels in the target tissue has been increased due to disease conditions such as in tumors. Such "enhanced permeability and retention" has been observed in many cases [282, 283], showing increased accumulation of drug in those (mostly peripheral) areas. Unfortunately, drug delivery to the brain by enhanced permeability and retention is not effective in treating human brain diseases.

Enhanced drug delivery to the brain has been achieved in various other ways also. One is the osmotic disruption/shrinking of the BBB by intracarotid administration of a hypertonic mannitol solution. By subsequent administration of drug, substantial increased concentrations can be achieved in brain or tumor tissue. However, because the BBB is temporarily opened under such conditions, which has to be done under anesthesia, it has the disadvantage also that neurons may be damaged permanently due to unwanted blood components entering the brain [284]. Therefore, this procedure is only applicable in life-threatening brain diseases (e.g., tumors) [186].

A less "aggressive" approach seems to be the intracarotid administration of alkylglycerol [285], which enhances mainly drug transport by the paracellular route. In rats with brain implanted C_6-glioma, increased tissue fluorescence was found in both tumor tissue and brain surrounding the tumor following coadministration of FITC-dextran (40 kDa). Similar data on brain tissue were observed following coadministration of methotrexate to nude mice. However, anesthesia is needed to perform this type of administration, which limits its applicability to life-threatening brain diseases like brain tumors. In addition, no human data are available yet.

Another procedure is the application of a bradykinin-analogue (RMP-7) that has been shown to increase BBB permeability by opening of the tight junctions via a receptor-mediated mechanism (Ceroport®), which resulted in an enhanced uptake of carboplatin in C_6-glioma implanted in rat brain [286]. However, a Phase II study could not show improved carboplatin efficacy in combination with RMP-7 [287]. In addition, a Phase III study with RMP-7 and carboplatin with radiotherapy was stopped because of no increased efficacy.

At last, a general aspect about these agents is the possibility that besides opening of the BBB and the associated brain disturbances, application in the treatment of brain tumors could also cause an enhanced incidence of tumor dissemination via vascular spread of tumor cells [288].

Enhanced delivery can be achieved also by application of so-called protein transduction domains (PTDs) (for reviews see Refs. 289 and 290). These PTDs are typical amino acid sequences that are capable of enhancing delivery of large molecules into cells. Typical examples are the Tat-PTD [291], the homeodomain of Antennapedia [292], SynB-vectors [293], and others [294, 295]. These peptides are basic molecules (and therefore cations) that are able to enhance protein uptake by cells mainly by increased adsorptive-mediated endocytosis. Toxicity profiles of the various PTDs are an important issue [296] but because this approach lacks cell or tissue selectivity it seems to be particularly suitable for local drug delivery. Clinical proof of principle has recently been demonstrated with SynB-vectors to enhance the transport of morphine-6-glucuronide to the brain (www.syntem.com).

Recently, therapeutic gene silencing of apolipoprotein B has been demonstrated in mice following administration of a high dose (50 mg/kg) of modified siRNAs [297]. This was achieved by coupling cholesterol to siRNA. Increased uptake by liver, heart, kidney, adipose, and lung tissue was seen but not by brain. The uptake into these tissues was mainly established by lipophilization of the siRNA by cholesterol and the resulting increase in plasma half-life from 6 min (naked siRNA) to 95 min (chol-siRNA).

A similar approach has been applied by coupling lipophilic and amphiphilic groups (stearoyl groups or Pluronic block copolymers) to polypeptides to enhance the uptake of these compounds by the brain. However, no selectivity in brain uptake has been demonstrated by applying such modifications [298].

In conclusion, all these approaches are able to enhance more or less the uptake into various tissues but lack selective/specific homing devices that are needed to target drugs to the brain and to selectively/specifically increase drug delivery to the brain.

Global Brain Delivery by Active Vascular Receptor-Mediated (Nonviral) Drug Targeting

Active physiological or disease-induced drug targeting strategies involve the application of a homing device or technology to apply endogenous transport mechanisms for site selective/specific delivery in the body [273, 275, 299]. With respect to the BBB, this particularly involves receptor-mediated transcytosis systems at the BBB to reach extracellular or intracellular targets in the brain. The advantage of active targeting is the increase of the amount of drug in the target tissue, thereby increasing the pharmacological response and reducing (peripheral) side effects. However, when the homing device is not specific, side effects can still occur. Interestingly, targeting efficiency can be increased when the target is disease-induced such as occurs for the diphtheria toxin receptor under inflammatory disease conditions (see following paragraphs). The focus of the following paragraphs is on active targeting by receptor-mediated transcytosis, and several examples of receptor-mediated transcytosis that have successfully been employed to target drugs to the brain are reviewed.

In general, receptor-mediated transcytosis occurs in three steps: receptor-mediated endocytosis of the compound at the luminal (blood) side, movement through the endothelial cytoplasm, and exocytosis of the drug at the abluminal (brain) side of the brain capillary endothelium [12]. Upon receptor–ligand internalization, chlathrin-coated vesicles are formed, which are approximately 120 nm in diameter [300, 301]. These vesicles may transport their content to the other side of the cell or go into a route leading to (protein) degradation. Indeed, at least two important routes for degrading proteins have been identified including the lysosomal and the ubiquitin-proteasome route [302–304]. Nevertheless, protein delivery to the brain has been shown to be effective. Therefore, receptor-mediated transcytosis allows the specific delivery/targeting of larger drug molecules or drug-carrying particles (like liposomes or nanoparticles) to the brain.

Transferrin Receptor   The most widely characterized receptor-mediated transcytosis system for the targeting of drugs to the brain is the transferrin receptor (TfR). TfR is a transmembrane glycoprotein consisting of two 90 kDa subunits. A disulfide bridge links these subunits and each subunit can bind one transferrin molecule [305]. The TfR is expressed mainly on hepatocytes, erythrocytes, intestinal cells, and monocytes, as well as on endothelial cells of the BBB [306, 307]. Furthermore, in the brain the TfR is expressed on choroid plexus epithelial cells and neurons [305]. The TfR mediates cellular uptake of iron bound to transferrin.

Drug targeting to the TfR can be achieved by either using the endogenous ligand, transferring, or using an antibody directed against the TfR (OX-26 anti-rat TfR). Each of these targeting vectors has its advantages and disadvantages. For transferrin, the *in vivo* application is limited due to high endogenous concentrations of transferrin in plasma and the likely overdosing with iron when one tries to displace the endogenous transferrin with exogenously applied transferrin-containing systems. However, recent studies in our group [309] have shown that liposomes tagged with transferrin are suitable for drug delivery to BBB endothelial cells *in vitro*, even in the presence of serum. OX-26 does not bind to the transferrin binding site and is therefore not displaced by endogenous transferrin.

The TfR is responsible for iron transport to the brain. So far, the intracellular trafficking of transferrin and OX-26 upon internalization via the TfR has not yet been elucidated. Some literature reports suggest transcytosis of transferrin across the BCECs, while others claim endocytosis of transferrin, followed by an intracellular release of iron and a subsequent return of apo-transferrin to the apical side of the BCEC [268, 309, 310]. Moos and Morgan [305] have shown that the transcytosis of iron exceeds the transcytosis of transferrin across the BBB, supporting the second theory. Furthermore, these authors have proposed a new theory in which the TfR–transferrin complex is transcytosed to the basolateral side of the BCEC, where transferrin remains bound to the TfR, but iron is released into the brain extracellular fluid [311]. Subsequently apo-transferrin bound to the TfR will recycle back to the apical side of the BBB. This theory is supported by data from Zhang and Pardridge [309], who found a 3.5-fold faster efflux from brain to blood of apo-transferrin than holo-transferrin. In addition, in a recent publication Deane et al. [312] illustrated that free iron is rapidly taken up by brain capillaries and subsequently released into the brain extracellular fluid and CSF at controlled moderate to slow rates.

The mechanism of transcytosis of OX-26 is not yet fully elucidated either. Pardridge and colleagues have shown efficient drug targeting and delivery to the brain *in vivo* by applying OX-26 (examples can be found in [265, 313–315]. In contrast, Broadwell et al. [316] have shown that both transferrin and OX-26 are able to cross the BBB, but that the transcytosis of transferrin is more efficient. Furthermore, Moos and Morgan [317] have shown that OX-26 mainly accumulates in the BCECs and not in the postcapillary compartment. In addition, iron deficiency did not increase OX-26 uptake in rats. Our data as well as literature reports show that iron deficiency causes an increase in TfR expression [306, 318, 319]. Therefore, it is expected that the uptake of OX-26 would increase as well. The data by Moos and Morgan [317] suggest that OX-26 transcytosis might result from a high-affinity accumulation by the BCECs, followed by a nonspecific exocytosis at the basolateral side of the BCECs. In addition, these authors found a periventricular localization of OX-26, which suggests that OX-26 probably also is transported across the BCSFB.

Although the mechanism of transcytosis of transferrin and OX-26 may not yet be fully elucidated, it is important to realize that drug delivery to the brain via the TfR is efficient. By these means, vasoactive intestinal peptide (VIP), brain-derived neurotrophic factor (BDNF), basic fibroblast growth factor (bFGF), epidermal growth factor (EGF), and peptide nucleic acids, as well as pegylated immunoliposomes containing plasmid DNA encoding for β-galactosidase, tyrosine hydroxylase, and short hairpin RNAs, have all been made available to the brain [320]. However, OX-26 is an antibody against the rat TfR and does not bind to the human TfR, making it impossible to translate this technology to the clinic. Moreover, rat antibodies will cause immunogenic reactions in humans, unless they are humanized. The preparation of humanized or chimeric antibodies is difficult and in some cases this may lead to a loss of affinity for the target receptor [321]. In addition, one can argue that the administration of antibodies directed against such an important uptake mechanism involved in iron homeostasis poses a risk for human application.

Still, preferably, a targeting vector directed to the TfR would be small and nonimmunogenic and should initialize internalization of the TfR upon binding. Xu et al. [322] have used a single-chain antibody Fv fragment against the human TfR, which was tagged with a lipid anchor for insertion into a liposomal bilayer [323]. The molecular weight of this antibody fragment, including the lipid anchor, was approximately 30 kDa. In addition, Lee et al. [323] have used a phage-display technique to find small peptide ligands for the human TfR. They obtained 7 mer and 12 mer peptides that bind to a different binding site than transferrin and are internalized by the TfR. Although these small peptides can also exert immunogenic reactions in humans, they are promising ligands for drug targeting to the human TfR on the BBB.

Insulin Receptor   Another widely characterized, classical, receptor-mediated transcytosis system for the targeting of drugs to the brain is the insulin receptor. Again, just as for the TfR system, Pardridge and colleagues have documented use of the insulin receptor for the targeted delivery of drugs to the brain.

The insulin receptor is a large 300 kDa protein and is a heterotetramer of two extracellular α and two transmembrane β subunits. Each β chain contains a tyrosine kinase activity in its cytosolic extension. The α and β subunits are coded by a single gene and are joined by disulfide bonds to form a cylinder structure. Primarily, insulin binds and changes shape of the receptor to form a tunnel to allow entry of molecules such as glucose into the cells. The insulin receptor is a tyrosine kinase receptor and induces a complex cellular response by phosphorylating proteins on their tyrosine residues. The binding of a single insulin molecule into a pocket created by the two α chains effects a conformational change in the insulin receptor, so that the β chains approximate one another, and carries out transphosphorylation on tyrosine residues. This autophosphorylation is necessary for the receptor to internalize into endosomes. The endosomal system has been shown to be a site where insulin signaling is regulated, but also the degradation of endosomal insulin occurs there. Most of the insulin is degraded, but less so in endothelial cells [324], whereas the receptors are largely recycled to the cell surface. Endocytosis is not necessary for insulin action but probably is important for removing the insulin from the cell, so the target cell for insulin responds in a time-limited fashion to the hormone. This endocytosis mechanism of the insulin receptor has been exploited for the targeting of drugs to the brain.

As for transferrin, the *in vivo* application of insulin as the carrier protein is limited, mainly due to the high concentrations of insulin needed and the resulting lethal overdosing with insulin. Therefore, drug or gene delivery, for instance, to rhesus monkeys is performed with the murine 83–14 MAb that binds to the exofacial epitope on the α subunit of the human insulin receptor. The MAb has a BBB permeability surface area (PS) product in the primate that is ninefold greater than murine MAbs to the human TfR [325]. By using this MAb, Pardridge and co-workers have successfully made available to the brain of primates radio-labeled amyloid-β peptide$_{1-40}$ (Aβ_{1-40}), serving as a diagnostic probe for Alzheimer disease, and pegylated immunoliposomes containing plasmid DNA encoding for β-galactosidase [325].

Unfortunately, the 83-14 MAb cannot be used in humans owing to immunogenic reactions to this mouse protein. However, genetically engineered, effective, forms of the MAb have now been produced, which may allow for drug and gene delivery to the human brain [326]. Still, one can argue that the administration of antibodies directed against such an important mechanism involved in glucose homeostasis poses a risk for human application.

LRP1 and LRP2 Receptors   During the past few years, the LRP1 and LRP2 (also known as megalin or glycoprotein 330) receptors have been exploited to target drugs to the brain in a similar fashion as the transferrin and insulin receptors. Both LRP1 and LRP2 receptors belong to the structurally closely related cell surface LDL receptor gene family. Both receptors are multifunctional, mutiligand scavenger and signaling receptors. A large number of substrates are shared between the two receptors, like lipoprotein lipase (LPL), α_2-macroglobulin (α_2M), receptor-associated protein (RAP), lactoferrin, tissue- and urokinase-type plasminogen activator (tPA/uPA), plasminogen activator inhibitor (PAI-1), and tPA/Upa:PAI-1 complexes. More specific ligands for the LRP1 receptor are melanotransferrin (or P97), thrombospondin 1 and 2, hepatic lipase, factor VIIa / tissue-factor pathway inhibitor (TFPI), factor VIIIa, factor IXa, Aβ_{1-40}, amyloid-β precursor protein (APP), C1 inhibitor, complement C3, apolipoprotein E (apo E), *Pseudomonas* exotoxin A, HIV-1 Tat protein, rhinovirus, matrix metalloproteinase 9 (MMP-9), MMP-13 (collagenase-3), sphingolipid activator protein (SAP), pregnancy zone protein, antithrombin III, heparin cofactor II, α_1-antitrypsin, heat shock protein 96 (HSP-96), and platelet-derived growth factor (PDGF, mainly involved in signaling) [327–331], where apolipoprotein J (apo J, or clusterin), Aβ bound to apo J and apo E, aprotinin, and very low density lipoprotein (VLDL) are more specific for the LRP2 receptor [332, 333].

The group of Richard Béliveau first reported that melanotransferrin/P97 was actively transcytosed across the BBB and suggested that this was mediated by the

LRP1 receptor [331]. Melanotransferrin is a membrane-bound transferrin homolog that can also exist in a soluble form and is highly expressed on melanoma cells compared to normal melanocytes. Intravenously applied melanotransferrin delivers the majority of its bound iron to the liver and kidney, where only a small part was taken up by the brain [334]. After conjugation to melanotransferrin, the group of Béliveau was able to successfully deliver doxorubicin to brain tumors in animal studies [335, 336]. This melanotransferrin-mediated drug targeting technology (now designated NeuroTrans™) is currently further developed by BioMarin Pharmaceuticals Inc. (Novato, CA, USA) for the delivery of enzyme replacement therapies to the brain. Interestingly, together with researchers from BioMarin, Pan et al. [337] recently reported on the efficient transfer of RAP across the BBB by means of the LRP1/LRP2 receptors, suggesting a novel means of protein-based drug delivery to the brain. RAP is a 39kDa protein that functions as a specialized endoplasmic reticulum chaperone assisting in the folding and trafficking of members of the LDL receptor family. In yet unpublished results, the group of Béliveau have now filed a patent application on the use of the LRP2-specific ligand aprotinin, and more specifically on functional derivatives thereof (e.g., angio-pep1), thereby providing a noninvasive and flexible method and a carrier for transporting a compound or drug across the BBB [338]. Aprotinin (Trasylol®) is known as a potent inhibitor of serine proteases such as trypsin, plasmin, and tissue and plasma kallikrein and is the only pharmacologic treatment approved by the U.S. Food and Drug Administration to reduce blood transfusion in coronary artery bypass grafting [339].

In addition to being a tumor marker protein, melanotransferrin is also associated with brain lesions in Alzheimer disease and is a potential marker of the disorder [340]. In addition, the proposed receptor for melanotransferrin, LRP1, has genetically been linked to Alzheimer disease and may influence APP processing and metabolism and Aβ uptake by neurons through α_2M (α_2M is one of the Aβ carrier proteins next to, e.g., apo E, apo J, transthyretin, and albumin) [332, 341]. Furthermore, a close relationship with RAGE (receptor for advanced glycation end products) in shuttling Aβ across the BBB has been described [332, 341]. In addition, the LRP2 receptor has also been described to mediate the uptake of Aβ complexed to apo J and apo E across the BBB [333, 342, 343]. This complex interaction with Alzheimer disease makes the safety of the use of the LRP1/LRP2 receptors for the targeting of drugs to the brain difficult to predict in human application; especially when one considers that the complex signaling function of these receptors is included in the assessment (e.g., the control of permeability of the BBB, vascular tone, and the expression of MMPs [327]), as well as the fact that both receptors are critically involved in the coagulation-fibrinolysis system. On top of that, melanotransferrin was also reported to be directly involved in the activation of plasminogen [344], and high plasma concentrations of melanotransferrin are needed to deliver drugs to the brain, resulting perhaps in dose limitations because of the high iron load in the body.

The same line of reasoning for the interactions at the level of the uptake receptors may apply to the use of RAP and aprotinin (derivatives). On the other hand, the latter has already been successfully applied to humans usually without severe side effects, indeed making the peptide derivatives potentially safe drug carriers. As for RAP, though, no results on the efficacy or capacity of the aprotinin peptides as carrier for drugs have been made available yet.

Diphtheria Toxin Receptor   Recently, our group has identified a novel human applicable carrier protein (known as CRM197) for the targeted delivery of conjugated proteins across the BBB [345, 346]. Uniquely, CRM197 has already been used as a safe and effective carrier protein in human vaccines for a long time [347] and recently also as a systemically active therapeutic protein in anticancer trials [348]. This has resulted in a large body of prior knowledge on the carrier protein, including its transport receptor and mechanism of action, receptor binding domain, conjugation and manufacturing process, and kinetic and safety profile both in animals and humans. CRM197 delivers drugs across the BBB by the well characterized, safe, and effective mechanism called receptor-mediated transcytosis. From the literature, it was already known that CRM197 uses the membrane-bound precursor of heparin-binding epidermal growth factor-like growth factor (HB-EGF) as its transport receptor [349]. This precursor is also known as the diphtheria toxin receptor (DTR). In fact, CRM197 is a nontoxic mutant of diphtheria toxin. Membrane-bound HB-EGF is constitutively expressed on the BBB, neurons, and glial cells [350]. Moreover, HB-EGF expression is strongly upregulated on cerebral blood vessels by ischemic stroke and in gliomas [351, 352], which may lead to a site-selective improvement of the therapeutic efficacy of the targeted drugs in the brain.

By means of a dynamic cell culture model of the BBB, our group was able to demonstrate the functional expression of the DTR, safety of the CRM197 carrier protein, and specific transport efficacy of CRM197 carrier protein conjugated to a 40 kDa enzyme (horseradish peroxidase, HRP, serving as a "model" protein drug) and DTR-targeted pegylated liposomes containing HRP. In addition, the *in vivo* proof-of-principle with this novel brain drug targeting technology was demonstrated by the specific brain uptake of DTR-targeted HRP in guinea pigs [345, 346].

Although HB-EGF is expressed in species including human, monkey, rat, and mouse with a similar tissue distribution, only rats and mice are resistant to diphtheria toxin because of an amino acid substitution in the receptor-binding domain on HB-EGF that reduces binding of diphtheria toxin to rodent HB-EGF [346, 353]. Fortunately, a transgenic mouse (conditionally) expressing the human DTR was recently generated by Cha and co-workers [354], allowing researchers to specifically study the brain drug delivery technology in mice as well.

Another known complication of the bacterial CRM197 protein is that neutralizing antibodies against diphtheria toxin may develop or may already be present in serum of the recipient because of earlier vaccinations, thereby reducing the efficacy of the drug delivery system. There are, however, several lines of evidence that such an immune response to CRM197 can occur, but, most importantly, that it is not really a problem in the clinic, at least not for the treatment of acute indications. In fact, the clinical studies performed by Buzzi et al. [348] indicate that preexisting levels of neutralizing antibodies were rather decreased 30 days after repeated treatment with CRM197.

Another interesting aspect of the DTR is the fact that this receptor is strongly upregulated under inflammatory disease conditions [346] such as occur in many brain diseases like Alzheimer disease, Parkinson disease, multiple sclerosis, ischemia, encephalitis, epilepsy, and tumors [351]. On the one hand, such a situation may enhance the therapeutic effect by disease-induced targeting. On the other hand, this may be used to image (inflammatory) disease areas in the brain. For instance, it has already been shown that the DTR is upregulated in the brain following seizures [355]. By applying CRM197-coated liposomes loaded with an MRI-enhancing agent (e.g., gadolinium), it would be possible to image such disease areas, as has been done for the glucose receptor [356]. In particular, this would be helpful to investigate the extent of damage/recovery and disease progression/therapy in time of many brain diseases, particularly epilepsy, ischemia, and brain tumors.

11.5   CONCLUSION

There is still an unmet need for the treatment of brain diseases. In addition to the presently applied small molecular drugs, there are many good biopharmaceutical drugs that, unfortunately, cannot enter the brain in sufficient quantities to be effective. Therefore, (new) technologies have to be applied and developed to accomplish this. In this chapter we have tried to give insight into the present *in vitro* [357] and *in vivo* [358] techniques to study and improve drug absorption and distribution of biopharmaceutical drugs (e.g., proteins, RNAi, and genes) to the brain.

In vitro techniques to study BBB drug transport and BBB functionality should use an endothelial/astrocyte coculture system for establishing a tight and functional BBB system. Some systems with BBB barrier enhancers (e.g., cAMP, phosphodiesterase inhibitors, glucocorticoids) could be used to estimate BBB drug transport but may lack BBB functionality. From the *in vivo* methods, the noninvasive MRI techniques seem to be very promising and impressive advancements have been made to image (diseased) brain by application of MRI contrast-enhancing agents. The development of technologies to actively target such agents to the (diseased) brain will open a wide area for diagnostic investigations and the possibility to monitor disease progression in the brain.

With respect to the therapeutic treatment of brain diseases, the only human applied technology to deliver (biopharmaceutical) drugs to the brain is by viral delivery. Up to now viral delivery to the brain has to be performed by direct injection/infusion into the brain because of insufficient brain targeting due to the lack of a homing device, which makes it only sufficient for local delivery. Therefore, the most promising technology in our opinion is active vascular nonviral receptor-mediated targeting. Vascular nonviral active targeting has been shown to be effective and selective for global delivery of drugs to the brain in several animals. By using antibodies against receptors (e.g., transferrin and insulin receptor), it has been demonstrated that proteins (enzymes), RNAi, and genes could be targeted to the brain. However, these applications cannot be transferred directly to the human situation: first, because the antibodies used in animals cannot (without humanization) directly be applied in humans; and second, antibodies are meant to stick to their counterpart, which means that administration of these will reduce the availability of receptors at the BBB and in the brain. Moreover, several of these receptors (insulin receptor and the multiligand LRP1 and LRP2 receptors) are involved in signaling too [27, 359]. Therefore, brain targeting by such antibodies may interfere with both the transport of endogenous ligands (e.g., insulin, transferrin) and brain signaling and cause downregulation of receptors; and therefore these antibodies should not be used for chronic administration. Furthermore, the melanotransferrin receptor seems to be involved in the release of plasmin [344] and therefore with the blood clotting cascade, while the LRP1 receptor seems to be involved with apolip-rotein J transport in a complex with Alzheimer's amyloid-β [343]. Interference with such transport systems poses a potential hazard. In this respect, the DTR seems to be a human applicable, safe, and effective uptake receptor for the targeting of drugs to the brain. Moreover, the DTR does not have an endogenous ligand, so there is no competition for transport. Furthermore, CRM197 is already safely applied to humans (illustrating that binding to the DTR *per se* does not result in serious side effects), where other carrier systems involve potential safety hazards in human application. However, even though specific brain uptake of DTR-targeted enzyme was already established in guinea pigs, the technology now awaits further *in vivo* validation in terms of kinetics of brain distribution and efficacy of targeted drugs in relevant disease models of the CNS.

REFERENCES

1. Ehrlich P. *Das Sauerstoff-Bedurfnis des Organismus: eine farbenanalytische Studie.* Berlin: Hirschwald; 1885.
2. Goldman EE. Vitalfarbung am Zentralnervensystem. *Abh Preuss Akad Wiss Phys Math KI* 1913;1:1–60.
3. Abbott NJ. Dynamics of CNS barriers: evolution, differentiation, and modulation. *Cell Mol Neurobiol* 2005;25(1):5–23.
4. Begley DJ, Brightman MW. Structural and functional aspects of the blood–brain barrier. *Prog Drug Res* 2003;61:39–78.
5. Hawkins BT, Davis TP. The blood–brain barrier/neurovascular unit in health and disease. *Pharmacol Rev* 2005;57(2):173–185.
6. Abbott NJ. Inflammatory mediators and modulation of blood–brain barrier permeability. *Cell Mol Neurobiol* 2000;20(2):131–147.
7. Gaillard PJ, de Boer AG, Breimer DD. Pharmacological investigations on lipopolysac-charide-induced permeability changes in the blood–brain barrier *in vitro*. *Microvasc Res* 2003;65(1):24–31.
8. Pardridge WM. Molecular biology of the blood–brain barrier. *Mol Biotechnol* 2005;30(1): 57–70.
9. de Vries HE, Kuiper J, de Boer AG, van Berkel ThJC, Breimer DD. The role of the blood–brain barrier in neuroinflammatory diseases. *Pharmacol Rev* 1997;49(2):143–155.
10. Begley DJ. Delivery of therapeutic agents to the central nervous system: the problems and the possibilities. *Pharmacol Ther* 2004;104(1):29–45.
11. Pardridge WM. Blood–brain barrier biology and methodology. *J Neurovirol* 1999;5(6): 556–569.
12. Pardridge WM. Drug targeting, drug discovery, and brain drug development. In Pardridge WM, Ed. *Brain Drug Targeting—The Future of Brain Drug Development*. New York: Cambridge University Press; 2001, pp 1–12.
13. Keep RG, Jones HC. A morphometric study on the development of the lateral ventricle choroids plexus, choroids plexus capillaries and ventricular ependyma in the rat. *Brain Res Dev Brain Res* 1990;56:47–53.
14. Rubin LL, Staddon JM. The cell biology of the blood–brain barrier. *Annu Rev Neurosci* 1999;22:11–28.

15. Pardridge WM. Overview of blood–brain barrier transport biology and experimental methodologies. In Pardridge WM, Ed. *Peptide Drug Delivery to the Brain*. New York: Raven Press; 1991, pp 52–98.

16. Janzer RC, Raff MC. Astrocytes induce blood–brain barrier properties in endothelial cells. *Nature* 1987;325(6101):253–257.

17. Gaillard PJ, van der Sandt IC, Voorwinden LH, Vu D, Nielsen JL, de Boer AG, Breimer DD. Astrocytes increase the functional expression of P-glycoprotein in an *in vitro* model of the blood–brain barrier. *Pharm Res* 2000;17(10):1198–1205.

18. Lai CH, Kuo KH. The critical component to establish *in vitro* BBB model: pericyte. *Brain Res Brain Res Rev* 2005 [Epub ahead of print].

19. Abbott NJ. Astrocyte-endothelial interactions and blood–brain barrier permeability. *J Anat* 2002;200(6):629–638.

20. Brightman MW, Reese TS. Junctions between intimately apposed cell membranes in the vertebrate brain. *J Cell Biol* 1969;40(3):648–677.

21. Reese TS, Karnovsky MJ. Fine structural localization of a blood–brain barrier to exogenous peroxidase. *J Cell Biol* 1967;34(1):207–217.

22. Minn A, Ghersi-Egea J-F, Perrin R, Leinigner B, Siest G. Drug metabolizing enzyme in the brain and cerebral microvessels. *Brain Res Rev* 1991;16:65–82.

23. el-Bacha RS, Minn A. Drug metabolizing enzymes in cerebrovascular endothelial cells afford a metabolic protection to the brain. *Cell Mol Biol (Noisy-le-grand)* 1999;45(1): 15–23.

24. Ghersi-Egea JF, Leininger-Muller B, Cecchelli R, Fenstermacher JD. Blood–brain interfaces: relevance to cerebral drug metabolism. *Toxicol Lett* 1995;82–83:645–653.

25. Wekerle H. Immune protection of the brain—efficient and delicate. *J Infect Dis* 2002; 186(Suppl 2):S140–S144.

26. Biessels GJ, Bravenboer B, Gispen WH. Glucose, insulin and the brain: modulation of cognition and synaptic plasticityin health and disease: a preface. *Eur J Pharmacol* 2004; 490(1–3):1–4.

27. Herz J, Strickland DK. LRP: a multifunctional scavenger and signaling receptor. *J Clin Invest* 2001;108(6):779–784.

28. Debault LE, Cancilla PA. gamma-Glutamyl transpeptidase in isolated brain endothelial cells: induction by glial cells *in vitro*. *Science* 1980;207(4431):653–655.

29. Hendry SH, Jones EG, Beinfeld MC. Cholecystokinin-immunoreactive neurons in rat and monkey cerebral cortex make symmetric synapses and have intimate associations with blood vessels. *Proc Natl Acad Sci USA* 1983;80(8):2400–2404.

30. Balabanov R, Dore-Duffy P. Role of the CNS microvascular pericyte in the blood–brain barrier. *J Neurosci Res* 1998;53(6):637–644.

31. Kim JA, Tran ND, Li Z, Yang F, Zhou W, Fisher MJ. Brain endothelial hemostasis regulation by pericytes. *J Cereb Blood Flow Metab* 2005; Jul 13 [Epub ahead of print].

32. Cordon-Cardo CJ, O'Brien JP, Casals D, Rittman-Grauer L, Biedler JL, Melamed MR, Bertino JR. Multidrug-resistance gene P-glycoprotein is expressed by endothelial cells at blood–brain barrier sites. *Proc Natl Acad Sci USA* 1989;86:695–698.

33. Schinkel AH, Wagenaar E, van Deemter L, Mol CAAM, Borst P. Absence of the mdr1a P-glycoprotein in mice affects tissue distribution and pharmacokinetics of dexamethasone, digoxin, and cyclosporin A. *J Clin Invest* 1995;96(4):1698–1705.

34. Borst P, Evers R, Kool M, Wijnholds J. The multidrug resistance protein family. *Biochem Biophys Acta* 1999;1461:347–557.

35. Borst P, Evers R, Kool M, Wijnholds J. A family of drug transporters: the multidrug resistance-associated proteins. *J Natl Cancer Inst* 2000;92:1295–1302.

36. de Boer AG, van der Sandt IC, Gaillard PJ. The role of drug transporters at the blood–brain barrier. *Annu Rev Pharmacol Toxicol* 2003;43:629–656.

37. Lee G, Dallas S, Hong M, Bendayan R. Drug transporters in the central nervous system: brain barriers and brain parenchyma considerations. *Pharmacol Rev* 2001;53(4):569–596.

38. Loscher W, Potschka H. Role of drug efflux transporters in the brain for drug disposition and treatment of brain diseases. *Prog Neurobiol* 2005;76(1):22–76.

39. Abbott NJ. Physiology of the blood–brain barrier and its consequences for drug transport to the brain. International Congress Series 1277, *Proceedings of the Esteve Foundation Symposium*, Volume *11*. Amsterdam: Elsevier; 2005, pp 3–18.

40. Begley DJ. ABC transporters and the blood–brain barrier. *Curr Pharm Des* 2004;10(12): 1295–1312.

41. Lo EH, Singhal AB, Torchilin VP, Abbott NJ. Drug delivery to damaged brain. *Brain Res Brain Res Rev* 2001;38(1–2):140–148.

42. Johanson CE, Duncan JA, Stopa EG, Baird A. Enhanced prospects for drug delivery and brain targeting by the choroid-plexus-CSF route. *Pharm Res* 2005;22(7):1011–1037.

43. Emerich DF, Skinner SJM, Borlongan CV, Vasconcellos AF, Thanos CG. The choroids plexus in the rise, fall and repair of the brain. *BioEssays* 2005;27:262–274.

44. Strazielle N, Khuth ST, Ghersi-Egea J-F. Detoxification systems, passive and specific transport for drugs at the blood–CSF barrier in normal and pathological situations. *Adv Drug Deliv Res* 2004;56:1717–1740.

45. Shen DD, Artru AA, Adkinson KK. Principles and applicability of CSF sampling for the assessment of CNS drug delivery and pharmacodynamics. *Adv Drug Deliv Rev* 2004;56:1825–1857.

46. Chodobski A, Szmydynger-Chodobska J. Choroid plexus, target for polypeptides and site of their synthesis. *Microsc Res Tech* 2001;52:65–82.

47. Abbott NJ. Evidence for bulk flow of brain interstitial fluid: significance for physiology and pathology. *Neurochem Int* 2004;45(4):545–552.

48. Faraci FM, Kinzenbaw D, Heistad DD. Effect of endogenous vasopressin on blood flow to choroids plexus during hypoxia and intracranial hypertension. *Am J Physiol* 1994;266: H393–H398.

49. Joó F. The blood–brain barrier *in vitro*: ten years of research on microvessels isolated from the brain. *Neurochem Int* 1985;7:1–25.

50. Joó F. The cerebral microvessels in culture, an update. *J Neurochem* 1992;58:1–17.

51. Joó F. The blood–brain barrier *in vitro*: the second decade. *Neurochem Int* 1933;23(6):499–521.

52. Takakura Y, Audus KL, Borchardt RT. Blood–brain barrier: transport studies in isolated brain capillaries and in cultured brain endothelial cells. *Adv Pharmacol* 1991;22:137–165.

53. Eddy EP, Maleef BE, Hart TK, Smith PL. *In vitro* models to predict blood–brain barrier permeability. *Adv Drug Deliv Rev* 1997;23(1–3):185–198.

54. de Boer AG, Breimer DD. Reconstitution of the blood–brain barrier in cell culture for studies of drug transport and metabolism. *Adv Drug Deliv Rev* 1996;22:251–264.

55. Cecchelli R, Dehouck B, Descamps L, Fenart L, Buée-Scherrer V, Duhem C, Lundquist S, Rentfel M, Torpier G, Dehouck MP. *In vitro* model for evaluating drug transport across the blood–brain barrier. *Adv Drug Deliv Rev* 1999;36:165–178.

56. Pardridge WM. Blood–brain barrier biology and methodology. *J Neurovirol* 1999;5(6): 556–569.

57. Bradbury MWB. The blood–brain barrier. Transport across the cerebral endothelium. *Circ Res* 1985;57:213–222.

58. Gumbleton M, Audus KL. Progress and limitations in the use of *in vitro* cell cultures to serve as a permeability screen for the blood–brain barrier. *J Pharm Sci* 2001;90(11):1681–1698.

59. Cucullo L, Aumayr B, Rapp E, Janigro D. Drug delivery and *in vitro* models of the blood–brain barrier. *Curr Opin Drug Discov Dev* 2005;8(1):89–99.

60. Reichel A, Begley DJ, Abbott NJ. An overview of *in vitro* techniques for blood–brain barrier studies. *Methods Mol Med* 2003;89:307–324.

61. Weksler BB, Subileau EA, Perriere N, Charneau P, Holloway K, Leveque M, Tricoire-Leignel H, Nicotra A, Bourdoulous S, Turowski P, Male DK, Roux F, Greenwood J, Romero IA, Couraud PO. Blood–brain barrier-specific properties of a human adult Brain endothelial cell line. *FASEB J* 2005; [Epub ahead of print].

62. de Boer AG, Gaillard PJ, Breimer DD. The transference of results between blood–brain barrier cell culture systems. *Eur J Pharm Sci* 1999;8(1):1–4.

63. Youdim KA, Avdeef A, Abbott NJ. *In vitro* trans-monolayer permeability calculations: often forgotten assumptions. *Drug Discov Today* 2003;8(21):997–1003.

64. de Boer AG, Sutanto W, Eds. *Drug Transport Across the Blood–Brain Barrier: New Experimental Strategies*. Amsterdam: Harwood Scientific Publisher; 1997.

65. Audus KL, Borchardt RT. Characterization of an *in vitro* blood–brain barrier model system for studying drug transport and metabolism. *Pharm Res* 1986;3:81–87.

66. Audus KL, Rose JM, Wang W, Borchardt RT. In Pardridge W, Ed. *An Introduction to the Blood–Brain Barrier: Methodology and Biology*. New York: Cambridge University Press; 1998, p 86.

67. Dehouck M-P, Méresse S, Delorme P, Fruchart J-C, Cecchelli R. An easier, reproducible, and mass-production method to study the blood–brain barrier *in vitro*. *J Neurochem* 1990;54:1798–1801.

68. Rubin LL, Hall DE, Parter S, Barbu K, Cannon C, Horner HC, Janatpour M, Liaw CW, Manning K, Morales J, Tanner LI, Tomaselli KJ, Bard F. A cell culture model of the blood–brain barrier. *J Cell Biol* 1991;115(6):1725–1735.

69. Gaillard PJ, Voorwinden LH, Nielsen JL, Ivanov A, Atsumi R, Engman H, Ringbom C, de Boer AG, Breimer DD. Establishment and functional characterization of an *in vitro* model of the blood–brain barrier, comprising a co-culture of brain capillary endothelial cells and astrocytes. *Eur J Pharm Sci* 2001;12:215–222.

70. Janzer RC, Raff MC. Astrocytes induce blood–brain barrier properties in endothelial cells. *Nature* 1987;325:253–257.

71. Meresse S, Dehouck MP, Delorme P, Bensaid M, Tauber JP, Delbart C, Fruchart JC, Cecchelli R. Bovine brain endothelial cells express tight junctions and monoamine oxidase activity in long-term culture. *J Neurochem* 1989;53(5):1363–1371.

72. Gaillard PJ, van der Sandt ICJ, Voorwinden LH, Vu D, Nielsen JL, de Boer AG, Breimer DD. Astrocytes increase the functional expression of P-glycoprotein in an *in vitro* model of the blood–brain barrier. *Pharm Res* 2000;17(10):1198–1205.

73. Augustin HG, Kozian DH, Johnson RC. Differentiation of endothelial cells: analysis of the constitutive and activated endothelial cell phenotypes. *BioEssays* 1994;16(12):901–906.

74. Parkinson FE, Friesen J, Krizanac-Bengez L, Janigro D. Use of a three-dimensional *in vitro* model of the rat blood–brain barrier to assay nucleoside efflux from brain. *Brain Res* 2003;980(2):233–241.

75. Coisne C, Dehouck L, Faveeuw C, Delplace Y, Miller F, Landry C, Morissette C, Fenart L, Cecchelli R, Tremblay P, Dehouck B. Mouse syngenic *in vitro* blood–brain barrier model: a new tool to examine inflammatory events in cerebral endothelium. *Lab Invest* 2005;85(6):734–746.

76. Ramsauer M, Kunz J, Krause D, Dermietzel R. Regulation of a blood–brain barrier-specific enzyme expressed by cerebral pericytes (pericytic aminopeptidase N/ pAPN) under cell culture conditions. *J Cerebral Blood Flow Metab* 1998;18:1270–1281.

77. Mukhtar M, Pomerantz RJ. Development of an *in vitro* blood–brain barrier model to study molecular neuropathogenesis and neurovirologic disorders induced by human immunodeficiency virus type 1 infection. *J Human Virol* 2000;3:324–334.

78. Tahti H, Nevala H, Toimela T. Refining *in vitro* neurotoxicity testing—the development of blood–brain barrier models. *Altern Lab Anim* 2003;31(3):273–276.

79. Hurst RD, Fritz IB. Properties of an immortalised vascular endothelial/glioma cell co-culture model of the blood–brain barrier. *J Cell. Physiol* 1996;167:81–88.

80. de Boer AG, Gaillard PJ. Unpublished results, 2005.

81. Tan KH, Dobbie MS, Felix RA, Barrand MA, Hurst RD. A comparison of the induction of immortalized endothelial cell impermeability by astrocytes. *Neuroreport* 2001;12(7): 1329–1334.

82. Franke H, Galla H-J, Beuckmann CT. An improved low-permeability *in vitro*-model of the blood–brain barrier: transport studies on retinoids, sucrose, haloperidol, caffeine and mannitol. *Brain Res* 1999;818:65–71.

83. Sobue K, Yamamoto N, Yoneda K, Hodgson ME, Yamashiro K, Tsuruoka N, Tsuda T, Katsuya H, Miura Y, Asai K, Kato T. Induction of blood–brain barrier properties in immortalized bovine brain endothelial cells by astrocytic factors. *Neurosci Res* 1999;35(2):155–164.

84. Reuss B, Dono R, Unsicker K. Functions of fibroblast growth factor (FGF)-2 and FGF-5 in astroglial differentiation and blood–brain barrier permeability: evidence from mouse mutants. *J Neurosci* 2003;23(16):6404–6412.

85. de Boer AG, de Vries HE, Gaillard PJ, Breimer DD. In de Boer AG, Sutanto W, Eds. *Drug Transport Across the Blood–Brain Barrier: New Experimental Strategies.* Amsterdam: Harwood Scientific Publisher; 1997.

86. Garberg P. Alternatives to laboratory animals. *Altern Lab Anim* 1998;26(6):821–825.

87. Takakura Y, Audus KL, Borchardt RT. Blood–brain barrier: transport studies in isolated brain capillaries and in cultured brain endothelial cells. *Adv Pharmacol* 1991;22:137–165.

88. Gaillard PJ, de Boer AG. Relationship between permeability status of the blood–brain barrier and *in vitro* permeability coefficient of a drug. *Eur J Pharm Sci* 2000;12:95–102.

89. Prieto P, Blaauboer BJ, de Boer AG, Boveri M, Cecchelli R, Clemedson C, Coecke S, Forsby A, Galla HJ, Garberg P, Greenwood J, Price A, Tahti H, European Centre for the Validation of Alternative Methods. Blood–brain barrier *in vitro* models and their application in toxicology. The report and recommendations of ECVAM Workshop 49. *Altern Lab Anim* 2004;32(1):37–50.

90. Garberg P, Ball M, Borg N, Cecchelli R, Fenart L, Hurst RD, Lindmark T, Mabondzo A, Nilsson JE, Raub TJ, Stanimirovic D, Terasaki T, Oberg JO, Osterberg T. *In vitro* models for the blood–brain barrier. *Toxicol In Vitro* 2005;19(3):299–334.

91. Schinkel AH. P-glycoprotein, a gatekeeper in the blood–brain barrier. *Adv Drug Deliv Rev* 1999;36(2–3):179–194.

92. Tamai I, Tsuji A. Transporter-mediated permeation of drugs across the blood–brain barrier. *J Pharm Sci* 2000;89(11):1371–1388.

93. Jaehde U, Masereeuw R, de Boer AG, Fricker G, Nagelkerke JF, Vonderscher J, Breimer DD. Quantification and visualization of the transport of octreotide, a somatostatin analogue, across monolayers of cerebrovascular endothelial cells. *Pharm Res* 1994;11(3): 442–448.

94. Sorensen M, Steenberg B, Knipp GT, Wang W, Steffansen B, Frokjaer S, Borchardt RT. The effect of beta-turn structure on the permeation of peptides across monolayers of bovine brain microvessel endothelial cells. *Pharm Res* 1997;14(10):1341–1348.

95. Gaillard PJ, van der Meide PH, de Boer AG, Breimer DD. Glucocorticoid and type I interferon interactions at the blood–brain barrier: relevance for drug therapies for multiple sclerosis. *NeuroReport* 2001;12(10):2198–2193.

96. Fenart L, Buee-Scherrer V, Descamps L, Duhem C, Poullain MG, Cecchelli R, Dehouck MP. Inhibition of P-glycoprotein: rapid assessment of its implication in blood–brain barrier integrity and drug transport to the brain by an *in vitro* model of the blood–brain barrier. *Pharm Res* 1998;15(7):993–1000.

97. van der Sandt ICJ, Gaillard PJ, Voorwinden LH, de Boer AG, Breimer DD. P-glycoprotein inhibition leads to enhanced disruptive effects by anti-microtubule cytostatics at the *in vitro* blood–brain barrier. *Pharm Res* 2001;18(5):587–592.

98. Barrand MA, Robertson KJ, von Weikersthal SF. Comparisons of P-glycoprotein expression in isolated rat brain microvessels and in primary cultures of endothelial cells derived from microvasculature of rat brain, epididymal fat pad and from aorta. *FEBS Lett* 1995;374(2):179–183.

99. Zhang Y, Han H, Elmquist WF, Millen DW. Expression of various multidrug resistance-associated protein MRP homologues in brain microvessel endothelial cells. *Brain Res* 2000;876:148–153.

100. Durieu-Trautmann O, Fooignant-Chaverot N, Perdomo J, Gounon P, Strosberg AD, Couraud PO. Immortalization of brain capillary endothelial cells with maintenance of structural characteristics of the blood–brain barrier endothelium. *In Vitro Cell Dev Biol* 1991;27(A):771–778.

101. Sobue K, Yamamoto N, Yoneda K, Hodgson ME, Yamashiro K, Tsuroika N, Tsuda T, Katsuya H, Miuara Y, Asai K, Kato T. Induction of blood–brain barrier properties in immortalized bovine brain endothelial cells by astrocytic factors. *Neurosci Res* 1999;35: 155–164.

102. Stins MF, Prasadarao NV, Zhou J, Arditi M, Kim KS. Bovine brain microvascular endothelial cells transfected with SV40-large T antigen: development of an immortalized cell line to study pathophysiology of CNS disease. *In Vitro Cell Dev Biol Anim* 1997;33:243–247.

103. Kido Y, Tamai I, Okamoto M, Suzuki F, Tsuji A. Functional clarification of MCT1-mediated transport of monocarboxylic acids at the blood–brain barrier using *in vitro* cultured cells and *in vivo* BUI studies. *Pharm Res* 2000;17(1):55–62.

104. Terasaki T, Hosoya K. Conditionally immortalized cell lines as a new *in vitro* model for the study of barrier functions. *Biol Pharm Bull* 2001;24(2):111–118.

105. Roux F, Durieue-Trautmann O, Chaverot N, Claire M, Mailly P, Bourre JM, Strosberg AD, Couraud PO. Regulation of gamma-glutamyl transpeptidase and alkaline phosphatase activities in immortalized rat brain microvessel endothelial cells. *J Cell Physiol* 1994;159:101–113.

106. Lechardeur D, Schwartz B, Paulin D, Scherman D. Induction of blood–brain barrier differentiation in a rat brain-derived endothelial cell line. *Exp Cell Res* 1995;220(1): 161–170.

107. Mooradian DL, Diglio CA. Production of a transforming growth factor-beta-like growth factor by RSV-transformed rat cerebral microvascular endothelial cells. *Tumour Biol* 1991;12:171–181.

108. Regina A, Romero IA, Greenwood J, Adamson P, Bourre JM, Couraud PO, Roux F. Dexamethasone regulation of P-glycoprotein activity in an immortalized rat brain endothelial cell line, GPNT. *J Neurochem* 1999;73:1954–1963.

109. Pham YT, Regina A, Farinotti R, Couraud PO, Wainer IW, Roux R, Gimeniz F. Interactions of racemic mefloquine and its enantiomers with P-glycoprotein in an immortalised rat brain capillary endothelial cell line, GPNT. *Biochem Biophys Acta* 2000;1524:212–219.

110. Greenwood J, Pryce G, Devine L, Male DK, Dos Santos WLC, Calder VL, Adamson P. SV40 large T immortalised cell lines of the rat blood–brain and blood–retinal barriers retain their phenotypic and immunological characteristics. *J Neuroimmunol* 1996;71:51–63.

111. Asaba H, Hosoya K, Takanaga H, Ohtsuki S, Tamura E, Takizawa T, Terasaki T. Blood–brain barrier is involved In the efflux transport of a neuroactive steroid, dehydroepiandrosterone sulphate, via organic anion transporting polypeptide 2. *J Neurochem* 2000;75:1907–1916.

112. Tatsuta T, Naito M, Oh-hara T, Sugawara I, Tsuruo T. Functional involvement of P-glycoprotein in blood–brain barrier. *J Biol Chem* 1992;267:20383–20393.

113. Wijsman JA, Shivers RR. Immortalized mouse brain endothelial cells are ultrastructurally similar to endothelial cells and respond to astrocyte-conditioned medium. *In Vitro Cell Dev Biol Anim* 1998;34:777–784.

114. Teifel M, Friedl P. Establishment of the permanent microvascular endothelial cell line PBMEC/C1–2 from porcine brains. *Exp Cell Res* 1996;228:50–57.

115. Muruganandam A, Herx LM, Monette R, Durkin JP, Stanimirovic DB. Development of immortalized human cerebromicrovascular endothelial cell line as an *in vitro* model of the human blood–brain barrier. *FASEB J* 1997;11:1187–1197.

116. Prudhomme JG, Sherman IW, Land KM, Moses AV, Stenglein S, Nelson JA. Studies of *Plasmodium falciparum* cytoadherence using immortalized human brain capillary endothelial cells. *Int J Parasitol* 1996;26:647–655.

117. Xiao L, Yang C, Dorovinin-Zis K, Tandon NN, Ades E, Lal AA, Udhayakumar V. *Plasmodium falciparum*: involvement of additional receptors in the cytoadherence of infected erythrocytes to microvascular endothelial cells. *Exp Parasitol* 1996;84:42–55.

118. Beuckmann CT, Dernbach K, Hakvoort A, Galla HJ. A new astrocytic cell line which is able to induce a blood–brain barrier property in cultured brain capillary endothelial cells. *Cytotechnology* 1997;24(1):11–17.

119. Raub TJ. Signal transduction and glial cell modulation of cultured brain microvessel endothelial cell tight junctions. *Am J Physiol* 1996;271:C495–C503.

120. Lagrange P, Romero IA, Minn A, Revest PA. Transendothelial permeability changes induced by free radicals in an *in vitro* model of the blood–brain barrier. *Free Radic Biol Med* 1999;27(5–7):667–672.

121. Stanness KA, Guateo E, Janigro D. A dynamic model of the blood–brain barrier "*in vitro.*" *Neurotoxicology* 1996;17(2):481–496.

122. Tetsuka K, Hosoya K, Ohtsuki S, Takanaga H, Yanai N, Ueda M, Obinata M, Terasaki T. Acidic amino acid transport characteristics of a newly developed conditionally immortalized rat type 2 astrocyte cell line (TR-AST). *Cell Structure and Function* 2001;26(4):197–203.

123. Veronesi B. Characterization of the MDCK cell line for screening neurotoxicants. *NeuroToxicology* 1996;17(2):433–443.

124. Oldendorf WH. Measurement of brain uptake of radiolabeled substances using a tritiated water internal standard. *Brain Res* 1970;24:372–376.

125. Oldendorf WH. Blood–brain barrier permeability to drugs. *Annu Rev Pharmacol* 1974;14:239–248.

126. Kakee A, Terasaki T, Sygiyama Y. Brain efflux index as a novel method of analyzing efflux transport at the blood–brain barrier. *J Pharmacol Exp Ther* 1996;277:1550–1559.

127. Kakee A, Terasaki T, Sugiyama Y. Selective brain to blood efflux transport of para-aminohippuric acid across the blood–brain barrier: *in vivo* evidence by use of the brain efflux index method. *J Pharmacol Exp Ther* 1997;283(3):1018–1025.

128. Brodie BB, Kurz H, Shanker LS. The importance of dissociaton constant and lipid-solubility in influencing the passage of drugs into the cerebrospinal fluid. *J Pharmacol Exp Ther* 1960;130:20–25.

129. Ohno K, Pettigrew KD, Rapoport SI. Lower limits of cerebrovascular permeability to nonelectrolytes in the conscious rat. *Am J Physiol* 1978;235:H299–H307.

130. Preston E, Haas N. Defining the lower limits of blood–brain barrier permeability: factors affecting the magnitude and interpretation of permeability-area products. *J Neursci Res* 1986;16:709–719.

131. Smith QR. In Neuwelt EA, Ed. *Implications of the Blood–Brain Barrier and Its Manipulation, Volume 1: Basic Science Aspects*. New York: Plenum Publishing Corp; 1989, pp 85–118.

132. Smith QR. A review of blood–brain barrier transport techniques. *Methods Mol Med* 2003;89:193–208.

133. Patlak CS, Blasberg RG, Fenstermacher JD. Graphical evaluation of blood-to-brain transfer constants from multiple-time uptake data. *J Cerebral Blood Flow Metab* 1983;3:1–7.

134. Crone C, Levitt DG. In Renkin EM, Michel CC, Eds. *Handbook of Physiology*. Bethesda, MD: American Physiological Society; 1984, Vol 4, Part I, pp 411–466.

135. Patlak CS, Blasberg RG. Graphical evaluation of blood-to-brain transfer constants from multiple-time uptake data. Generalizations. *J Cerebral Blood Blow Metab* 1985;5: 584–590.

136. Takasato Y, Rapoport SI, Smith QR. An *in situ* brain perfusion technique to study cerebrovascular transport in the rat. *Am J Physiol* 1984;247:H484–H493.

137. Zlokovic BV, Begley DJ, Djuricic BM, Mitrovic DM. Measurement of solute transport across the blood–brain barrier in the perfused guinea pig brain: method and application to *N*-methyl-alpha-aminoisobutyric acid. *J Neurochem* 1986;46:1444–1451.

138. Vaughan DP, Dennis M. Mathematical basis of point-area deconvolution method for determining *in vivo* input functions. *J Pharm Sci* 1978;67:663–665.

139. Langenbucher F. Numerical convolution/deconvolution as a tool for correlating *in vitro* with *in vivo* drug availability. *Pharm Ind* 1982;44:1166–1172.

140. Langenbucher F. Improved understanding of convolution algorithms correlating body response with drug input. *Pharm Ind* 1982;44:1275–1278.

141. van Bree JBMM, Baljet AV, van Geyt A, de Boer AG, Danhof M, Breimer DD. The unit impulse response procedure for the pharmacokinetic evaluation of drug entry into the central nervous system. *J Pharmacokinet Biopharm* 1989;17:441–462.

142. Hendrikse NH, Schinkel AH, De Vries EGE, Fluks E, Van der Graaf WTA, et al. Complete *in vivo* reversal of P-glycoprotein pump function in the blood–brain barrier visualized with positron emission tomography. *Br J Pharmacol* 1998;124(7):1413–1418.

143. Davson H. A comparative study of the aqueous humour and cerebrospinal fluid in the rabbit. *J Physiol Lond* 1955;129:111–133.

144. Hendrikse NH, Franssen EJ, van der Graaf WT, Vaalburg W, De Vries EG. Visualization of multidrug resistance *in vivo. Eur J Nucl Med* 1999;26(3):283–293.

145. Hendrikse NH, de Vries EG, Eriks-Fluks L, van der Graaf WT, Hospers GA, Willemsen AT, Vaalburg W, Franssen EJ. A new *in vivo* method to study P-glycoproteIn transport In tumors and the blood–brain barrier. *Cancer Res* 1999;59(10):2411–2416.

146. Campbell D. Track autoradiography with iron-59 and sulphur-35 with quantitative evaluation. *Nature* 1951;167(4242):274–275.

147. de Lange ECM, de Boer AG, Breimer DD. Methodological issues in microdialysis sampling for pharmacokinetic studies. *Adv Drug Deliv Rev* 2000;45:125–148.

148. de Lange ECM, Zurcher C, Danhof M, de Boer AG, Breimer DD. Repeated microdialysis perfusions: periprobe tissue reactions and BBB permeability. *Brain Res* 1995;702:261–265.

149. de Lange ECM, de Boer AG, Breimer DD. Microdialysis for pharmacokinetic analysis of drug transport to the brain. *Adv Drug Deliv Rev* 1999;36:211–227.

150. Sawchuk RJ, Elmquist WF. Microdialysis in the study of drug transporters in the CNS. *Adv Drug Deliv Rev* 2000;45(2–3):295–307.

151. Xie R, Hammerlund-Udenaes M, de Boer AG, de Lange ECM. The role of P-glycoprotein in blood–brain barrier transport of morphine: transcortical microdialysis studies in mdr1a (−/−) and mdr1a (+/+) mice. *Br J Pharmacol* 1999;128:563–568.

152. Lonnroth P, Jansson PA, Smith U. A microdialysis method allowing characterization of intercellular water space in humans. *Am J Physiol* 1987;253:E228–E231.

153. Olson RJ, Justice JB. Quantitative microdialysis under transient conditions. *Anal Chem* 1993;65:1017–1022.

154. Jenkins BG, Chen YI, Kuestermann E, Makris NM, Nguyen V, et al. An integrated strategy for evaluation of metabolic and oxidative defects in neurodegenerative illness using magnetic resonance techniques. *Ann NY Acad Sci* 1999;893:214–242.

155. Del Sole A, Falini A, Ravasi L, Ottobrini L, De Marchis D, Bombardieri E, Lucignani G. Anatomical and biochemical investigation of primary brain tumours. *Eur J Nucl Med* 2001;28:1851–1872.

156. Barkhof F, van Walderveen M. Characterization of tissue damage in multiple sclerosis by nuclear magnetic resonance. *Philos Trans R Soc Lond B Biol Sci* 1999;354(1390):1675–1686.

157. Bradley WG Jr. Magnetic resonance imaging of the central nervous system. *Neurol Res* 1984;6(3):91–106.

158. Moller HE, Ullrich K, Weglage J. *In vivo* proton magnetic resonance spectroscopy in phenylketonuria. *Eur J Pediatr* 2000;159(Suppl 2):S121–S125.

159. Weglage J, Wiedermann D, Denecke J, Feldmann R, Koch HG, et al. Individual blood–brain barrier phenylalanine transport determines clinical outcome in phenylketonuria. *Ann Neurol* 2001;50(4):463–467.

160. McDonald WI. Rachelle Fishman–Matthew Moore Lecture. The pathological and clinical dynamics of multiple sclerosis. *Neuropathol Exp Neurol* 1994;53(4):338–343.

161. Simone IL, Tortorella C, Federico F. The contribution of (1)H-magnetic resonance spectroscopy in defining the pathophysiology of multiple sclerosis. *Ital J Neurol Sci* 1999;20(5 Suppl):S241–S245.

162. Ederoth P, Tunblad K, Bouw R, Lundberg CJ, Ungerstedt U, Nordstrom CH, Hammarlund-Udenaes M. Blood–brain barrier transport of MorphIne In patients with severe brain trauma. *Br J Clin Pharmacol* 2004;57(4):427–435.

163. Thakur ML, Lentle BC, SNM. Radiological Society of North America (RSNA) Joint SNM/RSNA Molecular Imaging Summit Statement. *J Nucl Med* 2005;46(9):11N–13N, 42N.

164. Pirko I, Fricke ST, Johnson AJ, Rodriguez M, Macura SI. Magnetic resonance imaging, microscopy, and spectroscopy of the central nervous system in experimental animals. *NeuroRx* 2005;2(2):250–264.

165. Jasanoff A. Functional MRI using molecular imaging agents. *Trends Neurosci* 2005;28(3): 120–126.

166. Koretsky AP. New developments in magnetic resonance imaging of the brain. *NeuroRx* 2004;1(1):155–164.

167. Rudin M, Rausch M, Stoeckli M. Molecular imaging in drug discovery and development: potential and limitations of nonnuclear methods. *Mol Imaging Biol* 2005;7(1):5–13.

168. Inglese M, Ge Y. Quantitative MRI: hidden age-related changes in brain tissue. *Top Magn Reson Imaging* 2004;15(6):355–363.

169. Gothelf D, Furfaro JA, Penniman LC, Glover GH, Reiss AL. The contribution of novel brain imaging techniques to understanding the neurobiology of mental retardation and developmental disabilities. *Ment Retard Dev Disabil Res Rev* 2005;11(4):331–339.

170. Jacobs AH, Kracht LW, Gossmann A, Ruger MA, Thomas AV, Thiel A, Herholz K. Imaging in neurooncology. *NeuroRx* 2005;2(2):333–347.

171. Sipkins DA, Gijbels K, Tropper FD, Bednarski M, Li KC, Steinman L. ICAM-1 expression in autoimmune encephalitis visualized using magnetic resonance imaging. *J Neuroimmunol* 2000;104(1):1–9.

172. Liu X, Chen C. Strategies to optimize brain penetration in drug discovery. *Curr Opin Drug Discov Dev* 2005;8(4):505–512.

173. Nicholson C, Sykova, E. Extracellular space structure revealed by diffusion analysis. *Trends Neurosci* 1998;21(5):207–215.

174. Fenstermacher J, Kaye T. Drug "diffusion" within the brain. *Ann N Y Acad Sci* 1988;531: 29–39.

175. Aird RB. A study of intrathecal, cerebrospinal fluid-to-brain exchange. *Exp Neurol* 1984;86(2):342–358.

176. Rall DP. Transport through the ependymal linings. *Prog Brain Res* 1968;29:159–172.

177. Yan Q, Matheson C, Sun J, Radeke MJ, Feinstein SC, Miller JA. Distribution of intracerebral ventricularly administered neurotrophins in rat brain and its correlation with trk receptor expression. *Exp Neurol* 1994;127(1):23–36.

178. Nagaraja TN, Patel P, Gorski M, Gorevic PD, Patlak CS, Fenstermacher JD. In normal rat, intraventricularly administered insulin-like growth factor-1 is rapidly cleared from CSF with limited distribution into brain. *Cerebrospinal Fluid Res* 2005;26:2–5.

179. Nutt JG, Burchiel KJ, Comella CL, Jankovic J, Lang AE, Laws ER Jr, Lozano AM, Penn RD, Simpson RK Jr, Stacy M, Wooten GF, ICV GDNF Study Group. Implanted intracerebroventricular, glial cell line-derived neurotrophic factor. Randomized, double-blind trial of glial cell line-derived neurotrophic factor (GDNF) in PD. *Neurology* 2003;60(1):69–73.

180. Patel NK, Bunnage M, Plaha P, Svendsen CN, Heywood P, Gill SS. Intraputamenal infusion of glial cell line-derived neurotrophic factor in PD: a two-year outcome study. *Ann Neurol* 2005;57(2):298–302.

181. Slevin JT, Gerhardt GA, Smith CD, Gash DM, Kryscio R, Young B. Improvement of bilateral motor functions in patients with Parkinson disease through the unilateral intraputaminal infusion of glial cell line-derived neurotrophic factor. *J Neurosurg* 2005;102(2):216–222.

182. Amgen Press Release. 11 Feb 2005.

183. Mardor Y, Rahav O, Zauberman Y, Lidar Z, Ocherashvilli A, Daniels D, Roth Y, Maier SE, Orenstein A, Ram Z. Convention-enhanced dud delivery increased efficacy and magnetic resonance image monitoring. *Cancer Res* 2005;65(15):6858–6863.

184. Ohata K, Marmarou A. Clearance of brain edema and macromolecules through the cortical extracellular space. *J Neurosurg* 1992;77:387–396.

185. Chen MY, Lonser RR, Morrison PF, Governale LS, Oldfield EH. Variables affecting CED to the striatum: a systemic examination of rate of infusion, cannula size, infusate concentration, and tissue–cannula sealing time. *J Neurosurg* 1999;90:315–320.

186. Kroll RA, Neuwelt EA. Outwitting the blood–brain barrier for therapeutic purposes: osmotic opening and other means. *Neurosurgery* 1998;42:1083–1100.

187. Wells DJ. Opening the floodgates: clinically applicable hydrodynamic delivery of plasmid DNA to skeletal muscle. *Mol Ther* 2004;10(2):207–208.

188. Wolff JA, Budker V. The mechanism of naked DNA uptake and expression. *Adv Genet* 2005;54:3–20.

189. Krewson CE, Klarman ML, Saltzman WM. Distribution of nerve growth factor following direct delivery to brain interstitium. *Brain Res* 1995;680(1–2):196–206.

190. Davidson BL, Breakefield XO. Viral vectors for gene delivery to the nervous system. *Nat Rev Neurosci* 2003;4(5):353–364.

191. Snyder RO, Francis J. Adeno-associated viral vectors for clinical gene transfer studies. *Curr Gene Ther* 2005;5(3):311–321.

192. Deglon N, Hantraye P. Viral vectors as tools to model and treat neurodegenerative disorders. *J Gene Med* 2005;7(5):530–539.

193. de Lima MC, Da Cruz MT, Cardoso AL, Simoes S, de Almeida LP. Liposomal and viral vectors for gene therapy of the central nervous system. *Curr Drug Targets CNS Neurol Disord* 2005;4(4):453–465.

194. Fountaine TM, Wood MJ, Wade-Martins R. Delivering RNA interference to the mammalian brain. *Curr Gene Ther* 2005;5(4):399–410.

195. Kootstra NA, Verma IM. Gene therapy with viral vectors. *Annu Rev Pharmacol Toxicol* 2003;43:413–439.

196. Kay MA, Glorioso JC, Naldini L. Viral vectors for gene therapy: the art of turning infectious agents into vehicles of therapeutics. *Nat Med* 2001;7(1):33–40.

197. Chen H, McCarty DM, Bruce AT, Suzuki K. Oligodendrocyte-specific gene expression in mouse brain: use of a myelin-forming cell type-specific promoter in an adeno-associated virus. *J Neurosci Res* 1999;55(4):504–513.

198. Niwa H, Yamamura K, Miyazaki J. Efficient selection for high-expression transfectants with a novel eukaryotic vector. *Gene* 1991;108(2):193–199.

199. Klein RL, Meyer EM, Peel AL, Zolotukhin S, Meyers C, Muzyczka N, King MA. Neuron-specific transduction in the rat septohippocampal or nigrostriatal pathway by recombinant adeno-associated virus vectors. *Exp Neurol* 1998;150(2):183–194.

200. Fu H, Samulski RJ, McCown TJ, Picornell YJ, Fletcher D, Muenzer J. Neurological correction of lysosomal storage in a mucopolysaccharidosis IIIB mouse model by adeno-associated virus-mediated gene delivery. *Mol Ther* 2002;5(1):42–49.

201. Peel AL, Zolotukhin S, Schrimsher GW, Muzyczka N, Reier PJ. Efficient transduction of green fluorescent protein in spinal cord neurons using adeno-associated virus vectors containing cell type-specific promoters. *Gene Ther* 1997;4(1):16–24.

202. Paterna JC, Moccetti T, Mura A, Feldon J, Bueler H. Influence of promoter and WHV post-transcriptional regulatory element on AAV-mediated transgene expression in the rat brain. *Gene Ther* 2000;7(15):1304–1311.

203. Zhang Y, Schlachetzki F, Zhang YF, Boado RJ, Pardridge WM. Normalization of striatal tyrosine hydroxylase and reversal of motor impairment in experimental parkinsonism with intravenous nonviral gene therapy and a brain-specific promoter. *Hum Gene Ther* 2004;15(4):339–350.

204. Mandel RJ, Rendahl KG, Spratt SK, Snyder RO, Cohen LK, Leff SE. Characterization of intrastriatal recombinant adeno-associated virus-mediated gene transfer of human tyrosine hydroxylase and human GTP-cyclohydrolase I in a rat model of Parkinson's disease. *J Neurosci* 1998;18(11):4271–4284.

205. Owen R, Mandel RJ, Ammini CV, Conlon TJ, Kerr DS, Stacpoole PW, Flotte TR. Gene therapy for pyruvate dehydrogenase E1alpha deficiency using recombinant adeno-associated virus 2 (rAAV2) vectors. *Mol Ther* 2002;6(3):394–399.

206. Donello JE, Loeb JE, Hope TJ. Woodchuck hepatitis virus contains a tripartite post-transcriptional regulatory element. *J Virol* 1998;72(6):5085–5092.

207. Loeb JE, Cordier WS, Harris ME, Weitzman MD, Hope TJ. Enhanced expression of transgenes from adeno-associated virus vectors with the woodchuck hepatitis virus post-transcriptional regulatory element: implications for gene therapy. *Hum Gene Ther* 1999;10(14):2295–2305.

208. Trojan J, Blossey BK, Johnson TR, Rudin SD, Tykocinski M, Ilan J, Ilan J. Loss of tumorigenicity of rat glioblastoma directed by episome-based antisense cDNA transcription of insulin-like growth factor I. *Proc Natl Acad Sci USA* 1992;89(11):4874–4878.

209. Zhang Y, Zhang YF, Bryant J, Charles A, Boado RJ, Pardridge WM. Intravenous RNA interference gene therapy targeting the human epidermal growth factor receptor prolongs survival in intracranial brain cancer. *Clin Cancer Res* 2004;10(11):3667–3677.

210. Snudden DK, Smith PR, Lai D, Ng MH, Griffin BE. Alterations in the structure of the EBV nuclear antigen, EBNA1, in epithelial cell tumours. *Oncogene* 1995;10(8):45–52.

211. Blau HM, Rossi FM. Tet B or not tet B: advances in tetracycline-inducible gene expression. *Proc Natl Acad Sci USA* 1999;96(3):7–9.

212. Kafri T, van Praag H, Gage FH, Verma IM. Lentiviral vectors: regulated gene expression. *Mol Ther* 2000;1:516–521.

213. Pfeifer A, Brandon EP, Kootstra N, Gage FH, Verma IM. Delivery of the Cre recombinase by a self-deleting lentiviral vector: efficient gene targeting *in vivo*. *Proc Natl Acad Sci USA* 2001;98(20):450–455.

214. Daly TM. Overview of adeno-associated viral vectors. *Methods Mol Biol* 2004;246:157–165.

215. Burger C, Nash K, Mandel RJ. Recombinant adeno-associated viral vectors in the nervous system. *Hum Gene Ther* 2005;16(7):1–91.

216. Gao G, Alvira MR, Somanathan S, Lu Y, Vandenberghe LH, Rux JJ, Calcedo R, Sanmiguel J, Abbas Z, Wilson JM. Adeno-associated viruses undergo substantial evolution in primates during natural infections. *Proc Natl Acad Sci USA* 2003;100(10):81–86.

217. Grimm D, Kay MA. From virus evolution to vector revolution: use of naturally occurring serotypes of adeno-associated virus (AAV) as novel vectors for human gene therapy. *Curr Gene Ther* 2003;3(4):1–304.

218. McCown TJ, Xiao X, Li J, Breese GR, Samulski RJ. Differential and persistent expression patterns of CNS gene transfer by an adeno-associated virus (AAV) vector. *Brain Res* 1996;713(1–2):99–107.

219. Muzyczka N, Berns KI. Parvoviridae: the viruses and their replication. In Knipe DM, Howley PM, Eds. *Field's Virology*. New York: Lippincott, Williams; 2001, pp 2327–2360.

220. Lu Y. Recombinant adeno-associated virus as delivery vector for gene therapy—a review. *Stem Cells Dev* 2004;13(1):3–45.

221. Fitzsimons HL, Bland RJ, During MJ. Promoters and regulatory elements that improve adeno-associated virus transgene expression in the brain. *Methods* 2002;28(2):7–36.

222. Davidson BL, Paulson HL. Molecular medicine for the brain: silencing of disease genes with RNA interference. *Lancet Neurol* 2004;3(3):5–9.

223. Somia N, Verma IM. Gene therapy: trials and tribulations. *Nat Rev Genet* 2000;1(2): 1–9.

224. Hsich G, Sena-Esteves M, Breakefield XO. Critical issues in gene therapy for neurologic disease. *Hum Gene Ther* 2002;13(5):9–604.

225. Tang G, Chiocca A. Gene transfer and delivery in central nervous system disease. *Neurosurg Focus* 1997;3(3):e2.

226. Latchman DS, Coffin RS. Viral vectors in the treatment of Parkinson's disease. *Mov Disord* 2000;15(1):17.

227. Ruitenberg MJ, Blits B, Dijkhuizen PA, te Beek ET, Bakker A, van Heerikhuize JJ, Pool CW, Hermens WT, Boer GJ, Verhaagen J. Adeno-associated viral vector-mediated gene transfer of brain-derived neurotrophic factor reverses atrophy of rubrospinal neurons following both acute and chronic spinal cord injury. *Neurobiol Dis* 2004; 15(2):4–406.

228. Kirik D, Georgievska B, Burger C, Winkler C, Muzyczka N, Mandel RJ, Bjorklund A. Reversal of motor impairments in parkinsonian rats by continuous intrastriatal delivery of L-dopa using rAAV-mediated gene transfer. *Proc Natl Acad Sci USA* 2002;99(7):8–13.

229. Shen Y, Muramatsu SI, Ikeguchi K, Fujimoto KI, Fan DS, Ogawa M, Mizukami H, Urabe M, Kume A, Nagatsu I, Urano F, Suzuki T, Ichinose H, Nagatsu T, Monahan J, Nakano I, Ozawa K. Triple transduction with adeno-associated virus vectors expressing tyrosine hydroxylase, aromatic-L-amino-acid decarboxylase, and GTP cyclohydrolase I for gene therapy of Parkinson's disease. *Hum Gene Ther* 2000;11(11):9–19.

230. Passini MA, Watson DJ, Vite CH, Landsburg DJ, Feigenbaum AL, Wolfe JH. Intraventricular brain injection of adeno-associated virus type 1 (AAV1) in neonatal mice results in complementary patterns of neuronal transduction to AAV2 and total long-term correction of storage lesions in the brains of beta-glucuronidase-deficient mice. *J Virol* 2003;77(12):34–40.

231. Desmaris N, Verot L, Puech JP, Caillaud C, Vanier MT, Heard JM. Prevention of neuropathology in the mouse model of Hurler syndrome. *Ann Neurol* 2004;56(1):8–76.

232. Kordower JH, Emborg ME, Bloch J, Ma SY, Chu Y, Leventhal L, McBride J, Chen EY, Palfi S, Roitberg BZ, Brown WD, Holden JE, Pyzalski R, Taylor MD, Carvey P, Ling Z, Trono D, Hantraye P, Deglon N, Aebischer P. Neurodegeneration prevented by lentiviral vector delivery of GDNF in primate models of Parkinson's disease. *Science* 2000; 290(5492):767–773.

233. Consiglio A, Quattrini A, Martino S, Bensadoun JC, Dolcetta D, Trojani A, Benaglia G, Marchesini S, Cestari V, Oliverio A, Bordignon C, Naldini L. *In vivo* gene therapy of metachromatic leukodystrophy by lentiviral vectors: correction of neuropathology and protection against learning impairments in affected mice. *Nat Med* 2001;7(3):310–316.

234. Mandel RJ, Snyder RO, Leff SE. Recombinant adeno-associated viral vector-mediated glial cell line-derived neurotrophic factor gene transfer protects nigral dopamine neurons after onset of progressive degeneration in a rat model of Parkinson's disease. *Exp Neurol* 1999;160(1):205–214.

235. Bosch A, Perret E, Desmaris N, Heard JM. Long-term and significant correction of brain lesions in adult mucopolysaccharidosis type VII mice using recombinant AAV vectors. *Mol Ther* 2000;1(1):63–70.

236. Dodge JC, Clarke J, Song A, Bu J, Yang W, Taksir TV, Griffiths D, Zhao MA, Schuchman EH, Cheng SH, O'riordan CR, Shihabuddin LS, Passini MA, Stewart GR. Gene transfer of human acid sphingomyelinase corrects neuropathology and motor deficits in a mouse model of Niemann–Pick type A disease. *Proc Natl Acad Sci USA*, 2005;Nov 21 [Epub ahead of print].

237. Xu J, Ma C, Bass C, Terwilliger EF. A combination of mutations enhances the neurotropism of AAV-2. *Virology* 2005;341(2):203–214.

238. Wang X, Kong L, Zhang GR, Sun M, Geller AI. Targeted gene transfer to nigrostriatal neurons in the rat brain by helper virus-free HSV-1 vector particles that contain either a chimeric HSV-1 glycoprotein C-GDNF or a gC-BDNF protein. *Brain Res Mol Brain Res* 2005;139(1):88–102.

239. Jooss K, Chirmule N. Immunity to adenovirus and adeno-associated viral vectors: implications for gene therapy. *Gene Ther* 2003;10(11):955–963.

240. Barkats M, Bilang-Bleuel A, Buc-Caron MH, Castel-Barthe MN, Corti O, Finiels F, Horellou P, Revah F, Sabate O, Mallet J. Adenovirus in the brain: recent advances of gene therapy for neurodegenerative diseases. *Prog Neurobiol* 1998;55(4):333–341.

241. Lowenstein PR, Castro MG. Inflammation and adaptive immune responses to adenoviral vectors injected into the brain: peculiarities, mechanisms, and consequences. *Gene Ther* 2003;10(11):946–954.

242. Thomas CE, Storm TA, Huang Z, Kay MA. Rapid uncoating of vector genomes is the key to efficient liver transduction with pseudotyped adeno-associated virus vectors. *J Virol* 2004;78(6):3110–3122.

243. Landles C, Bates GP. Huntington and the molecular pathogenesis of Huntington's disease. Fourth in molecular medicine review series. *EMBO Rep* 2004;5(10):958–963.

244. Thomas CE, Schiedner G, Kachaned S, Castro MG, Loewenstein PR. Peripheral infection with adenovirus causes unexpected long-term brain inflammation in animals injected intracranially with first-generation, but not with high capacity adenovirus vectors: toward realistic long-term neurological gene therapy for chronic diseases. *Proc Natl Acad Sci USA* 2000;97:7482–7487.

245. Schlachetzki F, Zhang Y, Boado RJ, Pardridge WM. Gene therapy of the brain: the transvascular approach. *Neurology* 2004;62(8):1275–1281.

246. Abordo-Adesida E, Follenzi A, Barcia C, Sciascia S, Castro MG, Naldini L, Lowenstein PR. Stability of lentiviral vector-mediated transgene expression in the brain in the presence of systemic antivector immune responses. *Hum Gene Ther* 2005;16(6):741–751.

247. Tsuji D, Kuroki A, Ishibashi Y, Itakura T, Itoh K. Metabolic correction in microglia derived from Sandhoff disease model mice. *J Neurochem* 2005;94(6):1631–1638.

248. Kobayashi H, Carbonaro D, Pepper K, Petersen D, Ge S, Jackson H, Shimada H, Moats R, Kohn DB. Neonatal gene therapy of MPS I mice by intravenous injection of a lentiviral vector. *Mol Ther* 2005;11(5):776–789.

249. Fjord-Larsen L, Johansen JL, Kusk P, Tornoe J, Gronborg M, Rosenblad C, Wahlberg LU. Efficient *in vivo* protection of nigral dopaminergic neurons by lentiviral gene transfer of a modified Neurturin construct. *Exp Neurol* 2005;195(1):49–60.

250. Georgievska B, Jakobsson J, Persson E, Ericson C, Kirik D, Lundberg C. Regulated delivery of glial cell line-derived neurotrophic factor into rat striatum, using a tetracycline-dependent lentiviral vector. *Hum Gene Ther* 2004;15(10):934–944.

251. Ralph GS, Radcliffe PA, Day DM, Carthy JM, Leroux MA, Lee DC, Wong LF, Bilsland LG, Greensmith L, Kingsman SM, Mitrophanous KA, Mazarakis ND, Azzouz M. Silencing mutant SOD1 using RNAi protects against neurodegeneration and extends survival in an ALS model. *Nat Med* 2005;11(4):429–433.

252. Vezzani A. Gene therapy in epilepsy. *Epilepsy Curr* 2004;4(3):87–90.

253. Crozet C, Lin YL, Mettling C, Mourton-Gilles C, Corbeau P, Lehmann S, Perrier V. Inhibition of PrPSc formation by lentiviral gene transfer of PrP containing dominant negative mutations. *J Cell Sci* 2004;117(Pt 23):5591–5597.

254. Steffens S, Tebbets J, Kramm CM, Lindemann D, Flake A, Sena-Esteves M. Transduction of human glial and neuronal tumor cells with different lentivirus vector pseudotypes. *J Neurooncol* 2004;70(3):281–288.

255. Wong LF, Ralph GS, Walmsley LE, Bienemann AS, Parham S, Kingsman SM, Uney JB, Mazarakis ND. Lentiviral-mediated delivery of Bcl-2 or GDNF protects against excitotoxicity in the rat hippocampus. *Mol Ther* 2005;11(1):89–95.

256. Pardridge WM. Drug and gene delivery to the brain: the vascular route. *Neuron* 2002;36(4):555–558.

257. Bradbury MW. *The Concept of a Blood–Brain Barrier*. Chichester: Wiley; 1979.

258. Pardridge WM. Transport of small molecules through the blood–brain barrier: biology and methodology. *Adv Drug Deliv Rev* 1995;15:5–36.

259. Stein WD. *The Movement of Molecules Across Cell Membranes*. New York: Academic Press; 1967.

260. Abraham MH, Chadha HS, Mitchell RC. Hydrogen bonding. 33. Factors that influence the distribution of solutes between blood and brain. *J Pharm Sci* 1994;83(9):1257–1268.

261. Lipinski CA, Lombardo F, Dominy BW, Feeney PJ. Experimental and computational approaches to estimate solubility and permeability in drug discovery and development settings. *Adv Drug Deliv Rev* 2001;46(1–3):3–26.

262. Bickel U, Yoshikawa T, Pardridge WM. Delivery of peptides and proteins through the blood–brain barrier. *Adv Drug Deliv Rev* 2001;46(1–3):247–279.

263. Vorbrodt AW. Ultracytochemical characterization of anionic sites in the wall of brain capillaries. *J Neurocytol* 1989;18(3):359–368.

264. Lockman PR, Koziara JM, Mumper RJ, Allen DD. Nanoparticle surface charges alter blood–brain barrier integrity and permeability. *J Drug Target* 2004;12(9–10):635–641.

265. Abbott NJ, Romero IA. Transporting therapeutics across the blood–brain barrier. *Mol Med Today* 1996;2(3):106–113.

266. Tamai I, Tsuji A. Transporter-mediated permeation of drugs across the blood–brain barrier. *J Pharm Sci* 2000;89(11):1371–1388.

267. Tsuji A, Tamai II. Carrier-mediated or specialized transport of drugs across the blood–brain barrier. *Adv Drug Deliv Rev* 1999;36(2–3):277–290.

268. Smith QR. Drug delivery to brain and the role of carrier mediated transport. *Adv Exp Med Biol* 1993;331:83–93.

269. Duffy KR, Pardridge WM. Blood–brain barrier transcytosis of insulin in developing rabbits. *Brain Res* 1987;420(1):32–38.

270. Moos T, Morgan EH. Transferrin and transferrin receptor function in brain barrier systems. *Cell Mol Neurobiol* 2000;20(1):77–95.

271. Pardridge WM, Eisenberg J, Yang J. Human blood–brain barrier transferrin receptor. *Metabolism* 1987;36(9):892–895.

272. Dehouck B, Fenart L, Dehouck MP, et al. A new function for the LDL receptor: transcytosis of LDL across the blood–brain barrier. *J Cell Biol* 1997;138(4):877–889.

273. Bjorbaek C, Elmquist JK, Michl P, et al. Expression of leptin receptor isoforms in rat brain microvessels. *Endocrinology* 1998;139(8):3485–3491.

274. Duffy KR, Pardridge WM, Rosenfeld RG. Human blood–brain barrier insulin-like growth factor receptor. *Metabolism* 1988;37(2):136–140.

275. Loscher W, Potschka H. Drug resistance in brain diseases and the role of drug efflux transporters. *Nat Rev Neurosci* 2005;6(8):591–602.

276. Loscher W, Potschka H. Role of drug efflux transporters in the brain for drug disposition and treatment of brain diseases. *Prog Neurobiol* 2005;76(1):22–76.

277. van der Sandt IC, De Boer AG, Breimer DD. Implications of Pgp for the transport and distribution of drugs into the brain. In Sharma HS, Wesman J, Eds. *Blood–Spinal Cord and Brain Barriers in Health and Disease.* San Diego, CA: Elsevier Academic Press; 2004, pp 63–72.

278. Zhang Y, Han H, Elmquist WF, Miller DW. Expression of various multidrug resistance-associated protein (MRP) homologues in brain microvessel endothelial cells. *Brain Res* 2000;876(1–2):148–153.

279. Yokoyama M. Drug targeting with nano-sized carrier systems. *J Artif Organs* 2005;8(2):77–84.

280. Kreuter J. Influence of the surface properties on nanoparticle-mediated transport of drugs to the brain. *J Nanosci Nanotechnol* 2004;4(5):484–488.

281. Marcucci F, Lefoulon F. Active targeting with particulate drug carriers in tumor therapy: fundamentals. *Drug Discov Today* 2004;9(5):219–228.

282. Matsumura Y, Maeda H. A new concept for macromolecular therapeutics in cancer chemotherapy: mechanism of tumoritropic accumulation of proteins and the antitumor agent smancs. *Cancer Res* 1986;46(12 Pt 1):6387–6392.

283. Gabizon A, Papahadjopoulos D. Liposome formulations with prolonged circulation time in blood and enhanced uptake by tumors. *Proc Natl Acad Sci USA* 1988;85(18):6949–6953.

284. Miller G. Drug targeting. Breaking down barriers. *Science* 2002;297(5584):1116–1118.

285. Erdlenbruch B, Alipour M, Fricker G, Miller DS, Kugler W, Eibl H, Lakomek M. Alkyl-glycerol opening of the blood–brain barrier to small and large fluorescence markers in normal and C6 glioma-bearing rats and isolated rat brain capillaries. *Br J Pharmacol* 2003;140:1201–1210.

286. Matsukado K, Inamura T, Nakano S, Fukui M, Bartus RT, Black KL. Enhanced tumor uptake of carboplatin and survival in glioma-bearing rats by intra-carotid infusion of bradykinin analog, RMP-7. *Neurosurgery* 1996;39:125–133.

287. Prados MD, Schold SC Jr, Fine HA, Jaeckle K, Hochberg F, Mechtler L, Fetell MR, Phuphanich S, Feun L, Janus TJ, Ford K, Graney W. A randomized, double-blind, placebo-controlled, phase 2 study of RMP-7 in combination with carboplatin administered intravenously for the treatment of recurrent malignant glioma. *Neuro-oncol* 2003;5(2):96–103.

288. Packer RJ, Krailo M, Mehta M, Warren K, Allen J, Jakacki R, Villablanca JG, Chiba A, Reaman G. Phase 1 study of concurrent RMP-7 and carboplatin with radio-therapy for children with newly diagnosed brainstem gliomas. *Cancer* 2005;104(6):1281–1287.

289. Dietz GP, Bahr M. Delivery of bioactive molecules into the cell: the Trojan horse approach. *Mol Cell Neurosci* 2004;27(2):85–131.

290. Lindgren M, Hallbrink M, Prochiant A, Langel U. Cell-penetrating peptides. *Trends Pharmacol Sci* 2000;21(3):99–103.

291. Jeang KT, Xiao H, Rich EA. Multifaceted activities of the HIV-1 transactivator of transcription, *Tat. J Biol Chem* 1999;274(41):28837–28840.

292. Perez F, Joliot A, Bloch-Gallego E, Zahraoui A, Triller A, Prochiantz A. Antennapedia homeobox as a signal for the cellular internalization and nuclear addressing of a small exogenous peptide. *J Cell Sci* 1992;102(Pt 4):717–722.

293. Rousselle C, Clair P, Lefauconnier JM, Kaczorek M, Scherrmann JM, Temsamani J. New advances in the transport of doxorubicin through the blood–brain barrier by a peptide vector-mediated strategy. *Mol Pharmacol* 2000;57(4):679–686.

294. Langedijk JP, Olijhoek T, Schut D, Autar R, Meloen RH. New transport peptides broaden the horizon of applications for peptidic pharmaceuticals. *Mol Divers* 2004;8(2):101–111.

295. Wender PA, Mitchell DJ, Pattabiraman K, Pelkey ET, Steinman L, Rothbard JB. The design, synthesis, and evaluation of molecules that enable or enhance cellular uptake: peptoid molecular transporters. *Proc Natl Acad Sci USA* 2000;97(24):13003–13008.

296. Saar K, Lindgren M, Hansen M, Eiriksdottir E, Jiang Y, Rosenthal-Aizman K, Sassian M, Langel U. Cell-penetrating peptides: a comparative membrane toxicity study. *Anal Biochem* 2005;345(1):55–65.

297. Soutschek J, Akinc A, Bramlage B, Charisse K, Constien R, Donoghue M, Elbashir S, Geick A, Hadwiger P, Harborth J, John M, Kesavan V, Lavine G, Pandey RK, Racie T, Rajeev KG, Rohl I, Toudjarska I, Wang G, Wuschko S, Bumcrot D, Koteliansky V, Limmer S, Manoharan M, Vornlocher HP. Therapeutic silencing of an endogenous gene by systemic administration of modified siRNAs. *Nature* 2004;432(7014):173–178.

298. Batrakova EV, Vinogradov SV, Robinson SM, Niehoff ML, Banks WA, Kabanov AV. Polypeptide point modifications with fatty acid and amphiphilic block co-polymers for enhanced brain delivery. *Bioconjug Chem* 2005;16(5):793–802.

299. Laakso T, Andersson J, Artursson P, Edman P, Sjoholm I. Acrylic microspheres *in vivo*. X. Elimination of circulating cells by active targeting using specific monoclonal antibodies bound to microparticles. *Life Sci* 1986;38(2):183–190.

300. Conner SD, Schmid SL. Regulated portals of entry into the cell. *Nature* 2003; 422(6927):37–44.

301. Gumbleton M, Abulrob AG, Campbell L. Caveolae: an alternative membrane transport compartment. *Pharm Res* 2000;17(9):1035–1048.

302. Sachse M, Urbe S, Oorschot V, Strous GJ, Klumperman J. Bilayered clathrin coats on endosomal vacuoles are involved in protein sorting toward lysosomes. *Mol Biol Cell* 2002;13(4):1313–1328.

303. Cuervo AM. Autophagy: many paths to the same end. *Mol Cell Biochem* 2004; 263(1–2):55–72.

304. Ciechanover A. Proteolysis: from the lysosome to ubiquitin and the proteasome. *Nat Rev Mol Cell Biol* 2005;6(1):79–87.

305. Moos T, Morgan EH. Transferrin and transferrin receptor function in brain barrier systems. *Cell Mol Neurobiol* 2000;20(1):77–95.

306. Morgan EH. Iron metabolism and transport. In Zakin D, Boyer TD, Eds. *Hepatology. A Textbook of Liver Disease*. Philadelpia: Saunders; 1996, pp 526–554.

307. Ponka P, Lok CN. The transferrin receptor: role in health and disease. *Int J Biochem Cell Biol* 1999;31(10):1111–1137.

308. Visser CC, Stevanovic S, Voorwinden LH, van Bloois L, Gaillard PJ, Danhof M, Crommelin DJ, de Boer AG. Targeting liposomes with protein drugs to the blood–brain barrier *in vitro*. *Eur J Pharm Sci* 2005;25(2–3):299–305.

309. Zhang Y, Pardridge WM. Rapid transferrin efflux from brain to blood across the blood–brain barrier. *J Neurochem* 2001;76(5):1597–1600.

310. Pardridge WM, Buciak JL, Friden PM. Selective transport of an anti-transferrin receptor antibody through the blood–brain barrier *in vivo*. *J Pharmacol Exp Ther* 1991;259(1):66–70.

311. Moos T, Morgan EH. The significance of the mutated divalent metal transporter (DMT1) on iron transport into the Belgrade rat brain. *J Neurochem* 2004;88(1):233–245.

312. Deane R, Zheng W, Zlokovic BV. Brain capillary endothelium and choroid plexus epithelium regulate transport of transferrin-bound and free iron into the rat brain. *J Neurochem* 2004;88(4):813–820.

313. Pardridge WM, Boado RJ, Kang YS. Vector-mediated delivery of a polyamide ("peptide") nucleic acid analogue through the blood–brain barrier *in vivo*. *Proc Natl Acad Sci USA* 1995;92(12):5592–5596.

314. Shi N, Boado RJ, Pardridge WM. Receptor-mediated gene targeting to tissues *in vivo* following intravenous administration of pegylated immunoliposomes. *Pharm Res* 2001;18(8):1091–1095.

315. Zhang YF, Boado RJ, Pardridge WM. Absence of toxicity of chronic weekly intravenous gene therapy with pegylated immunoliposomes. *Pharm Res* 2003;20(11):1779–1785.

316. Broadwell RD, Baker-Cairns BJ, Friden PM, Oliver C, Villegas JC. Transcytosis of protein through the mammalian cerebral epithelium and endothelium. III. Receptor-mediated transcytosis through the blood–brain barrier of blood-borne transferrin and antibody against the transferrin receptor. *Exp Neurol* 1996;142(1):47–65.

317. Moos T, Morgan EH. Restricted transport of anti-transferrin receptor antibody (OX26) through the blood–brain barrier in the rat. *J Neurochem* 2001;79(1):119–129.

318. Van Gelder W, Huijskes-Heins MI, Cleton-Soeteman MI, Van Dijk JP, Van Eijk HG. Iron uptake in blood–brain barrier endothelial cells cultured in iron-depleted and iron-enriched media. *J Neurochem* 1998;71(3):1134–1140.

319. Visser CC, Voorwinden LH, Crommelin DJ, Danhof M, De Boer AG. Characterization and modulation of the transferrin receptor on brain capillary endothelial cells. *Pharm Res* 2004;21(5):761–769.

320. Pardridge WM. Drug and gene targeting to the brain via blood–brain barrier receptor-mediated transport systems. *Int Congress Series* 2005;1277:49–59.

321. Pardridge WM. Vector discovery: genetically engineered Trojan horses for drug targeting. In Pardridge WM, Ed. *Brain Drug Targeting—The Future of Brain Drug Development*. New York: Cambridge University Press; 2001, pp 126–154.

322. Xu L, Tang WH, Huang CC, et al. Systemic p53 gene therapy of cancer with immunolipoplexes targeted by anti-transferrin receptor scFv. *Mol Med* 2001;7(10):723–734.

323. Lee JH, Engler JA, Collawn JF, Moore BA. Receptor mediated uptake of peptides that bind the human transferrin receptor. *Eur J Biochem* 2001;268(7):2004–2012.

324. Bottaro DP, Bonner-Weir S, King GL. Insulin receptor recycling in vascular endothelial cells. Regulation by insulin and phorbol ester. *J Biol Chem* 1989;264(10):5916–5923.

325. Wu D, Yang J, Pardridge WM. Drug targeting of a peptide radiopharmaceutical through the primate blood–brain barrier *in vivo* with a monoclonal antibody to the human insulin receptor. *J Clin Invest* 1997;100(7):1804–1812.

326. Coloma MJ, Lee HJ, Kurihara A, et al. Transport across the primate blood–brain barrier of a genetically engineered chimeric monoclonal antibody to the human insulin receptor. *Pharm Res* 2000;17(3):266–274.

327. Herz J, Strickland DK. LRP: a multifunctional scavenger and signaling receptor. *J Clin Invest* 2001;108(6):779–784.

328. Herz J. LRP: a bright beacon at the blood–brain barrier. *J Clin Invest* 2003;112(10):1483–1485.

329. Boucher P, Gotthardt M, Li WP, Anderson RG, Herz J. LRP: role in vascular wall integrity and protection from atherosclerosis. *Science* 2003;300(5617):329–332.

330. Yepes M, Sandkvist M, Moore EG, et al. Tissue-type plasminogen activator induces opening of the blood–brain barrier via the LDL receptor-related protein. *J Clin Invest* 2003;112(10):1533–1540.

331. Demeule M, Poirier J, Jodoin J, et al. High transcytosis of melanotransferrin (P97) across the blood–brain barrier. *J Neurochem* 2002;83(4):924–933.

332. Deane R, Wu Z, Zlokovic BV. RAGE (yin) versus LRP (yang) balance regulates Alzheimer amyloid beta-peptide clearance through transport across the blood–brain barrier. *Stroke* 2004;35(11 Suppl 1):2628–2631.

333. Chun JT, Wang L, Pasinetti GM, Finch CE, Zlokovic BV. Glycoprotein 330/megalin (LRP-2) has low prevalence as mRNA and protein in brain microvessels and choroid plexus. *Exp Neurol* 1999;157(1):194–201.

334. Richardson DR, Morgan EH. The transferrin homologue, melanotransferrin (p97), is rapidly catabolized by the liver of the rat and does not effectively donate iron to the brain. *Biochim Biophys Acta* 2004;1690(2):124–133.

335. Gabathuler R, Kolaitis G, Brooks RC, et al. WO0213843 (2002).

336. Gabathuler R, Arthur G, Kennard M, et al. Development of a potential vector (NeuroTrans) to deliver drugs across the blood–brain barrier. *Int Congress Series* 2005; 1277:171–184.

337. Pan W, Kastin AJ, Zankel TC, et al. Efficient transfer of receptor-associated protein (RAP) across the blood–brain barrier. *J Cell Sci* 2004;117(Pt 21):5071–5078.

338. Béliveau R, Demeule M. WO2004060403 (2004).

339. Sedrakyan A, Treasure T, Elefteriades JA. Effect of aprotinin on clinical outcomes in coronary artery bypass graft surgery: a systematic review and meta-analysis of randomized clinical trials. *J Thorac Cardiovasc Surg* 2004;128(3):442–448.

340. Jefferies WA, Food MR, Gabathuler R, et al. Reactive microglia specifically associated with amyloid plaques in Alzheimer's disease brain tissue express melanotransferrin. *Brain Res* 1996;712(1):122–126.

341. Deane R, Du Yan S, Submamaryan RK, et al. RAGE mediates amyloid-beta peptide transport across the blood–brain barrier and accumulation in brain. *Nat Med* 2003;9(7):907–913.

342. Zlokovic BB. Cerebrovascular transport of Alzheimer's amyloid beta and apolipoproteins J and E: possible anti-amyloidogenic role of the blood–brain barrier. *Life Sci* 1996;59(18):1483–1497.

343. Zlokovic BV, Martel CL, Matsubara E, et al. Glycoprotein 330/megalin: probable role in receptor-mediated transport of apolipoprotein J alone and in a complex with Alzheimer disease amyloid beta at the blood–brain and blood–cerebrospinal fluid barriers. *Proc Natl Acad Sci USA* 1996;93(9):4229–4234.

344. Demeule M, Bertrand Y, Michaud-Levesque J, et al. Regulation of plasminogen activation: a role for melanotransferrin (p97) in cell migration. *Blood* 2003;102(5):1723–1731.

345. Gaillard PJ, Brink A, De Boer AG. Diphtheria toxin receptor-targeted brain drug delivery. *Int Congress Series* 2005;1277:185–195.

346. Gaillard PJ, Brink A, De Boer AG. WO2004069870 (2004).

347. Anderson P. Antibody responses to *Haemophilus influenzae* type b and diphtheria toxin induced by conjugates of oligosaccharides of the type b capsule with the nontoxic protein CRM197. *Infect Immun* 1983;39(1):233–238.

348. Buzzi S, Rubboli D, Buzzi G, et al. CRM197 (nontoxic diphtheria toxin): effects on advanced cancer patients. *Cancer Immunol Immunother* 2004;53(11):1041–1048.

349. Raab G, Klagsbrun M. Heparin-binding EGF-like growth factor. *Biochim Biophys Acta* 1997;1333(3):F179–F199.

350. Mishima K, Higashiyama S, Nagashima Y, et al. Regional distribution of heparin-binding epidermal growth factor-like growth factor mRNA and protein in adult rat forebrain. *Neurosci Lett* 1996;213(3):153–156.

351. Mishima K, Higashiyama S, Asai A, et al. Heparin-binding epidermal growth factor-like growth factor stimulates mitogenic signaling and is highly expressed in human malignant gliomas. *Acta Neuropathol (Berl)* 1998;96(4):322–328.

352. Tanaka N, Sasahara M, Ohno M, et al. Heparin-binding epidermal growth factor-like growth factor mRNA expression in neonatal rat brain with hypoxic/ischemic injury. *Brain Res* 1999;827(1–2):130–138.

353. Mitamura T, Higashiyama S, Taniguchi N, Klagsbrun M, Mekada E. Diphtheria toxin binds to the epidermal growth factor (EGF)-like domain of human heparin-binding EGF-like growth factor/diphtheria toxin receptor and inhibits specifically its mitogenic activity. *J Biol Chem* 1995;270(3):1015–1019.

354. Cha JH, Chang MY, Richardson JA, Eidels L. Transgenic mice expressing the diphtheria toxin receptor are sensitive to the toxin. *Mol Microbiol* 2003;49(1):235–240.

355. Opanashuk LA, Mark RJ, Porter J, Damm D, Mattson MP, Seroogy KB. Heparin-binding epidermal growth factor-like growth factor in hippocampus: modulation of expression by seizures and anti-excitotoxic action. *J Neurosci* 1999;19(1):133–146.

356. Luciani A, Olivier JC, Clement O, Siauve N, Brillet PY, Bessoud B, Gazeau F, Uchegbu IF, Kahn E, Frija G, Cuenod CA. Glucose-receptor MR imaging of tumors: study in mice with PEGylated paramagnetic niosomes. *Radiology* 2004;231(1):135–142.

357. de Boer AG, Gaillard PJ. *In vitro* models of the blood–brain barrier: when to use which? *Curr Med Chem Central Nervous Syst Agents* 2002;2(3):203–209.

358. de Boer AG, Gaillard PJ. *In vivo* methods to estimate drug transport to the brain across the blood–brain barrier. *Med Chem Rev Online* 2005;2(2):127–131.

359. Plum L, Schubert M, Brüning JC. The role of insulin receptor signaling in the brain. *Trends Endocrinol Metab* 2005;16(2):59–65.

12

TRANSPORTER INTERACTIONS IN THE ADME PATHWAY OF DRUGS

YAN ZHANG[1] AND DONALD W. MILLER[2]

[1]*Drug Metabolism and Biopharmaceutics, Incyte Corporation, Wilmington, Delaware*
[2]*University of Manitoba, Winnipeg, Manitoba, Canada*

Contents

12.1   INTRODUCTION

Approximately 30% of the human genome encodes membrane proteins [1]. It has been estimated that as many as 1200 of these genes code for potential drug transporters [2]. Given the number of transport proteins expressed on cell membranes,

Preclinical Development Handbook: ADME and Biopharmaceutical Properties,
edited by Shayne Cox Gad
Copyright © 2008 John Wiley & Sons, Inc.

it stands to reason that interactions of therapeutic agents with endogenous transporter systems could have a major impact on the absorption, distribution, metabolism, and excretion (ADME) properties of drugs. Transporter interactions can impact on the ADME pathway in two distinct and important ways. First, if a drug is a substrate for a specific transporter involved in absorption, distribution, or elimination, the transporter can influence the ADME properties of the drug itself. Examples of this include increased intestinal absorption of cephalosporins through transport by a peptide transporter in the intestine [3, 4], and decreased intestinal absorption of taxol by the efflux transporter, P-glycoprotein [5, 6]. Second, a drug may act as either an inhibitor or inducer of a selective transporter involved in the ADME properties, thereby altering the ADME properties of another drug. In this case, the result would be a drug–drug interaction that changes the pharmacokinetics of the drug. Athough such interactions were in the past considered to be entirely drug metabolism (cytochrome P450-mediated) related, it is now recognized that transporters may also be involved [7, 8].

Identification of the transport properties of compounds during the drug discovery process is essential for optimization of the ADME properties of therapeutic agents. In this regard, the pharmaceutical scientist has a variety of tools with which to probe transporter interactions of compounds. These include cell-based uptake, absorption and transport assays, *in situ* models that can isolate the pertinent absorption, distribution, or elimination tissues, and computational models that can simulate and/or predict transporter interactions. In addition, transgenic mouse models have made it possible to examine the impact of selected transport systems on the ADME process at the whole animal level. This chapter identifies some of the more important transporters that can influence the ADME properties of drugs. In addition, a strategy for evaluating compounds for transporter interactions is discussed that incorporates *in silico*-based modeling and *in vitro* and *in vivo* transporter studies.

12.2 TRANSPORT SYSTEMS IMPACTING DRUG ADME

There are several types of transport systems involved in moving solutes and macromolecules across cellular barriers. These include primary active transport systems that rely directly on ATP hydrolysis to move solutes across the membrane. Examples include the drug efflux transporters such as P-glycoprotein (P-gp), multidrug resistance associated protein (MRP), and breast cancer resistant protein (BCRP). Transporters in this group belong to the ATP binding cassette (ABC) superfamily of proteins [9–11]. In general, these transporters consist of 6–17 membrane spanning domains, one or more nucleotide binding domains, and one or more drug binding domains [10–12]. As these transporters rely directly on ATP hydrolysis, they have the capability of transporting the solutes and macromolecules against a concentration gradient. In mammalian cells, the direction of transport is usually directed toward removing compounds from the cell (i.e., outwardly directed).

Drug efflux transporters have been closely linked with the development of drug resistance in cancer [9, 10], bacterial [13], and parasitic [14] cells. These same drug efflux transporters are also present in normal tissue such as epithelial cells of the intestine, liver, and kidney, and endothelial cells forming the blood–brain barrier [15–18]. While the drug efflux transporters serve an important protective function, preventing the absorption and distribution and speeding the elimination of potentially toxic xenobiotics, due to their rather promiscuous nature (i.e., ability to transport a wide variety of chemical compositions), they also have a substantial impact on the ADME properties of drugs. P-glycoprotein, the most widely studied drug efflux transporter, contributes to the low oral bioavailability of several drugs [19]. Furthermore, even those drugs that can overcome P-gp efflux in the intestine are still subject to restricted tissue distribution and increased clearance [20]. For these reasons, much effort has been placed on the identification of potential drug efflux transporter interactions early in the drug development process.

Another type of transport system present in the cell is secondary active transporters. In contrast to primary active transporters that rely on ATP hydrolysis, the secondary active transporters utilize electrochemical gradients to supply the energy required to move the solutes into or out of the cell. Thus, the "energy" for these transporters comes from the movement of ions, typically either sodium or hydrogen, down their concentration gradient. Examples of secondary active transporters include the sodium-dependent amino acid transporters found in the intestine and blood–brain barrier [21, 22], and the hydrogen ion-dependent peptide transporters (PepT1 and PepT2) found in the intestine, kidney, lung, and blood–cerebrospinal fluid barrier [23–25].

From a drug transport perspective, PepT1 and PepT2 deserve special mention. Both of these transporters were the first mammalian transporters identified that use the electrochemical proton gradient as a driving force [26]. The "preferred" substrates for PepT1 and PepT2 are di- and tripeptides [27]. This property of PepT transporters has been exploited to aid in the absorption of peptide and peptidomimetic agents in the intestine and lung [28, 29]. An example of this is the angiotensin converting enzyme (ACE) inhibitors [28]. However, unlike many of the solute and nutrient transporters that have relatively rigid structural requirements for transport substrates, the PepT transporters accommodate a wide variety of compounds. Consequently, not only are PepT1 and PepT2 able to aid in the intestinal absorption (PepT1) and kidney reabsorption (PepT2) of peptidomimetic drugs [28], but they can also influence the ADME properties of antibiotics such as cephalosporin [3, 4], and nucleoside-based antiviral prodrugs such as valacyclovir [30]. Although PepT1 and PepT2 share the same set of substrates, they differ in their affinity and capacity. Whereas PepT1 is a low affinity, high capacity transporter, PepT2 has high affinity and low capacity for the same substrates [23]. In addition, the presence of PepT2 on pulmonary epithelial cells [24, 29, 31] and epithelial cells of the choroid plexus, which form the blood–cerebrospinal fluid barrier [25], suggests this transporter could also influence drug distribution of selected therapeutic agents in these tissues.

A third type of transporter class is the solute carriers that allow the passage of compounds across the cellular barrier through a process involving facilitated diffusion [32]. In facilitated diffusion, the transported molecule interacts with the protein carrier, and through conformational changes in the protein, the molecule is allowed to pass through the lipid membrane. Cellular uptake of many nutrients such as glucose [33], various nucleotides [34, 35], and creatine [36] are known to occur through facilitated diffusion processes. These carriers display the same characteristics of saturability and solute selectivity as observed with the active transporters. However, unlike primary or secondary active transport systems, the carriers involved in facilitated diffusion processes are not sensitive to metabolic inhibitors. In addition, the carriers involved in facilitated diffusion are bidirectional in that the solute will follow a concentration gradient whether that is directed into or out of the cell. While such carriers are important for nutrient absorption and distribution, the impact of facilitated diffusion on ADME properties of drugs is minimal, due in large part to the stringent structural requirements for these transporters.

12.3 COMPUTATIONAL MODELING OF TRANSPORTER INTERACTIONS

A number of criteria have to be met to successfully develop a drug-like compound. It has to be absorbed into the bloodstream and be distributed and bound to targeted tissues. Furthermore, in order to avoid toxic effects, many drugs require biotransformation for efficient elimination from the body. All of these aspects are significantly mediated or influenced, at some level, by transporter proteins. This has made the identification of transporter interactions a very important part of the ADME process. The following section summarizes the various options available for examining transport-mediated influences in the ADME pathway.

Prediction of the passive permeability of a compound using computational modeling is relatively straightforward and is aided by a very large training set of compounds with established physicochemical properties (i.e., lipophilicity, H-bonding potential, solubility, and stability) with which to generate the computer simulations. However, prediction of permeability when transporter interactions are involved is much more difficult. Indeed, when correlating actual permeability as accessed in either cell based or *in vivo* systems, to that predicted by computer modeling, it is often the outliers that have either metabolism or transport issues influencing permeability. Despite the added complexity, computational modeling of transporter interactions is an area of intense interest. Numerous efforts have been made to characterize various transporter/carrier proteins, including the PepT1, and the drug efflux pumps such as P-gp and MRP. However, little is known about these proteins at the molecular level due to the limited availability of high resolution crystal structures. Determination of crystal structure for transport proteins is important not only for understanding the function of these transporters but also for defining the structure–activity properties required for compounds transported by specific systems. The two general approaches used to model drug transporter systems include transporter-based modeling and substrate-based modeling [37]. Each of these approaches to computer modeling of transporter interactions is described.

12.3.1 Transporter-Based Modeling

The transporter-based approach focuses on the three-dimensional structure of the transport protein to assist in understanding the drug transport process. This approach uses the known or predicted three-dimensional structure of the protein to map out the topography of the transporter in the cell membrane. As would be predicted, the better the information is concerning the three-dimensional structure of the transporter being examined, the better the resulting computational model will be. However, complete knowledge of the three-dimensional structure is not essential as a transporter-based approach can be applied when the target transporter shares the same number of transmembrane domains (TMDs) and an adequate level (generally >30%) of amino acid sequence identity with a second transporter, that has a known crystal structure available. This approach can be used even when the two transporters are not functionally related. For example, modeling of the apical sodium-dependent bile acid transporter (ASBT) was based on the crystal structure of bacteriorhodopsin [38]. In addition, the three-dimensional structure of the human facilitative glucose transporter (GLUT1) was predicted by using the crystal structure of a bacterial transporter, glycerol-3-phosphate transporter (GlpT), as a template [39]. Furthermore, important insights regarding the functionality of a target transporter can still be generated by modeling partial domains of the transporter when there is an absence of appropriate templates for a full-length transporter [37]. In studying the sulfate transporter, Rouached et al. [40] avoided modeling the transmembrane domains in their entirety because of the lack of appropriate templates. However, they identified the bacterial SpoIIAA protein as a template for the functionally unknown C-terminal sulfate transporter and anti-sigma antagonist (STAS) domain and directly generated a three-dimensional model for this domain [40].

In the transporter-based approach, the structure of a target transporter can be calculated using homology modeling techniques, including several commercially available programs, such as Modeller [41], InsightII homology [42], and ICM (MolSoft, San Diego, CA) [37]. Among these, Modeller is the most widely applied program. It follows four general steps, including template selection, sequence alignment, model generation, and model validation. These four steps are repeated as a cycle until no further improvements to the model are observed. Among the four steps, validation is an essential process to ensure accuracy of the generated model. Modeller generates several models based on the sequence alignment, which are, in turn, evaluated by internal self-consistency checks and external programs that verify structural protein quality. Examples of external programs used to verify protein structures are Procheck [43] and WHAT IF [44]. Generally, these programs develop rules and parameters extracted from available crystal structures and apply these to the model structure. The fitness that is represented by a "fit score" indicates the compatibility of the model to the available crystal structures [37]. The transporter-based modeling approach now enables the elucidation of three-dimensional structures for a large number of transporters that would otherwise not be available to scientists. Examples include the glucose transporter (GLUT1) [39], P-gp [45], and MRP1 [46].

Both P-gp and MRP1 belong to the ABC superfamily of transporters that have been extensively studied. The initial models of both P-gp and MRP are based on the crystal structures of bacterial transporters. P-gp was initially modeled using the crystal structure of the *Escherichia coli* lipid A transporter (MsbA), which shares ~30% homology with P-gp [45]. Subsequently, Stenham and colleagues [47] constructed an atomic detail model for P-gp based on assessment of the crystal structure of MsbA in relation to their disulfide cross-linking data. The two diverging models of P-gp were later harmonized in accordance with a theory proposed by Lee et al. [48], who postulated that P-gp could exist in two dynamic conformations—an open conformation [45] and a closed conformation [47]. Similarly, MRP1 was modeled based on the crystal structure of *Vibrio cholerae* MsbA [46]. The model implied that Phe594 forms a hydrophobic pocket with four residues, therefore successfully predicting the functional importance of the Phe594 in transmembrane helix 11 of the MRP1 [46].

The transporter-based approach provides detailed protein structural information. Based on the topographical characterization of the protein, one can identify potential areas/pockets where substrate and/or inhibitor interact with the transporter proteins. It should be noted that this approach is not feasible for proteins without a suitable TMD template. To date, this approach has been applied mostly to transporters possessing 7 or 12 TMDs with the exception of MRP1, which has 17 TMDs [37]. For those transporters for which no suitable TMD template is available, techniques such as substrate-based methods that do not require knowledge of transporter structure can be applied.

12.3.2   Substrate-Based Modeling

Substrate-based modeling correlates biological activity of a series of substrates or inhibitors for a transporter with their molecular descriptors or chemical features. Based on the compiled properties of the substrates and inhibitors, the models can then predict potential transporter interactions. This approach has been applied successfully to generate pharmacophore (the spatial arrangement of the hydrophobicity, hydrogen bonding status, charged state, and other features of a compound) and quantitative structure–activity relationship (QSAR) models for many membrane transporter proteins, such as P-gp [49], MRP2 [50], human peptide transporter 1 (hPEPT1) [51, 52], organic cation transporters (OCTs) [53], organic anion transporter polypeptides (OATPs) [54], and nucleoside transporter [55, 56].

Several substrate-based computational programs are commercially available to generate these modelings. The most widely used programs include CATALYST (Accelrys Inc., San Diego, CA) and distance comparison (DISCO) [57] for pharmacophore generation. For more quantitative structure–activity relationship (QSAR) predictions, comparative molecular field analysis (CoMFA) [58] and comparative molecular similarity index analysis (CoMSIA) [59] are commercially available modeling programs. Both CATALYST and DISCO programs attempt to determine common features based on the superposition of active compounds (i.e., transporter substrates or inhibitors) using different algorithms [37]. For example, HIPHOP is one of the algorithms of CATALYST which generates a pharmacophore based on common chemical features among active molecules. In an effort to identify novel hPEPT1 inhibitors, Ekins and co-sworkers [52] used three relatively high affinity ligands—Gly-Sar, bestatin, and enalapril—to generate a common features (HIPHOP) pharmacophore. This consisted of two hydrophobic features, a hydrogen bond donor, acceptor, and a negative ionizable feature. The pharmacophore was then used to search the Comprehensive Medicinal Chemistry (CMC) database of more than 8000 drug-like molecules and retrieved 145 virtual hits mapping to the pharmacophore features. Furthermore, the pharmacophore was also able to identify known hPEPT1 substrates and inhibitors in further database mining of more than 500 commonly prescribed drugs [52]. In contrast to pharmacophore modeling, a 3D-QSAR model consists of a mathematical equation describing potency as a function of 3D interaction fields around aligned training set compounds [60]. Both CoMFA and CoMSIA are commonly used algorithms for 3D-QSAR generation. They are based on the assumption that changes in binding affinities of ligands are related to changes in molecular properties, represented by interaction fields [58, 59]. Recently, Biegel et al. [61] determined the structural requirements for the substrates of the renal type peptide transporter (PEPT2) by 3D-QSAR using the CoMSIA program. The model was built based on 83 compounds (including dipeptides, tripeptides, and β-lactam antibiotics) covering a wide range of affinity constants. An analysis of the contour maps provided by the CoMSIA method gave insights into the requirements for high affinity substrates of PEPT2. Furthermore, an additional 3D-QSAR model based on the same compounds was generated and correlated with affinity data of the intestinal peptide transporter (PEPT1). By comparing the CoMSIA contour plots, differences in substrate selectivity between PEPT1 and PEPT2 were determined [61].

Substrate-based modeling can often provide insight in the ligand–protein binding or inhibition process and assist in the identification of other molecules that contain the same pharmacophore features. Furthermore, the correlation between the variations in ligand or inhibitor binding affinities and the variations in their respective structural features can assist in the design of more potent inhibitors or substrates with higher affinity. However, disadvantages are also present in the substrate-based modeling approach. First, the training datasets that the models are based on are generated from different sources, that is, different cell type, species, and laboratories. Therefore, the data are often not directly comparable, and the quality and consistency of the data might also be in question. Second, although a large body of literature involving the QSAR of various transporters can be found, it is often based on datasets comprised of transport inhibitors, not necessarily transport substrates. This is especially true for the QSAR modeling of P-gp and MRP, as much of the early work was aimed at finding compounds that could inhibit these transporters and thus reverse multidrug resistance [62]. The major reason inhibition data is frequently used to establish the computational models is because generation of this data is relatively higher throughput and simpler in experimental design compared to determination of the kinetic data (K_m, V_{max}) for transported substrates [37].

12.3.3 Applied Computer Modeling Systems in ADME

Within the ADME process, absorption and elimination (especially through metabolic pathways) have been the most extensively modeled. With respect to absorption, most of the current computational approaches used to predict absorption are based on the assumption that absorption is a passive process. In contrast, computer models for predicting elimination pathways place more emphasis on active processes such as enzyme–drug interactions. Thus, examination of both processes provides a very diverse exposure to the computational models currently employed in early ADME studies.

One of the simplest and most widely used computational approaches to estimate passive absorption or permeation was developed by Lipinski and co-workers in 1997 [63]. The authors selected a compound library consisting of 2287 drug candidates with good absorption properties according to the data of intestinal epithelial permeability and solubility. Based on the physicochemical properties of these compounds, the authors proposed the "rule of five" (ROF), taking into account hydrogen bonding, molecular weight, and lipophilicity.

Although the ROF allows quick screening of many NCEs and provides an initial indication of human intestinal absorption (HIA) of those compounds, there are some weaknesses associated with this model. First, the ROF does not apply to compounds that are subject to active transport processes. For example, therapeutic classes, such as antibiotics, antifungals, vitamins, and cardiac glycosides, consistently fall outside the ROF parameter cutoffs [63] and yet are effectively absorbed in the GI system via various transport systems. Second, the model was created using those compounds with high absorption as its database; only a limited number of compounds with a low absorption were included.

While the ROF is a model more based on the physicochemical properties of a compound, there are several physiological based models that also have great potential for use within both the early and later stages of drug discovery. Two examples of these models are iDEA™ (*in vitro* determination for the estimation of ADME) and GastroPlus™. GastroPlus was developed by Simulations Plus, Inc. (Lancaster, CA; http://www.simulations-plus.com/). It simulates GI absorption and pharmacokinetics for drugs dosed orally or intravenously in humans and animals. The simulation is based on the advanced compartmental absorption and transit (ACAT) model [64], which is an advanced version of the one originally reported by Yu and Amidon [65]. The ACAT model is a flexible physiologically based simulation with nine compartments corresponding to different segments of the digestive tract including stomach, seven small intestinal compartments, and colon. Each compartment is modeled with accurate physiological information regarding volumes, transit times, length, and radius [64]. This model takes into account pH dependency of basic parameters, solubility and permeability, transport of drug material through the GI tract, and absorption of drug through the intestinal wall into the portal vein. In addition to these, GastroPlus provides the ability for customization by allowing absorption constants to be set individually for each intestinal compartment [66]. With this physiologically based simulation software program, the rate, extent, and gastrointestinal location of oral drug absorption can be predicted [67]. For predictions based on measured permeability, the GastroPlus model has been trained to accept values for human jejunal permeability as input. The determination for human permeability (P_{eff}) is based on a combination of experimental data inputs from both *in vivo* human values and *in situ* rat or dog intestinal permeability values. These values then further convert to human values using a built-in correlation [67, 68]. However, because there is no relation between the Caco-2 data and the human P_{eff} with this model, human P_{eff} cannot be predicted using Caco-2 data [67]. Therefore, a preliminary step is transformation based on a correlation when Caco-2 data is used. Normally, a correlation of human P_{eff} against Caco-2 permeability can be built using reference compounds by users before the simulation. By doing this, the Caco-2 permeability is converted to effective human jejunal permeability, P_{eff}, based on the established correlation [68].

Another computational model for the simulation of absorption is iDEA, a predictive ADME simulation system developed by Lion Bioscience Inc. (San Diego, CA; http://www.lionbioscience.com/). This particular model was developed based on a proprietary database that coupled oral bioavailability data from human clinical trials with preclinical *in vitro* data characterizing various parameters of the drug including solubility, Caco-2 permeability, protein binding, and metabolic stability in human cryopreserved hepatocytes. This model can simulate human physiology and accounts for regional variations in intestinal permeability, solubility, surface area, and fluid movement [66, 68]. iDEA is based on the STELLA (Structural Thinking Experimental Learning Laboratory with Animation) simulation software and comprises structure-based Caco-2 and absorption modules (SBM) and a physiologically based (PBM) absorption module [69, 70]. Therefore, it allows the prediction of Caco-2 permeability or the fraction of dose absorbed (F_a) of drugs from their structures. It also predicts the rate and extent of human oral drug absorption, by taking into account physiological parameters such as intestinal pH, transit time, and blood flow. Since there are large interlaboratory differences in the absolute values of Caco-2 permeability, it may be necessary to "customize" the simulation package to the individual laboratory. This is done by determining the Caco-2 permeability of several marker compounds for comparison the Caco-2 values used in the simulation software package. In doing this, one can determine how Caco-2 permeability values from Lion Bioscience Inc. correlate with the in-house Caco-2 permeability data and modify the simulation model accordingly.

Overall, the computational approaches for predicting oral drug absorption are still in their infancy. Neither the GastroPlus nor the iDEA system has been evaluated completely. Part of the issues with evaluating the extent to which either model predicts drug absorption in the GI tract is the limited access to a large data bank for fraction of dose absorbed. While such information is often available in-house, public access is limited by most pharmaceutical companies due to issues of confidentiality. An inherent limitation with the iDEA system is that compounds suspected to be metabolized or substrates of active transporters or carriers in the intestine have been excluded from model building [67]. To this extent, GastroPlus shows strengths in its ability to integrate additional data, including transport/efflux processes and intestinal metabolism [68]. Recently, Tubic et al. [71] demonstrated that P-gp was involved in the talinolol nonlinear dose-dependent absorption using GastroPlus simulation modeling. Furthermore, it was observed that the results predicted from the model were comparable to the finding of a Phase I dose escalation study [71].

Compared to GastroPlus, iDEA has a simpler operating structure. Once the server is installed, it runs as a web application on the corporate Intranet. Therefore, the deployment is simple and training is not a big issue. In this respect, iDEA could be aimed at use by non-DMPK specialists (e.g., medicinal chemists), who could access the absorption potential of compounds with a quick and easy tool. In contrast to the iDEA system, GastroPlus is well designed and suitable for those scientist dealing on a day-to-day basis with intestinal absorption issues. Because of the more complex modeling parameters, GastroPlus requires more thorough training compared to the iDEA system [68].

12.4 *IN VITRO* SYSTEMS FOR IDENTIFICATION OF TRANSPORTER INTERACTIONS

Identification of transporter interactions with drugs and determination of their impact on the ADME profile at an early stage in drug development has resulted in increased emphasis being placed on relatively high throughput *in vitro* screening methods. Commonly used cell-based approaches for examining transporter

TABLE 12.1   Cell-Based Approaches for Examining Transporter Interactions in the ADME Process

Cell System	ADME Property	Transporter Applications	Experimental Design
Intestinal brush border membrane vesicles	Intestinal absorption	• Identification of substrates/inhibitors • Determination of transporter kinetics	• Uptake studies
Caco-2 cell line	Intestinal absorption	• Identification of substrates/inhibitors • Determination of transporter kinetics • Determination of transporter polarity	• Uptake studies • Permeability studies • Bidirectional permeability studies
Isolated brain microvessel endothelial cells	Blood–brain barrier (brain distribution)	• Identification of substrate/inhibitors • Determination of transporter kinetics	• Uptake studies
Cultured brain microvessel endothelial cells	Blood–brain barrier (brain distribution)	• Identification of substrate/inhibitors • Determination of transporter kinetics • Determination of transporter polarity	• Uptake studies • Permeability studies • Bidirectional permeability studies
Liver canalicular membrane vesicles	Hepatic/biliary excretion	• Identification of substrates/inhibitors • Determination of transporter kinetics	• Uptake studies
Cultured hepatocytes	Hepatic/biliary excretion	• Identification of substrate/inhibitors • Determination of transporter kinetics • Determination of transporter polarity	• Uptake studies • Permeability studies • Bidirectional permeability studies
Madin–Darby canine kidney (MDCK) cell line	General absorption, distribution, and excretion	• Identification of substrate/inhibitors • Determination of transporter kinetics • Determination of transporter polarity	• Uptake studies • Permeability studies • Bidirectional permeability studies

interactions and their applications in ADME processes are listed in Table 12.1. These include isolated cell or membrane preparations from various tissues. Examples are the use of isolated brain microvessel endothelial cells to study transporters at the blood–brain barrier [72, 73] and the use of membrane vesicles prepared from the brush-border membrane of intestinal epithelial cells [74] or the canalicular membrane of liver hepatocytes [75] to study transporter processes in the intestine and liver, respectively. While isolated cell and cell membranes typically have the highest levels of transporter expression, use of these preparations requires a great deal of starting tissue and determination of actual permeability and polarized transport is difficult. In addition, assay validation with the isolated cell and cell membrane preparations is difficult. Thus, efforts have been made to develop cell culture systems to model the different ADME transport and permeability barriers (see Table 12.1). The advantages of cell culture systems are that one can examine polarized transporter processes and actually evaluate both cellular accumulation and permeability across confluent monolayers. Thus, the influence of transporters on the actual permeability of a compound can be determined. For those cell culture systems that utilize established, immortalized cells lines (i.e., Caco-2, MDCK) there are the added advantages of reproducibility and low interassay variability. In addition, the cell lines can also be transfected to express specific transporters of interest. Examples are the MDCK cell lines that have been transfected with MDR1, MRP1, or MRP2 drug efflux transporters [76–78]. The availability of the transfected cell lines provides important research tools for honing in on transporter dynamics and function.

12.4.1 *In Vitro* Accumulation Assays for Identification of Transporter Processes

Experiments examining the transport properties of compounds in cell-based systems fall into three major categories. These include studies based on cell or vesicle accumulation, unidirectional transport, or bidirectional transport. Studies examining the cellular or membrane vesicle accumulation of a compound can provide a fast and reliable method for identifying both transporter substrates and inhibitors. An example of this is the use of various membrane vesicle preparations to identify the transporter-mediated uptake and efflux of the lipid lowering drug pitavastatin [79]. These studies examined both the acid and lactone forms of pitavastatin. In the case of the acid form, uptake into the cell was dependent on multiple solute transporters, including members of the organic anion transporter (OAT) and the organic anion transporter polypeptide (OATP) family. In contrast, the lactone form was not a substrate for transport into the cell [79]. With regard to transporter-mediated efflux from the cell, the lactone form of pitavastatin was a substrate for P-gp, while the acid form displayed BCRP efflux activity [79]. These studies are a prime example of how vesicular and cellular accumulation can be used to delineate the structure–activity requirements for transport processes.

Cell accumulation assays are also helpful for identification of compounds that can inhibit drug transport. An example is the use of isolated brain capillaries and cultured brain microvessel endothelial cells in drug screening assays for drug efflux transporters [73, 80]. In these studies, changes in the cellular accumulation of fluorescent probes for P-gp and MRP were used to quantitatively assess the inhibitor properties of a series of compounds. Identification of potential inhibitors of drug efflux transport proteins, especially P-gp, are increasingly part of the early testing in the drug development process. This is due to the emphasis placed on knowing whether a compound is a P-gp inhibitor and/or inducer at the time a new drug application (NDA) is filed with the Food and Drug Administration (FDA). In addition, since many inhibitors of drug transport can also act as substrates, cellular accumulation assays are often used as a first screen for potential transporter interactions of compounds. Those agents showing activity can then be examined for substrate properties.

A final application for the cellular accumulation assays is quantitative determination of transporter kinetics. Using the cellular accumulation of fluorescent probes for P-gp and MRP transport, Bachmeier et al. [81] determined and compared the Michaelis–Menten kinetics of these drug efflux transporters in primary cultured brain microvessel endothelial cells, MDR1 transfected MDCK cells, and freshly isolated brain microvessels. In these studies, P-gp related transport displayed similar K_m values across the different BBB models; however, V_{max} was significantly higher in the freshly isolated brain microvessels [81]. For MRP related transport, differences in both K_m and V_{max} were noted in the various BBB models [81].

12.4.2   *In Vitro* Permeability Assays for Identification of Transporter Processes

Drug interactions with transport systems can also be evaluated using actual cell monolayer permeability. These studies can be performed unidirectionally with and without various transport inhibitors to determine the impact of the transport system on actual permeability of the compound. This type of experiment typically examines the absorptive, distributional, or excretory transport. As with the cellular accumulation assays, transported compounds will display concentration-dependent monolayer permeability. An example is the permeability studies for the amino acid phenylalanine in Caco-2 monolayers [82]. These studies showed that the transport of L-phenylalanine from the apical to basolateral side of Caco-2 cells was concentration dependent. The transport process was saturable with a very high affinity ($K_m =$ 0.019 mM) to the amino acid transporter in Caco-2 cells [82]. Studies performed in the presence of specific transport inhibitors will also influence permeability. For absorptive transporters such as PepT, inhibition of the transporter results in reduced permeability in cell expression of PepT [82]. For drug efflux transporters, such as P-gp, inhibitors will increase the absorptive or distributive permeability of substrates [72, 78]. Alternatively, bidirectional permeability studies can be performed to identify potential transport systems. In these studies permeability is assessed in the apical-to-basolateral (A-B) direction and also in the basolateral-to-apical (B-A). By examining the resulting B-A/A-B ratio of the permeability coefficients, one can determine whether absorptive/uptake transporters (ratios significantly less than 1) or efflux transporters (ratios significantly greater than 1) are involved. Bidirectional permeability studies in either Caco-2 or MDCK MDR1 cells have been very useful for identifying those compounds that are transported by drug efflux transport proteins [83, 84]. While most commonly used to identify secretory transport systems, bidirectional permeability studies are also useful for the identification of absorptive transport properties as well. Studies by Li and colleagues [85] used bidirectional permeability in Caco-2 cell monolayers to aid in the identification of amino acid prodrugs of the antiviral levovirin, which utilize the PepT system. These studies were able to identify ester-based amino acid prodrugs with PepT substrate and inhibitor properties. Such compounds are anticipated to result in improved oral bioavailability for levovirin.

12.5   *IN VIVO* METHODS FOR ASSESSING TRANSPORT INTERACTIONS

Examination of drug transporter interactions at the whole animal level is much more complex than cell-based assays. However complex, ultimate determination of

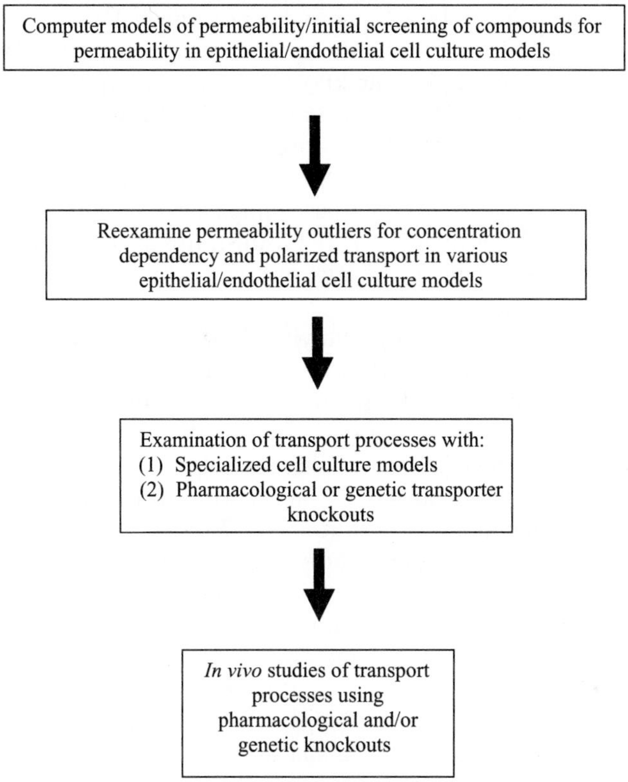

Computer models of permeability/initial screening of compounds for permeability in epithelial/endothelial cell culture models

Reexamine permeability outliers for concentration dependency and polarized transport in various epithelial/endothelial cell culture models

Examination of transport processes with:
(1) Specialized cell culture models
(2) Pharmacological or genetic transporter knockouts

In vivo studies of transport processes using pharmacological and/or genetic knockouts

FIGURE 12.1 Experimental process for determining transporter-related processes in ADME.

the impact that transporters have on the ADME properties of a drug require whole animal studies. Thus, *in vivo* studies examining transporter influences on the ADME properties of a drug are typically performed after extensive *in vitro* evaluation of the transport properties of the lead compound(s) (see Fig. 12.1). The exception to this is the cassette dosing of drugs to rodents during the early drug development stage. In these studies, a series of compounds are administered together, to obtain an early glimpse of the ADME properties in the *in vivo* setting [86–88]. However, it should be noted that performing the cassette dosing at both low and high doses of the compounds can provide preliminary indications of drug transporter interactions, as drugs that are substrates for transporters will demonstrate concentration dependency [88].

The advantage to performing *in vivo* studies during the final stages of the preclinical development of a drug is that a great deal of information concerning drug transporter interactions has already been identified. This allows the *in vivo* studies to hone in on the appropriate transporter using either pharmacological or genetic inhibition of transport properties. In the past, *in vivo* demonstration of transport relied on dose dependency and the use of pharmacological agents that inhibited transport processes. However, through advances in molecular biology, researchers now have the ability to selectively "knock out" drug transporters either through creation of transgenic animals [89] or, more recently, through the use of small inhibitory RNA (siRNA) [90], to transiently knock down transporter expression. An example of the power that transgenic knockouts bring to *in vivo* studies of transporter interactions in the ADME process can be found in the MDR1 transgenic knockout mice [89, 91]. Studies with these mice have established quite conclusively the influence that P-glycoprotein has in the oral absorption, brain penetration, and elimination of selected drugs [91]. Similar examples can be found with the PEPT2 knockout mice, where levels of model PEPT2 substrates have been reduced in blood and cerebral spinal fluid owing to the lack of transporter at the kidney and blood–cerebrospinal fluid barriers [92].

The use of transgenic animals for studying ADME processes is not without its limitations. This is especially true when dealing with transporters. The main problems with transgenic animals in the study of ADME properties of a drug revolve around the related issues of transporter promiscuity and transporter compensation. For many transporters, there are various subtypes or homologs. Examples include the MRP drug efflux transporter family with over nine different homologs [93–95], and the organic anion transporter (OAT) with at least five homologs in humans [96]. Given the overlapping substrate and inhibitor properties of these transporters [17, 95] it is no wonder that transgenic knockout mice for single homologs of *mrp* have not yielded the dramatic results observed with *mdr1* knockout mice [97, 98]. The other issue to keep in mind is the upregulation of compensatory transport systems in the various transgenic knockout models. For example, *mdr1* knockout mice deficient in P-gp appear to have enhanced BCRP transport. This is suggested by the studies of Salama and colleagues [99], which evaluated the tissue accumulation of the HIV protease inhibitor nelfinavir, in wild-type and *mdr1* knockout mice. While significant increases in the brain accumulation of nelfinavir were observed in the *mdr1* knockout mice compared to wt controls, an even greater increase was observed when the P-gp/BCRP inhibitor GF120918 was administered to the knockout mice. As these mice had no P-gp, the increased brain accumulation of nelfinavir in the *mdr1* knockout mice exposed to GF120918 is likely due to inhibition of BCRP. These findings are consistent with the studies of Cisternino and colleagues [100] that show an increased expression of BCRP in brain microvessel endothelial cells from *mdr1* knockout mice compared to wt mice, and suggest compensatory increases in BCRP can occur in selected tissues as a result of P-gp deficiency.

In vivo application of siRNA to selectively knockdown transporter expression is relatively new. The technique involves the introduction of single chain oligonucleotides into the cell that bind to specific single chain RNA sequences preventing transcription into protein [90]. The use of siRNA to knock down the expression of a variety of protein targets has been demonstrated in cell culture systems [90]. While there are reports in the literature of successful use of siRNA technology *in vivo*, applications to transporter relevant topics are lacking. The main obstacle to application of siRNA technology for the study of ADME-related transport processes is the effective delivery of siRNA to the relevant tissue/organs [101]. However, as methods for the efficient introduction of siRNA into targeted tissue improve, it is highly likely that this technique will have future applications for ADME-related studies in the whole animal.

12.6   CONCLUSION

The increasing cost of drug development is partially due to the failure to identify undesirable compounds at an early enough stage of the drug discovery process. Therefore, development of tools capable of predicting the ADME (absorption, distribution, metabolism, and excretion) properties of the new chemical entities (NCEs) becomes a significant way to reduce the cost for drug failure and to improve the chances of designing drugs with optimal ADME characteristics. In this regard, *in vitro* models capable of screening large numbers of compounds and computational (*in silico*) based models have greatly streamlined the early ADME process. This is especially true for identification of transporter interactions at the early stages of drug development. Using a rationale approach, such as that outlined in Fig. 12.1, that incorporates early *in silico* and cell-based assays to identify potential compounds that interact with transport systems coupled with *in vivo* studies of the ADME properties of identified compounds, one can optimize the identification of transporter-related issues and evaluate their potential impact on the ADME properties of drugs in the developmental pipeline.

REFERENCES

1. Yeh AP, McMillan A, Stowell MH. Rapid and simple protein-stability screens: application to membrane proteins. *Acta Crystallogr D Biol Crystallogr* 2006;62:451–457.
2. Sakaeda T, Nakamura T, Okumura K. Pharmacogenetics of drug transporters and its impact on the pharmacotherapy. *Curr Top Med Chem* 2004;4:1385–1398.
3. Boll M, Markovich D, Weber WM, Korte H, Daniel H, Murer H. Expression cloning of a cDNA from rabbit small intestine related to proton-coupled transport of peptides, beta-lactam antibiotics and ACE-inhibitors. *Pflugers Arch* 1994;429:146–149.
4. Ganapathy ME, Prasad PD, Mackenzie B, Ganapathy V, Leibach FH. Interaction of anionic cephalosporins with the intestinal and renal peptide transporters PEPT 1 and PEPT 2. *Biochim Biophys Acta* 1997;1324:296–308.
5. Malingre MM, Richel DJ, Beijnen JH, Rosing H, Koopman FJ, Ten Bokkel Huinink WW, Schot ME, Schellens JH. Coadministration of cyclosporine strongly enhances the oral bioavailability of docetaxel. *J Clin Oncol* 2001;19:1160–1166.
6. Chiou WL, Wu TC, Ma C, Jeong HY. Enhanced oral bioavailability of docetaxel by coadministration of cyclosporine: quantitation and role of P-glycoprotein. *J Clin Oncol* 2002;20:1951–1952; author reply 1952.
7. Christians U, Schmitz V, Haschke M. Functional interactions between P-glycoprotein and CYP3A in drug metabolism. *Expert Opin Drug Metab Toxicol* 2005;1:641–654.
8. Holtzman CW, Wiggins BS, Spinler SA. Role of P-glycoprotein in statin drug interactions. *Pharmacotherapy* 2006;26:1601–1607.
9. Gottesman MM, Pastan I. Biochemistry of multidrug resistance mediated by the multidrug transporter. *Annu Rev Biochem* 1993;62:385–427.
10. Barrand MA, Bagrij T, Neo SY. Multidrug resistance-associated protein: a protein distinct from P-glycoprotein involved in cytotoxic drug expulsion. *Gen Pharmacol* 1997;28:639–645.
11. Bates SE, Robey R, Miyake K, Rao K, Ross DD, Litman T. The role of half-transporters in multidrug resistance. *J Bioenerg Biomembr* 2001;33:503–511.

12. Borst P, Evers R, Kool M, Wijnholds J. A family of drug transporters: the multidrug resistance-associated proteins. *J Natl Cancer Inst* 2000;92:1295–1302.

13. van Veen HW, Konings WN. Multidrug transporters from bacteria to man: similarities in structure and function. *Semin Cancer Biol* 1997;8:183–191.

14. Klokouzas A, Shahi S, Hladky SB, Barrand MA, van Veen HW. ABC transporters and drug resistance in parasitic protozoa. *Int J Antimicrob Agents* 2003;22:301–317.

15. Thiebaut F, Tsuruo T, Hamada H, Gottesman MM, Pastan I, Willingham MC. Cellular localization of the multidrug-resistance gene product P-glycoprotein in normal human tissues. *Proc Natl Acad Sci USA* 1987;84:7735–7738.

16. Cordon-Cardo C, O'Brien JP, Casals D, Rittman-Grauer L, Biedler JL, Melamed MR, Bertino JR. Multidrug-resistance gene (P-glycoprotein) is expressed by endothelial cells at blood–brain barrier sites. *Proc Natl Acad Sci USA* 1989;86:695–698.

17. Borst P, Evers R, Kool M, Wijnholds J. The multidrug resistance protein family. *Biochim Biophys Acta* 1999;1461:347–357.

18. Seetharaman S, Barrand MA, Maskell L, Scheper RJ. Multidrug resistance-related transport proteins in isolated human brain microvessels and in cells cultured from these isolates. *J Neurochem* 1998;70:1151–1159.

19. Chan LM, Lowes S, Hirst BH. The ABCs of drug transport in intestine and liver: efflux proteins limiting drug absorption and bioavailability. *Eur J Pharm Sci* 2004;21:25–51.

20. Lin JH. Drug–drug interaction mediated by inhibition and induction of P-glycoprotein. *Adv Drug Deliv Rev* 2003;55:53–81.

21. Smith QR, Stoll J. Blood–brain barrier amino acid transport. In Pardridge WM, Ed. *Introduction to the Blood–Brain Barrier.* Cambridge: Cambridge University Press; 1988, pp 188–197.

22. Castagna M, Shayakul C, Trotti D, Sacchi VF, Harvey WR, Hediger MA. Molecular characteristics of mammalian and insect amino acid transporters: implications for amino acid homeostasis. *J Exp Biol* 1997;200:269–286.

23. Daniel H, Herget M. Cellular and molecular mechanisms of renal peptide transport. *Am J Physiol* 1997;273:F1–F8.

24. Groneberg DA, Nickolaus M, Springer J, Doring F, Daniel H, Fischer A. Localization of the peptide transporter PEPT2 in the lung: implications for pulmonary oligopeptide uptake. *Am J Pathol* 2001;158:707–714.

25. Teuscher NS, Novotny A, Keep RF, Smith DE. Functional evidence for presence of PEPT2 in rat choroid plexus: studies with glycylsarcosine. *J Pharmacol Exp Ther* 2000;294:494–499.

26. Paulsen IT, Skurray RA. The POT family of transport proteins. *Trends Biochem Sci* 1994;19:404.

27. Leibach FH, Ganapathy V. Peptide transporters in the intestine and the kidney. *Annu Rev Nutr* 1996;16:99–119.

28. Shu C, Shen H, Hopfer U, Smith DE. Mechanism of intestinal absorption and renal reabsorption of an orally active ace inhibitor: uptake and transport of fosinopril in cell cultures. *Drug Metab Dispos* 2001;29:1307–1315.

29. Groneberg DA, Fischer A, Chung KF, Daniel H. Molecular mechanisms of pulmonary peptidomimetic drug and peptide transport. *Am J Respir Cell Mol Biol* 2004;30: 251–260.

30. Ganapathy ME, Huang W, Wang H, Ganapathy V, Leibach FH. Valacyclovir: a substrate for the intestinal and renal peptide transporters PEPT1 and PEPT2. *Biochem Biophys Res Commun* 1998;246:470–475.

31. Groneberg DA, Eynott PR, Doring F, Dinh QT, Oates T, Barnes PJ, Chung KF, Daniel H, Fischer A. Distribution and function of the peptide transporter PEPT2 in normal and cystic fibrosis human lung. *Thorax* 2002;57:55–60.

32. Stein WD. Facilitated diffusion: the simple carrier. In Stein WD, Ed. *Transport and Diffusion Across Cell Membranes*. New York: Academic Press; 1986, pp 231–362.

33. Wright EM, van Os CH, Mircheff AK. Sugar uptake by intestinal basolateral membrane vesicles. *Biochim Biophys Acta* 1980;597:112–124.

34. Wohlhueter RM, Marz R, Plagemann PG. Thymidine transport in cultured mammalian cells. Kinetic analysis, temperature dependence and specificity of the transport system. *Biochim Biophys Acta* 1979;553:262–283.

35. Harley ER, Paterson AR, Cass CE. Initial rate kinetics of the transport of adenosine and 4-amino-7-(beta-D-ribofuranosyl)pyrrolo[2,3-d]pyrimidine (tubercidin) in cultured cells. *Cancer Res* 1982;42:1289–1295.

36. Ku CP, Passow H. Creatine and creatinine transport in old and young human red blood cells. *Biochim Biophys Acta* 1980;600:212–227.

37. Chang C, Swaan PW. Computational approaches to modeling drug transporters. *Eur J Pharm Sci* 2006;27:411–424.

38. Zhang EY, Phelps MA, Banerjee A, Khantwal CM, Chang C, Helsper F, Swaan PW. Topology scanning and putative three-dimensional structure of the extracellular binding domains of the apical sodium-dependent bile acid transporter (SLC10A2). *Biochemistry* 2004;43:11380–11392.

39. Salas-Burgos A, Iserovich P, Zuniga F, Vera JC, Fischbarg J. Predicting the three-dimensional structure of the human facilitative glucose transporter glut1 by a novel evolutionary homology strategy: insights on the molecular mechanism of substrate migration, and binding sites for glucose and inhibitory molecules. *Biophys J* 2004;87:2990–2999.

40. Rouached H, Berthomieu P, El Kassis E, Cathala N, Catherinot V, Labesse G, Davidian JC, Fourcroy P. Structural and functional analysis of the C-terminal STAS (sulfate transporter and anti-sigma antagonist) domain of the Arabidopsis thaliana sulfate transporter SULTR1.2. *J Biol Chem* 2005;280:15976–15983.

41. Sali A, Blundell TL. Comparative protein modelling by satisfaction of spatial restraints. *J Mol Biol* 1993;234:779–815.

42. Greer J. Comparative modeling methods: application to the family of the mammalian serine proteases. *Proteins* 1990;7:317–334.

43. Laskowski RA, MacArthur MW, Moss DS, Thornton JM. PROCHECK: a program to check the stereochemical quality of protein structures. *J Appl Crystallogr* 1993;26:283–291.

44. Vriend G. WHAT IF: a molecular modeling and drug design program. *J Mol Graph* 1990;8:52–56, 29.

45. Seigneuret M, Garnier-Suillerot A. A structural model for the open conformation of the mdr1 P-glycoprotein based on the MsbA crystal structure. *J Biol Chem* 2003;278:30115–30124.

46. Campbell JD, Koike K, Moreau C, Sansom MS, Deeley RG, Cole SP. Molecular modeling correctly predicts the functional importance of Phe594 in transmembrane helix 11 of the multidrug resistance protein, MRP1 (ABCC1). *J Biol Chem* 2004;279:463–468.

47. Stenham DR, Campbell JD, Sansom MS, Higgins CF, Kerr ID, Linton KJ. An atomic detail model for the human ATP binding cassette transporter P-glycoprotein derived from disulfide cross-linking and homology modeling. *FASEB J* 2003;17:2287–2289.

48. Lee JY, Urbatsch IL, Senior AE, Wilkens S. Projection structure of P-glycoprotein by electron microscopy. Evidence for a closed conformation of the nucleotide binding domains. *J Biol Chem* 2002;277:40125–40131.

49. Yates CR, Chang C, Kearbey JD, Yasuda K, Schuetz EG, Miller DD, Dalton JT, Swaan PW. Structural determinants of P-glycoprotein-mediated transport of glucocorticoids. *Pharm Res* 2003;20:1794–1803.

50. Ng C, Xiao YD, Lum BL, Han YH. Quantitative structure–activity relationships of methotrexate and methotrexate analogues transported by the rat multispecific resistance-associated protein 2 (rMrp2). *Eur J Pharm Sci* 2005;26:405–413.

51. Gebauer S, Knutter I, Hartrodt B, Brandsch M, Neubert K, Thondorf I. Three-dimensional quantitative structure–activity relationship analyses of peptide substrates of the mammalian H^+/peptide cotransporter PEPT1. *J Med Chem* 2003;46:5725–5734.

52. Ekins S, Johnston JS, Bahadduri P, D'Souza VM, Ray A, Chang C, Swaan PW. *In vitro* and pharmacophore-based discovery of novel hPEPT1 inhibitors. *Pharm Res* 2005;22:512–517.

53. Suhre WM, Ekins S, Chang C, Swaan PW, Wright SH. Molecular determinants of substrate/inhibitor binding to the human and rabbit renal organic cation transporters hOCT2 and rbOCT2. *Mol Pharmacol* 2005;67:1067–1077.

54. Chang C, Pang KS, Swaan PW, Ekins S. Comparative pharmacophore modeling of organic anion transporting polypeptides: a meta-analysis of rat Oatp1a1 and human OATP1B1. *J Pharmacol Exp Ther* 2005;314:533–541.

55. Chang C, Swaan PW, Ngo LY, Lum PY, Patil SD, Unadkat JD. Molecular requirements of the human nucleoside transporters hCNT1, hCNT2, and hENT1. *Mol Pharmacol* 2004;65:558–570.

56. Hu H, Endres CJ, Chang C, Umapathy NS, Lee EW, Fei YJ, Itagaki S, Swaan PW, Ganapathy V, Unadkat JD. Electrophysiological characterization and modeling of the structure–activity relationship of the human concentrative nucleoside transporter 3 (hCNT3). *Mol Pharmacol* 2006;69:1542–1553.

57. Martin YC, Bures MG, Danaher EA, DeLazzer J, Lico I, Pavlik PA. A fast new approach to pharmacophore mapping and its application to dopaminergic and benzodiazepine agonists. *J Comput Aided Mol Des* 1993;7:83–102.

58. Cramer RD 3rd, Patterson DE, Bunce JD. Recent advances in comparative molecular field analysis (CoMFA). *Prog Clin Biol Res* 1989;291:161–165.

59. Klebe G, Abraham U, Mietzner T. Molecular similarity indices in a comparative analysis (CoMSIA) of drug molecules to correlate and predict their biological activity. *J Med Chem* 1994;37:4130–4146.

60. Chang C, Ray A, Swaan P. *In silico* strategies for modeling membrane transporter function. *Drug Discov Today* 2005;10:663–671.

61. Biegel A, Gebauer S, Brandsch M, Neubert K, Thondorf I. Structural requirements for the substrates of the H^+/peptide cotransporter PEPT2 determined by three-dimensional quantitative structure–activity relationship analysis. *J Med Chem* 2006;49:4286–4296.

62. Stouch TR, Gudmundsson O. Progress in understanding the structure–activity relationships of P-glycoprotein. *Adv Drug Deliv Rev* 2002;54:315–328.

63. Lipinski CA, Lombardo F, Dominy BW, Feeney PJ. Experimental and computational approaches to estimate solubility and permeability in drug discovery and development settings. *Adv Drug Deliv Rev* 1997;23:3–25.

64. Agoram B, Woltosz WS, Bolger MB. Predicting the impact of physiological and biochemical processes on oral drug bioavailability. *Adv Drug Deliv Rev* 2001;50(Suppl 1): S41–S67.

65. Yu LX, Amidon GL. A compartmental absorption and transit model for estimating oral drug absorption. *Int J Pharm* 1999;186:119–125.

66. Boobis A, Gundert-Remy U, Kremers P, Macheras P, Pelkonen O. *In silico* prediction of ADME and pharmacokinetics. Report of an expert meeting organised by COST B15. *Eur J Pharm Sci* 2002;17:183–193.

67. Bohets H, Annaert P, Mannens G, Van Beijsterveldt L, Anciaux K, Verboven P, Meuldermans W, Lavrijsen K. Strategies for absorption screening in drug discovery and development. *Curr Top Med Chem* 2001;1:367–383.

68. Parrott N, Lave T. Prediction of intestinal absorption: comparative assessment of GASTROPLUS and IDEA. *Eur J Pharm Sci* 2002;17:51–61.

69. Grass GM. Simulation models to predict oral drug absorption from *in vitro* data. *Adv Drug Deliv Rev* 1997;23:199–219.

70. Norris DA, Leesman GD, Sinko PJ, Grass GM. Development of predictive pharmaco-kinetic simulation models for drug discovery. *J Control Release* 2000;65:55–62.

71. Tubic M, Wagner D, Spahn-Langguth H, Bolger MB, Langguth P. *In silico* modeling of non-linear drug absorption for the P-gp substrate talinolol and of consequences for the resulting pharmacodynamic effect. *Pharm Res* 2006;23:1712–1720.

72. Batrakova EV, Li S, Miller DW, Kabanov AV. Pluronic P85 increases permeability of a broad spectrum of drugs in polarized BBMEC and Caco-2 cell monolayers. *Pharm Res* 1999;16:1366–1372.

73. Bachmeier CJ, Miller DW. A fluorometric screening assay for drug efflux transporter activity in the blood–brain barrier. *Pharm Res* 2005;22:113–121.

74. Hashimoto T, Nomoto M, Komatsu K, Haga M, Hayashi M. Improvement of intestinal absorption of peptides: adsorption of B1-Phe monoglucosylated insulin to rat intestinal brush-border membrane vesicles. *Eur J Pharm Biopharm* 2000;50:197–204.

75. Shilling AD, Azam F, Kao J, Leung L. Use of canalicular membrane vesicles (CMVs) from rats, dogs, monkeys and humans to assess drug transport across the canalicular membrane. *J Pharmacol Toxicol Methods* 2006;53:186–197.

76. Zhang Y, Benet LZ. Characterization of P-glycoprotein mediated transport of K02, a novel vinylsulfone peptidomimetic cysteine protease inhibitor, across MDR1-MDCK and Caco-2 cell monolayers. *Pharm Res* 1998;15:1520–1524.

77. Bakos E, Evers R, Szakacs G, Tusnady GE, Welker E, Szabo K, de Haas M, van Deemter L, Borst P, Varadi A, Sarkadi B. Functional multidrug resistance protein (MRP1) lacking the N-terminal transmembrane domain. *J Biol Chem* 1998;273:32167–32175.

78. Evers R, Kool M, van Deemter L, Janssen H, Calafat J, Oomen LC, Paulusma CC, Oude Elferink RP, Baas F, Schinkel AH, Borst P. Drug export activity of the human canalicular multispecific organic anion transporter in polarized kidney MDCK cells expressing cMOAT (MRP2) cDNA. *J Clin Invest* 1998;101:1310–1319.

79. Fujino H, Saito T, Ogawa S, Kojima J. Transporter-mediated influx and efflux mechanisms of pitavastatin, a new inhibitor of HMG-CoA reductase. *J Pharm Pharmacol* 2005;57:1305–1311.

80. Bubik M, Ott M, Mahringer A, Fricker G. Rapid assessment of P-glycoprotein-drug interactions at the blood–brain barrier. *Anal Biochem* 2006;358:51–58.

81. Bachmeier CJ, Trickler WJ, Miller DW. Comparison of drug efflux transport kinetics in various blood–brain barrier models. *Drug Metab Dispos* 2006;34:998–1003.

82. Yamashita S, Hattori E, Shimada A, Endoh Y, Yamazaki Y, Kataoka M, Sakane T, Sezaki H. New methods to evaluate intestinal drug absorption mediated by oligopeptide transporter from *in vitro* study using Caco-2 cells. *Drug Metab Pharmacokinet* 2002;17: 408–415.

83. Troutman MD, Thakker DR. Novel experimental parameters to quantify the modulation of absorptive and secretory transport of compounds by P-glycoprotein in cell culture models of intestinal epithelium. *Pharm Res* 2003;20:1210–1224.

84. Wang Q, Rager JD, Weinstein K, Kardos PS, Dobson GL, Li J, Hidalgo IJ. Evaluation of the MDR-MDCK cell line as a permeability screen for the blood–brain barrier. *Int J Pharm* 2005;288:349–359.

85. Li F, Hong L, Mau CI, Chan R, Hendricks T, Dvorak C, Yee C, Harris J, Alfredson T. Transport of levovirin prodrugs in the human intestinal Caco-2 cell line. *J Pharm Sci* 2006;95:1318–1325.

86. Korfmacher WA, Cox KA, Ng KJ, Veals J, Hsieh Y, Wainhaus S, Broske L, Prelusky D, Nomeir A, White RE. Cassette-accelerated rapid rat screen: a systematic procedure for the dosing and liquid chromatography/atmospheric pressure ionization tandem mass spectrometric analysis of new chemical entities as part of new drug discovery. *Rapid Commun Mass Spectrom* 2001;15:335–340.

87. Raynaud FI, Fischer PM, Nutley BP, Goddard PM, Lane DP, Workman P. Cassette dosing pharmacokinetics of a library of 2,6,9-trisubstituted purine cyclin-dependent kinase 2 inhibitors prepared by parallel synthesis. *Mol Cancer Ther* 2004;3:353–362.

88. Smith NF, Hayes A, Nutley BP, Raynaud FI, Workman P. Evaluation of the cassette dosing approach for assessing the pharmacokinetics of geldanamycin analogues in mice. *Cancer Chemother Pharmacol* 2004;54:475–486.

89. Schinkel AH, Smit JJ, van Tellingen O, Beijnen JH, Wagenaar E, Van Deemter L, Mol CA, Van der Valk MA, Robanus-Maandag EC, te Riele HP, et al. Disruption of the mouse *mdr1a* P-glycoprotein gene leads to a deficiency in the blood–brain barrier and to increased sensitivity to drugs. *Cell* 1994;77:491–502.

90. Toub N, Malvy C, Fattal E, Couvreur P. Innovative nanotechnologies for the delivery of oligonucleotides and siRNA. *Biomed Pharmacother* 2006;60:607–620.

91. Schinkel AH, Mol CA, Wagenaar E, van Deemter L, Smit JJ, Borst P. Multidrug resistance and the role of P-glycoprotein knockout mice. *Eur J Cancer* 1995;31A:1295–1298.

92. Ocheltree SM, Shen H, Hu Y, Keep RF, Smith DE. Role and relevance of peptide transporter 2 (PEPT2) in the kidney and choroid plexus: *in vivo* studies with glycylsarcosine in wild-type and PEPT2 knockout mice. *J Pharmacol Exp Ther* 2005;315:240–247.

93. Kool M, de Haas M, Scheffer GL, Scheper RJ, van Eijk MJ, Juijn JA, Baas F, Borst P. Analysis of expression of cMOAT (MRP2), MRP3, MRP4, and MRP5, homologues of the multidrug resistance-associated protein gene (MRP1), in human cancer cell lines. *Cancer Res* 1997;57:3537–3547.

94. Kool M, van der Linden M, de Haas M, Baas F, Borst P. Expression of human MRP6, a homologue of the multidrug resistance protein gene MRP1, in tissues and cancer cells. *Cancer Res* 1999;59:175–182.

95. Kruh GD, Guo Y, Hopper-Borge E, Belinsky MG, Chen ZS. ABCC10, ABCC11, and ABCC12. *Pflugers Arch* 2007;453:675–684.

96. Anzai N, Kanai Y, Endou H. Organic anion transporter family: current knowledge. *J Pharmacol Sci* 2006;100:411–426.

97. Sun H, Johnson DR, Finch RA, Sartorelli AC, Miller DW, Elmquist WF. Transport of fluorescein in MDCKII-MRP1 transfected cells and mrp1-knockout mice. *Biochem Biophys Res Commun* 2001;284:863–869.

98. Sugiyama D, Kusuhara H, Lee YJ, Sugiyama Y. Involvement of multidrug resistance associated protein 1 (Mrp1) in the efflux transport of 17beta estradiol-D-17beta-glucuronide ($E_2$17betaG) across the blood–brain barrier. *Pharm Res* 2003;20:1394–1400.

99. Salama NN, Kelly EJ, Bui T, Ho RJ. The impact of pharmacologic and genetic knockout of P-glycoprotein on nelfinavir levels in the brain and other tissues in mice. *J Pharm Sci* 2005;94:1216–1225.

100. Cisternino S, Mercier C, Bourasset F, Roux F, Scherrmann JM. Expression, up-regulation, and transport activity of the multidrug-resistance protein Abcg2 at the mouse blood–brain barrier. *Cancer Res* 2004;64:3296–3301.

101. Aigner A. Delivery systems for the direct application of siRNAs to induce RNA interference (RNAi) in vivo. *J Biomed Biotechnol* 2006:1–15.

13

ACCUMULATION OF DRUGS IN TISSUES

KRISHNAMURTHY VENKATESAN,[1] DEEPA BISHT,[1] AND MOHAMMAD OWAIS[2]

[1]*National JALMA Institute for Leprosy and Other Mycobacterial Diseases, Agra, India*
[2]*Aligarh Muslim University, Aligarh, India*

Contents

Preclinical Development Handbook: ADME and Biopharmaceutical Properties, edited by Shayne Cox Gad
Copyright © 2008 John Wiley & Sons, Inc.

429

13.1   INTRODUCTION

In order to exert desirable pharmacological action, drugs need to achieve an adequate concentration in their target tissues. The term pharmacokinetics refers to absorption, distribution, metabolism, excretion, and toxicity. This chapter deals, in detail, with the aspects concerned with drug distribution and disposition.

The two fundamental processes that determine the concentration of a drug at any moment and in any region of the body are (1) translocation of the drug molecules and (2) the chemical transformations they undergo due to metabolic action. Drug molecules move around the body in two ways: bulk flow transfer (i.e., in the bloodstream) and diffusional transfer. The chemical nature of the drug makes no difference to its transfer by bulk flow as the cardiovascular system provides a very fast long-distance distribution system. In contrast, diffusional characteristics differ markedly between different drugs. In particular, ability to cross hydrophobic diffusion barriers is strongly influenced by lipid solubility of the drug molecule. Aqueous diffusion is also part of the overall mechanism of drug transport since it is this process that delivers drug molecules to and from the nonaqueous barriers.

Once the drug reaches the bloodstream, it is distributed to all organs including tissues that are not relevant to its pharmacological or therapeutic effect. Thus, after absorption, the drug may not only get reversibly associated with its site of action (receptor) but may get bound to plasma proteins or may accumulate in various storage sites or may enter into tissues that are not involved in its primary action (although they may be involved in metabolism, and excretion). This part of pharmacokinetics, which deals with distribution, metabolism, and excretion, is termed drug disposition because these three phases precisely decide the fate of a drug after absorption. The drug may be evenly, or unevenly, or selectively distributed in different body compartments, which are physiological in character rather than anatomical entities.

13.2   MOVEMENT OF DRUG MOLECULES ACROSS CELL BARRIERS

Plasma membrane limits the boundary of a cell from the rest of the body parts including aqueous compartments. In fact, a single layer of membrane separates intracellular and extracellular compartments. An epithelial barrier such as the gastrointestinal mucosa or renal tubule consists of a layer of cells tightly connected with each other so that molecules traverse at least two cell membranes—inner and outer. Vascular epithelium is still more complicated, with its variation in anatomical disposition and vascular flow between tissues. In some organs, especially the central nervous system and placenta, there are tight junctions between the cells and the endothelium is covered with an impermeable layer of periendothelial cells. In organs such as the liver and spleen, the endothelium is discontinuous, allowing free passage between cells.

There are four main ways by which small molecules cross cell membranes—(1) by diffusing directly through the lipids of the plasma membrane; (2) by diffusing through aqueous pores formed by special proteins that traverse the lipid bilayer; (3) by combining with a transmembrane carrier protein that binds a drug molecule on one side of the membrane, then changes conformation and releases it on the other; or (4) by pinocytosis. Of these four ways, diffusion through lipid and carrier-mediated transport are very important in relation to pharmacokinetic mechanisms. There is yet another mechanism of transport, by which some drugs are actively transported into the cell by energy-dependent pumps [1]. In some cases, two or more drugs may share the same pump, giving rise to drug–drug interactions A different energy-dependent efflux pump may also pump them out of the cell. It is thought that multidrug resistance (mdr) transporter may play a role in lowering intracellular drug concentrations via an efflux mechanism. Increased expression of P-glycoprotein is often associated with lower intracellular accumulation of certain drugs due to efflux of the drug from the cells [2–5].

13.3   ABSORPTION OF DRUGS

Absorption is defined as the passage of a drug from the site of administration into the plasma. Absorption is therefore important for all routes of administration, except intravenous injection. The main routes of administration are oral, sublingual, rectal, topical application to other epithelial surfaces (e.g., skin, cornea, vagina, and nasal mucosa), inhalation, and injection—subcutaneous, intramuscular, intravenous, and intrathecal [6].

13.3.1   Oral, Sublingual, and Rectal Administration

Oral Administration   Although most drugs are swallowed by the oral route, little absorption occurs until the drug reaches the small intestine. The mechanism of drug absorption is the same as for other epithelial barriers, namely, the passive diffusion at a rate determined by the ionization and lipid solubility of the drug molecules. In a few instances intestinal absorption depends on carrier-mediated transport rather than simple lipid diffusion. Examples of the drugs under this category are levodopa and fluorouracil. In general, iron is absorbed via specific carriers in the surface membranes of the jejunal mucosa, and calcium is absorbed by means of vitamin D-dependent carrier systems. The biochemical properties of the drug such as molecular weight, particle size, and pH, along with local factors such as food, intestinal motility, and blood flow, all affect gastrointestinal (GI) absorption. The presence of agents that may affect gastric pH or motility or interact with the drug to produce binding will prevent or slow the absorption. Examples of these agents and the absorption factors affected are antacids (pH), vasodilators (GI perfusion), cathartics (GI motility), and calcium (binding). Some drugs are given to patients as prodrugs since the absorption of the prodrug may be superior to the parent drug (hence increased bioavailability). Examples of prodrugs are levodopa and azarabine, prodrugs of dopamine and azauridine, respectively. The term *bioavailability* indicates the proportion of the drug that passes into the systemic circulation after oral administration, taking into consideration both absorption and metabolic degradation in the gut wall or liver before reaching the systemic circulation.

Sublingual Administration   A few drugs are placed under the tongue (taken sublingually) for their direct absorption into the small blood vessels that lie underneath the tongue. The absorption is rapid and the drug enters the systemic circulation without entering the portal system and so escapes first-pass metabolism. The sublingual route is especially good for nitroglycerin, which is used for treatment of angina.

Rectal Administration   Rectal administration is useful for drugs that are required both to produce a local effect (e.g., anti-inflammatory drugs for treating ulcerative colitis) and to produce systemic effects. The spatial positioning of the rectal suppositories avoiding the upper hemorrhoidal vein can avoid the *first-pass effect*, as the encapsulated drug molecules will be directly released into the inferior vena cava. Nevertheless, the popularity of this mode of route has abated because of erratic absorption behavior and also a great deal of advancement in parenteral preparations.

13.3.2   Application to Epithelial Surfaces

Cutaneous Administration   Cutaneous administration is used when a local effect on the skin is required (e.g., topically applied steroids). Appreciable absorption may nonetheless occur and lead to systemic effects. Most drugs are absorbed very poorly through unbroken skin. Transdermal dosage forms in which the drug is incorporated as a stick-on patch applied in the area of thin skin are increasingly used. Several drugs are available in this form, for example, estrogen for hormone replacement.

Nasal Sprays   Some drugs like peptide hormone analogues (e.g., antidiuretic hormone, gonadotropin-releasing hormone, and calcitonin), if given orally, will be inactive as they will quickly be destroyed in the gastrointestinal tract, and so they are administered in nasal sprays so that adequate absorption takes place through nasal mucosa. Intranasal administration has advantages in several cases. For example, clinical experience suggests that intranasal sumatriptan (a potent serotonin $5HT_{1B/1D}$ agonist widely used in the treatment of migraine) has more advantages over oral and subcutaneous administration, such as more rapid onset of the effect and use in patients with gastrointestinal complaints [7].

Eye Drops   Many drugs are applied as eye drops and they get absorbed through the epithelium of the conjunctival sac. Systemic side effects are not caused while desirable local effects are best achieved. One example is dorzolamide (a carbonic anhydrase inhibitor), which is given as eye drops to lower ocular pressure in glaucoma patients. In some cases administration of eye drops may result in unwanted side effects on account of delivery of absorbed material from the eye to the systemic circulation.

13.3.3   Administration by Inhalation

This route is best used for volatile and gaseous anesthetics and the lung serves as the route of administration and elimination. Rapid absorption on account of large surface area and high vascularity of the lung tissue makes it possible to achieve rapid adjustments of plasma concentration of the drugs. Drugs used for their effects on the lung are also given by inhalation, usually as an aerosol. Inhalation therapy is commonly used in the treatment of asthma as it results in a high concentration of active drug at the site of action. The degree of lung deposition of an inhaled drug is influenced by several factors—the one most important is the inhalation maneuvers. Other possible factors are related to the properties of the formulation, such as particle size and hygroscopic nature. Glucocorticoids (e.g., beclomethasone) and bronchodilators (e.g., salbutamol) are given by this route, which results in high local concentration in the lung while minimizing systemic side effects. Minimizing the systemic absorption by chemical modification of a drug will reduce the side effects. For example, ipatropium, a muscarinic receptor antagonist, a quaternary ammonium ion analogue of atropine, is poorly absorbed into systemic circulation.

13.3.4 Administration by Injection

Intravenous Injection   This is the fastest and the most certain route of drug administration. Bolus injection produces a very high concentration of drug first in the right heart and lungs, and then in the systemic circulation. The rate of injection of the drug decides the peak concentration reaching the tissues. Steady intravenous infusion avoids the uncertainties of absorption from other sites while avoiding high peak plasma concentrations resulting from bolus injection. Several antibiotics and anesthetics such as propofol and diazepam, used for treatment of patients with status epilepticus, are administered intravenously for better bioavailability of the drug.

Subcutaneous or Intramuscular Injection   Subcutaneous or intramuscular injection of drugs usually produces a faster effect than oral administration, but the rate of absorption depends on the site of injection and on local blood flow. Diffusion through the tissue and removal of the injected drug by local blood flow are the rate-limiting factors.

Intrathecal (Intraspinal) Injection   Injection of a drug into the subarachnoid space via a lumbar puncture needle is often used for some specialized purposes. Methotrexate is administered intrathecally in the treatment of certain childhood leukemias. Regional anesthesia can be produced by intrathecal administration of a local anesthetic, such as bupivacaine. Some antibiotics (e.g., aminoglycosides) cross the blood–brain barrier very slowly and in rare cases of nervous system infections they are given intrathecally.

13.4 DRUG DISTRIBUTION

Following absorption from the gastrointestinal tract or direct administration through another route, the drug is distributed to the tissues and organs throughout the body. Most drugs do not localize to one particular site, but are distributed to a number of organs and tissues. Distribution refers to both rate of distribution and extent of distribution. The rate of distribution depends on the membrane permeability and the blood perfusion, while the extent of distribution is influenced by factors such as lipid solubility of the drug, pH–pK_a, plasma protein binding, and intracellular binding [8, 9].

13.4.1 Rate of Distribution

Membrane Permeability   Membrane permeability refers to the ability of a drug to cross the cell membranes. This may occur by passive diffusion, where the drug simply moves from an area of higher concentration to one of lower concentration. Nonpolar drug molecules dissolve freely in the lipid bilayer of the membrane and are translocated across it by diffusion. The permeability coefficient, P, and the concentration gradient across the membrane will determine the number of drug molecules that will cross per unit area in unit time. In general, two physicochemical factors that significantly contribute to the permeability coefficient are solubility of the drug and its diffusivity across the membrane. Solubility is expressed as a partition coefficient for the substance to be distributed between the membrane phase (lipid environment) and the aqueous environment and the diffusivity is a measure of the mobility of the molecules within membrane lipid and is expressed as a diffusion coefficient. Since the diffusion coefficient varies only slightly among different drug molecules, the partition coefficient remains as the most important variable influencing drug diffusion. Lipid solubility is one of the important determinants of the pharmacokinetic characteristics of a drug. Many properties, such as rate of absorption from the gut, penetration into brain and the other tissues, and the extent of renal elimination, can be predicted from the drug's solubility profile.

Lipid-soluble compounds pass trough the cell membranes very rapidly, whereas water-soluble compounds penetrate more slowly at a rate dependent on their size. Low molecular weight drugs pass through by simple diffusion. The transfer is slow for drugs with molecular diameter above 100 Å. There are two deviations to the typical capillary structure, which result in variation from normal drug permeability. First, the permeability is greatly increased in the renal capillaries by pores in the membrane of the endothelial cells and also in specialized hepatic capillaries (sinusoids), where a complete lining is generally lacking. This results in more extensive transfer of drugs out of the capillary bed. Second, the brain capillaries seem to have impermeable walls restricting the transfer of molecules from blood to brain tissue (blood–brain barrier). Lipid-soluble compounds can readily be transferred but the transfer of polar compounds is severely restricted by the barrier.

The transfer rate of ionizable drugs across the capillary membrane depends on the pK_a of the drug molecule as well as the pH of the blood. Many drugs are weak acids or bases and therefore exist in the un-ionized as well as the ionized form. The ratio of un-ionized to ionized or vice versa will depend on the pH of the environment. The ionized species has very low lipid solubility and is virtually unable to permeate membrane except where a specific transport mechanism exists. The lipid solubility of the un-ionized species will depend on the chemical nature of the drug. Most of the un-ionized drug molecules are adequately lipid soluble. There are, however, exceptions to this rule while dealing with many drug molecules. For example, aminoglycoside antibiotics are sufficiently hydrophilic in the uncharged form, here the presence of hydroxyl groups (electronegative oxygen) in the sugar molecules of the drug that plays an important role in imparting solubility to polar solvents like water.

Ionization affects not only the rate of drug permeation across membranes but also the steady-state distribution of the drug molecules between two or more aqueous compartments like plasma, urine, and gastric juice, if a pH difference exists between them. Within each compartment the ratio of ionized to un-ionized species of the drug, as determined by the pK_a of the drug and the pH of the environment, will be different and acidic drug will be concentrated in the compartment with high pH and vice versa. This is called ion trapping. The larger the pH difference between two aqueous compartments, the greater will be the concentration gradient produced by ion trapping.

13.4.2 Blood Perfusion

Membrane permeability tends to restrict the transfer and distribution of drugs once they are delivered to the tissue. The other major factor that determines the rate of drug distribution is blood perfusion. The rate at which blood perfuses to different organs varies widely. Total blood flow is greatest to brain, kidneys, liver, and muscle with highest perfusion rates to brain, kidney, liver, and heart. Hence total drug concentration would rise most rapidly in these organs. Highly perfused organs, namely, heart, liver, kidney, and brain, usually receive drug within minutes after its absorption. Distribution to tissues like muscle, fat, and skin may require longer periods of time (minutes to hours). Certain organs such as the adrenals also have large perfusion rates. The relative restriction/contribution of the twin factors of membrane permeability and blood perfusion to drug distribution can better be understood with examples of transfer of thiopental and penicillin to brain and muscle. Thiopental gets into the brain faster than muscle, while penicillin gets into muscle more quickly than it gets into brain. Thiopental is only partly ionized and passes into the brain or muscle easily. But since brain has a perfusion rate approximately 20 times higher than muscle, thiopental transfers in and out of brain more quickly. On the other hand, penicillin, which is quite polar, transfers faster in muscle than brain on account of lesser restriction of muscle capillaries to the drug.

There is growing evidence that the reduction of blood flow in soft tissues is closely associated with the significant impairment of the rate of tissue penetration by antimicrobial agents. For example, in patients with peripheral arterial occlusive disease, it has been demonstrated that the peak concentrations are significantly lower in the interstitium of ischemic soft tissue in comparison with that in healthy and well perfused tissue.

13.4.3 Extent of Drug Distribution

Several physiological barriers influence the extent of drug distribution. Chemicophysical properties, molecular weight, degree of plasma protein binding, and intracellular binding are among the most important intrinsic characteristics that condition the extent of drug distribution in the body [10, 11]. Besides its ability to bind with plasma protein, the size and degree of ionization as well as lipid solubility of a drug molecule specifically regulate its extravascular transfer. Host-related factors such as site of infection, presence of biological barriers (blood–brain barrier, placental barrier, blood–CSF barrier, prostate, ocular membranes), and local pH may contribute to the pharmacological action of drug molecules. Sometimes these factors can inhibit a particular drug molecule as well. Inactivation of the antibacterial agent in the tissue can occur at infection sites by binding to interstitial fluid proteins, soluble intracellular proteins, or subcellular structures (nucleic acids, leukocytic chromatin cell membranes, and mucopolysaccharides).

13.4.4   Physiological Barriers and Reservoirs Influencing Drug Distribution

Blood–Brain Barrier   A major problem in drug delivery to brain is the presence of the blood–brain barrier (BBB), which is now well established as a unique membranous barrier that tightly segregates the brain from the blood influx. Endothelial cells of brain capillaries differ from most other capillaries of the body, as they are very tightly joined and lack intracellular pores. In addition, these brain capillaries are also enveloped by less permeable glial cells. Morphologically, this constitutes the *blood–brain barrier* [12, 13]. Anatomically, there exists a dual barrier in the CNS: the blood–brain barrier and blood–CSF barrier (located in the choroid plexus). The BBB places certain constraints on the passage of drugs from the blood to the brain and the CSF. As a rule only lipid-soluble nonionized forms of drugs penetrate more easily into brain as compared to water-soluble ionized forms of drugs [14, 15]. The volatile anesthetics like ether and chloroform, ultrashort acting barbiturates like thiopental, narcotic analgesics like morphine and heroin, dopamine precursor like L-dopa, sympathomimetics like amphetamine and ephedrine, and drugs like diazepam and propranolol can pass through the BBB, while polar compounds like dopamine, serotonin, and streptomycin and quaternary substances like *d*-tubocurarine, hexamethonium, neostigmine, and acetylcholine do not penetrate the BBB. The following five regions of the brain, on account of their relative permeability, do not form part of the BBB—pituitary gland, pineal body, area prostrema near the floor of the fourth ventricle, median eminence, and choroid plexus capillaries. The BBB is further reinforced by a high concentration of P-glycoprotein (P-gp) active drug efflux transporter protein in the luminal membranes of the cerebral capillary endothelium. This efflux transporter actively removes a broad range of drug molecules from the endothelial cell cytoplasm before they cross into the brain parenchyma [13].

Blood–CSF Barrier   The second barrier that a systemically administered drug encounters before entering the central nervous system (CNS) is known as the blood–CSF barrier (BCB). Since CSF can exchange molecules with the interstitial fluid of the brain parenchyma, the passage of drug molecules from the blood into the CSF is also carefully regulated by the BCB. Physiologically, the BCB is found in the epithelium of choroid plexus, which are arranged in a manner that limits the passage of molecules and cells into the CSF. The choroid plexus and the arachnoid membrane act together at the barriers between the blood and the CSF. [13]. Only nonionizable lipid-soluble drugs can pass from blood to the CSF as in the case of the BBB where the epithelial cells of choroid plexuses are lined by occluding zonulae. But the brain–CSF barrier is composed of epithelial cells lining the ventricles and occluding zonulae do not connect these. Hence the CSF–brain barrier is extremely permeable to drug molecules from the CSF to brain cells [16]. The significance of this fact is that drugs like penicillin that have poor penetration through the BBB can cross the brain–CSF barrier if given by the intrathecal route and reach the brain tissue in sufficient concentration. In the clinical setting, drug concentrations in CSF are sometimes used as a surrogate for drug concentrations at the target site within the brain. But multiplicity of compartments of the brain and involvement of several factors in the transport of dugs from plasma into the brain and distribution within the brain limit the applicative value of CSF drug levels in prediction of brain target concentrations [17].

Placental Barrier The placental membrane readily allows the transfer of nonpolar lipid-soluble drugs mainly by passive diffusion. However, the other transport mechanisms like active transport and pinocytosis are also operative. Thus, lipid-soluble nonionizable drugs like hypnotics, narcotics, general anesthetics, cardiac glycosides, alcohol, neuroleptics, and certain antibiotics can readily cross the placental barrier, while nonionizable and very high molecular weight substances cannot cross the barrier. Antihypertensive drugs that are lipid soluble bind with proteins to lesser extent, and when in un-ionized form generally pass through the placental barrier with ease [18].

Special Compartments for Drug Distribution Besides plasma proteins, the tissues of the body can also act as reservoirs for drugs, but usually the sites where drugs accumulate are not those where they exert their physiological action. These stored drugs are in equilibrium with the drug in plasma and are only slowly released from these storage sites to provide enough circulating drug to produce biological effects. Consequently, this type of storage, unlike plasma protein binding, represents "a site of loss" rather than "a depot" for continued drug action.

Cellular Reservoir A drug may have a great affinity for plasma proteins, yet primarily be distributed in tissue if the tissue has an even higher affinity for the drug. This affinity could be due to several reasons, for example, binding to tissue proteins (albumin) or top nucleoproteins. Examples are digoxin and emetine to skeletal muscle, heart, liver, kidney (bound to muscle proteins), and retina (nucleoproteins); cadmium, lead, and mercury in kidney (muscle protein, metallothionein); and chlorpromazine in eye (affinity to retinal pigment melanin).

Fat Reservoir Highly lipid-soluble drugs like thiopentone, DDT, and phenoxybenzamine get selectively accumulated in fat and adipose tissue. The fat, however, is a sluggish reservoir due to lesser blood flow; but if body fat starts depleting, as occurs during starvation, the stored drug may be mobilized and toxicity may occur.

Transcellular Reservoir Aqueous humor (e.g., chloramphenicol and prednisolone), CSF (e.g., amino sugars and sucrose), endolymph, joint fluid (e.g., ampicillin), and pleural (e.g., imipramine and methadone), pericardial, and peritoneal sacs can also serve as drug reservoirs.

Bone and Connective Tissue Reservoirs Many drugs and substances like tetracycline, cisplatin, lead, arsenic, and fluorides form a complex with bone salts and get deposited in nails, bones, and teeth. The antifungal drug griseofulvin has an affinity for keratin precursor cells and is selectively accumulated in the skin and fingernails. Bone may become a reservoir for the slow release of toxic substances like lead and arsenic and for the anticancer drug cisplatin into the blood.

Biliary Reservoir The lipophilic drugs with relatively high molecular weight (~325 Da in rats and greater than 500 Da in humans) are generally metabolized in liver and eventually accumulate in bile. Subsequent biliary excretion of such drugs can significantly impact their systemic exposure, which in turn regulates their pharmacological effect on the one hand and their toxicity on the other. Drugs (such as mycophenolic acid and digoxin) excreted into bile often undergo some degree of reabsorption along the gastrointestinal tract [19, 20]. Enterohepatic recycling is also a very important physiological process for bile salt homeostasis. In humans, more than 95% of the bile salt is reabsorbed in the distal ileum [21]. The biliary clearance of a drug would be extremely valuable in elucidating the potential mechanism operative in hepatobiliary toxicity, predicting drug–drug interaction, and identifying enterohepatic versus enteroenteric recirculation. Several clinical studies have shown that drug–drug interaction can result in changes in drug absorption due to inhibition of transport proteins. For example, inhibition of P-glycoprotein results in increased absorption of talinolol [22]. The liver plays a central role in the biotransformation and removal of xenobiotics and endogenous compounds from the blood; while the majority of small, lipophilic compounds flow through the space of Disse and enter the hepatocyte via the basolateral membrane by simple diffusion. On the other hand, more polar and bulky molecules require transport systems to cross the sinusoidal membrane. After reaching the hepatocyte, drugs can be transported into bile either as an uncharged species or as more hydrophilic metabolites produced after phase I and phase II biotransformation, or they can be excreted into the bloodstream by basolateral transport proteins. In addition to bile salt transport, hepatic transport proteins facilitate excretion of end products of metabolism, such as bilirubin or xenobiotics, into bile for subsequent removal via the intestine.

Plasma Protein Binding as Reservoir Although some drugs are simply dissolved in plasma water, most of them get bound to plasma components, such as albumin, globulin, transferrin, and ceruloplasmin (and also through the BBB), get metabolized, and are excreted in urine, saliva, CSF, and milk. As the free or unbound drug is eliminated from the body, more drug dissociates from the drug–plasma protein complex, glycoproteins, and α- and β-lipoproteins to replenish the free drug levels in plasma. Drugs usually are bound to plasma and cellular proteins in a reversible manner and in dynamic equilibrium, according to the law of mass action [23]. Thus, extensive plasma protein binding may serve as a circulating drug reservoir. But it is only the free fraction of the drug that is pharmacologically active, while the protein bound component is inert. Similarly, it is the free fraction of the drug that diffuses through the capillary wall (and also through the BBB), gets metabolized, and is excreted in urine, saliva, CSF, and milk.

13.5 IMPORTANT PROTEINS THAT CONTRIBUTE TO DRUG BINDING

1. *Albumin.* Of the plasma proteins, albumin is the major drug binding and transport protein of the circulatory system. Drug binding to plasma albumin occurs to a variable extent. It consists of three homologous domains. Each domain consists of two subdomains, A and B. The principal sites of ligand binding to HSA are located in hydrophobic cavities in subdomains IIA and IIIB. HSA is known to undergo different pH-dependent conformational transitions, the N-F transition between pH 5.0 and 3.5, the F-E transition between pH 3.5 and 1.2, and the N-B transition

between pH 7.0 and 9.0. The N-F isomerization involves unfolding and separation of domain III from the rest of the molecule without significantly affecting the rest of the molecule. The I state is characterized by unfolding of domain III together with partial but significant loss of native conformation of domain I. The domain II of HSA remains unaffected in the intermediate state. That the N-B transition has physiological significance is suggested by the fact that under increased Ca^{2+} concentration in blood plasma, the B isomer predominates. Moreover, it is believed that the transport function of albumin is controlled through this transition or akin to it.

Most of the acidic drugs (such as warfarin, penicillin, sulfonamides, phenylbutazone, and salicylic acid), in principle, bind to albumin. Two binding sites for acidic drugs have been identified on human serum albumin. Although less specific, domain I can bind with a variety of structurally unrelated drugs like acenocoumarin, warfarin, dicoumarol, phenylbutazone, phenytoin, valproic acid, sulfonamides, and endogenous substances like bilirubin. On the other hand, site II is more specific. With the exception of benzodiazepines, acidic drugs such as ibuprofen, naproxen, and analogues of probenecid, clofibric acid, cloxacillin, and endogenous substances like tryptophan bind to this site. Some drugs bind to both the sites with different affinities, and examples are salicylic acid, tolubutamide, and indomethacin [24–26].

2. *α_2-Acid Glycoprotein.* While acidic drugs primarily bind to albumin, many lipophilic basic drugs, such as quinidine, imipramine, lidocaine, chlorpromazine, propranolol and its analogues, and spinperidol bind avidly to α_2-acid glycoprotein (AAG). The drug binding to AAG in health and disease has been extensively reviewed by Kremer et al. [27].

3. *Lipoproteins.* The role of lipoproteins as a transport system for drugs has been largely overlooked compared to the extensive reports on drug binding with albumin and AAG. However, there are reports that lipoproteins could be implicated in the binding process; for example, propofol binds extensively to all lipoprotein fractions [28, 29].

4. *Tissue Proteins and Nucleoproteins.* Some drugs, particularly those having high apparent volume of distribution, specifically bind to tissue proteins (e.g., digoxin, emetine, and chloroquine). The steroidal drugs can bind to specific receptor and nuclear proteins present on nucleus.

5. *Miscellaneous Binding Proteins.* Only a few drugs are significantly bound to other special proteins; for example, corticosteroids are bound to steroid binding globulin, transcortin; thyroxine to α-globulin; and antigens to γ-globulin.

13.6 VOLUME OF DISTRIBUTION

The distribution of drugs in the body depends on their lipophilicity and protein binding. Low plasma binding or high tissue binding or high lipophilicity means an extensive tissue distribution. In pharmacokinetics, the distribution is described by the parameter V_d, the apparent volume of distribution [10]. The apparent volume of distribution, V_d, is defined as the volume of fluid required to contain the total amount, Q, of drug in the body at the same concentration as that present in the plasma, C_p.

$$V_d = Q/C_p$$

Values of V_d for many drugs have been measured. The drugs with high plasma protein binding remain largely restricted to the vascular compartment and tend to have lower volumes of distribution. Some drugs are confined to the plasma compartment. The plasma volume is about 0.05 L/kg body weight. A few drugs such as heparin (V_d of 0.05–0.1 L/kg) are confined to plasma volume because the molecule is so large that it cannot cross the capillary wall easily. More often, the retention of a drug in the plasma following a single dose reflects the strong binding to plasma protein. However, the free drug in the interstitial fluid only exerts a pharmacological effect.

Following multiple dosing, equilibration occurs with an ensuing increase in V_d values. Drugs such as warfarin, sulfamethoxazole, glibenclamide, and atenolol are confined to the plasma compartment. Few drugs are distributed in the extracellular compartment, which has a volume of about 0.2 L/kg and many polar compounds such as vecuronium, gentamicin, and carbenicillin show an approximate V_d of 0.2 L/kg. These drugs cannot easily enter cells because of their low lipid solubility and they do not traverse the blood–brain or placental barriers easily. Drugs like tubocurarine (V_d 0.2–0.4 L/kg) and theophylline (V_d 0.4–0.7 L/kg) are also distributed in the extracellular fluid. Some other drugs are distributed throughout the body water. Total body water represents about 0.55 L/kg, which approximates the distribution volume of relatively lipid-soluble drugs that cross cell membranes, such as phenytoin and ethanol. There are many drugs with the volume of distribution greater than the total body volume on account of binding of drug outside the plasma compartment, or partitioning into body fat. Examples are morphine, tricyclic antidepressants, and haloperidol.

13.7   INFLUENCE OF LIPOPHILICITY AND LYSOSOMAL ACCUMULATION ON TISSUE DRUG DISTRIBUTION

Distribution of a drug in the body is dependent on the permeation properties, the blood flow rates in various tissues, and plasma and tissue uptake. The distribution of drugs *in vivo* is largely determined by uptake competition among individual tissues [30, 31]. The lipophilic drugs are characterized by extensive accumulation in tissues, which leads to a high volume of distribution. Nonspecific binding to cellular membrane (phospholipids) and uptake by acidic compartments (mainly lysosomes) are responsible for such a distribution pattern [32]. Lysosomal trapping is an important mechanism of distribution of basic psychotropic drugs [33]. Lysosomal trapping has been reported to contribute to the uptake of despiramine and chloroquine in various tissues [34]. Basic drugs are distributed widely in various tissues in the following order: lung, fat, heart, kidney, brain, gut, muscle, and bone. The fat volume in the body influences the deposition kinetics. There is a good correlation in various tissues between the tissue–plasma concentration ratio and the octanol–water coefficient among various drugs.

13.8   PARTITION OF THE DRUG INTO FAT AND OTHER TISSUES

Drug accumulation or concentration in a tissue or biological fluid occurs when the influx of a drug is greater than the efflux. However, concentration gradients do not govern the rate of active transport. Thus, active transport can play a part in accumulation. Fat represents a large nonpolar compartment. In practice, this is important only for a few drugs mainly because the effective fat–water partition coefficient is relatively low for most drugs. For example, sequestration of morphine by body fat is of little importance as the drug's lipid–water partition coefficient is only 0.4, although the drug is sufficiently lipophilic to cross the blood–brain barrier. On the other hand, a drug such as thiopental, with a fat–water partition coefficient of about 10, accumulates substantially in body fat. The second factor that limits the sequestration of a drug in body fat is the amount of blood supply. Since fat receives less than 2% of cardiac output, drugs are delivered to body fat rather slowly. But some drugs like clofazimine (a riminophenazine with anti-inflammatory properties), used in the treatment of leprosy and other mycobacterial infections, extensively accumulates in fatty tissues and organs with in the reticuloendothelial system and the drug is retained for a long time even after stopping administration of the drug [35]. Sequestration also involves either drug ionization or drug binding to proteins and other macromoleules, preventing efflux by diffusion or active transport.

13.9   SPECIAL DRUG DELIVERY SYSTEMS

Several approaches are being explored to improve drug delivery. Some of these are polymeric carriers [36], biologically erodable microspheres [37], nanoparticles [38, 39], prodrugs [40, 41], antibody–drug conjugates, liposomes, and coated implantable devices [42, 43].

Many drugs can be formulated using simple vehicles; however, a large number of chemical entities pose problems because of the dose and poor solubility in simple solvents and cosolvent systems. As a result, there is a need for advanced formulations that will permit the administration of challenging drugs efficiently. For that purpose, drugs can be attached to the polymeric carriers or dispersed in suitable (colloidal) vehicles. In the past, surfactant systems that solubilized the drug and thereby provided a transparent product for injection were in use; for example, cremophor was a material of choice—unfortunately, it has been associated with anaphylactic reactions. Workers in the field hence sought alternative lipid carriers such as liposomes and lipid emulsions. Although fat emulsions have been in trend for decades for parenteral nutrition and these systems have been used with success as drug carriers, yet they are avoided, as such preparations allowed the drugs to rapidly exit the system and reach the bloodstream, hence limiting the possibilities of drug targeting [44]. Successful homing of drugs to the desired biological compartment of the host depends on the intrinsic properties of the drug, or it can also be achieved by manipulation of the carrier/delivery system, as little can be done to influence the target and its surroundings. Liposomes have been developed as carriers for the delivery of therapeutic and diagnostic agents against various infectious diseases. Incidentally, the particulate nature of the vesicles may facilitate passive homing of the entrapped drug molecules to the macrophages, which harbor many of the important pathogens in their intracellular compartments such as *Mycobacterium, Leishmania,* and *Candida* species, belonging to three different major classes of microbes, namely, bacteria, protozoans, and fungi, respectively. Moreover, macrophages upon interaction with particulate drug delivery vehicles may act as the secondary depot for them, thereby helping in targeted delivery of entrapped drug molecules.

Particulate novel drug delivery vehicles such as liposomes, microspheres, and niosomes deliver entrapped material to macrophages and dendritic cells mainly. Liposomes have been documented as microscopic vesicles composed of phospholipid bilayers surrounding aqueous compartments. Liposomes have been used extensively as drug carriers. Potential applications of this delivery system include cancer chemotherapy, enzyme therapy, immunomodulation, antimicrobial therapy, metal detoxification, diagnostics, and topical therapy [45–49].

Injecting drugs encapsulated in liposomes has an advantage: since they are colloidal in nature, they are recognized as foreign particles and can readily be taken up by phagocytic cells of the immune system (cf. macrophages); thus, the drugs rapidly accumulate in the mononuclear phagocyte system (MPS). The inherent tendency of the liposomes to concentrate in MPS can be exploited in enhancing the nonspecific host defense against various intracellular pathogens by entrapping chemotactic or immunomodulatory chemical entities in them besides using them as carriers of antibiotics against various intracellular infections. Liposomal systems have been optimistically considered as "magic bullets" for more than three decades. Drug delivery with liposomes as the carrier system provides options and opportunities for designing biostable and/or site-specific drug therapy. Engineered or tailored versions of liposomes that offer the potentials of exquisite levels of specificity for drug targets are receiving much attention these days. Depending on the site of targeting, liposomes may be modified by either grafting chemotactic ligands such as peptides, polysaccharides, or affinity ligands like antibodies to the liposomal surface directly or may be coated via poly(ethylene glycol) anchors [50–52].

The delivery of diagnostic, therapeutic, and immunomodulatory agents to lymph nodes is mandatory for treatment of diseases with lymphatic involvement [53–55]. Saccharide modified liposomes showed enhanced absorption from the injection site and enhanced lymph node uptake compared to control liposomes [56]. Liposomes coated with nonspecific human antibodies injected subcutaneously showed a modestly increased lymphatic absorption and lymph node uptake compared to liposomes without the coating [57]. For example, administration of anti-HLA-DR bearing immunoliposomes resulted in a threefold higher accumulation in regional lymph nodes [58]. Poly(ethylene glycol) (PEG) coated liposomes were found to avoid uptake by the lymphatic system as compared to the plain liposomes [59, 60]. A novel method to enhance lymph node uptake of biotin-coated liposomes has been explored to facilitate the uptake of the drug-bearing liposomes [61].

The amino-phospholipids are generally confined to the inner leaflet of the plasma membrane. Translocation of phosphatidylserine (PS) to the outer leaflet serves as a signal for triggering recognition by macrophages [62]. Studies on the interaction between liposomes and macrophages have shown that larger particles may be phagocytosed more efficiently by macrophages than smaller liposomes [63]. Similarly, grafting of tetrapeptide tuftsin on the liposome surface would therefore enable us not only to "home" the liposomized drug to macrophages but also to stimulate these cells nonspecifically against infections [64–69].

Analysis of the intracellular trafficking patterns of the liposomal antigens reveals that after being phagocytosed by macrophages, liposomal antigen readily escapes from the endosomes into the cytoplasm of the macrophages [70]. Moreover, liposomes made up of lipids with fusogenic properties have been shown to deliver their entrapped molecules in the cytosol of the target cells more efficiently than conventional forms of liposomes. The membrane lipid composition of microorganisms exhibits a large amount of anionic phospholipids that play a pivotal role in membrane–membrane fusion [71]. Liposomes made up of lipids from various microorganisms have been used for targeting to macrophages as well as dendritic cells [72–75]. Recently, we have demonstrated that antigen entrapped in liposomes made up of lipids from *Escherichia coli* and edible yeast generate strong humoral as well as cell-mediated responses far better then conventional egg PC liposomes [76–78]. Moreover, sterically stabilized liposomes have been found to possess increased stability and to play a major role in CD8$^+$ T-cell response by targeting mature as well as immature dendritic cells. In a more recent study, PorA, a major antigen of *Neisseria meningitidis*, was purified and reconstituted in different types of targeted liposomes, by using mannose or phosphatidylserine as targeting moieties, or with positively charged liposomes for targeting dendritic cells (DCs). The use of targeted PorA liposomes resulted in an improved uptake by and activation of DCs and an increased localization in draining lymph nodes [79].

The interaction of liposomes with phagocytic cells is followed by either stable adsorption to the cell surface or cellular uptake of intact vesicles by an energy-dependent mechanism leading to lysosomal degradation of the liposomes and their contents. Liposome adsorption to the cell surface seems to be the rate-limiting step, since it can be assumed that stably adsorbed vesicles are more susceptible to subsequent uptake than vesicles that are loosely attached to the cell surface. Several prerequisites have to be successfully met that eventually enable liposomes to deliver biologically active agents to macrophages. Essentially, liposomes must readily bind to and be phagocytosed by free and fixed phagocytes; they must prevent degradation of entrapped drug; they must retain the encapsulated agent for delivery to the intracellular compartment of RES cells; and they must localize to macrophages in organs where metastasis or macrophage-associated disorders occur. Moreover, it has been shown that liposome with specific lipid composition or those harboring fusogenic peptide on their surface can specifically fuse with the target cells.

In general, liposomes are the most widely studied carrier in drug targeting to macrophages. However, the extent of liposome binding and subsequent ingestion by macrophages depends on a number of features of the lipid vesicles. These include composition, type, size, and surface properties of liposomes. For example, PS containing negatively charged liposomes can associate more effectively and deliver the liposomal content more efficiently to the macrophages than PS containing neutral liposomes [80–83]. Similarly, smaller liposomes deliver drugs more effectively than larger ones; presumably they are internalized more efficiently [84]. Some studies implied that positively charged and large sized liposomes could, however, improve liposome uptake in comparison with their counterparts [85, 86].

It was also observed that liposome uptake increased linearly with the incubation time and concentration. Higher uptake was observed with smaller and negatively charged liposomes. Inclusion of increasing amounts of cholesterol and sphingomyelin resulted in a decrement in the uptake by macrophages. The same study also revealed that the uptake of liposomes differed considerably in different mouse strains [80–83].

The fatty acyl chains of the phospholipids used in the preparation of liposomes can regulate their *in vivo* stability. The efficacy of a liposomal formulation of a drug can be affected by the composition of liposomes [87]. Encapsulation of ampicillin in vesicles of solid liposomes—prepared from distearoylphosphatidylcholine (DSPC) and dipalmitoylphosphatidylglycerol (DPPG)—as compared with fluid type liposomes (composed of cholesterol, PC, and PS) resulted in delay of intracellular killing of *Listeria monocytogenes*. Besides charge, size and lamellarity of the liposomes are important characteristics that regulate their uptake by macrophages. Systematic evaluation of multilamellar vesicles (MLVs) with different phospholipid composition reveals that certain classes of phospholipids are recognized preferentially by macrophages. Inclusion of negatively charged phospholipids, such as phosphatidylserine (PS) or phosphatidylglycerol, in MLVs consisting of phosphatidylcholine (PC) greatly enhances their binding to and phagocytosis by macrophages. In contrast, neutral MLVs composed exclusively of PC are not efficiently taken up by macrophages. Such enhancement of phagocytosis has been shown to occur in mouse peritoneal macrophages, mouse Kupffer cells, rodent alveolar macrophages, human peripheral blood monocytes, and human alveolar macrophages [88]. Normal rat alveolar macrophages were incubated with two different types of liposomes—MLV (<5 lamellae) and REV (reverse evaporation vesides) (<5 lamellae)—and adjusted to contain equal amounts of lipid and entrapped muramyldipeptide. Similarly, it was found that the extent of tumoricidal activity was higher in the case of MLV than that of REV. Recently developed poly(ethylene glycol)-coated liposomes, known as Stealth liposomes, are not readily taken up by the macrophages in the reticuloendothelial system; however, they do stay in the circulation for a relatively long period of time [89–91]. It is simply because of the fact that long PEG chains impart steric hindrance in the interaction of liposomes with lipoproteins. In addition, it has been shown that incorporation of different polymers into liposomes can enhance liposome circulation time in a concentration-dependent manner. On the other hand, peptide-grafted liposomes were found to be more leishmanicidal than its ungrafted counterpart. This is because the peptide-grafted liposomes are phagocytosed more efficiently by macrophages [92]. Recently, it has been demonstrated that incorporation of a peptide from HIV-1 can also facilitate intracellular delivery of protein drugs [93].

Macrophages possess various receptors such as Fc receptors, complement, fibronectin lipoprotein, mannosyl, galactosyl, and many other receptors. These macrophage surface receptors determine the control of activities such as activation, recognition, endocytosis, and secretion. A useful approach for promoting the uptake of liposomal content by macrophages is to incorporate ligands capable of interacting with macrophage surface receptors [94]. Various research groups showed that uptake of ligand-incorporatcd liposomes was significantly higher than liposomes without ligands [95–101]. For example, mannose receptors on the macrophage surface have been exploited by developing neoglycoprotein and mannose residue on the surface of interacting drug carriers [101–103]. Studies on the interaction of mannosylated liposomes with macrophages indicate that targeted liposomes present much higher affinity for those cells than the unconjugated vesicles.

Liposomes composed of mannosylated *myo*-inositol (extracted from the cell wall of microorganisms) have been shown to be taken up by peritoneal macrophages.

Liposomes were composed of egg phosphatidylcholine, cholesterol, and dicetyl-phosphate with or without monoarachidic acid esters (MAEs). The liposomes with MAEs were rapidly eliminated from blood. More than 60% of the eliminated liposomes were recovered in the liver and spleen [98]. The modification did not, however, affect the distribution to the other tissues. The modified liposomes are taken up by Kupffer cells of the liver and resident macrophages of the spleen via mannose receptor-mediated binding endocytosis. Moreover, both *in vitro* and *in vivo* uptake of liposomes have been increased extraordinarily by targeting these carriers through Fc surface receptors of macrophages. Coupling of rabbit immunoglobulin with liposomes increases the uptake by rat liver macrophages more than five times compared with control liposomes [103–105]. *In vivo* study demonstrated that 80–85% of the coupled liposomes were accumulated in the liver within 1 h of the injection. This was because of the presence of the Fc moiety in immunoglobulin-coupled liposomes. Mouse monoclonal antibody modified with W-succinimidyl-3-(2-pyridyldithio) propionate in order to conjugate with liposomes containing dideoxycytidine triphosphate by covalent bonding was found to home entrapped material to the macrophages. The uptake of antibody-conjugated liposomes was four to six times higher than that of plain liposomes. This increase in uptake was thought to be due to the Fc receptor-mediated binding [105].

In a manner similar to liposomes, size, surface property, composition, concentration, and hydrophilicity or lipophilicity of microspheres and nanoparticles play a significant role in the uptake by macrophages. The events of phagocytosis include contact with pseudopods of macrophages followed by their engulfment into the cytoplasm by lamellipods [106]. Hydrophobic and relatively large microspheres are more susceptible to phagocytosis than their hydrophilic counterparts. Likewise, nanoparticles with lipophilic coating are taken up by macophages more readily as compared to their hydrophilic counterparts. Coating the particle surface with opsonic materials and activating macrophages with various activating factors can improve the extent of phagocytosis. Incubation time and dose of the vehicles can also control the process of phagocytosis.

The influence of surface charge and size of microspheres on their phagocytosis by mouse peritoneal macrophages was studied by using polystyrene and phenylated polyacrolein microspheres of different diameter as well as modified cellulose microspheres with different surface charge [107]. It was found that efficiency of uptake was maximum when size range of microsphere was on the order of 1–2 μm. For both negatively and positively charged particles, the extent of phagocytosis was increased with increasing zeta potentials, and was the lowest when zeta potential was zero [108]. However, there was no significant difference in the phagocytosis between the cationic and anionic surfaces when compared at a zeta potential of the same absolute value. Modified cellulose microspheres were allowed to incubate with macrophages in order to study the influence of the hydrophobicity on macrophage phagocytosis. Hydrophobic microspheres prepared from benzoyl cellulose were the most susceptible to phagocytosis and the nonionic hydrophilic ones were the least susceptible. It was observed that an optimal surface hydrophobicity is necessary for the microspheres to be phagocytosed [109].

Similarly, nanoparticles made from polyalkylcyanoacrylate and polymethylmethacrylate and human serum albumin microspheres have been used to study the influence of various parameters that can regulate uptake by human macrophages. The incorporation of lipophilic polymethylmethacrylate in nanoparticles was found to result in better phagocytosis, when compared with polyalkylcyanoacrylate nanoparticles of similar size range [109]. Polybutylcyanoacrylate nanoparticles coated with lipophilic Pluronic F68—a biocompatible poloxamer—increased phagocytosis by nearly 50%, while Pluronic F108 had no influence. Nanoparticles of the same material were phagocytosed to a larger extent if they were of larger diameter. For example, phagocytosis of nanoparticles made from human serum albumin of 1.5 μm in diameter was higher than that of 200 nm diameter nanoparticles. Recently, it was found that poly(ethylene glycol)-distearate-incorporated microspheres can modify the extent of the phagocytosis depending on the concentration of the excipient used in their preparation [110]. It seems that microsphere association or uptake by macrophages might be a saturable process. For a given cell density, uptake of particles into macrophages was also dose dependent. In one study, the most avid uptake was observed with a microsphere dose of 1 mg/L; however, there was a gradual reduction in the uptake as microsphere dose was increased further [111].

In a manner that is typical of a particulate delivery system, coating of microspheres with opsonic materials and amphiphiles can modify significantly the extent of phagocytosis by macrophages, depending on the state of macrophage activation. Several proteins such as γ-globulin, human fibronectin, bovine tuftsin, and gelatin enhance the phagocytosis, while bovine serum albumin reduces the phagocytosis of cellulose microspheres [112]. It was also observed that the presence of fetal calf serum increases the phagocytosis of gelatin-grafted cellulose microspheres, while showing no effect on other protein-grafted microspheres. The influence of cross-linking and concentration of gelatin microspheres on the phagocytosis by mouse peritoneal macrophages has also been studied. Glutaraldehyde-mediated cross-linking of gelatin microspheres was found to facilitate interferon targeting to macrophages [113]. The study showed that phagocytosis of microspheres decreased with decreasing concentration of gelatin and glutaraldehyde and was proportional to the amount of microspheres added, until a saturation of phagocytosis was observed at higher doses of microspheres. It was also demonstrated that precoating or surface immobilization with gelatin was the most effective method to enhance the phagocytosis among all other opsonic proteins. Phagocytic uptake of poly styrene microspheres, coated with a series of perfluoroalkylated amphiphiles derived from phosphocholine and poly(ethylene glycol), was studied in the presence or absence of serum and peritoneal macrophages were used as phagocytic cells [114]. Phagocytic uptake tests carried out at 37 °C showed that microspheres coated with any surfactants cause a decrement in the phagocytosis under both conditions—either in the presence or absence of serum. However, the extent of decrease varied among the surfactants, and in most instances, the presence of serum had no influence on the phagocytosis when microspheres were coated with the same surfactant.' Microspheres from some biodegradable substances such as copolymers of polylactic acid and polyglycolic acid, cross-linked potato starch, hydroxyethyl starch, dextran, lichenan, and mannan are found to be successfully phagocytosed by macrophages [115–119].

When encapsulation materials produced from nanoparticles in the 1–100 nm size range have a larger surface area for the same volume, smaller pore size improved both solubility and structural properties. Hence, the drug nanoparticles, irrespective of the method of production, represent a technology that may overcome solubility problems and bioavailability problems of all poorly soluble drugs. The transformation of any drug into drug nanoparticles, leading to an increase in saturation solubility and dissolution velocity and providing the general feature of an increased adhesiveness to surfaces, is one of the most important achievements. Surface modification of the drug nanocrystals can further increase the benefits, by producing mucoadhesive nanosuspensions for oral application (e.g., targeting to the stomach or colon) or surface-modified site-specific nanoparticles for intravenous injection (e.g., targeting to the brain or bone marrow). A fusion of the novel nanosuspension technology with the traditional dosage forms (e.g., incorporating drug nanoparticles into pellets or tablets for oral delivery) is also a noteworthy advantage.

ACKNOWLEDGMENTS

The authors thank Prashant Sharma, research scholar, for his help in the preparation of the manuscript for this chapter. We are also grateful to the coordinator of the unit, Prof. M. Saleemuddin, for the facilities provided to complete this task.

REFERENCES

1. Jones K, Hoggard PG, Sales SD, Khoo S, Davey R, Back DJ. Differences in the intracellular accumulation of HIV-protease inhibitors *in vitro* and the effect of active transport. *AIDS* 2001;15:675–681.

2. Leveque D, Jehl F. P-glycoprotein and pharmacokinetics. *Anticancer Res* 1995;15: 331–336.

3. Sadeque AJ, Wandel C, He H, Shah S, Wood AJ. Increased drug delivery to the brain by P-glycoprotein inhibition. *Clin Pharmacol Ther* 2000;68:231–237.

4. Taylor EM. The impact of efflux transporters in the brain on the development of drugs for CNS disorders. *Clin Pharmacokinet* 2002;41:81–92.

5. Meaden ER, Hoggard OG, Newton P, Tjia JF, Aldam D, Cornforth D, Lloyd J, Williams J, Back DJ, Khoon SH. P-glycoprotein and MRP1 expression and reduced ritonavir and saquinavir accumulation in HIV-infected individuals. *J Antimicrob Chemother* 2002;50:583–588.

6. http://www.merck.com. Introduction: administration and kinetics of drugs. Merck Manual Home Edition: Updated 1 Feb 2003.

7. Fuseau E, Petricoul O, Moore KHP, Barrow A, Ibbotson T. Clinical pharmacokinetics of intranasal sumatriptan. *Clin Pharmacokinet* 2002;41:801–811.

8. Peterson L, Gerding D. Influence of protein binding of antibiotics in serum pharmacokinetics and extra-vascular penetration: clinically useful concepts. *Rev Infect Dis* 1980;2:340–348.

9. http://www.boomer.org/c/p/1/Ch18/Ch1803.html. Factors affecting drug distribution.

10. Oie S. Drug distribution and binding. *J Clin Pharmacol* 1986;26:583–586.

11. Mendell GL. Uptake, transport delivery and intracellular activity of antimicrobial agents. *Pharmacotherapy* 2005;25:130S–133S.

12. Abbon NJ, Romero JA. Transporting therapeutics across the blood–brain barrier. *Mol Med Today* 1996;2:106–113.

13. Misra A, Ganesh S, Shahiwala A, Shah SP. Delivery to the central nervous system: a review. *J Pharm Pharmaceut Sci* 2003;6:252–273.

14. Audus KL, Chikhale PJ, Miller DW, Thompson SE, Borchadt RT. Brain uptake of drugs: chemical and biological factors. *Adv Drug Res* 1992;23:1–64.

15. Oldendorf WH. Lipid solubility and drug penetration of the blood–brain barrier. *Proc Exp Biol Med* 1974;14:813–816.

16. Barling RWA, Selkont JB. The penetration of antibiotics into cerebrospinal fluid and brain tissue. *J Antimicrob Chemother* 1992;4:203–227.

17. de Lange ECM, Danhof M. Considerations in the use of cerebrospinal fluid pharmaco-kinetics to predict brain target concentrations in the clinical setting: implications of the barriers between blood and brain. *Clin Pharmacokinet* 2002;10:691–703.

18. Khedun SM, Maharaj B, Moodley J. Effects of antihypertensive drugs on the unborn child: what is known, and how should this influence prescribing? *Pediatr Drugs* 2000;2:419–436.

19. Bullingham RE, Nicolls AJ, Kamm BR. Clinical pharmacokinetics of mycophenolate mofetil. *Clin Pharmacokinet* 1998;34:429–455.

20. Roberts MS, Magnusson BM, Burczynski FJ, Weiss M. Enterohepatic circulation: physiological, pharmacokinetics and clinical implications. *Clin Pharmacokinet* 2002;41:751–790.

21. Pauli-Magnus C, Stiegar B, Meier Y, Kullak-Ublick GA, Meier PJ. *J Hepatol* 2005;43:342–357.

22. Schwarz UI, Gramatte T, Krappweis J, Oertel R, Kirch W. P-glycoprotein inhibitor erythromycin increases oral bioavailability of talinolol in humans. *Int J Clin Pharmacol Ther* 2000;38:161–167.

23. Curry SH. Binding to plasma protein. In Curry SH, Ed. *Drug Disposition and Pharma-cokinetics with a Combination of Pharmacological and Clinical Relationships*, 3rd ed. Oxford, UK: Blackwell Scintific Publications; 1980.

24. Tillement JP, Zini R, d'Athis P, Vassent G. Binding of certain acidic drugs to human albumin: theoretical and practical estimation of fundamental parameters. *Eur J Clin Pharmacol* 1974;7:307–313.

25. Koch-Weser J, Sellers EM. Binding of drugs to serum albumin (2 parts) *N Engl J Med* 1976;294:311–316, 526–531.

26. Urien S, Nguyen P, Berlioz S, Bree F, Vacherot F, Tillement JP. Characterization of dis-crete classes of binding sites of human serum albumin by application of thermodynamic principles. *Biochem J* 1994;302:69–72.

27. Kremer JMH, Wilting J, Janssen LMH. Drug binding to human α_2-acid glycoprotein in health and disease. *Pharmacol Rev* 1988;40:1–47.

28. Lemaire M, Urien S, Albengres E, et al. Lipoprotein binding of drugs. In Reidenberg MM, Erill S, Eds. *Drug Protein Binding*. New York: Praeger, 1986, pp 93–108.

29. Zamacona MK, Suarez E, Garcia E, Aguirre C, Calvo R. The significance of lipoproteins in serum binding variations of propofol. *Anasth Analg* 1998;87:1147–1151.

30. Barza M. Principles of tissue penetration antibiotics. *J Antimicrob Chemother* 1981;3:45–65.

31. Craig WA. Tissue binding of antimicrobials: a brief review. *Infection* 1976;4(Suppl 2):S160–S163.

32. Yogokawa K, Ishizaki J, Ohkuma S, Miyamoto K. Influence of lipophilicity and lyso-somal accumulation on tissue distribution kinetics of basic drugs: a physiologically based pharmacokinetic model. *Methods Find Exp Clin Pharmacol* 2002;24:81–93.

33. Daniel WA. Mechanisms of cellular distribution of psychotropic drugs. Significance for drug action and interactions. *Prog Neuro-psychopharmacol Biol Psychiatr* 2003;27:66–73.

34. Daniel WA, Bickel MH, Honegger UE. The contribution of lysosomal trapping in the uptake of desipramine and chloroquine by different tissues. *Pharmacol Toxicol* 1995;77: 402–406.

35. Venkatesan K. Clinical pharmacokinetic considerations in the treatment of patients with leprosy. *Clin Pharmacokinet* 1989;16:365–386.

36. Langer R. 1994 Whittacker lecture: polymers for drug delivery and tissue engineering. *Annu Biomed Eng* 1995;23:101–111.

37. Mathiovitz E, Jacob JS, Jong YS, et al. Biologically erodable microspheres as potential oral drug delivery systems. *Nature* 1997;386:410–414.

38. Lobenberg R, Araujo L, Kreuter J. Body distribution of azidothymidine bound to nanoparticles after oral administration. *Eur J Pharm Biopharmt* 1997;44:127–132.

39. Lobenbeg R, Kreuter J. Macrophage targeting of azidothymidine: a promising strategy for AIDS therapy. *AIDS Res Hum Retroviruses* 1996;12:1709–1715.

40. Bodor N, Kaminski JJ. Prodrugs and site-specific chemical delivery systems. *Annu Rep Med Chem* 1987;22:303–313.

41. Lambert DM. Rationale and applications of lipids as prodrug carriers. *Eur J Pharm Sci* 2000;11:S15–S27.

42. Chonn A, Cullis PR. Recent advances in liposomal drug delivery systems. *Curr Opin Biotechnol* 1995;6:698–708.

43. Lian T, Rodney J, Ho Y. Trends in developing liposome drug delivery systems. *J Pharm Sci* 2001;90:667–680.

44. Gregoriadis G, Ed., *Liposomes as Drug Carriers, Recent Trends and Progress*. Chichester: Wiley; 1988.

45. Martin IJ. Specialized drug delivery systems, manufacturing and production technology. In Tyle P, Ed., *Drugs and Pharmaceutical Series*. Volume 41. New York: Marcel Dekker; 1990, pp 267–316.

46. Alving CR. Liposomes as carriers of antigens and adjuvants. *J Immunol Methods* 1991;140:1–13.

47. Fidler IJ, Kleinerman ES. Clinical application of liposomes containing macrophage activators for therapy of cancer metastasis. *Adv Drug Deliv Rev* 1994;13:325–340.

48. Gregoriadis G, Gursel M, McCormack B. Liposomes as immunological adjuvants and vaccine carriers. *J Control Release* 1996;41:49–56.

49. Bendas G. Immunoliposomes: a promising approach to targeting cancer therapy. *Biodrugs* 2001;15:215–224.

50. Muggia PM. Liposomal encapsulated anthracyclines: new therapeutic horizons. *Curr Oncol Rep* 2001;3:156–162.

51. Vyas SP, Sihorkar V. Endogenous ligands and carriers in non-immunogenic site-specific drug delivery. *Adv Drug Deliv Rev* 2000;43:101–164.

52. Sunamoto J, Sakai K, Sato T, Kondo H. Molecular recognition of polysaccharide-anchored liposomes. Importance of sialic acid moiety on liposomal surface. *Chem Lett* 1988;43:1781–1784.

53. Puri N, Weyland EH, Abdel-Rahman SM, Sinko PJ. An investigation of the intradermal route as an effective means of immunization for microparticulate vaccine delivery systems. *Vaccine* 2000;18:2600–2612.

54. Muranishi S, Takuya F, Murakami M, Yamamoto A. Potential for lymphatic targeting of peptides. *J Control Release* 1997;46:157–164.

55. Harvie P, Desormeaux A, Gagne N, Tremblay M, Poulin L, Beauchamp D, Bergeron MG. Lymphoid tissue targeting of liposome-encapsulated 29,39-dideoxyinosine. *AIDS* 1995;9: 701–707.

56. Wu MS, Robbins JC, Bugianesi RL, Ponpipom MM, Shen TY. Modified *in vivo* behaviour of liposomes containing synthetic glycolipids. *Biochim Biophys Acta* 1981;674:19–29.

57. Mangat S, Patel H. Lymph node localization of nonspecific antibody coated liposomes. *Life Sci* 1985;36:1917–1925.

58. Dufresne I, Desormeaux A, Bestman-Smith I, Gourde P, Tremblay MJ, Bergeron MG. Targeting lymph nodes with liposomes bearing anti-HLA-DR Fab2 fragments. *Biochim Biophys Acta* 1999;1421:284–294.

59. Oussoren C, Storm G. Lymphatic uptake and biodistribution of liposomes after subcutaneous injection. III Influence of surface modification with poly(ethyleneglycol). *Pharm Res* 1997;14:1479–1484.

60. Allen TM, Hansen CB, Guo LSS. Subcutaneous administration of liposomes: a comparison with the intravenous and intraperitoneal routes of injection. *Biochim Biophys Acta* 1993;1150:9–16.

61. Phillips WT, Klipper R, Goins B. Novel method of greatly enhanced delivery of liposomes to lymph nodes. *Pharm Exp Ther* 2000;295:309–313.

62. Schwartz RS, Tanaka Y, Fidler IJ, Chiu DT, Lubin B, Schroit AJ. Increased adherence of sickled and phosphatidylserine-enriched human erythrocytes to cultured human peripheral blood monocytes. *J Clin Invest* 1985;75:1965–1972.

63. Senior J. Fate and behaviour of liposomes *in vivo*: a review of controlling factors. *Ther Drug Carrier Syst* 1987;3:123–193.

64. Owais M, Ahmed I, Krishnakumar K, Jain RK, Bachhawat BK, Gupta CM. Tuftsin-bearing liposomes as drug vehicles in treatment of experimental aspergillosis. *FEBS Lett* 1993;326:56–58.

65. Masood AK, Faisal SM, Haque W, Owais M. Immunomodulator tuftsin augments antifungal activity of amphotericin B against experimental murine candidiasis. *J Drug Target* 2002;10:185–192.

66. Masood A, Khan TH, Nasti Khanam S, Mallick AI, Ahmad FirozHaq W, Ahmed N, Owais M. Co-administration of tuftsin and liposomized nystatin can combat less susceptible *C albicans* in neutropenic mice. *FEMS Immunol Med Micobiol* 2004;42:249–258.

67. Singhal A, Bali A, Jain RK, Gupta CM. Specific interactions of liposomes with PMN leukocytes upon incorporating tuftsin in their bilayers. *FEBS Lett* 1984;178:109–113.

68. Gupta CM, Puri A, Jain RK, Bali A, Anand N. Protection of mice against *Plasmodium berghei* infection by a tuftsin derivative. *FEBS Lett* 1986;205:351–354.

69. Guru PY, Agrawal AK, Singha UK, Singhal A, Gupta CM. Drug targeting in *Leishmania donovani* infections using tuftsin-bearing liposomes as drug vehicles. *FEBS Lett* 1989;245:204–208.

70. Alving CR. Liposomal vaccines: clinical status and immunological presentation for humoral and cellular immunity. *Ann NY Acad Sci* 1995;754:143–152.

71. Pluschke G, Overath P. Influence of changes in polar head group composition on the lipid phase transition and characterization of a mutant containing only saturated phospholipid acyl-chains. *J Biol Chem* 1981;268:3207–3212.

72. Owais M, Gupta CM. Liposome mediated cytosolic delivery of macromolecules and its possible use in vaccine development. *Eur J Biochem* 2000;267:3946–3956.

73. Ahmad N, Masood AK, Owais M. Fusogenic potential of prokaryotic membrane lipids: implication in vaccine development. *Eur J Biochem* 2001;268:5667–5675.

74. Sproitt GD, Dicaire CJ, Gurnani K, Deschatelets LA, Krishnan L. Liposome adjuvants prepare from the total polar lipids of *Haloferax volcanii, Planococcus* spp. *and Bacillus*

firmus differ in ability to elicit and sustain immune responses. *Vaccine* 2004;22:2154–2162.

75. Krishnan L, Dicaire CJ, Patel GB, Sprott GD. Archeosome vaccine adjuvants induce strong humoral, cell mediated and memory responses: comparison to conventional liposome and alum. *Infect Immun* 2000;68:54–63.

76. Faisal MS, Masood AK, Tahseen HN, Nadeem A, Owais M. Antigen entrapped in the escheriosomes leads to the generation of CD4+ helper and CD8+ cytotoxic T-cell response. *Vaccine* 2003;21:2383–2393.

77. Owais M, Khan MA, Agrewala JN, Bist D, Gupta CM. Use of liposomes as an immunopotentiating delivery system: in perspective of vaccine development. *Scand J Immunol* 2001;54:125–132.

78. Agrewala JN, Owais M, Gupta CM, Mishra GC. Antigen incorporation into liposomes results in the enhancement of IL-4 and IgG1 secretion: evidence for preferential expansion of Th-2 cells. *Cytokines Mol Ther* 1996;2:59–65.

79. Arigita C, Bevaart L, Everse LA, Koning GA. Liposomal meningococcal B vaccination: role of dendritic cell targeting in the development of a protective immune response. *Infect Immun* 2003;71:5210–5218.

80. Duzgunes N, Pretzer E, Simoes S, Slepushkin V, Konopka K, Flasher D, de Lima MC. Liposome-mediated delivery of antiviral agents to human immunodeficiency virus-infected cells. *Mol Membr Biol* 1999;16:111–118.

81. Raz A, Bucana C, Fogler WE, Poste G, Fidler IJ. Biochemical, morphological and ullrastructural studies on the uptake of liposomes by murine macrophages. *Cancer Res* 1981;41:487–494.

82. Hsu MJ, Juliano RL. Interactions of liposome with reticulo-endothelial system. II. Nonspecific and receptor mediated uptake of liposomes by mouse peritoneal macrophages. *Biochim Biophys Acta* 1982;720:411–419.

83. Heath TD, Lopez NG, Papahadjospoulous D. The effect of liposome size and surface charge on liposome mediated delivery of methotrexate–aspartate to cells *in vitro*. *Biochim Biophys Acta* 1985;820:74–84.

84. Allen TM, Austin GA, Chonn A, Lin L, Lee KC. Uptake of liposomes by cultured mouse bone marrow macrophages: influence of liposome composition and size. *Biochim Biophys Acta* 1991;106:56–64.

85. Schwendener RA, Lagocki PA, Rahman YH. The effects of charge and size on the interaction of unilamnellar liposomes with macrophages. *Biochim Biophys Acta* 1984;772:93–101.

86. Rahman YE, Cerny EA, Patel KR, Lau EH, Wright BJ. Differential uptake of liposomes varying in size and lipid composition by parenchymal and Kupffer cells of mouse liver. *Life Sci* 1982;31:2061–2071.

87. Bakker-Woudenbcrg IAJM, Lokerse AF, Roerdink FH. Effect of lipid composition on the activity of liposome-entrapped ampicillin against intracellular Listeria monocytogenes. *Antimicrob Agents Chemother* 1988;32:1560–1564.

88. Maruyama K. Liposomal technology in cancer therapy. *Biother Jpn* 1998;12:1051–1058.

89. Torchilin VP, Trabetskoy VS, Whiteman KR, Caliceti P, Femiti P, Veronese PM. New synthetic amphiphilic polymers for steric protection of liposomes *in vivo*. *J Pharm Sci* 1995;84:1049–1053.

90. Torchilin VP. Polymer coated long circulating microparticulate pharmaceuticals. *J Microencaps* 1998;15:1–19.

91. Torchilin VP. Affinity liposomes *in vivo*: factors influencing target accumulation. *J Mol Recogn* 1996;9:335–346.

92. Banerjee G, Medda S, Basu MK. A novel peptide-grafted liposomal delivery system targeted to macrophages. *Antimicrob Agents Chemother* 1998;42:348–351.

93. Torchilin VP, Rammohan R, Weissig V, Levchenko TS. TAT peptide on the surface of liposomes affords their efficient intracellular delivery even at low temperature and in the presence of metabolic inhibitors. *Proc Natl Acad Sci USA* 2001;15:8786–8791.

94. Kaneda Y. Virosomes: evolution of the liposomes as a targeted drug delivery system. *Adv Drug Deliv Rev* 2000;43:197–205.

95. Gregoriadis G. Liposome as immunological adjuvants: approaches to immunopotentiation including ligand-mediated targeting to macrophages. *Res Immunol* 1992;143:178–185.

96. Aramaki Y, Murai M, Tsuchiya S. Activation of Fc receptor mediated phagocytosis by mouse peritoneal macrophages following the intraperitoneal administration of liposomes. *Pharm Res* 1994;11:518–521.

97. Dutta M, Bandyopadhyay R, Basu MK. Neoglycosylated liposomes as efficient ligand for the evaluation of specific sugar receptors on macrophages in health and in experimental leishmaniasis. *Parasitology* 1994;109:139–147.

98. Yachi K, Kikuchi H, Yamauchi H, Hirota S, Tomikawa M. Distribution of liposomes containing mannobiose esters of fatty acid in rats. *J Microencaps* 1995;12:377–388.

99. Shao J, Ma JKH. Characterization of mannosylated liposome system for drug targeting to alveolar macrophages. *Drug Deliv* 1997;4:43–48.

100. Muller CD, Schuber F. Neo-mannosylated liposomes: synthesis and interaction with mouse Kupffer cells and resident peritoneal macrophages. *Biochim Biophys Acta* 1989;986:97–105.

101. Kole L, Sarkar K, Mahato SB, Das PK. Neoglycoprotein conjugated liposomes as macrophage specific drug carrier in the therapy of leishmaniasis. *Biochem Biophys Res Commun* 1994;200:351–358.

102. Barrat G, Term JP, Yapo A, Petit JF. Preparation and characterisation of liposome containing mannosylated phospholipids capable of targeting to macrophages. *Biochim Biophys Acta* 1986;862:153–164.

103. Derksen JTP, Morselt HWM, Kalicharan D, Hul-staert CE, Scherphof GL. Interaction of immunoglobul in-coupled liposomes with rat liver macrophages *in vitro*. *Exp Cell Res* 1987;167:105–115.

104. Derksen JTP, Morselt HWM, Scherptiof GL. Uptake and processing of immunogliobulin-coated liposomes by sub-populations of rat liver macrophages. *Biochim Biophys Acta* 1988;971:127–136.

105. Bettageri GV, Black CDV, Szebeni J, Wahl LM, Weinstein JN. Fc-receptor-mediated targeting of antibody-bearing liposomes containing dideoxycytidine triphosphate to human monocyte/macrophage. *J Pharm Pharmacol* 1993;45:48–53.

106. Schafer V, Briesen HV, Riibsamen-Waigmann H, Steffan AM, Royer C, Kreuter J. Phagocytosis and degradation of human serum albumin microspheres and nanoparticles in human macrophages. *J Microencaps* 1994;11:261–269.

107. Tabata Y, Ikada Y. Effect of the size and surface charge of polymer microspheres on their phagocytosis by macrophage. *Biomaterials* 1988;9:356–362.

108. Roser M, Fischer D, Kissel T. Surface-modified biodegradable albumin nano- and microspheres. II: Effect of surface charges on *in vitro* phagocytosis and biodistribution in rats. *Eur J Pharm Biopharm* 1998;4:255–263.

109. Schafer V, von Briesen H, Andreesen R, Steffan AM, Royer C, Troster S, Kreuter J, Waigmann HR. Phagocytosis of nanoparticles by human immunodeficiency virus

(HIV)-infected macrophages: a possibility for antiviral drug targeting. *Pharm Res* 1992;9:541–546.

110. Lacasse FX, Filion MC, Phillips NC, Escher E, McMullen JN, Hildgen P. Influence of surface properties at biodegradable microsphere surfaces: effects of plasma protein adsorption and phagocytosis. *Pharm Res* 1998;15:312–317.

111. Akhtar S, Lewis KJ. Antisense oligonucleotide delivery to cultured macrophages is improved by incorporation into sustained-release biodegradable polymer microspheres. *Int J Pharm* 1997;151:57–67.

112. Ikada Y, Tabata Y. Phagocytosis of bioactive microspheres. *J Bioact Compat Polym* 1986;1:32–46.

113. Tabata Y, Ikada Y. Synthesis of gelatin microspheres containing interferon. *Pharm Res* 1989;6:422–427.

114. Privitera N, Naon R, Riess VIG. Phagocytic uptake by peritoneal macrophages of microspheres coated with phosphocholine or polyethylene glycol phosphate-derived perfluoro alkylated surfactants. *Int J Pharm* 1995;120:73–82.

115. D'Souza M, DeSouza P. Site specific microencapsulated drug targeting strategies—liver and gastro-intestinal tract targeting. *Adv Drug Deliv Rev* 1995;17:247–254.

116. Mullerad J, Apte RN, Cohen S. Delivery of IL-1 microspheres to tumor macrophages. *Proc Int Symp Control Release Bioact Mater* 1995;22:512–513.

117. Okawa T, Ichimal H, Ishida T, Kawata M, Kaguba S, Mamba K, Makita T. Implication of activation of intraperitoneal macrophages with biodegradable microspheres. *Cell Biol Int Rep* 1989;13:547–553.

118. Kanke M, Geissler RG, Deborah P, Kaplan A, DeLuca PP. Interaction of microspheres with blood constituents. *J Parent Sci Technol* 1988;42:157–165.

119. Artursson P, Arro Edman P, Ericsson JLE, Sjoholm I. Biodegradable microspheres V: stimulation of macrophages with microparticles made of various polysaccharides. *J Pharm Sci* 1987;76:127–133.

14

SALT AND COCRYSTAL FORM SELECTION

ANN W. NEWMAN, SCOTT L. CHILDS, AND BRETT A. COWANS

SSCI, Inc., West Lafayette, Indiana

Contents

14.1 INTRODUCTION

Form selection is critical to the successful development of an active pharmaceutical ingredient (API) [1–5]. A number of physical properties vary with the solid form (a partial list is given in Table 14.1) and several properties such as crystallinity, solubility, and stability need to be measured and evaluated to determine whether a candidate will be acceptable for development [6, 7]. If other options are needed, a different crystalline form, a different salt, or a cocrystal may be explored. It has been estimated that approximately half of all administered drugs are formulated as salts [8]. With more poorly soluble drugs being found and developed, form selection can

Preclinical Development Handbook: ADME and Biopharmaceutical Properties,
edited by Shayne Cox Gad
Copyright © 2008 John Wiley & Sons, Inc.

TABLE 14.1   Properties that Can Vary with Solid Form

Bioavailability
Hygroscopicity
Dissolution rate
Solubility
Physical stability
Chemical stability
Compressibility
Chargeability
Filterability
Flow
Millability
Melting point
Color
Excipient compatibility
Morphology
Density
Taste
Toxicology
Levels of gastric irritation
Clinical results

improve properties, such as solubility and ultimately bioavailability, and increase the potential viability of a candidate. Form selection is therefore an integral part of the drug development process.

Various approaches to form selection exist during development. One general approach is to perform sufficient work initially in order to choose a good candidate early (before the Investigational New Drug (IND) application is filed and clinical trials are started). This approach is believed to reduce the time to market. Another approach is to initially limit the time and money spent choosing a form early in development since many compounds will be eliminated. For this latter scenario, a form is chosen that is believed to be adequate for early trials, knowing that changing forms later will have the added cost and time commitment for bridging studies. In practice, the actual approach will be some combination of these two extremes.

Clearly, the risk assessment for each compound must be evaluated based on the information available for the drug being developed. The dosage form to be developed also needs to be considered when choosing the form, since the desired properties for an oral dosage form will be significantly different from those needed for a suspension or an IV formulation. For most compounds, a complete picture for form selection and an understanding of the solid-state properties should be developed and presented at the end of Phase II clinical trials.

It should be noted that form selection also influences intellectual property position. Crystalline forms including salts and cocrystals are patentable. Additional form selection studies may be carried out late in development for intellectual property protection on improved products. Understanding the solid-state properties of the API is critical to these endeavors.

This chapter discusses solid form screening and the selection process for pharmaceutical compounds with the main focus on salts and cocrystals. Information on counterion/guest selection, preparation, characterization, and property evaluation are also presented. The need for polymorph screening as part of the selection process is included, and the role of quantitative methods to determine the solid forms present in API and drug product is also discussed.

14.2   SALTS AND COCRYSTALS

When ionizable groups are present in an API molecule, a salt can be formed which often provides better physical properties, such as increased water solubility or melting point. In addition, nonionizable compounds and salts may form cocrystals with the desired properties. Working definitions for these materials are given below and the concepts are shown schematically in Fig. 14.1.

Salt. Acid/base chemistry creates a new species; a free acid or free base is needed for salt formation. An acid–base complex is formed that contains the API along with additional nontoxic molecular species (counterion) in the same crystal structure.

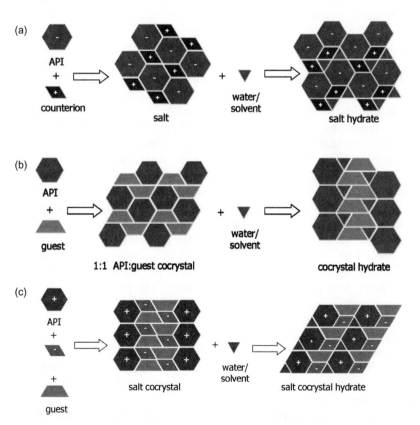

FIGURE 14.1 Schematic of salt and cocrystal formation: (a) salt and salt hydrate/solvate, (b) cocrystal and cocrystal hydrate/solvate, and (c) salt cocrystal and salt cocrystal hydrate/solvate.

Cocrystal. A crystalline molecular complex of an API or a salt of an API; it consists of two or more components, with each component being an atom, ionic compound, or molecule.

Salts are commonly produced and used as drug substances in the pharmaceutical industry, and numerous studies of salts and salt selections have been reported [9–13]. Cocrystals are comparatively new to the pharmaceutical industry but have been studied and used in other industries for years [14]. As a solid form, cocrystals perform essentially the same function as salts according to the regulatory definition of an active moiety [15]: "the molecule or ion, excluding those appended portions of the molecule that cause the drug to be an ester, salt (including a salt with hydrogen or coordination bonds), or other noncovalent derivative (such as a complex, chelate, or clathrate) of the molecule, responsible for the physiological or pharmacological action of the drug substance." For all compounds, including cocrystals, the regulatory requirement is not the categorization of the particular form; rather, it is to adequately and accurately characterize the system, to understand scientifically the form that is being developed, and to transfer this information to the regulatory agency. From this perspective, salts, hydrates, and cocrystals are identical in that they all contain the essential active moiety plus additional ions or molecules that are present primarily to impart specific physical properties on the solid form containing the active moiety.

A number of variables need to be considered when selecting a form, such as target solubility, dosage form to be developed, loading in the dosage form, physical and chemical stability, and amount of material available. It should be emphasized that there is more than one way to select a salt or cocrystal since numerous factors should be considered in the selection process. A tiered approach to salt/cocrystal selection is helpful when screening a number of possible candidates. Common properties used to evaluate materials include crystallinity, hygroscopicity, solubility, melting point, density, and stability. An example of a decision tree designed to select a material for an oral dosage form is given in Fig. 14.2a. The variables included in this selection include crystallinity, hygroscopicity, solubility, and polymorphism. These decision trees can be modified for different situations. Properties needed for an injectable formulation are usually different from those required for an oral dosage form, as shown in Fig. 14.2b. Because the properties needed for the selection process cover a broad range, it is imperative that a multidisciplinary approach be used to choose the solid form. The three main departments that deal directly with the solid form issues are chemical development (to produce the API with the desired properties), analytical (for testing of materials), and pharmaceutics (for preformulation and formulation development). Other groups, such as discovery, toxicology, and pharmacokinetics may also provide useful information during the selection process.

Salt/cocrystal selection involves experimentally identifying and characterizing a variety of different multicomponent solids by incorporating a number of secondary molecular species into the lattice with the active moiety. By taking a broader view concerning the types of secondary molecules that are experimentally investigated and not limiting the counterions tested based on pK_a, a wider variety of solid forms with potentially useful properties can be considered in the process of form selection. The cocrystal discussion in this chapter is intended to act as a guide in the expansion of the targeted multicomponent solids that are investigated during form selection.

(a)

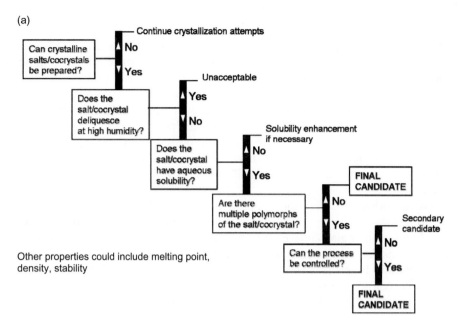

(b)

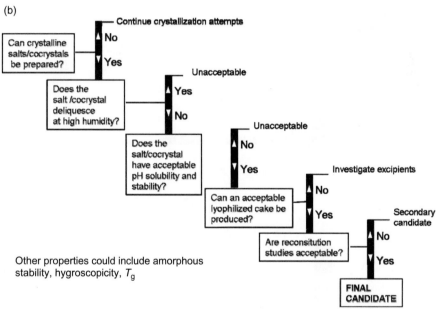

FIGURE 14.2   Decision trees for salt/cocrystal selection: (a) example for an oral dosage form and (b) example for an injectable formulation.

14.3   FORM SELECTION PROCESS

The form selection process is divided into five sections: counterion/guest selection, formation, characterization, evaluation, and polymorph screening. Each section provides an overview of common methodologies used.

14.3.1   Counterion/Guest Selection

Pharmaceutically acceptable counterions and cocrystal guests are often used to simplify the regulatory concerns surrounding the product, since information about the materials is already known and has been filed previously with the regulatory agency. The list of pharmaceutically acceptable compounds typically includes molecules that are readily found in marketed products. Figure 14.3 shows the most common counterions found in marketed products based on databases compiled in our laboratory; the results are similar to those reported elsewhere [8]. If acceptable toxicology can be demonstrated for a new entity and it provides significant property improvement, a strong case can be made for using a new substance as a guest or counterion.

There are other considerations when determining a list of possible counterions and guests. For instance, the loading in the drug product may make a high molecular weight counterion or guest unacceptable. Commonly, sodium or potassium are used as counterions for acidic APIs when high loading is a factor, but small organic species may still be preferable over inorganic ions. The type of dosage form also needs to be considered since there will be limitations for injectable, ocular, and inhalation formulations that may be different from those encountered with oral

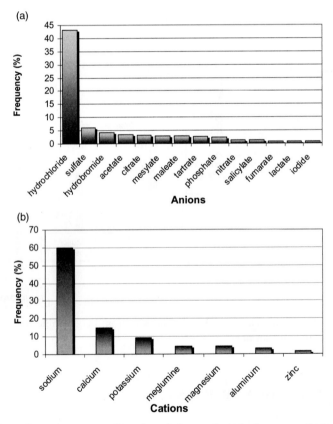

FIGURE 14.3   Common counterions found in marketed pharmaceutical products: (a) anions and (b) cations.

formulations [8]. The indication expected for the API may also have limitations regarding other components that can be present.

For salts, the pK_a of the relevant functional groups on the drug molecule is considered initially. A two to three unit separation between the pK_a values of the functional groups on the API and the counterion is commonly invoked when making salts [16]. This is fine as a guideline, but salts and cocrystals can be formed outside this range based on the decreased solubility of the salt formed. Hydrochloride (HCl) salts are commonly produced for pharmaceutical bases, but there are issues that should be considered when using HCl [8, 17]. Some issues to consider for an HCl salt include the common ion effect *in vivo*, corrosive properties during production, and loss of HCl during processing. Many companies have a list of acceptable counterions that are used for every salt selection. Although this is an acceptable place to start, many of the counterions on the list may not be ideal for the molecule being developed. It is important to look at the chemistry and the solid-state aspects of salts and cocrystals while compiling a list of possible counterions and guests that are to be empirically evaluated.

A cocrystal screen is an empirical exercise but can be guided by an analysis of the API in order to determine the potential for cocrystallization and to gather information to assist in the selection of the most appropriate guest molecules. The number and arrangement of the hydrogen bond donors and acceptors, salt forming ability, size and conformational flexibility, stability of the homomeric structure, physical properties, and solubility requirements are all considered during the initial evaluation. Crystal engineering also relies heavily on information contained in the Cambridge Structural Database [18]. The crystal engineering approach used to design an effective cocrystal screen is based on academic studies [19–21] and the application of this methodology to pharmaceuticals has generated a number of recent successes [22].

The ability of the selected guests to form hydrogen bonded synthons with the API that are energetically more favorable than the homomeric intermolecular interactions can be an important consideration in guest selection [23]. This is consistent with the observation that after the intramolecular hydrogen bonds form, the strongest remaining hydrogen bond donors typically interact with the best acceptor sites [24]. If these groups are on the same molecule, then a homomeric form is favored; however, by choosing API:guest combinations that place the strongest donor and acceptor on different molecular species, the potential for cocrystallization is increased.

It should be noted that many of the compounds used as counterions in salt selections can also be used as guests for cocrystals. We find that pharmaceutically acceptable, weak carboxylic acids typically used in salt screens are particularly useful guest molecules. One of the most effective ways for a company to initiate cocrystal screening is by using these carboxylic acids to extend the range of a traditional salt screen of a basic API. By removing the traditional limitations on counterion selection based on pK_a values, the potential for finding stable solid forms that meet the physical property requirements is increased. The concern over whether a solid is a cocrystal or a salt should be secondary to the consideration of the properties of the solid form.

Pharmaceutically "unacceptable" compounds may be employed if cocrystal formation is used initially as a purification or isolation step. The cocrystal can then be broken to isolate the API [25]. The API can be used upon isolation/crystallization or a cocrystal or salt with a pharmaceutically acceptable guest could be produced for development.

Although finding cocrystals can be challenging, the unique benefits of cocrystals outweigh the possible difficulties because they provide a screening option for APIs that cannot form salts. Until now, nonionizable or poor salt-forming APIs typically have had no recourse for crystalline solid form variation other than the adventitious formation of hydrates or solvates. Cocrystallization provides a systematic approach to form selection for these APIs.

14.3.2   Salt/Cocrystal Formation

After selecting a list of possible counterions and guests, the crystallization experiments to be performed need to be planned. There are a number of issues to consider when producing salts and cocrystals. This section outlines some of these issues, such as solvent choice, solution crystallization experiments, nonsolvent options, and possible stoichiometries.

One of the first considerations in salt or cocrystal formation from solvents is the solubility of the API as well as the counterions or guests. A common solvent or miscible solvent system with acceptable solubility must be found for the experiments. This appears to be straightforward, but it can become a major issue for poorly soluble drugs. This is especially problematic for cocrystal formation. When a strong salt forms, charge balance requirements necessitate the crystallization of the anion and cation together and the effects of solubility of either of the individual ions (and conjugate acid/base) are minimized compared to the analogous situation of cocrystallizing two independent nonionized components. It has been shown that the phase diagram for a cocrystal is related to the solubility of the individual components [26]. For example, experiments that involve solvent systems in which the guest is very soluble and the API has very low solubility are less likely to produce a solid phase containing both components.

Other considerations are methods of preparation and the type of screening methods used. Automated methods using 96 well plates, for example, screen a large number of counterions or guests with less material [27, 28]. The amount of each sample produced is determined by the solubilities of the components and is typically small (1–3 mg). Due to the small sample size, characterization is usually limited to optical microscopy, X-ray powder diffraction (XRPD), and/or Raman spectroscopy. Crystallization conditions are limited to solvent based experiments, such as evaporations or cooling when solubility permits, and a limited temperature range is available for most plates. If solids are not formed initially, recrystallization attempts may be more difficult because of experimental limitations with the plate. Crystalline materials that are produced in the plates need to be produced on a larger scale for further characterization to confirm stoichiometry and volatile content. Traditional (manual) preparation methods typically screen a smaller number of counterions or guests and will use more material per experiment. These methods produce adequate material for preliminary characterization or additional recrystallization attempts if necessary. The use of automated versus manual techniques is a decision that is usually based on material availability and known properties.

Numerous solvent methods have been used to produce salts and cocrystals. Commonly, both the API and counterion/guest are dissolved and the solutions added together. Parameters such as the order of acid/base addition, temperature, or rate of addition can all play an important role in salt or cocrystal formation. For cocrystal experiments, the solubility of the API is often lower than that of the guest compounds being screened. This can lead to the preferential nucleation of a homomeric API solid phase instead of cocrystal formation. To reduce the effects of solubility differences, yet still retain the advantages of high throughput methods, slurry experiments are often employed in the screening process.

Salt exchanges in solution or with the aid of a resin are also possible choices depending on the properties of the API [29]. Gases, such as HCl or HBr (hydrogen bromide), have also been bubbled into API solutions to produce salts [30]. Preparation techniques such as precipitation and evaporation are commonly used to produce the solid. If precipitation does not readily occur once the components are mixed, other methods may be needed to produce solids, such as concentration of the solution, antisolvent addition, lower temperatures, or a combination of these procedures.

Nonsolvent methods can also be used. Fusion methods based on Kofler techniques have been reported for a variety of systems [31]. More recently, solid-state grinding, with or without small amounts of solvent, has been used successfully for cocrystal and salt formation [32]. Even though these, or even some solvent based methods, may not be suitable for a large scale process, the seeds obtained from these experiments can be used to produce larger amounts of the desired material.

Stoichiometry is another consideration in salt and cocrystal formation. More than one acidic or basic site may be present for the API. If more than one site is available on the API, control of stoichiometry may be an issue if the pK_a values are similar. Diacid counterions, such as fumarate and malate, can also be used to investigate different stoichiometries in salts or cocrystals. An example of a system with two basic sites with similar pK_a values is given in Table 14.2. Two different stoichiometries of a hydrobromide (HBr) salt were targeted. Based on the yield and elemental data, it was obvious that the disalt was formed in both cases, regardless of the targeted stoichiometry. Additional XRPD data showed that both experiments produced the same crystal form of the disalt.

In general, there are common solvents and procedures, such as evaporation, that are used for salt and cocrystal formation, but they will not work in every case. It is

TABLE 14.2   Characterization Data on a Hydrobromide Salt

Assay	1:1 HBr:API	2:1 HBr:API	Expected Values for Disalt
C	49.77	49.92	49.48
H	4.05	3.97	3.97
N	14.83	14.91	15.05
Br	28.86	29.20	28.63
Yield	Poor yield	Good yield	—
XRPD	Form A	Form A	—

important to consider the properties of the API and design experiments that are appropriate and have the greatest chance of success. A variety of methods will also produce a wider range of crystalline solids to choose from during form selection and development.

14.3.3   Characterization

Characterization is essential for identification of the solid produced during the screen and provides the information necessary to determine if the new material can easily be developed. Information from several techniques is often required to confirm that a salt or cocrystal was prepared and to determine the chemical and physical properties. Numerous references are available that describe solid-state characterization techniques for new salts and cocrystals [1, 12, 13, 33, 34]. The theory and instrumentation of commonly used techniques are not reviewed in this section, but these techniques are discussed in terms of the information provided on new salts/cocrystals.

X-ray powder diffraction (XRPD) is often used to determine if the material is crystalline and to identify the solid form. A unique XRPD pattern does not always indicate that a new salt or cocrystal was formed and the data should be compared to the XRPD patterns of known forms of the API and the counterion/guest. As shown in Fig. 14.4, an HCl salt preparation experiment (diethyl ether fast evaporation) using Form A of the free amine resulted in the formation of a new solid form of the free amine (Form B). The HCl salt was produced from acetone using a combination of slow cool and slow evaporation techniques. The presence, or absence, of the HCl was confirmed using elemental analysis.

Raman spectroscopy is another fast and efficient tool used to determine salt or cocrystal formation [35]. Unique spectra obtained on any new material should be compared to the spectra obtained on the initial components, as shown in Fig. 14.5. In this case, the Raman spectrum indicates that a cocrystal of theophylline and salicylic acid was formed and was confirmed by other methods of analysis. Infrared (IR) spectroscopy can also be used to determine salt formation. Shifts in the carbonyl bands will indicate salt formation but can also indicate a different crystal form, so comparison with known forms is critical. The presence of NH_2 peaks in an IR spectrum can confirm that the ionized species is present in the new material. Amorphous materials usually exhibit broad IR or Raman peaks, but they can also exhibit a unique spectrum that can make interpretation more difficult.

Solid-state nuclear magnetic resonance (ssNMR) spectroscopy is a powerful tool for studying solid forms of salts or cocrystals [36, 37]. Solid-state NMR can confirm that a salt or cocrystal was formed and provide structural or conformational information [38, 39]. Solvated forms can be identified as well. In some cases, ssNMR can distinguish solid forms that are indistinguishable by other techniques [40].

Solution nuclear magnetic resonance (NMR) spectroscopy can provide a variety of information on new solids. In many cases, a solution proton NMR can reveal if a salt is formed, even if the counterion or guest is not directly observable. The chemical shift of protons that are at or near the site of charge transfer or complex formation will change compared to the chemical shift of those protons in the neutral or uncom-

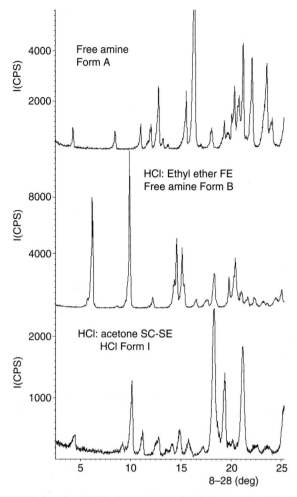

FIGURE 14.4 XRPD data for HCl salt attempts: (top) free amine Form A, (middle) HCl salt attempt from ethyl ether fast evaporation that resulted in free amine Form B, and (bottom) HCl salt attempt from acetone slow cool/slow evaporation that resulted in HCl salt Form I. The presence or absence of HCl was confirmed by other methods.

plexed species. An example is given in Fig. 14.6, which compares the spectral region of interest for an acetate salt and the free base. The NH resonance of the secondary amine at approximately 1.9 ppm in the free base spectrum is shifted to approximately 9.5 ppm (inset) as the protons of the ammonium salt. In addition, methylene proton resonances alpha to the ammonium ion have shifted approximately 0.2 ppm downfield compared to the position of those resonances in the free base.

The stoichiometry of an organic counterion or guest can be determined as well. A stoichiometry of approximately 1:1 acetate:API was determined from the peak integration for the acetate salt (Fig. 14.6). If an organic solvent is present, the amount can be determined and indicates whether the material is a solvate or not. This type of information is crucial in determining the developability of the new solid and can easily be obtained on a few milligrams of material.

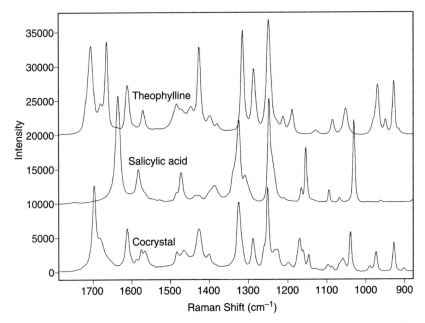

FIGURE 14.5   Raman spectra of (top) theophylline, (middle) salicylic acid, and (bottom) theophylline:salicylic cocrystal.

Differential scanning calorimetry (DSC) can also be used for the characterization of new solids if the free base or acid has a distinct thermal curve [11, 12]. DSC can be very sensitive to small amounts of the initial material depending on the strength of the melting endotherm. An example is given in Fig. 14.7. The free base exhibits a melting endotherm at approximately 228 °C while the salt exhibits a melting endotherm at approximately 250 °C. There is an additional broader endotherm observed for the salt at approximately 149 °C, which later proved to be due to the volatization of solvent from the crystalline material.

Other characterization can also be performed depending on the amount of material available. Confirming the stoichiometry with elemental analysis is a common practice. Measuring the chemical purity with HPLC is important for many API materials that may be prone to degradation under acidic or basic conditions. Determining the solvent content using NMR, gas chromatography (GC), thermogravimetry (TG), TG-IR, KF, or other methods is critical in assessing the developability of a new salt or cocrystal.

14.3.4   Evaluation

Once acceptable salts or cocrystals are found based on the characterization data, other properties need to be evaluated to choose the best compound for development. This assessment is performed as the latter part of the tiered flowchart, as shown in the examples in Fig. 14.2. Any number of factors can be investigated during this period and they should be tailored to the known issues of the API as well as the anticipated dosage form.

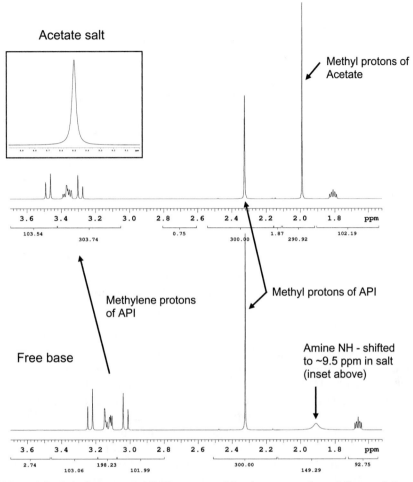

FIGURE 14.6 Solution proton NMR spectra of (top) acetate salt and (bottom) free base. Shifting observed for methylene and amine protons in acetate salt spectrum is due to salt formation. Stoichiometry of the acetate salt can also be estimated by integration of the methyl proton resonances for the acetate and the API.

A wide range of acceptable values are possible for the properties identified as important, and they depend on the development plan and dosage form [9]. In general, a solubility of 0.1–10 mg/mL is targeted for a solid oral dosage form and greater than 10 mg/mL for parenteral formulations. A pH range of 3–10 for an aqueous solution is targeted for intravenous delivery. A melting point of greater than 100 °C is usually desired for acceptable processing, especially if drying or grinding steps are anticipated. Hygroscopicity can be acceptable if the material does not deliquesce at 60–75% RH or if minimal water uptake occurs during normal processing relative humidity conditions (typically 30–75% RH). Hygroscopicity is commonly evaluated by the amount of water sorbed by the material, but other changes, such as hydrate formation, should also be investigated when assessing

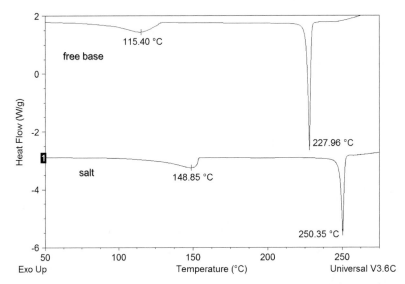

FIGURE 14.7 DSC curves of a pharmaceutical (top) free base and (bottom) salt. High temperature peaks are melting endotherms and low temperature broad endotherms are due to volatilization.

hygroscopicity [41]. Chemical and physical stability can be determined using accelerated stability conditions, such as 40 °C/75% RH over 1–2 weeks. Chemical stability can be evaluated by HPLC determination of impurities and physical stability can be evaluated by XRPD to determine a change in crystal structure. Crystal size and shape can be important to handling properties in processing and manufacturing, and an early assessment of these properties can save significant development time. The propensity of a salt or cocrystal to exist as multiple crystal forms can be evaluated at this stage with an abbreviated polymorph screen. Information on the formation of crystalline solvates from certain solvents can be used as an early guide for the crystallization step and will narrow the possible solvent choices. It should be noted that even salts or cocrystals with numerous forms can easily be developed once a controlled process is in place to produce the desired form.

This type of tiered approach was reported for BMS-180431 [11]. Seven crystalline salts were initially prepared: sodium, calcium, zinc, magnesium, potassium, lysine, and arginine. Tier 1 tested the hygroscopicity and three salts moved on to the next tier (magnesium, lysine, and arginine). Tier 2 encompassed solubility and crystal form changes and two salts, arginine and lysine, exhibited acceptable properties. The last tier tested stability (4 week evaluation) and excipient compatibility. The arginine salt was found to be the best candidate with the lysine salt as the alternate choice. The entire process was completed in approximately 6 weeks.

The evaluation process can be as simple or as complex as needed for the development of a particular compound. Numerous factors need to be considered when choosing the best salt or cocrystal for development, and it needs to be tailored to the compound. In some cases, there may not be a salt or cocrystal that exhibits all the desired attributes. When this occurs, a risk assessment must be performed to determine what extra considerations may be needed to develop the compound. If a compound is hygroscopic above 30% RH but the other attributes are acceptable, a decision needs to be made whether controlling manufacturing conditions below this level is feasible and cost effective. These types of decisions require a multidisciplinary approach among numerous groups.

14.3.5 Polymorph Screen

Once a salt or cocrystal is chosen, a more extensive polymorph screen should be performed to find the best crystal form for development [42]. Based on screens performed in our lab, it was found that 87% of the compounds investigated resulted in more than one form including amorphous material (Fig. 14.8a) [43]. Multiple polymorphs, defined as forms having the same chemical composition, were found in 51% of the cases, and hydrates were found in 37% of the screens. As shown in Fig. 14.8b, two to four forms were found for the largest number of compounds, but many cases exist where significantly more forms were obtained.

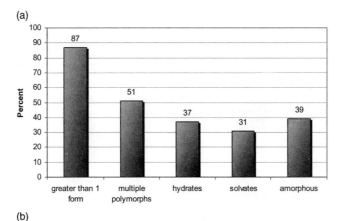

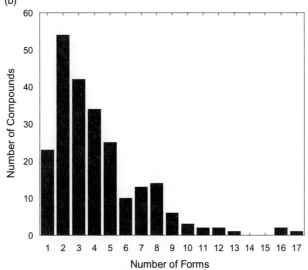

FIGURE 14.8 Forms observed in polymorph screens.

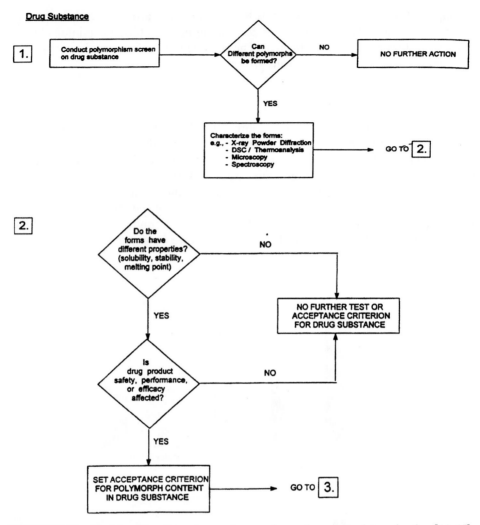

FIGURE 14.9   Decision trees for polymorph screening and property determination [44, 45].

A polymorph screen is recommended by regulatory agencies. The U.S. Food and Drug Administration (FDA) has recommended guidelines for polymorph screens [44, 45] and these decision trees are presented in Fig. 14.9. The purpose of a polymorph screen is to find multiple forms of a compound and it can be considered as a search for seeds. The decision trees are available to help guide the development of an API that can exist as more than one form. Issues such as stability, solubility, and performance in the dosage form need to be addressed for different forms of an API.

Polymorph screens can and should be performed at various stages of the development process, depending on the type of information that is required [46]. One automated screen early in development is not always sufficient to find the relevant forms for development. Possible screens and when they could be performed are summarized in Table 14.3 and Fig. 14.10. The screen should be tailored to the type

TABLE 14.3   Possible Polymorph Screens During Development

Type of Screen	Goal
Early	• Propensity for polymorphism • Indication of most stable forms • Indication of stable hydrates
Full	• Most stable form (enantiotropy) • Most stable hydrate • Other forms
Focused	• Selected form studied under GMP manufacturing conditions
Comprehensive	• Increase certainty of knowing most stable form • Find form giving improved drug product • Patent protection of all forms • Find noninfringing forms • Reduce patent costs by finding new forms at one time

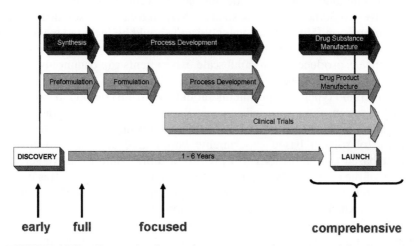

FIGURE 14.10   Types of polymorph screens at various stages of development.

of information required at that stage of development and, as the API progresses, additional information may be needed. The number and type of screens performed for an API will be determined based on the properties of the drug substance, the dosage form, and special issues that may come up during development.

Common steps in a polymorph screen are:

1. Characterize starting material.
2. Generate solid samples.
3. Collect XRPD data on solids produced.
4. Classify the XRPD patterns.
5. Scale up if needed.
6. Characterize each form.
7. Compare properties.
8. Determine relative thermodynamic stability.
9. Select form.

A wide range of crystallization techniques used in polymorph screens have been reported and reviewed [47, 48]. The majority of them are solvent based. A variety of factors are considered when choosing solvent systems for a screen, including solubility of the API, solvents to be used in manufacturing, a range of polarities and functionalities, and a range of water activities. Choices should not be limited to Class 3 solvents at this stage of the selection process. Crystallization experiments can include evaporations, slurries, cools, diffusion (vapor or liquid), solvent drop grinding, and antisolvent addition. The solubility of the API in organic solvents can help guide the type of crystallization experiments to perform. Material that is poorly soluble in most solvents would lend itself to slurry experiments or elevated temperature experiments with subsequent cooling. Material that is highly soluble may oil out at concentrations that are too high. Crystallizations covering both thermodynamic and kinetic conditions should be included since manufacturing processes commonly employ kinetic crystallization conditions (such as antisolvent addition). Experiments intended to influence the nucleation event should also be considered [49]. Nonsolvent based experiments, such as thermal treatment, sublimation, grinding, and compression [50], are also valuable and should be included whenever possible. Crystallization conditions used in a screen do not have to mimic manufacturing conditions. Seeds produced from small scale experiments can commonly be used to make larger amounts of desired forms.

The number and types of experiments should vary from compound to compound since crystallization conditions will change with the properties of the API. The choice of manual versus automated experiments also needs to be determined. A combination of solvent based experiments (automated and manual) along with nonsolvent based crystallizations will provide a more comprehensive screen and cover more of the crystallization space for the compound of interest. It is not necessary, and is sometimes counterproductive, to perform thousands of the same type of experiment, which will cover a limited portion of the crystallization space.

Analysis of the solids produced during the screen is the next step. A variety of techniques are used to characterize new materials, such as XRPD, thermal methods, and spectroscopic methods. A multidisciplinary approach is needed to understand the polymorphic system of an API. One technique will not provide all the necessary information on new crystal forms of the material and how they relate to one another. Numerous references are available that describe characterization of new forms [13, 32, 42, 46]. Analytical techniques in this section are discussed in terms of the information provided on new solids obtained during a polymorph screen.

XRPD is commonly used to determine if the samples are crystalline and it is a direct measurement of the crystal form. Once data are collected, the patterns are classified into different groups that may represent different forms of the material. At this stage, a different pattern may represent a pure material, preferred orientation, or a mixture of forms. Additional characterization information is needed on a representative sample to determine if a pure phase has been produced.

Once crystallinity has been established, determining the presence of solvents is important. Crystal forms can be solvated or unsolvated. In many cases, solvated forms are dismissed in a screen because they cannot readily be used as an API. However, solvates can play an important role in processing and crystallization development and can help explain the formation of one form over another from a certain solvent or process. Solvates would usually not be chosen for development, but upon drying a new unsolvated form may be produced that has all the properties required for the targeted product. Hydrates can be considered a subset of solvates, with water being the solvent incorporated into the lattice. Various types of hydrates have been characterized and discussed [51]. Two common types are stoichiometric and variable hydrates. Stoichiometric hydrates contain water in molar ratios. Those that are stable over a wide range of relative humidity conditions are possible candidates for development. Others may be unstable and unsuitable for further consideration. Variable hydrates typically contain water in nonstoichiometric amounts and the amount of water readily changes with relative humidity conditions. These types of hydrates are difficult to characterize, control, and develop.

Melting point can be a factor during development and should be determined for the various forms. DSC, hot-stage microscopy, or a melting point apparatus can be used to measure this property. A higher melting solid, generally greater than 100 °C, is desirable. A low melting material is more difficult to dry, mill, or compress. DSC data can also provide information on high temperature crystal form changes that may impact development [42], as well as information on physical purity of the sample. Other data can be invaluable in determining if a sample is a pure form or a physical mixture of two or more forms. Solid-state NMR has been used to characterize many pharmaceutical materials and can commonly provide information on mixtures that is difficult to obtain by other methods [35, 36]. IR spectroscopy and Raman spectroscopy are also commonly used to differentiate crystalline forms [32].

Once the forms have been characterized, it is important to understand the relationship between the forms. A schematic, such as the one given in Fig. 14.11 [52], can be constructed to visualize changes in the forms during development. An early

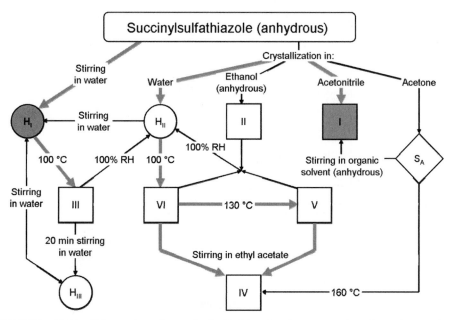

FIGURE 14.11 Schematic of succinylsulfathiazole forms produced under various conditions [52].

understanding of possible form changes during processing, such as upon drying or exposure to water, will help to design acceptable processes that will minimize form changes [53, 54].

The thermodynamically most stable form should be identified if more than one acceptable unsolvated form is found in the screen [46, 55, 56]. The most stable crystalline form is defined as that with the lowest free energy and it will also exhibit the lowest solubility. In a monotropic system, the relative free energy for the two forms remains the same along the entire temperature range, as shown in the energy–temperature diagram in Fig. 14.12a. The heat of fusion curves show that the more stable form has the higher melting point and the greater heat of fusion. In an enan-

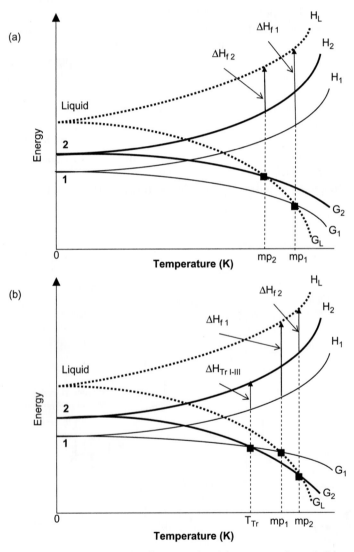

FIGURE 14.12 Energy–temperature diagrams for (a) monotropic and (b) enantiotropic systems.

TABLE 14.4   Burger and Ramburger Rules to Determine the Thermodynamically Stable Form [57]

Rule	Description
Heat of transition rule	If an endothermic transition is observed at some temperature below the melting point, it may be assumed that there are two forms related enantiotropically.
	If an exothermic transition is observed below the melting point, it may be assumed that there are two forms related monotropically or the transition temperature is higher.
Heat of fusion rule	If the higher melting form has the lower heat of fusion, the two forms are usually enantiotropic; otherwise they are monotropic.
IR rule	If the first absorption band in the infrared spectrum of a hydrogen-bonded molecular crystal is higher for one modification than for the other, that form may be assumed to have the larger entropy.
Density rule	If one modification of a molecular crystal has a lower density than the other, it may be assumed to be less stable at absolute zero.

tiotropic system, the relative stabilities change at a temperature defined as the transition temperature, as shown in Fig. 14.12b. In energy–temperature diagrams, the free energy curves can cross, but the enthalpy curves do not. Based on this, the more stable form below the transition temperature in an enantiotropic system will exhibit the lower melting point and the higher heat of fusion. There are four rules proposed by Burger and Ramburger to determine the type of relationship between forms [57] and these are summarized in Table 14.4. Other methods to determine the stability include plotting solubility data at different temperatures in a van't Hoff plot [58] as well as eutectic mixtures [59]. This information is important for crystallization processes since crystallization above the transition temperature will favor one form and below the transition temperature will favor the other. It is also critical for long term stability since the metastable form may transform to the more stable form over time. A metastable form with sufficient stability to provide an acceptable shelf life is another option to consider.

At this stage, other factors need to be considered in the form selection process. Information on solubility, intrinsic solubility, modified absorption potential [60], and chemical and physical stability will help in selection of the best candidate for development.

14.3.6   Crystallization and Quantitation

Once a crystal form is found, crystallization method development will be needed to determine the best conditions to produce material with optimal characteristics, with crystal form being only one consideration. Crystallization conditions to produce the salt or cocrystal directly are the best option. However, a recrystallization step may be needed to produce the desired crystal form with acceptable purity and yield. Numerous factors, such as crystallization equipment, solvent, temperature, cooling rate, antisolvent addition, and other parameters, will need to be investigated [61].

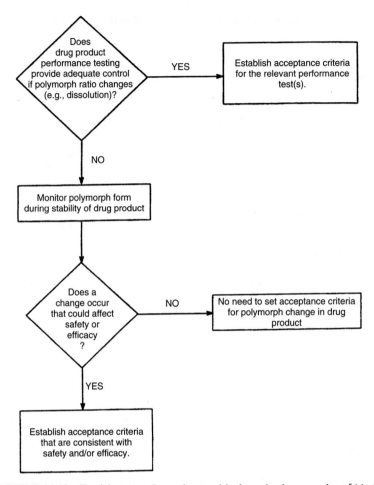

FIGURE 14.13   Decision tree for polymorphic form in drug product [44, 45].

Seeding is also a good option for many systems. Knowing the transition temperature for an enantiotropic pair will be necessary to determine the best crystallization conditions.

When multiple forms are known, the process needs to be controlled to make the desired form of the API consistently. An assay, qualitative or quantitative, may be needed for confirmation, as outlined in Fig. 14.9. Quantitation of forms may also need to be addressed for the drug product as shown in the flowchart in Fig. 14.13. Common analytical techniques used to quantitate the forms in solid samples include XRPD, DSC, IR and Raman spectroscopy, and NMR. Moisture balance data can also be used to quantitate amorphous materials in crystalline solids. Specificity needs to be determined for the technique being used for method development. Guidelines for quantitative method development have been reported [62] and the parameters to be investigated include specificity, linearity, range, accuracy, precision, detection limit, and quantitation limit. Different types of quantitative methods can be developed, as summarized in Table 14.5. Different assays can be used at various stages of development and to obtain suitable data for specific situations. An assay

TABLE 14.5 Summary of Solid-State Quantitative Assays

Quantitative Method	Scope of Assay	Result
Limit test	A limit of detection for a technique is determined (such as 2%)	Result is specified as "less than 2% Form B present"
Specification assay	An assay limit is determined for a technique (such as 95%)	Result is specified as "greater than 95% Form A present"
Full quantitative method	A minimum quantifiable limit (MQL) (such as 2%) and linear range (such as 2–25%) are determined	"X% of Form B" if within the quantitation range of 2–25%, or "less than 2% Form B" if below MQL, or "greater than 25% Form B" if above linear range

may be needed to show that a new process is producing the desired form and may eventually be sunsetted after control is established over a period of time.

14.4 CONCLUSION

Significant information is needed to select a form for development. Making salts and cocrystals of the API for evaluation is a small part of the form selection process. Characterization of physical properties and understanding the interaction of various forms in a solid system are critical for the success of a formulated product and can significantly reduce time to market. A qualitative or quantitative assay may be needed for the API and/or drug product if multiple forms are found. The information obtained during form selection can be used for regulatory and intellectual property documentation and can help extend the life of an important franchise.

REFERENCES

1. Byrn SR, Pfeiffer RR, Stowell JG. *Solid-State Chemistry of Drugs*, 2nd ed. West Lafayette, IN: SSCI Inc; 1999.
2. Clas SD. The importance of characterizing the crystal form of the drug substance during drug development. *Curr Opin Drug Discov Dev* 2003;6:550–560.
3. Curatolo W. Physical–chemical properties of oral drug candidates in the discovery and exploratory development settings. *Pharm Sci Technol Today* 1998;1:387–393.
4. Gardner CR, Walsh CT, Almarsson O. Drugs as materials: valuing physical form in drug discovery. *Nat Rev Drug Discov* 2004;3:926–934.
5. Venkatesh S, Lipper RA. Role of the development scientist in compound lead selection and optimization. *J Pharm Sci* 2000;89:145–154.
6. Fiese EF. General pharmaceutics—the new physical pharmacy. *J Pharm Sci* 2003;92(7): 1331–1342.
7. Huang LF, Tong WQ. Impact of solid state properties on developability assessment of drug candidates. *Adv Drug Deliv Rev* 2004;56:321–334. Kibbey CE, Poole SK, Robinson

B, Jackson JD, Durham D. An integrated process for measuring the physicochemical properties of drug candidates in a preclinical discovery environment. *J Pharm Sci* 2001;90:1164–1175. Wenlock MC, Austin RP, Barton P, Davis AM, Leeson PD. A comparison of physiochemical property profiles of development and marketed oral drugs. *J Med Chem* 2003;46:1250–1256.

8. Stahl PH, Wermuth CG, Eds. *Handbook of Pharmaceutical Salts*. Hoboken, NJ:Wiley-VCH; 2002.

9. Balbach S, Korn C.. Pharmaceutical evaluation of early development candidates "the 100 mg-approach." *Int J Pharm* 2004;275:1–12.

10. Bastin RJ, Bowker MJ, Slater BJ. Salt selection and optimisation procedures for pharmaceutical new chemical entities. *Org Proc Res Dev* 2000;4:427–435.

11. Morris KR, Fakes MG, Thakur AB, Newman AW, Singh AK, Venit JJ, Spagnuolo CJ, Serajuddin ATM. An integrated approach to the selection of optimal salt form for a new drug candidate. *Int J Pharm* 1994;105:209–217.

12. Giron D. Characterisation of salts of drug substances. *J Thermal Anal Calorimetry* 2003;73:441–457.

13. Newman AW, Stahly GP. Form selection of pharmaceutical compounds. In: Ohannessian L, Ed. *Handbook of Pharmaceutical Analysis, Volume 117*. New York: Marcel Dekker; 2001, pp 1–57.

14. Braga D, Brammer L, Champness NR. New trends in crystal engineering. *Crystengcomm* 2005;7:1–19. Erk P, Hengelsberg H, Haddow MF, van Gelder R. The innovative momentum of crystal engineering. *Crystengcomm* 2004;6:474–483. Hulliger J, Roth SW, Quintel A, Bebie H. Polarity of organic supramolecular materials: a tunable crystal property. *J Solid State Chem* 2000;152:49–56. Iimura N, Ohashi Y, Hirata H. Complex formation of perfumes with cationic surfactants and the enhanced thermal stability. *Bull Chem Soc Jpn* 2000;73:1097–1103. Wong MS, Pan F, Bosshard C, Guenter P. Supramolecular synthesis of molecular co-crystals with highly optimized chromophoric orientation for second-order nonlinear optics. *Polym Mater Sci Eng* 1996;75:132–133. Wong MS, Pan F, Gramlich V, Bosshard C, Gunter P. Self-assembly of an acentric co-crystal of a highly hyperpolarizable merocyanine dye with optimized alignment for nonlinear optics. *Adv Materials* 1997;9:554–557.

15. 21 CFR 314.108(a) and Draft Guidance *Applications Covered by Section 505(b)(2)*, http://www.fda.gov/cder/guidance/2853dft.htm.

16. Gould PL. Salt selection of basic drugs. *Int J Pharm* 1986;33:201–217.

17. Miyazaki S, Oshiba M, Nadai T. Precaution on use of hydrochloride salts in pharmaceutical formulation. *J Pharm Sci* 1981;70(6):594–596.

18. Bruno IJ, Cole JC, Lommerse JPM, Rowland RS, Taylor R, Verdonk ML. IsoStar: a library of information about nonbonded interactions. *J Comput Aided Mol Des* 1997; 11(6):525–537. Chisholm J, Pidcock E, Van De Streek J, Infantes L, Motherwell S, Allen FH. Knowledge-based approaches to crystal design. *Crystengcomm* 2006;8:11–28. Gillon AL, Feeder N, Davey RJ, Storey R. Hydration in molecular crystals—a Cambridge Structural Database analysis. *Crystal Growth Des* 2003;3:663–673. Steiner T. The hydrogen bond in the solid state. *Angew Chem Int Ed* 2002;41:48–76.

19. Aakeroy CB, Salmon DJ. Building co-crystals with molecular sense and supramolecular sensibility. *Crystengcomm* 2005;7:439–448.

20. Anthony A, Desiraju GR, Jetti RKR, Kuduva SS, Madhavi NNL, Nangia A, Thaimattam R, Thalladi VR. Crystal engineering: some further strategies. *Mater Res Bull* 1998;1–18.

21. Desiraju GR. Supramolecular synthons in crystal engineering—a new organic-synthesis. *Angew Chem Int Ed Engl* 1995;34:2311–2327.

22. Childs SL, Chyall LJ, Dunlap JT, Smolenskaya VN, Stahly BC, Stahly GP. Crystal engineering approach to forming cocrystals of amine hydrochlorides with organic acids. Molecular complexes of fluoxetine hydrochloride with benzoic, succinic, and fumaric acids. *J Am Chem Soc* 2004;126:13335–13342. Fleischman SG, Kuduva SS, McMahon JA, Moulton B, Walsh RDB, Rodriguez-Hornedo N, Zaworotko MJ. Crystal engineering of the composition of pharmaceutical phases: multiple-component crystalline solids involving carbamazepine. *Crystal Growth Des* 2003;3:909–919.McMahon JA, Bis JA, Vishweshwar P, Shattock TR, McLaughlin OL, Oswald MJ, Allan DR, McGregor PA, Motherwell WDS, Parsons S, Pulham CR. The formation of paracetamol (acetaminophen) adducts with hydrogen-bond acceptors. *Acta Crystallogr B Struct Sci* 2002;58:1057–1066.Remenar JF, Morissette SL, Peterson ML, Moulton B, MacPhee JM, Guzman HR, Almarsson O. Crystal engineering of novel cocrystals of a triazole drug with 1,4-dicarboxylic acids. *J Am Chem Soc* 2003;125:8456–8457.Rodriguez-Spong B, Price CP, Jayasankar A, Matzger AJ, Rodriguez-Hornedo N. General principles of pharmaceutical solid polymorphism: a supramolecular perspective. *Adv Drug Deliv Rev* 2004;56:241–274.Trask AV, Motherwell WDS, Jones W. Pharmaceutical cocrystallization: engineering a remedy for caffeine hydration. *Crystal Growth Des* 2005;5:1013–1021.Walsh RDB, Bradner MW, Fleischman S, Morales LA, Moulton B, Rodriguez-Hornedo N, Zaworotko MJ. Crystal engineering of the composition of pharmaceutical phases. *Chem Commun* 2003;186–187.

23. Aakeroy CB, Desper J, Helfrich BA. Heteromeric intermolecular interactions as synthetic tools for the formation of binary co-crystals. *Crystengcomm* 2004;6:19–24.

24. Etter MC. Hydrogen-bonds as design elements in organic-chemistry. *J Phys Chem* 1991;95:4601–4610.

25. Amos JG, Indelicato JM, Pasini CE, Reutzel SM. US patent 6,001,996. 1999.

26. Nehm SJ, Rodriguez-Spong B, Rodriguez-Hornedo N. Phase solubility diagrams of cocrystals are explained by solubility product and solution complexation. *Crystal Growth Des* 2006;6:592–600.

27. Monissette SL, Almarsson O, Peterson ML, Remenar JF, Read J, Lemmo AV, Ellis S, Cima MJ, Gardner CR. High-throughput crystallization: polymorphs, salts, co-crystals and solvates of pharmaceutical solids. *Adv Drug Deliv Rev* 2004;56:275–300. Remenar JF, MacPhee JM, Larson BK, Tyagi VA, Ho JH, McIlroy DA, Hickey MB, Shaw PB, Almarsson O. Salt selection and simultaneous polymorphism assessment via high-throughput crystallization: the case of sertraline. *Org Proc Res Dev* 2003;7:990–996. Ware EC, Lu DR. An automated approach to salt selection for new unique trazodone salts. *Pharm Res* 2004;21:177–184.

28. Stephenson GA. Applications of X-ray powder diffraction in the pharmaceutical industry. *Rigaku J* 2005;22(1):2–15.

29. Kondritzer AA, Ellin RI, Edberg LJ. Investigation of methyl pyridinium-2-aldoxime salts. *J Pharm Sci* 1961;50(2):109.

30. Koehler HM, Hefferren JJ. Mineral salts of lidocaine. *J Pharm Sci* 1964;53(9):1126.

31. Childs SL, Chyall LJ, Dunlap JT, Coates DA, Stahly BC, Stahly GP. A metastable polymorph of metformin hydrochloride: isolation and characterization using capillary crystallization and thermal microscopy techniques. *Crystal Growth Des* 2004;4:441–449. Rai RN, Varma KBR. Phase diagram and dielectric studies of binary organic materials. *Mater Lett* 2000;44:284–293. Zalac S, Khan MZI, Gabelica V, Tudja M, Mestrovic E, Romih M. Paracetamol-propyl phenazone interaction and formulation difficulties associated with eutectic formation in combination solid dosage forms. *Chem Pharm Bull* 1999;47:302–307. Kuhnert-Brandstatter M, Geiler M, Wurian I. *Sci Pharm* 1983;51:34–41. Kofler A, Kolsek J. *Mikrochimi Acta* 1969;2:408–435.

32. Pedireddi VR, Jones W, Chorlton AP, Docherty R. Creation of crystalline supramolecular arrays: a comparison of co-crystal formation from solution and by solid state grinding. *Chem Commun* 1996;987–988. Shan N, Toda F, Jones W. Mechanochemistry and co-crystal formation: effect of solvent on reaction kinetics. *Chem Commun* 2002;2372–2373. Trask AV, Haynes DA, Motherwell WDS, Jones W. Screening for crystalline salts via mechanochemistry. *Chem Commun* 2006;51–53. Trask AV, van de Streek J, Motherwell WDS, Jones W. Achieving polymorphic and stoichiometric diversity in cocrystal formation: importance of solid-state grinding, powder X-ray structure determination, and seeding. *Crystal Growth Des* 2005;5:2233–2241.

33. Brittain HG, Ed. *Physical Characterization of Pharmaceutical Solids.* New York: Marcel Dekkar; 1995.

34. Brittain HG, Bogdanowich SJ, Bugay DE, DeVincentis J, Lewen G, Newman AW. Physical characterization of pharmaceutical solids. *Pharm Res* 1991;8(8):963–973.

35. Mehrens SM, Kale UJ, Qu XG. Statistical analysis of differences in the Raman spectra of polymorphs. *J Pharm Sci* 2005;94:1354–1367.

36. Tishmack PA, Bugay DE, Byrn SR. Solid-state nuclear magnetic resonance spectroscopy—pharmaceutical applications. *J Pharm Sci* 2003;92:441–474.

37. Stephenson GA, Forbes RA, Reutzel-Edens SM. Characterization of the solid state: quantitative issues. *Adv Drug Deliv Rev* 2001;48:67–90.

38. Padden BE, Zell MT, Dong ZD, Schroeder SA, Grant DJW, Munson EJ. Comparison of solid-state ^{13}C NMR spectroscopy and powder X-ray diffraction for analyzing mixtures of polymorphs of neotame. *Anal Chem* 1999;71(16):3325–3331.

39. Reutzel-Edens SM, Bush JK. Solid-state NMR spectroscopy of small molecules: from NMR crystallography to the characterization of solid oral dosage forms. *Am Pharm Rev* 2002;5/2:112–115.

40. Stahly GP, Bates S, Andres MC, Cowans BA. Discovery of a new polymorph of dehydroepiandrosterone (prasterone) and solution of its crystal structure from X-ray powder diffraction data. *Crystal Growth Des* 2006;6:925–932.

41. Reutzel-Edens SM, Newman AW. The physical characterization of hygroscopicity in pharmaceutical solids. In Hilfiker R, Ed. *Polymorphism.* Weinheim:Wiley-VCH; 2006, pp 235–258.

42. Giron D, Mutz M, Garnier S. Solid-state of pharmaceutical compounds—impact of the ICH Q6 guideline on industrial development. *J Thermal Anal Calorimetry* 2004;77:709–747. Singhal D, Curatolo W.. Drug polymorphism and dosage form design: a practical perspective. *Adv Drug Deliv Rev* 2004;56:335–347. Raw AS, Furness MS, Gill DS, Adams RC, Holcombe FO, Yu LX.. Regulatory considerations of pharmaceutical solid polymorphism in abbreviated new drug applications (ANDAs). *Adv Drug Deliv Rev* 2004;56:397–414. Yu LX, Furness MS, Raw AS, Outlaw KPW, Nashed NE, Ramos E, Miller SPF, Adams RC, Fang F, Patel RM, Holcombe FO, Chiu YY, Hussain AS.. Scientific considerations of pharmaceutical solid polymorphism in abbreviated new drug applications. *Pharm Res* 2003;20:531–536.

43. Stahly GP. Polymorphism in crystals: fundamentals, predications and industrial practice. Presented at the American Chemical Society ProSpectives Meeting, Tampa, FL, 23–26 Feb 2003.

44. Q6A Specifications, Test procedures and acceptance criteria for new drug substances and new drug products: chemical substances. *Fed Reg* 1997;62:62889–62910.

45. Byrn SA, Pfeiffer R, Ganey M, Hoiberg C, Poochikian G. *Pharm Res* 1995;12:945–954.

46. Blagden N, Davey RJ. Polymorph selection: Challenges for the future? *Crystal Growth Des.* 2003;3:873–885.

47. Guillory JK. Generation of polymoprhs, hydrates, solvates, and amorphous solids. In Brittain HG, Ed. *Polymorphism in Pharmaceutical Solids*. New York: Marcel Dekker; 1999, Ch 5, pp 183–226.

48. Bernstein J. *Polymorphism in Molecular Crystals*. London:Oxford Science Publications; 2002.

49. Gracin S, Uusi-Penttila M, Rasmuson AC. Influence of ultrasound on the nucleation of polymorphs of *p*-aminobenzoic acid. *Crystal Growth Des* 2005;5:1787–1794. Davey RJ, Allen K, Blagden N, Cross WI, Lieberman HF, Quayle MJ, Righini S, Seton L, Tiddy GJT. Crystal engineering—nucleation, the key step. *Crystengcomm* 2002;257–264.

50. Fabbiani FPA, Allan DR, David WIF, Moggach SA, Parsons S, Pulham CR. High-pressure recrystallisation—a route to new polymorphs and solvates. *Crystengcomm* 2004;6:505–512.

51. Morris KM, Rodriquez-Hornedo N. Hydrates. In Swarbrick J, Boylan JC, Eds. *Encyclopedia of Pharmaceutical Technology, Volume 7*. New York: Marcel Dekker; 1993, pp 393–440.

52. Burger A, Grießer UJ. The polymorphic drug substances of the European Pharmacopoeia. Part 7: Physical stability, hygroscopicity and solubility of succinylsulfathiazole crystal forms. *Eur J Pharm Biopharm* 1991;37:118–124.

53. Herbstein FH. Diversity amidst similarity: a multidisciplinary approach to phase relationships, solvates, and polymorphs. *Crystal Growth Des* 2004;4:1419–1429.

54. Morris KR, Griesser UJ, Eckhardt CJ, Stowell JG. Theoretical approaches to physical transformations of active pharmaceutical ingredients during manufacturing processes. *Adv Drug Deliv Rev* 2001;91–114.

55. Miller JM, Collman BM, Greene LR, Grant DJW, Blackburn AC. Identifying the stable polymorph early in the drug discovery–development process. *Pharm Dev Technol* 2005;10:291–297.

56. Grunenberg A, Henck J-O, Siesler HW. Theoretical derivation and practical application of energy/temperature diagrams as an instrument in preformulation studies of polymorphic drug substances. *Int J Pharm* 1996;129:147–158.

57. Burger A, Ramburger R. On the polymorphism of pharmaceuticals and other molecular crystals. I. *Mikrochim Acta (Wien) II* 1979;259–272. Burger A, Ramburger R. On the polymorphism of pharmaceuticals and other molecular crystals. II. *Mikrochim Acta (Wien) II* 1979;273–316.

58. Behme RJ, Brooke D. Heat of fusion measurement of a low melting polymorph of carbamazepine that undergoes multiple-phase changes during differential scanning calorimetry analysis. *J Pharm Sci* 1991;80(10):986–990. Behme RJ, Brooke D, Farney RF, Kensler TT. Characterization of polymorphism of gepirone hydrochloride. *J Pharm Sci* 1985;74(10):1041–1046.

59. Yu L, Stephenson GA, Mitchell CA, Bunnell CA, Snorek SV, Bowyer JJ, Borchardt TB, Stowell JG, Byrn SR. Thermochemistry and conformational polymorphism of a hexamorphic crystal system. *J Am Chem Soc* 2000;122(4):585–591.

60. Sanghvi T, Ni N, Yalkowsky SH. A simple modified absorption potential. *Pharm Res* 2001;18(12):1794–1796. Anderson NG. *Practical Process Research and Development*. San Diego, CA: Academic Press; 2000.

61. International Conference on Harmonisation; Q2B validation of analytical procedures: methodology. *Fed Reg* 1997;62:27464.

62. Newman AW, Byrn SR. Solid-state analysis of the active pharmaceutical ingredient in drug products. *Drug Discov Today* 2003;8(9):898–905.

15

DISSOLUTION

A.K. Tiwary, Bharti Sapra, and Subheet Jain
Punjabi University, Patiala, Punjab, India

Contents

15.1 INTRODUCTION

Dissolution of the active ingredients is of paramount importance for the successful performance of a dosage form. Dissolution testing is a convenient tool for ensuring intra- and interbatch performance compliance of dosage forms. Furthermore, the release profiles obtained from *in vitro* dissolution tests can be used for predicting *in vitro–in vivo* correlation models. Thus, carefully conducted dissolution tests are useful for ensuring dosage form functionality.

Preclinical Development Handbook: ADME and Biopharmaceutical Properties,
edited by Shayne Cox Gad
Copyright © 2008 John Wiley & Sons, Inc.

The physicochemical characteristics of a drug and its site of action/absorption together dictate the type of dosage form to be developed. The plethora of additives and technologies available in the hands of the product development scientist make it possible to design a dosage form possessing the predetermined drug release attributes. Great strides in the excipient and technology arena, however, make it imperative to critically evaluate their influence on *in vitro* drug dissolution during the preformulation phase. This involves proper selection of dissolution media, dissolution apparatus, operation variables, and interpretation of generated data. Although a preliminary estimate of the dosage form's *in vivo* performance can be gauged by applying *in vitro–in vivo* correlation models, it is essential to test the dosage form in animals to demonstrate its efficacy and safety. Therefore, the functionality of dosage form is first demonstrated in appropriate animal model(s) during the preclinical phase before testing it in human beings. Figure 15.1 gives a schematic representation of the steps to be followed during the course of dosage form development with respect to dissolution testing of a dosage form.

15.2   FACTORS INFLUENCING DRUG DISSOLUTION FROM DOSAGE FORMS

Dissolution of drug from a dosage form is unequivocally the most important indicator of its anticipated *in vivo* performance. Both nature of formulation ingredients and methods of incorporating them influence drug release from dosage forms. Therefore, formulation and process variables demand careful evaluation during the initial product development phase in order to achieve the predetermined drug dissolution profile.

15.2.1   Formulation Variables

A variety of excipients are available for use in solid dosage forms. Functional differences in excipients are known to exist depending on the material and usage and it is difficult to generalize findings for all the drugs. Therefore, the potential of these excipients to modify drug release from dosage forms should be critically evaluated during formulation. Although a detailed discussion on all excipients would not be possible, a few categories needing special attention are discussed next.

Diluents   Diluents are used in solid dosage forms as main bulk forming agents. Being present in large quantities, they can exert profound influence on the stability of the active ingredient, ease of manufacturing, drug release, and bioavailability profile. Table 15.1 lists important diluents used for direct compression and wet granulation. It is evident from this table that an excipient influences compression kinetics, tablet properties, and eventually functionality of the dosage form.

Furthermore, the effect of precompression, which is often used for reworking tablet/capsule granules, on drug release should be evaluated especially while attempting dry granulation. The quality of tablets containing a combination of microcrystalline cellulose and lactose was found to increase after reworking when the proportion of spray dried lactose was increased. However, the tablet weight uniformity decreased [5]. Generally, recompression reduces tablet strength and this

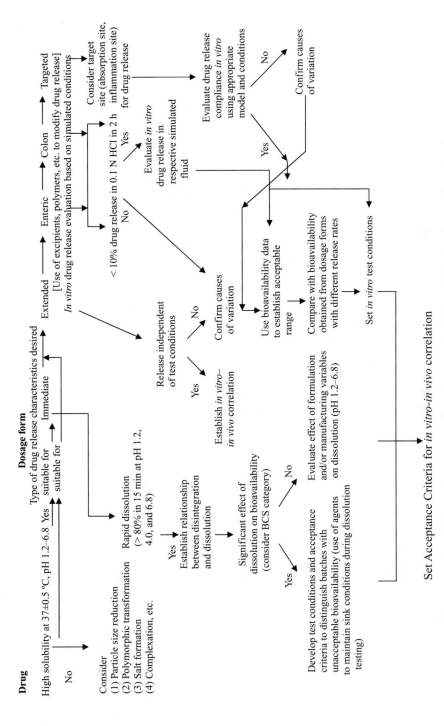

FIGURE 15.1 Schematic representation of steps to be followed during dosage form development.

TABLE 15.1 A Few Important Diluents and Their Properties

Excipient (Trade Name)	Properties		Suitable for	Effect on Drug Dissolution	References
	Advantages	Disadvantages			
Microcrystalline cellulose (Avicel, PH-101)	Good compressibility, forms hard tablets at low pressure, fast tablet disintegration, available in different particle sizes for use in different types or tablets	Fair flowability, costly	• Direct compression • Wet granulation • With nonaqueous binding system • Higher carrying capacity • Hard tablet at low applied pressure • Controlled release when combined with lactose, starch, etc.	Capillarity explains the penetration of water into tablet, thereby destroying cohesive bonds between particles	1–3
Powdered cellulose	Little inherent lubrication property, inexpensive	Poor flowability, poor compressibility, poor binding, high dilution potential	• Wet granulation	Tablets often disintegrate readily; but chances of physical entrapment are also there, which may lead to delayed dissolution	1, 2
Dicalcium phosphate	Fairly good compressibility, excellent flow property	Soluble in acidic pH of stomach	• Direct compression • Wet granulation with nonaqueous binding system	Negative effect on dissolution by using increased proportions with microcrystalline cellulose; because of hydrophobic nature, may limit the dispersion of drug particles, hence may lead to slow dissolution	1, 2

Excipient	Properties	Limitations	Method	Effect on dissolution	Ref.
Spray dried lactose	Good compressibility, excellent flow property, low hygroscopicity, low reactivity with active ingredient; excellent physical, chemical, and microbiological stability	Browning due to the presence of 5-hydroxy methyl 2-furaldehyde when combined with amines, moisture, lactates, phosphates; has relatively poor dilution potential	• Direct compression • Wet granulation with nonaqueous binding system	Aids in dissolution	1, 2, 4
Starch directly compressible (Sta-Rx-1500)	Acts as local desiccant to help stabilize moisture sensitive drugs, free flowing, self lubricating	Tablets with high content are soft and may be difficult to dry, susceptible to softening when combined with 0.5% magnesium stearate	• Direct compression	Starch granules swell in dissolution media forming a viscous matrix that retards dissolution medium penetration and hence decrease the dissolution	1, 2
Compressible sugar (invert sugar, malt dextrins)	Highly compressible, inexpensive nonhygroscopic (invert sugar is hygroscopic at elevated temperature and high humidity)	Readily soluble, calorigenic, not acceptable for diabetes	• Tablet at high moisture content requires high ejection force • Low lubricant requirement		1, 2

TABLE 15.1 *Continued*

Excipient (Trade Name)	Properties			Suitable for	Effect on Drug Dissolution	References
	Advantages	Disadvantages				
Mannitol	Nonhygroscopic, needs combination with other directly compressible excipients for good compression, relatively inert with high heat stability	Poor flowability and requires high lubricant addition, expensive		• Mouth dissolving • Buccal tablet • Chewable tablet • Generally wet granulated using auxillary binder to produce compressible granules	Not relevant	1, 2
Ethyl cellulose (TOEC-Aqualon)	High ethoxyl content and low viscosity, excellent flowability, drug release triggered by circumferential failure of the coat, greater lag time (3–16h) by increasing coating compression force (5-L5KN) than other grades	Relatively expensive		• Compression coating	May have a serious retardant effect on disintegration and drug dissolution release	1, 2
Pregelatinized starch (PCS PC-10)	Free flowing, good binding ability, good disintegrating capacity, high dilution potential, some lubricant action, good oil absorption capacity	Requires high pressure to produce hard table; binding gets reduced by lubricants; magnesium stearate softens the tablet		• Direct compression	Effect is concentration dependent, generally improves dissolution	1, 2

488

reduction becomes more significant when initial compression is carried out at higher pressure. Hence, these tablets can be expected to exhibit faster drug release.

Directly Compressible Vehicles   Direct compression is preferred over wet granulation as it requires fewer unit operations and less space, saves time, and labor costs, and hence is more economical. Tablets prepared by direct compression exhibit less variation in dissolution profile after storage [6]. In addition, as directly compressed tablets disintegrate, discrete drug particles are released—unlike granules from wet granulation—which ensures faster as well as complete drug dissolution. It is well known that if fragmentation predominates during compression, an increase in specific surface area leads to enhanced dissolution. However, if consolidation is the predominating phenomenon, an increase in compression pressure decreases dissolution. Therefore, it is essential to evaluate the compression behavior of compressible vehicles before using them as diluents in solid dosage forms.

LACTOSE   Lactose exhibits polymorphism depending on crystallization conditions. Crystalline lactose undergoes fragmentation while amorphous lactose undergoes plastic deformation during compression. Tablets prepared from amorphous lactose show greater hardness with increasing water content [7].

α-Lactose monohydrate (100#) is generally used in direct compression due to its good flow property. It undergoes fragmentation during compression and exhibits poor binding [8] and the tablet strength decreases with increase in particle size [9]. Tablets prepared by combining microcrystalline cellulose and α-lactose exhibit greater hardness with an increase in proportion of the former [9]. α-Lactose monohydrate exhibits good flowability, compressibility, and hardness when mixed with polyethylene glycol 6000 [10]. A multifunctional coprocessed, directly compressible diluent containing lactose, polyvinyl pyrrolidone, and croscarmellose sodium was found to exhibit better flow properties, compressibility, and disintegration than lactose monohydrate [11]. The binding capacity of α-lactose monohydrate increases considerably after dehydration, wherein it changes from single crystals to aggregates of anhydrous α-lactose particles [12]. Tablets containing anhydrous α-lactose show slow disintegration and dissolve during disintegration [5]. Anhydrous β-lactose monohydrate is 10-fold more soluble than α-lactose monohydrate. The slowing effect is suggested to be due to the presence of small pore diameters and precipitation of anhydrous α-lactose as α-lactose monohydrate in these pores. The smaller initial solubility of α-lactose monohydrate produces this effect and the tablets exhibit higher dissolution [13].

Spray dried lactose contains a mixture of crystals of lactose monohydrate and spherical agglomerates of small crystals bound together by glassy or amorphous material. The hardness of tablets was found to increase with decrease in particle size [14]. Furthermore, disintegration time is reported to increase with an increase in compression force [15]. Addition of lubricant to spray dried lactose prolongs the disintegration time and drug dissolution [16].

The granulated form of α-lactose monohydrate (agglomerated lactose) possesses good flow and binding property but not as good as spray dried lactose. The presence of increasing amounts of β-lactose in agglomerated lactose is suggested to impart strong intergranular cohesion [17].

CELLULOSE DERIVATIVES   Microcrystalline cellulose (MCC) finds wide application in the formulation of tablets by both direct compression and wet granulation. MCC possesses good flow property, hardness, and friability. It is available in different grades depending on physical state, powder (PH-101) and granular (PH-102) as well as particle size. It can be used for controlling the release of both water-soluble and water-insoluble drugs when combined with other diluents like lactose, starch, and dibasic calcium phosphate [18]. The granular form (PH-102) is reported to exhibit better flow [15]. The denser versions of PH-101 or PH-102—PH-301 and PH-302, respectively—have improved flowability but reduced compressibility [19]. Tablets containing higher proportion of PH-101 were found to exhibit higher crushing strength and lower disintegration time, while those containing PH-102 and PH-200 exhibited lower crushing strength and shorter disintegration time [20]. An increase in the ratio of length to diameter of particles (Celous KR 801) yields tablets with higher tensile strength [21]. Similarly, presence of cellulose II polymorph in Avicel PH-102 gives more elasticity to particles than Avicel PH-102 that contains cellulose I polymorph [22].

SUGARS   Sucrose is widely used in the manufacture of chewable tablets [23]. However, its use is restricted due to concerns regarding microbial growth, high calorie contribution, and moisture sensitivity. Di-Pac consists of 97% sucrose and 3% modified dextrin [24]. It is directly compressible but tends to cake and lose its fluidity at high moisture level. Due to cocrystallization of sucrose and dextrin, Di-Pac undergoes plastic deformation and produces harder tablets that dissolve slower than those obtained from sucrose alone [25]. Mannitol is water soluble and nonhygroscopic and is an important ingredient in chewable tablets due to its negative heat of solution that produces a cooling effect in the buccal cavity. Emdex is produced by hydrolysis of starch and consists of aggregates of dextrose microcrystals intermixed with higher molecular weight sugars. Theophylline tablets prepared with emdex were found to exhibit higher mechanical strength, rapid disintegration, and faster drug release than the tablets prepared with maltodextrin M 450 [26]. The rate of release of water-insoluble drug was found to be significantly affected by addition of lubricants in tablets prepared from maltodextrin (M 700, M 500, and M 150) while the release of water-soluble drug remained unaffected [27].

Starch may be obtained from corn, wheat, potatoes, tapioca, or rice. Tablets containing a high concentration of starch are usually soft. An increase in starch content and precompression force and a decrease in granule size was found to enhance the dissolution rate of salicylic acid tablets [28]. Presence of high initial moisture content in starch often leads to poor tablet properties. Therefore, directly compressible varieties are used for improving processing characteristics.

Sta-Rx-1500, a partially gelatinized cornstarch, is free flowing and directly compressible. If compressed alone, it is self-lubricating. However, on addition of 5–10% ingredient that does not possess lubricating property, it requires additional lubricant, usually a glidant, such as colloidal silicone. It softens on mixing with magnesium stearate [29]. Compressible starch gives faster dissolution as compared to other normal starches [20, 30]. Rice starch (Era Tab) produced tablets of terfenadine with higher crushing strength and lower friability than those produced from Sta-Rx-1500, dicalcium phosphate, or Avicel PH-101 [31]. Uni-pure, a fully gelatinized maize starch, was found to possess strong binding properties with faster dissolution and disintegration [32].

DICALCIUM PHOSPHATE   Dicalcium phosphate dihydrate is the most common inorganic material used as a diluent in direct compression. The slightly alkaline nature (pH 7.0–7.4) makes it less suitable for use with drugs that are prone to alkali degradation [33]. Emcompress, containing aggregates of dicalcium phosphate, is directly compressible. However, it requires addition of a large quantity of lubricant for easy ejection from dies. Because Emcompress undergoes fragmentation during consolidation, the added lubricant significantly reduces dissolution of drugs [34].

Coprocessed Diluents for Direct Compression   Coprocessing of well established diluents is a method that is used for obtaining an integrated product, which possesses superior functionality. A few well known coprocessed, directly compressible diluents are summarized in Table 15.2. Although improved functionality depends on the specific purpose related to drug delivery, all directly compressible diluents, in general, need careful evaluation with respect to flowability, tablet characteristics, and reworkability [35].

COPROCESSED LACTOSE   Ludipress consists of α-lactose monohydrate (93.4%), polyvinyl pyrrolidone (3.2%), and crospovidone (3.4%). In spite of the presence of disintegrant, tablets containing Ludipress take more time to disintegrate than those containing α-lactose monohydrate, Tablettose, or anhydrous β-lactose [36]. Although addition of lubricant is essential, the mixing time was not found to influence the crushing strength of tablets [37]. The disintegration time of tablets compressed using Ludipress at 100 MPa pressure did not change, whereas that for Cellactose tablets got prolonged [38, 39]. Cellactose contains α-lactose monohydrate (75%) and cellulose (25%). Good compressibility is attributed to synergistic effect by fragmentation of lactose and plastic deformation of cellulose [40, 41]. Investigators have reported better compressibility of Cellactose as compared to Ludipress, Fast Flo Lactose, Tablettose, Di-Pac, anhydrous lactose [37, 42], and a mixture of Avicel PH-101 and Tablettose [43]. Reduction in compression pressure, which does not eliminate macropores, was reported to decrease the disintegration time of Cellactose tablets [44]. Tablets prepared from granules containing lactose coprocessed with microcrystalline cellulose and dextrin [45], dicalcium phosphate, and microcrystalline cellulose [46] were found to exhibit satisfactory properties.

Pharmatose DCL 40 contains β-lactose (95%) and anhydrous lacitol (5%). It is spherical in shape, exhibits good flowability, and is comparatively stable on exposure to high humidity [23].

StarLac is produced by spray drying of α-lactose monohydrate and maize starch [47]. Its tablets exhibited very good flow behavior, acceptable crushing force due to presence of lactose, rapid disintegration due to starch, and rapid release of theophylline [48].

COPROCESSED MICROCRYSTALLINE CELLULOSE   A codried mixture of microcrystalline cellulose and β-cyclodextrin was found to exhibit improved flowability and compressibility [49]. However, coprocessing microcrystalline cellulose with sodium lauryl sulfate by ultrasonic homogenization followed by spray drying yielded a product that was inferior to microcrystalline cellulose for tableting paracetamol [50]. The PH-M series of microcrystalline cellulose is reported to be suitable for rapidly disintegrating tablets of acetaminophen and ascorbic acid [51]. The tensile strength of tablets prepared from coprocessed granules containing microcrystalline cellulose

TABLE 15.2 A Few Important Commercially Available Coprocessed Diluents and Their Functionality

Brand Name	Adjuvants	Properties
Cellactose	Coprocessed lactose and microcrystalline cellulose (MCC)	Among directly compressible fillers, MCC is the most compressible and has the highest dilution potential because of its high binding and good disintegrating properties. MCC is of interest when combined with other less compressible excipients as an added component in coprocessed direct tableting excipients.
XyliTab	Directly compressible xylitol and sodium CMC	Xylitab granulates provide the convenience of direct compression. Use of Xylitab avoids the need for lengthy traditional granulation processes and allows dry mixing of tablet components.
Ludipress	β-Lactose and crospovidone, PVP	Direct compression auxiliary with medium porosity and good flow properties.
Starlac	Lactose and maize starch	Direct compression excipient, improved flowability, rapid disintegration of tablets, increases crushing strength.
Pharmatose DCL 11	Anhydrous lactose, maize starch	Excellent flow properties and porous surface structure ensure excellent mixing properties as a consequence; DCL 11 permits very low tablet weight variation and high drug content uniformity; DCL 11 is only slightly affected by the level of lubrication.
Pharmatose DCL 14	Mixture of fine crystals of lactose monohydrate and amorphous lactose	Directly compressible product, better compaction properties, uniform particle size, high degree of flowability.
Avicel CE 15	MCC and guar gum	Incorporates particle-engineered products and process technology; provides excellent control of sensory factors that affect palatability; imparts such pleasing sensory features to chewable tablets that the perceived taste of drugs is remarkably altered; produces comparably softer tablets that are less friable and disintegrate rapidly.
Carbofarma GS 12	Calcium carbonate (90%) and pregelatinized starch (10%)	High fluidity (easy workability at high speeds), high density (allows high calcium dosage in small tablets), excellent palatability (no awful feeling especially in chewable formulations).
Carbofarma GM 11	Calcium carbonate (90%) and maltodextrin (10%)	High fluidity, high density, and excellent palatability.
Plasdone S-630	Vinyl acetate and vinyl pyrrolidone	Versatile wet granulation tablet binder, viscosity modifier, crystal growth inhibitor, and solubilizer in liquid dosage forms; available in pyrogen-free "C" grade suitable for parenteral and ophthalmic applications; soluble in water and all pharmaceutically acceptable solvents; protective colloid/stabilizer, demulcent, and lubricant in ophthalmic solutions, solubilizer by complexation.
BarcroftTM CS90	Spray dried calcium carbonate and starch	Highly compressible and free flowing. Simply adjusting the compression force used can allow one to make both chewable and conventional tablets.
Di-Pac	Sucrose and dextrin	Excellent flowability, high compressibility, low hygroscopicity, sweet and nonreactive.
Advantose FS 95	Codried fructose	Turns fructose into an excellent excipient for pharmaceutical, nutraceuticals, and chewable vitamin tablets, improved flow properties, excellent compressibility.

and calcium carbonate decreases with an increase in the amount of calcium carbonate [52].

Prosolv contains microcrystalline cellulose (98%) coprocessed with colloidal silicone dioxide (2%). It has better flowability and compressibility [19, 53] and the tablets maintain tensile strength even in the presence of magnesium stearate, unlike microcrystalline cellulose [54]. A marked enhancement in disintegration time was observed in tablets coated with Prosolv as compared to Avicel [55].

Low crystallinity cellulose is prepared by reacting cellulose with 85% w/w phosphoric acid fumes at room temperature for 1 h, then at 50 °C until a viscous solution is formed. This is poured into water to obtain a fine powder [56–58]. Kumar et al. [59] found that tablets obtained by compressing low crystallinity cellulose (LCPC) were intact even after 6 h, whereas those obtained by compressing LCPC-2000 disintegrated in 4 min. LCPC-4000 was found to be the most ductile material and exhibited the highest compression and compaction characteristics [59].

Lubricants Lubricants are used for reducing the friction between granules and the die wall during compression. Antiadherents prevent sticking to the punch, while glidants improve the flowability of granules. They act by either fluid (hydrodynamics) lubrication by providing a continuous layer of fluid lubricant or by boundary lubrication that results from adherence of polar portions of molecules with carbon chains to metallic surfaces. Additional mechanisms by which antiadherents and glidants improve granule properties relate to electrostatic charge, gas adsorption, and van der waals forces [60, 61].

Lubricants are hydrophobic in nature. Their presence on the granule/tablet surface may decrease the area of contact between the particles and interfere in particle–particle bonding, thereby providing a less cohesive tablet [62]. Furthermore, the coating of lubricant on particles renders the surface hydrophobic and may increase the disintegration time while decreasing the dissolution rate.

An increase in concentration of calcium stearate, glyceryl monostearate, magnesium stearate, or stearic acid from 0.1% to 5% was observed to decrease the dissolution rate of salicylic acid and aspirin, whereas no effect was observed when talc was used [63]. It is important to ascertain whether the lubricant exhibits interaction with excipients or not. Although magnesium stearate possesses higher specific surface area than sodium stearyl fumarate, its adhesion to drug–crospovidone agglomerates results in a decrease in dissolution rate [64]. The negative effect of lubricants on dissolution can be counteracted by choosing diluents that possess both high solubility and fragmentation [65]. The deleterious effect of magnesium stearate (0.5%) on dissolution of ketorolac tromethamine was alleviated by hydrophobic anionic surfactants (sodium *N*-lauroyl sarcosinate, sodium stearoyl 2-lactylate, and sodium stearate), nonionic surfactants (polaxmer 188), and cationic surfactant (cetyl pyridinium chloride). However, lipophilic surfactant (glyceryl monostearate) was ineffective in counteracting the effect of magnesium stearate [66]. The deleterious effect of lubricant on drug dissolution can also be overcome by including superdisintegrants in the formulation [67].

The effect of lubricant on dissolution depends on the aqueous solubility of the drug. Magnesium stearate did not influence the dissolution rate of hydrochlorothiazide, sorivudine, and aztreonam capsules stored at 50 °C for six months. Although caking was observed in capsules of all the drugs on storage at 40 °C/75% RH, the

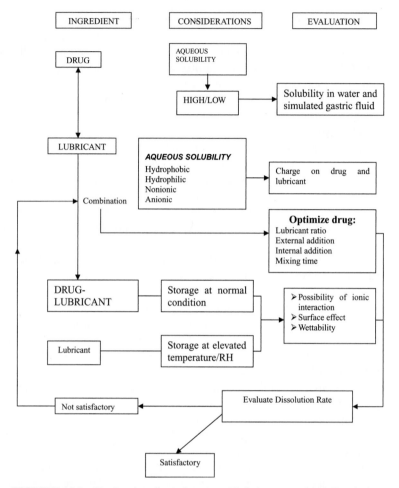

FIGURE 15.2   Evaluating the influence of lubricant on drug dissolution.

decrease in dissolution rate of only sorivudine could be attributed to this effect. On the other hand, aztreonam, due to its inherent high aqueous solubility, did not exhibit any discernible effect on dissolution [68].

The addition of lubricants is known to decrease tablet hardness and results in incomplete drug dissolution [64, 69–72]. External addition of magnesium stearate was found to produce tablets that disintegrated immediately and rapidly released trypsin as compared to those containing internally added lubricant. This was ascribed to higher water penetration rate in tablets prepared by external addition of magnesium stearate [73]. This aspect becomes important when a high dose of poorly wettable drug has to be incorporated in tablet formulation [74]. A decision tree for evaluating the influence of lubricants on drug dissolution during preformulation phase is depicted in Fig. 15.2.

Disintegrants   The dissolution of a solid dosage form depends to a large extent on its mode of disintegration. The properties of disintegrant and diluent together dictate the disintegration as well dissolution of a solid dosage form. Disintegrants acting by swelling mechanism generally increase the dissolution efficiency with an increase in compression pressure [74]. The fragmentation at high compression pressure was suggested to be responsible for increasing dissolution rate of tablets containing starch [75]. Slightly swelling disintegrant (potato starch) containing diazepam tablets were found to exhibit more disintegration time with an increase in mixing time with magnesium stearate. On the other hand, tablets containing strongly swelling disintegrant (sodium starch glycolate) were not significantly affected. Furthermore, *in vitro* dissolution of potato starch containing tablets could be correlated with *in vivo* absorption by employing a high stirring rate [76]. This suggests an overwhelming role of swelling capacity of disintegrant in influencing drug dissolution from dosage forms.

Systems containing high quantity of hydrophobic drug possess an area with pronounced hydrophobicity where wetting acts as the rate-limiting step in dissolution. In such systems, the incorporation of disintegrant does not affect drug dissolution [77]. An increase in hydrophobicity of tablet formulation decreases the efficiency of superdisintegrants [78]. Storage of wet granulated tablets containing superdisintegrants revealed a decrease in dissolution efficiency, with the effect being more pronounced for croscarmellose than for crospovidone or sodium starch glycolate [79]. This is due to slow loss of swelling capacity of disintegrants upon storage of wet granulated tablets.

Incorporation of a large concentration of superdisintegrant reduces the release of poorly soluble drugs due to formation of a viscous layer around the granules during the dissolution process [80]. Lundqvist et al. [81] reported a reduction in disintegration and an increase in friability time when the amount of disintegrant pellets compressed into tablets was increased. However, disintegrants possessing a higher true particle density enhance the disintegration time of pellets. Furthermore, although barium sulfate or calcium carbonate were more effective than magnesium oxide or ferric oxide, use of higher concentration produced an adverse effect due to the large increase in pellet density [81]. Therefore, both the type and concentration of superdisintegrant seem to be critical for obtaining optimum drug release characteristics.

Furthermore, the performance of a disintegrant varies with the pH of the medium. Significant differences in dissolution of acetaminophen from tablets containing sucrose and Primogel or Ac-Di-Sol are attributed to the depressed functioning of Primogel coupled with stronger binding of sucrose in acidic medium than that in neutral medium [82]. Similarly, tablets of terfenadine showed improved disintegration/dissolution with superdisintegrants in the order Crospovidone > Ac-Di-Sol > Primogel > low substituted hydroxypropyl cellulose. Starch decreases dissolution rate by forming a barrier in the form of swollen grains around the particles [83].

It is important to note that the solubility of the major component (diluent) in a tablet formulation can significantly affect disintegration and dissolution. Water-soluble materials tend to dissolve rather than disintegrate, while insoluble materials produce a rapidly disintegrating tablet if an appropriate quantity of disintegrant is included in the formulation [78]. For soluble formulations, the development of disintegration force could be hindered [84]. In addition, the role of soluble excipients like lactose that possibly act passively by hydrogen bond annihilation cannot be ruled out when present in tablet formulations [5]. As the quantity of water penetrating into a tablet is limited, the soluble excipients can be expected to partially consume the available water, leaving only a part of it for development of disintegration force. Lopez-Solis and Villafuerte-Robles [85] found greater dissolution improvement of norfloxacin when tablets contained a dissolving diluent, Pharmatose DCL 11 and less hygroscopic disintegrant PVP XL 10, as compared to tablets containing more hygroscopic disintegrant like croscarmellose or starch 1500. Both sodium starch glycolate and croscarmellose sodium showed significantly reduced water uptake than crospovidone in 0.1 N HCl. Tablets containing the former disintegrant revealed significant increase in disintegration time for slowly disintegrating (lactose based) tablets as compared to rapidly disintegrating (dicalcium phosphate based) tablets. The dependence of dissolution rate of hydrochlorothiazide on both water uptake and solubility of ingredients in the testing medium suggests the importance of swelling capacity of disintegrants in determining drug release from tablets [86].

Furthermore, the surface area of disintegrated agglomerates during dissolution needs to be critically considered while judging drug dissolution from tablets. Difference in dissolution rate of aspirin from tablets containing different superdisintegrants was attributed to their behavior in promoting disintegration. Video images of the dynamic process indicated Ac-Di-Sol, Primogel, or Polyplasdone XL 10 promote, respectively, rapid disintegration, slow disintegration, and rapid disintegration but into large agglomerates [87].

Therefore, drug release from tablets is intimately connected with the performance of disintegrant present in the formulation. Solubility of diluent, water uptake, swelling behavior, development of disintegration force, and disintegration behavior of disintegrant are critical parameters to be considered while optimizing a tablet dosage form with respect to drug dissolution.

Release Modifiers   Polymers are used for modifying the release of drugs from solid dosage forms. They may be employed in matrix form or as a coating for this purpose. Furthermore, the physical form (tablets, granules, beads, pellets, etc.) of the dosage form may vary. Figure 15.3 gives an overview of the decision making process while selecting a release modifier for solid dosage forms. The choice of polymer(s) for modifying drug release depends on many factors, as summarized in Table 15.3. The drug release characteristics from dosage forms become more complex when combinations of release modifiers are used. It would not be possible to discuss all the release modifiers here with respect to their mechanism of drug release. Hence, a few important factors that may influence drug dissolution in the presence of release modifiers are discussed next.

Polymer Characteristics   The desired drug release profile governs the choice of release modifier(s). Polymers possessing pH-independent solubility (Carbopol and HPC) provide continuous drug release in acidic as well as alkaline buffer media. Polymers that have pH-dependent solubility (Eudragits) are suitable for achieving drug release at a particular pH or site in the gastrointestinal tract. Polymers that are insoluble at all pH values (ethyl cellulose) need to be combined with other polymers to obtain the desirable drug release profile. Such polymers may be combined with pH-sensitive polymers to obtain drug release at specific pH values [88] or with polysaccharides to obtain drug release in the colon [89].

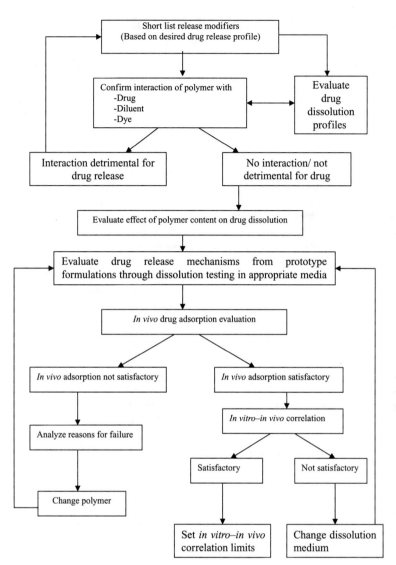

FIGURE 15.3 Decision tree for evaluating the influence of release modifiers on drug dissolution.

Polymer Content The selected polymer or polymer combination is developed into the prototype formulation and evaluated for drug release profile through dissolution testing. Usually, preparation of a series of formulations with different polymer contents exhibiting different dissolution profiles [90] helps in elucidating the drug release mechanism(s). The drug release rate from a tablet formulated using polymer(s) depends on the molar ratio of polymer(s) [91, 92]. Chiao and Price [93] observed that release rate of propranolol hydrochloride from cellulose acetate butyrate microspheres increased with higher drug to polymer ratio and decreased with increasing diameter.

TABLE 15.3   Dissolution as a Tool for Accessing Functionality of Release Modifiers

Purpose (Dosage Form)	Polymer Characteristic Desired	Dissolution Behavior Desired	Correlation with Absorption[a]
Release in stomach	Good solubility in 0.1 N HCl	Drug level detectable immediately. Peak level corresponds to disintegration.	Drug detectable in plasma soon after ingestion. Concentration falls depending on t_{50}
Continuous release in stomach (floating)	Restricted solubility in 0.1 N HCl; swells in acidic medium, thereby delaying drug release.	Drug released with little delay; concentration rises continuously.	Drug detectable with little delay and with continuous rise for 3–5 h (fed state trial essential)
Sustained release	pH-independent solubility. Continuous release over extended time period irrespective of pH.	Drug released slowly with delay. Release continues at constant rate in pH-progression media.	Drug detectable in blood with little delay. Constant concentration maintained over prolonged period.
Colon release	Not soluble in both acidic and alkaline pH; degradation due to bacteroids present in cecal contents.	No/little (<10%) drug released on sequential exposure to 0.1 N HCl (2 h) and pH 7.5 (3 h). Total release in pH 6.8 containing cecal contents.	No drug detectable until 2 h after oral ingestion; abrupt rise in concentration after 5 h. (Assurance of no effect of pH on drug release essential.)
Site-specific release	Soluble at pH of the site.	Drug released only after exposure to particular pH.	No drug detected until dosage form reaches the desired site.
Time release	Slow erosion over the desired time interval.	Very little drug released over a particular time interval; abrupt release after that.	Negligible drug in blood until a few hours after ingestion; abrupt increase thereafter. (Assurance of no effect of pH, gastric emptying, and dietary factors essential.)

[a]Assuming high solubility, high gastrointestinal permeability, and passive absorption.

The absolute amount of polymers also influences drug release. Extended release tablets of cephalexin showed reduced release in the presence of higher amounts of HPMC [94]. Release of ascorbic acid from tablets revealed that t_{50} and t_{90} was delayed from 1 h to 1.4 h and from 4.55 h to 7.2 h, respectively, when the total polymer content was increased to 60 g/500 g in comparison to 45 g/500 g. Similar results were obtained when Kollicoat SR 30D was used in formulating ibuprofen granules [95]. However, slight modification in HPMC concentration does not significantly affect drug release rate [96].

Polymer–Drug Interaction Various interactions taking place between the drugs and polymers may lead to change in drug release pattern, where drug solubility in external medium as well as its diffusion capacity within the polymer network play an important role. The ability of Eudragit polymers to adsorb acidic drugs from a solution at pH 7.4 is well known. The ionized acid molecules carry a negative charge to ammonium groups linked to polymer backbone. This allows electrostatic binding to take place [97, 98]. This phenomenon occurs when the pH of the dissolution medium is higher than the pK_a of the drug [97]. In the case of tris-HCl buffer (pH 7.4), chloride ions compete with drug molecule anions for active sites in the polymer backbone, thus resulting in a lower adsorption rate of drugs [99].

Many acids have been used to prepare chitosan based controlled release drug delivery systems. Such conditions may not be desirable for some drugs, especially for an acid labile drug [100]. It was further confirmed by Nunthanid et al. [101] that the drug release behavior was sustained from high molecular weight chitosan acetate films. In addition, they observed sustained release of theophylline from tablets prepared with spray dried chitosan and as its amount increased, the drug release occurred at a much slower rate [101].

Polymer–Diluent Interaction Like other factors, polymer–diluent interaction may also affect drug release. Microcrystalline cellulose allowed rapid penetration of aqueous medium, resulting in rapid erosion of polymer matrices. Lactose played an important role in imparting a physical barrier affecting diclofenac release kinetics by reducing tortuosity of diffusion pathway [102]. Anionic dyes like erythrosine, panceau 4 R, sunset yellow, and tartrazine are immiscible with chitosan citrate. But brilliant blue and green FS at concentrations of 0.02–1.0% w/w are miscible with chitosan. This could be due to reduced interaction because of the presence of positive charge on these dye molecules. Drug dissolution with these coated tablets was pH dependent and also corresponded to the ability of chitosan to protonate in the medium. Faster drug dissolution occurs from coated tablets colored with brilliant blue than from those colored with green FS. This is due to the fact that brilliant blue exhibits more water solubility due to the presence of more SO_3H groups [103]. In another study, the miscibility of dye and chitosan was found to depend on the molecular configuration and ionic group of dye molecule. Drug dissolution from tablets coated with green FS is slightly slower than that from tablets coated with plain films and core tablet, respectively [104].

Polymer–Excipient Interaction Drug–excipient, excipient–excipient, and polymer–excipient interactions are of major preformulation consideration in the pharmaceutical industry and usually they can be predicted at early stages of product development. Interactions in the liquid state are more complicated than in the solid state, as sometimes predictions can be complicated by the dispersion medium, change in pH of the medium, ionic strength, a difference in the solubility parameter of the drug, or temperature fluctuations [98]. It is reported that PEG 6000 and Eudragit L-30 D have similar solubility parameters. This increases their affinity toward each other [105]. Chances of interaction of Eudragit L-30D with PEG 6000 increase in an acidic medium due to hydrogen bonding between the ether oxygen of the oxyethylene groups of PEG 6000, resulting in faster dissolution [98]. PEG usually interacts with molecules that have hydrogen bonding functions as polymethacrylic acid polymers [105, 106].

Physicochemical Characteristics of Drug   The physicochemical properties of pharmaceuticals, including solubility and dissolution rate, can be influenced by the degree of crystallinity, solvation rate, crystal form, particle size/surface area, and so on. The solubility of a drug is influenced by many factors, which in turn affect the dissolution behavior. The rate of dissolution assumes great importance if it is lower than the rate of diffusion to the site of absorption or the rate of absorption of the drug. In such cases, there is a need for manipulating the drug characteristics in order to achieve the required dissolution profile.

Decreasing the particle size is the most common approach for increasing the solubility of a drug. However, the role of particle size should be considered for drugs exhibiting solubility of 0.1 mg/mL or less. This is because the chances of toxic effects associated with faster dissolution of a drug often increase with an increase in the drug solubility [107]. It is important to note that decreasing the particle size of a hydrophobic drug, phenytoin, actually decreases the proportion of particles in contact with dissolution medium. Furthermore, the small particles have air adsorbed on their surface due to which they float on the surface of the dissolution medium, thereby exhibiting lower dissolution [108]. The stability of different salts/coprecipitates in the gastro intestinal fluids needs to be critically evaluated. The most soluble sodium salt of penicillin is the least bioavailable form as it is most unstable in the digestive fluids [109].

Deaggregation of the drug particles is necessary to aid faster dissolution as evidenced by significantly different plasma concentrations obtained after administration of different brands of chloramphenicol capsules [108].

The availability of the weakly acidic drug para amino-salicylic acid is only 77% of that of its salt forms. A correlation in the rank order of availability of its potassium, calcium, or sodium salt forms indicated the pivotal role of their respective drug solubility in influencing the absorption of para amino-salicylic acid [108].

The beneficial effect of modifying the nonionized drugs into salt forms was reported for tetracycline and tolbutamide. The dissolution rate of weakly basic drug (tetracycline) decreases, whereas for the weakly acidic drug (tolbutamide) it increases as the pH of the dissolution medium is increased. However, the dissolution of salt forms of aluminum acetyl salicylate, sodium warfarin, or pamoate salt of benzamphetamine was found to be lower than that of their nonionized forms. This was suggested to be due to precipitation of an insoluble particle or film on the surface of the tablet rather than in bulk solution, which decreased the effective surface area by preventing deaggregation of the particles. Furthermore, the properties of the inactive ingredients present in the dosage form may also be influenced by the pH of the dissolution medium and may exert profound influence on dissolution characteristics of drugs (phenytoin, nitrofurantoin) [108]. Table 15.4 lists a few drugs whose dissolution is known to be influenced by physicochemical properties. In view of the above, it seems essential to compare the solubility and dissolution profile of the active ingredient/salt form with that of the dosage form in an

TABLE 15.4 Influence of Physicochemical Factors on Dissolution Rate of Drugs

Drug	Characteristic Feature Influencing Dissolution	Remarks	References
Folic acid	Particle size	Formulations made from 9.0 μm particles release higher amount at 60 min as compared to formulations containing 24.4 μm sizes. Difference not statistically significant.	110
Griseofulvin	Particle size	Unmodified griseofulvin is required to dissolve NLT 70% and micronized griseofulvin is required to dissolve NLT 85% of stated amount in presence of 4% or 0.54% w/v SLS.	111
Nitrofurantoin	Particle size	Particles smaller than 10 μm are more rapidly and completely absorbed from tablet dosage form than macro-crystalline form (74–177 μm) from capsule.	108
Phenacetin	Particle size	Dissolution rate increased with increasing size. Addition of Tween-80 to dissolution medium increases the dissolution rate as particle size is decreased.	108
Para amino-salicylic acid (PAS)	Salt form	Solubility of nonionized PAS = 1 g/600 mL Potassium PAS = 1 g/10 mL Calcium PAS = 1 g/7 mL Sodium PAS = 1 g/2 mL Salt forms are more rapidly available than nonionized drug.	108
Tolbutamide	pH effect	As pH increases, dissolution rate increases.	108
Tetracycline	pH effect	As pH increases, dissolution rate decreases.	108
Ampicillin, glutethemide, theophylline	Anhydrous forms (solvate form)	At room temperature anhydrous forms exhibit higher dissolution rate than their corresponding hydrates due to difference in free energy of hydration.	112
Azetazolamide, carbamazepine, indomethacin	Metastable forms (phase transformations)	Because of the higher free energy they dissolve more rapidly than their corresponding stable forms.	113
Diclofenac sodium	Solid–solid transition	Anhydrous form dissolves faster than hydrated form. Storage under uncontrolled environment conditions (RH ≤ 60%, 25 °C) transforms the anhydrous form to hydrous form; adverse effect is anticipated during dosage form manufacturing too.	114
Chloramphenicol palmitate (polymorphic forms: A and B)	Polymorphism	As percentage of polymorph B increases, extent and rate of availability also increase due to increase in rate of dissolution. But since polymorph B is less stable, the less soluble polymorphic form A is used in formulations.	108
Diclofenac	Complexation (with cyclodextrin)	Time for dissolving 50% of drug is decreased. Dissolution efficiency of complex is 40.31 as compared to 1.21 of drug alone.	115
Triamterene	Complexation (with cyclodextrin)	95% of drug dissolves in 2 h, whereas complexed drug dissolves within 10 min.	116

appropriate medium in order to discern the effect of factors other than the inherent characteristics of the drug molecule.

15.2.2 Process Variables

Granulation Procedure

Wet/Dry Granulation   The type of granulation process can influence the dissolution rate of tablets [117]. A wet granulation process imparts hydrophilic properties to granules and hence is known to improve the dissolution rate of poorly soluble drugs [118]. Tablets of cephalexin formulated by a dry granulation process exhibited slower dissolution than those formulated by using a wet granulation technique. This was attributed to slow penetration of dissolution medium into tablets prepared by dry granulation [94]. On the other hand, dissolution of naproxen sodium tablets was fastest when they were manufactured by a direct compression method. The exothermic reaction during wet granulation produced the hydrate form of naproxen, which dissolved at a slower rate [119].

HPMC swells in contact with dissolution medium [120, 121] and forms a thick gel, which in turn may decrease the pore size and hence reduce drug release. However, in the presence of PVP (highly water-soluble additive) tablets prepared by wet granulation may undergo faster dissolution due to contact of the dissolution medium inside the swollen HPMC [94]. The dissolution rate of ticlopidine hydrochloride was improved by incorporating cornstarch in wet granulated tablets as compared to dry granulation. This could be attributed to better bonding and better homogeneity of starch disintegrant within the tablets [122]. Phenylpropanolamine tablets prepared with different granulation techniques resulted in different dissolution profiles. Partial melt and melt granulated tablets resulted in slower drug release than that obtained after dry blending or wet grinding. This was perhaps due to formation of different matrix structures from different methods. Furthermore, insufficient heat generated during compression does not seem enough to melt the wax and does not form internal structure similar to that produced in melt granulated and partial melt granulated tablets [123]. Faster dissolution of phenobarbital sodium was obtained from tablets prepared by compression with Avicel than that from tablets prepared by wet granulation with gelatin [124]. Tablets prepared by wet granulation using ethyl cellulose and lactose, acacia mucilage and lactose, or starch paste and lactose released the drug in the order: acacia mucilage and lactose = starch paste and lactose > acacia mucilage and lactose [117]. Therefore, the type of additive seems to play an important role in influencing drug dissolution besides the method of granulation.

Granulating Solvent   Ghorab and Adeyeye [125] granulated ibuprofen with β-cyclodextrin using water, ethanol (95%), and isopropanol as the granulating solvents. Isopropanol and water, as granulating solvents, enhanced the dissolution of the oven-dried batches more than ethanol [125].

Drying Process   A significant effect on particle size as well as on release rate of ibuprofen from microspheres was observed when the cooling time from 65 °C to room temperature was varied between 2 min and 100 min. The drug release was maximum when drying was rapid. Granules prepared by a faster cooling process seemed to be more porous and had a less smooth surface [126].

Granule Size   Granule size is not of considerable importance while studying dissolution rate of a drug, especially when the granules are softer [127, 128]. The effects of granule size and concentration of magnesium stearate as lubricant on the dissolution rate of paracetamol tablets were studied. The results obtained show that dissolution rate was increased as the granule size of the tablet was increased for tablets prepared with 1.5% magnesium stearate as lubricant. However, tablets prepared with different granule size exhibited no pronounced effect on the dissolution characteristics when the concentration of magnesium stearate used was 0.75% [129].

Mixing   Some physical interactions between drug and excipient can take place during the dry blending phase of powders/granules. Blending with lubricants/glidants/antiadherents results in their absorption on particle surfaces, thereby increasing the hydrophobicity of drug particles. This decreases drug dissolution [2]. The dissolution rate of prednisolone was found to depend on the length of time for which ingredients were mixed with magnesium stearate [130].

Compression Force   The relationships between compression force and dissolution can be of four types:

1. Dissolution rate is increased as compression force is increased (e.g., use of starch paste as granulating agent).
2. Dissolution is slowed as the compressional force is increased (e.g., use of methylcellulose as granulating agent).
3. Dissolution rate is faster as compression force is increased to a maximum value. After this, the dissolution rate decreases with increase in compression force (e.g., use of gelatin solution as granulating agent).
4. Dissolution rate is slowed down as compression force is increased. However, further increase in compression pressure leads to an increase in dissolution rate [131].

Generally, an increase in compression force should decrease the bonding of particles because of crushing or cleavage of particles that in turn may increase the dissolution rate. Investigations on spironolactone tablets employed a granulated mixture of calcium carbonate and starch. The effect of manufacturing variables like compression force, crushing strength, or friability was studied by using tablets having the same composition but prepared under different conditions. The tablets compressed from each mixture exhibited a significant relationship between compression force and crushing strength or friability. Tablet strength increased linearly with increase in applied pressure. However, tablets prepared from large granulates showed an increase in disintegration time with increase in compression force, whereas those prepared from smaller granulates exhibited no dependence on compression force. In addition, disintegration times were shorter for the latter type of tablets. Furthermore, tablets prepared from smaller granulates required less time to dissolve [132].

Compression alters the size of drug particles, which in turn can affect the dissolution rate [133]. In a study conducted by Ganderton et al. [134], the dissolution rate of prednisolone tablets was examined at different compressional pressures. The dissolution rate of prednisolone from tablets prepared at low pressure was less compared to tablets manufactured at high pressures. With further increase in pressure, depressed dissolution rates were observed. This could be attributed to reduced breakage of tablets compressed at low pressure and release of stress along with loss of small air bubbles leading to disruption in tablets compressed at very high pressure. However, rebonding of material in tablets compressed at very high pressure produced stronger and denser tablets, which were not readily penetrated by dissolution medium [134]. A difference in pellet density of 19% was observed after compression at different pressures. The dissolution rate for the lot with lowest density made at lowest compression was significantly greater than other lots. This could be due to "channeling" that occurs within the pellet, thereby increasing the effective dissolving surface [135]. A study conducted by Chiao and Price [93] revealed faster release of propranolol hydrochloride from compressed tablets than from uncompressed microspheres. This may be attributed to rupture of microspheres at higher compression pressure. A compression force $<200\,\text{kg/cm}^2$ to the inner core tablet influenced the release behavior of drug but a force $>200\,\text{kg/cm}^2$ delayed the lag time [136]. Hence, it could be concluded that the effect of compression pressure is dependent on the pressure range evaluated and on the properties of drug, filler, binder, and so on. Therefore, it is rather difficult to predict the effect of compression pressure on the dissolution rate. Nevertheless, compression does influence drug release and this could be evaluated in relation to the properties of other formulation components.

15.3   DISSOLUTION TEST DESIGNING

Drug dissolution testing is a fundamental part of drug product development and manufacturing and is also employed as a quality control tool to monitor batch-to-batch consistency of drug release from a product. The dissolution test has extensively been used as a test to reflect the bioavailability of a drug product in humans. The advancements made for obtaining better correlation between dissolution and systemic availability include use of different media, evaluation of entire drug release profile, use of dialysis membrane, and flow through cell.

Drug classification based on permeability as well as solubility is gaining recognition and may be extremely useful during the early stages of dissolution methodology development. Changing the dissolution medium allows for testing the dosage form under conditions similar to the gastrointestinal tract. For a commercial product, dissolution testing is primarily used (1) to confirm manufacturing and product consistency, (2) to evaluate product quality during its shelf life, (3) to assess post-approval changes, and (4) to minimize the need for bioequivalency studies [137].

While developing a dissolution test for poorly soluble compounds during the early drug development phase, the process should focus on assessing relevant physical and chemical properties and dosage form design, as these play a major role in selecting the dissolution medium and apparatus. However, the strategy for designing dissolution tests depends on availability of additional data as well.

15.3.1 Media Selection

The choice of medium depends on the purpose of dissolution test. For batch-to-batch quality testing, selection of dissolution medium is based partially on the solubility data and the dose range of drug in the product to ensure that sink conditions may be justifiable, if it is shown to be more discriminating or if it provides reliable data, which otherwise can only be obtained with the addition of surfactants. On the other hand, when a dissolution test is used for evaluating the biopharmaceutical properties of a dosage form, it is more important that the proposed biorelevant test closely simulates the gastrointestinal environment rather than necessarily producing sink conditions [138].

The dissolution characteristics of oral conventional formulations should first be evaluated using test media within the physiological pH range (pH 1.2–6.8) and between pH 1.2 and 7.5 for modified release formulations. During method development, it may be useful to measure the pH of a test medium before and after the run to observe whether the pH changes during the test. An aqueous medium without surfactants is preferred, but an aqueous medium with surfactants may be used either to increase the probability of establishing an *in vivo* relationship or to increase the drug solubility in case of low solubility compounds [139, 140]. Table 15.5 highlights this aspect because different pharmacopoeias utilize different surfactants for testing drug release. The need for surfactants as well as their type and concentration need to be justified [143, 144]. The amount of surfactant needed depends on the critical micelle concentration of surfactant and the degree to which the compound partitions into the surfactant micelles. Furthermore, the critical micelle concentration of

TABLE 15.5 Use of Different Surfactants at Various Concentrations During Dissolution Testing of Tablets [111, 141, 142]

Surfactant	Concentration	Drug Product (Tablet)	Official in
Sodium lauryl sulfate	0.5% w/v	Medroxypyrogesterone acetate	USP
	1% w/v	Megestrol	USP
	0.09% w/v	Norethindone and ethinyl estradiol	USP
	0.09% w/v	Norethindone and mestranol	USP
	0.02% w/v	Norethindone acetate	USP
	0.05% w/v	Penicillamine	USP
	0.2% w/v	Praziquantel	USP
	0.1% w/v	Spironolactone	USP
	0.1% w/v	Spironolactone and hydrochlorothiazide	USP
	4% w/v	Griseofulvin	USP, IP
	1% w/v	Carbamazepine	USP
	0.3% w/v	Estradiol	USP
	0.54% w/v	Ultramicrosize griseofulvin	USP
Polysorbate 80	5 ppm in water	Levonorgesterol and ethinyl estradiol	USP
Polysorbate 20	1% v/v	Lacidipine	BP
Sodium dodecyl sulfate	0.07% w/v	Cyproterone	BP
	1.5% w/v	Griseofulvin	BP
	0.1% w/v	Spironolactone	BP
	0.3% w/v	Nimodipine	BP

surfactant depends on the characteristics of the surfactants and the ionic strength of the dissolution medium.

Development of medium for colon-specific drug delivery systems is a great challenge. This is due to the diversity in rationale behind developing a delivery system. In addition, inadequate understanding of the colon's hydrodynamics and motility complicates the development of *in vitro* evaluation. USP dissolution methods using multiple-pH media are employed for such products [145].

Simple aqueous media such as simulated gastric fluid without pepsin (SGFsp) can be satisfactorily used for BCS-I (high solubility, high permeability) drugs. Milk as a biorelevant medium may be useful for detecting special food-formulation interactions. However, for BCS-II drugs (low solubility, high permeability), the choice of dissolution medium shall depend on the ionization behavior of the drug. For neutral BCS-II drugs, the presence of solubility enhancers seems to be necessary. However, for weakly basic BCS-II compounds, whose dissolution in stomach is of prime importance, the use of SGFsp medium seems to be important while assessing the initial dissolution. Furthermore, comparison of dissolution behavior in fluids that simulate conditions in the proximal small intestine in the fed state and also in fluids that simulates condition in the proximal small intestine in the fasted state is needed to establish the effect of meals on absorption of these drugs [146].

15.3.2 Apparatus Selection

Physical and chemical properties of a drug as well as formulation play an important role in selection of dissolution test apparatus, especially in the case of poorly soluble compounds. Sometimes, the existing dissolution apparatus may need modifications to accommodate new release mechanisms; for example, in the case of a nondisintegrating dosage form, there is a requirement of delivery orifice. On the other hand, a disintegrating delivery system faces problems as there is the requirement of transferring the dosage form (without losing any portion) to a different medium. In the case of modified release delivery systems, the challenging task is to change the medium to obtain a pH gradient or simulation of fed and fasted conditions. Both USP apparatus III (reciprocating cylinder) and apparatus IV (flow through cell) are useful when the drug release from the dosage form is to be tested in different media [111, 147, 148]. However, it is important to note that both type and purpose of using a particular dissolution apparatus are often different in USP, BP, and IP (Table 15.6). Despite these differences, each pharmacopoeia aims to closely mimic the *in vivo* conditions. Still, endeavors are needed to achieve similarity in dissolution testing apparatus for various dosage forms among different pharmacopoeias.

In addition, modifications in existing apparatus can be done depending on its applicability to the type of dosage forms. Burns et al. [149] found the modified paddle (BP type II paddle) method best for studying the dissolution release profile of floating propanolol capsules. In this apparatus paddle blades were set at the surface of the dissolution medium [149].

The surface area of a pure drug may be held constant in order to evaluate the dissolution rate. Agitation intensity is another alternative, where alteration of stationary film thickness surrounding the particles is reflected in a change in dissolution rate constant and should be carefully controlled.

TABLE 15.6 Critical Differences in Dissolution Rate Test Apparatus Used in Various Pharmacopoeias [111, 141, 142]

Dissolution Apparatus	Used for Dosage Form			Critical Differences		
	USP	BP	IP	USP	BP	IP
1	Coated tablet Uncoated tablet Delayed release Extended release	Conventional	Conventional Coated Uncoated	Basket	Basket	Paddle
2	Conventional Enteric coated Extended release	Conventional Extended release Delayed release	Conventional Coated Uncoated	Paddle	Paddle	Basket
3	Extended release Modified release dosage form Bead type	Modified release dosage form	(Not official)	Reciprocating cylinder	Flow through cell apparatus	(Not official)
4	Modified release (especially when active ingredient has limited solubility/soft gelatin, bead products, suppositories/ poorly soluble drugs)	(Not official)	(Not official)	Flow through cell apparatus	(Not official)	(Not official)
5	Transdermal	(Not official)	(Not official)	Paddle over disk	(Not official)	(Not official)
6	Transdermal	(Not official)	(Not official)	Cylinder	(Not official)	(Not official)
7	Non disintegrating modified release dosage form Transdermal	(Not official)	(Not official)	Reciprocating holder	(Not official)	(Not official)

15.3.3 Dissolution Apparatus Operating Parameters

The operating parameters of dissolution testing apparatus also need to be evaluated critically before finalizing the dissolution conditions for a drug product. These parameters include medium volume, temperature, aeration/deaeration, sinker evaluation, sampling time point specification (single point or multiple point), and agitation speed.

Volume of Dissolution Medium   Table 15.7 lists pharmacopoeial dissolution testing requirements of a few drugs representing the biopharmaceutical classification scheme (Classes I–IV).

It is evident from this table that the recommended volume of dissolution medium varies from 500 to 1000 mL. A volume of 900 mL is the most common volume, while using apparatus 1 and apparatus 2 according to USP, BP, and IP specifications. The volume can be increased to 2–4 L in special cases (e.g., in the case of low solubility compounds) and then the standard vessels are rejected and large vessels are used for conducting dissolution testing. The volume can be decreased to 100–250 mL in the case of highly potent and low dose dosage forms [150, 151]. Hence, in both cases, proper justification is required for increasing/decreasing the volume of the testing medium.

Temperature of Dissolution Medium   The standard temperature conditions for dissolution testing of conventional oral (to be swallowed) dosage forms is $37 \pm 0.5\,°C$ [111, 141, 142]. Drug solubility is temperature dependent. Hence, control of temperature during the dissolution testing is very crucial. However, for products that are intended to be dissolved/dispersed in water and then administered orally, a temperature of $17.5 \pm 2.5\,°C$ needs to be employed [111]. A comparison of dissolution profiles of HALO™ at $36.5\,°C$ and $37\,°C$ indicated a considerable decrease in release (54% after 60 min at $36.5\,°C$, 63% after 60 min at $37\,°C$). Similarly, release of propranolol was observed to be 73% at $37 \pm 0.2\,°C$ as compared to 84% at $37 \pm 0.5\,°C$ after 300 min. Therefore, proper control of temperature during dissolution testing seems to be important [149].

Aeration/Deaeration   The dissolved gas/air in the dissolution medium can influence dissolution of drug particles. Dissolved air can lead to a change in the pH of the dissolution medium. Furthermore, air bubbles may act as a barrier for dissolution if they are present on the dosage form or in the mesh of the basket. In addition, aeration can retard dissolution as it can push the particles away from the center and toward the walls of the dissolution vessel [152, 153].

Sinker Selection   USP recommends some nonreactive material wire when the dosage forms tend to float [111]. The sinker should be evaluated for its ability to maintain the dosage form at the bottom of the vessel without inhibiting drug release. Paddle apparatus tablet sinkers were used by Cappola to prevent tablets from sticking to the bottom of the dissolution vessel. Overall, dissolution for all tablets with sinkers showed more rapid and complete drug release than tablets without sinkers [154].

TABLE 15.7   Pharmacopoeial Dissolution Requirements of a Few Drug Products Belonging to the Biopharmaceutical Classification Scheme (Classes I–IV)

Drug product	Pharmacopoeial Requirements		
	USP	BP	IP
		BCS Class I	
Aspirin (acetyl salicylic acid)	0.05 M acetate buffer (pH 4.5), 500 mL, apparatus 1 (50 rpm), NLT 80% of Q^a dissolved in 30 min.	Acetate buffer (pH 4.5), apparatus 1 (50 rpm), NLT 70% of Q dissolved in 45 min.	Not recommended.
Aspirin tablet (delayed release)	Apparatus 1 (100 rpm), 90 min (buffer stage).	0.1 N HCl, 1000 mL, apparatus 1 (100 rpm), NLT 5% of Q in 2 h; mixed phosphate buffer (pH 6.8), 900 mL, NLT 70% of Q in 45 min.	Not recommended.
Digoxin tablet	0.1 N HCl, 500 mL, apparatus 1 (120 rpm), NLT 805 of Q dissolved in 60 min (average of 12 tablets has LT 75% of Q in 60 min). If amount dissolved in 60 min is MT 95% for any individual tablet, amount dissolved in 15 min is NMT 90% for each tablet.	Water, 600 mL, 120 rpm, basket apparatus, NLT 75% of Q is dissolved in 60 min.	Water, 600 mL, 120 rpm, basket apparatus, NLT 75% of Q is dissolved in 60 min.
Prednisolone tablet	Water, 900 mL, apparatus 2 (50 rpm), NLT 70% of Q is dissolved in 30 min.	Water, 900 mL, apparatus 2 (50 rpm), NLT 70% of Q is dissolved in 45 min.	Water, 900 mL, paddle (50 rpm), NLT 70% of Q is dissolved in 30 min.
Quinine SO$_4$ tablet	0.1 N HCl, 900 mL, apparatus 1 (100 rpm), NLT 85% of Q is dissolved in 30 min.	0.1 N HCl, 900 mL, basket apparatus (100 rpm), NLT 70% of Q is dissolved in 45 min.	0.1 N HCl, 900 mL, apparatus 2 (100 rpm), NLT 70% of Q is dissolved in 30 min.
Quinine SO$_4$ ER tablet	0.1 N HCl (900 mL), apparatus 1 (100 rpm) 20–50% dissolved in 0.125 D h; 43–73% dissolved in 0.5 D hNLT 70% dissolved in 1.5 D h	Not recommended.	Not recommended.
Quinine BiSO$_4$ ER tablet	Not recommended.	0.1 N HCl (900 mL), basket (100 rpm), NLT 70% of Q is dissolved in 45 min.	Not recommended.
Warfarin (sodium) tablet	Water, 900 mL, apparatus 2 (50 rpm), NLT 80% of Q is dissolved in 30 min.	0.68% w/v potassium dihydrogen orthophosphate (pH 6.8), 900 mL, basket (100 rpm), NLT 70% of Q is dissolved in 45 min.	0.68% w/v potassium dihydrogen orthophosphate (pH 6.8), 900 mL, paddle (100 rpm), NLT 70% of Q is dissolved in specific time.

TABLE 15.7 *Continued*

Drug product	Pharmacopoeial Requirements		
	USP	BP	IP
Levodopa tablet	0.1 N HCl, 900 mL, apparatus 1 (100 rpm), NLT 75% of Q is dissolved in 30 min.	0.1 N HCl, 900 mL, apparatus 1 (100 rpm), NLT 70% of Q is dissolved in 45 min.	0.1 N HCl, 900 mL, apparatus 2 (75 rpm), NLT 75% of Q is dissolved in 30 min.
Lithium carbonate tablet	Water, 900 mL, apparatus 1 (100 rpm), NLT 60% of Q is dissolved in 30 min.	Not recommended.	Water, 900 mL, paddle (100 rpm), NLT 60% of Q is dissolved in 30 min.
Paracetamol tablet	Not recommended.	Phosphate buffer (pH 5.8), 900 mL, apparatus 2 (50 rpm), NLT 70% of Q is dissolved in 45 min.	Phosphate buffer (pH 7.6), 900 mL, paddle (50 rpm), NLT 80% of Q is dissolved in 30 min.
Diazepam tablet	0.1 N HCl, 900 mL, apparatus 1 (100 rpm), NLT 85% of Q is dissolved in 30 min.	0.1 N HCl (900 ml), apparatus 1 (100 rpm), NLT 70% of Q is dissolved in 45 min.	Water (900 mL), paddle apparatus (100 rpm), NLT 85% of Q is dissolved in 45 min.
Theophylline tablet	Water, 900 mL, apparatus 2 (50 rpm), NLT 80% of Q is dissolved in 45 min.	Not recommended.	Not recommended.
BCS Class II			
Griseofulvin tablet	Water, 4% sodium lauryl sulfate (SLS), 1000 mL, apparatus 2 (100 rpm), NLT 70% of Q is dissolved in 60 min.	Water, 1.5% sodium dodecyl sulfate, 1000 mL, apparatus 2 (100 rpm), NLT 70% of Q is dissolved in 45 min.	Water, 4% SLS, 900 mL, paddle apparatus (100 rpm), NLT 70% of Q is dissolved in 60 min.
Dapsone tablet	Dilute HCl (2 in 100), 1000 mL, apparatus 1 (100 rpm), NLT 70% of Q is dissolved in 60 min.	0.1 M HCl, 900 mL, apparatus 1 (100 rpm), NLT 70% of Q is dissolved in 45 min.	2% v/v HCl, 900 mL, paddle apparatus (100 rpm), NLT 70% of Q is dissolved in 60 min.
Ibuprofen	Phosphate buffer (pH 7.2), 900 mL, apparatus 1 (150 rpm), NLT 75% of Q is dissolved in 30 min.	Not recommended.	Phosphate buffer (pH 7.2), 900 mL, paddle apparatus (100 rpm), NLT 50% of Q is dissolved in 30 min.
Naproxen tablet	Phosphate buffer (pH 7.4), 900 mL, apparatus 2 (50 rpm), NLT 80% of Q is dissolved in 45 min.	Phosphate buffer (pH 7.4), 900 mL, apparatus 2 (50 rpm), NLT 70% of Q is dissolved in 45 min.	Not recommended.
Naproxen enteric coated	Not recommended.	0.1 N HCl, 900 mL, apparatus 2 (50 rpm), 2h in acid stage, NLT 5% in acid stage. Buffer stage: 900 mL, 45 min, NLT 70% of Q in buffer stage.	Not recommended.

Trimethoprim	0.01N HCl, 900mL, apparatus 2 (50rpm), NLT 75% of Q is dissolved in 45min.	Not recommended.	Not recommended.
		BCS Class III	
Acyclovir tablet	Not recommended	0.1M HCl, 900ml, apparatus 2 (50rpm), NLT 70% of Q is dissolved in 45min.	Not recommended.
Chlorpromazine HCl tablet	0.1N HCl, 900mL, apparatus 1 (50rpm), NLT 80% of Q is dissolved in 30min.	0.1M HCl, 900mL, apparatus 2 (50rpm), NLT 70% of Q is dissolved in 45min.	Not recommended.
Rythromycin stearate tablet	Phosphate buffer 0.05M (pH 6.8), 900mL, apparatus 2 (100rpm), NLT 75% of Q is dissolved in 120min.	2.722% Sodium acetate (pH 5.0), 900mL, apparatus 2 (50rpm), NLT 70% of Q is dissolved in 45min.	Not recommended.
Hydrochlorothiazide tablet	0.1N HCl, 900mL, apparatus 1 (100rpm), NLT 60% of Q is dissolved in 60min.	Not recommended.	0.1M HCl, 900mL, paddle apparatus (100rpm), NLT 60% of Q is dissolved in 45min.
		BCS Class IV	
Acetazolamide tablet	0.1N HCl, 900mL, apparatus 1 (100rpm), NLT 75% of Q is dissolved in 60min.	Not recommended.	Not recommended.
Cefixime tablet	Potassium phosphate buffer 0.05M (pH 7.2) 900mL, apparatus 1 (100rpm), NLT 75% of Q is dissolved in 45min.	Not recommended.	Not recommended.
Furosemide	Phosphate buffer (pH 5.8), 900mL, apparatus 2 (50rpm), NLT 80% of Q is dissolved in 60min.	Phosphate buffer (pH 5.8), 900mL, apparatus 2 (50rpm), NLT 80% of Q is dissolved in 45min.	Not recommended.
Hydralazine tablet	0.1N HCl, 900mL, apparatus 1 (100rpm), NLT 60 % of Q is dissolved in 30min.	Not recommended.	Not recommended.
Sulfasalazine tablet	Phosphate buffer (pH 7.5), 900mL, apparatus 1 (100rpm), NLT 85% of Q is dissolved in 60min.	Not recommended.	Not recommended.

Q, stated/labeled amount.

Sampling Time Point Specification   Sampling at early time points is used to show that there is little/no probability of dose dumping/accumulation. Drug release during the initial period should not be more than the specified amount. An intermediate time point is chosen to evaluate the *in vitro* drug release profile. Lastly, the final time point is used to explain almost complete release of drug from the respective dosage form. In the case of products with more than one active ingredient, drug release is determined at different time intervals for different active ingredients of the drug product [152]. Single point sampling during dissolution does not yield an estimate of the dissolution pattern of drug from a dosage form. Table 15.8 summarizes a few important drug products that are required to undergo single/multiple time point sampling. It is evident that multiple sampling assumes more importance while testing a modified release dosage form because it becomes essential to evaluate the entire dissolution profile rather than only the extent of drug dissolved.

Rotational Speed   Variation in the amount of drug dissolved can be due to variation of the hydrodynamics in the vicinity of a tablet. Fluctuations in flow can affect shearing of the tablet surface, deagglomeration of particles, mass transfer from solid to liquid, and mixing of tablet fragments and thus eventually influencing the hydrodynamics. The literature reveals that a change in rotational speed can alter the dissolution rate [28, 155]. Kukura et al. [156] showed that increasing the stirring from 50 to 100 rpm increased the intensity of shear force exerted by the fluid but did not improve the homogeneity of the spatial distribution of shear. Dissolution testing of carbamazepine tablets using the paddle method in hydroalcoholic medium was conducted at 100 rpm and 75 rpm. The results showed a decrease in the amount of carbamazepine dissolved at lower rotation speed [157]. An increase in rate and extent of ranitidine dissolved was observed along with less individual tablet variability when the basket method at 30 rpm was used instead of the paddle method at 500 rpm [154].

Altered Dissolution Environment   To study the impact of slight variations in vessel dimensions, a metal strip was placed to simulate altered dissolution environment. During testing, the metal strip is expected to force the product/product-deaggregates to remain off center, resulting in a large surface area for dissolution. In addition, the contact of dissolution fluid with product should also increase as the distance from the center increases. However, results with or without a metal strip were observed to be dependent, which could be due to product sensitivity to the density of disintegrated particles or gradual change in available surface of the dissolution vessel. Nondisintegrating tablets showed higher dissolution than disintegrating tablets with a metal strip in place due to production and settling of denser particles at the bottom [158]. Hence, slight modifications in the dimensions/shape of dissolution vessels do not seem to exert a remarkable influence on drug release rate provided there is no appreciable change in the hydrodynamics inside the vessel.

Viscosity of Medium   Dissolution rate decreases with an increase in the viscosity of the dissolution medium especially when the dissolution process is diffusion controlled [159].

TABLE 15.8 A Few Examples of Single Point and Multiple Point Correlation

Drug Product	Dissolution Condition	Recommended Units Sampling			Official in
Aspirin tablet	0.05 M acetate buffer, 500 mL, pH 4.5, apparatus 1, 50 rpm, 30 min.	NLT 80% of Q is dissolved in 30 min.			USP
Buffered aspirin tablet	0.05 M acetate buffer, 500 mL, pH 4.5, apparatus 2, 75 rpm, 30 min.	NLT 80% of Q is dissolved in 30 min.			USP
Aspirin ER tablet	Test 1: 0.1 N HCl, 900 mL, apparatus 2, 60 rpm, time 1 h; 4 h.	Tolerance time	Amount dissolved		USP
		1 h	20–55%		
		4 h	NLT 80%		
Diazepam capsule	0.1 N HCl, 900 mL, apparatus 1, 100 rpm, time 45 min.	NLT 85% of Q is dissolved in 45 min.			USP
Diazepam ER capsule	Simulated gastric fluid TS (without enzymes), 900 mL, apparatus 1, 100 rpm, 0.042 D h, 0.167 D h, 0.333 D h, 0.5 D h.	Time (h)	Amount dissolved		USP
		0.042 D	15–27%		
		0.167 D	49–66%		
		0.333 D	76–96%		
		0.5 D	85–115%		
Methylphenidate HCl tablet	Water, 900 mL, apparatus 1, 100 rpm, 45 min.	NLT 755 of Q is dissolved in 45 min.			USP
Methylphenidate HCl ER tablet	Water, 500 mL, apparatus 2, 50 rpm 0.125 D h, 0.25 D h, 0.438 D h, 0.625 D h, 0.875 D h.	Time (h)	Amount dissolved		
		0.125	20% and 50%		
		0.25	35% and 70%		
		0.438	53% and 83%		
		0.625	70% and 95%		
		0.875	NLT 80% amount dissolved		

TABLE 15.8 *Continued*

Drug Product	Dissolution Condition	Recommended Units Sampling	Official in
Oxprenolol HCl tablet	0.1 N HCl, 900 mL, apparatus 1, 100 rpm, 30 min.	NLT 80% of Q is dissolved in 30 min.	USP
Oxprenolol HCl ER tablet	Acid medium (0.1 N HCl), 900 mL. Dissolution medium (simulated intestinal fluid Ts: without enzyme), 900 mL, apparatus 1, 100 rpm, 1 h in acid.	Time — Amount dissolved 1 (acid medium) — Between 15% and 45% 1 (dissolution medium) — Between 30% and 60% 3 (dissolution medium) — Between 50% and 80% 7 (dissolution medium) — NLT 75%	USP
Procainamide HCl tablet	0.1 N HCl, 900 mL, apparatus 1, 100 rpm, 75 min.	NLT 80% of Q in 75 min.	USP
Procainamide HCl ER tablet	Test 1: 0.1 N HCl, 900 mL, apparatus 2, 50 rpm, time 1, 4, 6 hr Test 2: acid stage (1 h), buffer stage (0.05 M, pH 7.5, PO₄ buffer), NLT 8 h Test 3: medium same as in test 2; apparatus 2, 50 rpm; time 1, 3, 6, 8 h	Time — Amount dissolved 1 — Between 30% and 60% 4 — Between 60% and 90% 6 — NLT 75% Time — Amount dissolved 1 — Between 30% and 60% 4 — Between 60% and 90% 8 — NLT 80% Time — Amount dissolved 1 — Between 25% and 50% 3 — Between 40% and 75% 6 — Between 65% and 90% 8 — NLT 80%	USP

Ionic Strength   Ionic strength of the dissolution medium plays an important role in the dissolution process [160]. Dissolution behavior of extended release dosage forms that use hydrophilic gel forming polymers seems to be significantly affected by small changes in the ionic strength of the dissolution medium. Certain ionic salts and drugs are reported to cause failure of HPMC based extended release products [161]. HPMC based extended release diclofenac sodium tablets had significantly different release profiles in dissolution media of the same pH but different ionic strengths. The dissolution rate of theophylline from extended release granules prepared using HPMC as a retarding agent was observed to increase with increasing ionic strength of the dissolution medium whereas an initial decrease followed by an increase in the dissolution rate of theophylline was observed from commercially available extended release matrix tablet formulation with an increase in the ionic strength of the dissolution medium [162, 163]. Alterations in dissolution profiles may be due to changes in thermal gelation point (critical temperature that determines the sol to gel transition of polymers in aqueous media) of the polymers [161], increased surface erosion leading to dissolution of polymer chains, increased osmotic pressure [161, 162], and/or lower polymer solubility [164].

pH of Medium   pH of the dissolution medium influences solubility of the drug. In addition, it can affect the solubility/stability of the excipients. Both factors may produce an entirely different dissolution profile if the pH of the dissolution medium is not selected carefully. Furosemide tablets were observed to dissolve faster as the pH of the medium was increased. The tablet brand that dissolved poorly at pH 4.6 also exhibited poor bioavailability [165]. The intrinsic dissolution rate of piroxicam increased with an increase in pH of the medium [144]. Thus, careful selection of pH and buffers composing the dissolution medium seems to be essential for *in vitro* dissolution studies as well as for prediction of bioavailability.

15.4   ANALYSIS OF DISSOLUTION DATA

Whenever a new solid dosage form is developed or produced, it is necessary to ensure that drug dissolution occurs in an appropriate manner. In addition, for a pharmaceutical company to obtain approval for a generic product, there are a series of criteria that must be addressed to demonstrate that the product is bioequivalent to a proprietary counterpart. Under certain conditions, one of these criteria is to demonstrate that the dissolution curves of the two products are similar. The *in vivo* bioavailability study investigates the rate and extent of drug absorption in humans. The fact that drug absorption depends on the dissolved state of the drug has encouraged pharmaceutical companies to explore the relationship between *in vivo* drug bioavailability and *in vitro* dissolution. It has been suggested that *in vitro* dissolution testing can be used as a surrogate for *in vivo* bioequivalence studies to assess equivalence between the test and reference formulations, and for postapproval changes. If dissolution profile similarity is demonstrated for the formulations before and after the changes, then expensive *in vivo* bioequivalence testing can be waived off. Various procedures have been proposed to compare dissolution profile data (Fig. 15.4). The utility of these methods is briefly discussed next.

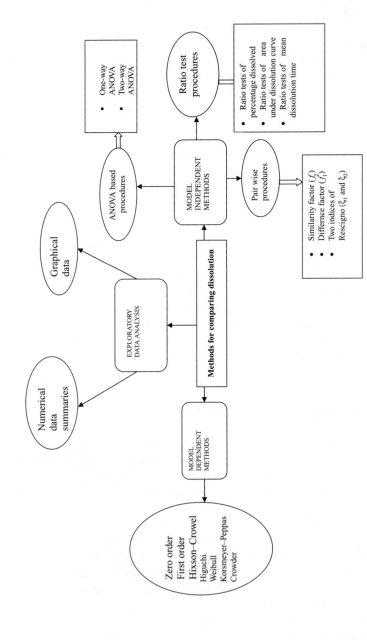

FIGURE 15.4 Various methods used for evaluating dissolution data.

Exploratory Data Analysis   As a first step, it is useful to perform exploratory data analysis to compare dissolution profile data. The U.S. FDA does not currently endorse these methods. In this method the dissolution profile data are illustrated graphically by plotting mean dissolution profile data for each formulation with error bars extending to two standard errors at each dissolution time point. Then the data are summarized numerically and 95% confidence intervals are evaluated in mean dissolution profiles at each dissolution time point. This method is useful in obtaining an improved understanding of dissolution data. It can also be used as a first step to compare the dissolution profile data (in a graphical as well as numerical manner). However, the analysis of dissolution profiles becomes difficult if the error bars for two formulations overlap (graphically as well as numerically) [166, 167].

Statistical Methods (Model-Independent Methods)   Using one-way ANOVA, statistical comparisons of the mean dissolution data at each dissolution time point are performed. One-way ANOVA is equivalent to the *t*-test in the case where the dissolution profile data of two formulations is compared. This method takes the variability in the dissolution profile data into account while comparing each time point. Two-way ANOVA is used in data analysis when both formulation and time are class variables (in the case of immediate release data when one-way ANOVA is not applicable). But the major limitation is that this method ignores the correlation between the dissolution time points [168, 169].

Multivariate Approach (MANOVA) Methods   These are based on repeated measures, where time is the repeated factor and percent drug dissolved is the dependent variable. The method is more precise as it takes into account the variability as well as the correlation structure in data. However, this method may not be too informative, because it doesn't contain information about the nature of differences between mean dissolution profiles. In addition, it is difficult to implement this method tactically [170].

Chow–Ki Method   This is another statistical method, which is comparable to the approach used for assessing the average bioequivalence of two formulations. Equivalence limits for similarity at each dissolution time point are derived from Q (as defined in USP). It uses the concept of local and global similarity to assess closeness of test to reference dissolution profiles. This method is relatively easy to implement. Correlation between successive time points is accounted for by using an autoregressive time series model. Power and Type I error of this method are unknown at this stage. Type I error is the probability of concluding that the test and reference mean profiles are different when in fact they are similar. Type II error is the probability of concluding that the test and reference mean profiles are the same when they are actually different [168].

Model-Independent Method   This uses the dissolution data in their native form. Two mathematical methods are described in this method. The first is the difference factor equation, which is also called the f_1 equation, and the second is the similarity factor, also called the f_2 equation. The FDA approves both equations for dissolution profile comparison but the similarity equation is preferred.

$$f_1 = \left(\frac{\sum\limits_{t=1}^{n} |R_t - T_t|}{\sum\limits_{t=1}^{n} R_t} \right) \times 100$$

$$f_2 = 50 \log_{10} \left\{ \left(1 + \frac{1}{n} \sum_{t=1}^{n} w_t (R_t - T_t)^2 \right)^{-0.5} \times 100 \right\}$$

where n is the number of dissolution sample time points; w_t is the optional weighting factor, and R_t and T_t are the mean percent drug dissolved at each time point, respectively, for each reference and test product. Evaluation requires the use of a minimum of three time points (except zero), not less than 12 individual values for every time point for each formulation, and the standard deviation should not be more than 10% from the second to the last time point. When the calculated values of f_1 lie between 0 and 15 and those of f_2 lie above 50, the dissolution profiles are interpreted to be similar. In f_2 estimation, bias could take place due to the contribution of variances in the percentage of drug dissolved in test and reference preparations measured at a particular time point. Unbiased similarity factor (f_2^*) is calculated to determine the effect of variances of the percentage of drug dissolved from test and reference products at particular time points on f_2:

$$f_2^* = 50 \left(\log_{10} \left\{ 1 + \left(\frac{1}{n} \right) \left[\sum_{t=1}^{n} (R_t - T_t)^2 - \sum_{t=1}^{n} (S_r^2 - S_t^2)/N \right] \right\}^{-0.5} \times 100 \right)$$

where $S_r^2 - S_t^2$ is the variance in the percentage of drug dissolved measured at any time point of reference and test preparations and N is the number of units on which dissolution is conducted. By this method it is easy to compare the data. In addition, it also provides a single number to describe the comparison of dissolution profile data. However, it is not possible to know the Type I and Type II errors [171–173].

Rescigno's Indices   Rescigno's indices have been developed for comparing blood-plasma concentration functions. ξ_i and ξ_2 are considered analogous to f_1 and f_2:

$$\xi_i = \left[\frac{\int_0^{t_n} |R_t - T_t|^i \, dt}{\int_0^{t_n} |R_t + T_t|^i \, dt} \right]^{1/i}$$

where R_t and T_t are the mean percentages of drug dissolved, respectively, for reference and test formulations at each time point and t_n is the final dissolution time point. ξ_i can be thought of as a function of the weighted average of the vertical distances between test and reference mean profiles at each time point. More precisely, ξ_i is the absolute value of vertical distance and ξ_2 is the square of vertical distance.

The denominator of ξ_i is a scaling factor. The main advantage of this method is that, unlike f_1, the value of ξ_i remains unchanged if reference and test are interchanged. But this method does not take into account variability and correlation structure data like f_1 and f_2 equations, and also it is difficult to calculate Rescigno's indices. Moreover, there is no definite criterion for concluding difference or similarity data profile [174].

Korsmeyer–Peppas Model   This is a simple, semiempirical model relating exponentially the drug release to the elapsed time. This model uses the following equation for evaluation of dissolution data:

$$f_t = at^n$$

where a is a constant incorporating structural and geometric characteristics of the dosage form and n is a release exponent indicative of the drug release mechanism. This equation can be written

$$f_t = \frac{M_t}{M_\infty} \quad \text{(fractional release of drug)}$$

where M_t/M_∞ is a function of t (fractional release of drug). Modifying the above equation to accommodate lag time generates the following equation:

$$\frac{M(t-l)}{M_\infty} = a(t-l)^n$$

where l is the lag time.

In the case of a burst effect, the equation becomes

$$\frac{M_t}{M_\infty} = at^n + b$$

In the absence of lag time or burst effect, at^n is used and the resulting model, also known as the power law, has been used, very frequently, to describe the drug release from several modified release dosage forms [175, 176].

It is a simple and empirical model and describes drug release from modified release dosage forms [175, 177, 178]. This model assumes that the rate-limiting step to drug release is erosion of matrix. The time-dependent diffusional resistance to eroding matrix is hypothesized not to influence drug release [179].

Crowder Model   This is a mechanistic model. It uses repeated measures regression analysis techniques for comparing data from different formulations. It is considered superior to other modeling based approaches and takes covariance structure into account while statistically comparing the data. However, its practical utility is limited because it may be difficult to analyze the data using conventional statistical packages [180].

Baker–Lonsdale Model   This has been developed from the Higuchi model:

$$f_t = \frac{3}{2}\left[1-\left(1-\frac{M_t}{M_\infty}\right)^{2/3}\right]-\frac{M_t}{M_\infty} = Kt$$

where K is the release rate constant (slope), and M_t; and M_∞ are the amounts of drug released, respectively, at time t and infinite period. This model has been utilized for linearizing release data from several formulations of microcapsules or microspheres [181–183].

The Hopfenberg model utilizes the following equation to describe the dissolution data:

$$\frac{M_t}{M_\infty} = 1-\left(1-\frac{K_0 t}{c_0 a_0}\right)^n$$

where M_t is the amount of drug dissolved in time t; M_∞ is the total amount of drug dissolved when dosage form is exhausted; M_t/M_∞ is the fraction of dose dissolved; K_0 is the erosion rate constant; C_0 is the initial drug concentration in matrix; and A_0 is the initial radius of spheres/cylinder/half-thickness of the slab, where on A value of 1, 2, or 3 is used for a slab, a cylinder, or a sphere, respectively. This model is generally useful while studying release from surface eroding devices (slab, cylinder, sphere) [184].

Higuchi Model   Higuchi developed several theoretical models to study the release of water-soluble and poorly soluble drugs incorporated in semisolid and/or solid matrixes. Generally, a simplified equation is used for analyzing dissolution data:

$$Q_t = K_H t$$

where K_H is the Higuchi dissolution constant. This model is widely used to describe drug dissolution from modified release dosage forms [185–187].

Hixson–Crowell Model   This has been used to describe the release profile by considering the diminishing surface of the drug particles during dissolution:

$$Q_0^{1/3} - Q_t^{1/3} = K_s t$$

where K_s is the constant incorporating the surface–volume relationship; Q_0 and Q_t are, respectively, the initial amount of drug and the remaining amount of drug in the dosage form at time t. Upon simplification, the equation can be written

$$(1-f_t)^{1/3} = 1-K_\beta t$$

where $f_t = 1-(Q_t/Q_0)$, and f_t represents the rug-dissolved fraction at time t and K_β is the release constant. This model is applied to dosage forms (e.g., tablets) where the dissolution occurs in planes that are parallel to the drug surface—that is, if tablet dimensions diminish proportionally in such a way that the geometrical form remains constant all the time. The major assumption made is that the release rate is limited by the drug particles' dissolution rate and not by diffusion through the polymeric matrix [188].

Weibull Function   This is a modeling based method used for evaluating the dissolution data profiles:

$$m = 1 - \exp\left(\frac{-(t - Ti)^b}{a}\right)$$

where a defines the time scale of the process, T_i is the lag time before the onset of the dissolution or release process (in most cases zero), b is the shape parameter, m is the accumulated fraction of drug, and t is the solution time of the drug.

Upon rearranging, this equation becomes

$$\log[-\ln(1-m)] = b\log(t - T_i) - \log a$$

On the basis of this equation, the plot between log of dissolved amount of drug versus log of time will be linear for dosage forms. The main limitation of this model is the lack of a kinetic basis for its use due to the nonphysical nature of the parameters. In addition, it cannot characterize the dissolution kinetic properties of a drug. Furthermore, there is no single parameter related to the intrinsic dissolution rate of the drug. Lastly, it is of limited use for establishing *in vitro–in vivo* (IVIV) correlation [189–191].

Order of Drug Release Analysis   Zero order and first order kinetics and ratio test procedures are modeling based methods. Drug dissolution from dosage forms that do not disaggregate and release the drug slowly is characterized by zero order kinetics (assuming that area doesn't change):

$$Q_t = Q_0 + K_0 t$$

where Q_t is the amount of drug dissolved in time t, Q_0 is the initial amount of drug in solution, and K_0 is the zero order release rate constant. This method can be used to describe drug dissolution of modified release dosage forms [192, 193].

First order drug release can be represented by

$$\ln Q_t = \ln Q_0 + K_1 t$$

where K_1 is the first order release constant. This equation is modified to yield the following equation:

$$\ln Q_t = \ln Q_0 + K_1 t S$$

where S is the solid area accessible to dissolution [192].

Ratio Test Procedures   These compare dissolution profiles of two formulations at a particular time point. Ratio tests of percentage dissolved can be performed to give a 90% confidence interval for the mean ratio of percentage dissolved [194].

15.5   *IN VITRO–IN VIVO* CORRELATION

Ethical constraints make it imperative to generate pharmacological and toxicological data in laboratory animals and *in vitro* systems before human testing can begin. Two fundamental challenges faced by pharmaceutical scientists pertain to scaling up of pharmacokinetic data from animals to humans and extrapolation of the *in vitro* data to the *in vivo* situation.

15.5.1   Physiological Concerns

Drug absorption is influenced by physicochemical characteristics of the drug as well as physiological factors. While physicochemical factors are species independent, physiological factors are species dependent. Therefore, it is essential to examine the bioavailability of a drug in animals with respect to the physiological differences with human beings. Often, the knowledge of different absorption or first-pass metabolism in animals helps in reasonably extrapolating the absorption of drugs to that in human beings (Table 15.9). Furthermore, differences in the gastrointestinal physiology of monkeys and dogs with respect to human beings play a significant role in addressing the differences observed in dosage form performance (Table 15.10). It is evident from Table 15.11 that solution is emptied from the stomach within 1 h and it is only slightly influenced by feeding. t_{lag}, t_{max}, and MAT of tablet were much longer than those of solution. The gastric emptying of tablets in the fed state is delayed more than the solution dosage forms. It is noteworthy that agitation intensity in the gastrointestinal tract of monkeys is closer to that in humans than that in dogs. This leads to approximately similar gastric emptying time of solid dosage forms in monkeys and humans [207].

The rate of distribution of a drug to the organs or tissues is determined by the rate of blood flow and ease with which the drug molecules cross the capillary wall and penetrate the cells. Like most physiological parameters, blood flow and circulation time can be extrapolated across species by use of an allometric equation [210, 211]:

$$y = aw^b$$

where y is the blood flow, a is the allometric coefficient, b is the allometric exponent, and w is the body weight. The allometric relationship between blood circulation time (seconds) and total body weight is $21\,w^{0.21}$ [212].

The smaller animal species deliver drugs faster and more frequently to organs of elimination. This is expected to result in rapid elimination of drugs in smaller animals than in humans [210, 211]. Furthermore, differences in amino acid sequences and the presence of different isoforms and enzymes in different species may lead to significantly different patterns of drug metabolism (Table 15.12). Drugs and their metabolites are usually eliminated from the body via urine and bile. The relative contribution of biliary and urinary excretion to overall elimination of drugs depends

TABLE 15.9   A Few Examples of Interspecies Differences in Drug Bioavailability

Drug	Bioavailability				Remarks	References
	Dog	Rat	Monkey	Human		
Indinavir (solution)	72%	24%	19%	40–60%	Decreased bioavailability in rat and monkey due to extensive hepatic first-pass metabolism.	195
L-365,260: cholecystokinin receptor antagonist (suspension)	9%	14%	—	—	Limited bioavailability was attributed to poor absorption as a result of low aqueous solubility.	196
L-365,260: cholecystokinin receptor antagonist (solution in PEG 600)	70%	50%	—	—	Improved bioavailability due to greater amount of drug soluble in PEG 6000.	196
Melatonin (oral dose 10 mg/kg) Intraperitoneal dose	100% 74%	53.5%	100%	—	Suggested lack of substantial hepatic first-pass of melatonin in rats. However, the oral bioavailability of melatonin in dogs decreased to 16.9% following a 1 mg/kg oral dose, indicating dose-dependent bioavailability in dogs.	197

on the nature of the drugs and is significantly affected for molecules possessing molecular weight greater than 7500 kDa [220]. Many drugs are excreted unchanged by the kidneys. The rate of renal excretion depends on renal blood flow, glomerular filteration rate (GFR), tubular secretion, and reabsorption [201]. Both GFR and number of nephrons show a good allometric relationship. Like GFR, renal excretion of drugs also shows a good allometric relationship across species. Thus, the renal clearance of drugs in humans can be extrapolated from animal data by use of an allometric approach. But this approach requires at least four or five animal species in order to obtain a proper allometric relationship. An alternative to predict human renal clearance is to use the ratio of GFR between rats and humans. The ratio of renal clearance of various drugs between rats and humans is roughly equal to the ratio of GFR between these two species [221].

TABLE 15.10 Summary of Physiological Parameters that May Influence Drug Bioavailability in Different Species

Species	Biliary Excretion Rate (of Organic Chemicals)	Plasma Volume (L/kg)	Body Weight (kg)	Maximum Life Period (years)	Relative Length of Small Intestine (%)	Average Absolute Length of Small Intestine (m)	pH of Small Intestine	Transit Time	Glomerular Filteration Rate (mL/min/kg)	References
Rabbit	Relatively poor	0.0314	3.0	8.0	60	1.51	6–8	a	4.8	198–200
Pig	a	a	a	a	78	14.16–18.29	6–7.5 (fasted)	a	a	198, 199
Mouse	Good	a	0.02	2.7	a	a	a	a	10	201
Monkey	Relatively poor	0.0448	3.5	20	a	a	5.6–9 (fasted)	a	a	199, 201, 202
Dog	Good	0.0515	12.5	20	85	2.48–4.14	6.2–7.5, 4.5–7.5 (fasted)	0.5–2h	4.0	198, 199, 203, 204
Rat	Good	0.0313	0.25	4.7	64	0.82	6.5–7.1	1.5h	8.7	198, 203, 205
Human	Relatively poor	0.0436	70	93	79	6.25	6.8–8.6, 5–7 (fasted)	2.7–8.5h	1.8	198, 201, 202, 205, 206

aNot found.

TABLE 15.11 Gastric Emptying Time of Dosage Forms Under Fasted and Fed State in Animals and Humans

Type of Dosage Form	Parameter	Human		Monkeys		Dog		References
		Fasting	Fed	Fasting	Fed	Fasting	Fed	
Solution	MAT (h)	1.3 ± 0.3	2.6 ± 0.2	0.8 ± 0.4	1.8 ± 1.4	0.7 ± 0.4	1.3 ± 0.6	207, 208
	$t$lag (h)	0.1 ± 0.1	0.4 ± 0.1	0.1 ± 0.0	0.0 ± 0.0	0.2 ± 0.2	0.3 ± 0.1	
	$t$max (h)	1.0	3.0	1.0 ± 0.2	1.8 ± 1.3	1.0	1.0	
Controlled release tablet	MAT (h)	3.4 ± 0.5	6.0 ± 1.6	3.6 ± 2.0	Plasma concentration rose rapidly, $t$lag was delayed	2.1 ± 0.6	Not calculated, delayed compared to human	207, 208
	$t$lag (h)	1.7 ± 0.6	3.3 ± 0.8	2.3 ± 1.5		1.2 ± 0.5		
	$t$max (h)	2.0	6.0	3.7 ± 2.1		3.0		
Coumarin (solution)	$t$max (h)	0.2	—	0.21 ± 0.03	—	—	—	209
Rolipram (suspension)	$t$max (h)	0.38 ± 0.22	—	1.7 ± 0.9	—	—	—	209
Zomepira (solution)	$t$max (h)	0.6 ± 0.3	—	1.2 ± 0.8	—	—	—	209

TABLE 15.12 Summary of Drug Metabolizing Enzymes Present in Liver of Different Species

Species	Gender/Strain	Liver Weight	Enzyme	References
Dog	Mixed/beagle	360 g (sd = 20)	Cytochrome P450 (CYP) CYP1A1/1A2; ethoxyresorufin O-deethylation	213–216
			CYP1A2; phenacetin O-deethylation	
			CYP2A6; coumarin 7-hydroxylation	
			CYP2B6; pentoxyresorufin O-dealkylation	
			CYP2C9; phenytoin p-hydroxylation	
			CYP3A4; human 3A4 antibodies	
			CYP2E1; human 2E1 antibodies	
			CYP2C9; human 2C9 antibodies	
			CYP3A/2B; ethylmorphine N-demethylation	
Rat	Female and male/Sprague–Dawley	10.6 g (sd = 3)	Cytochrome P450 (CYP)	216
			CYP3A/2B; ethylmorphine N-demethylation	
			CYP3A4/5; nifedipine oxidation	
			CYP3A4/5; erythromycin N-demethylation	
			CYP3A4; benzphetamine N-demethylation	
			CYP2E1; aniline p-hydroxylation	
			CYP2D6; bufuralol 1-hydroxylation	
			CYP2C19; S-mephenytoin 4'-hydroxylation	
			CYP2C9; phenytoin p-hydroxylation	
			CYP2B6; pentoxyresorufin O-dealkylation	
			CYP2A6; coumarin 7-hydroxylation	
			CYP1A2; phenacetin O-deethylation	

Species	Strain/sex	Weight	Activity	References
Mouse	Mixed/ICR	Not found		217
Human	Mixed	1700 g	GST; chlorodinitrobenzene glutathione transferase Cytochrome P450 (CYP) t CYP1A1/1A2; ethoxyresorufin O-deethylation CYP1A2; phenacetin O-deethylation CYP2A6; coumarin 7-hydroxylation CYP2B6; pentoxyresorufin O-dealkylation CYP2C8/2C9; tolbutamide hydroxylation CYP2C9; phenytoin p-hydroxylation CYP2C19; S-mephenytoin 4'-hydroxylation CYP2D6; bufuralol 1'-hydroxylation CYP2E1; aniline p-hydroxylation CYP3A; chlorpromazine S-oxygenation CYP3A4; benzphetamine N-demethylation CYP3A4/5; nifedipine oxidation CYP3A/2B; ethylmorphine N-demethylation	213–216, 218
Rabbit	Mixed/New Zealand white	Not found	GST; chlorodinitrobenzene glutathione transferase GST; dichloronitrobenzene glutathione transferase GST; ethacrynic acid glutathione transferase	217, 219
Monkey	Male/cynomolgus	62.5 g	Cytochrome P450 (CYP) content CYP1A2; phenacetin O-deethylation CYP2A6; coumarin 7-hydroxylation CYP2D6; dextromethorphan O-demethylation CYP2E1; chlozoxazone 6-hydroxylation CYP2E1; ethoxycoumarin O-deethylation	213

15.5.2   Correlation

The development and subsequent validation of an *in vitro–in vivo* correlation (IVIVC) is an increasingly important component of dosage form optimization. An IVIVC is a relationship (preferably linear) between a biological parameter (C_{max}, t_{max}, or AUC) produced by a dosage form and an *in vitro* characteristic (e.g., *in vitro* dissolution data). The IVIVC guidance developed by the U.S. FDA states that the main objective of developing and evaluating an IVIVC is to enable the dissolution test to serve as a surrogate for *in vivo* bioavailability studies. An IVIVC has been defined as "a predictive mathematical model describing the relationship between an *in vitro* property of a dosage form and an *in vivo* response." Generally, rate or extent of drug dissolution is the *in vitro* property while plasma drug concentration/amount of drug absorbed is the *in vivo* property.

The development of correlation usually involves three steps: (1) formulation development with different release rates, (2) obtaining *in vitro* dissolution profiles and *in vivo* plasma concentration profiles for these formulations, and (3) estimation of *in vivo* absorption or *in vitro* dissolution time course using an appropriate technique for each formulation.

Level A correlations are the most common type of correlation submitted to the FDA. It is usually estimated by a two-stage procedure comprising deconvolution followed by comparison of the fraction of drug absorbed to the fraction of drug dissolved. A correlation of this type is generally linear and represents a point-to-point relationship between the *in vitro* and *in vivo* input rate. In a linear correlation, the *in vitro* and *in vivo* data curves are superimposable or may be made superimposable with the help of a scaling factor. One of the alternative approaches to develop Level A correlation is a convolution procedure that models the relationship between *in vitro* dissolution and plasma concentration in a single step.

Level B correlation uses the principles of statistical moment analysis. The mean *in vitro* dissolution time is compared to either the mean residence time or the mean *in vivo* dissolution time. It also uses all of the *in vitro* and *in vivo* data, but it is not considered to be a point-to-point correlation. Level B correlation does not reflect the actual *in vivo* plasma level curve.

Level C correlation establishes a single point relationship between a dissolution parameter like t_{50} and a pharmacokinetic parameter like AUC. It does not reflect the complete shape of the plasma concentration time curve, which is an essential factor.

Multiple Level C correlates one or several pharmacokinetic parameters ofinterest to the amount of drug dissolved at several time points of the dissolution profile [222, 223].

The USP recognizes these levels of IVIVC. However, the applicability of IVIVC depends on the inherent permeability of the molecules across the gastrointestinal membrane. Table 15.13 summarizes the possibility of IVIVC for immediate as well as extended release oral products on the basis of the biopharmaceutical classification scheme (BCS).

A successful IVIVC utilizes (1) *in vitro* values to evaluate different batches of a pharmaceutical product as a quality control check to ensure the desired physiologic performance, and (2) *in vitro* values as a tool for developing a series of dosage forms to obtain a desired *in vivo* performance. These objectives can only be fulfilled if a

TABLE 15.13   Possibility of IVIVC of IR and ER Dosage Forms According to BCS [223]

Type of Formulation	Class	Solubility	Permeability	IVIVC (Possible/ Not Possible)
Immediate release (IR)	I	High	High	May not be possible
	II	Low	High	May not be possible
	III	High	Low	May not be possible
	IV	Low	Low	May be possible
Extended release (ER)	Ia	High + site dependent	High + site dependent	Level A
	Ib	High + site dependent	Site dependent with narrow absorption window	Level C
	IIa	Low + site dependent	High + site dependent	Level A
	IIb	Low + site dependent	Site dependent with narrow absorption window	May not be possible
	Va	Variable	Variable	May not be possible
	Vb	Variable	Variable	Level A

relationship between *in vitro* and *in vivo* parameters is confirmed. The approaches for IVIVC are summarized in Fig. 15.5.

IVIVCs can be divided into nonquantitative and quantitative correlations. In the case of nonquantitative correlations, the two variables are not related to each other mathematically as observed in rank order correlation (not popular now) [224–226]. In the case of quantitative correlations, the variables correlate with each other through a linear or nonlinear equation. A quantitative correlation can be established by using well known estimated values of important *in vitro* dissolution processes and *in vivo* parameters; for instance, amount dissolved at a specific time point can be correlated with fraction absorbed or absorption rate constant. These correlations can be categorized as single point correlations/or multiple point correlations.

Single point correlations are not very informative and sometimes they are not easy to apply practically [227, 228]. On the other hand, point-to-point or multiple point correlations are informative and are established in two ways. In the first case, a relationship is established between the actual time course of the *in vitro* dissolution and the time course of dissolution in the lumen or arrival in the general circulation, which is estimated by using a deconvolution method (observed concentration in the bloodstream versus time profile). In the second case, the relationship between actual plasma concentrations versus time profile is evaluated. In both cases, there is a requirement of intravenous or oral solution data or in the case of extended release product of high solubility, oral data from immediate release solid dosage form is required. In the case of multiple point correlation, *in vitro* dissolution

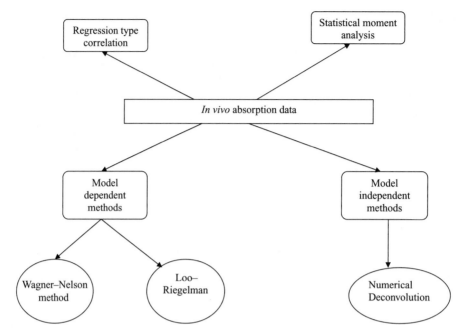

FIGURE 15.5   Approaches for *in vivo* data analysis.

datasets must be compared with each other at the time of evaluation as well as application [222, 229]. In addition to the well recognized methods of IVIVC, a few useful methods are summarized in Table 15.14.

15.5.3 Biowaivers for Changes in the Manufacture of a Drug Product

1. *Biowaivers Without an IVIVC.* For formulations consisting of beads in capsules, with the only difference between strengths being the number of beads, approval of lower strengths without an IVIVC is possible, provided bioavailability data are available for the highest strength.

2. *Biowaivers Using an IVIVC.* Nonnarrow therapeutic Index Drugs: If an IVIVC is developed with the highest strength, any lower strengths may be granted approval if these strengths are proportional or qualitatively the same. Furthermore, the *in vitro* dissolution profiles of all strengths should be similar, and all strengths should have the same release mechanisms. In addition, changes in release controlling excipients in the formulations should be within the range of release controlling excipients of established correlations.

3. *Biowaivers Using an IVIVC.* Narrow therapeutic Index Drugs: If external predictability of IVIVC is established, following waivers are likely to be granted, if the release rate of at least two formulations have been studied for IVIVC development. If an IVIVC is developed with the highest strength, any lower strength may be granted approval if the strengths are proportional or qualitatively the same. Furthermore, the *in vitro* dissolution profiles of all strengths should be similar and

TABLE 15.14 A Few Methods of IVIVC with Respect to Time Profile

Correlation Method	Remarks	References
Characterization of time profile		
Distribution functions (e.g., Weibull function)	Represented by *in vitro* and *in vivo* time profiles, for example, (a) *in vitro* release profile corresponds to distribution of drug released at time *t* and the corresponding probability distribution function profile characterizes the release rate; (b) plasma concentration profile represents drug distribution in plasma at any time and its cumulative distribution function represents the drug absorbed and already eliminated.	230–232
Semi-invariants (moments)	Area (K_0), mean (K_1), variance (K_2), skewness (K_3), and kurtosis (K_4) are semi-invariants. All semi-invariants are defined in terms of integrals of time profile between $t = 0$ and $t = \infty$. Variance, skewness, and kurtosis are called higher rate semi-invariants.	230–232
Comparison of time profiles		
General aspects	Model-independent techniques compare data pairs observed at corresponding time values, where time is only a class effect (e.g., paired *t*-test, ANOVA). Model-dependent techniques are better as they assume that observed data pairs belong to a general distribution function.	230–232
Model-dependent/-independent comparison		
Horizontal/vertical comparison	Vertical comparison represents the value obtained at a given time (i.e., extent characteristics of the process) and horizontal comparison represents the time required to reach a certain ordinate value (i.e., rate aspect of process).	230–232
Comparison by semi-invariants	For the comparison of two differential plasma concentration profiles the index of bioequivalence is used (discussed in data analysis).	230–232
Rescigno's indices (ξ_1 and ξ_2)		
Model-independent indices		230–232
Moore–flanner index (f_1)	$$f_1 = \frac{\sum |R - T|}{\sum R}$$	
Moore–flanner index (f_2)	$$f_2 = 50\log\left\{\frac{100}{\left(\sqrt{1 + \sum(R^\wedge - T^\wedge)2}\right)/N}\right\}$$	
Statistical consideration	Statistical comparisons are performed in terms of dissimilarity rather than similarity. If computed statistics or indices exceed a predefined decision limit, both samples are considered as different.	230–232
Decision intervals and limits	The Chow–Ki model, multivariate aspects, and bootstrap techniques are used.	

531

all strengths should have the same release mechanism. Biowaiver for the approval of new strengths is applicable to strengths lower than the highest strength, within the dosing range that has been established to be safe and effective, provided that the new strengths are proportional or qualitatively the same, have the same release mechanisms, have similar *in vitro* dissolution profiles, and are manufactured using the same type of equipment and the same process at the same site as other strengths that have bioavailability data available. The generic products can also qualify for this biowaiver (a) if bioequivalence has been established for all strengths of reference listed products, (b) if dose proportionality has been established for reference listed products, and (c) if bioequivalence is established between the generic product and reference listed products and all strengths are compositionally proportional or qualitatively the same and have a similar release mechanism as well as *in vitro* dissolution profiles.

4. *Biowaivers When in Vitro Dissolution Is Independent of Dissolution Test Conditions.* Narrow and nonnarrow therapeutic Index Drugs: Biowaivers may be granted if dissolution data are submitted in compendial medium and in three other media (water, 0.1 N HCl, USP buffer pH 6.8). In addition, if *in vitro* dissolution should be shown to be independent of dissolution test conditions after change is made in drug product manufacturing, biowaivers may be granted.

5. *Situations for Which IVIVC Is Not Recommended.* IVIVC is not recommended (a) for approval of a new formulation (extended release) of an approved drug product when the new formulation has a different release mechanism, (b) for approval of a dosage strength higher/lower than doses that have been shown to be safe and effective in clinical trials, (c) for approval of another sponsor's product, even with the same release controlling mechanism, and (d) for approval of a formulation change involving a nonrelease controlling excipient in the drug product that may significantly affect drug absorption [222, 233, 234].

REFERENCES

1. Czeisler JL, Perlman KP. *Encyclopedia of Pharmaceutical Technology*, Volume 4. New York: Marcel Dekker; 1991, pp 40–52.

2. Scolk KGV, Zogiio M, Carstensen JT. *Pharmaceutical Dosage Forms: Tablets*, Volume I. New York: Marcel Dekker; 1980, pp 73–105.

3. Shah MA, Wilson RG. Some effects of humidity and heat on the tableting properties of microcrystalline cellulose formulations. I. *J Pharm Sci* 1968;57:181–182.

4. Brownley CA, Lachman L. Browning of spray-processed lactose. *J Pharm Sci* 1964;53:452–454.

5. Van Kamp HV, Bolhuis GK, Kussendrager KD, Lerk CF. Studies on tableting properties of lactose. IV. Dissolution and disintegration properties of different types of crystalline lactose. *Int J Pharm* 1986;28:229–238.

6. Shangraw RF. Direct compression tableting. In *Encyclopedia of Pharmaceutical Technology*, Volume 4 2nd ed. New York: Marcel Dekker; 1980, pp 85–160.

7. Lerk CF. Consolidation and compaction of lactose. *Drug Dev Ind Pharm* 1993;19:2359–2398.

8. Roberts RJ, Rowe RC. Effect of punch velocity on the compaction of a variety of materials. *J Pharm Pharmacol* 1985;37:377–384.

9. Fell JT, Newton JM. The tensile strength of tablets. *J Pharm Sci* 1968;20:657–658.

10. Gohel MC, Patel LD, Amin AF, Jogani PD, Bajaj SB, Patel GJ. Studies in improvement of flow and compressional characteristics of lactose. *Int J Pharm Excipients* 1999;1: 86–92.

11. Gohel MC, Jogani PD. Functionality testing of a multifunctional directly compressible adjuvant containing lactose, polyvinyl pyrrolidone, and croscarmellose sodium. *Pharm Technol* 2002;25:64–82.

12. Wong DY, Wright P, Aulton ME. Deformation of alpha-lactose monohydrate and anhydrous alpha-lactose monocrystals. *Drug Dev Ind Pharm* 1988;14:2109–2126.

13. Shukla AJ, Price JC. Effect of moisture content on compression properties of directly compressible high beta-content anhydrous lactose. *Drug Dev Ind Pharm* 1991; 17:2067–2081.

14. Alpar O, Hersey JA, Shotton E. The compression properties of lactose. *J Pharm Pharmacol* 1970;22:1S–7S.

15. Bolhuis GK, Lerk CF. Comparative evaluation of excipients for direct compression. Part 1. *Pharma Weekb* 1973;108:469–481.

16. Vromans H, Bolhuis GK, Lerk CF, Kussendrager KD. Studies on tableting properties of lactose. VIII. The effect of variations in primary particle size, percentage of amorphous lactose and addition of a disintegrant on the disintegration of spray-dried lactose tablets. *Int J Pharm* 1987;39:201–206.

17. Bolhuis GK, Zuurman K. Tableting properties of experimental and commercially available lactose granulations for direct compression. *Drug Dev Ind Pharm* 1995;21: 2057–2071.

18. Bavitz JF, Schwartz JB. Direct compression vehicles, part II. *Drug Cosmetic Ind* 1976;118(4):60–77.

19. Hwang R, Peck GR. A systematic evaluation of the compression and tablets characteristics of various types of microcrystalline cellulose. *Pharm Technol* 2001;24:112–132.

20. Obae K, Iijima H, Imada K. Morphological effect of microcrystalline cellulose particles on tablet tensile strength. *Int J Pharm* 1999;182:155–164.

21. Lahdenpaa E, Niskanen M, Yliruusi J. Crushing strength, disintegration time and weight variation of tablets compressed from three Avicel pH grades and their mixtures. *Eur J Pharm Biopharm* 1997;43:315–322.

22. Reus-Medina M, Lanz M, Kumar V, Leuenberger H. Comparative evaluation of the powder properties and compression behaviour of a new cellulose based direct compression excipient and Avicel PH 102. *J Pharm Pharmacol* 2004;56:951–956.

23. Bolhuis GK, Chowhan ZT. *Materials for direct Compression, Pharmaceutical Powder Compaction Technology*, Volume 7. New York: Marcel Dekker; 1996, pp 419–499.

24. Shangraw RF. Direct compression tableting. In *Encyclopedia of Pharmaceutical Technology*, Volume 4, 2nd ed. New York: Marcel Dekker; 1988, pp 85–160.

25. Rizzuto AB, Chen AC, Veiga ME. Modification of the sucrose crystal structure to enhance pharmaceutical properties of excipient and drug substances. *Pharm Technol* 1984;8:32–39.

26. Olmo IG, Ghaly ES. Evaluation of two dextrose-based directly compressible excipients. *Drug Dev Ind Pharm* 1998;24:771–778.

27. Papadimitriou E, Efentakis M, Choulis NH. Evaluation of maltodextrins as excipients for direct compression and tablets and their influence on the rate of dissolution. *Int J Pharm* 1992;86:131–136.

28. Levy G. Effect of certain tablet formulation factors on dissolution rate of the active ingredient I. *J Pharm Sci* 1963;52:1039–1046.

29. Manudhane KS, Contractor AM, Kim HY, Shangraw RF. Tableting properties of a directly compressible starch. *J Pharm Sci* 1969;61:616–620.

30. Underwood TW, Cadwallader DE. Influence of various starches on dissolution rate of salicylic acid from tablets. *Pharm Sci* 1972;58:239–243.

31. Hsu SH, Tsai TR, Chuo WH, Cham TM. Evaluation of era-tab as direct compression excipients. *Drug Dev Ind Pharm* 1997;23:711–716.

32. Heinze F. Starch—the natural excipient choice. *Manufacturing Chemist* 2002;73:40–42.

33. Rees JE, Rue PJ. Time dependent deformation of some direct compression excipients. *J Pharm* 1978;30:601–607.

34. Khan KA, Rhodes, CT. Effect of variation in compaction force on properties of six direct compression tablet formulation. *J Pharm Sci* 1976;65:1835–1837.

35. Gohel MC. A review of co-processed directly compressible excipients. *J Pharm Pharm Sci* 2005;8:76–93.

36. Whiteman M, Yarwood RJ. Evaluation of six lactose-based materials as direct compression tablet excipients. *Drug Dev Ind Pharm* 1988;14:1023–1040.

37. Plaizier-Vercammen JA, Van Den Bossche H. Evaluation of the tableting properties of a new excipient for direct compression. *Drugs Made in Germany* 1993;36:133–137.

38. Schmidt PC, Rubensdorfer CJ. Evaluation of ludipress as a multipurpose excipient for direct compression. Part 1. Powder characteristics and tableting properties. *Drug Dev Ind Pharm* 1994;20:2899–2925.

39. Schmidt PC, Rubensdorfer CJ. Evaluation of ludipress as a multipurpose excipient for direct compression. Part II: Inactive blending and tableting with micronized glibenclamide. *Drug Dev Ind Pharm* 1994;20:2927–2952.

40. Garr JS, Rubinstein MH. Compaction properties of a cellulose-lactose direct compression excipient. *Pharm Tech Int* 1991;3:24–27.

41. Armstrong NA, Roscheisen G, Al-Aghbar MR. Cellactose as a tablet diluent. *Manufacturing Chemist* 1996;67:25–26.

42. Reimerdes D. The near future of tablet excipients. *Manufacturing Chemist* 1993; 64:14–15.

43. Belda PM, Mielck JB. The tabletting behaviour of cellactose compared with mixtures of celluloses with lactoses. *Eur J Pharm Biopharm* 1996;42:325–330.

44. Casalderrey M, Souto C, Concheiro A, Gomea-Amoza JL, Martinez-Pacheco RA. Comparison of cellactose with two ad hoc processed lactose–cellulose blends as direct compression excipients. *Chem Pharm Bull* 2000;48: 458–463.

45. Gohel MC, Modi CJ, Jogani PD. Functionality testing of a coprocessed diluent containing lactose and microcrystalline cellulose. *Pharm Technol* 1999;22:40–46.

46. Gohel MC, Bariya S, Jogani PD. Investigation in direct compression characteristics of coprocessed adjuvant containing lactose, microcrystalline cellulose and dicalcium phosphate. *Pharm Dev Technol* 2003;8:143–152.

47. Meggle AG. Technical information at www.megglepharma.de/en/product/uebersich/starlac.

48. Hauschild K, Picker KM. Evaluation of new coprocessed compound based on lactose and maize starch for tablet formulation. *AAPS PharmSci* 2004;6:1–12.

49. Tsai T, Wu J, Ho H, Sheu M. Modification of physical characteristics of microcrystalline cellulose by codrying with β-cyclodextrin. *J Pharm Sci* 1998;87:117–122.

50. Levis SR, Deasy PB. Pharmaceutical applications of size reduced grades of surfactant co-processed microcrystalline cellulose. *Int J Pharm* 2001;230:25–33.

51. Ishikawa T, Mukai B, Shiraishi S, Utoguchi N, Fujii M, Matsumoto M, Watanaba Y. Preparation of rapidly disintegrating tablet using new types of microcrystalline cellulose (PH-M Series) and low substituted-hydroxypropylcellulose or spherical sugar granules by direct compression method. *Chem Pharm Bull* 2001;49:134–139.

52. Lourdes Garzo'n M, Villafuerte L. Compactibility of mixtures of calcium carbonate and microcrystalline cellulose. *Int J Pharm* 2002;231:33–41.

53. Luukkonen P, Schaefer T, Hellen L, Juppo AM, Yliruusi J. Rheological characterization of microcrystalline cellulose and silicified microcrystalline cellulose wet masses using a mixer torque rheometer. *Int J Pharm* 1999;188:181–192.

54. Allen JD. Improving DC with SMCC. *Manufacturing Chemist* 1996:67:19–23.

55. Kachimanis K, Nikolakakis I, Malamataris S. Tensile strength and disintegration of tableted silicified microcrystalline cellulose: influences of interparticle bonding. *J Pharm Sci* 2003;92:1489–1501.

56. Wei S. Preparation and physical/mechanical evaluation of new crystallinity forms of cellulose as pharmaceutical excipients. Minneapolis, MN: University of Minnesota; 1991.

57. Banker GS, Wei S. Low crystallinity cellulose. U.S. patent 5417984. 23 May 1995.

58. Wei S, Kumar V, Banker GS. Phosphoric acid mediated depolymerization and decrystallinization of cellulose. Preparation of low crystallinity cellulose—a new pharmaceutical excipient. *Int J Pharm* 1996;142:175–191.

59. Kumar V, Kothari SH, Banker GS. Effect of agitation rate on the generation of low crystallinity cellulose from phosphoric acid. *J Appl Polym Sci* 2001;82:2624–2628.

60. Jones TM. *Symposium On Powders*. Dublin: Society of Cosmetic Chemists of Great Britain; 1969.

61. Peleg M, Mannheim CH. Effect of conditioners on the flow properties of powdered sucrose. *Powder Technol* 1973;7:45–50.

62. Matsuda Y, Minamida Y, Hayashi S. Comparative evaluation of tablet lubricants: effect of application method on tablet hardness and ejectability after compression. *J Pharm Sci* 1976;65:1155–1160.

63. Iranlove TA, Parrot EL. Effects of compression force, particle size, and lubricants on dissolution rate. *J Pharm Sci* 1978;67:535–539.

64. Chowhan ZT, Chi LH. Drug–excipient interactions resulting from powder mixing. IV: Role of lubricants and their effect on *in vitro* dissolution. *J Pharm Sci* 1986; 75:542–545.

65. Westerberg M, Nystrom C. Physicochemical aspects of drug release. XII. The effect of some carrier particle properties and lubricant admixture on drug dissolution from tableted ordered mixtures. *Int J Pharm* 1991;69:129–141.

66. Ong JTH, Chowhan ZT, Samuels JG. Drug–excipient interactions resulting from powder mixing. VI. Role of various surfactants. *Int J Pharm* 1993;96:231–242.

67. Desai DS, Rubitski BA, Varia SA, Newman AW. Physical interactions of magnesium stearate with starch derived disintegrants and their effects on capsule and tablet dissolution. *Int J Pharm* 1993;91:217–226.

68. Desai DS, Rubitski BA, Bergum JS, Varia SA. Effect of various fomulation factors on dissolution stability of aztreonam, hydrochlorothiazide, and sorivudine capsules. *Drug Dev Ind Pharm* 1994;110:249–255.

69. Shah AC, Mlodozeniec AR. Mechanism of surface lubrication: influence of duration of lubricant excipient mixing on processing characteristics of powders and properties of compressed tablets. *J Pharm Sci* 1997;66:1377–1382.

70. Chowhan ZT, Chi LH. Drug–excipient interactions resulting from powder mixing. V: Role of sodium lauryl sulphate. *Int J Pharm* 1986;60:61–78.

71. Otsuka M, Gao J, Matsuda Y. Effects of mixer and mixing time on the pharmaceutical properties of theophylline tablets containing various kinds of lactose as diluents. *Drug Dev Ind Pharm* 1993;19:333–348.

72. Kikuta J, Kitamori N. Effect of mixing time on the lubricating properties of magnesium stearate and the final characteristics of the compressed tablet. *Drug Dev Ind Pharm* 1994;20:343–355.

73. Otsuka M, Sato M, Matsuda Y. Comparative evaluation of tableting compression behaviours by methods of internal and external lubricant addition: inhibition of enzymatic activity of trypsin preparation by using external lubricant addition during the tableting compression process. *AAPS PharmSci* 2001;3:1–11.

74. Khan KA, Rooke DJ. Effect of disintegrant type upon the relationship between compressional pressure and dissolution efficiency. *J Pharm Pharmacol* 1976;28:633–636.

75. Zhang Y, Law Y, Chakrabarti S. Physical properties and compact analysis of commonly used direct compression binders. *AAPS PharmSci* 2003;4(article 62):1–11.

76. Proost JH, Bolhuis GK, Lerk CF. The effect of the selling capacity of disintegrants on the *in vitro* and *in vivo* availability of diazepam tablets, containing magnesium stearate as a lubricant. *Int J Pharm* 1983;13:287–296.

77. Sjokvist E, Nystrom C, Alden M. Physicochemical aspects of drug release. IX: Investigation of some factors that impair dissolution of drugs from solid particulate dispersion systems. *Int J Pharm* 1989;54:161–170.

78. Johnson JR, Wang LH, Gordon MS, Chowhan ZT. Effect of formulation solubility and hygroscopicity on disintegrant efficiency in tablets prepared by wet granulation, in terms of dissolution. *J Pharm Sci* 1991;80:469–471.

79. Gordan MS, Rudrarju VS, Rhie JK, Chowhan ZT. The effect of aging on the dissolution of wet granulated tablets containing super disintegrants. *Int J Pharm* 1993;97:119–131.

80. Bolhuis GK, Zuurman K, Wierik GHP. Improvement of dissolution of poorly soluble drugs by solid deposition on a super disintegrant. II. The choice of super disintegrants and effect of granulation. *Eur J Pharm BioPharm* 1997;5:63–69.

81. Lundqvist AEK, Podczeck F, Newton JM. Influence of disintegrant type and proportion on the properties of tablets produced from mixtures of pellets. *Int J Pharm* 1997;147:95–107.

82. Chen CR, Cho SL, Lin CK, Lin YH, Chiang ST, Wu HL. Dissolution difference between acidic and neutral media of acetaminophen tablets containing a super disintegrant and a soluble excipient. II. *Chem Pharm Bull* 1998;46:478–481.

83. Sallam E, Ibrahim H, Dahab RA, Shubair M, Khalil E. Evaluation of fast disintegrants in terfenadine tablets containing a gas evolving disintegrant. *Drug Dev Ind Pharm* 1998;24:501–507.

84. Carmella C, Colombo P, Conte U, La Manna A. Tablet disintegrate update; the dynamic approach. *Drug Dev Ind Pharm* 1987;13:2111–2145.

85. Lopez-Solis J, Villafuerte-Robles L. Effect of disintegrants with different hygroscopicity on dissolution of Norfloxacin/Pharmatose DCL 11 tablets. *Int J Pharm* 2001;216:127–135.

86. Zao N, Augsburger LL. The influence of swelling capacity of superdisintegrants in different pH media on the dissolution of hydrochlorothiazide from directly compressed tablets. *AAPS PharmSci* 2005;6:E120–E126.

87. Zao N, Augsburger LL. Functionality comparison of 3 classes of superdisintegrants in promoting aspirin tablet disintegration and dissolution. *AAPS PharmSci* 2005;6:E634–E640.

88. Cheng G, An F, Zou MJ, Sun J, Hao XH, He YX. Time- and pH-dependent colon-specific drug delivery for orally administered diclofenac sodium and 5-aminosalicylic acid. *World J Gastroenterol* 2004;10:1769–1774.

89. Wakerly Z, Fell JT, Attwood D, Parkins D. Pectin/ethylcellulose film coating formulations for colonic drug delivery. *Pharm Res* 1996;13:1210–1212.

90. Prabakaran D, Singh P, Kanaujia P, Mishra V, Jaganathan KS, Vyas SP. Controlled porosity osmotic pumps of highly aqueous soluble drug containing hydrophilic polymers as release retardants. *Pharm Dev Technol* 2004;9:435–442.

91. Rao VM, Haslam JL, Stella VJ. Controlled and complete release of a model poorly water-soluble drug, prednisolone, from hydroxypropyl methylcellulose matrix tablets using (SBE) (7m)-beta-cyclodextrin as a solubilizing agent. *J Pharm Sci* 2001;90: 807–817.

92. Tiwari D, Sause R, Madan PL. Evaluation of polyxyethylene homopolymers for buccal bioadhesive drug delivery device formulations. *AAPS PharmSci* 1999;1(article 13):1–8.

93. Chiao CS, Price JC. Formulation, preparation and dissolution characteristics of propranolol hydrochloride microspheres. *J Microencapsulation* 1994;11:153–159.

94. Saravanan M, Natraj KS, Ganesh KS. Hydroxypropyl methylcellulose based cephalexin extended release tablets: influence of tablet formulation, hardness and storage on *in vitro* release kinetics. *Chem Pharm Bull* 2003;51:978–983.

95. Bordaweka MS, Zia H. Evaluation of polyvinyl acetate dispersion as a sustained release polymer for tablets. *Drug Deliv* 2006;13:121–131.

96. Bravo SA, Lamas MC, Salomon CJ. *In-vitro* studies of diclofenac sodium controlled-release from biopolymeric hydrophilic matrices. *J Pharm Pharm Sci* 2002;5:213–219.

97. Pignatello R, Ferro M, Puglisi G. Preparation of solid dispersions of nonsteroidal anti-inflammatory drugs with acrylic polymers and studies on mechanisms of drug-polymer interactions. *AAPS PharmSci* 2002;3(article 10):1–11.

98. Adeyeye MC, Mwangi E, Katondo B, Jain A, Ichikawa H, Fukumori Y. Dissolution stability studies of suspensions of prolonged-release diclofenac microcapsules prepared by the Wurster process: I. Eudragit-based formulation and possible drug-excipient interaction. *J Microencapsulation* 2005;22:333–342.

99. Jenquin MR, McGinity JW. Characterization of acrylic resin matrix films and mechanisms of drug–polymer interactions. *Int J Pharm* 10:23–34.

100. Karlsen J. Excipient properties of chitosan. *Manufacturing Chemist* 1991;62:18–19.

101. Nunthanid J, Laungtana-anan M, Sriamornsak P, Limmatvapirat S, Puttipipatkhachorn S, Lim, LY, Khor E. Characterization of chitosan acetate as a binder for sustained release tablets. *J Control Release* 2004;99:15–26.

102. Gao P, Nixon P, Skoug J. Diffusion in HPMC gels. II. Prediction of drug release rates from hydrophilic matrix extended-release dosage forms. *Pharm Res* 1995;12:965–971.

103. Phaechamud T, Koizumi T, Ritthidej GC. Chitosan citrate as film former: compatibility with water-soluble anionic dyes and drug dissolution from coated tablets. *Int J Pharm* 2000;198:97–111.

104. Ritthidej GC, Phaechamud TW. Effect of anionic water-soluble dyes on film coating properties of chitosan acetate. *Drug Dev Ind Pharm* 2003;29:585–594.

105. Breikkreutz J. Leakage of enteric (Eudragit L)-coated dosage forms in simulated gastric juice in the presence of poly(ethylene glycol). *J Control Release* 2000;67:79–88.

106. Mathur A V, Hammonds KF, Klier J, Scranton AB. Equilibrium swelling of poly(methacrylic acid-ethylene glycol) hydrogels: effect of swelling medium and synthesis conditions. *J Control Release* 1998;54:177–184.

107. Chasseaud LF, Taylor T. Bioavailability of drugs from formulations after oral administration. *Annu Rev Pharmacol* 1974;14:35–46.

108. Bourne DWA, Dittert LW. *Modern Pharmaceutics* 4th ed. New York: Marcel Dekker; 1996, pp 122–153.

109. Banakar UV, Makoid MC. *Drug Development Process: Increasing Efficiency and Cost-Effectiveness.* New York: Marcel Dekker Taylor & Francis CRC; 1996, pp 117–168.

110. Du J, Hoag SW. Characterization of excipient and tableting factors that influence folic acid dissolution, friability and breaking strength of oil- and water-soluble multi vitamin with minerals tablets. *Drug Dev Ind Pharm* 2003;29:1137–1147.

111. *United States Pharmacopoia* 24 and *National Formulary 19.* USP publishers. Rockville, MD: US Pharmacopoeia; 2001.

112. Urakami K, Shono Y, Higashi A, Umemoto K, Godo M. A novel method for estimation of transition temperature for polymorphic pairs in pharmaceuticals using heat of solution and solubility data. *Chem Pharm Bull* 2002;50:263–267.

113. Hancock BC, Parks M. What is the true solubility advantage of amorphous pharmaceuticals? *Pharm Res* 2001;17:397–404.

114. Bartolomei M, Bertocchi P, Antoniella E, Rodomonte A. Physicochemical charaterization and intrinsic dissolution study of new hydrate form of diclofenac sodium: comparison with anhydrous form. *J Pharm Biomed Anal* 2006;40:1105–1113.

115. Manca ML, Zaru M, Ennas G, Valenti D, Sininco C, Loy G, Fadda AM. Diclofenac-β-cyclodextrin binary system: physicochemical characterization and *in vitro* dissolution and diffusion study. *AAPS PharmSci Tech* 2005;6(article 58):E464–E472.

116. Mukne AP, Nagarsenker MS. Triamterene-β-cyclodextrin systems: preparation, characterization and *in vivo* evaluation. *AAPS PharmSci Tech* 2004;5(article 19):1–9.

117. Marlowe E, Shangraw RF. Dissolution of sodium salicylate from tablet matrices prepared by wet granulation and direct compression. *J Pharm Sci* 1967;56:498–504.

118. Abdou HM. *Remington's Pharmaceutical Sciences,* 17th ed. Easton, PA: Mack Publishing; 1986, pp 653–666.

119. Bansal P, Haribhakti K, Subramanian V, Plakogiannis F. Effect of formulation and process variables on the dissolution profile of naproxen sodium from tablets. *Drug Dev Ind Pharm* 1994;20:2151–2156.

120. Mitchell K, Ford JL, Armstrong DJ, Elliott PNC, Hogan JE, Rostron C. The influence of the particle size of hydroxypropylmethylcellulose K15M on its hydration and performance in matrix tablets. *Int J Pharm* 1999;100:175–179.

121. Gao P, Meury RH. Swelling of hydroxypropyl methylcellulose matrix tablets. 1. Characterization of swelling using a novel optical imaging method. *J Pharm Sci* 1996;85: 725–731.

122. Chowhan ZT, Yang IC. Effect of intergranular versus intragranular cornstarch on tablet friability and *in vitro* dissolution. *J Pharm Sci* 1983;72:983–988.

123. Zhang YE, Tchao R, Schwartz JB. Effect of processing methods and heat treatment on the formation of wax matrix tablets for sustained drug release. *Pharm Dev Technology* 2001;6:131–144.

124. Finholt P. In Leeson LJ, Carstenson JT, Eds. *Dissolution Technology.* Industrial Pharmaceuticals Technology Section. Washington DC: Apha; 1974, pp 136–137.

125. Ghorab MK, Adeyeye MC. Enhancement of ibuprofen dissolution via wet granulation with beta-cyclodextrin. *Pharm Dev Technol* 2001;6:305–304.

126. Al-Kassas RS, Gilligan CA, Po ALW. Processing factors affecting particle size and *in vitro* drug release of sustained release ibuprofen microspheres. *Int J Pharm* 1993;94: 59–67.

127. Kanig JL, Rudnic EM. The mechanism of disintegrant action. *Pharm Technol* 1984; 8:50–62.

128. Levy G, Gumtow RH. Effect of certain formulation factors on dissolution rate of the active ingredient III: tablet lubricants. *J Pharm Sci* 1963;52:1139–1144.

129. Basak SC, Sivakamasundari T, Shivagamasundari S, Manavalan R. Influence of granule size and lubricant concentration on the dissolution of paracetamol tablets. *Indian J Pharm Sci* 2003;65:299–301.

130. Lerk CF, Bolhuis GK, Smallenbroek AJ, Zuurman K. Interaction of tablet disintegrants and magnesium stearate during mixing II. Effect on dissolution rate. *Pharm Acta Helv* 1982;57:282–286.

131. Van Oudtshoorn MC, Potgieter FJ, de Blaey CJ, Polderman J. The influence of compression and formulation on the hardness, disintegration, dissolution, absorption and excretion of sulphadimidine tablets. *J Pharm Pharmacol* 1971;23:583–586.

132. Massimo G, Santi P, Colombo G, Nicoli S, Zani F, Colombo P, Bettini R. The suitability of disintegrating force kinetics for studying the effect of manufacturing parameters on spironolactone tablet properties. *AAPS PharmSci* 2003;4(article17):1–7.

133. Tuladhar MD, Carless JE, Summers MP. The effects of polymorphism, particle size and compression pressure on the dissolution rate of phenylbutazone tablets. *J Pharm Pharmacol* 1983;35:269–274.

134. Ganderton D, Hadgraft JW, Rispin WT, Thompson AG. The breakup and dissolution of phenindione tablets. *Pharm Acta Helv* 1967;42:152–162.

135. Kent JS. Implant pellets I: effects of compression pressure on *in vivo* dissolution of delmadinone acetate pellets. *J Pharm Sci* 1976;65:89–92.

136. Lin KH, Lin SY, Li MJ. Compression forces and amount of outer coating layer affecting the time-controlled disintegration of the compression-coated tablets prepared by direct compression with micronized ethylcellulose. *J Pharm Sci* 2001;90:2005–2009.

137. Food and Drug Administration. Guidance for Industry: Immediate release solid oral dosage forms; scale-up and postapproval changes: chemistry, manufacturing, and controls, *in vitro* dissolution testing, and *in vivo* bioequivalance documentation. Rockville, MD: FDA Nov 1995.

138. Prabhu S, Jacknowitz AI, Stout PJ. A study of factors controlling dissolution kinetics of zinc complexed protein suspensions in various ionic species. *Int J Pharm* 2001;217: 71–78.

139. Tang L, Khan SU, Muhammad NA. Evaluation and selection of biorelevant dissolution media for a poorly water soluble new chemical entity. *Pharm Dev Technol* 2001; 6:531–540.

140. Noory C, Tran N, Ouderkirk L, Shah V. Steps for development of a dissolution test for sparingly water soluble drug products. *Dissolution Technol* 2000;Article 3:1–5.

141. *British Pharmacopoeia*. London: British Pharmacopoeia Commission Bernan Press; 2003.

142. Government of India Ministry of Health and Family Welfare. *The Pharmacopoeia of India*. Delhi, India: Controller of Publication; 1996.

143. Crison JR, Weiner ND, Amidon GL. Dissolution media for *in vitro* testing of water insoluble drugs: effect of surfactant purity and electrolyte on *in vitro* dissolution of carbamazepine in aqueous solutions of sodium lauryl sulphate. *J Pharm Sci* 1997;86: 384–388.

144. Jinno J, Oh D, Crison JR, Amidon GL. Dissolution of ionizable water insoluble drugs: the combined effect of pH and surfactant. *J Pharm Sci* 2000;89:268–274.

145. Li J, Yang L, Ferguson SM, Hudson TJ, Watanabe S, Katsuma M, Fix JA. *In vitro* evaluation of dissolution behaviour for a colon specific drug delivery system (CODES™) in multi-pH media using United States Pharmacopeia apparatus II and III. *AAPS Pharm-SciTech* 2002;3(article 33):1–9.

146. Galia E, Nicolaides E, Hörter D, Löbenberg R, Reppas C, Dressman JB. Evaluation of various dissolution media for predicting *in vivo* performance of class I and II drugs. *Pharm Res* 1998;15:698–705.

147. Crison JR. Developing dissolution test for modified release dosage form: general considerations. http://wwwdissolutiontechcom/Dtresour/299articlesCrison,htm.

148. Moller H, Wirbitzki E. Regulatory aspects of modified release dosage form: special cases of dissolution testing using the flow-through system. *Bollettino Chim Farma* 1993;132:105–115.

149. Burns SJ, Corness D, Hay G, Higginbottom S, Whelan I, Attwood D, Barnwell SG. Development and validation of an *in vitro* dissolution method for a floating dosage form with biphasic release characteristics. *Int J Pharm* 1995;121:37–44.

150. Crail DJ, Tunis A, Dansereau R. Is the use of a 200 ml vessel suitable for dissolution of low dose drug products? *Int J Pharm* 2004;269:203–209.

151. Yu LX, Carlin AS, Amidon GL, Hussain AS. Feasibility studies of utilizing disk intrinsic dissolution rate to classify drugs. *Int J Pharm* 2004;270:221–227.

152. Banakar UV. *Pharm Dissolution Testing*. New York: Marcel Dekker; 1992, pp 107–187.

153. Sarapu A, Clark J. Elimination of tablet air entrapment using USP 1 rotating-basket dissolution apparatus. *J Pharm Sci* 1980;69:129.

154. Cappola ML. A better dissolution method for ranitidine tablets USP. *Pharm Dev Technol* 2001;6:11–17.

155. Hamlin WE, Nelson E, Ballard BE, Wagner JG. Loss of sensitivity in distinguishing real differences in dissolution rates due to increasing intensity of agitation. *J Pharm Sci* 1962;51:432–435.

156. Kukura J, Baxter JL, Muzzio FJ. Shear distribution and variability in the USP apparatus 2 under turbulent conditions. *Int J Pharm* 2004;279:9–17.

157. Shah VP, Konecny JJ, Everett RL, McCullough B, Noorizadeh AC, Skelly JP. *In vitro* dissolution profile of water insoluble drug dosage forms in the presence of surfactants. *Pharm Res* 1989;6:612–618.

158. Qureshi SA, Shabnam J. Cause of high variability in drug dissolution testing and its impact on setting tolerances. *Eur J Pharm Sci* 2001;12:271–276.

159. Wurster DE, Polli GP. Investigation of drug release from solids. V. Simultaneous influence of adsorption and viscosity on the dissolution rate. *J Pharm Sci* 1964;53:311–314.

160. Bodmeier R, Guo X, Sarabia RE, Skultety PF. The influence of buffer species and strength on diltiazem HCl release from beads coated with aqueous cationic polymer dispersions. Eudragit RS, RL 30D. *Pharm Res* 1996;13:52–56.

161. Fagan PG, Harrison PJ, Shankland N. A correlation between cloud point and disintegration of hydroxyalkylcellulose controlled release matrices. *J Pharm Pharmacol* 1989;41:25.

162. Jalil R, Ferdous AJ. Effect of viscosity increasing agent and electrolyte concentration on the release rate of theophylline from HPMC based sustained release capsules. *Drug Dev Ind Pharm* 1993;19:2637–2643.

163. Li WPA, Wong LP, Gilligan CA. Characterization of commercially available theophylline sustained or controlled-release systems: *in vitro* drug release profiles. *Int J Pharm* 1990;66:111–130.

164. Bonferoni MC, Rossi S, Ferrari F, Stavik F, Pena-Romero A, Caramella C. Factorial analysis of the influence of dissolution medium on drug release from carrageenan–diltiazem complexes. *AAPS PharmSciTech* 2000;1(article 15):1–8.

165. Prasad VK, Rapaka RS, Knight PW, Cabana BE. Dissolution medium—a critical parameter to identify bioavailability problems of furosemide tablets. *Int J Pharm* 1982;11:81–90.

166. O'Hara TO, Dunne A, Butler J, Devane J. A review of methods used to compare dissolution profile data. *AAPS PharmSciTech* 2000;1(article 15):214–223.

167. Demirtürk E, Öner L. Evaluation of *in vitro* dissolution profile comparison methods of immediate release gliclazide tablet formulations. *Hacettepe Univ J Faculty Pharm* 2005;25:1–10.

168. Chow SC, Ki FYC. Statistical comparison between dissolution profiles of drug products. *J BioPharm Stat* 1997;7:241–258.

169. Qazi S, Samuel NKP, Venkatachalam TK, Uckun FM. Evaluating dissolution profiles of an anti-HIV agent using ANOVA and non-linear regression models in JMP software. *Int J Pharm* 2003;252:27–39.

170. Tsong Y, Hammerstorm T, Sathe P, Shah VP. Statistical assessment of mean difference between two dissolution data sets. *Drug Info J* 1996;30:1105–1112.

171. Sathe P, Tsong Y, Shah VP. *In vitro* dissolution profilee comparison: statistics and analysis, model dependent approach. *Pharm Res* 1996;13:1799–1803.

172. Shah VP, Tsong Y, Sathe P, Liu JP. *In vitro* dissolution profile comparison and analysis of the similarity factor, f_2. *Pharm Res* 1998;15:889–896.

173. Peh KK, Wong CF. Application of similarity factor in development of controlled release diltiazem tablet. *Drug Dev Ind Pharm* 2000;26:723–730.

174. Rescigno R. Bioequivalence. *Pharm Res* 1992;9:925–928.

175. Lin SY, Yang JC. *In vitro* dissolution behaviour of some sustained release theophylline dosage forms. *Pharm Acta Helv* 1989;4:236–240.

176. Sangali ME, Giunchedi P, Maggi L, Conte U, Gazzaniga A. Inert monolithic device with a central hole for constant drug release. *Eur J Pharm Sci* 1994;40:370–373.

177. Korsmeyer RW, Gurny R, Doelker EM, Buri P, Peppas NA. Mechanism of solute release from porous hydrophilic polymers. *Int J Pharm* 1983;15:25–35.

178. Kim H, Fassihi R. Application of binary polymer system in drug release rate modulation. 2. Influence of formulation variables and hydrodynamic conditions on release kinetics. *J Pharm Sci* 1997;86:323–328.

179. El-Arini SK, Leuenberger H. Dissolution properties of praziquantel–PVP systems. *Pharm Acta Helv* 1998;73:89–94.

180. Crowder MJ. Keep timing the tablets: statistical analysis of pill dissolution rates. *Appl Stat* 1996;45:323–334.

181. Baker RW, Losdale HS. *Controlled Release: Mechanisms and Rates*. New York: Plenum Press, 1974, pp 15–71.

182. Jun HW, Lai JW. Preparation and *in vitro* dissolution tests of egg albumin microcapsules of nitrofurantoin. *Int J Pharm* 1983;16:65–77.

183. Shukla AJ, Price JC. Effect of drug (core) particle size on the dissolution of theophylline from microspheres made from low molecular weight cellulose acetate propionate. *Pharm Res* 1989;6:418–421.

184. Hopfenberg HB. In Paul DR, Harris FW. Eds. *Controlled Release Polymeric Formulations*. ACS Symposium Series 33. Washington DC: American Chemical Society; 1976, pp 26–31.

185. Higuchi T. Mechanism of sustained action medication. Theoretical analysis of rate of release of solid drugs dispersed in solid matrices. *J Pharm Sci* 1963;52:1145–1149.

186. Desai SJ, Singh P, Simonelli AP, Higuschi WI. Investigation of factors influencing release of solid drug dispersed in inert matrices. III. Quantitative studies involving the polyethylene plastic matrix. *J Pharm Sci* 1966;55:1230–1234.

187. Desai SJ, Singh P, Simonelli AP, Higuschi WI. Investigation of factors influencing release of solid drug dispersed in inert matrices. IV. Some studies involving the polyvinyl chloride matrix. *J Pharm Sci* 1966;55:1235–1239.

188. Niebergall PJ, Milosovich G, Goyan JE. Dissolution rate studies. II. Dissolution of particles under conditions of rapid agitation. *J Pharm Sci* 1963;52:236–241.

189. Langenbucher F. Linearization of dissolution rate curves by the Weibull distribution. *J Pharmacol* 1972;24:979–981.

190. Pedersen PV, Myrick JW. Versatile kinetic approach to analysis of dissolution data. *J Pharm Sci* 1978;67:1450–1455.

191. Christensen FN, Hansen FY, Bechgaard H. Physical interpretation of parameters in the Rosin–Rammler–Sperling–Weibull distribution for drug release from controlled release dosage forms. *J Pharm Pharmacol* 1980;32:580–582.

192. Costa P, Lobo JMS. Modeling and comparison of dissolution profiles. *Eur J Pharm Sci* 2001;13:123–133.

193. Varelas CG, Dixon DG, Steiner C. Zero order release from biphasic polymer hydrogels. *J Control Release* 1995;34:185–192.

194. Polli JE, Rekhi GS, Shah VP. Methods to compare dissolution profiles. *Drug Info J* 1996;30:1113–1120.

195. Lin JH, Chiba M, Balani SK, Chen I-W, Kwei GY-S, Vastag KJ, Nishine JA. Species differences in the pharmacokinetics and metabolism of indinavir, a potent HIV protease inhibitor. *Drug Metab Dispos* 1996;24:1111–1120.

196. Lin JH, Storey DE, Chen I-W, Xu X. Improved absorption of L-365,260, a poorly soluble drug. *Biopharm Drug Dispos* 1996;17:1–16.

197. Yeleswara K, McLaughlin LG, Knipe JO, Schabdach D. Pharmacokinetics and oral bioavailability of exogenous melatonin in preclinical animal models and clinical implications. *J Pineal Res* 1997;22:45–51.

198. Clemens ET, Stevens CE. A comparison of gastrointestinal transit time in ten species of mammal. *J Agric Sci* 1980;94:735–737.

199. Kararli TT. Comparison of the gastrointestinal anatomy, physiology, and biochemistry of humans and commonly used laboratory animals. *Biopharm Drug Dispos* 1995;16:351–380.

200. Obach RS, Baxter JG, Liston TE, Silber M, Jones BC, MACintyre F, Rance DJ, Wastall P. The prediction of human pharmacokinetic parameters from preclinical and *in vitro* metabolism data. *J Pharmacol Exp Ther* 1997;283:46–58.

201. Renkin EM, Gilmore JP. *Handbook of Physiology—Renal Physiology*. Baltimore, MD: Williams and Wilkins; 1973, pp 185–248.

202. Dressman JB, Yamada K. *Pharmaceutical Bioequivalence*. New York: Marcel Dekker; 1991, pp 235–266.

203. Davies B, Morris T. Physiological parameters in laboratory animals and humans. *Pharmaceutical Research*, 10, 1093–1095.

204. Miyabayashi T, Morgan JP, Atitola MAO, Muhumuza L. Small intestinal emptying time in normal beagle dogs. A contrast radiographic study. *Vet Radiol* 1986;27:197–209.

205. Ilet KF, Tee LBG, Reeves PhT, Minchin RF. Metabolism of drugs and other xenobiotics in the gut lumen and wall. *Pharmacol Ther* 1990;46:67–93.

206. Degen LP, Phillips SF. Variability of gastrointestinal transit in healthy women and men. *Gut* 1996;39:299–305.

207. Ikegami K, Tagawa K, Narisawa S, Osawa T. Suitability of the cynomolgus monkey as an animal model for drug absorption studies of oral dosage forms from the viewpoint of gastrointestinal physiology. *Biol Pharm Bull* 2003;1442–1447.

208. Kaniwa N, Aoyagi N, Ogata H, Ejima A. Gastric emptying rates of drug preparations. I. Effects of size of dosage form, food and species on gastric emptying rates. *J Pharmco-bioDynam* 1988;11:563–570.

209. Chiou1 WL, Buehler1 PW. Comparison of oral absorption and bioavailability of drugs between monkey and human. *Pharm Res* 2002;19:868–873.

210. Edwards NA. Scaling of renal function in mammals. *Comp Biochem Physiol* 1975;52A:63–66.

211. Boxenbaum H. Interspecies variation in liver weight, hepatic blood flow, and antipyrin intrinsic clearance in extrapolation of benzodiazepines and phenytoin. *J Phamacokinet Biopharm* 1980;8:165–176.

212. Stahl WR. Scaling of respiratory variable in mammals. *J Appl Physiol* 1969;22:453–460.

213. Knaak JB, Al-Bayati MA, Raabe OG, Blancatos JN. Development of *in vitro* V_{max} and K_m values for the metabolism of isofenphos by P-450 liver enzymes in animals and human. *Toxicol Appl Pharmacol* 1993;120:106–113.

214. Sharer JE, Shipley LA, Vandenbranden MR, Binkley SN, Wrighton SA. Comparisons of phase I and phase II *in vitro* hepatic enzyme activities of human, dog, rhesus monkey, and cynomolgus monkey. *Drug Metab Dispos* 1995;23:1231–1241.

215. Chauret N, Gauthier A, Martin J, Nicoll-Griffith D. *In vitro* comparison of cytochrome P450-mediated metabolic activities in human, dog, cat, and horse. *Drug Metab Rev* 1997;25:1130–1136.

216. Shimida T, Mimura M, Inoue K, Nakamura S, Oda H, Ohmori S, Yamazaki H. Cytochrome P450-dependent drug oxidation activities in liver microsomes of various animal species including rats, guinea pigs, dogs, monkeys, and humans. *Arch Toxicol* 1997;71:401–408.

217. Igarashi T, Tomihari N, Ohmori S, Ueno K, Kitagawa H, Satoh T. Comparison of glutathione *S*-transferase in mouse, guinea pig, rabbit and hamster liver cytosol to those in rat liver. *Biochem Int* 1986;13:641–648.

218. Stevens JC, Shipley LA, Cashman JR, Vandenbranden M, Wrighton SA. Comparison of human and rhesus monkey *in vitro* phase I and phase II hepatic drug metabolism activities. *Drug Metab Rev* 1993;21:753–759.

219. Puri S, Kohli KK. Differences in hepatic drug metabolizing enzymes and their response to lindane in rat, rabbit and monkey. *Pharmacol Toxicol* 1995;77:136–141.

220. Kobayashi S, Murray S, Watson D, Sesardic D, Davies DS, Boobies AB. The specificity of inhibition of debrisoquine 4-hydroxylase activity in quinidine and quinine in rat is the reverse of that in man. *Biochem Pharmacol* 1989;38:2795–2799.

221. Lin JH. Species similarities and differences in pharmacokinetics. *Drug Metab Dispos* 1995;17:221–223.

222. Guidance for Industry. Extended release oral dosage forms: development, evaluation and application of *in vitro/in vivo* correlations. Washington DC: Food and Drug Administration CDER; Sept 1997.

223. Young D, Davane JG, Butler J. *In Vitro–In Vivo Correlations*. New York: Plenum Press; 1997.

224. Nelson E. Comparative dissolution rates of weak acid and their sodium salts. *J Am Pharm Assoc* 1958;47:297–300.

225. Schirmer RE, Kleber JW, Black HR. Correlation of dissolution, disintegration and bio-availability of aminosalicylic acid tablets. *J Pharm Sci* 1973;62:1270–1274.

226. Needham TE, Shah K, Kotzan J, Zia H. Correlation of aspirin excretion with parameter from different dissolution methods. *J Pharm Sci* 1978;67:1070–1073.

227. Fairweather WR. Investigating relationships between *in vivo* and *in vitro* pharmacological variables for the purpose of prediction. *J Pharmacokinet BioPharm* 1977;5:405–418.

228. Concherio A, Vila-Jato JL, Martinez-Pacheco R, Seijo B, Ramos T. *In vitro-in vivo* correlations of eight nitrofurantoin tablet formulations: effect of various technological factors. *Drug Dev Ind Pharm* 1987;13:501–516.

229. Wagner JG. *Pharmacokinetics for the Pharmceutical Scientist*. New York: Technomic Publishing; 1993, pp 259–269.

230. Bennett CA, Franklin NL. *Statistical Analysis in Chemistry and the Chemical Industry*. Hoboken, NJ: Wiley; 1963.

231. Johnson NL, Leone FC. *Statistics and Experimental Design in Engineering and the Physical Sciences*. Hoboken, NJ: Wiley; 1977.

232. Dressman J, Krämer J. *Pharmaceutical Dissolution Testing*. New York: Taylor & Francis Group; 2005.

233. *Guidance for Industry*. Waiver of *in vivo* bioavailability and bioequivalance studies for immediate-release solid oral dosage forms based on a biopharmaceutics classification system. Washington DC: Food and Drug Administration CDER, Aug 2000.

234. Burgess DJ, Hussain AS, Ingallinera TS, Chen ML. Assuring quality and performance of sustained and controlled release parenterals: workshop report. *AAPS PharmSci* 2002;4(article 7):1–11.

16

STABILITY: PHYSICAL AND CHEMICAL

Eric M. Gorman,[1] Brian E. Padden,[2] and Eric J. Munson[1]

[1]*The University of Kansas, Lawrence, Kansas*
[2]*Schering-Plough Research Institute, Summit, New Jersey*

Contents

Preclinical Development Handbook: ADME and Biopharmaceutical Properties,
edited by Shayne Cox Gad
Copyright © 2008 John Wiley & Sons, Inc.

16.1   INTRODUCTION

The pharmaceutical properties of a drug, such as solubility, dissolution, and toxicology, can change dramatically when a drug undergoes chemical or physical degradation. This can severely limit the drug's efficacy and safety. After a compound is synthesized it must undergo several steps before being used by the patient. Some of these steps include formulation into the final product, storage during manufacturing and distribution, and dispensing to the patient. Understanding the stability of a potential drug is a vital component to the pharmaceutical development process because if the drug changes during any one of these steps it may not have the desired pharmaceutical effects. Therefore, the evaluation of drug stability becomes part of the development process as early as candidate selection and continues for the lifetime of the product. For the purposes of this chapter, however, we only consider drug stability up to and through the formulation process.

There are four main reasons to study the stability of drugs [1]:

1. *Quantitation of Drug Loss.* It is essential to know how fast the drug degrades so that an accurate shelf life can be determined.
2. *Identification and Quantitation of Degradation Products.* It is important to know what the degradation products are, as they may be toxic, and to know at what levels they are produced.
3. *Change in Aesthetic Properties Upon Degradation.* If a drug product changes notably in its aesthetic appearance it is presumed adulterated, even if by all other criteria the drug product is perfectly safe for use. This typically occurs if one of the degradation products either has an offensive odor or is highly colored. An example is tetracycline degrading to form epianhydrotetracycline, which is red [2, 3].
4. *Degradation of Drug After Administration.* Even if the drug is stable in its formulation, it is important to know how it will degrade under physiologic conditions; for example, degradation at low pH for an orally administered drug.

There have been numerous articles and books published on the subject of stability. The best way to begin a stability study is to perform a thorough search of the literature to find similar compounds that have been studied previously, which may provide some insight into potential reaction mechanisms and products. In doing this, a foundation is laid for the studies that are to be performed on the new compound.

16.2 SOLUTION STABILITY

Stability studies on new drug candidates are typically performed in the solution state. These studies are used as an aid in candidate selection and are intended to identify compounds that would likely pose a significant challenge during the drug development process. Solution stability is also important as a guide for the formulation process. For example, if a drug is very sensitive to low pH then an enteric-coated tablet may be required for oral drug delivery.

16.2.1 Chemical Stability

Chemical stability is a measure of the susceptibility of a compound to undergo a chemical reaction in which atoms are rearranged via bond breakage and bond formation to produce a different chemical entity. Drugs have a myriad of different chemical structures and are thus subject to a variety of different possible mechanisms of degradation. Most drugs degrade by one or more of the following mechanisms: hydrolysis, dehydration, isomerization, racemization, decarboxylation, elimination, oxidation, or photodegradation [1, 4, 5]. It may also be possible to have reactions between two drug molecules [6] or between a drug molecule and an excipient within a formulation [7].

Hydrolysis is one of the most frequent degradation mechanisms observed in pharmaceuticals for two main reasons. First, drugs are typically dissolved in media primarily composed of water, which results in a relative abundance of water that is available to react. Second, ester and amide functional groups degrade primarily via hydrolysis and these are two very common functional groups in pharmaceuticals.

Proteins and peptides are steadily becoming more popular as pharmaceuticals. These biopharmaceuticals, as they are called, are subject to the same degradation reactions as "traditional" small molecule pharmaceuticals, and in some cases these reactions are given specific names to describe both the reaction type and the amino acid that is involved [8, 9]. For example, the hydrolysis of the amino acid asparagine to form aspartate and isoaspartate is referred to as deamidation. Biopharmaceuticals are inherently more complex than small molecules because of their increased size and higher levels of organization (primary, secondary, tertiary, and quaternary structure), which leads to significantly increased complexity when the stability of these compounds is considered [9–13].

16.2.2 Physical Stability

Physical stability is a measure of the propensity of a compound to undergo changes that do not involve the breaking or formation of covalent bonds. In this case the compound has the exact same chemical structure but the physical state has changed in some way. For small molecules, two potential physical stability problems in solution are precipitation and aggregation [14, 15]; however, these are both relatively rare when compared with chemical degradation mechanisms of small molecules. On the other hand, physical stability is a major concern in the case of biopharmaceuticals. If the protein/peptide denatures (typically through the loss of quaternary and tertiary structure) then it can adsorb to surfaces (such as glass or plastic), aggregate, and precipitate [16]. In the case of biopharmaceuticals, in particular, these physical changes typically are not easily reversed [10, 17]. One additional mechanism of physical degradation is vaporization. If the drug has a sufficiently high vapor pressure it can evaporate from the formulation whether it is in the solution or solid state. This phenomenon has been observed in nitroglycerin and can result in large variability in the drug content of tablets after being stored in the same container [18].

16.3   SOLID-STATE STABILITY

Pharmaceuticals are typically formulated in the solid state for several reasons. One major advantage is increased patient compliance, because it is easy to dose the pharmaceutical. It is also discreet, meaning that a patient can use it in a social setting and not draw the attention of other people while doing so. Another advantage is that it is typically cheaper than developing and producing a sterile product for parenteral administration. One of the main reasons for formulating a pharmaceutical in the solid state is that typically the compound is more stable in the solid state compared to the solution state. However, the solid state presents its own unique challenges.

16.3.1   Physical Stability

In the solid state a compound can be either amorphous or crystalline. A solid is amorphous if it lacks long-range order in the arrangement of the molecules. Amorphous materials can exist in one of two states: glassy or rubbery. The glassy state (low temperature state) is a more rigid state while the rubbery state (high temperature state) is a much more mobile state and hence is less stable. An amorphous material has a characteristic glass transition temperature (T_g), which is the temperature at which the material changes from the glassy to the rubbery state, or vice versa [19, 20].

   If the molecules in the solid state are packed in a regular pattern with long-range order, then the solid is said to be crystalline. The different conformations or orientations in which molecules are able to pack are referred to as crystal forms. If the molecules pack in one crystalline form the material may be called Form I and if the molecules pack in a different crystalline form the material may be called Form II. The naming of these crystal forms is arbitrary and usually reflects the order in which they were discovered. They are usually represented by either Roman numerals (e.g., I, II, III, IV), letters of the Latin alphabet (e.g., A, B, C, D), letters of the Greek alphabet (e.g., α, β, γ, δ), or Arabic numerals (e.g., 1, 2, 3, 4). These different crystalline forms must be chemically identical in order to be called polymorphs. If the solid also contains solvent molecules in the crystal structure then it is referred to as a solvate, and if that solvent is water then it is specifically called a hydrate. The stoichiometry of the water molecules present in the crystal structure is represented by the name (e.g., a monohydrate has one molecule of water per molecule of the compound of interest, a dihydrate has two molecules of water, etc.). On the other hand, if the crystal structure contains no water then it is referred to as an anhydrate. If multiple anhydrous forms of the same compound exist they are said to be polymorphs. Additionally, if multiple monohydrate forms of the same compound exist they are also said to be polymorphs. Other terms (such as solvatomorphs and pseudopolymorphs) have been used to describe solvates, but these are less favorable because their definitions are not as clear. Crystal habits are another phenomenon of crystalline solids, where crystals have the same internal structure (molecular packing) but have different external shapes or morphologies (e.g., needles, plates), which leads to differences in their pharmaceutical properties, including mixing, flowability, and dissolution [21].

The stability of a polymorph is represented by its free energy. The free energy of a polymorph is proportional to its solubility. Since polymorphs have different free energies, they will also have different solubilities [19]. Therefore, the solubility of polymorphs can be used to determine their relative stability. Only the form with lowest free energy at a specified temperature and pressure is said to be stable. All other forms are said to be metastable relative to that form. If at any temperature the relative solubility difference between two polymorphs is maintained, as shown in Fig. 16.1a, then the polymorphs are said to be related monotropically. However, if at some temperature the relative solubility of the polymorphs inverts, as shown in Fig. 16.1b, then they are said to be enantiotropically related. Unfortunately, solubility studies have their drawbacks when it comes to identifying monotropic and enantiotropic systems. One of the major problems is a limited temperature range over which the measurements can be made. While many times the data is linear on a van't Hoff plot (as in Fig. 16.1), the extrapolation of this data outside the experimental range is often prone to large errors [21]. Differential scanning calorimetry (DSC) can be a very useful tool in identifying monotropic and enantiotropic systems, because it provides heats of transition and fusion for polymorphs and polymorphic conversions. These values can then be interpreted using the rules developed by Burger and Ramberger [22, 23]:

1. *Heat (or Enthalpy) of Transition Rule.* If a solid–solid transition is endothermic then the polymorphs are related enantiotropically; if the transition is exothermic then they are related monotropically.

2. *Heat (or Enthalpy) of Fusion Rule.* If a polymorph has a lower heat of fusion but a higher melting point than another polymorph, then the two forms are related enantiotropically; if not, the relationship is monotropic.

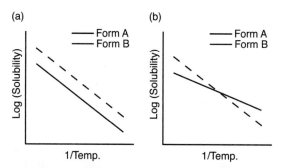

FIGURE 16.1 Theoretical van't Hoff plots showing relative water solubility of two polymorphs related (a) monotropically and (b) enantiotropically.

Figure 16.2a shows the heat of transition rule. In the monotropic system, the metastable Form B converts, at some temperature, to the stable Form A; since Form A has a lower enthalpy (H_A) the conversion is an exothermic process. This also holds true for the enantiotropic system if Form B converts to Form A before the crossover temperature, where Form B becomes the stable form and Form A becomes metastable. On the other hand, if Form A converts to Form B in the enantiotropic system, at a temperature above the crossover temperature, then since Form B has a higher enthalpy (H_B) the conversion will be endothermic. Figure 16.2b shows the heat of fusion rule. The point at which the free-energy curve of each polymorph crosses the liquid line in the energy–temperature diagrams is the temperature at which it melts. In the monotropic system the metastable Form B melts at a lower temperature and has a smaller heat of fusion ($\Delta_F H$) than the stable Form A, which has a higher

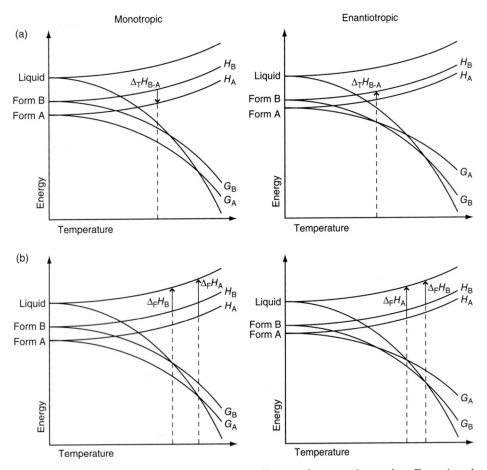

FIGURE 16.2 Theoretical energy–temperature diagrams for two polymorphs—Form A and Form B—showing the enthalpy (H) and free energy (G) of each polymorph as a function of temperature. (a) Energy–temperature diagrams illustrating the heat of transistion ($\Delta_T H$) rule for both a monotropic and an enantiotropic system. (b) Energy–temperature diagrams illustrating the heat of fusion ($\Delta_F H$) rule for both a monotropic and enantiotropic system.

melting temperature and a larger $\Delta_F H$. Conversely, in the enantiotropic system, Form A melts at a lower temperature with a higher $\Delta_F H$ and Form B melts at a higher temperature with a lower $\Delta_F H$. This occurs because the free-energy lines cross but the enthalpy lines do not cross. Additionally, different polymorphs may have different rates of dissolution.

Occasionally, the solubility of the stable form is too low for the drug to reach therapeutic levels when administered to patients. This may require the use of a metastable form with a higher solubility to be used in a formulation. Typically, an amorphous material will have a significantly higher solubility and dissolution rate than any crystalline form of a material and thus is also less stable. Caution must be used when developing a formulation because many of the processing techniques that are used in the pharmaceutical industry can cause polymorphic conversions or other changes to the physical state of a solid, making it vital to identify and control these properties throughout the development process and especially in the final formulated product. One rule of thumb is that if an amorphous material is stored 50 °C below its T_g, then its mobility will be sufficiently low to prevent crystallization or other degradation [19, 20, 24, 25].

One example of the consequences of polymorphic change in a formulation is ritonavir [26], a protease inhibitor, that was discovered in 1992 at Abbott Laboratories and was given FDA approval in 1996. It was formulated and marketed as a semisolid capsule (containing a nearly saturated solution) and a liquid formulation. Despite attempts to produce and identify other crystal forms, only one (Form I) was known to exist. Then in 1998 the semisolid formulation began failing dissolution tests because the drug was precipitating in the formulated product. When the precipitate was analyzed it was found to be in a previously unknown crystal form (Form II) and this new form was found to be more thermodynamically stable and thus less soluble. Form II spread throughout their production facilities and eventually they were only able to produce the new less soluble form.

While small molecules are almost always more stable in a crystalline form, the same is not necessarily true for biopharmaceuticals. Pikal and Rigsbee [27] showed that insulin is actually more stable when it is amorphous.

16.3.2 Chemical Stability

All of the chemical reactions that are possible in the solution state are also possible in the solid state. Reactions in crystalline solids are governed by the topochemical postulate [28], which states that reactions will occur with a minimum of atomic and molecular movement. In the solid state, functional groups on a molecule or neighboring molecules may be held closer or farther away from one another than they are in the solution state, which may change the rates of the reactions or even the degradation products that are formed [29]. Additionally, polymorphs and solvates may have different reactivities because of the differences in their crystal structures.

16.3.3 Identifying True Solid-State Chemical Reactions

Water is often present in the solid state, whether it is atmospheric, in the excipients of the formulation, or in the drug itself (e.g., a hydrate). This raises the question of

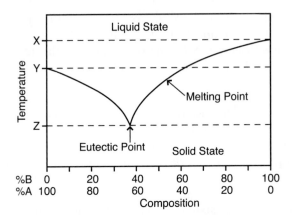

FIGURE 16.3 Phase diagram depicting how the melting point of the material changes as the hypothetical degradation of A proceeds to Form B. (Adapted from Ref. 21.)

whether a reaction actually occurs in the solid state or a solution state, where the molecules actually dissolve in the water, react, and then precipitate back out of solution. Five criteria have been developed to identify true solid-state reactions [21].

A reaction occurs in the solid state if:

1. In solution the reaction is slower or does not occur.
2. Pronounced differences are found in the reactivity of compounds with very similar chemical structures when they are in the solid state.
3. Reaction products are different from those observed in solution.
4. Different crystalline forms of the same compound have different reactivities or yield different reaction products.
5. The reaction occurs at a temperature below the eutectic point of a mixture of the starting material and products.

The fifth criterion is illustrated in Fig. 16.3, where A reacts to form B. A has a melting point of Y and B has a melting point of X. As B is formed it depresses the observed melting point because it acts as an impurity in A. At some critical composition (eutectic point) the melting point begins to rise again because A begins to be the impurity in B. The fifth criterion is fulfilled if the reaction occurs at a temperature below Z.

16.4 KINETICS

In the most general sense drug stability is a very simple concept. A drug reacts via some mechanism, at some rate, and produces a product. However, reactions can become very complex when variables such as temperature, pH, physical state, and so on are taken into account.

16.4.1 Kinetic Models

A chemical reaction can be represented by a rate expression, such as

$$\frac{-d[A]}{dt} = k[A]^x[B]^y[C]^z \cdots \tag{16.1}$$

The order of the reaction is given by the sum of the powers $(x, y, z, \ldots)$ in the rate expression. In the simplest system the rate of the reaction does not depend on the concentration of any of the reactants. This is called a zero-order reaction and is given by

$$\frac{-d[A]}{dt} = k \tag{16.2}$$

The integrated form of this equation is

$$[A]_t = [A]_0 - kt \tag{16.3}$$

Equation 16.4 represents a first-order reaction and Eq. 16.5 gives the integrated form:

$$\frac{-d[A]}{dt} = k[A] \tag{16.4}$$

$$[A]_t = [A]_0 e^{-kt} \tag{16.5}$$

Equation 16.6 represents one example of a second-order reaction and Eq. 16.7 gives the integrated form:

$$\frac{-d[A]}{dt} = k[A]^2 \tag{16.6}$$

$$\frac{1}{[A]_t} = kt + \frac{1}{[A]_0} \tag{16.7}$$

The order of a reaction is determined by observing the reaction over time and then fitting it to the models to determine which one fits the observed data. Most reactions will be zero, first, or second order. However, if several reactions are occurring simultaneously the model may become more complex. Once the order of the reaction is determined it is important to verify that the order matches the mechanism. For example, hydrolysis reactions should depend on the concentration of both the drug and the water. However, these reactions often appear to follow first-order kinetics because the media in which they occur are composed primarily of water. The concentration of water is so large that it does not change significantly over the course of the reaction, so the rate of the reaction only depends on the concentration of the drug because there is essentially an infinite supply of water for the reaction.

Since this reaction is second order, but appears to be first order, it is referred to as a pseudo-first-order reaction.

Solid-state reactions often display more complicated kinetics, which leads to difficulties in understanding the kinetics of the system. There are four main steps in a solid-state reaction [21].

1. *Loosening of Molecules.* This step occurs at nucleation/defect sites, which are imperfections in the crystal that typically form during the crystallization process or during processing (e.g., grinding) and allow sufficient mobility for the reaction to occur.
2. *Molecular Change.* This step is the actual reaction of interest and is typically slower than the same reaction in solution due to the restricted motion.
3. *Solid Solution Formation.* Early in the reaction only a small amount of the product has been formed and is randomly mixed with the reactant (this mixture is the solid solution), eventually enough product forms and the reactants and products separate.
4. *Separation of Product.* When the product separates from the reactant it forms a new phase that can be amorphous or crystalline.

It is often difficult to fully understand the kinetics of a reaction in the solid state. Several models are commonly used (shown in Table 16.1) and they can be grouped

TABLE 16.1   Solid-State Kinetic Models

Name	Equation^a
Prout–Tompkins	$\ln\left(\dfrac{\alpha}{1-\alpha}\right) = kt + c$
Avrami–Erofe'ev	$[-\ln(1-\alpha)]^n = kt \quad n = \dfrac{1}{4}, \dfrac{1}{3}, \dfrac{1}{2}, \dfrac{2}{3}$, or 1
One-dimensional phase boundary (zero order)	$1 - \alpha = kt$
Two-dimensional phase boundary (contracting area)	$1 - (1-\alpha)^{1/2} = kt$
Three-dimensional phase boundary (contracting volume)	$1 - (1-\alpha)^{1/3} = kt$
Diffusion-controlled one-dimensional	$\alpha^2 = kt$
Diffusion-controlled two-dimensional	$(1-\alpha)\ln(1-\alpha) + \alpha = kt$
Diffusion-controlled three-dimensional	$1 - \dfrac{2}{3}\alpha - (1-\alpha)^{2/3} = kt$
Jander equation	$[1 - (1-\alpha)^{1/3}]^2 = kt$
Power law	$a^n = kt \quad n = \dfrac{1}{4}, \dfrac{1}{3}, \dfrac{1}{2}$, 1, or 2
First order	$\ln(\alpha) = kt$
Second order	$\dfrac{1}{1-\alpha} = kt$

$^a\alpha$ = fraction decomposed, k = rate constant, t = time, and c = constant.

into four types: reactions involving nucleation, reactions controlled by phase boundaries, diffusion-controlled reactions, and other reactions [21].

The two models that fall into the nucleation category are the Prout–Tompkins and Avrami–Erofe'ev equations. Prout and Tompkins [30, 31] developed an equation that assumes a solid-state reaction begins at a nucleation site, branches out in chains, and is terminated more rapidly as the number of nuclei increase. This can be likened to a polymer chain reaction in which there is an initiation, propagation, and termination step. The Avrami–Erofe'ev equation [32–34] also assumes that the reaction starts at nuclei; however, it assumes that the nuclei grow and engulf other nuclei and the directionality of this growth is interpreted from the value of n.

If a reaction begins on the surface of a crystal and advances toward the interior, then it falls into the phase boundary category. There are three equations in this group and each represents a different dimensionality of the growth. The one-dimensional or zero-order rate equation (identical to the solution-state zero-order rate equation) assumes that the reaction only moves in one direction across the crystal (e.g., in a rod-shaped crystal the reaction begins at one or both ends and the reaction front travels down the crystal to the opposite end). If the reaction progresses in two dimensions (e.g., in a rod-shaped crystal the reaction initiates on the circumference and then travels radially toward the long axis of the rod) then it is represented by the two-dimensional or contracting area equation [35]. Finally, if the reaction travels in three dimensions (e.g., in a rod-shaped crystal the reaction initiates on both the ends and the circumference and then travels toward the center of the rod) then it can be modeled by the three-dimensional or contracting volume equation [35].

The third group contains the diffusion-controlled reactions and, as the name implies, these equations describe reactions in which two reactants must come together to form the product. As with the phase boundary equations there are three equations that describe the dimensionality of the diffusion: one-, two-, and three-dimensional diffusion-controlled rate equation [35–39]. The Jander equation also falls into this category and it is a simplified form of the three-dimensional diffusion-controlled rate equation.

The final group is composed of all the other equations that are used but do not have any physical interpretation. The power-law equation has been used in solid-state kinetic studies; however, it has no theoretical basis for interpretation except that when $n = 2$ it is identical to the one-dimensional diffusion equation. The first- and second-order rate equations are sometimes used to describe solid-state reactions; however, the order of a reaction in the solid state is not understood or defined as well as it is in the solution state and therefore it has little interpretive value. On the other hand, the zero-order (one-dimensional phase boundary) equation does have a physical meaning in the solid state.

Typically in solid-state kinetic studies the data is fit to each of the equations described earlier, and in the case of the Avrami–Erofe'ev and power-law equations, where n can have multiple values, all of the possible values of n are used to fit the data. This results in approximately 19 different fits of the same set of data and for most fits the correlation will be very good ($R^2 > 0.9$). If information is known about the reaction mechanism, then it can be used to narrow the possible fits to use. For example, if it is known that the reaction does involve two reactants that are not held closely in the crystal structure, then it is likely that one of the diffusion models would be more representative of the reaction rate. However, typically these distinctions cannot be made and the models with the best fits ($R^2 > 0.98$) are analyzed to see if they can yield some information about the mechanism of the reaction. For example, do the nucleation equations seem to fit better or do the phase boundary equations seem to fit better? One model is then chosen and used to measure the degradation rates in the subsequent stability studies.

16.4.2   Temperature

Drugs must be stable enough to be stored for long periods of time (~2 years); however, when trying to develop a stable formulation it is not desirable to wait for a long period of time to find out if the formulation will be stable enough to survive storage. Therefore, a method for speeding up stability measurements is needed. It is well known that the Arrhenius equation (Eq. 16.8) describes the relationship between the activation energy (E_a) of a reaction and the rate of the reaction (k) at a given temperature (T), where A is a frequency term and R is the gas constant. The Arrhenius equation can also be linearized (Eq. 16.9) to simplify data fitting and analysis.

$$k = A\exp\left(\frac{-E_a}{RT}\right) \tag{16.8}$$

$$\ln(k) = \ln(A) + \left(\frac{-E_a}{RT}\right) \tag{16.9}$$

Therefore, if the rate of degradation is measured at multiple temperatures it is possible to measure E_a for the reaction by plotting $\ln(k)$ versus $1/T$ to produce an Arrhenius plot, and determine E_a from the slope ($-E_a/R$). The stability of the formulation can then be predicted at room temperature or any other storage conditions such as refrigeration (assuming that the reaction mechanism does not change [40]). While E_a and A are typically assumed to be constants, in theory they are not. The Eyring equation (Eq. 16.10) can be used to account for the temperature dependency of both E_a and A, and as with the Arrhenius equation it can be linearized (Eq. 16.11) to simplify data analysis.

$$k = \left[\frac{k_B T}{h}\exp\left(\frac{\Delta S^{\ddagger}}{R}\right)\right]\exp\left(\frac{-\Delta H^{\ddagger}}{RT}\right) \tag{16.10}$$

$$\ln\left(\frac{k}{T}\right) = \left[\ln\left(\frac{k_B}{h}\right) + \left(\frac{\Delta S^{\ddagger}}{R}\right)\right] + \left(\frac{-\Delta H^{\ddagger}}{RT}\right) \tag{16.11}$$

The Eyring plot is produced by plotting $\ln(k/T)$ versus $1/T$, where $\Delta H^{\ddagger}$ can be obtained from the slope and used to predict the stability at lower temperatures (although the Arrhenius plot is much more commonly used for this purpose). The Arrhenius and Eyring equations form the basis for the accelerated stability tests that are used to evaluate and compare potential formulations in the development process (for more information see Section 16.5).

TABLE 16.2   Sensitivity of Rate Constants to Changes in Temperature

	k_2/k_1	
E_a (kcal/mol)	$\Delta T = 1\,^\circ\text{C}$	$\Delta T = 0.1\,^\circ\text{C}$
10	1.058	1.006
20	1.119	1.011
30	1.184	1.017

When studying stability it is important to maintain a constant temperature because, as shown by the Arrhenius and Eyring equations, if the temperature changes the rate constant will change. The relevant degradation reactions that most pharmaceuticals undergo in the solution state have an E_a between 10 and 30 kcal/mol and Table 16.2 shows how sensitive the rate constant of a reaction with an E_a in this range is to changes in the temperature.

Table 16.2 demonstrates the need for accurate temperature control during stability studies. If the reaction being studied has an E_a of 30 kcal/mol, the measured degradation rate can be off by as much as 18.4% if the temperature is off by only 1 °C. Therefore, ovens that are used for stability studies should have the ability to maintain temperatures as accurately as possible.

In the solid state it is usually assumed that reactions will exhibit Arrhenius kinetics (linear Arrhenius plot); however, this is not always the case. One potential reason for non-Arrhenius kinetics is a change in the mechanism of degradation. Additionally, the physical state of the material may change. For example, an amorphous material may not exhibit Arrhenius kinetics if the temperature range being studied spans the T_g of the material [41], or the material may even crystallize at higher temperatures. Also, a crystalline material may undergo a polymorphic conversion to a different crystalline form at some temperature in the range that is being studied [40].

16.4.3   pH

Hydrogen (H^+) and hydroxide ions (OH^-) can act as catalysts in reactions. Therefore, the observed rate of a reaction (k_{obs}) is actually the sum of the multiple of the rate constants of each reaction mechanism and the concentration (or more accurately the activity) of the corresponding catalyst:

$$k_{obs} = k_{H^+}[H^+] + k_{H_2O} + k_{OH^-}[OH^-] \tag{16.12}$$

The observed rate of degradation can be measured at numerous pH values and then plotted, as in Fig. 16.4, to yield a pH–rate profile. Buffers are typically employed to maintain a constant pH during the stability studies; however, they can dramatically affect the results if not properly accounted for (see Section 16.4.4 on buffers). These profiles can be very simple as they are in Fig. 16.4a–e, or very complex as in Fig. 16.4f. If there is no catalysis ($k_{H^+} \ll k_{H_2O} \gg k_{OH^-}$; Fig. 16.4a) the pH–rate profile should just be a flat line parallel to the x-axis (no change in rate). However, if hydrogen ions catalyze the reaction ($k_{H^+} \geq k_{H_2O} \gg k_{OH^-}$; Fig. 16.4b) then the left side

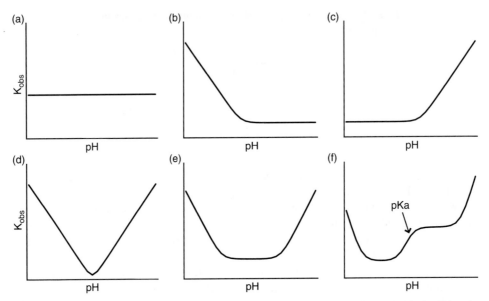

FIGURE 16.4 Theoretical pH–rate profiles showing (a) no acid or base catalysis, (b) only acid catalysis, (c) only base catalysis, (d) acid and base catalysis in V-shaped profile, (e) acid and base catalysis in U-shaped profile, and (f) acid and base catalysis of a weak base.

of the profile should curve up, and if hydroxide ions catalyze the reaction ($k_{H^+} \ll k_{H_2O} \leq k_{OH^-}$; Fig. 16.4c) then the right side of the profile should curve up. Subsequently, if both ions catalyze the reaction then both ends should curve up, and in this case there are two types of profiles that are possible: the V shaped and the U shaped. In the V shape (Fig. 16.4d) the k_{H^+} and k_{OH^-} are significantly larger than the k_{H_2O} such that the two sloped regions meet at a point and the profile resembles the letter V. However, in the U shape (Fig. 16.4e) all three rate constants are much closer to the same value so that the center of the profile is flattened and the entire profile resembles the letter U. If the molecule that is being studied is a weak acid or a weak base (Fig. 16.4f), the neutral and the ionized forms can have different reactivities and the H^+ and OH^- may have different abilities to catalyze the reactions of the two forms. This results in a much more complex equation to describe k_{obs} (Eq. 16.13) where k is the rate of the reaction of the ionized form and k' is the rate of the neural form and f_{DH^+} and f_D are the fractions of the ionized and neutral forms of a weak base, respectively.

$$k_{obs} = (k_{H^+}[H^+] + k_{H_2O} + k_{OH^-}[OH^-])f_{DH^+} + (k'_{H^+}[H^+] + k'_{H_2O} + k'_{OH^-}[OH^-])f_D \quad (16.13)$$

$$f_{DH^+} = \frac{[H^+]}{K_a + [H^+]} \quad (16.14)$$

$$f_D = \frac{K_a}{K_a + [H^+]} \quad (16.15)$$

It is possible to show that $k_{H_2O} f_{DH^+}$ and $k'_{H^+}[H^+] f_D$ are mathematically equivalent and that $k_{OH^-}[OH^-] f_{DH^+}$ and $k'_{H_2O} f_D$ are also mathematically equivalent; therefore, Eq. 16.13 can be simplified to produce Eq. 16.16:

$$k_{obs} = k_{H^+}[H^+] f_{DH^+} + k_{H_2O} f_{DH^+} + k'_{H_2O} f_D + k'_{OH^-}[OH^-] f_D \qquad (16.16)$$

When examining a pH–rate profile the regions of acid and base catalysis should have a slope of −1 and +1, respectively. If the slopes are closer to zero then the reaction may be pH dependent but not acid or base catalyzed. The individual rate constants can be determined manually or the pH–rate profile can be fit to an equation, such as Eq. 16.16, that appropriately describes k_{obs} using a software program that is capable of performing nonlinear regression analysis. If a software program is used to fit the profile the data should be weighted because the [H⁺] can span as many as 12 orders of magnitude.

When it comes to the solid state, pH has no definition. However, differences have been observed in the solid state when proteins are prepared from solutions of different pH values. Therefore, effective pH or "pH" has been defined as the pH of a solution before it is converted to a solid (typically by lyophilization) or after the solid is reconstituted. While the physical basis of this "pH" is not yet fully understood it can be a very helpful parameter when trying to develop a solid formulation for peptides and proteins [41].

The pH– and "pH"–rate profiles play a very important role in formulation development. It provides an easy mechanism by which an appropriate formulation pH or "pH" can be identified visually and it provides an idea of how vital pH control is. For example, if a drug has a V-shaped pH–rate profile it may be vital to buffer the formulation because a small change in the pH may result in a large change in the degradation rate; however, if the drug has a U-shaped profile the formulation could be prepared near the center of the flat region and it may not require buffering since a small change in the pH will result in little to no change in the stability.

16.4.4 Buffers

As stated previously, buffers are commonly used in stability studies to maintain the pH of the solution over the course of the experiment, since the k_{obs} is dependent on the concentration of the H⁺ and OH⁻. However, the buffer can also catalyze (k_{cat}) the reaction through general acid or general base catalysis; although different ionized or un-ionized states of the buffer may have more or less catalytic activity. If this occurs then more terms must be added to the k_{obs} equation (Eq. 16.12) to account for this catalysis:

$$k'_{obs} = k_{obs} + k_{cat}[\text{Buffer}]_{total} \qquad (16.17)$$

$$k_{cat} = k_{BH^+} f_{BH^+} + k_B f_B \qquad (16.18)$$

In this example the buffer is a weak base with a single ionized state. When the pH is changed to study the stability at another pH, the k_{cat} will also change because the fractions of the ionized (f_{BH^+}) and neutral (f_B) buffer components will change.

Therefore, it is necessary to determine the k_{obs} so that the buffer catalysis does not impact the pH–rate profile. By increasing the concentration of the buffer while maintaining the pH, it is possible to extrapolate the k_{obs} from a plot of k'_{obs} versus the total concentration of the buffer (Fig. 16.5), where the y-intercept is k_{obs} and the slope is k_{cat}. The k_{obs} of studies at different pH values can then be combined to create a pH–rate profile. The k_{cat} can also be plotted versus the fraction of one of the ionized forms of the buffer (e.g., f_B) to determine the k_{BH^+} and k_B (Fig. 16.6); this may help in identifying which buffer to use in a formulation by helping to determine

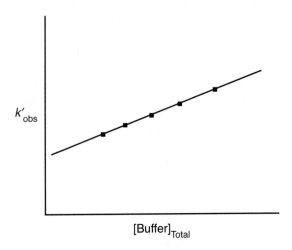

FIGURE 16.5 Theoretical plot of k'_{obs} versus total buffer concentration showing the effects of general acid/base catalysis on k'_{obs} when buffer concentration is changed.

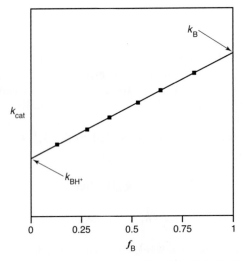

FIGURE 16.6 Theoretical plot of k_{cat} versus the fraction of the buffer that is in the neutral form, showing that the ionized form of the buffer is less catalytic than the neutral form.

which buffers do not catalyze the degradation or which do so only slightly. Note that ionic strength can also affect the rate of degradation; therefore, it is also important that the ionic strength be kept constant as the pH and the buffer concentration are changed.

16.4.5 Relative Humidity

In the solution state a drug is already dissolved in a solvent and thus water vapor has little to no interaction with the drug. However, solids can interact with water vapor in multiple ways. The interaction can be a physical one in which the solid takes up the water. If the solid is amorphous the water could increase the mobility of the matrix since water acts as a plasticizer to decrease the T_g of amorphous materials, or if the mobility increases sufficiently the drug may be able to crystallize [20]. On the other hand, a crystalline solid, either anhydrous or hydrated, could take up water stoichiometrically to form a hydrate or a higher order hydrate, respectively. Conversely, a hydrated form could lose water to the atmosphere if the humidity drops below a particular level. Water can also be involved in chemical reactions in the solid state. In the case of a hydrolysis reaction, the water from the atmosphere could diffuse into the solid and then react with the drug. The water may also produce a physical change, such as an increase in mobility, which may subsequently lead to the increased rate of a chemical reaction due to the increased mobility of the drug molecule. Additionally, there is a possibility that the water may form a thin layer on the surface of the particles in which the drug could dissolve and then degrade [42–44].

Since water can play such a vital role in the degradation of drugs in the solid state it is vital to characterize how water vapor interacts with solid materials. This is typically performed by water vapor sorption analysis in which the material is stored at multiple relative humidities while the temperature is held constant until the material reaches equilibrium. The water content of the material stored at each relative humidity is then measured and plotted against the corresponding relative humidity to form a water vapor sorption isotherm. The isotherm provides important information concerning the stability of different polymorphs or amorphous material to relative humidity. For example, if a drug has two anhydrate forms (A and B) by comparing their isotherms at 25 °C it can be seen that at 20% relative humidity Form A takes up 1 mole of water for every mole of drug and thus forms a monohydrate, and subsequently at 75% relative humidity this monohydrate produced from Form A takes up another mole of water for every mole of drug to produce a dihydrate. Form B does not take up any significant amount of water and remains anhydrous at all relative humidities. This information can be very important when preparing to develop a formulation. If Form B could not be used in the formulation, the consequences of the formation of the mono- and dihydrates must be considered (i.e., differences in the stability, solubility, or dissolution rate of Form A and the hydrates).

Deliquescence occurs when a solid, typically amorphous, adsorbs enough water vapor to liquefy. Conversely, if water evaporates to leave behind a solid this process is called efflorescence. When these processes occur the material is not simply labeled deliquescent or efflorescent; instead the temperature and relative humidity at which the water gain or loss occurs should be reported [21].

16.5   ACCELERATED STABILITY TESTING

The degradation of drugs means that eventually they will no longer be effective because too much of the drug will have degraded and the delivered dose will be too small. Therefore, drugs are given a shelf life that indicates how long they can be stored and still be guaranteed effective. For some drugs, this lifetime is defined as the amount of time that it takes for 10% of the drug to degrade or the t_{90}. However, occasionally the degradation of the drug produces a toxic compound, and the amount of this toxic substance that is produced will determine the shelf life of the formulation [40, 45]. The t_{90} for a first-order degradation reaction can be determined from the rate constant using

$$t_{90} = \frac{-\ln(0.9)}{k} \tag{16.19}$$

However, when determining if a potential formulation will be stable enough it is undesirable to wait for a year or longer to see if more than 10% of the drug has degraded. Thus, accelerated stability studies are used to stress the formulation (increased temperature and relative humidity) in an effort to predict the shelf life of the formulation under typical storage conditions. By stressing the formulation the study can be completed in several months and then, once an appropriate formulation is found, an extended stability study (~2 years) under typical storage conditions can be performed to verify the predictions.

While the principles are the same for accelerated stability testing in the solution and solid states, it is important to note that additional complications can arise in solids. For example, the drug may have polymorphs that are related enantiotropically and either some or all of the temperatures used may be above the crossover temperature; therefore, the accelerated stability testing may be done on one polymorph while the study is meant to predict the stability of the other polymorph. Also, the polymorphs could be related monotropically and some or all of the temperatures may be above the temperature at which the metastable form converts to the more stable form. However, it is not common to develop a formulation that contains a metastable polymorph, but it could be formed unintentionally in the processing steps used to produce the formulation. Additionally, it is possible that, when performing an accelerated stability study on an amorphous material, the material may be in its rubbery state and under normal storage conditions it would be in the glassy state, depending on the T_g of the material. In all of these cases, the accelerated stability study would give erroneous results and would not correctly predict the stability under normal storage conditions. It would not be possible to detect these errors unless the stability is studied under normal storage conditions, which may take a year or longer. Therefore, it is vital to thoroughly characterize solid-state systems before performing accelerated stability studies [46].

16.5.1   Isothermal Kinetics

Isothermal kinetics studies rely on the relationships between temperature and rate constant (as shown previously in Eq. 16.8 and 16.10) to predict the shelf life of a formulation. These studies are termed isothermal because the temperature is held constant to measure the rate constant of the degradation. The rate constant is measured at multiple temperatures and subsequently fit to the Arrhenius equation (Eq. 16.9) to obtain the E_a of the reaction. The E_a of the reaction can subsequently be used to predict the rate of degradation and thus the t_{90} at lower temperatures using Eq. 16.8. This can be used to determine if the formulation is sufficiently stable or if a change must be made to increase the stability.

16.5.2 Nonisothermal Kinetics

Nonisothermal kinetics studies were first proposed by Rogers [47] as a way to simplify stability studies. In a nonisothermal kinetics study the temperature is increased throughout the course of the study. This allows the E_a to be determined from only one experiment and eliminates the need for measuring the degradation rate at multiple temperatures. The degradation of a drug that follows first-order kinetics can be described by Eq. 16.20 [47], which is achieved by substituting Eq. 16.8 into Eq. 16.5:

$$[D]_t = [D]_0 \exp[-tA\exp(-E_a/RT)] \tag{16.20}$$

$[D]_t$ and $[D]_0$ are the concentrations of the drug at the time t and zero, respectively; t is the time; A is the frequency term from the Arrhenius equation; R is the gas constant; and T is the temperature. However, Eq. 16.20 describes the isothermal degradation kinetics; King et al. [48] derived Eq. 16.21, which can be fit via nonlinear regression to directly estimate both E_a and t_{90}.

$$[D]_t = [D]_0 \exp\left\{-t\left(\frac{0.1054}{t_{90}}\right)\exp\left[\left(\frac{E_a}{R}\right)\left(\frac{1}{298} - \frac{1}{T(t)}\right)\right]\right\} \tag{16.21}$$

In this equation $T(t)$ is the temperature at time t. One major drawback to this method is that the quality of the prediction depends on the experimental design; thus, significant care must be taken to choose the correct experiment length, sampling interval, and temperature program (rate of temperature change) in order to get accurate predictions [49]. Unfortunately, isothermal studies are needed to obtain the correct variables for accurate nonisothermal studies. In practice, there is very little, if any, gain from performing nonisothermal studies. For this reason, these studies are not routinely performed. They do occasionally experience a resurgence in popularity due to their potential to reduce the number of experiments that are required. Additionally, nonisothermal kinetics also require very accurate temperature control but have the added requirement that the oven also be able to precisely increase the temperature according to a predefined program.

16.6 IMPROVING STABILITY

There are several ways to produce a stable formulation when the drug that it contains is inherently unstable. In general, this is accomplished by either adding excipients or making chemical modifications to the drug. If the drug is moderately stable and only a slight increase in stability is needed, then excipients will probably be sufficient, although they will only slow the degradation. However, if the molecule is extremely unstable, it will probably require changes to its chemical structure to obtain sufficient stability.

Aside from the previously mentioned excipients (e.g., buffers to control pH, desiccants to control humidity), there are many excipients that can be used to increase stability. The drug may undergo photodegradation. If so, the formulation can be protected from light by being placed in an opaque container, a photoprotective coat can be applied to the outside of a tablet, or a colorant can be added to the formulation to absorb the light. Exposure to light can also cause the formation of compounds that can oxidize drug molecules. If the drug is sensitive to oxidation, an antioxidant (e.g., α-tocopherol, butylated hydroxyanisole, ascorbic acid, thioglycolic acid) could be added to the formulation to reduce the oxidation rate of the drug. Additionally, oxygen adsorbent can be used to reduce the oxygen concentration and thereby reduce the concentration of the reactive oxygen species [1].

Some drugs can be stabilized either by forming a complex or partitioning into another environment. There are several ways that a ligand can protect a drug molecule when forming a complex: the ligand can act as a barrier that blocks a reactant from reaching the drug molecule or it can restrict the freedom of the drug molecule and hold it in a more stable conformation. Cyclodextrins, in particular, have proved to be very useful in their ability to complex with and stabilize drugs; however, cyclodextrins can be toxic and therefore cyclodextrin derivatives are typically used instead [50]. In some cases liposomes or micelles can be used in a formulation to increase the stability of a drug, either through interactions at the "oil–water" interface or by the partitioning of the drug into the lipid phase [1].

In some cases excipients are not able to adequately stabilize a drug. In these cases chemical modification of the drug will likely be required, thereby creating a new chemical entity and requiring that the entire stability testing process be repeated. One potential solution is to develop a prodrug that will be converted to the active pharmaceutical after it is administered to the patient. Additionally, it may be necessary to remove the unstable functional group in the drug. This may create problems if that functional group is also needed for the pharmacological activity; if this is the case, it may be necessary to identify a similar functional group that will still result in the necessary pharmacological activity but is less reactive. Even if the unstable functional group is removed, the drug will almost certainly still degrade, but the degradation would likely be much slower, and occur through another mechanism [1].

16.7   METHODS OF ANALYSIS

When performing stability studies it is necessary to use an analytical method that is capable of determining the extent of the reaction by following either the disappearance of the drug or appearance of its degradation products, or ideally both. This requires a method that can identify and quantify either the drug or its products in a mixture containing the drug, all of its degradation products, excipients, and any impurities [51].

Chemical stability is commonly measured using a chromatography technique, such as HPLC, to separate the reactants and products and is coupled with a detection method for identification and quantification, including electromagnetic spectroscopy (e.g., UV or visible light absorption), mass spectrometry, and electrochemical detection [51]. The only difference between studying the solution and solid states is that the solid must be dissolved before analysis. Since the studies typically can go for long periods of time (days to months), it is not uncommon to store the samples until the end of the experiment and then perform the analysis of all of the samples at once to help reduce the day-to-day variability of the instruments. The samples are typically stored by freezing; however, it is imperative that a control be performed to verify that no changes occur in the samples when they are frozen [52].

Physical stability requires a much broader set of techniques. For peptides and proteins there are several spectroscopic techniques that can be used to follow changes in the secondary and tertiary structure. Circular dichroism and infrared spectroscopy can be used to follow changes in the secondary structure, while intrinsic fluorescence can be used to follow changes in the tertiary structure. UV-Vis spectroscopy and DSC can be used to monitor denaturation [10]. Light scattering techniques and size exclusion chromatography are available to analyze aggregation.

When it comes to solids there are several techniques available to identify and track physical changes. X-ray diffractometry can be used to determine the crystal structure of a crystalline material, and to identify and quantitate polymorphs, solvates, and amorphous materials [21, 53]. Hot-stage microscopy can be used to follow changes in solids during heating by changes in birefringence [21, 54]. Thermogravimetric analysis (TGA) can be used to determine water or other volatile content (identify solvates and determine their stochiometry) and to follow stability to thermal decomposition to form gaseous products [21]. Additionally, Karl Fischer titration can be used to determine water content. DSC can provide a variety of information including melting points of polymorphs, T_g of amorphous material [20], and identification of monotropic versus enantiotropic systems [21]. Infrared and Raman spectroscopy can be utilized to identify and quantitate polymorphs and solvates [21]. Water vapor sorption can be used to characterize how different solid forms (polymorphs, solvates, and amorphous materials) interact with atmospheric water. Solid-state NMR spectroscopy can provide mobility information (such as T_g) and identify polymorphs, solvates, and amorphous materials [55]. Solid-state NMR spectroscopy is gaining popularity for several reasons, including that it is nondestructive, that it can often differentiate the drug from the excipients in a formulation when other techniques cannot, and that it can be used to study many dosage forms *in situ* [21]. Solid-state NMR spectroscopy can also provide crystal structure information, such as the number of crystallographically inequivalent sites [56].

16.8   REGULATORY GUIDELINES

In the pharmaceutical industry, stability testing is typically performed according to guidelines established by the International Conference on Harmonization of Technical Requirements for Registration of Pharmaceuticals for Human Use (ICH). The ICH groups "stability" among its "Quality Topics" and thus identifies each individual "Quality" guideline with a Q-code. Some of the relevant guidances are shown in Table 16.3 and are available online at http://www.ich.org.

TABLE 16.3   ICH Stability Guidelines

Q-Code	Topic
Q1A(R2)	Stability Testing of New Drug Substances and Products
Q1B	Stability Testing: Photostability Testing of New Drug Substances and Products
Q1C	Stability Testing for New Dosage Forms
Q1D	Bracketing and Matrixing Designs for Stability Testing of New Drug Substances and Products
Q1E	Evaluation of Stability Data
Q1F	Stability Data Package for Registration Applications in Climatic Zones III and IV

There are also national and regional guidelines on stability testing. In the United States, the U.S. Food and Drug Administration (FDA) is the regulatory body and the FDA's Center for Drug Evaluation and Research (CDER) issues stability guidances. These documents can be found online at http://www.fda.gov/cder/guidance/index.htm and http://www.fda.gov/cber/guidelines.htm.

16.9   FURTHER READING

Stability is a very broad topic that has been widely studied for many years due to the need to understand the degradation of every potential pharmaceutical before being approved by the FDA, and every new compound offers its own new and unique challenges. There have been countless articles and numerous books written on the subject; thus, it is impossible to condense all of this information into one chapter. The following articles and books are good resources for further information about specific topics that have been discussed in this chapter.

Yoshioka and Stella [1] have written a book that provides extensive information regarding the stability of drugs (both small molecules and biopharmaceuticals) primarily in the solution state. They provide many examples for each of the possible degradation mechanisms and present a thorough discussion of kinetics and the factors that affect the chemical stability of drugs. Additionally, they include the ICH guidelines on stability and photostability testing of new drug substances and products (Q1A and Q1B) and the major concerns that have been raised by the European Union, the United States, and Japan regarding these guidelines. However, note that the ICH guidelines are revised occasionally. Therefore, it is best to refer to the most up-to-date copies, which are available at the ICH website (www.ich.org).

Byrn, Pfeiffer, and Stowell [21] wrote a useful book concerning drugs in the solid state. In the book they provide a good introduction to solid-state chemistry along with some of the more common methods of analysis that are used to study solids: X-ray diffractometry, microscopy, DSC, TGA, solubility, dissolution, particle-size analysis, infrared spectroscopy, and solid-state NMR spectroscopy. They include extensive discussions and examples of both crystalline (polymorphs, hydrates, and solvates) and amorphous materials and the physical and chemical changes that can occur within them, complete with a discussion about solid-state kinetics.

In addition to the two books discussed above there are also many books and review articles that have been written about stability but are more focused on specific issues. The photodegradation of drugs and formulations is described in a book edited by Tønnesen [4], including information on how photostability testing is performed, how to treat and interpret data from photostability tests, and many other issues concerning the exposure of drugs to light. The book series entitled Pharmaceutical Biotechnology [11] contains several volumes concerning the stability and characterization of proteins and peptides. Additionally, Chi et al. [17] wrote a review paper discussing the physical stability of proteins in solution and the mechanism and driving forces for aggregation. There is another book series, Drugs and the Pharmaceutical Sciences, which also contains several volumes with very helpful information regarding the stability of drugs [12, 14, 18]. Connors, Amidon, and Kennon [57] wrote a book in which they discuss the kinetics of degradation and provide stability monographs of 30 drugs, including acetaminophen, aspirin, and vitamin A. There are also several review articles that discuss amorphous materials [19, 20], crystalline materials [53], polymorphism [58], the effects of water on drugs in the solid state [42, 44], and accelerated aging studies [40]. Finally, there are countless articles that have been published about the stability of specific compounds that may help to understand the degradation of a new drug. Therefore, a good stability study always begins with a thorough literature search.

ACKNOWLEDGMENTS

The authors thank Dr. Valentino J. Stella for his discussions regarding the stability of drugs in the solution state and for informing the authors of several of the examples provided in this chapter. The authors also thank Dr. Dewey H. Barich for his help in reviewing the manuscript for this chapter. EMG was supported by a Biotechnology Training Grant (NIH 29488) from the National Institute of General Medical Sciences. This material is based on work supported by the National Science Foundation under Grant No. 046214. Any opinions, findings, and conclusions or recommendations expressed in this chapter are those of the authors and do not necessarily reflect the views of the National Science Foundation.

REFERENCES

1. Yoshioka S, Stella VJ. *Stability of Drugs and Dosage Forms*. New York: Kluwer Academic/ Plenum Publishers; 2000, p 268.

2. Hoener BA, Sokoloski TD, Mitscher LA, Malspeis L. Kinetics of dehydration on epitetracycline in solution. *J Pharm Sci* 1974;63:1901–1904.

3. Sokoloski TD, Mitscher LA, Juvarkar JV, Hoener B. Rate and proposed mechanism of anhydrotetracycline epimerization in acid solution. *J Pharm Sci* 1977;66:1159–1165.

4. Moore DE. Standardization of photodegradation studies and kinetic treatment of photochemical reactions. In Tønnesen HH, Ed. *Photostability of Drugs and Drug Formulations*. Bristol, PA: Taylor & Francis; 1996, pp 63–82.

5. Greenhill JV, McLelland MA. Photodecomposition of drugs. In Ellis GP, West GB, Eds. *Progress in Medicinal Chemistry. Progress in Medicinal Chemistry Series*, Vol 27. Amsterdam: Elsevier Science; 1990, pp 51–121.

6. Bundgaard H. Polymerization of penicillins: kinetics and mechanism of di- and polymerization of ampicillin in aqueous solution. *Acta Pharma Suecica* 1976;13(1):9–26.

7. Bundgaard H, Larsen C. Piperazinedione formation from reaction of ampicillin with carbohydrates and alcohols in aqueous solutions. *Int J Pharm* 1979;3:1–11.

8. Pogocki D, Schoneich C. Chemical stability of nucleic acid-derived drugs. *J Pharm Sci* 2000;89(4):443–456.

9. Oliyai C, Schoneich C, Wilson GS, Borchardt RT. Chemical and physical stability of protein pharmaceuticals. *Top Pharm Sci 1991: Proc 51st Int Congr Pharm Sci FIP* 1992;23–46.

10. Krishnamurthy R, Manning MC. The stability factor: importance in formulation development. *Curr Pharm Biotechnol* 2002;3(4):361–371.

11. Meyer JD, Ho B, Manning MC. Effects of conformation on the chemical stability of pharmaceutically relevant polypeptides. In Carpenter JF, Manning MC, Eds. *Rational Design of Stable Protein Formulations. Pharmaceutical Biotechnology Series*, Vol 13. New York: Kluwer Academic/Plenum Publishers; 2002, pp 85–107.

12. McNally EJ, Lockwood CE. The importance of a thorough preformulation study. In McNally EJ, Ed. *Protein Formulation and Delivery. Drugs and the Pharmaceutical Sciences Series*, Vol 99. New York: Marcel Dekker; 2000, pp 111–138.

13. Wang W. Lyophilization and development of solid protein pharmaceuticals. *Int J Pharm* 2000;203(1–2):1–60.

14. Lucks J-S, Müller BW, Klütsch K. Parenteral fat emulsions: structure, stability, and applications. In Nielloud F, Marti-Mestres G, Eds. *Pharmaceutical Emulsions and Suspensions. Drugs and the Pharmaceutical Sciences Series*, Vol 105. New York: Marcel Dekker; 2000, pp 229–257.

15. Heurtault B, Saulnier P, Pech B, Proust J-E, Benoit J-P. Physico-chemical stability of colloidal lipid particles. *Biomaterials* 2003;24(23):4283–4300.

16. Yoshioka S, Aso Y, Izutsu K, Terao T. Aggregates formed during storage of β-galactosidase in solution and in the freeze-dried state. *Pharm Res* 1993;10(5):687–691.

17. Chi EY, Krishnan S, Randolph TW, Carpenter JF. Physical stability of proteins in aqueous solution: mechanism and driving forces in nonnative protein aggregation. *Pharm Res* 2003;20(9):1325–1336.

18. Guillory JK, Poust RI. Chemical kinetics and drug stability. In Banker GS, Rhodes CT, Eds. *Modern Pharmaceutics. Drugs and the Pharmaceutical Sciences Series*, Vol 121. New York: Marcel Dekker; 2002, pp 139–166.

19. Kaushal AM, Gupta P, Bansal AK. Amorphous drug delivery systems: molecular aspects, design, and performance. *Crit Rev Ther Drug Carrier Syst* 2004; 21(3):133–193.

20. Craig DQM, Royall PG, Kett VL, Hopton ML. The relevance of the amorphous state to pharmaceutical dosage forms: glassy drugs and freeze dried systems. *Int J Pharm* 1999;179(2):179–207.

21. Byrn SR, Pfeiffer RR, Stowell JG. *Solid-State Chemistry of Drugs*, 2nd ed. West Lafayette, IN: SSCI, Inc; 1999, p 576.

22. Burger A, Ramberger R. On the polymorphism of pharmaceuticals and other molecular crystals. I. Theory of thermodynamics rules. *Mikrochim Acta* 1979;72:259–271.

23. Burger A, Ramberger R. On the polymorphism of pharmaceuticals and other molecular crystals. II. Applicability of thermodynamic rules. *Mikrochim Acta* 1979;72:273–316.

24. Watanabe T, Wakiyama N, Kusai A, Senna M. Drug–carrier interaction in solid dispersions prepared by co-grinding and melt-quenching. *Ann Chim (Cachan, France)* 2004;29(1):53–66.

25. Hancock BC. Disordered drug delivery: destiny, dynamics and the Deborah number. *J Pharm Pharmacol* 2002;54(6):737–746.

26. Chemburkar SR, Bauer J, Deming K, Spiwek H, Patel K, et al. Dealing with the impact of ritonavir polymorphs on the late stages of bulk drug process development. *Org Process Res Dev* 2000;4(5):413–417.

27. Pikal MJ, Rigsbee DR. The stability of insulin in crystalline and amorphous solids: observation of greater stability for the amorphous form. *Pharm Res* 1997;14(10):1379–1387.

28. Cohen MD, Schmidt GMJ. Topochemistry. I. A survey. *J Chem Soc* 1964;June: 1996–2000.

29. Cohen MD, Schmidt GMJ, Sonntang FI. Topochemistry. II. The photochemistry of trans-cinnamic acids. *J Chem Soc* 1964;June:2000–2013.

30. Prout EG, Tompkins FC. Thermal decomposition of $KMnO_4$. *Trans Faraday Soc* 1944;40:488–498.

31. Brown ME. The Prout–Tompkins rate equation in solid-state kinetics. *Thermochim Acta* 1997;300:93–106.

32. Avrami M. Kinetics of phase change. II. Transformation–time relations for random distribution of nuclei. *J Chem Phys* 1940;8:212–224.

33. Avrami M. Kinetics of phase change. III. Granulation, phase change and microstructure. *J Chem Phys* 1941;9:177–184.

34. Erofe'ev BV. Generalized equation of chemical kinetics and its application in reactions involving solids. *C R Acad Sci. USSR* 1946;52:511–514.

35. Sharp JH, Brindley GW, Narahari Achar BN. Numerical data for some commonly used solid state reaction equations. *J Am Ceram Soc* 1966;49:379–382.

36. Holt JB, Cutler IB, Wadsworth ME. Rate of thermal dehydration of kaolinite in vacuum. *J Am Ceram Soc* 1962;45:133–136.

37. Ginstling AM, Brounshteĭn BI. The diffusion kinetics of reactions in spherical particles. *J Appl Chem USSR Engl Trans* 1950;23:1327–1338.

38. Valensi G. Kinetics of oxidation of metallic spherules and powders. *C R Acad Sci USSR* 1936;202:309–312.

39. Carter RE. Kinetic model for solid-state reactions. *J Chem Phys* 1961;34:2010–2015.

40. Waterman KC, Adami RC. Accelerated aging: prediction of chemical stability of pharmaceuticals. *Int J Pharm* 2005;293(1–2):101–125.

41. Lai MC, Topp EM. Solid-state chemical stability of proteins and peptides. *J Pharm Sci* 1999;88(5):489–500.

42. Stewart PJ, Tucker IG. Prediction of drug stability. Part 5: Physical stability. *Aust J Hosp Pharm* 1985;15(4):236–246.

43. Ahlneck C, Zografi G. The molecular basis of moisture effects on the physical and chemical stability of drugs in the solid state. *Int J Pharm* 1990;62(2–3):87–95.

44. Airaksinen S, Karjalainen M, Shevchenko A, Westermarck S, Leppänen E, et al. Role of water in the physical stability of solid dosage formulations. *J Pharm Sci* 2005;94: 2147–2165.

45. Stella VJ. Chemical and physical bases determining the instability and incompatiblity of formulated injectable drugs. *J Parent Sci Technol* 1986;40(4):142–163.

46. Lachman L. Physical and chemical stability testing of tablet dosage forms. *J Pharm Sci* 1965;54(10):1519–1526.

47. Rogers AR. An accelerated storage test with programmed temperature rise. *J Pharm Pharmacol* 1963;15(Suppl):101T–105T.

48. King S-YP, Kung M-S, Fung H-L. Statistical prediction of drug stability based on nonlinear parameter estimation. *J Pharm Sci* 1984;73(5):657–662.

49. Yoshioka S, Aso Y, Uchiyama M. Statistical evaluation of nonisothermal prediction of drug stability. *J Pharm Sci* 1987;76(10):794–798.

50. Albers E, Müller BW. Cyclodextrin derivatives in pharmaceutics. *Crit Rev Ther Drug Carrier Syst* 1995;12(4):311–337.

51. Mehta AC. Analytical issues in the chemical stability testing of drugs in solution. *Anal Proc (London)* 1995;32(2):67–70.

52. Chilamkurti RN. Formulation development of frozen parenteral dosage forms. *J Parent Sci Technol* 1992;46(4):124–129.

53. Datta S, Grant DJ. Crystal structures of drugs: Advances in determination, prediction and engineering. *Nat Rev Drug Discov* 2004;3(1):42–57.

54. Windram VA, Threlfall TL. Chemical microscopy in the pharmaceutical industry. *Anal Proc (London)* 1992;29(3):108–110.

55. Bugay DE. Solid-state nuclear magnetic resonance spectroscopy: theory and pharmaceutical applications. *Pharm Res* 1993;10(3):317–327.

56. Ripmeester JA. Application of solid state ^{13}C NMR to the study of polymorphs, clathrates and complexes. *Chem Phys Lett* 1980;74(3):536–538.

57. Connors KA, Amidon GL, Kennon L. *Chemical Stability of Pharmaceuticals. Hoboken.* NJ: Wiley; 1979, p 367.

58. Haleblain J, McCrone W. Pharmaceutical applications of polymorphism. *J Pharm Sci* 1969;58(8):911–929.

17

DOSAGE FORMULATION

Alexander V. Lyubimov

University of Illinois at Chicago, Chicago, Illinois

Contents

17.1   INTRODUCTION

17.1.1   Background

Advances in biotechnology have allowed the economical and large scale production of therapeutically important complex polymers of amino acids (peptides and proteins), nucleosides (antisense molecules), and other biological drugs to be used to combat poorly controlled diseases [1]. This rapid progress in molecular biology required substantial progress in the formulation and development of delivery systems for the next generation of drugs. Rational drug design does not necessarily mean rational drug delivery, which strives to incorporate into a molecule the properties necessary for optimal transfer between the site of administration and the pharmacological target site in the body [2]. In addition, the advent of high throughput screening has affected contemporary drug pipelines based in large part on the nature of the assay, which includes the evaluation of organic solutions (e.g., DMSO) of drug candidates in immobilized receptor matrices. As a result, new drug leads tend to be more lipophilic. On top of this, the hit to lead process reduces still further aqueous solubility, meaning that the formulator is often faced with significant challenges with regard to generating appropriately orally bioavailable dosage forms. Various new vehicles and delivery systems, such as liposomes, biodegradable microspheres, biopolymers, hydrogels, and bioavailability enhancers, have been introduced during the last decades to improve delivery and bioavailability of new chemical and biological drugs. Safety evaluation of new vehicles and excipients as well as their role on efficacy and toxicity of new drugs is an important part of new formulations assessment.

Drug formulation is a rapidly evolving field. The new formulations, their function and characterization, absorption mechanisms, and novel routes and modes of delivery are described in many journals including (but obviously not limited to) the following journals: *International Journal of Pharmaceutics* (http://www.sciencedirect.com/science/journal/03785173); *AAPS PharmSciTech; Journal of Control Release* (http://www.sciencedirect.com/science/journal/01683659); *AAPS PharmSciTech* (http://www.aapspharmscitech.org), an online-only journal of the American Association of Pharmaceutical scientists; *European Journal of Pharmaceutical Sciences* (http://sciencedirect.com/science/journal/092809870); *European Journal of Pharmaceutics and Biopharmaceutics* (http://www.sciencedirect.com/science/journal/09396411); and *Advanced Drug Delivery Reviews* (http://www.sciencedirect.com/science/journal/0169409X).

17.1.2   Objectives/Definitions

Formulation is a preparation of pharmaceutical product in various dosage forms containing a new active ingredient(s) (AI) [3]. The purpose of drug formulation is to determine experimentally all the variables necessary to develop an optimal formula and working directions for making the pharmaceutical product. Pharmaceutical technology applied to developing a drug formulation comprises selection of materials and procedures that are adaptable to various processes that lend themselves to inclusion in specific dosage forms (tablets, injections, capsules, ointments, etc.). Dosage formulations can include sterile products, tablets, capsules, topical preparations, and nonconventional products such as semisolid or sustained release preparations. Formulations can be developed to enhance drug solubility, improve bioavailability, enhance drug stability, target tissue delivery, and treat specific patient populations. Stability and release properties of formulations can be evaluated *in vitro* prior to their use in animals.

Clinical drug formulation is a very complex multistep process that is significantly simplified at the stage of preclinical dosage formulations. A dosage form for preclinical study should optimize chances for a compound to exert its pharmacological action, determine the ways of solubilizing the compound, and determine photosensitivity and other aspects of stability. In a preclinical toxicity study, it is important that the formulation does not change the toxic effect of the active ingredient (either mask or enhance it). It is very important because in many cases the final clinical formulations may be quite different in composition from the dosage forms used for safety assessment in animals.

Stability is one of the most important factors that determine whether a compound or mixture of compounds can be developed in a therapeutically useful product. The stability of a dosage formulation can be defined as its degree of resistance to chemical and physical changes. The efficacy of the preparation must remain constant (or changed only within the specified limits) until the date of expiration. The formulation must be chemically, physically, microbiologically, therapeutically, and toxicologically stable.

Drug stability may be influenced by internal and external factors.

Internal Factors. Potential drug–drug (when mixtures are used) or drug–excipient interactions.

External Factors. The test articles (drugs) and dosage formulations come into contact with containers or packaging materials. For example, alkali from the glass containers, heavy metals from the metal containers, components of cork or rubber stopper, and plastics can penetrate and react with preparations. Various storage conditions may indicate three types of changes: (1) physical and colloidal–physical changes, (2) chemical changes, and (3) microbiological changes. Proper storage conditions should be determined and followed to minimize these changes.

There are numerous types of potential undesired interactions between the drug and excipients, which can occur during the process of formulation preparation, storage, and administration. For example, solubility, ionization pH effects, formation of complexes, and degradation reactions are possible. These changes may be *intentional* (e.g., prolonged release or enhanced delivery) or *unintentional* (e.g., discoloration, precipitation, liquefaction). The second group is usually referred to as incompatibilities. Incompatibilities are undesired physical, chemical, colloidal, or biopharmaceutical processes that take place during preparation, storage, or administration of the drug formulation. Incompatibilities may take place in visible or hidden manners. Visible incompatibilities include the following processes: (1) changes in solubility or degree of dispersion, turbidity, precipitation, coagulation, aggregation, crystallization, or crystal growth; (2) changes involving viscosity, physical state, crystal form, liquefaction, solidification, separation of phases, and uptake or loss of moisture; and (3) discoloration or change in odor or taste due to chemical transformation such as oxidation, hydrolysis, or enzyme degradation [3].

Hidden incompatibilities may be the result of interactions between active ingredients and excipients or packing materials and environmental conditions and include chemical, physical, physicochemical, colloidal, technological, and biopharmaceutical interactions. Some typical chemical interactions include spatial rearrangements, hydrolysis, the formation of esters, oxidation and reduction, and polymerization and depolymerization. Incompatibilities may also be related to the electric charge of molecules (e.g., formation of new salts, double salts, and intermolecular associations and complexes as a result of the interaction of AI and excipients, which have opposite charge). Physical interactions include adhesion, absorption, molecular adhesion, and ionic absorption.

To assess stability of the dosage formulation in a preclinical safety study, usually purity of active ingredient in formulation is determined over time. A formulation is considered unstable when the purity of the active ingredient (AI) decreases more than 10%. This may depend on accuracy of the analytical method and type of formulation (e.g., diet formulations may be considered stable up to a 15–20% decrease of AI). When chromatographic methods are used for purity determination, the appearance of additional peaks may be another sign of AI decomposition over time. Stability of formulation under the storage and application conditions should be determined prior to any preclinical safety assessment. It is not acceptable to simply assume that the drug will be stable in the diet or ointment even if it is known to be stable for a long period of time at room temperature in a powder form. Mixing with the diet (for oral studies) or with "inert" excipient (e.g., Vaseline for dermal administration) or even with water can significantly shorten stability of very stable drugs. Stability at storage conditions of formulations determined prior to toxicological experiment will dictate how often formulations need to be prepared in a repeated dosing study. Stability at room temperature is important to know even in a single dose experiment to assure formulation stability throughout the time of administration, which may be long when a significant number of small animals per dose group are used (especially important for dermal applications and lengthy infusions).

17.2 GENERAL PRINCIPLES OF DOSAGE FORMULATION IN PRECLINICAL STUDIES

17.2.1 Dosage Formulation Preparation

The test article is rarely administered as a neat compound and in most cases a dosage formulation is prepared for dosing the animals. It may be as simple as a gelatin capsule filled with the drug for oral administration in dogs or a solution in water for gavage dosing of rodents. It can also be a complicated mixture of the drug, vehicle(s), surfactants, and so on. The desirable characteristics of the "ideal" formulation and its preparation are presented in Table 17.1. It is important to test solubility of dosage solutions or homogeneity/suspendability of suspensions prior to the dosing of animals. We suggest that the solubility/suspendability test be run with the proposed formulations several days prior to dosing. This will allow for adjustments of a formulation, if necessary. An example of the form to be completed to record the result of these tests is presented in Table 17.2.

TABLE 17.1   Desirable Characteristics of a Dosing Formulation and Its Preparation

1. Preparation of the formulation should not involve heating of the test material anywhere near to the point where its chemical or physical characteristics are altered.
2. If the material is a solid and it is to be assessed for dermal effects, its shape and particle size should be preserved.
3. Multicomponent test materials (mixtures) should be formulated so that the administered form accurately represents the original mixture (i.e., components should not be selectively suspended or taken into solution).
4. Formulation should preserve the chemical stability and identity of the test material.
5. Formulation should be such as to minimize total test volume. Use just enough solvent or vehicle.
6. Formulation should be easy to administer accurately.
7. The pH of dosing formulations should be between 5 and 9, if possible.
8. Acids or bases should not be used to divide the test material (for both humane reasons and to avoid pH partitioning in either the gut or the renal tubule).
9. If a parenteral route is to be employed, final solutions should be as nearly isotonic as possible.

Source: From Ref. 4, with permission.

The test substance can be administered to animals at a constant concentration across all dose levels (i.e., varying the dose volume) or at a constant dose volume (i.e., varying the dose concentration). The toxicity observed by administration of a constant concentration may be different from that observed for a constant dose volume. For instance, when a large volume of oil is given orally, gastrointestinal motility is increased, causing diarrhea and decreasing the time available for absorption of the test substance in the GI tract.

The volume of water or solvent–water mixture used to dissolve the chemical should be kept low, since excess quantities may distend the stomach and cause rapid gastric emptying. In addition, large volumes of water may carry the chemical through membrane pores and increase the rate of absorption. Thus, if dose-dependent absorption is suspected, it is important that the different doses are given in the same volume of solution [4].

Local irritation by a test substance generally decreases when the material is diluted. If the objective of the study is to establish systemic toxicity, the test substance should be administered in a constant volume to minimize gastrointestinal irritation that may, in turn, affect its absorption. If, however, the objective is to assess the irritation potential of the test substance, then it should be administered undiluted.

17.2.2   Role of the Route of Administration

The intended route of administration in humans dictates a route of administration in animals during preclinical studies. However, the drug formulations in animals are often different from the clinical formulations. The specific route of administration is a significant determinant of the commonly used formulations in preclinical testing. Specific types of formulations by route of administration are described in Section 17.3.

Generally, pharmaceutical companies prefer to develop an oral route of administration for a new chemical entity. Dosage forms associated with this route are

TABLE 17.2   Form for Preclinical Formulation Testing for Solubility/Suspensibility

<u>SOLUBILITY/SUSPENSION TESTING</u>

Chemical: _____

Performed By: _____

Date Performed: _____

The test article was mixed with the following vehicle(s):

Vehicle	Volume of Vehicle	Quantity of Test Article	Results
Water	_____	_____	_____
Corn Oil	_____	_____	_____
Peanut Oil	_____	_____	_____
_____	_____	_____	_____
_____	_____	_____	_____
_____	_____	_____	_____

Since the test article was not soluble in the above vehicles, it was suspended in the following vehicle(s):

Vehicle	Volume of Vehicle	Quantity of Test Article	Results
_____	_____	_____	_____
_____	_____	_____	_____
_____	_____	_____	_____

A = Test article was completely soluble.   D = Test article was adequately suspended.

B = Test article appeared partially soluble.   E = Test article was not adequately suspended.

C = Test article appeared insoluble.   — = Vehicle not utilized.

Comments: _____

_____

_____

Read and Reviewed by: _____   Date: _____

relatively cheap to manufacture, are simpler for patients to handle, and are widely accepted by the public. Because this is the preferred route of administration, it becomes crucial to evaluate the oral bioavailability of lead compounds in the earlier stage of the development process. Oral bioavailabilty of a compound can be a major selection criterion for the development candidate. Drawbacks of the low bioavailable compound from a pharmaceutical development standpoint are inherent variability in the oral bioavailablity, a requirement of large quantities of drug substance to establish a safety margin in preclinical safety studies, and, depending on the pharmacology of the molecule, a high dose to elicit the desired effect.

In contrast, with only a few exceptions, most new anticancer compounds are initially developed for intravenous (IV) use, despite some drawbacks such as the morbidity associated with gaining IV access; risk of IV catheter-related infection, thrombosis, and extravasation; and patients' preference for oral therapy when equally effective [5]. Important reasons for choosing IV use for initial drug development are the fact that usually less gastrointestinal toxicity occurs, there is immediate 100% bioavailability and instantaneous pharmacodynamic effects, and there is a possibility to modify the dosing rate or even halt the infusion if necessary. Solubility of the compound is a specific demand for IV administration, even for the newer chemotherapeutic agents, which are known to be poorly water soluble. Classical solubility approaches, which are discussed subsequently, include the use of colloidal systems, prodrug development, or solubilization techniques.

Colloidal systems such as liposomes, microcapsules, microspheres, nanoparticles, or macromolecule complexes may protect the anticancer drug from premature degradation or (chemical) inactivation within the systemic circulation. Prodrugs are inactive derivatives that release the active drug following spontaneous degradation or enzymatic reactions. Solubilization is the process of uptake of drugs through complex formation into, for example, oligomers of dextrose and fatty acids, through cosolvent systems (such as ethanol, polyethylene glycol, and glycerol), or through surfactant systems. The surfactant systems consist of amphoteric compounds (e.g., lecithin or gelatin), ionic surfactants (e.g., sodium palmitate), or nonionic surfactants (e.g., Tween 80 and Cremophor EL (CrEL)). Some of these solubilization approaches are discussed later in this chapter.

17.2.3 Role of Absorption/Enhancement of Oral Absorption

In the early stages of development, it is important to determine whether the dosage form targeted for clinical use has an acceptable level of bioavailability. To evaluate the dosage form in a clinical study is time consuming and costly. Large animals (e.g., dogs and monkeys) are used for assessment of bioavailability of different dosage formulations. Examples of the usefulness of such studies are presented in this volume in Chapter 32, Bioavailability and Bioequivalence Studies.

Oral administration is the most convenient mode of drug delivery and is associated with superior patient compliance as compared to other modes of drug intake. However, oral administration has only limited use for important drugs, from various pharmacological categories, that have poor oral bioavailability due to incomplete absorption and/or degradation in the gastrointestinal (GI) tract [6]. Some of these drugs are characterized by a narrow absorption window (NAW) at the upper part of the GI tract. This is because the proximal part of the small intestine exhibits extended absorption properties (including larger gaps between the tight junctions, and dense active transporters). Despite the extensive absorption properties of the duodenum and jejunum, the extent of absorption at these sites is limited because the passage through this region is rapid. Enhancing the gastric residence time (GRT) of a NAW drug may significantly improve the net extent of its absorption. To further increase the GRT of drugs, a gastroretentive dosage form (GRDF) can be developed. It is quite complex to achieve extensive retention of the GRDF since the natural activity of the stomach is to evacuate its contents into the intestine. The development of the GRDF has generated enormous interest and the pharmaceutical aspects of these developments are reviewed elsewhere [7, 8]. Controlled release (CR) dosage forms have been extensively used to improve therapy of many important medications. However, in the case of NAW drugs this pharmaceutical approach cannot be utilized since it requires sufficient colonic absorption of the drug (which is, by definition, not the case for NAW agents). On the other hand, incorporation of the drug in a controlled release gastroretentive dosage form (CR-GRDF) can yield significant therapeutic advantages due to a variety of pharmacokinetic (PK) and pharmacodynamic (PD) factors. Hoffman et al. [9] reviewed these aspects in rat and dog animal models in order to suggest rational selection of drugs for which CR-GRDF would be a beneficial strategy. These authors found that a CR-GRDF formulation was superior compared to other modes of administration for levodopa and riboflavin, but not for metformin.

Incomplete oral bioavailability has various causes. These include poor dissolution or low aqueous solubility, degradation of the drug in gastric or intestinal fluids, poor intestinal membrane permeation, and presystemic intestinal or hepatic metabolism. Absorption of peptides, peptide analogues, or other polar, high molecular weight drugs may be significantly enhanced by using excipients that increase intestinal permeability. For some compounds, permeation through the intestinal epithelium is hindered by their active transport from the enterocyte back into the intestinal lumen. The secretory transporters involved may include P-glycoprotein (P-gp), the family of multidrug resistance-associated proteins (MRPs), and possibly others. For substrates of these secretory transporters, inhibiting secretory transport can increase permeation in the absorptive direction. This can be accomplished with pharmacologically inactive excipients.

Before permeation-enhancing excipients are evaluated for a particular drug of interest, it is important to understand the cause of its low oral bioavailability. Ideally, first-pass metabolism and solubility are not limiting oral bioavailability. Furthermore, the role of secretory transport should be assessed, because excipients that increase absorption by inhibiting secretory transport are different from those that increase absorption by other mechanisms.

Several reviews address intestinal permeation-enhancing excipients and evaluate how far some of the more advanced technologies have come toward fulfilling these criteria [6, 9–13].

17.2.4   Role of Animal Species

The key issue of an assessment of new dosage formulations in animal studies is to extrapolate the results to humans. The bioavailability of drug formulation in animals and the ability to predict its bioavailability in humans is one of the most important factors. An important issue in determining the choice of animal species for bioavailability testing is its size. In most circumstances, it is not possible to administer intact, solid pharmaceutical formulations—tablets and capsules, for example—in small rodents such as mice, rats, or hamsters. If such dosage forms are to be tested, larger species, such as rabbits, dogs, and monkeys, are more appropriate.

Another problem associated with the use of smaller species is repetitive blood sampling. Urine measurements of drug excretion can be used for all animal species to determine bioavailability, overcoming many of the blood sampling difficulties. A reasonable proportion of the drug, however, must be excreted unchanged via kidney to make the results meaningful. In addition, extensive first-pass metabolism would preclude this approach if the total metabolite excretion is being used.

None of the animal models are ideal, and each has its advantages and disadvantages. Table 17.3 compares different animal species as a model for human bioavailability testing [14]. Nevertheless, many investigators have used animals for bioavailability testing and have obtained valuable information that has helped in their understanding of their product. The rabbit appears to be the least suitable animal model for bioavailability testing, despite its relatively large size (large enough to test solid formulations) and low cost. This is because it has a long gastric emptying time, and both its gastrointestinal pH and microflora bear little resemblance to those in humans. Table 17.4 presents gastric and intestinal pH values of common laboratory animals. The rat has the major disadvantage of being too small to test

TABLE 17.3 Advatages (+) and Disadvantages (−) of Different Animal Species as a Model for Humans in Bioavailability Testing

Parameters	Rat	Rabbit	Dog	Monkey
Cost	+	+	−	−
Ease of urine collection	+	+	+	−
Ease of blood sampling	−	+	+	+
Ease of handling	+	+	+	−
Intact solid formulation	−	+	+	+
Intestinal pH	+	−	+	+
Gastrointestinal transit time	−	−	−	−
Gastrointestinal microflora	−	−	+	+
Drug metabolism	−	(− +)	(− +)	+
Biliary excretion	−	+	−	+

Source: From Ref. 14, with permission.

TABLE 17.4 Gastric and Intestinal pH Values for Different Animal Species

Gastrointestinal section	pH Values					
	Rat	Guinea Pig	Rabbit	Dog	Monkey	Human
Stomach	3.3–5.5	4.1–4.5	1.9	3.5–5.5	2.8–4.8	1.5–3.5
Duodenum	6.5–6.7	7.6–7.7	6.0–6.8	6.2	5.8	5.0–7.0
Jejunum	6.7–6.8	7.7–8.1	6.8–7.5	6.2–6.6	5.8–6.0	6.0–7.0
Ilium	6.8–7.1	8.1	7.5–8.0	6.6–7.5	6.1	7.0
Colon	6.6	6.7	7.2	6.5	5.1	5.5–7.0

Source: From Ref. 14, with permission.

most solid formulations, as well as being difficult to obtain multiple blood samples from repetitive sampling. In addition, the gastrointestinal microflora is different from that of humans. This species does have the advantage of having a gastrointestinal pH similar to that in humans and, if urinary data are used for bioavailability testing, it is easy to obtain total urine collections using metabolism cages.

In most respects, the monkey offers the closest physiological and metabolic model for humans and would be the first choice if not for its extremely high cost and handling requirements. Additionally, the monkey is capable of transmitting several human pathogens, and care must be taken when handling analytical samples. Obviously, if primate facilities are available, the use of this species becomes more attractive. Dogs offer a reasonable compromise since (1) they are large enough to test solid dosage forms, (2) their gastrointestinal pH is similar to that in humans, (3) sampling is convenient, (4) they are easy to handle, and (5) special precautions are not needed when handling the biological samples after collection.

Throughout drug development, toxicology/safety studies are conducted in two species. As most drugs are intended for oral administration, the rat and dog are the primary species used for reasons of availability, costs, and long history of use. However, not all drugs are targeted for oral delivery and other routes (intravenous, dermal, etc.) and species (rabbit for reproductive toxicology, monkey) may be used.

The rat is the species most commonly used with oral administration—the route of choice—and is the primary rodent utilized in toxicology studies. Oral administration by gavage as a solution or suspension is the most frequently employed dosage form in rodents and is used in studies of up to 6–9 months duration. The primary consideration is the choice of vehicle. Solutions in water are chosen if the solubility of the drug is sufficient to deliver the highest dose proposed. For drugs of low or limited solubility, a dispersing agent for use in an aqueous milieu is selected. A vehicle of 0.5% aqueous Tween 80 (i.e., polysorbate 80) has a long history of use for a wide range of drugs. Cellulose and its derivatives (e.g., methyl-, carboxy-), starch, and different natural oils (e.g., corn, sesame) are often used as a vehicle for oral gavage formulations. For studies of greater duration than 9 months (i.e., lifetime carcinogenicity studies), oral drugs are usually administered as admixture in the diet of the rats. Dogs are often dosed with capsules.

Literature review of species differences in pharmacokinetics and bioavailabilty of different dosage formulations are presented in Section 32.2.5 of Chapter 32, Bioavailability and Bioequivalence Studies.

17.2.5   Protein/Peptide, DNA, Antisense Oligonucleotides (AS-ONs), siRNA, and Other Biological Formulations

Protein/Peptide Formulations   Protein pharmaceuticals have high specificity and activity at relatively low concentrations, in comparison with small chemical drugs. These features have made protein pharmaceuticals indispensable in combating human diseases. Currently, the U.S. Food and Drug Administration (FDA) has approved over 30 different recombinant DNA-derived proteins (e.g., erythropoietin, interferon α-2a/b, somatropin and follitropin β), and many more are in an advanced stage of development [15].

The most challenging task in the development of protein pharmaceuticals is to deal with physical and chemical instabilities of proteins. Protein instability is one of the major reasons why protein pharmaceuticals are administered traditionally through injection rather than taken orally like most small chemical drugs [16]. Problems such as acid catalyzed degradation in the stomach, proteolytic breakdown in the GI tract, poor permeability across the gastrointestinal mucosa, and first-pass metabolism during transfer across the absorption barrier and in the liver must be overcome for the efficient delivery of drugs into the bloodstream [17]. In order to achieve successful oral delivery of protein drugs, they need to be protected from the harsh environment in the stomach. For designing oral dosage forms, the formulator must consider that the natural pH environment of the GI tract varies from acidic (pH ~ 1.2) in the stomach to slightly alkaline in the intestine (pH ~ 7.4) [18]. The review by George and Abraham [19] describes the sources and physical and chemical properties of alginate and chitosan (naturally occurring biopolymers) that enable them to become suitable for protein delivery, the mechanisms of hydrogel formation, modifications that increase their protein encapsulation efficiency, and the recent trends in their application.

There are considerable hurdles to be overcome before practical use can be made of therapeutic peptides and proteins due to chemical and enzymatic instability, poor absorption through biological membranes, rapid plasma clearance, peculiar dose–response curves, and immunogenicity [1]. Many attempts have addressed these problems by chemical modifications or by coadministration of adjuvants to eliminate undesirable properties of peptides and proteins [20]. Cell permeant peptides and their delivery enhancement are reviewed by Ülo Langel [21]. Different types of protein/peptide formulations need to be developed based on clinical needs, patient compliance; delivery methods; drug stability, storage, and distribution; and market competitiveness. Having a clear vision of the type of formulation that is desired will allow one to design a better formulation. Liquid formulations have generally been preferred due to the convenience of manufacturing and use. However, protein drugs may not be stable enough to be handled as a liquid formulation. Dried formulations (e.g., lyophilized formulations) or suspension formulations have been successfully used to overcome stability problems. In addition, specific applications and/or delivery routes may demand an appropriate type of formulation such as a spray-dried formulation for pulmonary delivery.

Maximizing the stability of protein/peptide is one of the most important objectives of formulation optimization. Once the key degradation products, responsible stresses, and analytical methods are identified, the protein or peptide can be stabilized by optimizing various formulation variables. Often, well established scientific principles can be used to solve some stability problems. In other instances, solving stability issues can best be achieved through utilizing empirical approaches. When an optimized formulation does not provide sufficient stability, then alternative approaches like lyophilization are indicated. Table 17.5 provides some typical solutions for routine stability problems.

Gene Therapies   Gene delivery has been regarded as a powerful tool for curing disease by replacing defective genes, substituting missing genes, or silencing unwanted gene expression. Gene therapy holds great promise for treating various forms of diseases with a genetic origin including cystic fibrosis, different forms of cancer, and cardiovascular disorders. Basically, there are two types of gene carriers that deliver foreign DNA into the diseased target cell population. DNA delivery systems are viral and nonviral vectors [22]. Viral vectors are the most effective because of their evolutionary optimization for this purpose. However, recently

TABLE 17.5   Problems and Solutions of Protein and Peptide Drug Development

Problems	Solutions
Deamidation, cyclic imide formation	pH optimization
Aggregation, precipitation	pH optimization; addition of sugars, salts, amino acids, and/or surfactants
Truncation	pH optimization, protease removal
Oxidation	Excipient purity analysis, addition of free-radical scavengers (mannitol, sorbitol), use of a competitive inhibitor (methionine)
Surface denaturation, adsorption	Addition of surfactants or excipient proteins
Dehydration	Addition of sugars or amino acids

reported safety issues such as random recombination, oncogenic potential, and immunogenicity [23, 24] have set back the rapid development of viral vectors. As compared to viral vectors, nonviral systems have a low or absent immunogenicity, can relatively easily be scaled-up, and have great flexibility with regard to vector modification and DNA incorporation [25, 26]. Nonviral vectors are safe to use but less efficient. In light of safety concerns, nonviral delivery systems have been developed for gene therapy experiments. Among those, cationic liposomes are widely used for almost all animal cells because they have nonspecific ionic interaction and low toxicity properties [27–29]. However, there are some limitations for cationic liposomes. When they are used for *in vivo* transfection, they are unstable. Therefore, many polymeric cationic systems such as gelatin, polyethylenimine (PEI), poly(L-lysines), tetraaminofullerene, poly(L-histidine)-graft-poly(L-lysines), DEAE-dextrans, cationic dendrimers, and chitosan have been studied for *in vitro* as well as *in vivo* application [30, 31].

The clinical use of gene therapy treatments, however, is restricted, mainly because of the absence of safe and efficient gene delivery technologies [32–34]. In the past decade, nonviral approaches, particularly cationic lipid or polymer-based systems, have received rapidly growing interest, because they offer several advantages over the viral counterparts. Nevertheless, currently investigated gene delivery polymers like polyethylenimine (PEI), poly(L-lysine) (PLL), polyamidoamine dendrimers (PAMAM), and poly(2-(dimethylamino)ethyl methacrylate) (pDMAEMA) have not yet advanced to clinical evaluation, mainly due to their acute cytotoxicities and low *in vivo* transfection activity [24, 35–37].

Recently, biodegradable cationic polymers such as poly(4-hydroxy-L-proline ester) [38, 39], poly[α-(4-aminobutyl)-L-glycolic acid][40], poly(L-lysine) conjugates [41], linear poly(ester amine)s [42–45], poly(ester amine) networks [46], cationic polyphosphazenes [47], and degradable polyethylenimine [48, 49] have been investigated as nonviral carriers for gene delivery. Generally, polyplexes based on these polymers showed lower cytotoxicity and comparable *in vitro* transfection activities as compared to the nondegradable counterparts. Furthermore, the degradation properties of these polymeric vectors can be employed as a valuable tool to regulate the unpacking and release of the DNA inside the cells. Linear poly(ester amine)s as recently reported by Langer and co-workers are of particular interest because the applied synthesis is straightforward and polymers with a great variety of different structures and properties can readily be prepared [42, 43, 45]. Chitosan oligosaccharides (COSs) chemically modified with deoxycholic acid (DOCA) have low toxicity and possess a good transfection activity [50].

Zhong et al. [51] report a versatile family of degradable hyperbranched poly(ester amine)s that contain primary, secondary, and tertiary amino groups in their structures for nonviral gene delivery. These hyperbranched poly(ester amine)s could easily be synthesized in high yields by a Michael-type conjugate addition of trifunctional amines, containing both a primary and a secondary amino group to diacrylates [52]. As vectors for gene delivery, these hyperbranched polymers may have several advantages: (1) in general they exhibit much better solubility in water than their linear counterparts [53]; (2) primary amines present in the periphery of these hyperbranched polymers can interact more efficiently with the phosphate groups of DNA, resulting in the formation of nanosized polymer/DNA complexes, analogous to the behavior of hyperbranched PEI that was shown to condense DNA into a smaller size particle than linear PEI [54]; (3) the high density of secondary and tertiary amines will give rise to high buffering capacity over a wide pH range, facilitating endosomal escape of polymer/DNA complexes ("proton sponge hypothesis") [55]; and (4) due to their high functionality, the structure of hyperbranched polymers can easily be modified to further improve transfection efficacy and/or achieve targeted gene delivery *in vivo*. For example, hyperbranched PEI, consisting of 25%, 50%, and 25% of primary, secondary, and tertiary amines, is one of the most efficient polymeric gene carriers studied *in vitro* and *in vivo* [55–58].

A significant limitation in using nonviral gene therapy approaches for the treatment of disease has been poor delivery systems leading to poor cell transfection and protein expression [59]. Interest remains high in developing a robust nonviral system due to toxicity concerns associated with the alternative viral based approaches. The use of mechanical/physical delivery systems in combination with plasmid based vectors has produced encouraging results with regard to the high protein expression levels achieved [60–62]. These methodologies such as electroporation or hydrodynamic pressure are fairly complex in design and require special equipment and/or training; however, they are beginning to be clinically evaluated for various diseases and may ultimately prove to have therapeutic applicability [63]. Alternative nonviral approaches are directed at combining plasmid DNA with lipid or polymer based molecules that act to facilitate DNA uptake and expression by promoting interaction with cellular membranes, protecting DNA against endogenous nucleases and trafficking plasmid to the nucleus [64–66].

Polymeric gene carrier systems have been widely used for gene therapy applications and are emerging as a viable alternative to the current systems [35]. These systems are attractive because of ease of use and low cost. Furthermore, excellent molecular flexibility allows for sophisticated modifications and incorporation of novel chemistries with little difficulty [67, 68]. Use of polymers for gene therapy applications also offers the possibility of repeated injections in order to maximize and/or optimize the therapeutic applicability.

Polyethylenimine (PEI) as a gene delivery polymer has a distinct advantage over other nonviral gene delivery systems due to its inherent endosomolytic activity [69]. However, despite its use in animal studies, the clinical development of polyethylenimines has been sluggish due to molecular heterogeneity and acute toxicity [70, 71]. The transfection activity and cytotoxicity of PEI is directly related to its molecular size. Specifically, the larger the molecular size the higher the transfection activity and cytotoxicity. Different strategies have been described to improve polymer activity without compromising safety including incorporating degradable linkages into high molecular weight polymers to improve clearance [49] or incorporating biocompatible membrane-permeating moieties into low molecular weight polymers to improve activity [36, 72].

Fewell et al. [59] describe the chemical synthesis and the physical and chemical properties of a novel condensing lipopolymer based on a low molecular weight polyethylenimine covalently linked to cholesterol (CHOL) and methoxypolyethylene glycol (PEG) molecules forming PEG–PEI–CHOL (PPC). The polymer offers a high degree of protection against DNases and high *in vitro* and *in vivo* transfection activity. Lv et al. [73] discuss the toxicity of main cationic gene vectors (cationic lipids and cationic polymers); emphasis is placed on the relationship between toxicity and structure of these compounds. The authors evaluate the structural features of cationic compounds and discuss which groups may increase the toxicity, what kind of linkages have relatively short half-life, and how proper modifications will decrease the toxicity of cationic lipids and cationic polymers for gene delivery.

Antisense oligonucleotides (AS-ONs) are specific inhibitors of gene expression. As single strands of DNA, these molecules hybridize to complementary RNA and induce RNase H-mediated degradation of the target RNA [74, 75]. Initially introduced by Zamecnik and Stephenson [76] and Stephenson and Zamecnik [77], AS-ONs represent a promising tool in fighting viral, malignant, and inflammatory diseases. Since unmodified phosphodiester oligonucleotides are susceptible to degradation by exo- and endonucleases, the more stable phosphorothioate oligonucleotides (S-ONs) have become the most extensively used antisense agents. In these molecules, one of the nonbridging oxygens of the phosphate backbone is substituted by a sulfur atom [78]. Several clinical trials with S-ONs are in progress for treatment of chronic lymphocytic leukemia, multiple myeloma, malignant melanoma, pancreatic carcinoma, and non-small-cell lung carcinoma [79, 80]. However, a major problem for the development of antisense therapy is the ineffective cellular uptake of antisense molecules. Oligonucleotides are relatively large hydrophilic molecules with a molecular weight ranging from 5000 to 10,000 Da and do not passively diffuse across cell membranes. Conflicting theories for oligonucleotide transport into the cell have been reported: (1) receptor-dependent [81], (2) independent [82], (3) via pinocytosis [83], or (4) via unknown mechanism (e.g., caveolar or potocytotic) [84]. However, in order to be active, AS-ONs must preferentially be present either in the nucleus or in the cytoplasm. The intracellular localization of ONs is confined to the endocytotic compartments. Only a small portion of ONs are somehow released into the cytoplasm [85].

Improvement of cellular uptake is a major topic of ongoing antisense research. Numerous potential delivery systems such as viral capsid structures, nanoparticles, and liposomes have been explored for efficient antisense delivery [86–88]. Currently, most research focuses on liposomes. Anionic liposomes can be loaded with ONs and then be linked to specific antibodies for tissue targeting [89]. Unfortunately, for these liposomes encapsulation of ONs is quite inefficient. In contrast, incubation of ONs with cationic lipids results in the high efficient formation of liposome–ON complexes by electrostatic interaction. The cellular uptake of ONs with cationic liposomes is strongly enhanced by a factor of 15–25 over ON only, resulting in a 1000-fold overall increase in ON activity [90–92]. This tremendous increase in activity may be explained by the specific nuclear localization of ONs. In contrast to the cytoplasmic localization of noncomplexed ONs, ONs delivered by cationic liposomes accumulate predominantly in the cell nucleus [93].

Antisense oligonucleotides are being widely investigated for the downregulation of genes [94, 95]. To inhibit protein production, the ONs have to reach the cytoplasm or nucleus of the cells, where they act by specific binding to the target mRNA or DNA. In spite of this simple action mechanism, different barriers still limit the antisense activity. Actually, before the ONs can reach their target site, they first have to cross the cellular membrane, escape from the endosomal compartment, leave their pharmaceutical carriers (i.e., the delivery system), and hybridize to the target sequence [96].

Rapid degradation of phosphodiester ONs is known to be one of the factors limiting their success as therapeutics. One approach to improve antisense activity is to develop ONs with increased nuclease stability so that intracellular degradation should not be an issue [97]. However, modification of the ON backbone often induces undesirable features. The first generation of chemically modified ONs, namely, phosphothioate ONs, are known to frequently exhibit nonspecific, nonantisense effects, generally attributed to their increased nonspecific protein binding when compared to their phosphodiester analogues [98]. The second and third generation antisense compounds all work to some extent but have one or more problems such as solubility, delivery issues, lack of RNase H activation, or simply the cost of synthesis [99].

Another approach to improve the antisense activity of ONs is the development of suitable delivery systems [96, 100]. The delivery system, often composed of cationic lipids or cationic polymers, is designed to help the ONs enter the cell and escape from the endosomes. Clearly, in cases where (degradable) phosphodiester ONs (PO-ONs) are used, the protection of the ONs against nucleases, given by their carrier, becomes an important aspect. Ideally, the delivery system should protect the complexed ONs during the different steps of the trafficking pathway. In general, cationic carriers are believed to protect the complexed ONs against degradation. However, some carriers can establish an antisense effect with degradable phosphodiester ONs, while other carriers fail [101, 102]. The lack of antisense activity has been attributed to insufficient ON protection against nucleases with the carriers used, although no direct proof of this hypothesis was given.

RNAi is a recently developed technique to silence proteins in a sequence-specific manner by inhibiting mRNA and consequently reducing protein expression [103]. The functional mediator of RNA interference is a short dsRNA oligonucleotide called small interfering RNA (siRNA). A growing number of investigations are being reported on efforts to use siRNA as a candidate therapeutic agent [104]. To achieve therapeutic success, however, several hurdles must be overcome including rapid clearance, nuclease degradation, and inefficient intracellular localization. Most efforts reported to date are based on studies in rodents and rodent models of disease. With the exception of local administration into eye tissues, the results show low activity due to a strong dependence on methods for intracellular delivery, as found for antisense and gene therapy approaches. One surprising observation is that siRNA composed of unmodified RNA is rapidly cleared by the kidneys [105], indicating low binding to proteins or cells in the blood and a surprising lack of nuclease degradation as the major barrier. A delivery strategy for use of siRNA as a therapeutic modality should therefore firstly reduce glomerular filtration, and secondly optimize intracellular delivery to target cells, while also minimizing exposure to nuclease and distribution to nontarget tissues. Nanoparticle delivery systems developed with a ligand–polymer–polymer conjugate appear attractive to meet these needs and indeed neovasculature targeted forms, using a "cyclic" RGD peptide as the ligand, have produced successful results [106, 107].

Peptide nucleic acids (PNAs) are rapidly emerging as powerful tools in DNA hybridization and antisense techniques. PNAs are synthetic oligonucleotide analogues in which the natural nucleic acid backbone is replaced by an uncharged pseudopeptide backbone consisting of *N*-(2-aminoethyl)-glycine units linked to the natural purine and pyrimidine bases [108]. They form very stable complexes with complementary DNA or RNA strands with very high affinity, partially as a result of the neutrality and flexibility of the artificial backbone.

PNAs possess a strong resistance to enzymatic degradation in cells, fluids, and tissues, showing an exceptional stability in biological environments [109]. In addition, the unique chemical, physical, and biological properties of PNAs have been exploited to produce powerful biomolecular tools, antisense and antigene agents, molecular probes, and biosensors. Important new applications that could not be performed using natural oligonucleotides have emerged. Duplexes between PNA and DNA or RNA are in general thermally more stable than the corresponding DNA–DNA or DNA–RNA duplexes [109, 110]. The sequence dependence of the stability, however, is more complex than that found for DNA–DNA complexes because of the inherent asymmetry of the duplex. In fact, PNA–DNA duplexes show significantly increased stability when the purines are in the PNA strand. Thus, on top of the dependence on G–C content, the stability of PNA–DNA duplexes also depends on the purine fraction of the PNA strand [111]. In general, it is also observed that the thermal stability of PNA–PNA duplexes exceeds that of PNA–RNA duplexes, which again are more stable than PNA–DNA duplexes.

Very importantly, but not surprisingly, the stability of PNA–DNA duplexes is almost unaffected by the ionic strength of the medium (actually the stability decreases slightly with increasing Na^+ concentration due to counterion release upon duplex formation). This is in sharp contrast, of course, to the behavior of DNA–DNA (or RNA) duplexes, whose stability decreases dramatically at low ionic strength because of the required counterion shielding of the phosphate backbone [112].

PNA hybridization kinetics have also been studied by surface plasmon resonance (SPR) technology and the results, although they cannot be considered conclusive, indicate no major difference in PNA and DNA hybridization duplex formation [110]. Although it is not the intention to give an elaborate account of the ongoing development of gene therapeutic drugs based on PNA oligomers, it is fair to say that PNA does possess many of the properties desired for an antisense reagent. It binds strongly and with excellent sequence specificity to complementary mRNA, it has very high biological stability, and targeting of specific mRNAs with PNA has been shown to strongly inhibit its translation. This has been demonstrated in several biological systems *in vitro*, and the introduction of various novel methods for improved delivery of PNA to eukaryotic cells has recently also allowed good efficacy in cell culture *ex vivo* and, sometimes, *in vivo* [113–116]. In the last two years, PNA antisense and antigene technology has entered the realm of biological and preclinical studies. This is primarily due to the development of a number of methods able to improve PNA permeability across cell membranes [117–119] and to allow efficient delivery of PNA oligomers to eukaryotic cells. Two novel delivery systems based on polymeric core–shell microspheres and autologous loaded opsonized RBC systems were able to specifically inhibit the expression of COX-2 or iNOS proteins in murine macrophages at nanomolar concentration, that is, with 3 log lower concentration with respect to those required by PNA linked to hydrophobic peptide [120]. Authors concluded that core–shell polymeric microspheres and loaded RBC represent promising delivery strategies for *in vivo* targeting of antisense PNAs to macrophages during inflammatory processes.

17.2.6 Enhanced Delivery and Semisolid or Sustained Release Preparations (Micronization and Nanoparticles)

In order to improve the specific delivery and bioavailability of drugs with low therapeutic index, several drug carriers such as liposomes, microparticles, nanoassociates, nanoparticles, drug polymer conjugates, and polymeric micelles have been developed. In recent years, polymeric micelles have been the object of growing scientific attention [121].

Micelles One of the widely used techniques for augmenting the water solubility of drug candidates is through modification of the solubilization medium by using cosolvents, complexing agents (i.e., cyclodextrins), or surfactants [122, 123]. In an aqueous medium, above a given concentration termed the critical micellar concentration (CMC), surfactants self-assemble into a colloidal dispersion of molecular aggregates called micelles (<50–100 nm) [124] and have been shown to solubilize hydrophobic drugs inside the core formed by the lipophilic part of the surfactant. The hydrophilic moieties form the shell or corona of these nanocarriers [124–128]. In addition to the increase in drug solubility, micelles can protect the incorporated drugs by insulating them from the aqueous environment.

Besides classic surfactants, micelles can also be formed from amphiphilic polymers. These polymers often provide better kinetic and thermodynamic stability than conventional surfactants [124–128]. However, they exhibit a number of disadvantages including a complex manufacturing process, which requires organic solvents followed by a dialysis step or an evaporation process depending on polymer polarity [125–128]. These limitations were addressed by the introduction of self-assembling polymeric micelles such as mmePEG$_{750}$P(CL-*co*-TMC) (monomethyletherpoly(oxyethylene glycol$_{750}$)-poly(caprolactone-*co*-trimethylene carbonate)). This amphiphilic copolymer aggregates spontaneously into 20 nm micelles upon contact with water [129] and is intended for oral delivery of poorly soluble drugs.

Micelles as drug carriers are able to provide a set of unbeatable advantages—they can solubilize poorly soluble drugs and thus increase their bioavailability, they can stay in the body (in the blood) long enough to provide gradual accumulation in the required area, their size permits them to accumulate in body regions with leaky vasculature, they can be targeted by attachment of a specific ligand to the outer surface, and they can be prepared in large quantities easily and reproducibly [125]. Being in a micellar form, the drug (poorly soluble drug, first of all) is well protected from possible inactivation under the effect of biological surroundings, it does not provoke undesirable side effects, and its bioavailability is usually increased.

The micelle is structured in such a way that the outer surface of the micelle exposed to the aqueous surrounding consists of components that are hardly reactive toward blood or tissue components. This structural peculiarity allows micelles to stay in the blood (tissues) rather long without being recognized by certain proteins and/or phagocytic cells. This longevity is an extremely important feature of micelles as drug carriers. Long-circulating pharmaceuticals and pharmaceutical carriers currently represent a fast growing area of biomedical research; for example, see Refs. 130–134.

Micronization   Developing intravenous formulations of hydrophobic drugs is particularly challenging. Possessing intravenous formulations of drugs can open new markets for drugs like antibiotics that could often be initially prescribed in a hospital setting. In addition, intravenous formulations can expand the market for the oral dosage formulation because physicians typically prefer to discharge patients on the oral formulation of the same drug administered intravenously in the hospital.

Many hydrophobic drugs are comprised of particles that are relatively large and therefore have a limited surface area available for interaction with water. These hydrophobic drugs are often formulated in less than ideal ways in order to make them dissolve. It is possible to increase the dissolution rate of hydrophobic drugs by increasing their aggregate surface area. To accomplish this, many pharmaceutical companies use a process, called micronization, which entails grinding hydrophobic drugs into smaller microparticles. However, the drug particles produced by micronization are often still not small enough to adequately improve dissolution, or to be administered intravenously. New technologies have been developed that convert drugs that do not dissolve well in water—hydrophobic drugs—into microparticles or nanoparticles of the drugs embedded in small microparticles. Alternatively, oils like Cremophor are used to dissolve the drugs. However, these oils are often not well tolerated and can require prolonged infusion rather than rapid injections. In addition, some hydrophobic drugs can be formulated into soft gelatin capsules, but these are only suitable for oral administration and encapsulate only a small volume of drug, requiring the administration of many capsules. Sometimes development of these drugs must be terminated because no suitable formulation can be found.

A continuous basal insulin supply may help to improve the condition of diabetics. A body weight gain in diabetic rats was observed as fast as in normal rats after a single injection of insulin-loaded microspheres in 28 days [135]. *In vitro* release of insulin from poly(lactide-*co*-glycolide) (PLGA) microspheres was improved by physically mixing microspheres prepared by water-in-oil-in-water double emulsion and solid-in-oil-in-water emulsion methods [136]. In this study, insulin-loaded microspheres maintained basal insulin level in diabetic rabbits for 40 days. Histological evaluations suggested that the insulin-loaded microspheres were biocompatible.

Macromolecular drugs such as peptides and proteins are unable to overcome the mucosal barriers and/or are degraded before reaching the bloodstream. Among the approaches explored so far in order to optimize the transport of these macromolecules across mucosal barriers, the use of nanoparticulate carriers represents a challenging but promising strategy. Nanostructures based on the mucoadhesive polysaccharide chitosan-coated systems showed an important capacity to enhance the intestinal absorption of the model peptide, salmon calcitonin, as shown by the important and long-lasting decrease in the calcemia levels observed in rats [137].

Alonso [138] reviews recent advances in the design of polymeric nanosystems intended to be used as carriers for nasal vaccine delivery. The information accumulated regarding the *in vivo* behavior of these nanocarriers indicates that they are able to facilitate the transport of the associated antigen across the nasal epithelium, thus leading to efficient antigen presentation to the immune system. Furthermore, the results suggest that not only the size and surface properties but also the polymer composition and the structural architecture of the nanosystems are critical for the optimization of these antigen carriers.

Dendrimers   Dendrimers are one of the emerging delivery systems with the capability to present such hydrophobic agents in a formulation with better prospective [139]. Dendrimers are synthetic, highly branched, monodisperse macromolecules of nanometer dimensions. These dendritic macromolecules with a large number of surface terminal groups and interior cavities offer a better opportunity for delivery by becoming charged and acting as static covalent micelles [140]. Started in the mid-1980s, the research investigations into the synthetic methodology and physical and chemical properties of these macromolecules are increasing exponentially with growing interest in this field. Although dendrimer drug delivery is in its infancy and toxicity is still a problem, it offers several attractive features. It provides a uniform platform for drug attachment that has the ability to bind and release drugs through several mechanisms. Properties associated with these dendrimers such as uniform size, water solubility, modifiable surface functionality, and available internal cavities make them attractive for biological and drug delivery applications. These are biocompatible, nonimmunogenic, and water soluble and possess terminal functional groups for binding various targeted or guest molecules [141]. The host–guest properties of dendrimers based on hydrophobic and ionic interactions apart from physical entrapment have been thoroughly studied [142]. The involvement of dendrimer in enhancing solubility of acidic anti-inflammatory drug through ionic interaction has been explored [143]. Dendrimers have also been explored for intracellular delivery of the anti-inflammatory drug ibuprofen [144]. As the dendrimer has many end functional groups, these would determine their solubility and physical and chemical interaction in the immediate surrounding environment [145].

Liposomes   Liposomes are widely used as nanosized drug delivery vehicles for active and passive targeting [146]. Liposomes may also "plug" and "seal" the damaged myocyte membranes and protect cells against ischemic and reperfusion injury *in vitro* [147] and the delivery of the ATP into the ischemic myocytes at the same time [148, 149]. As a drug delivery system, liposomes can significantly alter the pharmacokinetics and pharmacodynamics of entrapped drugs, for example, by enhancing drug uptake, delaying rapid drug clearance, and reducing drug toxicity [150–152].

For example, pegylated liposomal formulation of 2′-deoxyinosine (a 5-fluorouracil modulator), through an optimized pharmacokinetic profile (near seven times clearance reduction as compared with the free form), displays a potent tumor reduction effect in xenografted mice [153].

17.2.7   Vehicles and Selection of Excipients

FDA guidance [154] means by *new excipients* any inactive ingredients that are intentionally added to therapeutic and diagnostic products, but that (1) we believe are not intended to exert therapeutic effects at the intended dosage, although they may act to improve product delivery (e.g., enhance absorption or control release of the drug substance); and (2) are not fully qualified by existing safety data with respect to the currently proposed level of exposure, duration of exposure, or route of administration. Examples of excipients include fillers, extenders, diluents, wetting agents, solvents, emulsifiers, preservatives, flavors, absorption enhancers, sustained release matrices, and coloring agents.

In addition to their intended use, excipient candidates should also be qualified as appropriate pharmaceutical ingredients. Generally, it is preferable to select excipients that have been used in marketed products with a relevant route of delivery. Furthermore, excipients that have been used with a similar dosing frequency, history of chronic use, and patient population are also preferable. Otherwise, the approval and safety of the excipients need to be carefully examined. If the excipient is known to be safe on the basis of solid science or has a proven clinical safety record, it can be considered equivalent to approved excipients. The list of excipients used for parenteral pharmaceuticals is available in the literature [155–157]. The current information from the Inactive Ingredient Database can be found at the FDA website at http://www.accessdata.fda.gov/scripts/cder/iig/index.cfm.

When it is necessary to introduce other excipients with minimal safety records, a significant risk associated with the excipients will be added to the product development process and additional preclinical and clinical studies may be needed. Not all excipients are inert substances; some have been shown to be potential toxicants. The Federal Food, Drug, and Cosmetic Act of 1938 (the Act) was enacted after the tragedy of the elixir of sulfanilamide in 1937 in which an untested excipient was responsible for the death of many children who consumed the pharmaceutical. The Act required manufacturers to perform safety testing of pharmaceuticals and submit new drug applications (NDAs) demonstrating safety before marketing. Since that time, the FDA has become aware that certain other excipients used in commerce can cause serious toxicities in consumers of prescription and over-the-counter (OTC) drug products in the United States and other countries.

The FDA's *Guidance for Industry: Nonclinical Studies for the Safety Evaluation of Pharmaceutical Excipients* [154] describes the types of toxicity data that the Agency uses in determining whether a potential new excipient is safe for use in human pharmaceuticals. It discusses recommended safety evaluations for excipients proposed for use in OTC and generic drug products, and describes testing strategies for pharmaceuticals proposed for short-term, intermediate, and long-term use. It also describes recommended excipient toxicity testing for pulmonary, injectable, and topical pharmaceuticals.

Another important requirement in qualifying an excipient is the purity of the raw material. Depending on its historical use as a pharmaceutical ingredient, excipients are available in several different pharmaceutical grades, for example, USP (U.S. Pharmacopoeia), Ph. Eur. (European Pharmacopoeia), and JP (Japan Pharmacopoeia). These pharmaceutical grade materials should be considered as a primary resource, but the quality provided may not be good enough for specific product development. For example, significant stability problems can be found with some impurities even at concentrations below their specification (e.g., metal ions, peroxides, protease, and reducing sugars). These problems are more prominent in low protein concentration products due to a high impurity/protein ratio, although problems like visible precipitation may be independent of protein concentration. If an adjustment to the existing specification is necessary, it is critical to look into the availability of GMP quality raw materials with modified specifications as early as possible once the potential problem is identified. The use of excipients derived from animals or humans should be avoided if possible due to the risks associated with transmissible diseases like bovine spongiform encephalopathy, Creutzfeldt–Jakob disease, hepatitis virus, and HIV. Numerous regulatory guidelines have been issued to discourage the use of animal/human derived excipients (Note for Guidance on Minimizing the Risk of Transmitting Animal Spongiform Encephalopathy Agents Via Medicinal Products—EMEA (4/99); Note for Guidance on Plasma-Derived Medicinal Products—EMEA (7/98); Development Pharmaceutics for Biotechnological and Biological Products. Annex to Note for Guidance on Development). When animal derived excipients have to be included in a product, the manufacturer will need to fulfill its responsibilities to justify their selection and implement adequate safety measures.

A review of commercially available oral and injectable solution formulations presented by Robert Strickley [158] reveals that the solubilizing excipients include *water-soluble organic solvents* (polyethylene glycol 300, polyethylene glycol 400, ethanol, propylene glycol, glycerin, *N*-methyl-2-pyrrolidone, dimethylacetamide, and dimethylsulfoxide), *nonionic surfactants* (Cremophor EL, Cremophor RH 40, Cremophor RH 60, *d*-α-tocopherol polyethylene glycol 1000 succinate, polysorbate 20, polysorbate 80, Solutol HS 15, sorbitan monooleate, poloxamer 407, Labrafil M-1944CS, Labrafil M-2125CS, Labrasol, Gellucire 44/14, Softigen 767, and mono- and di-fatty acid esters of PEG 300, 400, or 1750), *water-insoluble lipids* (castor oil, corn oil, cottonseed oil, olive oil, peanut oil, peppermint oil, safflower oil, sesame oil, soybean oil, hydrogenated vegetable oils, hydrogenated soybean oil, and medium-chain triglycerides of coconut oil and palm seed oil), *organic liquids/semisolids* (beeswax, *d*-α-tocopherol, oleic acid, medium-chain mono- and diglycerides), various *cyclodextrins* (α-cyclodextrin, β-cyclodextrin, hydroxypropyl-β-cyclodextrin, and sulfobutylether-β-cyclodextrin), and *phospholipids* (hydrogenated soy phosphatidylcholine, distearoylphosphatidylglycerol, 1-α-dimyristoylphosphatidylcholine, 1-α-dimyristoylphosphatidylglycerol). The chemical techniques to solubilize water-insoluble drugs for oral and injection administration include pH adjustment, cosolvents, complexation, microemulsions, self-emulsifying drug delivery systems, micelles, liposomes, and emulsions.

An excellent reference for excipient information is the APA's *Handbook of Pharmaceutical Excipients* [159]. A very extensive and detailed list of vehicles and excipients commonly used in preclinical animal studies is presented by S. Gad in his book *Drug Safety Evaluation* [4, pp. 494–500]. In addition to this, we present below in more detail three other commonly or more recently used vehicles—Cremophor, chitosan, and cyclodextrin.

Cremophor EL (Polyoxyethyleneglycerol Triricinoleate) The heterogeneous nonionic surfactant CrEL is a white to off-white viscous liquid with an approximate molecular weight of 3 kDa and a specific gravity (25 °C/25 °C) of 1.05–1.06, and it is produced by the reaction of castor oil with ethylene oxide at a molar ratio of 1:35 [160]. Castor oil is a colorless or pale yellow fixed oil obtained from the seeds of *Ricinus communis*, with an extremely high viscosity, and consists mainly of the glycerides of ricinoleic, isoricinoleic, stearic, and dihydroxystearic acids. CrEL is usually of highly variable composition, with the major component identified as

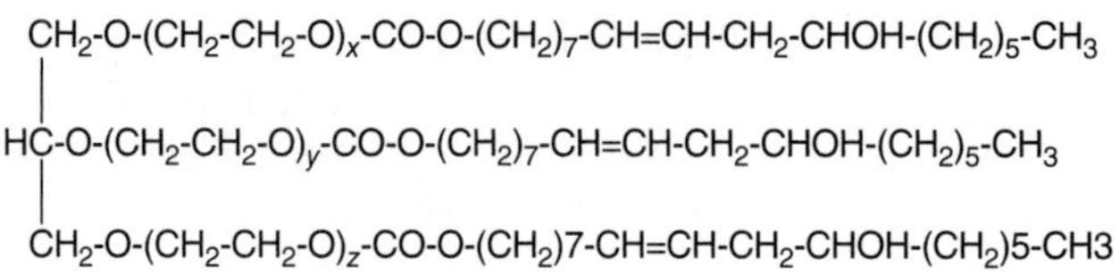

$$\text{CH}_2\text{-O-(CH}_2\text{-CH}_2\text{-O)}_x\text{-CO-O-(CH}_2)_7\text{-CH=CH-CH}_2\text{-CHOH-(CH}_2)_5\text{-CH}_3$$

$$\text{HC-O-(CH}_2\text{-CH}_2\text{-O)}_y\text{-CO-O-(CH}_2)_7\text{-CH=CH-CH}_2\text{-CHOH-(CH}_2)_5\text{-CH}_3$$

$$\text{CH}_2\text{-O-(CH}_2\text{-CH}_2\text{-O)}_z\text{-CO-O-(CH}_2)7\text{-CH=CH-CH}_2\text{-CHOH-(CH}_2)5\text{-CH3}$$

$$(x + y + z \approx 35)$$

FIGURE 17.1   Chemical structures of the main component of CrEL (polyoxyethyleneglycerol triricinoleate 35).

oxylated triglycerides of ricinoleic acid (i.e., polyoxyethyleneglycerol triricinoleate 35) (Fig. 17.1). Polyvinyl chloride (PVC)-free equipment for CrEL administration is obligatory, since CrEL is known to leach plasticizers from PVC infusion bags and polyethylene-lined tubing sets, which can cause severe hepatic toxicity [161]. CrEL is being used as a vehicle for the solubilization of a wide variety of hydrophobic drugs, including anesthetics, photosensitizers, sedatives, immunosuppressive agents, and (experimental) anticancer drugs. The amount of CrEL administered with these drugs averages 5 mL (range 1.5–10.3 mL), although paclitaxel is an exception as the amount of CrEL is much higher per administration, approximately 26 mL.

Recent investigations have revealed that CrEL, a widely used formulation vehicle, is a biologically and pharmacologically active ingredient of various commercially available drugs. For example, when used in paclitaxel administrations, an exceptionally large amount of CrEL is inevitably coadministered with the IV infusions, causing important biological events that can lead to serious acute hypersensitivity reactions and neurological toxicity, depending on the dose and duration of infusion [5, 162–164 for a review]. In addition, the substantial effects of CrEL on the disposition of other coadministered drugs (e.g., anthracyclines) with a narrow therapeutic window in polychemotherapeutic regimens also can be potentially hazardous to the patient [165]. In view of the inherent problems associated with the use of CrEL, it can be anticipated that there may be a therapeutic advantage from using paclitaxel formulations in which CrEL is absent [5]. Currently, a large variety of new (CrEL-free) formulation vehicles for paclitaxel are in (pre)clinical development, including cosolvent systems (Tween 80/ethanol/Pluronic L64), water-soluble polymers (e.g., polyethylene glycols), emulsions (e.g., triacetin), liposomes, albumin, cyclodextrins, nanocapsules, and microspheres (reviewed in Ref. 166).

In contrast, the *in vitro* and *in vivo* observations of myeloprotective effects related to the use of CrEL in combination with some agents, such as cisplatin, might be used to reformulate such agents with CrEL in order to achieve an optimization of their therapeutic window [167–169]. Iwase et al. [170, 171] have shown that Cremophor EL augments the cytotoxicity of hydrogen peroxide in rat thymocytes.

Based on our laboratory experience (data not published), we have seen some hypersensitivity reactions to CrEL in dogs and would recommend replacement of this vehicle with less toxic vehicles in preclinical dosage formulation, especially in dog studies.

Chitosan   Chitin is a copolymer of *N*-acetyl-glucosamine and *N*-glucosamine units randomly or block distributed throughout the biopolymer chain depending on the

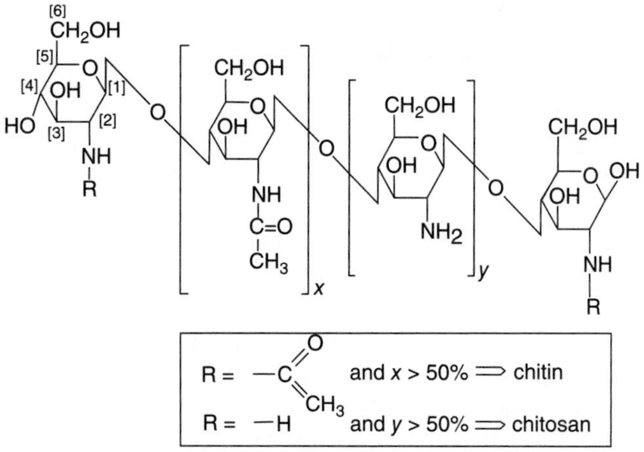

FIGURE 17.2 Schematic representation of the chitin and chitosan depicting the copolymer character of the biopolymers.

processing method used to derive the biopolymer (Fig. 17.2). When the number of N-acetyl-glucosamine units is higher than 50%, the biopolymer is termed chitin. Conversely, when the number of N-glucosamine units is higher, the term chitosan is used. Chitosan has been the better researched version of the biopolymer because of its ready solubility in dilute acids, rendering chitosan more accessible for utilization and chemical reactions.

Today, the production, chemistry, and applications of chitin and chitosan are well known. Commercially, chitin and chitosan are obtained from shellfish sources such as crabs and shrimps. It is likely that future sources of chitin and chitosan will come from biotechnology innovations, especially when medical applications are the focus.

Chitosan, a cationic polysaccharide obtained by alkaline N-deacetylation of chitin, is one of the most widely utilized polysaccharides. The sugar backbone of chitosan consists of β-1,4-linked d-glucosamine. In its structure, chitosan is very similar to cellulose, except for the amino group replacing the hydroxyl group on the C-2 position [172]. Recently, chitosan has been widely employed in pharmaceutical and biomedical fields owing to its unique properties such as nontoxicity, biocompatibility, and biodegradability [173, 174]. These characteristics make chitosan an excellent candidate for various biomedical applications such as drug delivery, tissue engineering, and gene delivery [173–178].

Chitosan has been investigated as an excipient in the pharmaceutical industry, to be used in direct tablet compression, as a tablet disintegrant, for the production of controlled release solid dosage forms, or for the improvement of drug dissolution [174]. Compared to traditional excipients, chitosan has been shown to have superior characteristics and especially flexibility in its use. Furthermore, chitosan has been used for production of controlled release implant systems for delivery of hormones over extended periods of time. Lately, the transmucosal absorption promoting characteristics of chitosan have been exploited, especially for nasal and oral delivery of polar drugs to include peptides and proteins and for vaccine delivery. These properties, together with the very safe toxicity profile, make chitosan an exciting and promising excipient for the pharmaceutical industry for present and future applications.

The transfection efficiency of low molecular weight chitosan (LMWC, molecular weight of 22 kDa) was significantly higher than naked DNA and higher than poly-L-lysine (PLL); it was also less cytotoxic than PLL [176]. For the further development of efficient gene carriers, highly purified chitosan oligosaccharides (COSs) were chemically modified with deoxycholic acid (DOCA). Owing to the amphiphilic characters, the DOCA-conjugated COSs (COSDs) formed self-aggregated nanoparticles in aqueous milieu. COSDs showed great potential as gene carriers with a high level of gene transfection efficiencies, even in the presence of serum. Considered with the negligible cytotoxic effects, DOCA-modified chitosan oligosaccharides can be considered as potential candidates for efficient nonviral gene carriers [50]. A vehicle containing 1.5% chitosan at pH 6.7 increased the bioavailability of intraduodenally administered buserelin in rats from 0.1% to 5.1% [179].

Cyclodextrins   Cyclodextrins (CDs) are cyclic oligosaccharides consisting of six or more glucose units linked by α-(1,4)-glycosidic bonds. α-, β-, and γ-Cyclodextrins (α-CD, β-CD, and γ-CD) are composed of six, seven, and eight unsubstituted glucose units, respectively (Fig. 17.3). In nature, cyclodextrins are produced as a storage form of carbohydrate (reserve substrate) by different microorganisms [180]. On an industrial scale, cyclodextrins are obtained by enzymatic hydrolysis of starch with cyclodextrin-glucosyltransferases. These amylolytic enzymes are produced by different strains of bacilli (e.g., *Bacillus macerans, Bacillus circulans*, and *Bacillus firmus*) and other organisms of other species (e.g., *Klebsiella oxytoca, Micrococcus* sp., and *Thermoanaerobacter* sp.). Cyclodextrin-glucosyltransferase (CGTase) cleaves the helical amylose molecule at regular intervals of six, seven, or eight glucose units, forming at the same time a ring by an intramolecular glucosyltransferase reaction [181].

Cyclodextrins have attracted the interest of the pharmaceutical, cosmetic, and—more recently—the food industry because they can entrap lipophilic compounds in the cavity of their torus-like structure [182–184]. Because of their larger ring, γ-CD and β-CD can host a wider range of molecules than α-CD. The usefulness of α-CD as a carrier and protectant of lipophilic molecules is therefore limited. However,

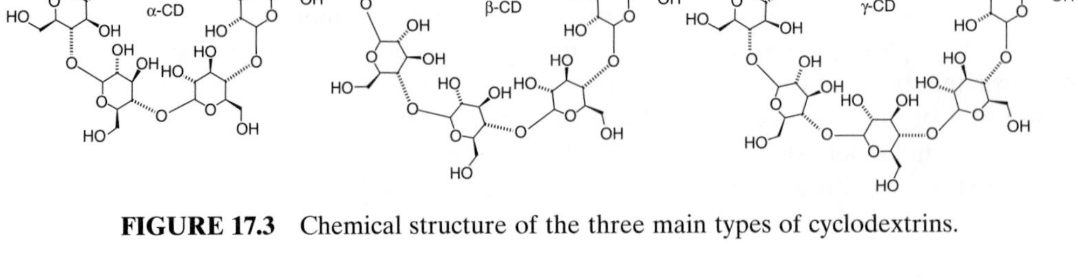

FIGURE 17.3   Chemical structure of the three main types of cyclodextrins.

α-CD merits interest as a potential food ingredient for a completely different reason. It has been found that α-CD is not digested by pancreatic amylase and therefore has the physiological properties of a water-soluble, dietary fiber. Consisting of α-(1,4)-linked glucose molecules, it structurally and metabolically resembles retrograded or crystalline nongranular starch ("resistant starch" of the RS3 type according to Englyst's classification) [185]. However, unlike resistant starch, α-CD is freely soluble in water (about 13 g/100 mL at 25 °C), yielding clear solutions with a low viscosity. Because of these properties, α-CD is very well suited for use as a dietary fiber not only in solid but also in semiliquid foods (e.g., yogurt) and all types of beverages.

The structural features of CDs are evaluated for their effect on complexation performance in pharmaceuticals [186]. Optimal specifications, quality production, and safety of each CD are presented. The current and future regulatory process facing excipients is summarized, and the current regulatory status of CDs in Japan, the United States, and Europe is presented.

Cyclodextrin complexation seems to be an attractive delivery system for proteins and peptides helping to overcome chemical and enzymatic instability, poor absorption through biological membranes, and rapid plasma clearance of these macromolecules [187]. The results from the study by Oda et al. [188] suggest that β-CD is considered as one of the most suitable solubilizing agents for evaluating poorly water-soluble drugs using *in situ* loop and perfusion techniques. The capacity to dissolve phenytoin was great in β-CD and hydroxypropyl β-cyclodextrin, followed by Tween 80. Those of methanol, dimethyl sulfoxide, dimethyl acetoamide, and polyethylene glycol 400 were much lower than expected.

However, CDs have been reported to interact with cell membrane constituents such as cholesterol, phospholipids, and phosphatidylinositols, resulting in the induction of hemolysis of RBCs [189–191]. Additionally, randomly methylated β-cyclodextrin (M-β-CD) disrupted the structures of lipid rafts and caveolae [192, 193], which are lipid microdomains formed by lateral assemblies of cholesterol and sphingolipids in the cell membrane, through extraction of cholesterol from the microdomains [194]. The magnitude of the hemolytic activity of the parent CDs is reported to increase in the order of γ-CD < α-CD < β-CD [189, 195]. Recently, various hydrophilic CD derivatives have been developed to improve aqueous solubility and complexation ability of parent CDs. Of the various hydrophilic CD derivatives, hydroxypropylated CDs, sulfobutyl ether CDs, and branched CDs are able to lower the hemolytic activity of each parent CD [196]. Conversely, methylation of the hydroxyl group at the 2 and 6 positions of a glucopyranose unit of β-CD is known to severely augment the hemolytic activity in high concentrations [197]. Arima et al. [198] and Motoyama et al. [199] reported that 2,6-di-*O*-methyl-α-CyD (DM-α-CyD) is predominantly likely to release CD14, a glycosylphosphatidylinositol (GPI)-anchored protein, from lipid rafts through the extractions of phospholipids from murine macrophages without cytotoxicity compared to α-CyD and 2-hydroxypropyl-α-cyclodextrin (HP-α-CyD). Recently, Motoyama et al. [200] showed that DM-α-CyD has higher hemolytic and morphological change activity than α-CyD and HP-α-CyD through more extraction of phospholipids including sphingomyelin and proteins, not cholesterol, from RBC membranes than α-CyD and HP-α-CyD. These toxicity reports for different types of cyclodextrins should be taken into account for their selection in dosage formulations.

17.3   TYPES AND CHARACTERISTICS OF DOSAGE FORMULATIONS BY ROUTE OF ADMINISTRATION

17.3.1   Oral Formulations

Pharmaceutical preparations for peroral administration form the majority of drug products most frequently administered. Within this group, availability for absorption usually decreases as solutions > suspensions > capsules > compressed tablets > coated tablets. Changes in this order may occur but are exceptions [201].

Solutions   This dosage form presents the drug component in a form most suitable for absorption. Hence, if there is no complexation or micellization with components of the formula, and if there is no degradation in the stomach, this dosage form will give maximal bioavailability and a rapid onset of action. The other advantage is that since solutions are homogeneous mixtures, the medication is uniformly distributed throughout the preparation. A number of drugs irritate the gastric mucosa when given in a concentrated form, such as a capsule or a tablet. This irritancy may be reduced by an adequate dilution factor if the drug is administered as a solution.

The disadvantage is that the solution form is bulky and hence requires increased costs for containers, handling, and storage. A drug in solution is usually the form most susceptible to degradation. Because solutions are, in many instances, fair to good microbiological growth media, adequate care must be taken to ensure a low initial bacterial count and prevention of growth during storage. The formulations are usually kept under refrigerated conditions to increase stability and decrease microbiological growth.

Emulsions   An emulsion is a thermodynamically unstable heterogeneous system consisting of at least one immiscible liquid intimately dispersed in another in the form of droplets. Oil emulsions (o/w) are usually manufactured to make the active oil phase easier to handle and sometimes more bioavailable. For example, griseofulvin, a poorly water-soluble drug, shows an increase in the rate and extent of absorption when dispersed in corn oil and then emulsified (o/w) [202]. The smaller amounts of drug present in the upper region of the small intestine at any particular time after oral administration of the corn oil emulsion, coupled with the inhibitory effect of lipid on proximal small intestine motility, allows the drug more time to dissolve in, and be absorbed from, the region of the intestinal tract where absorption is optimal. Also, the presence of emulsified corn oil in the intestinal tract stimulates bile excretion.

Emulsions, however, present problems with stability, not only of the emulsion itself, but also of the active ingredient. Changes in the solubility of emulsifiers and their hydrophilic–lipophilic balance, the viscosity of the emulsion, and partitioning of ingredients should always be considered.

Suspensions   A suspension is a two-phase system composed of a solid material dispersed in a liquid. A suspension may be considered the most desirable dosage form for a particular drug for a number of reasons. Certain drugs are chemically unstable when in solution but stable when a suitable salt or derivative is suspended. The suspension presents most of the advantages of the solution dose form: ease in swallowing, greater ease in administration of unusually large doses, and infinite variability of dosage. The disadvantages of suspensions are that they are heterogeneous systems: homogeneity of dose throughout the entire use period is difficult to maintain, or components may settle before the dose is measured. To overcome this problem, a suspending agent is usually added to increase viscosity and hence slow settling in the system.

Powders and Granules   Powders and granules, in general, provide a better environment for maintaining stability of the active drug than solutions, emulsions, and suspensions. They may be used to advantage in a number of different ways as follows:

1. The powder volume is usually less than an equivalent liquid volume.
2. The powder or granule could be administered by being mixed with the animal's food. Less common, the powder may be formulated as a soluble powder, to be added to drinking water.
3. There is good stability (may be difficult with some premix components) and easy tailoring of dose.
4. Specialized dosing equipment or unnecessary handling of the animal is not required.

A disadvantage would be that the dose actually consumed may vary widely, depending on the adequacy of the mix and the animal's eating/drinking habits. A medication that changes the odor and taste characteristics of the usual diet (or water) may cause problems with palatability.

Capsules   Capsules are the most common formulations used in dogs. Unlike other dosage forms, the capsule is a tasteless, easily administered and digested container for different materials such as powders, granules, pellets, suspensions, emulsions, or oils. There are two basic types of capsules. The hard gelatin capsule [203] is usually used for solid fill formulations and the soft gelatin capsule [204] for liquid or semisolid fill formulations. Soft gelatin capsules should be used in preference to hard gelatin capsules probably only if the fill is fluid or if bioavailability of the hard gelatin capsule formulation does not meet with requirements. The capsule offers an advantage in that the particle size and distribution of the original starting compound are rarely altered by the final filling process. Capsules are efficient in hiding the taste and odor of an unpleasant drug. Filling of the capsules takes time and labor costs are therefore high. The gelatin capsule does not offer protection from oxygen or moisture, although if it has an opaque shell, it will protect the contents from light. Hence, information on the stability and moisture sensitivity of the formulation must be known before the gelatin shell dosage form is selected.

Paste   Use of an oral paste formulation should be considered to overcome some of the dosing problems associated with other conventional dose delivery systems [205, 206]. A well formulated paste can provide accurate dose delivery, the dose being easily individually tailored to the animal's body weight. A paste affords a high degree of safety to both the administrator and animal.

TABLE 17.6   Advantages and Disadvantages of a Prolonged Release Delivery System

Advantages	Disadvantages
1. The maintenance of a relatively constant drug concentration in blood can reduce fluctuations of drug concentrations in tissue and at biological target sites for a more uniform pharmacological response.	1. Controlled release formulations are comparatively more costly to manufacture.
2. The incidence and intensity of side effects that might be caused by excessively high peak plasma concentrations resulting from the administration of conventional dosage forms may be reduced.	2. They do not permit termination.
3. The number and frequency of doses is decreased; hence, there is a reduction in labor costs and trauma to the animal.	3. Drugs with a low margin of safety may cause concern.
4. Slow accumulation (so-called enhanced permeability and retention effect, EPR) in pathological sites with affected and leaky vasculature (such as tumors, inflammations, and infarcted areas) and improved or enhanced drug delivery in those areas can be achieved.	4. A type of first-pass effect could be experienced.
5. Gradual release of a drug from a dosage form may reduce or prevent irritation to the gastrointestinal mucosa by drugs that are irritating to the tissue in high concentration.	

Tablets or Boluses   A tablet or bolus offers many advantages over other dose forms. The tablet offers relative ease of administration of an "accurate" dose and is readily adaptable to various dose sizes of medicinal substances. Tablets are portable and compact. They usually present the fewest problems with stability. However, the tablet form is usually not available in the early stages of preclinical safety drug assessment. Tablets also pose a problem because an animal can easily eject the tablet when out of sight of the doser, if the tablet has not been properly administered. To achieve optimal drug delivery to the intended site of absorption or action, the active ingredient should be protected from stomach function. Encapsulation or ptotective coating to achieve this should be considered. Gastric irritants, gastric degradable drugs, glandular products, and gastric nauseants, as well as drugs intended for action in the intestine, should be enteric coated to attain maximum effectiveness with least drug loss or side effects [205].

Controlled Release Pharmaceuticals   Long-circulating pharmaceuticals and new pharmaceutical carriers are rapidly developing. These dosage forms allow maintenance of a required level of a pharmaceutical agent in the blood for extended time intervals for better drug availability. The main advantages and disadvantages of prolonged release delivery are presented in Table 17.6.

17.3.2   Intravenous and Other Parenteral Formulations

The intravenous (IV) dosage form must be a solution and thus the physicochemical properties of the drug are taken into consideration. Once the formulation is established, its compatibility with blood must be determined to establish venous and perivenous tolerance. In addition, the duration of injection (or infusion) is

TABLE 17.7   Advantages and Disadvantages of Parenteral Therapy and Drug Formulations

Advantages	Disadvantages
1. The rate of onset of action can easily be controlled by the type of formulation and by the site of injection.	1. IV infusion warrants special apparatus (i.e., pumps) and sometimes animal surgery prior to dose (e.g., surgically implanted jugular catheter or VAP).
2. Nausea and vomiting are overcome.	2. The dosage form has to be administered by trained personnel (especially for IV) and requires strict adherence to aseptic technique.
3. Degradation of some drugs in the GI tract is avoided.	3. Once a drug is injected into the veins, tissue, or other body fluids, its removal is impossible.
4. Onset of action is faster and blood levels are more predictable.	4. Subcutaneous and intramuscular injections can produce severe local irritation and tissue necrosis.
5. Recommended for drugs that are poorly absorbed from the gastrointestinal tract.	5. Parenteral administrations (especially IV infusion) are time consuming.
6. Rapid onset of pharmacological effect.	6. Special care has to be taken in packaging parenterals.
7. When an animal is uncooperative or unconscious, parenteral administration is warranted.	
8. Parenteral administration can be used for local effects when desired (e.g., in anesthesiology).	

evaluated to establish the safety margin; however, it should be stated that this factor may not be applicable to human use because of anatomical and physiological differences.

Parenteral dose forms include aqueous, aqueous organic, and oily solutions, emulsions, suspensions, and solid forms for implantation. The parenterals should be sterile and pyrogen free; they are, if possible, buffered close to normal physiological pH and are preferably isotonic with body fluids [201]. The advantages and disadvantages of parenteral therapy should be considered and are presented in Table 17.7.

Severe local irritation and even tissue necrosis at the site of injection may be due to the solvent used [207, 208], or in many cases, the active drug results in a reaction. Rasmussen [209] has studied the tissue-damaging effect at the site of intramuscular injection of various preparations of antibiotics, other chemotherapeutic agents (sulfonamides, trimethoprim), certain drugs (lidocaine, diazepam, digoxin), and some vehicles. After intramuscular injection of physiological saline or sterile water, little or no tissue reaction was observed, while vehicles containing glycerol or propylene glycol caused severe damage at the injection site in swine, hens, and rabbits [210–212]. Pain is also likely to occur after intramuscular injection. Formulation techniques can often be used to overcome irritation and pain at the injection site.

17.3.3 Alternatives to Parenteral Administration (Nasal, Buccal, Transdermal, Rectal, and Vaginal)

Nasal Recent progress in biotechnology led to an enormous increase in the number of peptide and protein drugs that usually require parenteral administration to become therapeutically useful [213, 214]. Nonparenteral administration across mucosal surfaces (e.g., rectal, buccal, vaginal, nasal, and pulmonary epithelia) has been considered as an alternative route of application to replace parenteral injections [215, 216]. Among them, nasal delivery of peptides attracted strong interest because of its favorable biopharmaceutical properties. An overview is given by Gizurarson [217] on the relevance of the intranasal administration of drugs, peptides, and vaccines, and some physiological factors that present a barrier to the use of this route. The structure of the nasal epithelium, its high blood perfusion, and lower detrimental enzyme concentrations may result in higher bioavailabilities as compared to oral administration [218]. Nasal drug administration facilitates self-medication, thereby improving patient compliance. However, protein and peptide drugs show frequently low and variable bioavailabilities after nasal administration, for example, for insulin <1% [219]. Therefore, nasal insulin therapy necessitates coadministration of absorption enhancers such as surfactants, bile salts, fusidic acid derivatives, medium-chain fatty acids, chelators, or enzyme inhibitors to increase absorption and hence bioavailability [220, 221]. Although these absorption enhancers significantly increase transmucosal peptide transport, local tolerability, and safety concerns related to membrane damage, ciliary toxicity, mucus discharge, and epithelial disruption need to be overcome [222].

Consequently, the design of appropriate peptide carrier systems avoiding harmful additives has become a topic of intensive research. Nanoscale colloidal carriers from hydrophilic and biocompatible polymers, such as chitosan [223], were found to be useful for nasal vaccine [224] and insulin delivery [225] without employing additional penetration enhancers. Not only size and surface properties but also the polymer composition and architecture affected the functional properties of nanocarriers, such as transport of macromolecules across biological surfaces. In general, nanoscale dimensions favor transport of particles across mucosal epithelia [226, 227].

Moreover, nanocarriers with bioadhesive properties (e.g., nanoparticles (NP) coated with Carbopol) prevented rapid nasal clearance [228]. Increasing residence time in the nasal cavity was thought to improve drug absorption [229, 230]. Through the design of polymer properties, nanoparticle characteristics such as hydrophilicity and surface charge can be manipulated. In particular, polycations such as poly(L-lysine), protamine, polyethylene imine, chitosan, and dextran derivatives seem to increase mucosal permeability [231–233]. The combination of enhancing properties, mediated through cationic surface charges, with the formation of nanoparticulate carriers was achieved by encapsulating insulin into chitosan NP by ionotropic gelation, which yielded a significant blood glucose reduction in rabbits after nasal administration [225]. Recent study demonstrates that the nanocomplexes significantly enhanced insulin absorption, suggesting that amphiphilic biodegradable comb-polymers offer a promising approach for nasal peptide delivery [234].

In the development of a nasal drug delivery system (NDDS), formulation characteristics and device capabilities must be harmonized in order for consistent delivery into the nasal cavity. The approach to improve nasal bioavailability is the use of polymeric gel vehicles to increase nasal residence times and to control the rate of drug absorption. The aerosol droplet size distribution (DSD) is an important variable in defining the efficiency of aerosolized drugs. Low viscosity or shear-thinning vehicle systems were effectively atomized into small droplets using different nasal pump sprays, as previously reported [235]. There have been many reports that solutions of mixtures of certain polymers, surfactants, and excipients can exhibit molecular interactions that affect the rheological and physicochemical properties of the solutions [236]. The nature of these interactions can affect the ability of the solution to be aerosolized into small droplets and may alter the stability and liberation of the active components. The characteristic of nasal aerosol generation is dependent on a combination of actuation force, viscosity, rheological properties (e.g., changes in viscosity and appearance of the thixotropic system), surface tension, and pump design [235].

In the pharmaceutical industry, polymers are routinely used in the formulation of gels and in the stabilization of emulsions. In a recent publication, the insulin gel was formulated for intranasal administration using the combination of carbopol and hydroxypropyl methylcellulose as gelling agent [237]. The use of bioadhesive nasal gel containing insulin not only promoted the prolonged contact between the drug and the absorptive sites in the nasal cavity but also facilitated direct absorption of medicament through the nasal mucosa in rat and human studies. This study further demonstrates that administration of insulin intranasally in gel form is a pleasant and painless alternative to injectable insulin.

Buccal Among the various transmucosal routes, buccal mucosa has excellent accessibility, an expanse of smooth muscle, and relatively immobile mucosa, hence suitable for administration of retentive dosage forms. Direct access to the systemic circulation through the internal jugular vein bypasses drugs from the hepatic first-pass metabolism, leading to high bioavailability. Other advantages, such as low enzymatic activity, suitability for drugs or excipients that mildly and reversibly damage or irritate the mucosa, painless administration, easy drug withdrawal, facility to include permeation enhancer/enzyme inhibitor or pH modifier in the formulation, and versatility in designing multidirectional or unidirectional release systems for local or systemic actions, project buccal adhesive drug delivery systems as promising options for continued research [238, 239]. Morishita et al. [240] demonstrate in a rat model that 20% Pluronic PF-127 gels containing unsaturated fatty acids are potential formulations for the buccal delivery of insulin. Sudhakar et al. [239] discuss the implication of various approaches for buccal adhesive delivery strategies applied for the systemic delivery of orally less inefficient drugs, in addition to the widely used local drug delivery. The growth rate for transmucosal drug delivery systems is expected to increase 11% annually through 2007. Worldwide market revenues are at $3B with the United States at 55%, Europe at 30%, and Japan at 10%. However, the effect of salivary scavenging and accidental swallowing of the delivery system and the barrier property of buccal mucosa stand as major limitations in the development of buccal adhesive drug delivery systems.

An ideal buccal adhesive system must have the following properties:

1. Should adhere to the site of attachment for several hours.
2. Should release the drug in a controlled fashion.

3. Should provide drug release in a unidirectional way toward the mucosa.

4. Should facilitate the rate and extent of drug absorption.

5. Should not cause any irritation or inconvenience to the patient.

7. Should not interfere with normal functions, such as talking or drinking.

Buccal adhesive drug delivery systems using matrix tablets, films, layered systems, disks, microspheres, ointments, and hydrogels have been studied and reported by several research groups. However, limited studies exist on novel devices that are superior to those of conventional buccal adhesive systems for the delivery of therapeutic agents through buccal mucosa. A number of formulation and processing factors can influence properties of the buccal adhesive system. There are numerous important factors, including biocompatibility (both the drug–device and device–environment interfaces), reliability, durability, environmental stability, accuracy, delivery scalability, and permeability, to be considered while developing such formulations. Traditionally, pharmaceutically acceptable polymers were used to enhance the viscosity of products to aid their retention in the oral cavity. Dry mouth is treated with artificial saliva solutions that are retained on mucosal surfaces to provide lubrication. These solutions contain sodium CMC as bioadhesive polymer.

Several buccal adhesive delivery devices were developed at the laboratory scale by many researchers either for local or systemic actions. They are broadly classified into three groups presented in Table 17.8.

Selection of Animal Species for Buccal Studies   Apart from the specific methodology used to study buccal drug permeation characteristics, special attention is warranted for the selection of experimental animal species for such experiments. Many researchers have used small animals including rats and hamsters for permeability studies [241, 242]. But unlike humans, most laboratory animals have a totally keratinized oral lining and hence are not suitable. The rat has a buccal mucosa with a very thick, keratinized surface layer. The rabbit is the only laboratory rodent that has nonkeratinized mucosal lining similar to human tissue, but the sudden transition to keratinized tissue at the mucosal margins makes it hard to isolate the desired nonkeratinized region [243].

Among the larger experimental animals, monkeys are not practical models because of the difficulties associated with their maintenance. Dogs [244, 245] are easy to maintain and less expensive than monkeys [246] and their buccal mucosa is nonkeratinized and has a close similarity to that of the human buccal mucosa. However, we found in our laboratory that it is difficult to precisely deliver tablets intrabuccally to dogs as they tend to swallow tablets. Pigs also have nonkeratinized buccal mucosa similar to that of humans and their inexpensive handling and main-

TABLE 17.8   Classification of Buccal Adhesive Delivery Devices

Solid Buccal Adhesive Dosage Forms	Semisolid Buccal Adhesive Dosage Forms	Liquid Buccal Adhesive Dosage Forms
Tablets	Gels	Solutions
Microparticles	Patches/films	Suspensions
Wafers		
Lozenges		

tenance costs make them a highly suitable animal model for buccal drug delivery studies. In fact, the oral mucosa of pigs resembles that of humans more closely than any other animal in terms of structure and composition [247].

Adhesion of buccal adhesive drug delivery devices to mucosal membranes leads to an increased drug concentration gradient at the absorption site and therefore improved bioavailability of systemically delivered drugs. In addition, buccal adhesive dosage forms have been used to target local disorders at the mucosal surface (e.g., mouth ulcers) to reduce the overall dosage required and minimize side effects that may be caused by systemic administration of drugs. Researchers are now looking beyond traditional polymer networks to find other innovative drug transport systems. Much of the development of novel materials in controlled release buccal adhesive drug delivery is focusing on the preparation and use of a responsive polymeric system using a copolymer with desirable hydrophilic/hydrophobic interaction, block or graft copolymers, complexation networks responding via hydrogen or ionic bonding, and new biodegradable polymers especially from natural edible sources. At the current global scenario, scientists are finding ways to develop buccal adhesive systems through various approaches to improve the bioavailability of orally less inefficient drugs by manipulating the formulation strategies like inclusion of pH modifiers, enzyme inhibitors, and permeation enhancers. Novel buccal adhesive delivery systems, where drug delivery is directed toward buccal mucosa by protecting the local environment, is also gaining interest. Currently, solid dosage forms and liquids and gels applied to the oral cavity are commercially successful. The future direction of buccal adhesive drug delivery lies in vaccine formulations and delivery of small proteins/peptides. Microparticulate bioadhesive systems are particularly interesting as they offer protection to therapeutic entities as well as the enhanced absorption that results from increased contact time provided by the bioadhesive component. Exciting challenges remain to influence the bioavailability of drugs across the buccal mucosa. Many issues are yet to be resolved before safe and effective delivery through buccal mucosa. Successfully developing these novel formulations requires assimilation of a great deal of emerging information about the chemical nature and physical structure of these new materials.

Transdermal   In recent years, the development of transdermal dosage forms has been attracting increasing attention, owing to the several advantages that this administration route offers [248]. Transdermal delivery systems, when compared with conventional formulations, generally show a better control of blood levels, a reduced incidence of systemic toxicity, no hepatic first-pass metabolism, and higher patient compliance [249, 250]. In addition, the transdermal route provides sustained and controlled delivery [250]. It also allows continuous input of drugs with short biological half-lives and can eliminate pulsed entry into systemic circulation, which often causes undesirable side effects [251–254]. Release of drug from transdermal patches is controlled by the chemical properties of drug and delivery form as well as the physiological and physicochemical properties of the biological membrane [255]. Technological discoveries, over the last decade, have proved the feasibility of using several methodologies for enhancing transdermal drug delivery [256]. With a diverse set of tools to enhance skin permeability, the future of transdermal drug delivery looks brighter. The challenge now lies in converting these discoveries into useful products using newer excipients and technologies [257].

However, drug delivery via the skin is not an easy task because of the formidable barrier properties of the stratum corneum (SC). The majority of drugs do not appear to penetrate the skin at a sufficiently high rate to have therapeutic effectiveness. The feasibility of the transdermal route is thus limited to powerful actives presenting the appropriate features such as appropriate low molecular weight and high lipophilicity. Different approaches have been studied to overcome these limitations in order to develop efficient transdermal delivery systems [258–264].

The implication of skin permeation of drug on release rate profiles of the experimental formulations should not be ignored because the skin is known to have a substantial role in variation of release kinetics [265]. At an early stage and in a steady-state of skin permeation, diffusion of drug through appendages is considered to be significant. Selection of receptor fluid is also important for *in vitro* studies. A biphasic characteristic of the study fluid is desirable as the diffusion for the drug molecules through skin is routed through both aqueous and nonaqueous heterogeneous media. PEG 400 and water or normal saline are commonly selected to provide biphasic characteristics of the liquid [266].

The enhancement of skin flux with increase of drug concentrations may be due to accumulation of a greater amount of drug on the skin surface. The improvement in skin flux with the increase of PVP content may be owing to its antinucleating effect that converts the crystalline drug into an amorphous state, which generally possesses a high energy state with high solubility. The enhancement in drug solubility provides increased thermodynamic activity, which facilitates the skin permeation of drug [267].

One longstanding approach for improving transdermal drug delivery uses penetration enhancers (also called sorption promoters or accelerants), which penetrate into skin to reversibly decrease the barrier resistance [256]. Numerous compounds have been evaluated for penetration-enhancing activity, including sulfoxides (such as dimethylsulfoxide, DMSO), Azones (e.g., laurocapram), pyrrolidones (e.g., 2-pyrrolidone, 2P), alcohols and alkanols (ethanol or decanol), glycols (e.g., propylene glycol, PG, a common excipient in topically applied dosage forms), surfactants (also common in dosage forms), and terpenes. Different aspects of enhanced transdermal delivery are reviewed in Refs. 256 and 268.

Another way of enhancing transdermal delivery is iontophoresis. Iontophoresis involves application of small amounts of current to push charged drug molecules through skin, resulting in higher fluxes of the drug molecules for which permeation through skin is otherwise negligible. It provides the advantages of improved patient compliance, avoidance of first-pass metabolism, control rate of drug release from the patch, and the possibility of programmed delivery [269, 270]. The self-contained iontophoretic patches successfully delivered granisetron hydrochloride by iontophoresis and depot formation was observed in the dermal and subcutaneous structures in the skin [271]. In addition, the prodrug approach and, most recently, the use of colloidal carriers represent very promising strategies to improve transdermal delivery [260, 261].

Rectal   This route is used for local action on the rectum and lower colon. Glucose, digested proteins, and anesthetics are occasionally administered by high colonic irrigation to obtain systemic effect.

Vaginal   Vaginal tablets are ovoid or pear-shaped and prepared by granulation and compression. They can be formulated to exhibit two types of release mechanisms: (1) a slow release dissolution that retains the tablet's original shape; this tablet is ideal for drugs requiring low concentrations in the cavity for long periods; and (2) effervescent and disintegrating tablets that release quickly and ensure rapid distribution of the active drug for total local effect throughout the cavity. Both forms may often contain a buffer to maintain or change the vaginal pH to that required for normal physiologic vaginal flora.

Vaginal pessaries require specialized manufacturing equipment. The mass is usually a glycogelatin, theobroma oil, or synthetic base solid at room temperature but that dissolves or is fluid at body temperature. Pessaries pose special stability problems and should only be considered if the vaginal tablet does not give satifactory drug efficacy. Intravaginal and intrauterine drug delivery devices are often used.

17.3.4   Topical Formulations for Local Disorders (Dermal, Ocular, Ear)

Topical preparations may be used for local protective or therapeutic reasons (dusting powders, solutions, suspensions, lotions, liniments, creams, ointments, aerosols).

Dermal Formulations   Delivery of drugs to the skin is an effective and targeted therapy for local dermatological disorders. This route of drug delivery has gained popularity because it avoids first-pass effects, gastrointestinal irritation, and metabolic degradation associated with oral administration. Topical gel formulations provide a suitable delivery system for drugs because they are less greasy and can easily be removed from the skin. Percutaneous absorption of drugs from topical formulations involves the release of the drug from the formulation and permeation through skin to reach the target tissue. The release of the drug from topical preparations depends on the physicochemical properties of the vehicle and the drug employed. In order to enhance drug release and skin permeation, methods such as the selection of a suitable vehicle [271], coadministration of a chemical enhancer [268], and iontophoresis [272] have been studied.

The important considerations in the formulation of a dermatological preparation are, however, whether it is to be applied to a broken wound or an abrasion, whether it is to be rubbed into the affected area, whether it has to exhibit adhesiveness upon application to the skin, and whether it will deliver the active ingredient to the site required. Dusting powders, lotions, and aerosols are recommended formulations for application to abraded sites: lotions, liniments, creams, and ointments are best for unabraded sites.

For local therapeutic and systemic effects, the following should be considered: (1) the rate of dissolution of the drug in the vehicle, (2) the rate of diffusion of solubilized drug through the vehicle to the skin, and (3) the rate of permeation of the drug through the stratum corneum.

Formulation overcomes the problem of drug dissolution in the vehicle. Either the vehicle can be changed or the chemical structure of the active drug can be suitably altered (e.g., salt formation). The vehicle also governs the rate of diffusion and release of the drug to the stratum corneum. Thus, the vehicle is exceptionally important in determining topical bioavailability [273–278]. Nevertheless, vehicle design is often ignored in the development of a suitable delivery system.

In the design of a suitable delivery system, the following should be considered [201]:

1. Permeability of the stratum corneum may be increased if it is hydrated by a suitable vehicle (dimethyl sulfoxide can result in superhydration [279, 280]) or by occlusive dressings or vehicles. Transport in some species, however, may be via skin appendages; hence, agents promoting increased stratum corneum permeability may have no or even a negative effect [281].
2. The thermodynamic activity of the drug in the vehicle should be higher than in the stratum corneum [282].
3. The formulation should be buffered to a pH such that the active ingredient is in the un-ionized state.
4. Keratolytics, lipid and polar solvents (acetone and alcohol), surfactants after protracted use, and some vehicles may cause damage to the stratum corneum, thus increasing penetrability.
5. Viscosity of the medium is inversely related to flux.

There are various topical gel formulations on the market for both local and systemic delivery of drugs and several others are in clinical trials [283]. Various delivery systems, such as liposomes [284], biodegradable microspheres [285, 286], and hydrogels [287], have been investigated in order to circumvent the susceptibility of peptides to degradation during formulation, storage, and administration. Proteins and peptides are compatible with hydrogels, such as nonionic cellulose polymers and poloxamer gels, which are nontoxic and exhibit reversible thermal characteristics. Poloxamers have been reported as suitable gel systems for various proteins such as insulin [240], α-chymotrypsin, and lactate dehydrogenase [288] and peptides such as deslorelin and gonadotropin-releasing hormone (GnRH) [289]. Pluronic F127 (PF127), a type of poloxamer, has been shown to enhance the stability of proteins, such as urease, and interleukin-2 [290]. These formulations are targeted to deliver both small molecules and macromolecules. Spantide II, a neurokinin-1 receptor (NK-1R) antagonist, for the treatment of inflammatory skin disorders (e.g., dermatitis and psoriasis) showed significant retention in epidermis and dermis from lotion and gel formulations when the lotion and gel formulations contained N-methyl-2-pyrrolidone (NMP) as a penetration enhancer [291].

Recently, patch devices were introduced for local dermal (as well as systemic) drug delivery [292, 293]. The optimized bioadhesive patch device offered a more patient-compliant and convenient alternative to tetracaine percutaneous anesthetic gel, particularly where large areas of skin are to be treated [292].

Ocular Formulations Ophthalmic preparations are sterile aqueous or oily solutions, suspensions, emulsions, or ointments for topical administration by instillation. Ophthalmic solutions are usually isotonic and buffered to minimize irritation to the eye. All multiple-dose eye preparations must contain a bacteriostatic agent. These, however, cannot be used in the injured eye or during surgical intervention in the anterior eye chamber, because of possible irritation.

Solutions exhibit a fast drug pulse delivery: they produce an initial high dosage that rapidly lapses to very low concentrations. Ophthalmic suspensions should preferably have an aqueous vehicle containing the drug of low solubility. The suspension duration of action is more prolonged than in aqueous solution. Their disadvantage is the possibility of irritation due to suspended crystals or particles. Ointments remain in the eye longer than do solutions, both in the precorneal tear film and the conjunctival fornices, thereby increasing absorption of active ingredients [294]. The commonly used ointment bases may be toxic to the interior of the eye and should not be used when the cornea has been penetrated. Invasion of the ointment base into the internal chambers of the eye causes toxic endothelial damage, corneal edema, vascularization, and scarring [294].

Topical therapy with corticosteroids is quite common in the treatment of ocular inflammatory disorders. Many nonsteroidal anti-inflammatory drugs (NSAIDs) have been tested as ocular anti-inflammatory agents [295–297] so as to diminish the well documented ocular side effects caused by corticosteroids. Ketorolac tromethamine (KT), an aryl-acetic acid NSAID, is nonirritating to the eye at 0.5% wt/vol concentration [298]. Aqueous ocular drop of KT is an effective and safe anti-inflammatory agent for topical use following cataract surgery and intra ocular lens implantation [299–301].

Compared with aqueous drop, sesame and soybean oil drops of ketorolac provided higher ocular availability followed by ophthalmic ointment in rabbit ocular studies. The ointment formulation provided maximum sustained effect. Ketorolac aqueous drop with BAC and EDTA improved the rate of ocular absorption though not the extent of absorption [302]. Sesame and soybean oil drops containing 0.2% (wt/vol) ketorolac free acid and benzyl alcohol (0.5% vol/vol) and ophthalmic ointment containing 0.5% (wt/wt) KT (in dissolved state) showed higher *in vitro* transcorneal permeation with minimum corneal damage [303].

Iontophoresis as a noninvasive technique for ocular drug delivery has been investigated for many years. The technology of ocular iontophoresis has reached maturity in the aspect of device development. Therapeutic levels of drugs can be reached, in the anterior and posterior segments of the eye, after applying a convenient and noninvasive iontophoretic treatment [304]. It is clearly seen that ocular iontophoresis has clinical potential and importance as a local delivery system for many drugs. The iontophoretic treatment is already a promising tool for delivering anti-inflammatory and antibiotic drugs to the eye. Iontophoresis will soon be used in delivering chemotherapeutic agents for retinoblastoma and ocular melanomas or as home-use device for treating glaucoma. It is a matter of time until iontophoresis will routinely be used in the ophthalmic field [304].

Transscleral iontophoresis is a good potential alternative for multiple intravitreal injections or systemic therapy used for posterior ocular disorders, such as endophthalmitis, uveitis, retinitis, optic nerve atrophy, pediatric retinoblastoma, and age-related macular degeneration (AMD). The search for an alternative drug delivery system derives from the serious intraocular complications occurring after recurrent intravitreal injections including retinal detachment, vitreous hemorrhage, endophthalmitis, and cataract. One recent study [305] showed that compared to IV administration, transscleral Coulomb Control iontophoresis (CCI) achieved higher and more sustained tissue concentrations of methylprednisolone with negligible systemic absorption. These data demonstrate that high levels of methylprednisolone can safely be achieved in intraocular tissues and fluids of the rabbit eye, using CCI. Results from another study [306] suggest that focal delivery of carboplatin using subconjunctival injection or iontophoretic delivery transmits drug more effectively than intravenous delivery into the target tissues of the vitreous, choroid, retina, and optic nerve in the rabbit eye. Both focal applications resulted in significantly higher peak concentrations of carboplatin in the choroid, retina, optic nerve, and vitreous than those obtained after intravenous delivery. Focal chemotherapeutic delivery resulted in dramatically decreased carboplatin levels in the blood plasma compared with intravenous delivery.

Ear Formulations   Otic dosage forms are intended for administration either on the outer ear or into the auditory canal. They include a number of dosage forms: solutions, suspensions, ointments, otic cones, and powders. Their primary use is either to remove wax or supply local drug treatment. Direct delivery of new therapies for treatment of sensorineural hearing loss to the fluids of the inner ear is necessary because of the presence of a blood–labyrinth drug barrier, which is anatomically and functionally similar to the blood–brain barrier [307, 308]. Direct delivery also has significant potential advantages for therapeutic application. Drugs are largely unaltered by metabolic changes that inevitably occur with other routes of administration, and have ready access to the sensory cells of the inner ear (the hair cells) and the synaptic regions of hair cells [309]. Delivery directly to the inner ear can avoid undesirable systemic side effects that some drugs may produce. The performance of an extracorporeal reciprocating perfusion system in guinea pigs was recently described by Chen et al. [310].

17.3.5   Inhalation Formulations (Vapors and Aerosols)

Many biologically active peptides have been discovered recently and have attracted attention as new drugs. Because of transport and enzymatic barriers, clinical dosage forms of these peptides have been primarily parenteral forms [311]. Development of sustained release forms of these peptide drugs is also being actively researched [312–314] and the pulmonary route would seem to be a promising alternative for delivering them, because many drugs that are poorly absorbed from other mucosal sites are well absorbed from the lungs [315]. This route of administration offers several advantages over the conventional gastrointestinal pathway, including large surface area, extensive vasculature, easily permeable membrane, and low intracellular and extracellular enzymatic activity [316–319]. Recent clinical and preclinical reports reveal that delivery of peptide drugs such as leuprolide acetate and insulin is feasible through the pulmonary route [320–323]. However, the bioavailability of the drugs having relatively high molecular weight is still poor through the pulmonary route compared with the parenteral route.

Recent research is focused on the delivery of systemically acting drugs via the pulmonary route [324]. Dry powder inhalations are a promising application form for peptides and proteins for systemic delivery because they overcome the drawbacks of oral and invasive delivery forms [315].

The administration of liposome-encapsulated drugs by aerosols seems to be a feasible way of targeting these delivery systems to the lung. The tolerability and safety of liposome aerosols have previously been tested in animals as well as in human volunteers; no untoward effects have been recognized [325, 326]. Liposomes are also known to sustain the release of the entrapped drug(s) and to decrease the mucociliary clearance of the drug(s) because of their surface viscosity. Therefore, more effective and sustained systemic absorption of a drug would be attained by administering the drug containing liposomes in the respiratory tract. The developed liposomal dry powder inhaler of Leucinostatin demonstrated approximately 50% bioavailability compared with the SC route in rats [311]. This study justifies the role of the pulmonary route as a promising alternative to the presently available SC route. Green et al. [327] review the formulation process of inhalable drugs. They showed that high pressure media milling (HPMM) yields stable, fine-particle dispersion of medicament in hydrofluorocarbone propellant (HCP), which enhances a metered dose inhaler. HCP is currently mostly used for inhalation dose formulation as a more environmentally friendly product than previously used chlorofluorocarbons. However, eliminating chlorine from modern propellants introduced a solubility challenge for which the HPMM process helps to compensate.

17.4   CONCLUSION

Rapid developments in the field of molecular biology and gene technology resulted in generation of many macromolecular drugs including peptides, proteins, polysaccharides, and nucleic acids in great numbers and possessing superior pharmacological efficacy with site specificity and devoid of untoward and toxic effects. However, the main impediment for the oral delivery of these drugs as potential therapeutic agents is their extensive presystemic metabolism and instability in an acidic environment, resulting in inadequate and erratic oral absorption. This requires development of new drug delivery systems and increased usage of other routes of administration compared to the traditional oral and parenteral routes. These new therapies and new delivery systems require new formulations, which should be evaluated for toxicity and efficacy in preclinical studies using the proposed routes of administration.

REFERENCES

1. Irie T, Uekama K. Cyclodextrins in peptide and protein delivery. *Adv Drug Deliv Rev* 1999;36:101–123.
2. Pearlman R, Wang Y J, Eds. *Formulation, Characterization, and Stability of Protein Drugs*. New York: Plenum Press; 1996.
3. Ráscz I. In *Drug Formulation*. Hoboken, NJ: Wiley; 1989.
4. Gad SC, Ed. *Drug Safety Evaluation*. Hoboken, NJ: Wiley-Interscience; 2002.
5. Gelderblom H, Verweij J, Nooter K, Sparreboom A. Cremophor EL, the drawbacks and advantages of vehicle selection for drug formulation. *Eur J Cancer* 2001;37(13): 1590–1598.
6. Aungst BJ. Intestinal permeation enhancers. *J Pharm Sci* 2000;89(4):429–442.
7. Deshpande AA, Rhodes CT, Shah NH, Malick AW. Control-release drug delivery systems for prolonged gastric residence: an overview. *Drug Dev Ind Pharm* 1996;22: 531–539.

8. Hwang S-J, Park H, Park K. Gastric retentive drug-delivery systems. *Crit Rev Ther Drug Carrier Syst* 1998;15:243–284.

9. Hoffman A, Stepensky D, Lavy E, Eyal S, Klausner E, Friedman M. Pharmacokinetic and pharmacodynamic aspects of gastroretentive dosage forms. *Int J Pharm* 2004; 277(1–2):141–153.

10. Aungst BJ, Saitoh H, Burcham DL, Huang S-M, Mousa SA, Hussain MA. Enhancement of the intestinal absorption of peptides and non-peptides. *J Control Release* 1996;41: 19–31.

11. Fix JA. Strategies for delivery of peptides utilizing absorption-enhancing agents. *J Pharm Sci* 1996;85:1282–1285.

12. Hochman J, Artursson P. Mechanisms of absorption enhancement and tight junction regulation. *J Control Release* 1994;29:253–267.

13. Swenson ES, Curatolo WJ. Intestinal permeability enhancement for proteins, peptides and other polar drugs: mechanisms and potential toxicity. *Adv Drug Deliv Rev* 1992;8: 39–92.

14. Ings RMJ. In Smolen VF, Ball L, Eds. *Animal Studies and the Bioavailability Testing of Drug Products in Control Drug Bioavailability*. Hobohen, NJ: Wiley;1984, p 43.

15. Eriksson HJC, Hinrichs WLJ, van Veen B, Somsen GW, de Jong GJ, Frijlink HW. Investigations into the stabilisation of drugs by sugar glasses: I. Tablets prepared from stabilised alkaline phosphatase. *Int J Pharm* 2002;249: 59–70.

16. Wang W. Instability, stabilization, and formulation of liquid protein Pharmaceuticals. *Int J Pharm* 1999;185:129–188.

17. Xing L, Dawei C, Liping X, Rongquing Z. Oral colon-specific drug delivery for bee venom peptide: development of a coated calcium alginate gel beads-entrapped liposome. *J Control Release* 2003;93:293–300.

18. Shargel L, Yu A. In *Applied Biopharmaceutics and Pharmacokinetics*, 4th ed. New York: McGraw-Hill;1999, Ch 5.

19. George M, Abraham TE. Polyionic hydrocolloids for the intestinal delivery of protein drugs: alginate and chitosan—a review. *J Control Release* 2006;14(1):1–14.

20. Sayani AP, Chien YW. Systemic delivery of peptides and proteins across absorptive mucosae. *CRC Crit Rev Ther Drug Carrier Syst* 1996;13:85–184.

21. Langel Ü. In *Cell-Penetrating Peptides: Processes and Applications*. New York: CRC Press; 2002.

22. Weecharangsan W, Opanasopit P, Ngawhirunpat T, Rojanarata T, Apirakaramwong A. Chitosan lactate as a nonviral gene delivery vector in COS-1 cells. *AAPS PharmSciTech* 2006;7(3): Article 66.

23. De Smedt SC, Demeester J, Hennink WE. Cationic polymer based gene delivery systems. *Pharm Res* 2000;17:113–126.

24. Lundstrom K. Latest development in viral vectors for gene therapy. *Trends Biotechnol* 2003;21:117–122.

25. Li S, Huang L. Nonviral gene therapy: promises and challenges. *Gene Ther* 2000;7:31–34.

26. Luo D, Saltzman WM. Synthetic DNA delivery systems. *Nat Biotechnol* 2000;18:33–37.

27. Felgner JH, Kumar R, Sridhar CN, Wheeler CJ, Tsai YJ, Border R, Ramsey P, Martin M, Felgner PL. Enhanced gene delivery and mechanism studies with a novel series of cationic lipid formulations. *J Biol Chem* 1994;269:2550–2561.

28. Farhood H, Serbina N, Huang L. The role of dioleoyl phosphatidylethanolamine in cationic liposome mediated gene transfer. *Biochim Biophys Acta* 1995;1235:289–295.

29. Zabner J, Fasbender AJ, Moninger T, Poellinger KA, Welsh MJ. Cellular and molecular barriers to gene transfer by a cationic lipid. *J Biol Chem* 1995;270:18997–19007.

30. Lee KY, Kwon IC, Kim YH, Jo WH, Jeong SY. Preparation of chitosan self-aggregates as a gene delivery system. *J Control Release* 1998;51:213–220.

31. Mansouri S, Lavigne P, Corsi K, Benderdour M, Beaumont E, Fernandes JC. Chitosan–DNA nanoparticles as non-viral vectors in gene therapy: strategies to improve transfection efficacy. *Eur J Pharm Biopharm* 2004;57:1–8.

32. Thomas CE, Ehrhardt A, Kay MA. Progress and problems with the use of viral vectors for gene therapy. *Nat Rev Genet* 2003;4:346–358.

33. Pfeifer A, Verma IM. Gene therapy: promises and problems. *Annu Rev Genomics Hum Genet* 2001;2:177–211.

34. Anderson WF. Human gene therapy. *Nature* 1998;392:25–30.

35. Anwer K, Rhee BG, Mendiratta SK. Recent progress in polymeric gene delivery systems. *Crit Rev Ther Drug Carrier Syst* 2003;20:249–293.

36. Han S, Mahato RI, Sung YK, Kim SW. Water-soluble lipopolymer for gene delivery. *Bioconjug Chem* 2001;12:337–345.

37. Merdan T, Kopecek J, Kissel T. Prospects for cationic polymers in gene and oligonucleotide therapy against cancer. *Adv Drug Deliv Rev* 2002;54:715–758.

38. Lim YB, Choi YH, Park JS. A self-destroying polycationic polymer: biodegradable poly(4-hydroxy-l-proline ester). *J Am Chem Soc* 1999;121:5633–5639.

39. Putnam D, Langer R. Poly(4-hydroxy-l-proline ester): low-temperature polycondensation and plasmid DNA complexation. *Macromolecules* 1999;32:3658–3662.

40. Lim YB, Han SO, Kong HU, Lee Y, Park JS, Jeong B, Kim SW. Biodegradable polyester poly[alpha-(4 aminobutyl)-l-glycolic acid], as a non-toxic gene carrier. *Pharm Res* 2000; 17:811–816.

41. Bikram M, Ahn CH, Chae SY, Lee MY, Yockman JW, Kim SW. Biodegradable poly(ethylene glycol)-*co*-poly(L-lysine)-*g*-histidine multiblock copolymers for nonviral gene delivery. *Macromolecules* 2004;37:1903–1916.

42. Lynn DM, Langer R. Degradable poly(beta-amino esters):synthesis characterization and self-assembly with plasmid DNA. *J Am Chem Soc* 2000;122:10761–10768.

43. Anderson DG, Lynn DM, Langer R. Semi-automated synthesis and screening of a large library of degradable cationic polymers for gene delivery. *Angew Chem Int Ed Engl* 2003;42:3153–3158.

44. Liu Y, Wu DC, Ma YX, Tang GP, Wang S, He CB, Chung TS, Goh S. Novel poly(amino ester)s obtained from Michael addition polymerizations of trifunctional amine monomers with diacrylates: safe and efficient DNA carriers. *Chem Commun* 2003; 2630–2631.

45. Anderson DG, Akinc A, Hossain N, Langer R. Structure/property studies of polymeric gene delivery using a library of poly(beta-amino esters). *Mol Ther* 2005;11:426–434.

46. Lim YB, Kim SM, Suh H, Park JS. Biodegradable, endosome disruptive, and cationic network-type polymer as a highly efficient and nontoxic gene delivery carrier. *Bioconjug Chem* 2002;13:952–957.

47. Luten J, van Steenis JH, van Someren R, Kemmink J, Schuurmans-Nieuwenbroek NME, Koning GA, Crommelin DJA, van Nostrum CF, Hennink WE. Water-soluble biodegradable cationic polyphosphazenes for gene delivery. *J Control Release* 2003;89:483–497.

48. Ahn CH, Chae SY, Bae YH, Kim SW. Biodegradable poly(ethylenimine) for plasmid DNA delivery. *J Control Release* 2002;80:273–282.

49. Petersen H, Merdan T, Kunath F, Fischer D, Kissel T. Poly(ethylenimine-*co*-l-lactamide-*co*-succinamide): a biodegradable polyethylenimine derivative with an advantageous pH-dependent hydrolytic degradation for gene delivery. *Bioconjug Chem* 2002;13: 812–821.

50. Chae SY, Son S, Lee M, Jang M-K, Nah J-W. Deoxycholic acid-conjugated chitosan oligosaccharide nanoparticles for efficient gene carrier. *J Control Release* 2005;109(1–3): 330–344.

51. Zhong Z, Song Y, Engbersen JFJ, Lok MC, Hennink WE, Feijen J. A versatile family of degradable non-viral gene carriers based on hyperbranched poly(esteramine)s. *J Control Release* 2005;109(1–3):317–329.

52. Gao C, Tang W, Yan DY. Synthesis and characterization of water-soluble hyperbranched poly(ester amine)s from diacrylates and diamines. *J Polym Sci Polym Chem* 2002;40: 2340–2349.

53. Jikei M, Kakimoto M. Hyperbranched polymers: a promising new class of materials. *Prog Polym Sci* 2001;26:1233–1285.

54. Wightman L, Kircheis R, Rossler V, Carotta S, Ruzicka R, Kursa M, Wagner E. Different behavior of branched and linear polyethylenimine for gene delivery *in vitro* and *in vivo*. *J Gene Med* 2001;3:362–372.

55. Boussif O, Lezoualch F, Zanta MA, Mergny MD, Scherman D, Demeneix B, Behr JP. A versatile vector for gene and oligonucleotide transfer into cells in culture and in-vivo-polyethylenimine. *Proc Natl Acad Sci USA* 1995;92:7297–7301.

56. Abdallah B, Hassan A, Benoist C, Goula D, Behr JP, Demeneix BA. A powerful nonviral vector for *in vivo* gene transfer into the adult mammalian brain: polyethylenimine. *Hum Gene Ther* 1996;7:1947–1954.

57. Kircheis R, Wightman L, Wagner E. Design and gene delivery activity of modified polyethylenimines. *Adv Drug Deliv Rev* 2001;53:341–358.

58. Fischer D, Bieber T, Li YX, Elsasser HP, Kissel T. A novel non-viral vector for DNA delivery based on low molecular weight branched polyethylenimine: effect of molecular weight on transfection efficiency and cytotoxicity. *Pharm Res* 1999;16:1273–1279.

59. Fewell JG, Matar M, Slobodkin G, Han S-O, Rice J, Hovanes B, Lewis DH, Anwer K. Synthesis and application of a non-viral gene delivery system for immunogene therapy of cancer. *J Control Release* 2005;109:288–298.

60. Zhang G, Budker V, Williams P, Subbotin V, Wolff JA. Efficient expression of naked DNA delivered intraarterially to limb muscles of nonhuman primates. *Hum Gene Ther* 2001;12:427–438.

61. Fewell JG, MacLaughlin F, Mehta V, Gondo M, Nicol F, Wilson E, Smith LC. Gene therapy for the treatment of hemophilia B using PINC-formulated plasmid delivered to muscle with electroporation. *Mol Ther* 2001;3:574–583.

62. Herweijer H, Wolff JA. Progress and prospects: naked DNA gene transfer and therapy. *Gene Ther* 2003;10:453–458.

63. Database on Human Gene Transfer Trials (GeMCRIS). http://www4.od.nih.gov/oba/RAC/GeMCRIS_public.htm.

64. Ma H, Diamond SL. Non viral gene therapy and its delivery systems. *Curr Pharm Biotechnol* 2001;2:1–17.

65. Davis ME. Non-viral gene delivery systems. *Curr Opin Biotechnol* 2002;13:128–131.

66. Anwer K, Kao G, Rolland A, Driessen WH, Sullivan SM. Peptide-mediated gene transfer of cationic lipid/plasmid DNA complexes to endothelial cells. *J Drug Target* 2004;12: 215–221.

67. Wang DA, Narang AS, Kotb M, Gaber AO, Miller DD, Kim SW, Mahato RI. Novel branched poly(ethylenimine)–cholesterol water-soluble lipopolymers for gene delivery. *Biomacromolecules* 2002;3:1197–1207.

68. Furgeson DY, Cohen RN, Mahato RI, Kim SW. Novel water insoluble lipoparticulates for gene delivery. *Pharm Res* 2002;19:382–390.

69. Sonawane ND, Szoka FC Jr, Verkman AS. Chloride accumulation and swelling in endosomes enhances DNA transfer by polyamine–DNA polyplexes. *J Biol Chem* 2003;278: 44826–44831.

70. Chollet P, Favrot MC, Hurbin A, Coll JL. Side-effects of a systemic injection of linear polyethylenimine–DNA complexes. *J Gene Med* 2002;4:84–91.

71. Godbey WT, Wu KK, Mikos AG. Poly(ethylenimine) and its role in gene delivery. *J Control Release* 1999;60:149–160.

72. Furgeson DY, Chan WS, Yockman JW, Kim SW. Modified linear polyethylenimine–cholesterol conjugates for DNA complexation. *Bioconjug Chem* 2003;14:840–847.

73. Lv H, Zhang S, Wang B, Cui S, Yan J. Toxicity of cationic lipids and cationic polymers in gene delivery. *J Control Release* 2006;114(1):100–109.

74. Crooke ST. Molecular mechanisms of antisense drugs: RNase H. *Antisense Nucleic Acid Drug Dev* 1998;8:133–134.

75. Lindner LH, Brock R, Arndt-Jovin D, Eibl H. Structural variation of cationic lipids: minimum requirement for improved oligonucleotide delivery into cells. *J Control Release* 2006;110(210):444–456.

76. Zamecnik PC, Stephenson ML. Inhibition of Rous sarcoma virus replication and cell transformation by a specific oligodeoxynucleotide. *Proc Natl Acad Sci USA* 1978;75: 280–284.

77. Stephenson ML, Zamecnik PC. Inhibition of Rous sarcoma viral RNA translation by a specific oligodeoxyribonucleotide. *Proc Natl Acad Sci USA* 1978;75:285–288.

78. De Clercq E, Merigan TC. Requirement of a Stable Secondary Structure for the Antiviral Activity of Polynucleotides. *Nature* 1969;222:1148–1152.

79. Alberts SR, Schroeder M, Erlichman C, Steen PD, Foster NR, Moore DF Jr, Rowland KM Jr, Nair S, Tschetter LK, Fitch TR. Gemcitabine and ISIS-2503 for patients with locally advanced or metastatic adenocarcinoma: a North Central Cancer Treatment Group phase II trial. *J Clin Oncol* 2004;22:4944–4950.

80. Kim R, Emi M, Tanabe K, Toge T. Therapeutic potential of antisense Bcl-2 as a chemosensitizer for cancer therapy. *Cancer* 2004;101:2491–2502.

81. Loke SL, Stein CA, Zhang XH, Mori K, Nakanishi M, Subasinghe C, Cohen JS, Neckers LM. Characterization of oligonucleotide transport into living cells. *Proc Natl Acad Sci USA* 1989;86:3474–3478.

82. Wu-Pong S, Weiss TL, Hunt CA. Antisense c-myc oligodeoxyribonucleotide cellular uptake. *Pharm Res* 1992;9:1010–1017.

83. Yakubov LA, Deeva EA, Zarytova VF, Ivanova EM, Ryte AS, Yurchenko LV, Vlassov VV. Mechanism of oligonucleotide uptake by cells: involvement of specific receptors? *Proc Natl Acad Sci USA* 1989;86:6454–6458.

84. Zamecnik P, Aghajanian J, Zamecnik M, Goodchild J, Witman G. Electron micrographic studies of transport of oligrodeoxynucleotides across eukaryotic cell membranes. *Proc Natl Acad Sci USA* 1994;91:3156–3160.

85. Wagner RW, Matteucci MD, Lewis JG, Gutierrez AJ, Moulds C, Froehler BC. Antisense gene inhibition by oligonucleotides containing C-5 propyne pyrimidines. *Science* 1993;260:1510–1513.

86. Bertling WM, Gareis M, Paspaleeva V, Zimmer A, Kreuter J, Nurnberg E, Harrer P. Use of liposomes, viral capsids, and nanoparticles as DNA carriers. *Biotechnol Appl Biochem* 1991;13:390–405.

87. Gewirtz AM, Sokol DL, Ratajczak MZ. Nucleic acid therapeutics: state of the art and future prospects. *Blood* 1998;92:712–736.

88. Zobel HP, Junghans M, Maienschein V, Werner D, Gilbert M, Zimmermann H, Noe C, Kreuter J, Zimmer A. Enhanced antisense efficacy of oligonucleotides adsorbed to monomethylaminoethylmethacrylate methylmethacrylate copolymer nanoparticles. *Eur J Pharm Biopharm* 2000;49:203–310.

89. Zelphati O, Degols G, Loughrey H, Leserman L, Pompon A, Puech F, Maggio AF, Imbach JL, Gosselin G. Inhibition of HIV-1 replication in cultured cells with phosphory-lated dideoxyuridine derivatives encapsulated in immunoliposomes. *Antiviral Res* 1993;21:181–195.

90. Capaccioli S, DiPasquale G, Mini E, Mazzei T, Quattrone A. Cationic lipids improve antisense oligonucleotide uptake and prevent degradation in cultured cells and in human serum. *Biochem Biophys Res Commun* 1993;197:818–825.

91. Bennett CF, Chiang MY, Chan H, Shoemaker JE, Mirabelli CK. Cationic lipids enhance cellular uptake and activity of phosphorothioate antisense oligonucleotides. *Mol Pharmacol* 1992;41:1023–1033.

92. Weyermann J, Lochmann D, Zimmer A. Comparison of antisense oligonucleotide drug delivery systems. *J Control Release* 2004;100:411–423.

93. Lappalainen K, Urtti A, Soderling E, Jaaskelainen I, Syrjanen K, Syrjanen S. Cationic liposomes improve stability and intracellular delivery of antisense oligonucleotides into CaSki cells. *Biochim Biophys Acta* 1994;1196:201–208.

94. Sazani P, Kole R. Therapeutic potential of antisense oligonucleotides as modulators of alternative splicing. *J Clin Invest* 2003;112:481–486.

95. Remaut K, Lucas B, Braeckmans K, Sanders NN, Demeester J, De Smedt SC. Protection of oligonucleotides against nucleases by pegylated and non-pegylated liposomes as studied by fluorescence correlation spectroscopy. *J Control Release* 2005;110(1):212–226.

96. Shi F, Hoekstra D. Effective intracellular delivery of oligonucleotides in order to make sense of antisense. *J Control Release* 2004;97:189–209.

97. Agrawal S. Importance of nucleotide sequence and chemical modifications of antisense oligonucleotides. *Biochim Biophys Acta* 1999;1489:53–68.

98. Brown DA, Kang SH, Gryaznov SM, Dedionisio L, Heidenreich O, Sullivan S, Xu X, Nerenberg MI. Effect of phosphorothioate modification of oligodeoxynucleotides on specific protein-binding. *J Biol Chem* 1994;269:26801–26805.

99. Hogrefe RI. An antisense oligonucleotide primer. *Antisense Nucleic Acid Drug Dev* 1999;9:351–357.

100. Akhtar S, Hughes MD, Khan A, Bibby M, Hussain M, Nawaz Q, Double J, Sayyed P. The delivery of antisense therapeutics. *Adv Drug Deliv Rev* 2000;44:3–21.

101. Lucas B, Van Rompaey E, Remaut K, Sanders N, De Smedt S, Demeester J. On the biological activity of anti-ICAM-1 oligonucleotides complexed to non-viral carriers. *J Control Release* 2004;96:207–219.

102. Dheur S, Dias N, van-Aerschot A, Herdewijn P, Bettinger T, Remy JS, Helene C, Saison-Behmoaras ET. Polyethylenimine but not cationic lipid improves antisense activity of 3′-capped phosphodiester oligonucleotides. *Antisense Nucleic Acid Drug Dev* 1999;9:515–525.

103. Huppi K, Martin SE, Caplen NJ. Defining and assaying RNAi in mammalian cells. *Mol Cell* 2005;17:1–10.

104. Schiffelers RM, Mixson AJ, Ansari AM, Fens MHAM, Tang Q, Zhou Q, Xu J, Molema G, Lu PY, Scaria PV. Transporting silence: design of carriers for siRNA to angiogenic endothelium. *J Control Release* 2005;109(1–3):5–14.

105. Braasch DA, Paroo Z, Constantinescu A, Ren G, Oz OK, Mason RP, Corey DR. Biodistribution of phosphodiester and phosphorothioate siRNA. *Bioorg Med Chem Lett* 2004;14:1139–1143.

106. Schiffelers RM, Ansari A, Xu J, Zhou Q, Tang Q, Storm G, Molema G, Lu PY, Scaria PV, Woodle MC. Cancer siRNA therapy by tumor selective delivery with ligand-targeted sterically stabilized nanoparticle. *Nucleic Acids Res* 2004;32:149.

107. Kim B, Tang Q, Biswas PS, Xu J, Schiffelers RM, Xie FY, Ansari AM, Scaria PV, Woodle MC, Lu PY, Rouse BT. Inhibition of ocular angiogenesis by siRNA targeting vascular endothelial growth factor pathway genes: therapeutic strategy for herpetic stromal keratitis. *Am J Pathol* 2004;165:2177–2185.

108. Nielsen PE, Egholm M, Berg RH, Buchardt O. Sequence-selective recognition of DNA by strand displacement with a thymine-substituted polyamide. *Science* 1991;254:1497–1500.

109. Egholm M, Buchardt O, Christensen L, Behrens C, Freier SM, Driver DA, Berg RH, Kim SK, Norden B. PNA hybridizes to complementary oligonucleotides obeying the Watson–Crick hydrogen-bonding rules. *Nature* 1993;365:566–568.

110. Jensen KK, Orum H, Nielsen PE, Norden B. Kinetics for hybridization of peptide nucleic acids (PNA) with DNA and RNA studied with the BIAcore technique. *Biochemistry* 1997;36:5072–5077.

111. Giesen U, Kleider W, Berding C, Geiger A, Orum H, Nielsen PE. A formula for thermal stability prediction of PNA/DNA duplexes. *Nucleic Acids Res* 1998;26:5004–5006.

112. Tomac S, Sarkar M, Ratilainen T, Wittung P, Nielsen PE, Norden B, Graslund A. Ionic effects on the stability and conformation of peptide nucleic acid complexes. *J Am Chem Soc* 1996;118:5544–5552.

113. Eriksson M, Nielsen PE. PNA nucleic acid complexes. Structure, stability and dynamic. *Q Rev Biophys* 1996;29:369–394.

114. Pooga M, Soomets U, Hallbrink M, Valkna A, Saar K, Rezaei K, Kahl U, Hao JX, Xu XJ, Wiesenfeld-Hallin Z, Hokfelt T, Bartfai A, Langel U. Cell penetrating PNA constructs regulate galanin receptor levels and modify pain transmission *in vivo*. *Nat Biotechnol* 1998;16:857–861.

115. Hamilton SE, Simmons CG, Kathiriya IS, Corey DR. Cellular delivery of peptide nucleic acids and inhibition of human telomerase. *Chem Biol* 1999;6:343–351.

116. Fraser GL, Holmgren J, Clarke PBS, Wahlestedt C. Antisense inhibition of delta-opioid receptor gene function *in vivo* by peptide nucleic acids. *Mol Pharmacol* 2000;57:725–731.

117. Wittung P, Kajanus J, Edwards K, Nielsen P, Norden B, Malmstrom BG. Phospholipid membrane-permeability of peptide nucleic-acid. *FEBS Lett* 1995;365:27–29.

118. Buchardt O, Egholm M, Berg RH, Nielsen PE. Peptide nucleic-acids and their potential applications in biotechnology. *Trends Biotechnol* 1993;11:384–386.

119. Meier C, Engels JW. Peptide nucleic-acids (PNAs)—unusual properties of non-ionic oligonucleotide analogs. *Angew Chem Int Ed* 1992;31:1008–1010.

120. Chiarantini L, Cerasi A, Fraternale A, Millo E, Benatti U, Sparnacci K, Laus M, Ballestri M, Tondelli L. Comparison of novel delivery systems for antisense peptide nucleic acids. *J Control Release* 2005;109(1–3):24–36.

121. Sezgin Z, Yüksel N, Baykara T. Preparation and characterization of polymeric micelles for solubilization of poorly soluble anticancer drugs. *Eur J Pharm Biopharm* 2006;64(3): 261–268.

122. Strickley R. Solubilizing excipients in oral and injectable formulations. *Pharm Res* 2004;21:201–230.

123. Mathot F, van Beijsterveldt L, Préat V, Brewster M, Ariën A. Intestinal uptake and bio-distribution of novel polymeric micells after oral administration. *J Control Release* 2006;111(1–2):47–55.

124. Lavasanifar A, Samuel J, Kwon G. Poly(ethylene oxide)-*block*-poly(L-amino acid) micelles for drug delivery. *Adv Drug Deliv Rev* 2002;54:169–190.

125. Torchilin V. Structure and design of polymeric surfactant-based drug delivery systems. *J Control Release* 2001;73:137–172.

126. Jones M-C, Leroux J-C. Polymeric micelles—a new generation of colloidal drug carriers. *Eur J Pharm Biopharm* 1999;48:101–111.

127. Kataoka K, Harada A, Nagasaki Y. Block copolymer micelles for drug delivery: design characterization and biological significance. *Adv Drug Deliv Rev* 2001;47:113–131.

128. Kwon G, Okano T. Soluble self-assembled block copolymers for drug delivery. *Pharm Res* 1999;5:597–600.

129. Ould-Ouali L, Ariën A, Rosenblatt J, Nathan A, Twaddle P, Matalenas T, Borgia M, Arnold S, Leroy D, Dinguizli M, Rouxhet L, Brewster M, Préat V. Biodegradable self-assembling PEG-copolymer as vehicle for poorly water-soluble drugs. *Pharm Res* 2004;21:1581–1590.

130. Müller RH. In *Colloidal Carriers for Control Drug Delivery and Targeting*. Stuttgart Germany: Wissenschaftliche Verlagsgesellschaft Boca Raton, FL: CRC Press; 1991.

131. Lasic DD, Martin F, Eds. *Stealth Liposomes*. Boca Raton, FL: CRC Press; 1995.

132. Cohen S, Bernstein H, Eds. *Microparticulate Systems for the Delivery of Proteins and Vaccines*. New York: Marcel Dekker; 1996.

133. Torchilin VP, Trubetskoy VS. Which polymers can make nanoparticulate drug carriers long-circulating? *Adv Drug Deliv Rev* 1995;16:141–155.

134. Torchilin VP. How do polymers prolong circulation time of liposomes? *J Liposome Res* 1996;6:99–116.

135. Takenaga M, Yamaguchi Y, Kitagawa A, Ogawa Y, Mizushima Y, Igarashi R. A novel insulin formulation can keep providing steady levels of insulin for much longer periods *in-vivo*. *J Pharm Pharmacol* 2002;54:1189–1194.

136. Kang F, Singh J. Preparation, *in vitro* release *in vivo* absorption and biocompatibility studies of insulin-loaded microspheres in rabbits. *AAPS PharmSciTech* 2005;6(3): E487–E494.

137. Prego C, García M, Torres D, Alonso MJ. Transmucosal macromolecular drug delivery. *J Control Release* 2005;101(1–3):151–162.

138. Alonso MJ. Nanoparticles as carriers for nasal vaccine delivery. *Expert Rev Vaccines* 2005;4(2):185–196.

139. Asthana A, Chauhan AS, Diwan PV, Jain NK. Poly(amidoamine) (PAMAM) dendritic nanostructures for controled site-specific delivery of acidic anti-inflammatory active ingredient. *AAPS PharmSciTech* 2005;6(3):E536–E542.

140. Beezer AE, King ASH, Martin IK, Mitchel JC, Twyman LJ, Wain CF. Dendrimers as potential drug carriers; encapsulation of acidic hydrophobes within water soluble PAMAM derivatives. *Tetrahedron* 2003;59:3873–3880.

141. Patri AK Jr, Majoros IJ Jr, Baker JR Jr. Dendritic polymer macromolecular carriers for drug delivery. *Curr Opin Chem Biol* 2002;6:466–471.

142. Bosman AW, Janssen HM, Meijer EW. About dendrimers: structure physical properties, and applications. *Chem Rev* 1999;99:1665–1688.

143. Milhem OM, Myles C, McKeown NB, Attwood D, Emanuele AD. Poly-amidoamine starburst dendrimers as solubility enhancers. *Int J Pharm* 2000;197:239–241.

144. Kolhe P, Misra E, Kannan RM, Kannan S, Lieh-Lai M. Drug complexation *in vitro* release and cellular entry of dendrimers and hyperbranched polymers. *Int J Pharm* 2003;259:143–160.

145. Zeng F, Zimmerman SC. Dendrimers in supramolecular chemistry: from molecular recognition to self-assembly. *Chem Rev* 1997;97:1681–1712.

146. Lasic DD, Papahajopoulos D, Eds. *Medical Application of Liposomes*. Amsterdam, The Netherlands: Elsevier; 1998.

147. Khaw BA, Torchilin VP, Vural I, Narula J. Plug and seal: prevention of hypoxic cardiocyte death by sealing membrane lesions with antimyosin-liposomes. *Nat Med* 1995;1:1195–1198.

148. Liang W, Levchenko TS, Khaw BA, Torchilin VP. ATP-containing immunoliposomes specific for cardiac myosin. *Curr Drug Deliv* 2004;1:1–7.

149. Verma DD, Hartner WC, Levchenko TS, Bernstein EA, Torchilin VP. ATP-loaded liposomes effectively protect the myocardium in rabbits with an acute experimental myocardial infarction. *Pharm Res* 2005;22(12):2115–2120.

150. Kimelberg HK, Mayhew EG. Properties and biological effects of liposomes and their uses in pharmacology and toxicology. *CRC Crit Rev Toxicol* 1978;6:25–79.

151. Szoka F, Papahadjopoulos D. Liposomes: preparation and characterization. In Knight CG, Ed. *Liposomes: From Physical Structure to Therapeutic Applications*. New York: Elsevier/North-Holland Biomedical Press; 1981, pp 51–82.

152. Poznansky MJ, Juliano RL. Biological approaches to the Control delivery of drugs: a critical review. *Pharm Rev* 1984;36:277–336.

153. Fanciullino R, Giacometti S, Aubert C, Fina F, Martin P-M, Piccerelle P, Ciccolini J. Development of stealth liposome formulation of 2′-deoxyinosine as 5-fluorouracil modulator: *in vitro* and *in vivo* study. *Pharm Res* 2005;22(12):2051–2057.

154. FDA. *Guidance for Industry: Nonclinical Studies for the Safety Evaluation of Pharmaceutical Excipients*. FDA, Center for Drug Evaluation and Research (CDER) Center for Biologics Evaluation and Research (CBER); May 2005.

155. Powell MF, Nguyen T, Baloian L. Compendium of excipients for parenteral formulations. *PDA J Pharm Sci Technol* 1998;52:238–311.

156. Nema S, Washkuhn RJ, Brendel RJ. Excipients and their use in injectable products. *PDA J Pharm Sci Technol* 1997;51:166–171.

157. *Inactive Ingredient Guide: Inactive Ingredients for Currently Marketed Drug Products*. Rockville, MD: FOI Services Inc; 1996.

158. Strickley RG. Parenteral formulations of small molecules therapeutics marketed in the United States (1999). Part III. *PDA J Pharm Sci Technol* 2000;54(2):152–169.

159. Rowe RC, Sheskey PJ, Owen SC, Eds. *Handbook of Pharmaceutical Excipients*, 5th ed. Washington DC: American Pharmaceutical Association; 2005.

160. Hoffman H. Polyoxyethyleneglycerol triricinoleate 35 DAC 1979. *Pharm Zeit* 1984;129:730–733.

161. Goldspiel BR. Guidelines for administration. In McGuire WP, Rowinsky EK, Eds. *Paclitaxel in Cancer Treatment*. New York: Marcel Dekker; 1995, pp 175–186.

162. Windebank AJ, Blexrud MD, Groen PC. Potential neurotoxicity of the solvent vehicle for cyclosporine. *J Pharmacol Exp Ther* 1994;268:1051–1056.

163. Watkins J, Ward AM, Appleyard TN. Adverse reactions to intravenous anaesthetic induction agents. *Br Med J* 1997;2:1084–1085.

164. Szebeni J, Muggia FM, Alving CR. Complement activation by Cremophor EL as a possible contributor to hypersensitivity to paclitaxel: an *in vitro* study. *J Natl Cancer Inst* 1998;90:300–306.

165. Wandel C, Kim RB, Stein CM. "Inactive" excipients such as Cremophor can affect *in vivo* drug disposition. *Clin Pharmacol Ther* 2003;73:394–396.

166. van Zuylen L, Verweij J, Sparreboom A. Role of formulation vehicles in taxane pharmacology. *Invest New Drugs* 2001;19:125–141.

167. de Vos AI, Nooter K, Verweij J, Loos WJ, Brouwer E, De Bruijn P, Ruijgrok EJ, van der Burg ME, Stoter G, Sparreboom A. Differential modulation of cisplatin accumulation in leucocytes and tumor cell lines by the paclitaxel vehicle Cremophor EL. *Ann Oncol* 1997;8:1145–1150.

168. Ma J, Verweij J, Planting AST, Kolker HJ, Loos WJ, de Boer-Dennert M, van der Burg ME, Stoter G, Schellens JH. Docetaxel and paclitaxel inhibit DNA adduct formation and intracellular accumulation of cisplatin in human leukocytes. *Cancer Chemother Pharmacol* 1996;36:382.

169. Badary OA, Abdel-Naim AB, Khalifa AE, Hamada FMA. Differential alteration of cisplatin myelotoxicity by the paclitaxel vehicle Cremophor EL. *Naunyn-Schmiedeberg Arch Pharmacol* 2000;261:339–344.

170. Iwase K, Oyama Y, Tatsuishi T, Yamaguchi J, Nishimura Y, Kanada A, Kobayashi M, Maemura Y, Ishida S, Okano Y. Cremophor EL augments the cytotoxicity of hydrogen peroxide in lymphocytes dissociated from rat thymus glands. *Toxicol Lett* 2004;154: 143–148.

171. Yamaguchi J-Y, Nishimura Y, Kanada A, Kobayashi M, Mishima K, Tatsuishi T, Iwase K, Oyama Y. Cremophor EL, a non-ionic surfactant promotes Ca^{2+}-dependent process of cell death in rat thymocytes. *Toxicology* 2005;211(3):179–186.

172. Nah JW, Jang MK. Spectroscopic characterization and preparation of low molecular, water-soluble chitosan with free-amine group by novel method. *J Polym Sci Part A Polym Chem* 2002;40:3796–3803.

173. Thanou M, Verhoef JC, Junginge HE. Chitosan and its derivatives as intestinal absorption enhancers. *Adv Drug Deliv Rev* 2001;50(1):S91–S101.

174. Illum L. Chitosan and its use as a pharmaceutical excipient. *Pharm Res* 1998;15: 1326–1331.

175. Khor E, Lim LY. Implantable applications of chitin and chitosan. *Biomaterials* 2003;24:2339–2349.

176. Lee M, Nah JW, Kwon Y, Koh JJ, Ko KS, Kim SW. Water-soluble and low molecular weight chitosan-based plasmid DNA delivery. *Pharm Res* 2001;18:427–431.

177. Koping-Hoggard M, Tubulekas I, Guan H, Edwards K, Nilsson M, Varum KM. Chitosan as a nonviral gene delivery system. Structure–property relationships and characteristics compared with polyethylenimine *in vitro* and after lung administration *in vivo*. *Gene Ther* 2001;8:1108–1121.

178. Roy K, Mao HQ, Huang SK, Leong KW. Oral gene delivery with chitosan–DNA nanoparticles generates immunologic protection in a murine model of peanut allergy. *Nat Med* 1999;5:387–391.

179. Lueßen HL, de Leeuw BJ, Langemeÿer WE, de Boer AG, Verhoef JC, Junginger HE. Mucoadhesive polymers in peroral peptide drug delivery. VI. Carbomer and chitosan

improve the intestinal absorption of the peptide drug buserelin *in vivo*. *Pharm Res* 1996;13:1668–1672.

180. Lina BAR, Bär A. Subchronic oral toxicity studies with α-cyclodextrin in rats. *Regul Toxicol Pharmacol* 2004;39(1):14–26.

181. Schmid G. Cyclodextrin glycosyltransferase production: yield enhancement by overexpression of cloned genes. *TIBTECH* 1989;7:244–248.

182. Allegre M, Deratani A. Cyclodextrin uses: from concept to industrial reality. *Agro Food Industry Hi-Tech* 1994;5:9–17.

183. Le Bas G, Rysanek N. Structural aspects of cyclodextrins. In Duchêne D, Ed. *Cyclodextrins and Their Industrial Uses*. Paris: Editions de Santé; 1987, pp 105–130.

184. Schmid G. Preparation and application of γ-cyclodextrin. In Duchêne D, Ed. *New Trends in Cyclodextrins and Derivatives*. Paris: Editions Santé; 1991, pp 27–54.

185. Englyst HN, Kingman SM, Cummings JH. Classification and measurement of nutritionally important starch fractions. *Eur J Clin Nutr* 1992;46 Suppl (2):S33.

186. Thompson DO. Cyclodextrins—enabling excipients: their present and future use in pharmaceuticals. *Crit Rev Ther Drug Carrier Syst* 1997;14 (1):1–104.

187. Uekama K, Hirayama F, Irie T. Cyclodextrin drug carrier systems. *Chem Rev* 1998;98: 2045–2076.

188. Oda M, Saitoh H, Kobayashi M, Aungst BJ. β-Cyclodextrin as a suitable solubilizing agent for *in situ* absorption study of poorly water-soluble drugs. *Int J Pharm* 2004; 280(1–2):95–102.

189. Ohtani Y, Irie T, Uekama K, Fukunaga K, Pitha J. Differential effects of α-, β- and γ-cyclodextrins on human erythrocytes. *Eur J Biochem* 1989;186:17–22.

190. Debouzy JC, Fauvelle F, Crouzy S, Girault L, Chapron Y, Goschl M, Gadelle A. Mechanism of α-cyclodextrin induced hemolysis. 2. A study of the factors controlling the association with serine-, ethanolamine-, and choline-phospholipids. *J Pharm Sci* 1998;87: 59–66.

191. Fauvelle F, Debouzy JC, Crouzy S, Goschl M, Chapron Y. Mechanism of α-cyclodextrin-induced hemolysis. 1. The two-step extraction of phosphatidylinositol from the membrane. *J Pharm Sci* 1997;86:935–943.

192. Galbiati F, Razani B, Lisanti MP. Emerging themes in lipid rafts and caveolae. *Cell* 2001;106:403–411.

193. Simons K, Ehehalt R. Cholesterol, lipid rafts, and disease. *J Clin Invest* 2002;110: 597–603.

194. Anderson RG, Jacobson K. A role for lipid shells in targeting proteins to caveolae, rafts, and other lipid domains. *Science* 2002;296:1821–1825.

195. Irie T, Otagiri M, Sunada M, Uekama K, Ohtani Y, Yamada Y, Sugiyama Y. Cyclodextrin-induced hemolysis and shape changes of human erythrocytes *in vitro*. *J Pharmacobiodyn* 1982;5:741–744.

196. Irie T, Uekama K. Pharmaceutical applications of cyclodextrins. III. Toxicological issues and safety evaluation. *J Pharm Sci* 1997;86:147–162.

197. Uekama K, Otagiri M. Cyclodextrins in drug carrier systems. *Crit Rev Ther Drug Carrier Syst* 1987;3:1–40.

198. Arima H, Nishimoto Y, Motoyama K, Hirayama F, Uekama K. Inhibitory effects of novel hydrophilic cyclodextrin derivatives on nitric oxide production in macrophages stimulated with lipopolysaccharide. *Pharm Res* 2001;18:1167–1173.

199. Motoyama K, Arima H, Nishimoto Y, Miyake K, Hirayama F, Uekama K. Involvement of CD14 in the inhibitory effects of dimethyl-α-cyclodextrin on lipopolysaccharide signaling in macrophages. *FEBS Lett* 2005;579:1707–1714.

200. Motoyama K, Arima H, Toyodome H, Irie T, Hirayama F, Uekama K. Effect of 2,6-di-O-methyl-α-cyclodextrin on hemolysis and morphological change in rabbit's red blood cells. *Eur J Pharm Sci* 2006;29(2):111–119.

201. Pope DC, Baggot JD. The basis of selection of the dosage form. In Blodinger I, Ed. *Formulation of Veterinary Dosage Forms*. New York: Marcel Dekker; 1983, pp 1–70.

202. Bates TR, Sequeira JA. Bioavailability of micronized griseofulvin from corn oil-in-water emulsion, aqueous suspension and commercial tablet dosage forms in humans. *J Pharm Sci* 1975;64(5):793–797.

203. Jones BE. *Manuf Chem Aerosol News* 1969;40(2):25.

204. Lazor T. *Drug Cosmet Ind* 1974;114(3):42.

205. Pope DG. In Monkhouse, DC, Ed. *Animal Health Products, Design and Evaluation*. Washington DC: American Pharmaceutical Association; p 78.

206. Pope DG. *Aust Vet Pract* 1980;10:57.

207. Hem SL, Bright DR, Banker GS, Page JP. *Drug Dev Commun* 1974–75;1:471.

208. Spiegel AJ, Noseworthy MM. Use of nonaqueous solvents in parenteral products. *J Pharm Sci* 1963;52:917–927.

209. Rasmussen F. In Van Miert ASJPAM, Frens J, Van der Kreek FW, Eds. *Trends in Veterinary Pharmacology and Toxicology*. Amsterdam: Elsevier; 1980, p 27.

210. Rasmussen F, Svendsen O. Tissue damage and concentration at the injection site after intramuscular injection of chemotherapeutics and vehicles in pigs. *Res Vet Sci* 1976;20:55–60.

211. Blom L, Rasmussen F. Tissue damage at the infection site after intramuscular injection of drugs in hens. *Br Poult Sci* 1976;17:1–4.

212. Svendsen O, Rasmussen F, Nielson P, Steiness E. The loss of creatine phosphokinase (CK) from intramuscular injection sites in rabbits. A predictive tool for local toxicity. *Acta Pharmacol Toxicol (Copenhagen)* 1979;44:324–328.

213. Andersson L, Blomberg L, Flegel M, Lepsa L, Nilsson B, Verlander M. Large-scale synthesis of peptides. *Biopolymers* 2000;55:227–250.

214. Pontiroli AE. Peptide hormones: review of current and emerging uses by nasal delivery. *Adv Drug Deliv Rev* 1998;29:81–87.

215. Chetty DJ, Chien YW. Novel methods of insulin delivery: an update. *Crit Rev Ther Drug Carrier Syst* 1998;15:629–670.

216. Simon M, Kissel T. Away with the needle. Noninvasive administration routes for insulin: improved quality of life for diabetics. *Pharm Unserer Zeit* 2001;30:136–141.

217. Gizurarson S. The relevance of nasal physiology to the design of drug absorption studies. *Adv Drug Deliv Rev* 1993;11(3):329–347.

218. Gizurarson S, Bechgaard E. Study of nasal enzyme activity towards insulin *in vitro*. *Chem Pharm Bull* 1991;39:2155–2157.

219. Deurloo MJ, Hermens WA, Romeyn SG, Verhoef JC, Merkus FW. Absorption enhancement of intranasally administered insulin by sodium taurodihydrofusidate (STDHF) in rabbits and rats. *Pharm Res* 1989;6:853–856.

220. Hinchcliffe M, Illum L. Intranasal insulin delivery and therapy. *Adv Drug Deliv Rev* 1999;35:199–234.

221. Sanchez A, Ygartua P, Fos D. Role of surfactants in the bioavailability of intranasal insulin. *Eur J Drug Metab Pharmacokinet* 1991;3:120–124.

222. Chandler SG, Illum L, Thomas NW. Nasal absorption in the rats: II. Effect of enhancers on insulin absorption and nasal histology. *Int J Pharm* 1991;76:61–70.

223. Prego C, Garcia M, Torres D, Alonso MJ. Transmucosal macromolecular drug delivery. *J Control Release* 2005;101:151–162.

224. Koping-Hoggard M, Sanchez A, Alonso MJ. Nanoparticles as carriers for nasal vaccine delivery. *Expert Rev Vaccines* 2005;4:185–196.

225. Fernandez-Urrusuno R, Calvo P, Remunan-Lopez C, Vila-Jato JL, Alonso MJ. Enhancement of nasal absorption of insulin using chitosan nanoparticles. *Pharm Res* 1999;16:1576–1581.

226. Brooking J, Davis SS, Iluum L. Transport of nanoparticles across the rat nasal mucosa. *J Drug Target* 2001;9:267–279.

227. Vila A, Sanchez A, Evora C, Soriano I, McCallion O, Alonso MJ. PLA–PEG particles as nasal protein carriers: the influence of the particle size. *Int J Pharm* 2005;292:43–52.

228. Takeuchi H, Yamamoto H, Kawashima Y. Mucoadhesive nanoparticulate systems for peptide drug delivery. *Adv Drug Deliv Rev* 2001;47:39–54.

229. Dondeti P, Zia H, Needham T. Bioadhesive and formulation parameters affecting nasal absorption. *Int J Pharm* 1996;127:115–133.

230. Jimenez-Castellanos MR, Zia H, Rhodes CT. Mucoadhesive drug delivery systems. *Drug Dev Ind Pharm* 1993;19:143–194.

231. Granger DN, Kvielys PR, Perry MA, Taylor AE. Charge selectivity of rat intestinal capillaries—influence of polycations. *Gastroenterology* 1986;91:1443–1446.

232. Maitani Y, Machida Y, Nagai T. Influence of molecular weight and charge on nasal absorption of dextran and DEAE-dextran in rabbits. *Int J Pharm* 1992;76:43–49.

233. Illum L, Farraj NF, Davis SS. Chitosan as novel nasal delivery system for peptide drugs. *Pharm Res* 1994;11:1186–1189.

234. Simon M, Wittmar M, Kissel T, Linn T. Insulin containing nanocomplexes formed by self-assembly from biodegradable amine-modified poly(vinyl alcohol)-graft-poly(L-lactide): bioavailability and nasal tolerability in rats. *Pharm Res* 2005;22(11):1879–1886.

235. Dayal P, Shaik MS, Singh M. Evaluation of different parameters that affect droplet-size distribution from nasal sprays using the Malvern Spraytec. *J Pharm Sci* 2004;93:1725–1742.

236. Malmsten M, Ed. *Surfactants and Polymers in Drug Delivery*. Lancaster, PA: Marcel Dekker; 2002.

237. D'Souza R, Mutalik S, Venkatesh M, Vidyasagar S, Udupa N. Insulin gel as an alternate to parenteral insulin: formulation preclinical and clinical studies. *AAPS Pharm Sci Tech* 2005;6(2):E184–189.

238. Alur HH, Johnston TP, Mitra AK. Peptides and proteins: buccal absorption. In Superbrick J, Boylan JC, Eds. *Encyclopedia of Pharmaceutical Technology*. New York: Marcel Dekker; 2001, pp 193–218.

239. Sudhakar Y, Kuotsu K, Bandyopadhyay AK. Buccal bioadhesive drug delivery—a promising option for orally less efficient drugs. *J Control Release* 2006;114(1):15–40.

240. Morishita M, Barichello JM, Takayama K, Chiba Y, Tokiwa S, Nagai T. Pluronic F-127 gels incorporating highly purified unsaturated fatty acids for buccal delivery of insulin. *Int J Pharm* 2001;212(2):289–293.

241. Aungst BJ, Rogers NJ. Comparison of the effects of various transmucosal absorption promoters on buccal insulin delivery. *Int J Pharm* 1989;53:227–235.

242. Siegel IA, Gordon HP. Surfactant—induced increase of permeability Of rat oral mucosa to non-electrolytes *in vivo*. *Arch Oral Biol* 1985;30:43–47.

243. Squier CA, Wertz PW. In Rathbone MJ. Ed. *Structure and Function of the Oral Mucosa and Implications for Drug Delivery Oral Mucosal Drug Delivery*. New York: Marcel Dekker 1996, pp 1–26.

244. Ishida M, Machida Y, Nambu N, Nagai T. New mucosal dosage forms of insulin. *Chem Pharm Bull* 1981;84:810–816.

245. Barsuchn CL, Olanoff LS, Gleason DD, Olanoff EL, Gleason DD, Adkins EL, Ho NFH. Human buccal absorption of flubiprofen. *Clin Pharmacol Ther* 1988;44:225–231.

246. Mehta M, Kemppainen BW, Stafford RG. *In vitro* penetration of tritium labeled water (THO) and [^{3}H] Pb Tx-3 (a red tide toxin) through monkey buccal mucosa and skin. *Toxicol Lett* 1991;55:185–194.

247. Squier CA, Cox P, Wertz PW. Lipid content and water permeability of skin and oral mucosa. *J Invest Dermatol* 1991;96:123–126.

248. Puglia C, Filosa R, Peduto A, de Caprariis P, Rizza L, Bonina F, Blasi P. Evaluation of alternative strategies to optimize ketorolac transdermal delivery. *AAPS Pharm Sci Tech* 2006;7(3):Article 64.

249. Parikh DK, Ghosh TK. Feasibility of transdermal delivery of fluoxetine. *AAPS PharmSciTech* 2005;6:E144–E149.

250. Satturwar PM, Fulzele SV, Dorle AK. Evaluation of polymerized rosin for the formulation and development of transdermal drug delivery system: a technical note. *AAPS PharmSciTech* 2005;6(4):E649–E654.

251. Chien YW. Comparative Control skin permeation of nitroglycerin from marketed transdermal delivery systems. *J Pharm Sci* 1983;72:968–970.

252. Loftsson T, Gildersleeve N, Border N. The effect of vehicle additives on the transdermal delivery of nitroglycerin. *Pharm Res* 1987;4:436–444.

253. Corbo M, Liu JC, Chien YW. Bioavailability of propranolol following oral & transdermal administration in rabbits. *J Pharm Sci* 1990;79:584–587.

254. Aqil M, Sultana Y, Ali A. Matrix type transdermal drug delivery systems of metoprolol tartrate: *in vitro* characterization. *Acta Pharm* 2003;53:119–125.

255. Rao PR, Ramakrishna S, Diwan PV. Drug release kinetics from polymeric films containing propranolol hydrochloride for transdermal use. *Pharm Dev Technol* 2000;5:465–472.

256. Williams AC, Barry BW. Penetration enhancers. *Adv Drug Deliv Rev* 2004;56:603–618.

257. Bohme K. Buprenorphine in a transdermal therapeutic system—a new option. *Clin Rheumatol* 2002;21:S13–S16.

258. Foldvari M. Non-invasive administration of drugs through the skin: challenges in delivery system design. *Pharm Sci Technol Today* 2000;3:417–425.

259. Barry BW. Novel mechanisms and devices to enable successful transdermal drug delivery. *Eur J Pharm Sci* 2001;14:101–114.

260. Doh HJ, Cho WJ, Yong CS, Choi HG, Kim JS, Lee CH, Kim DD. Synthesis and evaluation of ketorolac ester prodrugs for transdermal delivery. *J Pharm Sci* 2003;92:1008–1017.

261. Alsarra IA, Bosela AA, Ahmed SM, Mahrous GM. Proniosomes as a drug carrier for transdermal delivery of ketorolac. *Eur J Pharm Biopharm* 2005;59:485–490.

262. Cho YA, Gwak HS. Transdermal delivery of ketorolac tromethamine: effects of vehicles and penetration enhancers. *Drug Dev Ind Pharm* 2004;30:557–564.

263. Tiwari SB, Udupa N. Investigation into the potential of iontophoresis facilitated delivery of ketorolac. *Int J Pharm* 2003;260:93–103.

264. Müller RH, Mäder K, Gohla S. Solid lipid nanoparticles for Controled drug delivery: a review of the state of the art. *Eur J Pharm Biopharm* 2000;50:161–177.

265. Johnson ME, Blankschtein D, Linger R. Evaluation of solute permeation through the stratum corneum: lateral bilayer diffusion as the primary transport mechanism. *J Pharm Sci* 1997;86:1162–1172.

266. Burger GT, Cheryl ML. Animal care and facilities. In Hayes AW, Ed. *Principles and Methods of Toxicology*, 2nd ed, New York: Raven Press Ltd; 1989, pp 521–552.

267. Rao PR, Diwan PV. Formulation and *in vitro* evaluation of polymeric films of diltiazem hydrochloride and indomethacin for transdermal administration. *Drug Dev Ind Pharm* 1998;24:327–336.

268. Marjukka ST, Bouwstra JA, Urtti A. Chemical enhancement of percutaneous absorption in relation to stratum corneum structural alterations. *J Control Release* 1999;59:149–161.

269. Guy RH, Kalia YN, Delgado-Charro MB, Merino V, Lopez A, Marro D. Iontophoresis: electrorepulsion and electroosmosis. *J Control Release* 2000;64:129–132.

270. Conjeevaram R, Banga AK, Zhang L. Electrically modulated transdermal delivery of fentanyl. *Pharm Res* 2002;19:440–444.

271. Behl C, Char HS, Patel SB, Mehta DB, Piemontese D, Malick AW. *In vivo* and *in vitro* skin uptake and permeation studies; critical considerations and factors, which affect them. In Shah BP, Maibach HI, Eds. *Topical Drug Bioavailability, Bioequivalence and Penetration*. New York: Plenum Press; 1993, pp 225–259.

272. Green PG, Flanagan M, Shroot B, Guy RH. Iontophoretic drug delivery. In Walters KA, Hadgraft J, Eds. *Pharmaceutical Skin Penetration Enhancement*. New York: Marcel Dekker; 1993, pp 311–333.

273. Malone T, Haleblian JK, Poulsen BJ, Burdick KH. Development and evaluation of ointment and cream vehicles for a new topical steroid fluclorolone acetonide. *Br J Dermatol* 1974;90:187–195.

274. Poulsen BJ, Young E, Coquilla V, Katz M. Effect of topical vehicle composition on the *in vitro* release of fluocinolone acetonide and its acetate ester. *J Pharm Sci* 1968;57:928–933.

275. Oishi J, Ushio Y, Narahara M, Takehara M, Nakagawa T. Effect of vehicles on percutaneous absorption. I. Characterization of oily vehicles by percutaneous absorption and trans-epidermal water loss test. *Chem Pharm Bull (Tokyo)* 1976;24:1765–1773.

276. Ostrenga J, Steinmetz C, Poulsen B. Significance of vehicle composition. I. Relationship between topical vehicle composition, skin penetrability and clinical efficacy. *J Pharm Sci* 1971;60:1175–1179.

277. Ostrenga J, Steinmetz C, Poulsen B, Yett S. Significance of vehicle composition. II Prediction of optimal vehicle composition. *J Pharm Sci* 1971;60:1180–1183.

278. Coldman MF, Poulsen BJ, Higuchi T. Enhancement of percutaneous absorption by the use of volatile: nonvolatile systems as vehicles. *J Pharm Sci* 1969;58:1098–1102.

279. Stoughton RB, Fritsch W. Influence of dimethylsulfoxide (DMSO) on human percutaneous absorption. *Arch Dermatol* 1964;90:512–517.

280. Maibach HT, Feldman RJ. The effect of DMSO on percutaneous penetration of hydrocortisone and testosterone in man. *Ann NY Acad Sci* 1967;141:423–427.

281. Pitman IH, Rostas SJ. Topical drug delivery to cattle and sheep. *J Pharm Sci* 1981;70:1181–1194.

282. Higuchi T. *J Soc Cosmet Chem* 1960;11:85.

283. Gordon RD, Peterson TA. Myths about transdermal drug delivery. *Drug Deliv Technol* 2003;3:1–4.

284. Tian J, Yin CH. *In vitro* and *in vivo* assessment of liposomes containing recombinant human interleukin-2. *Proc Int Symp Control Release Bioact Mate* 1998;25:439–440.

285. Hora MS, Rana RK, Nunberg JH, Tice TR, Gilley RM, Hudson ME. Control release of interleukin-2 from biodegradable microspheres. *Biotechnology (NY)* 1990;8:755–758.

286. Johnston TP, Punjabi MA, Froelich CJ. Sustained delivery of interleukin from poloxamer 407 gel matrix following intraperitoneal injection in mice. *Pharm Res* 1992;9:425–434.

287. Hennink W, Franssen EO, van Dijk-Wolthuis WNE, Talsma H. Dextran hydrogels for the Control release of proteins. *J Control Release* 1997;48:107–114.

288. Stratton LP, Dong A, Manning M, Carpenter JF. Drug delivery matrix containing native protein precipitates suspended in a poloxamer gel. *J Pharm Sci* 1997;86:1006–1010.

289. Wenzel JG, Balaji KS, Koushik K, Navarre C, Duran SH, Rahe CH, Kompella UB. Pluronic F127 gel formulations of deslorelin and GnRH reduce drug degradation and sustain drug release and effect in cattle. *J Control Release* 2002;85:51–59.

290. Wang P, Johnston TP. Enhanced stability of two model proteins in an agitated solution environment using poloxamer 407. *J Parenter Sci Technol* 1993;47:183–189.

291. Kikwai L, Babu RJ, Prado R, Kolot A, Armstrong CA, Ansel JC, Singh M. *In vitro* and *in vivo* evaluation of topical formulations of spantide II. *AAPS PharmSciTech* 2005;6(4):E565–E572.

292. Wolfson AD, McCafferty DF, Moss GP. Development and characterization of a moisture-activated bioadhesive drug delivery system for percutaneous local anaesthesia. *Int J Pharm* 1998;169(1):83–94.

293. Campbell CB. Ophthalmic agents: ointments or drops? *Vet Med Small Animal Clin* 1979;74:971–974.

294. McCarron PA, Donnelly RF, Zawislak A, Woolfson AD. Design and evaluation of a water-soluble bioadhesive patch formulation for cutaneous delivery of 5-aminolevulinic acid to superficial neoplastic lesions. *Eur J Pharm Sci* 2006;27(2–3):268–279.

295. Cooper CA, Bergamini MVW, Leopold IH. Use of flurbiprofen to inhibit corneal neovascularization. *Arch Ophthalmol* 1980;98:1102–1105.

296. Kraff MC, Sanders DR, Mcguigan L, Rannan MG. Inhibition of blood–aqueous humor barrier breakdown with diclofenac: a fluorometric study. *Arch Ophthalmol* 1990;108:380–383.

297. Searle AE, Pearce JL, Shaw DE. Topical use of indomethacin on the day of cataract surgery. *Br J Ophthalmol* 1990;74:19.

298. Mahoney JM, Waterbury LD. (±) 5 Benzoyl-1,2-dihydro-3H pyrrolo [1.2a] pyrrole-1-carboxylic acid (RS 37619): a non irritating ophthalmic anti-inflammatory agent. *Invest Ophthalmol Vis Sci* 1983;24:151–159.

299. Flach AJ, Kraff MC, Sanders DR, Tanenbaum L. The quantitative effect of 0.5% ketorolac tromethamine solution and 0.1% dexamethasone sodium phosphate solution on post surgical blood aqueous barrier. *Arch Ophthalmol* 1988;106:480–483.

300. Heier J, Cheetham JK, Degryse R. Ketorolac tromethamine 0.5% ophthalmic solution in the treatment of moderate to severe ocular inflammation after cataract surgery: a randomized vehicle–control clinical trial. *Am J Ophthalmol* 1999;127:253–259.

301. Solomen KD, Cheetham JK, Degryse R, Brint SF, Rosenthal A. Topical ketorolac tromethamine 0.5% ophthalmic solution in ocular inflammation after cataract surgery. *Ophthalmology* 2001;108:331–337.

302. Malhotra M, Majumdar DK. *In vivo* ocular availability of ketorolac following ocular instillations of aqueous, oil, and ointment formulations to normal corneas of rabbits: a technical note. *AAPS PharmSciTech* 2005;6(3):E523–E526.

303. Malhotra M, Majumdar DK. *In vitro* transcorneal permeation of ketorolac from oil based ocular drops and ophthalmic ointment. *Indian J Exp Biol* 1997;35:1324–1330.

304. Eljarrat-Binstock E, Domb AJ. Iontophoresis: a non-invasive ocular drug delivery. *J Control Release* 2006;110(3):479–489.

305. Behar-Cohen FF, El Aouni A, Gautier S, Davis GJ, Chapon P, Parel JM. Transscleral Coulomb-control iontophoresis of methylprednisolone into the rabbit eye: influence of duration of treatment current intensity and drug concentration on ocular tissue and fluid levels. *Exp Eye Res* 2002;74(1):51–59.

306. Hayden BC, Jockovich M-E, Murray TG, Voigt M, Milne P, Kralinger M, Feuer WJ, Hernandez E, Parel JM. Pharmacokinetics of systemic versus focal carboplatin chemotherapy in the rabbit eye: possible implication in the treatment of retinoblastoma. *Invest Ophthalmol Vis Sci* 2004;45:3644–3649.

307. Inamura N, Salt AN. Permeability changes of the blood–labyrinth barrier measured *in vivo* during experimental treatments. *Hear Res* 1992;61(1–2):12–18.

308. Juhn SK, Rybak LP. Labyrinthine barriers and cochlear homeostasis. *Acta Oto-Laryngol* 1981;91(5–6):529–534.

309. Tonndorf J, Duvall AJ, Reneau JP. Permeability of intracochlear membranes to various vital stains. *Ann Otol Rhinol Laryngol* 1962;71:801–841.

310. Chen Z, Kujawa SG, McKenna MJ, Fiering JO, Mescher MJ, Borenstein JT, Leary Swan EE, Sewell WF. Inner ear drug delivery via a reciprocating perfusion system in the guinea pig. *J Control Release* 2005;110(1):1–19.

311. Shahiwala A, Misra A. A preliminary pharmacokinetic study of liposomal leuprolide dry powder inhaler: a technical note. *AAPS PharmSciTech* 2005;6(3):E482–E486.

312. Jiang G, Qiu W, Deluca PP. Preparation and *in vitro/in vivo* evaluation of insulin-loaded poly(acryloyl-hydroxyethyl starch)-PLGA composite microspheres. *Pharm Res* 2003;20: 452–459.

313. Hildebrand GE, Tack JW. Microencapsulation of peptides and proteins. *Int J Pharm* 2000;196:173–176.

314. Haeckel S, Sachse S, Albayrak C, Müller RH. Preparation and characterization of insulin-loaded microcapsules produced by the induced phase separation method. In *Proceedings of the World Meeting, Association of Industrial Galenique Pharmacy/Association of Primate Veterinarians*; 25–28, May 1998, Paris France, pp 507–508.

315. Wall DA. Pulmonary absorption of peptides and proteins. *Drug Deliv* 1995;2:1–20.

316. Stanley SD. Delivery of peptide and non-peptide drugs through the respiratory tract. *Pharm Sci Tech Today* 1999;12:450–459.

317. Niven RW. Delivery of biotherapeutics by inhalation aerosol. *Crit Rev Ther Drug Carrier Syst* 1995;12:151–231.

318. Patton JS, Trinchero P, Platz RM. Bioavailability of pulmonary delivered peptide and protein: interferon alpha calcitonin and parathyroid hormones. *J Control Release* 1994;28:79–85.

319. Edwards DA, Hanes J, Caponetti G. Large porous particles for pulmonary drug delivery. *Science* 1997;276:1868–1871.

320. Berelowitz M, Becker G. Inhaled insulin: clinical pharmacology and clinical study results. *Respir Drug Deliv* 2000;7:151–154.

321. Clauson PG, Balent B, Okikawa J. PK-PD of four different doses of pulmonary insulin delivered with AERx Diabetes management system. *Respir Drug Deliv* 2000;7:155–161.

322. Adjel A, Hui J, Finley R, Lin T, Fort F. Pulmonary bioavailability of leuprolide acetate following multiple dosing to beagle dogs: some pharmacokinetic and pre-clinical issues. *Int J Pharm* 1994;107:57–66.

323. Garber RA, Cappelleri JC, Kourides IA, Gelgend RA, Chandler LP, Gorkin L. Improved patient satisfaction with inhaled insulin in subjects with Type I diabetes mellitus: results from a multi-center randomized Control trial. *Diabetes* 1999;48:A13.

324. Ganderton D. Targeted delivery of inhaled drugs: current challenges and future trends. *J Aerosol Med* 1999;12:3–8.

325. Saari M, Vidgren MT, Koskinen MO, Turjanmaa VMH, Nieminen MM. Pulmonary distribution and clearance of two beclomethasone liposome formulations in healthy volunteers. *Int J Pharm* 1999;181:1–9.

326. Waldrep JC, Gilbert BE, Knight CM. Pulmonary delivery of beclomethasone liposome aerosol in volunteers Tolerance and safety. *Chest* 1997;111:316–323.

327. Green J, Gommeren E, Creazzo J, Pharmaceutical K. Pharmaceutical aerosols: enhancing the metered dose inhaler. *Drug Delivery Technol* 2004;4(6):48–53.

18

CYTOCHROME P450 ENZYMES

EUGENE G. HRYCAY AND STELVIO M. BANDIERA
University of British Columbia, Vancouver, British Columbia, Canada

Contents

18.1   INTRODUCTION

The cytochrome P450 (CYP) enzymes, also known as the microsomal mixed function oxidase system, are the predominant biotransformation pathway in the body for lipid-soluble endogenous and xenobiotic compounds. CYP enzymes play a key role in the biotransformation of pharmaceutical agents and thus are major determinants of duration of action and clearance of drugs. CYP enzymes are also involved in complications arising from drug therapy, such as drug interactions, which may be caused by induction or inhibition of CYP enzymes. Moreover, CYP enzymes may contribute to disease states. For example, CYP enzymes are implicated in the etiology of some cancers because chemical procarcinogens require enzymatic conversion to carcinogens, a process that is mediated by CYP enzymes. This chapter presents aspects of the characterization, function, and regulation of CYP enzymes, in mammals generally and in humans specifically, that are relevant to our understanding of how CYP enzymes can metabolize a large variety of drugs.

CYP enzymes are membrane-bound proteins localized predominantly in the smooth endoplasmic reticulum of liver and other tissues and are quantitatively and qualitatively among the most important enzymes of the phase I pathway for xenobiotic biotransformation [1, 2]. CYP enzymes are responsible for oxidizing hydrophobic compounds to more polar metabolites for further biotransformation or subsequent excretion. CYP enzymes function as terminal oxidases of an electron transport chain in which one atom of oxygen from molecular oxygen is incorporated into the substrate and the other atom is reduced to water. The multicomponent electron transport chain also includes a flavoprotein, NADPH-dependent cytochrome P450 reductase, which serves to transfer reducing equivalents (electrons) supplied by NADPH (and sometimes NADH) to the CYP enzymes. CYP, as the terminal oxidase of the chain, is the enzyme active site, the oxygen- and substrate-binding site, and the determinant of substrate specificity (Fig. 18.1).

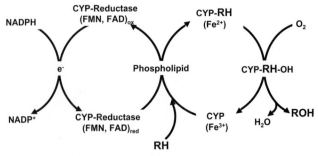

FIGURE 18.1   Electron transfer and metabolism of substrates by the microsomal CYP system. Electrons, transferred through a series of oxidation–reduction reactions from NADPH to CYP by NADPH-dependent CYP reductase, are used to reduce molecular oxygen with the concomitant oxidation of the substrate. FMN, flavin mononucleotide; FAD, flavin adenine dinucleotide; RH, substrate; ROH, oxidized product.

18.2   IDENTIFICATION OF CYP ENZYMES

18.2.1   Characterization of CYP Enzymes

CYP enzymes contain a heme prosthetic group, which gives the enzymes a reddish brown color. The heme group is iron protoporphyrin IX and is the same heme moiety found in hemoglobin. As is the case for hemoglobin, the iron protoporphyrin IX group in CYP enzymes has a strong affinity for molecular oxygen but binds carbon monoxide with higher affinity. The iron atom of the heme prosthetic group can exist in two oxidation states, Fe^{2+} (reduced) and Fe^{3+} (oxidized). The heme moiety bound to CYP enzymes is essential for activity, and loss of the heme group or "poisoning" by carbon monoxide is accompanied by loss of enzymatic activity.

In all CYP enzymes, the heme prosthetic group (iron protoporphyrin IX) is bound to a single polypeptide chain composed of approximately 500 amino acids. Considerable evidence indicates that the amino terminus of the apoprotein anchors CYP in the lipid membrane bilayer, with most of the enzyme including the active site exposed on the cytoplasmic side of the endoplasmic reticulum [3, 4]. The central iron atom of the heme group is bound noncovalently to the sulfur atom of a cysteine residue situated close to the C terminus of the apoprotein chain.

Interactions between the heme group and apoprotein produce unique spectral and magnetic properties. Normally, the iron in the heme prosthetic group of CYP is in the oxidized state, which exhibits low affinity for carbon monoxide and absorbs visible light with a spectral maximum at a wavelength of approximately 418 nm. However, if the iron is in the reduced state, it can then bind carbon monoxide with high affinity, and the resulting reduced carbon monoxide-bound CYP complex exhibits a large spectral maximum at 450 nm. This characteristic spectral property is a signature of CYP enzymes from which the name, cytochrome P450, was derived. Other heme proteins, such as hemoglobin, do not produce an absorbance at 450 nm when complexed with carbon monoxide.

Another essential component for CYP activity is NADPH-dependent CYP reductase, which is also located primarily on the surface of the phospholipid bilayer of the smooth endoplasmic reticulum in close proximity to the CYP enzymes. NADPH-dependent CYP reductase forms a temporary complex with CYP, permitting the flow of electrons to the heme prosthetic group and the resulting oxidation of the substrate. NADPH-dependent CYP reductase has two domains, one containing flavin adenine dinucleotide and the second containing flavin mononucleotide. Two electrons are acquired from NADPH and migrate from FAD to FMN, then to the heme group of CYP. In some cases, CYP enzymes can also accept electrons from cytochrome b_5, a small membrane-bound heme protein that receives electrons from NADH.

18.2.2   Detection and Isolation

Studies by Axelrod [5] and by Brodie and co-workers [6] in the mid-1950s revealed the existence of an enzyme system in liver that converted drugs and aromatic compounds into more polar metabolites and that required NADPH for the reaction. This enzyme system was subsequently identified as a carbon monoxide-binding pigment in liver microsomes by Klingenberg [7] and Garfinkel [8].

Microsomes is the name given to the endoplasmic reticulum membrane fraction, which can be isolated by breaking open and grinding cells to prepare a whole cell homogenate. If the homogenate is subjected to centrifugation at approximately 9000 g, cell debris, nuclei, and mitochondria spin down in the pellet. The resulting supernatant suspension, called the S9 fraction, contains both cytosolic and microsomal proteins. When the supernatant is spun at higher speed (e.g., 100,000 g), the resulting supernatant fraction contains the cytosolic fraction and the pellet contains the microsomal fraction. The pellet can be resuspended with 0.25 M sucrose or with 0.1 M potassium phosphate buffer containing 10% glycerol to give the microsomes, which can be stored at −80 °C for substantial periods of time. As long as the microsomal fraction is sufficiently concentrated (i.e., has a protein concentration >10 mg/mL), the CYP activity of the frozen microsomal fraction can be maintained for up to five years. The total CYP concentration of tissue preparations such as the S9 or microsomal fractions can be determined in a scanning spectrophotometer by measuring the height of the reduced carbon monoxide-bound CYP complex at 450 nm as reported by Omura and Sato [9].

The identity of CYP enzymes involved in the metabolism of a specific drug can be determined using a combination of approaches. Well characterized, specific inhibitory antibodies (either polyclonal or monoclonal) against various CYP enzymes are a valuable tool for identification of CYP enzymes in S9 and microsomal fractions. Chemical inhibitors (discussed later), especially highly selective inhibitors, can also be used. Finally, purified or recombinant enzymes can be used to determine the intrinsic ability of an individual or panel of CYP enzymes to catalyze a particular reaction or metabolize a specific drug. Once the CYP enzymes involved in the metabolism of a specific drug have been identified, it may be necessary to measure levels of the CYP enzymes in the liver or other relevant tissue. Immunological assays with specific antibodies, such as immunoblot analysis, are the preferred method for quantifying tissue levels of individual CYP enzymes.

18.2.3 Occurrence and Distribution

CYP enzymes are present in most organisms including mammals, birds, fish, reptiles, amphibians, insects, plants, fungi, and bacteria [10, 11]. The finding that CYP enzymes are found in every class of biota suggests that the diverse CYP enzymes identified to date have evolved from a single ancestral gene over a period of 1.36 billion years [12].

In humans and other mammals, CYP enzymes are found in almost all tissues including liver, intestine, lung, kidney, stomach, brain, adrenal gland, gonads, heart, nasal and tracheal mucosa, and skin [13, 14]. Concentrations and expression of individual CYP enzymes differ between tissues. Liver contains the largest number and the highest levels of CYP enzymes involved in drug biotransformation [2].

The endoplasmic reticular membrane is a structure with an extensive surface area in most cells. In rat liver, for example, the endoplasmic reticular membrane comprises 7–11 m^2/g of liver weight [15], and total microsomal protein represents 1.8–2% of liver wet weight. CYP enzymes comprise from 4% to 6% of total microsomal protein. This translates to a typical specific content of 0.8–1.1 nmol of total CYP per milligram of microsomal protein or approximately 20 nmol of total CYP per gram rat liver. In human liver, the total CYP content is lower, with CYP enzymes typically

TABLE 18.1   Total CYP Content in Various Human and Rat Organs

Organ	Human (nmol/mg microsomal protein)	Rat (nmol/mg microsomal protein)
Liver	0.30–0.60	0.8–1.1
Adrenal	0.23–0.54	0.5
Small intestine	0.03–0.21	0.02–0.13
Kidney	0.03	0.05–0.2
Lung	0.01	0.035–0.05
Brain	0.10	0.025–0.05
Testis	0.005	0.07–0.12
Skin	Not determined	0.05
Mammary	<0.001	0.001–0.003

Source: Compiled from Refs. 15–20.

comprising 1.5–3% of total microsomal protein, giving a specific content of 0.3–0.6 nmol of total CYP per milligram of microsomal protein (Table 18.1), or approximately 5 nmol of total CYP per gram human liver. For tissues other than liver, the CYP content, expressed in terms of microsomal protein or tissue weight, is lower (Table 18.1).

18.2.4   Nomenclature of CYP Enzymes

Multiple CYP enzymes have been identified in diverse species. Each CYP enzyme is encoded by a separate gene. To date, nearly 4000 CYP genes have been identified [21]. CYP enzymes are named and categorized according to their amino acid sequences. A systematic nomenclature has been developed to classify CYP enzymes into families and subfamilies based on the degree of similarity of their primary protein structure [22]. According to this system, CYP enzymes within the same family should exhibit at least 40% amino acid sequence identity, and CYP enzymes that share less than 40% identity in amino acid sequences are assigned to different families, which are designated using CYP as an abbreviation for cytochrome P450, followed by an Arabic numeral (e.g., CYP1, CYP2, CYP3, CYP4) [12]. Within a family, members that share more than 55% identity are assigned to the same subfamily, which is designated by a capital letter following the Arabic numeral (e.g., CYP2A, CYP2B, CYP2C) [12]. Individual enzymes are identified using a final number to specify the individual protein (e.g., CYP2A1, CYP2A2, CYP2B1).

To date, over 300 different CYP enzymes representing 50 families, 82 subfamilies, and 67 different species have been identified [12, 15]. In humans, 57 CYP genes belonging to 18 families and 42 subfamilies have been identified thus far [11, 23] (Table 18.2). In addition, more than 50 pseudogenes have been found. Pseudogenes are defective genes that do not produce functional proteins. They are thought to be relics of gene duplications in which one of the copies has degenerated and lost its function.

Although all members of the CYP superfamily possess highly conserved regions of amino acid sequences, there is variation in the primary sequences among individual CYP enzymes and among related enzymes across species. Small changes in amino acid sequences are reflected in profound differences in substrate specificity.

TABLE 18.2 Human CYP Enzymes

Family	Subfamily	Individual CYP Enzymes
CYP1	CYP1A	CYP1A1, CYP1A2
	CYP1B	CYP1B1
CYP2	CYP2A	CYP2A6, CYP2A7, CYP2A13
	CYP2B	CYP2B6
	CYP2C	CYP2C8, CYP2C9, CYP18, CYP19
	CYP2D	CYP2D6
	CYP2E	CYP2E1
	CYP2F	CYP2F1
	CYP2J	CYP2J2
	CYP2R	CYP2R1
	CYP2S	CYP2S1
	CYP2U	CYP2U1
	CYP2W	CYP2W1
CYP3	CYP3A	CYP3A4, CYP3A5, CYP3A7, CYP3A43
CYP4	CYP4A	CYP4A9, CYP4A11
	CYP4B	CYP4B1
	CYP4F	CYP4F2, CYP4F3, CYP4F8, CYP4F11, CYP4F12
	CYP4V	CYP4V2
	CYP4X	CYP4X1
	CYP4Z	CYP4Z1
CYP5	CYP5A	CYP5A1
CYP7	CYP7A	CYP7A1
	CYP7B	CYP7B1
CYP8	CYP8A	CYP8A1
	CYP8B	CYP8B1
CYP11	CYP11A	CYP11A1
	CYP11B	CYP11B1, CYP11B2
CYP17	CYP17	CYP17
CYP19	CYP19	CYP19
CYP20	CYP20	CYP20
CYP21	CYP21A	CYP21A1
CYP24	CYP24	CYP24
CYP26	CYP26A	CYP26A1
	CYP26B	CYP26B1
	CYP26C	CYP26C1
CYP27	CYP27A	CYP27A1
	CYP27B	CYP27B1
	CYP27C	CYP27C1
CYP39	CYP39	CYP39
CYP46	CYP46	CYP46
CYP51	CYP51	CYP51

Source: Adapted from D. Nelson website [396].

In addition, CYP enzymes differ in spectral, electrophoretic, and immunologic properties, modes of regulation, and inducibility.

Of the 18 CYP gene families identified in mammals thus far [12, 15], the major hepatic drug-metabolizing enzymes belong to families CYP1, CYP2, and CYP3. CYP enzymes belonging to families such as CYP5, CYP7, CYP8, CYP24, CYP27, and CYP51 are involved in the biosynthesis and catabolism of endogenous compounds.

The human CYP1 family, for example, consists of three enzymes, CYP1A1 and CYP1A2 in the CYP1A subfamily, and CYP1B1 in the CYP1B subfamily, although all three enzymes are not expressed in all tissues. Enzymes belonging to the CYP1 family are normally present in liver at very low levels but can be highly induced by treatment with planar halogenated and nonhalogenated aromatic compounds such as 3-methylcholanthrene, β-naphthoflavone, and 2,3,7,8-tetrachlorodibenzo-*p*-dioxin (TCDD) [15, 24–26].

The CYP2 family is represented by five major subfamilies, CYP2A, CYP2B, CYP2C, CYP2D, and CYP2E, in liver. CYP2E1, which is the only member of the CYP2E subfamily in various species and is involved in the metabolism of ethanol and other low molecular weight organic solvents, is induced by ethanol, acetone, and the antitubercular drug, isoniazid [24, 27]. The CYP2C enzymes, a quantitatively important group of enzymes in human and rodent liver, appear to be relatively refractory to induction by most drugs and other xenobiotics [27].

The CYP3 family is represented in liver by only one subfamily, CYP3A. CYP3A enzymes are inducible by glucocorticoids, phenobarbital, and macrolide antibiotics [15, 24, 28]. CYP3A enzymes are the most predominant CYP enzymes in human liver and intestine and are involved in the metabolism of a large percentage of therapeutic agents [1].

The CYP4 family, which is represented in liver by CYP4A and CYP4F subfamilies, is less important in xenobiotic metabolism. CYP4A and CYP4F enzymes catalyze the metabolism of fatty acids, leukotrienes, eicosanoic acids, and prostaglandins and are inducible by hypolipidemic agents, such as clofibrate, and by phthalates and other peroxisomal proliferators [15, 29].

In contrast to the CYP enzymes, NADPH-dependent CYP reductase is encoded by one gene. Thus the single form of NADPH-dependent CYP reductase, which exists in human liver, must be capable of interacting with the multiple CYP enzymes found in each cell. Moreover, NADPH-dependent CYP reductase is expressed at a lower level than CYP, with a reductase to CYP ratio of approximately 1:10 or less. NADPH-dependent CYP reductase is slightly inducible (a maximal two- to threefold increase) by some of the same compounds (e.g., 3-methylcholanthrene, phenobarbital, TCDD) that induce CYP enzymes.

A list of CYP enzymes that have been detected in human tissues is presented in Table 18.3.

18.2.5 Genetic Polymorphism

Genetic polymorphism is a common phenomenon in the CYP superfamily. A polymorphism arises from a single base change or multiple nucleotide base changes in a gene and leads to a variant form of the coded protein. The mutation can occur in both coding and noncoding regions of the gene. The variant form of the polymorphic CYP enzyme may have enzymatic activity that is identical to that of the native enzyme, or it may exhibit greater or lesser activity, or it may not be expressed. For example, more than 60 polymorphisms are known for CYP2D6 [44]. The different polymorphic variants are designated by the addition of an asterisk followed by a number to the CYP enzyme name. For example, CYP2D6*1 is a commonly

TABLE 18.3 CYP Enzymes Detected in Various Human Organs

Organ	CYP Genes Expressed (mRNA or Protein)
Liver[a]	CYP1A2, CYP2A6, CYP2B6, CYP2C8, CYP2C9, CYP2C18, CYP2C19, CYP2D6, CYP2E1, CYP3A4, CYP3A5, CYP3A7, CYP4A11
Small intestine[a,b]	CYP1A1 (5.6), CYP2C9 (8.4), CYP2C19 (1), CYP2D6 (0.5), CYP2J2 (0.9), CYP3A4 (43), CYP3A5 (16)
Nasal mucosa	CYP2A6, CYP2A13, CYP2B6, CYP2C, CYP2J2, CYP3A
Trachea	CYP2A6, CYP2A13, CYP2B6, CYP2C, CYP2J2, CYP2S1, CYP3A, CYP4X1
Lung	CYP1A1, CYP1A2, CYP1B1, CYP2A6, CYP2A13, CYP2B6, CYP2C8, CYP2C18, CYP2D6, CYP2E1, CYP2F1, CYP2J2, CYP3A4, CYP3A5, CYP4B1
Stomach	CYP1A1, CYP1A2, CYP2C, CYP2J2, CYP2S1, CYP3A4
Colon	CYP1A1, CYP1A2, CYP1B1, CYP2J2, CYP2S1, CYP3A4, CYP3A5, CYP4F12
Kidney	CYP1B1, CYP2A6, CYP2B6, CYP2E1, CYP2R1, CYP2S1, CYP3A5, CYP4A11, CYP4F2, CYP4F12
Skin	CYP1A1, CYP1A2, CYP1B1, CYP2A6, CYP2B6, CYP2C9, CYP2C18, CYP2C19, CYP2D6, CYP2E1, CYP2S1, CYP3A4, CYP3A5, CYP4A11
Brain	CYP1A1, CYP2B6, CYP2D6, CYP2E1, CYP2U1
Mammary	CYP1A1, CYP1B1, CYP2C, CYP2D6, CYP3A4, CYP3A5, CYP4Z1
Placenta	CYP1A1, CYP2E1, CYP2F1, CYP2S1, CYP3A4, CYP3A5, CYP4B1

[a]CYP enzyme levels in liver and small intestine were detected by protein expression, whereas CYP enzymes in other tissues were detected mainly by mRNA expression.
[b]CYP enzyme levels in the small intestine were determined by immunoblot analysis using intestinal microsomes from 31 individuals. The numbers shown in parentheses in the table are mean CYP enzyme levels, expressed as picomoles per milligram microsomal protein, in the small intestine [14]. Note: CYP1A1 was detected in 3, and CYP3A5 was detected in 11, of the 31 samples, and CYP1A2, CYP2A6, CYP2B6, CYP2C8, and CYP2E1 were below the limit of detection [14].
Source: Compiled from Refs. 2, 13, 14, and 30–43.

occurring variant of CYP2D6 that codes for an enzyme with high activity toward a number of substrates including debrisoquine and sparteine, whereas CYP2D6*9 codes for an enzyme with low activity. CYP2D6*4 and CYP2D6*5 are nonfunctional alleles, meaning that the CYP2D6 protein is not expressed. Although allelic variation can occur with any CYP gene, polymorphisms of CYP2A6, CYP2C9, CYP2C19, and CYP2D6 are the best characterized (Table 18.4) [45].

Enzyme polymorphism is inherited and is a major cause of interindividual and ethnic differences in the rates at which individuals metabolize drugs. The activities of the different polymorphic enzymes may vary by more than 100-fold when tested with the same drug substrate. Thus individuals bearing a nonfunctional allele such as CYP2D6*5 or an allele that codes for a CYP enzyme with low activity, such as CYP2D6*9, will metabolize debrisoquine, a drug that is hydroxylated at the 4-position by CYP2D6, more slowly than individuals bearing an allele that codes for a CYP enzyme with high activity, such as CYP2D6*1. People in the former group are classified as poor/slow metabolizers and people in the latter group are classified as extensive/fast metabolizers. Moreover, other people may have multiple copies of a variant allele, such as CYP2D6*2, and are classified as ultrarapid metabolizers [46].

TABLE 18.4   Human CYP Polymorphisms with Relatively High Population Frequency

CYP Enzyme	Allele[a]	Function
CYP2A6	*2	Inactive
	*4	Inactive
CYP2D6	*2	Decreased activity
	*3	Inactive
	*4	Inactive
	*5	Inactive
	*6	Inactive
	*7	Inactive
	*9	Decreased activity
	*10	Decreased activity
	*17	Decreased activity
	*2xN	Ultrarapid activity
CYP2C9	*2	Decreased activity
	*3	Decreased activity
CYP2C19	*2	Inactive
	*3	Inactive
	*4	Inactive
	*5	Inactive

[a]The *1 allele, which is not presented in the table, codes for CYP enzymes with high activity (i.e., represents the rapid/extensive metabolizer phenotype). The allelic variants listed in the table represent polymorphisms that occur with relatively high frequency and have functional relevance. Many more CYP allelic variants have been detected but are not listed in the table.

Source: Adapted from Ref. 45.

18.3   CYP ENZYME REACTIONS

18.3.1   CYP Substrates

The CYP enzyme system is capable of catalyzing the oxidative biotransformation of an almost limitless number of xenobiotics including drugs, solvents, anesthetics, dyes, petroleum products, pesticides, halogenated aromatic hydrocarbons such as polychlorinated biphenyls (PCBs), and plant products. An exhaustive list of substrates for the mammalian CYP enzymes is presented in Table 18.5. These substrates share a common feature in that most are lipid soluble and are converted by CYP into more water-soluble metabolites. This facilitates their eventual excretion from the body. Xenobiotics are metabolized by a relatively small number of CYP enzymes belonging to families CYP1, CYP2, and CYP3. Many lipid-soluble physiological compounds including fatty acids, steroids, eicosanoids, retinoids, and amino acids also serve as substrates of CYP1, CYP2, and CYP3 enzymes. A characteristic of the CYP1, CYP2, and CYP3 enzymes that contributes to their ability to metabolize such a diverse array of different substrates is that they possess broad and overlapping substrate selectivity.

By contrast, a large subset of CYP enzymes, especially those found in steroidogenic organs such as the adrenal gland and gonads, but also including enzymes present in the liver, are not involved in xenobiotic metabolism. These CYP enzymes

TABLE 18.5 Substrates for Mammalian CYP Enzymes[a]

Category/Subcategory of Substrates	Examples of Substrates[b]
Animal/Fungal/Plant Natural Products	
Alkaloids	Californine, protopine
Components of garlic	Diallyl disulfide, diallyl sulfide
Coumarins, furanocoumarins, psoralens	Bergamottin, BFC, coumarin, 7-ethoxycoumarin, methoxsalen
Drugs	Caffeine, cocaine, ipomeanol, morphine, nicotine, quinidine, quinine
Flavonoids	Aminoflavone, apigenin, 7,8-benzoflavone, biochanin A, daidzein, eriodictyol, flavanone, galangin, genistein, hesperetin, kaempferide, methoxyflavanone, naringenin, prunetin, tangeretin, tamarixetin
Flavorants, herbal constituents, spices	Aristolochic acids, capsaicin, glabridin
Indoles	Ibogaine, indole, 3-methylindole
Mycotoxins	Territrems A, B, C
Phytoalexins	Resveratrol
Retinoids	All-*trans*-retinoic acid, retinal, 9-*cis*-retinoic acid, 13-*cis*-retinoic acid
Safroles	Elemicin, myristicin
Terpenes and derivatives	Betulinic acid, eucalyptol, germander, limonenes, (R)-(+)-pulegone, verbenone
Vitamins	$1\alpha,25$-Dihydroxyvitamin D_3, 1α-hydroxyvitamin D_2, 1α-hydroxyvitamin D_3, vitamin A, vitamin B_2, vitamin D_2, vitamin D_3, vitamin E
Various natural products	Benzylisothiocyanate, odorants, oleuropein, pheromones, pyrrolizidine, tannins, tentoxin, yohimbine
Endogenous Compounds	
Amino acids, amines	Arginine, *N*-hydroxyarginine, octopamine, synephrine, tryptamine, tyramine
β-Carbolines	Methoxydimethyltryptamine, pinoline
Heme compounds	Bilirubin
Pineal hormones	Melatonin
Hydrocarbons	Acetone, acetol, H_2O_2
Lipids	Eicosanoic acids, fatty acids, leukotrienes, lipid peroxides, lipoxins, prostaglandins, thromboxanes
Steroid hormones and various steroids	Androgens, bile acids, cholesterol, estrogens, glucocorticoids, lanosterol, mineralocorticoids, progestins, steroid hydroperoxides
Xenobiotics	
Alcohols, aldehydes, alkanes, and related compounds	Acetal, acetoacetate, butanol, butanone, 3,4-dimethylhexane, ethanal, ethane, ethanol, glycerol, hexane, 2-hexanone, methanol, methyl-*t*-butyl ketone, *p*-nitrobenzaldehyde, pentane, pentanol, propanol, nonane, *p*-tolualdehyde

636

Category	Compounds
Alkenes, alkynes	Biphenyl acetylene, divinyl ether, ethene, fluroxene, propene
Amines and related compounds	Acetanilide, acetylhydrazine, aniline
Azo compounds, azoles	Azoxymethane, methylazoxymethanol, pyrazole
Benzene and derivatives	Benzene, bromobenzene, 2,6-di-t-butyl-4-methylphenol, nitrobenzene, phenol
Carcinogens[c]	
Alkaloids, alkenes, allylarenes, spices	β-Asarone, butadiene, estragole, isosafrole, methyleugenol, safrole, senecionine, styrene
Amines and derivatives	Acetylaminofluorene, aminoazotoluene, aminobiphenyl, benzidine, dimethylaminoazobenzene, Glu-P-1, Glu-P-2, HMP, IQ, MeIQ, MeIQx, 2-naphthylamine, PhIP, Trp-P-1, Trp-P-2
Carbamates, ethers	Diethylether, ethyl carbamate, methyl-t-butyl ether, vinyl carbamate
Estrogens	Diethylstilbestrol, 17β-estradiol
Halogenated hydrocarbons	Benzyl chloride, CCl$_4$, chloroform, bis(chloromethyl)ether, dibromochloropropane, 1,4-dichlorobenzene, dichloromethane, dichloropropane, dimethylcarbamoyl chloride, epichlorohydrin, ethylene dibromide, ethylene dichloride, methyl chloride, methylene chloride, MOCA, trichloroethane, trichloroethylene, Tris-BP, vinyl bromide, vinyl chloride, vinylidene chloride
Hydrazines, nitriles, triazenes	Acrylonitrile, agaritine, dimethylhydrazine, dimethylphenyltriazene, procarbazine
Mycotoxins	Aflatoxin B$_1$, aflatoxin G$_1$, aflatoxin M$_1$, ochratoxin A, sterigmatocystin
Nitro compounds	DEN, DMN, p-nitroanisole, 4-nitrobiphenyl, 2-nitrofluorene, nitrosodimethylmorpholine, nitrosomethylbenzylamine, NNAL, NNK, NNN
Polycyclic aromatics	Aminoanthracene, 6-aminochrysene, benzo[a]pyrene, chrysene, benzophenanthrene, dibenzanthracene, DMBA, MC, naphthalene, nitrobenzo[a]pyrene, 6-nitrochrysene, nitropyrene, phenanthrene
Catechols, hydroquinones	α-Methyldopa, m-AMSA
Fungicides	Furametpyr, o-phenylphenol
Halogenated hydrocarbons	Bromobenzene, chlorobenzene, 1,2-dichlorobenzene, enflurane, halothane, methoxyflurane, tetrachloroethane, tetrachloroethylene, trichlorobenzene
Heteroaromatics, nitroaromatics	Isaxonine, lasciocarpaine, p-nitrophenol, N-nitrosopyrrolidine, suprofen, thiophene, ticrynafen
Hydroperoxides	BOOH, t-butylhydroperoxide, cumene hydroperoxide, DBOOH, EBOOH, TMOOH
Insect repellents	N,N-Diethyl-m-toluamide
Oral contraceptives	Desogestrel, dienogest, ethinylestradiol, gestodene, medroxyprogesterone, mestranol, norethisterone
Organic solvents, petroleum products	CCl$_4$, chloroform, methylene chloride, pyridine, toluene, vinyl chloride, xylene
Pesticides	Aldrin, azobenzene, carbaryl, carbofuran, chlordanes, chlorpyrifos, chlortoluron, DCBN, DDT, diazinon, dieldrin, endosulfan, endrin, heptachlor, kepone, methiocarb, methoxychlor, parathion, phorate, pyrethrins, rotenone, strychnine
Plasticizers	Di-(2-ethylhexyl)phthalate

637

TABLE 18.5 *Continued*

Category/Subcategory of Substrates	Examples of Substrates[b]
Polyhalogenated aromatics	PBBs, PBDEs, PCBs, TCDD, TCDF
Sulfur compounds	Carbon disulfide, thioacetamide, thiobenzamide

Therapeutic/Pharmacologic Drugs[c,d]

Category/Subcategory of Substrates	Examples of Substrates[b]
Abortifacients	Mifepristone
Alcohol deterrents	Diethyldithiocarbamate, disulfiram
Analgesics	
Antimigraine drugs	Almotriptan, butalbital, divalproex, eletriptan, dihydroergotamine, ergotamine, flunarizine, lisuride, naratriptan, propranolol, valproic acid, zolmitriptan
Antineuralgia drugs	Capsaicin, carbamazepine, duloxetine
COX-3 inhibitors	Acetaminophen, aminopyrine, antipyrine
Opioid analgesics	Alfentanil, buprenorphine, codeine, dihydrocodeine, ethylmorphine, fentanyl, hydrocodone, hydromorphone, ketobemidone, meperidine, methadone, morphine, noralfentanil, oxycodone, pentazocine, phenazocine, propoxyphene, sufentanil, tramadol
Various analgesics	Acetaminophen, acetanilide, carisoprodol, phenacetin
Anesthetics, general	
Opioid anesthetics	Alfentanil, fentanyl, sufentanil
Fluorinated hydrocarbons	Desflurane, enflurane, fluroxene, halothane, isoflurane, methoxyflurane, sevoflurane
Various general anesthetics	Ketamine, phencyclidine, propofol, thiamylal, thiopental
Anesthetics, local	Bupivacaine, levobupivacaine, lidocaine, ropivacaine
Anorectic/antiobesity drugs	Dexfenfluramine, fenfluramine, phenmetrazine, phentermine, sibutramine
Antiacne drugs	Retinoic acid, erythromycin, metronidazole, salicylic acid, tazarotenic acid
Antiandrogenics	Bicalutamide, flutamide, finasteride, valproate
Anti-alopecia drugs	Finasteride, minoxidil
Anti-Alzheimer drugs	DMP543, donepezil, galantamine, milameline, tacrine
Anti-amyotrophic lateral sclerosics	Riluzole
Antiasthmatics/bronchodilators/ nasal decongestants	Flunisolide, fluticasone, methoxyphenamine, montelukast, paraxanthine, pseudoephedrine, salmeterol, theobromine, theophylline, tiaramide, zafirlukast, zileuton
Anti-ADHD drugs	d-Amphetamine, imipramine, methamphetamine, methylphenidate, nortriptyline, tamoxetine
Antibacterials	
Antileprotics	Dapsone, rifabutin
Anti-MAC drugs	Rifabutin
Antirickettsials	Chloramphenicol, rifampicin

Antituberculars	Isoniazid, rifabutin, rifalazil, rifampicin
Fluoroquinolones	Ciprofloxacin, grepafloxacin, pefloxacin
Macrolides	Azithromycin, clarithromycin, erythromycin, miocamycin, roxithromycin, troleandomycin
Various antibacterials	Chloramphenicol, clindamycin, rifabutin, metronidazole, sulfamethoxazole, sulfamidine, trimethoprim
Antibacterials, topical	Sulfadiazine silver
Anti-benign prostatic hyperplasia drugs	Alfuzosin, finasteride, prazosin, tamsulosin
Anticancer/antineoplastic drugs	All-*trans*-retinoic acid, aminoflavone, anastrozole, AQ4N, artemisinin, O^6-benzylguanine, berberine, bexarotene, bicalutamide, bropirimine, busulfan, *t*-butylhydroxyanisole, carmustine, coumarin, cyclophosphamide, dacarbazine, daidzein, DF203, docetaxel, doxorubicin, dutasteride, ellipticine, etoposide, exemestane, fadrozole, finasteride, ftorafur, gefitinib, genistein, hexamethyl-melamine, ifosfamide, imatinib, imiquimod, irinotecan, karenitecin, ketoconazole, letrozole, lonafarnib, mitotane, mitoxantrone, MMDX, oracin, paclitaxel, procarbazine, sirolimus, tamoxifen, targretin, tauromustine, tegafur, teniposide, thioguanine, 6-thiopurine, thioTEPA, toremifene, trofosfamide, urethane, valproic acid, vinblastine, vincristine, vindesine, vinorelbine
Antidepressants	
Monamine oxidase inhibitors	Amiflamine, brofaromine, iproniazid, moclobemide, phenelzine, tranylcypromine
NMRIs, tricyclic antidepressants	Amitriptyline, clomipramine, desipramine, doxepin, imipramine, medifoxamine, norclomipramine, nortriptyline, opipramol, trimipramine
SNRIs, S&NRIs, SSRIs	Citalopram, duloxetine, escitalopram, fluoxetine, fluvoxamine, maprotiline, milnacipran, norfluoxetine, paroxetine, reboxetine, sertraline, triazoledione, tomoxetine, venlafaxine
Various antidepressants	Adinazolam, bupropion, clonazepam, cotinine, gepirone, iprindole, iproclozide, mianserin, minaprine, mirtazapine, nefazodone, trazodone, triazoledione
Anti-dermatitis herpetiformis drugs	Dapsone
Antidiabetics	Acetohexamide, chlorpropamide, CPO, glibenclamide, gliclazide, glimepiride, glipizide, nateglinide, phenformin, pioglitazone, repaglinide, rosiglitazone, tolbutamide, troglitazone
Antiepileptics	Carbamazepine, clobazam, clomethiazole, clonazepam, diazepam, ethosuximide, felbamate, ganaxolone, losigamone, mephenytoin, mephobarbital, nimetazepam, phenobarbital, phenytoin, primidone, tiagabine, topiramate, trimethadione, valproic acid, zonisamide
Antierectile dysfunction drugs	Sildenafil, vardenafil, yohimbine
Antiestrogenics	Tamoxifen, toremifene
Antifungals	Clotrimazole, fluconazole, itraconazole, ketoconazole, miconazole, sirolimus, terbinafine, voriconazole
Antigout, uricosuric drugs	Benzbromarone, colchicine, dexamethasone, hydrocortisone, indomethacin, methylprednisolone, phenylbutazone, sulfinpyrazone, tienilic acid, zoxazolamine

TABLE 18.5 *Continued*

Category/Subcategory of Substrates	Examples of Substrates[b]
Antihistamines	Azelastine, brompheniramine, chlorpheniramine, cinnarizine, clemastine, cyproheptadine, diphenhydramine, doxylamine, ebastine, flunarizine, hydroxyzine, loratadine, medrylamine, mequitazine, orphenadrine, pheniramine, promethazine, rupatadine, tripelennamine
Antihyperlipoproteinemics	
Fibrates	Bezafibrate, ciprofibrate, clofibrate, fenofibrate, gemfibrozil
HMGRIs	Atorvastatin, cerivastatin, fluvastatin, lovastatin, pravastatin, simvastatin
Antihyperprolactinemics	Lisuride, terguride
Anti-inflammatory drugs	
COSAIDs	Budesonide, dexamethasone, fluticasone, mometasone, prednisolone
NSAIDs	
Anti-FMF drugs	Colchicine
COX-2 selective inhibitors	Celecoxib, etoricoxib, lumiracoxib, rofecoxib, valdecoxib
Various NSAIDs	Aceclofenac, acetylsalicylic acid, alclofenac, berberine, diclofenac, etodolac, flurbiprofen, ibufenac, ibuprofen, indomethacin, ketorolac, lisofylline, lornoxicam, mefenamic acid, meloxicam, naproxen, oxyphenbutazone, phenylbutazone, piroxicam, salicylate, suprofen, tazofelone, tenoxicam, tiaramide, tolmetin, zomepirac
Anti-malignant hyperthermia drugs	Dantrolene
Antimanics	Carbamazepine
Antinarcolepsy drugs	d-Amphetamine, methylphenidate, modafinil
Anti-OCD drugs	Clomipramine, fluoxetine, fluvoxamine, paroxetine, sertraline
Anti-opioid addiction drugs	Buprenorphine, methoxycoronaridine, vanoxerine
Anti-osteoporosis drugs	Raloxifene
Anti-parkinsonian drugs	Amantadine, benztropine, bromocriptine, lisuride, orphenadrine, procyclidine, rasagiline, ropinirole, terguride, tolcapone
Antiprogestins	Valproate
Antipruritics	Camphor, cyproheptadine, doxepin
Antipsoriatics	Bergapten, retinoic acid, methoxsalen, phenol, salicylic acid, tazarotenic acid
Antipyretics	Aceclofenac, acetaminophen, acetanilide, acetylsalicylic acid, alclofenac, aminopyrine, ibuprofen, indomethacin, naproxen, phenacetin, tiaramide
Antirheumatics	
Corticosteroids	Cortisone, dexamethasone, methylprednisolone, prednisolone
Various antirheumatics	Azathioprine, capsaicin, chloroquine, hydroxychloroquine sulfate, leflunomide
Antiseptics	Naphthalene, phenol, terpineol
Antithyroid drugs	Methimazole, methylthiouracil, propylthiouracil
Antitussives	Codeine, dextromethorphan, dihydrocodeine, dimemorfan, dropropizine, ethylmorphine, hydrocodone
Anti-urinary incontinence drugs	Oxybutynin, scopolamine, tolterodine

Antivirals	
Anti-influenza drugs	Amantadine, chloroquine
Anti-hepatitis B drugs	Pradefovir
Anti-herpetics	Valacyclovir
Anti-HIV drugs	Amprenavir, atazanavir, capravirine, delavirdine, efavirenz, indinavir, lopinavir, methoxycoronaridine, nelfinavir, nevirapine, ritonavir, saquinavir, tipranavir, zidovudine
Anti-papillomavirus drugs	Imiquimod, resiquimod
Anxiolytics/hypnotics/sedatives	Adinazolam, alpidem, alprazolam, brofaromine, brotizolam, buspirone, chlordiazepoxide, citalopram, clomethiazole, clomipramine, clonazepam, diazepam, escitalopram, fenobam, flunitrazepam, fluvoxamine, gespirone, imipramine, meprobamate, mexazolam, midazolam, nimetazepam, nordiazepam, opipramol, oxazepam, paroxetine, pimozide, sertraline, temazepam, triazolam, zaleplon, zolpidem, zopiclone
Anti-insomnials	Brotizolam, eszopiclone, zaleplon, zolpidem, zopiclone
Cardiovascular drugs	
ADR receptor agonists	Octopamine, synephrine
Antianginals	Amiodarone, amlodipine, bunitrolol, diltiazem, isosorbide dinitrate, metoprolol, nicardipine, nifedipine, oxprenolol, perhexiline, pronethalol, propranolol, ranolazine, timolol
Antiarrhythmics	Ajmaline, amiodarone, aprindine, azimilide, bepridil, bunitrolol, cibenzoline, digoxin, diltiazem, diprafenone, disopyramide, lidocaine, mexiletine, oxprenolol, phenytoin, procainamide, pronethalol, propafenone, propranolol, quinidine, sparteine, timolol, verapamil
Anticoagulants	Acenocoumarol, dicoumarol, phenprocoumon, warfarin
Antiglaucomics	Betaxolol, brinzolamide, dorzolamide, pilocarpine, pindolol, timolol
Antihypotensives	Desglymidodrine
Antihypertensives	
α-ADR receptor antagonists	Alfuzosin, indoramin, labetolol, prazosin, tamsulosin, yohimbine
β-ADR receptor antagonists	Betaxolol, bisoprolol, bufuralol, bunitrolol, bupranolol, carteolol, carvedilol, labetolol, metoprolol, nebivolol, oxprenolol, pindolol, pronethalol, propranolol, timolol
ACE inhibitors	Captopril, enalapril
AII receptor antagonists	Candesartan, irbesartan, losartan, tasosartan, valsartan

TABLE 18.5 *Continued*

Category/Subcategory of Substrates	Examples of Substrates[b]
Calcium channel blockers	Amlodipine, barnidipine, bepridil, diltiazem, felodipine, gallopamil, isradipine, lomerizine, mibefradil, nicardipine, nifedipine, niludipine, nilvaldipine, nimodipine, nisoldipine, nitrendipine, norverapamil, oxodipine, pranidipine, verapamil
Various antihypertensives	Ajmaline, debrisoquine, eplerenone, guanabenz, guanoxan, pargyline, pheniprazine
Antiplatelets	Acetylsalicylic acid, cilostazol, clopidogrel, seratrodast, sulfinpyrazone, ticlopidine
Cardiac inotropics	Digitoxin, digoxin, pimobendan, vesnarinone
Lipid peroxidase inhibitors	Tirilazad
Vasodilators	Bosentan, buflomedil, cinnarizine, dihydralazine, flosequinan, flunarizine, glyceryltrinitrate, hydralazine, isosorbide dinitrate, minoxidil, nimodipine, perhexiline
Diuretics	Caffeine, furosemide, perhexiline, tienilic acid, torasemide, triamterene
Estrogenics	17α-Ethinylestradiol
Gastrointestinal drugs	
Antidiarrheals	Berberine, loperamide
Antiemetics	Aprepitant, diphenidol, dolasetron, dronabinol, ezlopitant, granisetron, meclozine, metoclopramide, ondansetron, scopolamine, tropisetron, zatosetron
Antigastroenteritis drugs	Berberine
Antiulceratives	Cimetidine, esomeprazole, lansoprazole, omeprazole, pantoprazole, rabeprazole, ranitidine
Prokinetic drugs	Ecabapide, metoclopramide, mosapride
Immunosuppressants/ immunomodulators	Azathioprine, busulfan, cyclosporin A, imiquimod, laquinimod, lisofylline, mycophenolic acid, resiquimod, roquinimex, sirolimus, tacrolimus
Mucolytics	Ambroxol
Multidrug resistance modulators	Valspodar
Muscle relaxants	Carisoprodol, chlordiazepoxide, chlorzoxazone, cyclobenzaprine, dantrolene, diazepam, meprobamate, nimetazepam, orphenadrine, oxybutynin, tizanidine, tolterodine, zoxazolamine
Mydriatics	Atropine, scopolamine, yohimbine
Neuroleptics	Aripiprazole, bromoperidol, chlorpromazine, clozapine, etoperidone, fluperlapine, fluphenazine, haloperidol, harmaline, harmine, iloperidone, mazapertine, methoxyamphetamine, methoxyphenamine, olanzapine, perazine, perospirone, perphenazine, pimozide, protriptyline, quetiapine, remoxipride, risperidone, sertindole, thioridazine, tiospirone, trazodone, trifluperidol, ziprasidone, zotepine, zuclopenthixol
Nootropics	Nefiracetam, tacrine
Oxytocics	Sparteine

642

Parasiticides	
Anthelmintics	Albendazole, diethylcarbamazine, ivermectin, naphthalene, praziquantel, pyrantel, thiabendazole
Antimalarials	Amodiaquine, arteether, artelinic acid, artemether, artemisinin, artesunate, berberine, chloroquine, chlorproguanil, halofantrine, lumefantrine, mefloquine, primaquine, proguanil, pyrimethamine, quinidine, quinine, tafenoquine
Ectoparasiticides	Carbaryl, deltamethrin, lindane, malathion, methoxychlor, permethrin
Various parasiticides	Metronidazole, pentamidine, sulfamethoxazole, tinidazole
Photosensitizers	Methoxsalen, trioxsalen
Signal transduction inhibitors	Imatinib
Smoking cessation aids	Bupropion
Stimulants	
Hallucinogenics	Ibogaine, LSD, MBDB, MDA, MDE, MDMA, mescaline, methoxyamphetamine, phencyclidine, THC
Various stimulants	d-Amphetamine, benzphetamine, caffeine, methamphetamine, methylphenidate, modafinil
Topical keratolytics	Salicylic acid
Ultraviolet screens	p-Aminobenzoic acid

[a]Substrates presented in this Table are metabolized by CYP enzymes derived primarily from human and rodent species.

[b]Abbreviations: AII, angiotensin II; ACE, angiotensin converting enzyme; ADHD, attention-deficit hyperactivity disorder; ADR, adrenergic; AQ4N, 1,4-bis[[2-(dimethylamino-*N*-oxide)ethyl]amino]-5,8-dihydroxyanthracene-9,10-dione; BFC, 7-benzyloxy-4-trifluoromethylcoumarin; BOOH, 2-*t*-butyl-4-hydroperoxy-4-methyl-2,5-cyclohexadienone; CNS, central nervous system; COSAIDs, corticosteroidal anti-inflammatory drugs; COX, cyclooxygenase; CPO, 5-[4-[3-(4-cyclohexyl-2-propylphenoxy)propoxy]phenyl]-1,3-oxazolidine-2,4-dione; DBOOH, 2,6-di-*t*-butyl-4-methyl-4-hydroperoxy-2,5-cyclohexadienone; DCBN, 2,6-dichlorobenzonitrile; DDT, dichlorodiphenyltrichloroethane; DEN, diethylnitrosamine; DF203, 2-(4-amino-3-methylphenyl)benzothiazole; DMBA,7,12-dimethyl-benz[*a*]anthracene; DMN, dimethylnitrosamine; DMP543, 10,10-bis(2-fluoro-4-pyridinylmethyl)-9(10*H*)anthracenone; EBOOH, 2,6-di-*t*-butyl-4-ethyl-4-hydroperoxy-2,5-cyclohexadienone; FMF, familial Mediterranean fever; Glu-P-1, 2-amino-6-ethyldipyrido[1,2-*a*:3′,2′-*d*]imidazole; Glu-P-2, 2-aminodipyrido[1,2-*a*:3′,2′-*d*]imidazole; HIV, human immunodeficiency virus; HMGRIs, 3-hydroxy-3-methylglutarylcoenzyme A reductase inhibitors; HMP, hexamethylphosphoramide; IQ, 2-amino-3-methylimidazo[4,5-*f*]quinoline; LSD, lysergic acid diethylamide; MAC, *Mycobacterium avium* complex; MBDB, *N*-methylbenzodioxazolylbutanamine; MC, 3-methylcholanthrene; MDA, 3,4-methylenedioxyamphetamine; MDE, 3,4-methylenedioxyethylamphetamine; MDMA, 3,4-methylenedioxymethamphetamine; MeIQ, 2-amino-3,5-dimethylimidazo[4,5-*f*]quinoline; MeIQx, 2-amino-3,8-dimethylimidazo[4,5-*f*]quinoline; MMDX, methoxymorpholinodoxorubicin; MOCA, 4,4′-methylene-bis(2-chloroaniline); NMRIs, nonselective monamine reuptake inhibitors; NNAL, 4-(methylnitrosamino)-1-(3-pyridyl)-1-butanol; NNK, 4-(methylnitrosamino)-1-(3-pyridyl)-1-butanone; NNN, nornitrosonicotine; NSAIDs, nonsteroidal anti-inflammatory drugs; OCD, obsessive–compulsive disorder; PBBs, polybrominated biphenyls; PBDEs, polybrominated diphenyl ethers; PCBs, polychlorinated biphenyls; PhIP, 2-amino-1-methyl-6-phenylimidazo[4,5-*b*]pyridine; PPAR, peroxisome proliferator-activated receptor; SNRIs, selective noradrenaline reuptake inhibitors; S&NRIs, serotonin and noradrenaline reuptake inhibitors; SSRIs, selective serotonin reuptake inhibitors; TCDD, 2,3,7,8-tetrachlorodibenzo-*p*-dioxin; TCDF, 2,3,7,8-tetrachlorodibenzofuran; THC, Δ⁹-tetrahydrocannabinol; thioTEPA, triethylenethiophosphoramide; TOOH, 4-hydroperoxy-2,4,6-trimethyl-2,5-cyclohexadienone; Tris-BP, tris(2,3-dibromopropyl)phosphate; Trp-P-1, 3-amino-1,4-dimethyl-5H-pyrido[4,3-*b*]indole; Trp-P-2, 3-amino-1-methyl-5H-pyrido[4,3-*b*]indole.

[c]Some of the substrates listed as carcinogens or drugs are considered to be procarcinogens or prodrugs, respectively, and need to be bioactivated by CYP enzymes [15, 47–59].

[d]Therapeutic properties of the drugs were determined using human subjects. Drugs are listed under several alphabetically arranged categories/subcategories and are further classified under specific pharmacologic/chemical subheadings within a category. Certain drugs that are used for more than one indication are classified under more than one section. Drugs have been selected on the basis of past and present importance. Certain drugs are no longer marketed as therapeutic agents.

Source: Compiled from Refs. 10 and 60–108. A comprehensive listing of substrates for CYP enzymes can be found in book chapters [2, 15, 50, 53, 55], a review article [89], and websites [397, 398].

643

have much narrower substrate specificity and function exclusively in the biotransformation of physiological compounds. For example, CYP5 and CYP8A are involved in the production of thromboxane and prostacyclin. CYP11, CYP17, CYP19, and CYP21 play important roles in steroid biosynthesis. CYP7, CYP8B, and CYP27A are involved in the synthesis of bile acids, and CYP51 is involved in cholesterol biosynthesis. CYP24 and CYP27B metabolize vitamin D, while enzymes in the CYP26 family metabolize retinoic acid [23].

18.3.2   Types of Reactions Catalyzed by CYP Enzymes

CYP reactions are typically oxidative reactions that expose or add a functional group on to the substrate molecule. In addition to catalyzing the biotransformation of xenobiotics, CYP enzymes are also involved in the metabolism of endogenous compounds and the biosynthesis of signaling molecules used to control homeostasis and development [21].

Depending on the structure of the substrate, CYP enzymes catalyze a wide range of monooxygenase reactions (i.e., insertion of one atom of oxygen) including aromatic and aliphatic hydroxylations, N-, O-, and S-dealkylations, deaminations, N-, P-, and S-oxidations, and dehalogenations. Less commonly, CYP enzymes can catalyze reduction reactions under conditions of low oxygen tension (Table 18.6). CYP-catalyzed biotransformation often results in inactivation or a decrease in the biological activity of the substrate, although it can also lead to formation of chemically reactive metabolites that can bind to macromolecules such as proteins and DNA and initiate toxic, teratogenic, and carcinogenic events [47, 48]. Other products may be stable molecules possessing intrinsic biological activity that differs from that of the substrate.

It must be emphasized that one CYP enzyme may catalyze several pathways of drug metabolism, and one pathway may be catalyzed by several CYP enzymes. For example, human CYP3A4 can catalyze the hydroxylation of testosterone, N-demethylation of alfentanil, and N-oxidation of nifedipine, to name just a few reactions, and a drug such as acetaminophen can be metabolized by CYP1A2, CYP2E1, and CYP3A4. Furthermore, CYP enzymes often exhibit regio- and stereoselectivity toward a particular substrate. A good example is testosterone, which undergoes selective ring hydroxylation by various CYP enzymes at either the alpha or beta positions at carbons 2, 6, 7, and 16. Unfortunately, there is no relationship between various CYP enzymes and their abilities to catalyze specific types of reactions so that it is not possible, for example, to characterize an individual CYP enzyme as strictly an N-demethylase or an aromatic hydroxylase.

18.3.3   CYP Enzyme Marker Activities

An ideal marker enzyme activity should be catalyzed by a single CYP enzyme. However, in view of the versatile and nonspecific nature of CYP enzymes, it is difficult to find completely specific marker activities for individual CYP enzymes under all conditions.

Human and rodent liver contains more than 25 or 30 different CYP enzymes that can, under *in vitro* conditions, participate to varying degrees in the biotransformation of a given xenobiotic. However, at the concentration of substrates (e.g., drugs)

TABLE 18.6 Reactions Catalyzed by CYP Enzymes

Types of Reactions[a]	Examples of Substrates[a,b]	Product(s) Formed
Oxidative reactions		
Alicyclic carbon hydroxylation	Acetohexamide Cyclophosphamide Digitoxin Minoxidil	trans-4-Hydroxyacetohexamide 4-Hydroxycyclophosphamide Digoxin 4'-Hydroxyminoxidil
Aliphatic amine hydroxylation	Amantadine, benzylamphetamine, chlorphentermine, nicotine, phenmetrazine, phentermine	N-Hydroxy derivatives
Aliphatic carbon hydroxylation	n-Alkanes, barbiturates, bile acids, cyclohexane, fatty acids, prostaglandins, steroids, drugs (e.g., capsaicin, chlorpropamide, flutamide, glutethimide, ibuprofen, meprobamate, phenylbutazone, valproic acid)	ω- and (ω-1)-Hydroxylation; hydroxylation at other sites
Alkene epoxidation	Aflatoxin B_1 Carbamazepine Diethylstilbestrol Styrene	Aflatoxin B_1 2,3-oxide Carbamazepine 10,11-oxide Diethylstilbestrol oxide Styrene oxide
Aromatic amide hydroxylation	Acetaminophen, 2-acetylaminofluorene	N-Hydroxy derivatives
Aromatic carbon epoxidation	Benzene, benzo[a]pyrene, bromobenzene, DMBA, 4-ipomeanol, naphthalene, phenytoin	Epoxide derivatives
Aromatic carbon hydroxylation	Amphetamine, chlorpromazine, coumarins, diazepam, imipramine, lidocaine, lovastatin, mephenytoin, methadone, phenobarbital, polycyclic aromatics, promethazine, propranolol, salicylic acid, warfarin	Hydroxylation at different sites (certain reactions may proceed via an epoxide intermediate)
Aromatization	Felodipine, nicardipine, nifedipine	Aromatization derivatives
Arylamine hydroxylation	Aniline	Phenylhydroxylamine
	Dapsone	N-Hydroxydapsone
Cyclization	Proguanil	Cycloguanil

TABLE 18.6 *Continued*

Types of Reactions[a]	Examples of Substrates[a,b]	Product(s) Formed
N-Dealkylation	Aminopyrine	Monomethyl-4-aminoantipyrine
	Caffeine	1,7-Dimethylxanthine
	Diazepam	Nordiazepam
	Halofantrine	Desbutylhalofantrine
	Iproniazid	Isoniazid
	Lidocaine	Monoethylglycylxylidine
	(S)-Mephenytoin	Nirvanol
	Mephobarbital	Phenobarbital
	Methamphetamine	Amphetamine
	Promethazine	10-(2-Aminopropyl)phenothiazine
	Propranolol	Desisopropylpropranolol
	Sibutramine	Norsibutramine, dinorsibutramine
	Sildenafil	Norsildenafil
O-Dealkylation	Artelinic acid	Dihydroquinghaosu
	Astemizole	Desmethylastemizole
	Codeine	Morphine
	7-Ethoxycoumarin	7-Hydroxycoumarin
	Ethylmorphine	Morphine
	Methoxyamphetamine	Hydroxyamphetamine
	Phenacetin	Acetaminophen
	Reboxetine	Desethylreboxetine
S-Dealkylation	2-Benzylthio-5-trifluoromethylbenzoic acid	2-Thio-5-trifluoromethylbenzoic acid
	Methitural	Desmethylmethitural
	Methylmercaptan	Mercaptan
	6-Methylthiopurine	6-Thiopurine
Deamination	Amphetamine	Phenylacetone
	Bisdesmethylbrompheniramine	3-(p-Bromophenyl)-3-pyridyl-propionate
	(S)-(+)-α-Methyldopamine	3,4-Dihydroxyphenylacetone
	Propranolol	Desisopropylpropranolol
Dehalogenation	Chloramphenicol	Oxamic acid derivative
	Chloroform	Phosgene
	Dibromomethane	Hydrogen bromide
	Halothane	Trifluoroacetic acid

Reaction	Substrate	Product
Dehydrogenation	N-Methylformamide, valproic acid, zafirlukast	Dehydrogenated derivatives
Denitrification	2-Nitropropane	Nitrite, acetone
Denitrosation	N-Dimethylnitrosamine	Nitrite, methylamine
Descarbethoxylation	Loratadine	Descarboethoxyloratadine
Desulfuration	Chlorpyrifos, diazinon, parathion	Oxon derivatives
	Thiopental	Pentobarbital
Heterocyclic ring oxidation	Phenmetrazine	3-Oxophenmetrazine
N-Hydroxylation	Acetaminophen, acetylhydrazine, 6-aminochrysene, aminoglutethimide, amphetamine, isoniazid, phenacetin, phenmetrazine, phenytoin, riluzole	N-Hydroxy derivatives
Hydroxylation at allylic carbon atoms	Hexobarbital	3'-Hydroxyhexobarbital
	Pentazocine	trans- and cis-Hydroxypentazocine
	Quinidine	3-Hydroxyquinidine
	THC	7-Hydroxy-THC
Hydroxylation at benzylic carbon atoms	Amphetamine	α-Hydroxyamphetamine
	Methaqualon	2'-Hydroxymethylmethaqualon
	3-Methylcholanthrene	3-Hydroxymethylcholanthrene
	Metoprolol	α-Hydroxymetoprolol
	Tolbutamide	4-Hydroxytolbutamide
Hydroxylation of carbon atoms adjacent to a carbonyl or imine group	Diazepam	3-Hydroxydiazepam
	Flurazepam	3-Hydroxyflurazepam
	Glutethimide	4-Hydroxyglutethimide
	Nimetazepam	3-Hydroxynimetazepam
Hydroxylation of indole ring	Dolasetron, indole, ondansetron, tropisetron	Hydroxy derivatives
Isoxazole ring cleavage	Leflunomide	α-Cyanoenol derivative
Methyl hydroxylation	Dacarbazine, etoricoxib, ibuprofen, 3-methylindole, midazolam, montelukast, naproxen, omeprazole, terfenadine, tolterodine, triazolam, zolpidem	Hydroxymethyl derivatives
N-Oxidation	Dapsone, dolasetron, mephentermine, nifedipine, quinidine, senecionine, sparteine, trimethylamine	N-Oxidation derivatives
P-Oxidation	Diethylphenylphosphine	P-Oxidation derivative
S-Oxidation	Chlorpromazine, cimetidine, lansoprazole, metiamide, montelukast, promethazine, thioacetamide, thiobenzamide, thioguanine, thioridazine, zotepine	Sulfoxide derivatives

TABLE 18.6 *Continued*

Types of Reactions[a]	Examples of Substrates[a,b]	Product(s) Formed
Pyridine ester deesterification	Dehydrogenated pranidipine	OPC-13463
Ring formation	Pulegone	Menthofuran
Transannular dioxygenation	9,10-Dimethyl-1,2-benz[a]anthracene	9,10-Dimethyl-1,2-benz[a]anthracene -9,10-epidioxide
Reductive reactions		
t-Amine N-oxide reduction	AQ4N	AQ4
	N,N-Dimethylaniline N-oxide	N,N-Dimethylaniline
	Imipramine N-oxide	Imipramine
Arene oxide reduction	Benzo[a]pyrene-4,5-oxide	Benzo[a]pyrene
Azido reduction	Zidovudine	3'-Amino-3'-deoxythymidine
Azo reduction	Azobenzene	Aniline
	Azsulfidine	Sulfapyridine, p-aminosalicylic acid
	Prontosil	2,4-Diaminoaniline, sulfanilamide
Chromate reduction	Chromate (VI)	Chromate (III)
Hydroperoxide reduction	t-Butyl hydroperoxide, cumene hydroperoxide, H$_2$O$_2$, linoleic acid hydroperoxide, steroid hydroperoxides	Hydroxy derivatives, other products
Nitro reduction	Chloramphenicol	Dichloro-N-[2-hydroxy-1-(hydroxymethyl)-2-(4-aminophenyl) ethyl]acetamide
	Nitrobenzene	Aniline
	p-Nitrobenzoic acid	p-Aminobenzoic acid
Oxygen reduction	Oxygen	H$_2$O, H$_2$O$_2$, superoxide
Reductive dehalogenation	Carbon tetrachloride	Chloroform
	Halothane	Chlorodifluoroethylene
Reductive dehydrogenation	Hexachlorocyclohexane	Hexachlorocyclohexene
Reductive ring cleavage	Zonisamide	2-Sulfamoylacetylphenol

[a]The examples listed are not meant to be comprehensive but are meant to illustrate the diversity of types of reactions and substrates.

[b]Abbreviations: AQ4, 1,4-bis-[[2-dimethylamino)ethyl]amino]-5,8-dihydroxyanthracene-9,10-dione; AQ4N, 1,4-bis-[[2-(dimethylamino-N-oxide)ethyl]amino]-5,8-dihydroxyanthracene-9,10-dione; DMBA, 7,12-dimethylbenz[a]anthracene; OPC-13463, methyl-2,6-dimethyl-4-(3-nitrophenyl)-3-carboxy-5-pyridinecarboxylate; THC, Δ^9-tetrahydrocannabinol.

Source: Compiled from Refs. 15, 50–55, 60, 61, 89, and 109–122.

typically found in tissue after exposure, enzyme kinetics favors a single form of CYP as being the primary catalyst of metabolism for that substrate [27, 49]. Representative examples of CYP enzymes in human liver and their characteristic activities are presented in Table 18.7. The number of competing CYP enzymes, the amounts of individual enzyme present, and the catalytic efficiencies of each enzyme determine the rate and predominant pathway of metabolism of a compound.

TABLE 18.7 Marker Activities and Inhibitors of the Major Human Hepatic CYP Enzymes

CYP	Characteristic Marker Activities	Inhibitors[a]
CYP1A1	7-Ethoxyresorufin O-deethylation	9-Hydroxyellipticine
CYP1A2	7-Methoxyresorufin O-demethylation	7,8-Benzoflavone, fluvoxamine, furafylline
	Phenacetin O-deethylation	7,8-Benzoflavone, fluvoxamine, furafylline
CYP1B1	17β-Estradiol 4-hydroxylation	Propofol
CYP2A6	Coumarin 7-hydroxylation	Diethyldithiocarbamate, methoxsalen
CYP2B6	Bupropion hydroxylation	ThioTEPA, ticlopidine
	Efavirenz 8-hydroxylation	ThioTEPA
	7-Ethoxytrifluoromethylcoumarin O-deethylation	9-Ethynylphenanthrene
	(S)-Mephenytoin N-demethylation	ThioTEPA
CYP2C8	Amadiaquine N-deethylation	Quercetin
	Paclitaxel 6α-hydroxylation	Quercetin
CYP2C9	Celecoxib methyl hydroxylation	Sulfaphenazole
	Diclofenac 4'-hydroxylation	Sulfaphenazole, tienilic acid
	(S,R)-Flurbiprofen 4'-hydroxylation	Sulfaphenazole
	Naproxen O-demethylation	Sulfaphenazole, tienilic acid
	Tolbutamide p-methyl hydroxylation	Sulfaphenazole, tienilic acid
	Torasemide tolylmethyl hydroxylation	Sulfaphenazole
CYP2C19	(S)-Mephenytoin 4'-hydroxylation	Fluconazole, tranylcypromine
CYP2D6	Bufuralol 1'-hydroxylation	Quinidine
	Debrisoquine 4-hydroxylation	Ajmalicine, quinidine
CYP2E1	Chlorzoxazone 6-hydroxylation	Chlormethiazole, 4-methylpyrazole
	Lauric acid ω1-hydroxylation	Diethyldithiocarbamate
CYP3A4	Alfentanil N-dealkylation	Ketoconazole, troleandomycin
	Alprazolam 4-hydroxylation	Ketoconazole
	Midazolam 1'-hydroxylation	Ketoconazole
	Nifedipine N-oxidation	Gestodene, troleandomycin
	(S)-Quinidine 3-hydroxylation	Ketoconazole
	Testosterone 6β-hydroxylation	Troleandomycin
CYP4A11	Lauric acid ω-hydroxylation	10-(Imidazolyl)decanoic acid, TS-011

[a]Abbreviations: thioTEPA, triethylenethiophosphoramide; TS-011, [N-(3-chloro-4-morpholin-4-yl) phenyl-N-hydroxyimidoformamide].

Source: Compiled from Refs. 2, 15, 50, 51, 53, 55, 89, 123–149, and 398.

18.3.4   CYP Reaction Cycle

The fact that CYP enzymes have been conserved throughout evolution suggests that they serve a vital role in the preservation of life. Many believe the endogenous substrates of CYP enzymes are steroids or some as yet unidentified endogenous compounds [49, 150]. Alternatively, CYP enzymes may serve a critical protective role against the possible harmful effects of exogenous compounds ingested in the diet to which all organisms are exposed continually during their lifetimes. It has also been suggested that, from an evolutionary standpoint, the primary biological role of CYP can be considered to be the detoxification of molecular oxygen (O_2) in tissue to water [15]. This is accomplished by first activating oxygen with reducing equivalents supplied by NADPH, but the activation of oxygen is dangerous if not tightly regulated. The regulation is achieved by a mechanism that prevents CYP from activating oxygen unless a substrate molecule is bound to the enzyme to act as a recipient for the reactive oxygen insertion [15].

The basic aspects of the catalytic mechanism and the interactions of the components of the CYP system are generally agreed upon. The overall reaction for a typical CYP-mediated monooxygenation can be represented as follows:

$$RH + NAD(P)H + O_2 \rightarrow ROH + NAD(P) + H_2O$$

where RH is the substrate and ROH is the oxidized product (Fig. 18.1).

The catalytic cycle can be divided into several discrete steps but basically involves oxygen activation and oxygen insertion (Fig. 18.2). Binding of substrate to the CYP enzyme occurs in the first step. The substrate binds to a site on the enzyme in close proximity to the heme moiety, which results in displacement of the water molecule that normally occupies the sixth coordination site of the heme iron. Substrate binding also facilitates a change in spin state and a reduction of the heme iron, from the low spin ferric (Fe^{3+}) to the high spin ferrous (Fe^{2+}) state, by the addition of an electron from NADPH. Molecular oxygen is then able to bind to the high spin ferrous heme iron to form a dioxygen (Fe^{2+}—O_2) complex. The addition of a second electron results in conversion to a peroxoiron ($Fe^{2+}OOH$) complex. Protonation and cleavage of the O—O bond produces water and a reactive iron–oxo (FeO^{3+}) complex, which transfers its oxygen to the substrate [15, 21, 151–153]. The oxidized substrate is then released, permitting CYP to return to its initial state and repeat the cycle. Oxidation (oxygen insertion) of the substrate typically occurs at the most reactive carbon–hydrogen bond.

18.3.5   CYP Inhibitors

Many clinically important drug interactions involve the effect of one drug on the metabolism of another. Enzyme inhibition, specifically inhibition of CYP enzymes, is a very common mechanism behind drug interactions. Some CYP inhibitors and the CYP enzymes affected are listed in Table 18.7.

The effect of enzyme inhibition is to reduce the rate of metabolism of drugs, taken concurrently with the inhibitor, that are also substrates of the inhibited CYP enzyme. The affected drugs begin to accumulate in the body and their therapeutic activity and side effects are increased. For example, if erythromycin, an inhibitor of

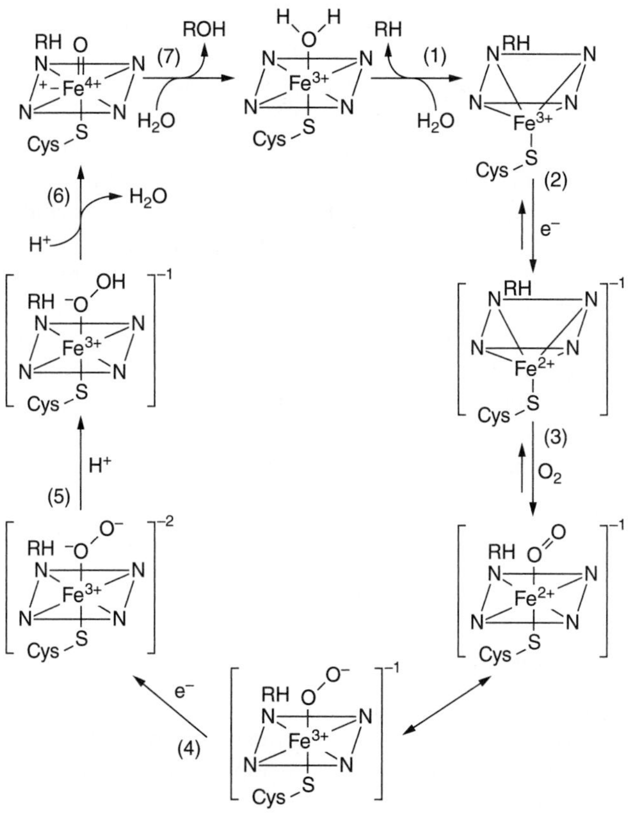

FIGURE 18.2 CYP catalytic cycle. Enzymatic steps by which CYP enzymes catalyze the hydroxylation of a substrate (RH) to a product (ROH). Adapted from Ref. 153.

CYP3A4, is taken by a patient who is also being treated with carbamazepine, which is extensively metabolized by CYP3A4, this may lead to toxicity due to higher concentrations of carbamazepine.

Inhibition is dose related, so that inhibition will not appear until a sufficient concentration of inhibitor is present in the liver. The effects are often maximal when steady-state plasma concentrations of the inhibitor are reached. Moreover, at low concentrations, the inhibitor may be relatively selective for a single CYP enzyme, whereas at high concentrations, the inhibitor may be relatively nonselective and several CYP enzymes will be inhibited.

There are several mechanisms by which drugs and other compounds inhibit CYP enzymes. The commonest mechanism is simple competition by two drugs for metabolism by the same CYP enzyme. The two drugs compete at the substrate binding site to produce reversible and rapid inhibition of the metabolism of one of the drugs, usually the drug with the lower affinity for the enzyme or the drug that is present at substantially lower concentration. Simple competitive inhibition is usually short-acting and is possible with any two drugs. A second more selective type of reversible inhibition is produced by drugs containing an azole group, such as the antifungal agents, ketoconazole, miconazole, and fluconazole, or by drugs containing an imidazole group, such as cimetidine. In this type of inhibition, a basic nitrogen atom of the azole or imidazole group interacts, via its free electron pair, with the iron in the heme group of CYP and forms a relatively stable but reversible substrate–enzyme complex. A more slowly reversible form of inhibition is produced when a drug is metabolized to a reactive metabolite that binds in a noncovalent fashion with the iron in the CYP heme group. Examples of drugs that produce this type of inhibitory metabolite (i.e., metabolism-dependent inhibitors) include nortriptyline, amiodarone, and the macrolide antibiotics such as erythromycin and clarithromycin. This type of inhibition often increases with repeated dosing and the effects may continue for several weeks after stopping the drug if the drug has a long half-life. Irreversible inhibition is relatively rare but the effects are long-lasting. Irreversible inhibitors such as gestodene, ethinyl estradiol, levonorgestrel, and spironolactone are metabolized to reactive metabolites that form covalent bonds with either the heme group or the apoprotein of CYP, a process that inactivates the enzyme and is only overcome when the inhibited CYP enzyme turns over (i.e., is destroyed and new enzyme is synthesized).

18.4 STRUCTURE AND REGULATION

18.4.1 Overview of Individual CYP Enzymes

The total CYP level in liver may vary two- to threefold, at most, among humans. However, there is considerably greater variation in the enzyme activities and protein levels of individual CYP enzymes within a population. Table 18.8 illustrates the variability and range of CYP enzyme levels that have been measured for 14 different enzymes in human liver microsomes. The interindividual variation in human

TABLE 18.8 CYP Enzyme Levels[a] in Human Liver Microsomes

CYP Enzyme	Content (pmol CYP/mg microsomal protein)	Percentage of Total CYP
CYP1A1	Not detected	0
CYP1A2	<1–45	<0.5–15
CYP1B1	Not detected	0
CYP2A6	<1–68	4–17
CYP2B6	1–39	<1–7
CYP2C8	1–60	12–15
CYP2C9	9–100	14–18
CYP2C18	<1	<0.5
CYP2C19	0.5–19	1–17
CYP2D6	1.5–10	1–4
CYP2E1	7–49	3–9
CYP3A4	40–140	18–29
CYP3A5	<1	<0.5
CYP4A11	Not determined	10

[a]CYP enzyme levels were compiled from Refs. 55, and 155–158. CYP enzyme levels were measured in individual human liver samples by immunoquantification. Values represent the approximate range of CYP levels reported.

hepatic CYP levels and activities is related to several factors including genetic polymorphism, enzyme inhibition, and enzyme induction.

18.4.2 CYP1 Family

Two CYP enzymes are present in the 1A subfamily, CYP1A1 and CYP1A2. These enzymes are highly conserved among species [15]. Human CYP1A1 and CYP1A2 share approximately 70% amino acid sequence identity.

CYP1A1 and CYP1A2 preferentially metabolize planar aromatic molecules but exhibit distinct substrate selectivity (Table 18.9). CYP1A1 and CYP1A2 both catalyze the O-dealkylation of 7-methoxyresorufin and 7-ethoxyresorufin and are involved in the bioactivation of chemical carcinogens [2, 159]. CYP1A1 preferentially catalyzes the hydroxylation of benzo[a]pyrene leading to the 7,8-epoxide intermediate, whereas CYP1A2 preferentially catalyzes the N-hydroxylation of aromatic amines including 4-aminobiphenyl, 2-naphthylamine, and 2-acetylaminofluorene [26, 51]. With respect to drug metabolism, CYP1A2 catalyzes the N-hydroxylation of acetaminophen, leading to formation of the reactive benzoquinoneimine metabolite, N3-demethylation of caffeine to paraxanthine, and O-dealkylation of phenacetin. Ellipticine is an inhibitor of human CYP1A1 and furafylline is a potent metabolism-dependent inhibitor of human CYP1A2 [2, 13].

CYP1A1 is not normally expressed in the liver of humans and most mammals but is detected in extrahepatic tissues such as lung and placenta in humans. CYP1A2 is expressed constitutively and almost exclusively in the liver [26, 158, 160]. Hepatic levels of CYP1A2 vary widely, exhibiting as much as a 40- to 100-fold difference, among individuals [155, 158].

CYP1B1 is the only member of the CYP1B subfamily. Recombinant CYP1B1 catalyzes the oxidation of 7,12-dimethylbenz[a]anthracene and the 4-hydroxylation of 17β-estradiol (Table 18.9). CYP1B1 protein has not been detected in liver [158] and is found primarily in extrahepatic tissues including thymus and the adrenal cortex [55]. CYP1B1 is linked to eye development as mutations in the human CYP1B1 gene are associated with congenital glaucoma [180].

CYP1A1, CYP1A2, and CYP1B1 are inducible enzymes, which are upregulated by the activation of the aryl hydrocarbon receptor (AhR) [26, 181]. In humans, CYP1A enzymes can be induced by polycyclic aromatic hydrocarbons found in charbroiled meat, cigarette smoke, and cruciferous vegetables. Omeprazole, a proton pump inhibitor, has also been shown to induce CYP1A enzymes [2]. In rodents, CYP1A1 levels increase from undetectable to approximately 40% of the total CYP content in the liver, following treatment with xenobiotic inducers such as 3-methylcholanthrene [160]. CYP1A1 levels in the lung, small intestine, and kidneys are also induced. CYP1A2 levels in the liver are increased but CYP1A2 remains undetectable in extrahepatic tissues following administration of inducers such as 3-methylcholanthrene [160].

18.4.3 CYP2 Family

The CYP2 family is the largest CYP family present in humans in terms of number of different CYP enzymes identified. CYP2 enzymes are responsible for steroid

TABLE 18.9   Substrates for Human CYP1 Enzymes[a]

CYP	Category of Substrates	Examples of Substrates[b]
CYP1A1	Benzene derivatives	o-Aminoazotoluene, toluene
	Carcinogens	
	Amino compounds	2-Acetylaminofluorene, 2-aminoanthracene, 4-aminobiphenyl, 6-aminochrysene, 2-aminofluorene, IQ, MeIQ, MeIQx, methoxyaminoazobenzene, NNK, PhIP, Trp-P-1, Trp-P-2
	Polycyclic aromatics	Benz[a]anthracene-3,4-diol, benzo[g]chrysene-11,12-diol, benzo[b]fluoranthene-9,10-diol, benzo[a]perylene, benzo[a]pyrene-7,8-diol, chrysene-1,2-diol, dibenz[a,h]anthracene, dibenzo[a,l]pyrene-11,12-diol, DMBA, DMBA-3,4-diol, 5,6-dimethylchrysene-1,2-diol, 1-ethylpyrene, 5-methylchrysene-1,2-diol, 6-nitrochrysene, 2-naphthylamine, 2-nitronaphthalene, nitropyrene, phenanthrene
	Various carcinogens	Aflatoxin B_1, diethylstilbestrol, 17β-estradiol, ochratoxin A
	Chloroaromatics	1,2,4-Trichlorobenzene, 1,2,3,5-tetrachlorobenzene
	Coumarins, resorufins	Coumarin, 7-ethoxycoumarin, ethoxyresorufin
	Endogenous compounds	Tryptamine, uroporphyrinogen
	Flavonoids	7,8-Benzoflavone, eriodictyol, galangin, genistein, hesperetin, kaempferide, methoxyflavanone
	Fungicides	Furametpyr
	Retinoids	All-trans-retinoic acid, retinal, retinol
	Steroids	Androstenedione, estrone, pregnenolone, progesterone, testosterone
	Drugs	Abecarnil, albendazole, aminopyrine, amiodarone, amodiaquine, benzydamine, bufuralol, caffeine, capsaicin, carvedilol, chloroquine, chlorzoxazone, cinnarizine, clomethiazole, dacarbazine, diclofenac, ellipticine, flunarizine, flutamide, fluvastatin, lisofylline, lisuride, MDE, nicardipine, nicotine, nifedipine, pentamidine, phenacetin, phencyclidine, pranidipine, propranolol, pyrantel, quinine, riluzole, ropivacaine, tegafur, terguride, theophylline, thiabendazole, tolbutamide, toremifene, troglitazone, warfarin, zotepine
CYP1A2	Benzene derivatives	o-Aminoazotoluene, toluene
	β-Carbolines	Harmaline, harmine
	Carcinogens	
	Amines and derivatives	2-Acetylaminofluorene, 2-aminoanthracene, aminoazotoluene, 4-aminobiphenyl, 6-aminochrysene, 2-aminofluorene, benzidine, dimethylaminoazobenzene, furylfuramide, Glu-P-1, Glu-P-2, IQ, MeIQ, MeIQx, methoxyaminoazobenzene, NNK, PhIP, Trp-P-1, Trp-P-2, 2-naphthylamine
	Polycyclic aromatics	Benz[a]anthracene-3,4-diol, benzo[a]pyrene-7,8-diol, 1,3-dinitropyrene, DMBA, DMBA-3,4-diol, 5-methylchrysene-1,2-diol, 1-methylpyrene, nitropyrene, naphthalene, 6-nitrochrysene, phenanthrene
	Various carcinogens	Aflatoxin B_1, butadiene, 1,4-dichlorobenzene, 17β-estradiol, methyleugenol, ochratoxin A

TABLE 18.9 *Continued*

CYP	Category of Substrates	Examples of Substrates[b]
	Chloroaromatics	Bromodichloromethane, 1,2-dichlorobenzene, 1,2,4-trichlorobenzene
	Coumarins, resorufins	BFC, coumarin, 7-ethoxycoumarin, methoxyresorufin
	Endogenous compounds	Arachidonic acid, linoleic acid, PGH_2, phosphatidylcholine, uroporphyrinogen
	Flavonoids	Aminoflavone, apigenin, biochanin A, daidzein, formononetin, galangin, genistein, hesperetin, kaempferide, kaempferol, methoxyflavanone, naringenin, prunetin, tangeretin, tamarixetin
	Fungicides	Furametpyr, *o*-phenylphenol
	Hormones	Estrone, melatonin, progesterone, testosterone
	Insect repellents	*N,N*-Diethyl-*m*-toluamide
	Pesticides	Ametryne, atrazine, chlorpyrifos, diazinon, methoxychlor, parathion
	Phytoalexins	Resveratrol
	Pneumotoxins, other toxins	3-Methylindole, myristicin
	Retinoids	Retinal, 13-*cis*-retinoic acid, retinol
	Xanthines	1,7-Dimethylxanthine, 8-ethylfurafylline, furafylline, paraxanthine
	Drugs	Acenocoumarol, acetaminophen, acetanilide, albendazole, aminopyrine, amiodarone, amitriptyline, amodiaquine, antipyrine, benzydamine, O^6-benzylguanine, bropirimine, bufuralol, bupivacaine, bupropion, caffeine, capsaicin, carbamazepine, carvedilol, chlordiazepoxide, chlorpromazine, chlorzoxazone, cilostazol, cinnarizine, ciprofloxacin, cisapride, clomipramine, clozapine, cyclobenzaprine, dacarbazine, dapsone, desipramine, diazepam, diclofenac, diethylcarbamazine, dihydralazine, doxepin, ellipticine, enoxacin, etoposide, fenfluramine, flunarizine, flunitrazepam, fluoxetine, flutamide, fluvoxamine, ftorafur, grepafloxacin, guanabenz, haloperidol, hydromorphone, iloperidone, imipramine, imiquimod, ipomeanol, leflunomide, lidocaine, lisofylline, maprotiline, MBDB, MDE, MDMA, (*S*)-mephenytoin, methadone, metoclopramide, mexiletine, mianserin, mirtazapine, naproxen, nicardipine, nicotine, nifedipine, nordiazepam, nortriptyline, olanzapine, ondansetron, pefloxacin, perazine, perphenazine, phenacetin, pimobendan, pimozide, pranidipine, praziquantel, primaquine, proguanil, propafenone, propofol, propranolol, ranitidine, rasagiline, resiquimod, riluzole, ritonavir, rofecoxib, ropinirole, ropivacaine, tacrine, tamoxifen, tauromustine, tegafur, terbinafine, theobromine, theophylline, thiabendazole, tizanidine, tolbutamide, tolcapone, toremifene, triamterene, verapamil, warfarin, zileuton, zolmitriptan, zolpidem, zotepine, zoxazolamine

TABLE 18.9   *Continued*

CYP	Category of Substrates	Examples of Substrates[b]
CYP1B1	Carcinogens	
	Amino compounds	2-Aminofluorene, IQ, MeIQ, MeIQx, methoxyaminoazobenzene, NNK, PhIP, Trp-P-1, Trp-P-2
	Polycyclic aromatics	2-Aminoanthracene, 6-aminochrysene, benz[a]anthracene-1,2-diol, benzo[g]chrysene-11,12-diol, benzo[b]fluoranthene-9,10-diol, benzo[c]phenanthrene-3,4-diol, benzo[a]pyrene, benzo[a]pyrene-7,8-diol, chrysene-1,2-diol, dibenzo[a,l]pyrene-11,12-diol, DMBA, DMBA-3,4-diol, 5,6-dimethylchrysene-11,12-diol, dinitropyrene, 9-hydroxybenzo[a]pyrene, 1-ethylpyrene, 5-methylchrysene, 5-methylchrysene-1,2-diol, 1-methylpyrene, 6-nitrochrysene, nitrofluoranthene, nitropyrene
	Various carcinogens	Aflatoxin B_1, 17β-estradiol
	Coumarins, resorufins	Coumarin, 7-ethoxycoumarin, ethoxyresorufin
	Flavonoids	Eriodictyol, genistein, hesperetin
	Steroid hormones	Estrone, progesterone, testosterone
	Fatty acids	Arachidonic acid
	Retinoids	Retinal, retinol
	Drugs	Albendazole, amodiaquine, artelinic acid, artemisinin, artesunate, bufuralol, caffeine, DF203, docetaxel, ellipticine, flutamide, nifedipine, pyrimethamine, theophylline, thiabendazole, tolbutamide

[a]Involvement of specific human CYP enzymes in the metabolism of substrates listed in Tables 18.9–18.12 was determined using *in vivo* and *in vitro* procedures. *In vivo* techniques included administering drugs and other substrates together with selective CYP inhibitors to human subjects and measuring metabolites in plasma and urine. *In vitro* studies included incubating human hepatic microsomes with substrate along with selective CYP inhibitors or antibodies and measuring inhibition of enzyme activity and product formation. Other *in vitro* studies included incubating purified human hepatic CYP enzymes, or a panel of cDNA expressed human CYP enzymes, with substrate and measuring product formation. Liver is the primary site of expression for the majority of CYP enzymes listed in Tables 18.9–18.12.
[b]Abbreviations: BFC, 7-benzyloxy-4-trifluoromethylcoumarin; DF203, 2-(4-amino-3-methylphenyl)benzothiazole; DMBA, 7,12-dimethylbenz[a]anthracene; Glu-P-1, 2-amino-6-methyldipyrido[1,2-a:3′,2′-d]imidazole; Glu-P-2, 2-aminodipyrido[1,2-a:3′,2′-d]imidazole; IQ, 2-amino-3-methylimidazo[4,5-f]quinoline; MBDB, N-methylbenzodioxazolylbutanamine; MDE, 3,4-methylenedioxyethylamphetamine; MDMA, 3,4-methylenedioxymethamphetamine; MeIQ, 2-amino-3,5-dimethylimidazo[4,5-f]quinoline; MeIQx, 2-amino-3,8-dimethylimidazo[4,5-f]quinoline; NNK, 4-(methylnitrosamino)-1-(3-pyridyl)-1-butanone; PGH₂, prostaglandin H₂; PhIP, 2-amino-1-methyl-6-phenylimidazo[4,5-b]pyridine; Trp-P-1, 3-amino-1,4-dimethyl-5H-pyrido[4,3-b]indole; Trp-P-2, 3-amino-1-methyl-5H-pyrido[4,3-b]indole.
Source: Compiled from Refs. 10, 51–56, 130, and 161–179. A comprehensive listing of substrates for CYP1 enzymes can be found in book chapters [2, 15, 50, 53, 55] and a review article [89].

hydroxylation and the biotransformation of a wide variety of drugs and xenobiotics, as well as many endogenous compounds (Table 18.10).

The CYP2A subfamily consists of three genes in humans, namely, CYP2A6, CYP2A7, and CYP2A13. CYP2A6, CYP2A7, and CYP2A13 exhibit >90% identity

TABLE 18.10 Substrates for Human CYP2 Enzymes

CYP	Category of Substrates	Examples of Substrates[a]
CYP2A6	Carcinogens	
	Amino compounds	6-Aminochrysene, PhIP
	Nitro compounds	p-Nitroanisole, DEN, DMN, NNAL, NNK, NNN
	Various carcinogens	Aflatoxin B_1, butadiene, chloroform, 17β-estradiol, MOCA, phenanthrene, safrole
	Components of garlic	Diallyl sulfide
	Coumarins	Coumarin, 7-ethoxycoumarin, psoralen
	Ethers, phenols	Ethyl t-butyl ether, methyl t-butyl ether, p-nitrophenol
	Fluorinated hydrocarbons	Halothane, methoxyflurane, sevoflurane
	Indoles, xanthines	1,7-Dimethylxanthine, indole, 3-methylindole, paraxanthine
	Insect repellants	N,N-Diethyl-m-toluamide
	Retinoids	All-trans-retinoic acid
	Steroid hormones	Progesterone, testosterone
	Terpenes	Verbenone
	Drugs	Acetaminophen, aminopyrine, amodiaquine, artelinic acid, artesunate, bupropion, chlorzoxazone, cinnarizine, cisapride, clomethiazole, clozapine, cotinine, cyclobenzaprine, cyclophosphamide, fadrozole, flunarizine, flunitrazepam, ftorafur, ifosfamide, letrozole, lidocaine, lisofylline, losigamone, medifoxamine, methoxsalen, mexiletine, naproxen, nicotine, nifedipine, omeprazole, phenacetin, primaquine, propofol, quinoline, ritonavir, tacrine, tamoxifen, tegafur, valproic acid, zidovudine
CYP2B6	Alkanes	Hexane
	Aromatic hydrocarbons	o-Phenylphenol, toluene
	Nitrosoamines	N-Nitrosomethylbutylamine, N-nitrosomethylethylamine, nitrosomorpholine
	Carcinogens	
	Polycyclic aromatics	6-Aminochrysene, benzo[a]pyrene, benzo[a]pyrene-7,8-diol, dibenzo[a]pyrene, DMBA, naphthalene, phenanthrene
	Various carcinogens	Aflatoxin B_1, butadiene, chloroform, 17β-estradiol, isoprene, DMN, NNK, styrene
	Coumarins, resorufins	Coumarin, 7-ethoxycoumarin, ethoxyresorufin, benzyloxyresorufin, pentoxyresorufin
	Fatty acids	Arachidonic acid, lauric acid
	Flavonoids	Flavanone, methoxyflavanone
	Fluorinated hydrocarbons	Chlorodifluoroethane, halothane, methoxyflurane, sevoflurane
	Insect repellents	N,N-Diethyl-m-toluamide

657

TABLE 18.10 *Continued*

CYP	Category of Substrates	Examples of Substrates[a]
	Pesticides	Acetochlor, ametryne, butachlor, chlorpyrifos, diazinon, endosulfan, methoxychlor, parathion, terbutryne
	Polychlorinated aromatics	2,4,5,2′,4′,5′-Hexachlorobiphenyl
	Retinoids	All-*trans*-retinoic acid
	Steroid hormones, sterols	5β-Cholestane-3α,7α,12α-triol, estrone, testosterone
	Terpenes	Verbenone
	Drugs	Alfentanil, aminopyrine, amitriptyline, antipyrine, arteether, artelinic acid, artemisinin, artesunate, benzphetamine, O^6-benzylguanine, bergamottin, bupropion, capsaicin, carteolol, cinnarizine, clobazam, clomethiazole, cyclophosphamide, diazepam, diclofenac, diethylcarbamazine, efavirenz, erythromycin, ethylmorphine, flunitrazepam, ifosfamide, ketamine, lidocaine, MDA, MDE, MDMA, (*S*)-mephenytoin, mephobarbital, mianserin, midazolam, nevirapine, nicotine, pentobarbital, primaquine, procainamide, promethazine, propofol, quinoline, ropivacaine, selegiline, seratrodast, sertraline, tamoxifen, tazofelone, temazepam, thioTEPA, tinidazole, trofosfamide, valproic acid, verapamil, zotepine
CYP2C8	Carcinogens	Benzo[*a*]pyrene, benzo[*a*]pyrene-7,8-diol, naphthalene, styrene
	Fatty acids	Arachidonic acid, 9,10-epoxystearic acid, leukotoxin
	Fluorescent probes	Dibenzylfluorescein
	Pesticides	Chlorpyrifos, diazinon, methoxychlor, parathion
	Retinoids	All-*trans*-retinoic acid, 13-*cis*-retinoic acid, retinol, tazarotenic acid
	Steroids	Androstenedione, testosterone
	Drugs	Albendazole, aminopyrine, amiodarone, amodiaquine, antipyrine, artelinic acid, benzphetamine, bufuralol, capsaicin, carbamazepine, cerivastatin, chloroquine, cisapride, clozapine, CPO, dapsone, diazepam, diclofenac, fluvastatin, ftorafur, gallopamil, halofantrine, karenitecin, lidocaine, lonafarnib, (*R*)-mephenytoin, mephobarbital, mirtazapine, mycophenolic acid, naproxen, omeprazole, paclitaxel, perospirone, phenprocoumon, phenytoin, pioglitazone, pyrantel, repaglinide, rosiglitazone, sulfadiazine, tegafur, temazepam, terbinafine, tiaramide, tienilic acid, tolbutamide, torasemide, trimethoprim, troglitazone, verapamil, warfarin, zidovudine, zopiclone

CYP2C9	Carcinogens	
	Polycyclic aromatics	Benzo[a]pyrene, benzo[a]pyrene-7,8-dihydrodiol, dibenzo[a]pyrene, naphthalene, phenanthrene
	Various carcinogens	Butadiene, 17β-estradiol, MeIQ, methyleugenol, safrole
	Components of garlic	Diallyl disulfide
	Coumarins	7-Ethoxycoumarin
	Fatty acids	Arachidonic acid, 9,10-epoxystearic acid, isoleukotoxin, leukotoxin, linoleic acid
	Flavonoids	Biochanin A, formononetin, tamarixetin
	Fluorescent probes	Dibenzylfluorescein
	Oral contraceptives	Desogestrel
	Retinoids	Retinoic acid, retinol
	Steroids	5α-Androstane-3α,17β-diol, testosterone
	Terpenes	Limonene
	Drugs	Aceclofenac, acenocoumarol, acetylsalicylic acid, albendazole, amitriptyline, antipyrine, artelinic acid, benzbromarone, bosentan, bufuralol, bupropion, candesartan, capsaicin, carvedilol, celecoxib, chloramphenicol, chlorpheniramine, cinnarizine, clozapine, cyclophosphamide, dapsone, dextromethorphan, diazepam, diclofenac, dicoumarol, dolasetron, dorzolamide, dronabinol, eletriptan, ellipticine, etodolac, etoricoxib, flunarizine, flunitrazepam, fluoxetine, flurbiprofen, fluvastatin, glimepiride, glipizide, hexobarbital, hydromorphone, ibuprofen, ifosfamide, imipramine, indomethacin, irbesartan, ketamine, ketobemidone, lornoxicam, losartan, lovastatin, lumiracoxib, mefenamic acid, meloxicam, (R)-mephenytoin, mirtazapine, moclobemide, montelukast, naproxen, nateglinide, nelfinavir, nevirapine, nicotine, ondansetron, perazine, perphenazine, phenobarbital, phenprocoumon, phenylbutazone, phenytoin, piroxicam, pravastatin, proguanil, propofol, pyrantel, ritonavir, rosiglitazone, selegiline, seratrodast, sertraline, sildenafil, simvastatin, sulfadiazine, sulfamethoxazole, sulfinpyrazone, suprofen, tafenoquine, tamoxifen, targretin, tauromustine, tegafur, temazepam, tenoxicam, terbinafine, THC, thiamylal, tiaramide, tienilic acid, tolbutamide, torasemide, trimethadione, trimethoprim, tropisetron, valproic acid, valsartan, venlafaxine, verapamil, voriconazole, warfarin, zafirlukast, zidovudine, zileuton, zopiclone
CYP2C18	Pesticides	Methoxychlor
	Retinoids	All-trans-retinoic acid
	Steroids	Progesterone
	Drugs	Aminopyrine, antipyrine, clobazam, diazepam, imipramine, lansoprazole, lidocaine, mephenytoin, naproxen, perphenazine, piroxicam, propofol, tienilic acid, tolbutamide, verapamil, warfarin

TABLE 18.10 *Continued*

CYP	Category of Substrates	Examples of Substrates[a]
CYP2C19	Carcinogens	Benzo[a]pyrene-7,8-dihydrodiol, benzo[a]pyrene-7,8-diol, chloroform, 17β-estradiol, methyleugenol
	Components of garlic	Diallyl disulfide
	Fatty acids	Arachidonic acid
	Hormones	Melatonin
	Indoles	Indole
	Insect repellents	*N,N*-Diethyl-*m*-toluamide
	Pesticides	Chlorpyrifos, diazinon, furametpyr, methoxychlor, parathion
	Prostaglandins	9,11-Epoxymethano-PGH$_2$, 11,9-epoxymethano-PGH$_2$, 9,11-diazo-15-deoxy-PGH$_2$
	Retinoids	Retinal, retinoic acid
	Steroids	Desogestrel, progesterone, testosterone
	Terpenes	Limonene
	Drugs	Acenocoumarol, adinazolam, albendazole, aminopyrine, amitriptyline, azelastine, benzbromarone, bufuralol, capsaicin, carisoprodol, chlorproguanil, citalopram, clobazam, clomethiazole, clomipramine, clozapine, CPO, dapsone, dextromethorphan, diazepam, diphenylhydantoin, divalproex, eletriptan, esomeprazole, etoricoxib, flunitrazepam, glibenclamide, hexobarbital, imipramine, lansoprazole, loratadine, (*R*)- and (*S*)-mephenytoin, mephobarbital, methadone, methoxycoronaridine, metoprolol, mianserin, moclobemide, naproxen, nelfinavir, nirvanol, nordiazepam, nortriptyline, omeprazole, pantoprazole, pentamidine, perazine, perphenazine, phenobarbital, phenytoin, piroxicam, praziquantel, proguanil, propranolol, pyrimethamine, quinine, rabeprazole, ranitidine, ritonavir, rofecoxib, selegiline, sertraline, tauromustine, temazepam, terbinafine, thalidomide, THC, tolbutamide, topiramate, valproic acid, venlafaxine, verapamil, voriconazole, warfarin, zidovudine, zotepine
CYP2D6	Amines	Octopamine, synephrine, tryptamine, tyramine
	β-Carbolines	Harmaline, harmine, methoxydimethyltryptamine, pinoline
	Carcinogens	Butadiene, 17β-estradiol, NNK, safrole
	Components of garlic	Diallyl disulfide
	Fungicides	*o*-Phenylphenol
	Insect repellents	*N,N*-Diethyl-*m*-toluamide
	Pesticides	Chlorpyrifos, diazinon, methoxychlor, parathion
	Steroids	Progesterone

	Drugs	Ajmaline, albendazole, alprenolol, amiflamine, aminopyrine, amitriptyline, amodiaquine, aprindine, aripiprazole, artemisinin, azelastine, barnidipine, benztropine, betaxolol, bisoprolol, brofaromine, bromoperidol, buflomedil, bufuralol, bunitrolol, bupranolol, capsaicin, captopril, carteolol, carvedilol, chloroquine, chlorpheniramine, chlorpromazine, cibenzoline, cinnarizine, citalopram, clemastine, clomipramine, clozapine, codeine, cyclobenzaprine, dapsone, debrisoquine, delavirdine, desglymidodrine, desipramine, desmethylcitalopram, dexfenfluramine, dextromethorphan, diazepam, diclofenac, diltiazem, diphenhydramine, diprafenone, dolasetron, donepezil, doxepin, doxylamine, duloxetine, efavirenz, eletriptan, encainide, ethylmorphine, etoricoxib, ezlopitant, fenfluramine, fentanyl, flecainide, flunarizine, fluoxetine, fluperlapine, fluphenazine, fluvastatin, fluvoxamine, galantamine, gallopamil, gepirone, guanoxan, haloperidol, hydrocodone, hydromorphone, hydroxyzine, ibogaine, imipramine, indinavir, indoramin, karenitecin, labetalol, lidocaine, lisuride, lopinavir, loratadine, lovastatin, maprotiline, MBDB, MDA, MDE, MDMA, meperidine, mequitazine, methadone, methamphetamine, methoxyamphetamine, methoxyphenamine, metoclopramide, metoprolol, mexiletine, mianserin, milameline, minaprine, mirtazapine, moclobemide, morphine, nebivolol, nefazodone, nelfinavir, nevirapine, norcodeine, norfluoxetine, nortriptyline, olanzapine, ondansetron, opipramol, oxycodone, oxyprenolol, paroxetine, pentazocine, perhexiline, perospirone, perphenazine, phenformin, pilocarpine, pimozide, pindolol, praziquantel, primaquine, procainamide, promethazine, propafenone, propoxyphene, propranolol, *N*-propylajmaline, pyrantel, quetiapine, quinidine, ranitidine, remoxipride, risperidone, ritonavir, rofecoxib, ropivacaine, selegiline, sertindole, sertraline, simvastatin, sparteine, sumatriptan, tamoxifen, tamsulosin, tauromustine, terguride, thebaine, thioridazine, timolol, tolterodine, tomoxetine, tramadol, trazodone, trifluperidol, trimipramine, tripelennamine, tropisetron, venlafaxine, yohimbine, zolpidem, zotepine, zuclopenthixol
CYP2E1	Alkanes and related compounds	Acetaldehyde, acetonitrile, diethylether, ethanol, glycerol
	Amides	Dimethylformamide, methylformamide
	Aromatic hydrocarbons	Aniline, naphthylhydrazine, *p*-nitrophenol, phenol, pyridine, toluene, xylene
	Carcinogens	
	Amine derivatives	DEN, DMN, NNAL, NNK, NNN
	Halogenated hydrocarbons	CCl₄, chloroform, 1,4-dichlorobenzene, dichloromethane, 1,2-dichloropropane, ethylene dibromide, ethylene dichloride, methyl chloride, methylene chloride, tetrachloroethane, trichloroethane, trichloroethylene, vinyl bromide, vinyl chloride
	Polycyclic aromatics	Benzo[*a*]pyrene-7,8-diol, 1-methylpyrene
	Various carcinogens	Acrylonitrile, benzene, butadiene, ethyl carbamate, isoprene, methyleugenol, *p*-nitroanisole, safrole, styrene, vinyl carbamate

661

TABLE 18.10 *Continued*

CYP	Category of Substrates	Examples of Substrates[a]
	Chloroaromatics	1,2-Dichlorobenzene, 1,2,4-trichlorobenzene, 1,2,3,5-tetrachlorobenzene, pentachlorobenzene
	Components of garlic	Diallyl disulfide, diallyl sulfide
	Coumarins	7-Ethoxycoumarin
	Endogenous compounds	Acetone, PGH_2, phosphatidylcholine
	Fatty acids	Lauric acid, linoleic acid, oleic acid
	Flavonoids	Genistein
	Fluorinated hydrocarbons	Desflurane, enflurane, halothane, isoflurane, methoxyflurane, sevoflurane
	Indoles	Indole, 3-methylindole
	Insect repellents	*N,N*-Diethyl-*m*-toluamide
	Pesticides	Methoxychlor, parathion
	Drugs	Acetaminophen, albendazole, artesunate, bupropion, caffeine, capsaicin, chloroquine, chlorzoxazone, dacarbazine, dapsone, disulfiram, dorzolamide, eszopiclone, felbamate, fluoxetine, isoniazid, ondansetron, phenobarbital, primaquine, quinoline, ritonavir, salicylate, sulfadiazine, tamoxifen, tegafur, theobromine, theophylline, thiamylal, tolcapone, trimethadione, vesnarinone, zidovudine
CYP2J2	Fatty acids	Arachidonic acid, linoleic acid
	Steroids	Testosterone
	Vitamins	1α-Hydroxyvitamin D_3, vitamin D_2, vitamin D_3
	Drugs	Astemizole, bufuralol, diclofenac, ebastine
CYP2R1	Vitamins	1α-Hydroxyvitamin D_2, 1α-hydroxyvitamin D_3, vitamin D_2, vitamin D_3

[a]Abbreviations: CPO, 5-[4-[3-(4-cyclohexyl-2-propylphenoxy)propoxy]phenyl]-1,3-oxazolidine-2,4-dione; DEN, diethylnitrosamine; DMN, dimethylnitrosamine; MBDB, *N*-methylbenzodioxazolylbutanamine; MDA, 3,4-methylenedioxyamphetamine; MDE, 3,4-methylenedioxyethylamphetamine; MDMA, 3,4-methylenedioxymethamphetamine; MeIQ, 2-amino-3,5-dimethylimidazo[4,5-*f*]quinoline; MOCA, 4,4′-methylene-bis(2-chloroaniline); NNAL, 4-(methylnitrosamino)-1-(3-pyridyl)-1-butanol; NNK, 4-(methylnitrosamino)-1-(3-pyridyl)-1-butanone; NNN, nornitrosonicotine; PGH_2, prostaglandin H_2; PhIP, 2-amino-1-methyl-6-phenylimidazo[4,5-*b*]pyridine; THC, Δ⁹-tetrahydrocannabinol; thioTEPA, triethylenethiophosphoramide.

Source: Compiled from Refs. 40, 112, and 182–252. A detailed listing of substrates for CYP2 enzymes can be found in book chapters [2, 15, 50, 53, 55] and a review article [89].

662

at the amino acid level [253]. CYP2A6 is expressed primarily in liver. CYP2A7, which was originally named CYP2A4, is considered nonfunctional. CYP2A13 is expressed mainly in the nasal mucosa, followed by the trachea and lung [13]. Expression of CYP2A6 is subject to genetic polymorphism (see Table 18.4), with four allelic variants having been described. CYP2A6 is involved in the metabolism of several compounds found in tobacco. For example, CYP2A6 catalyzes the C-oxidation of nicotine, hydroxylation of cotinine at the 3′-position, hydroxylation of N-nitrosonornicotine at the 5′-position, and oxidation of 4-(methylnitrosoamino)-1-(3-pyridyl)-1-butanone and N-nitrosodiethylamine [253]. In terms of drug substrates, CYP2A6 preferentially catalyzes the hydroxylation of coumarin at the 7-position, which serves as a marker activity for this enzyme. Methoxypsoralen (methoxsalen), a structural analogue of coumarin, is a potent inhibitor of CYP2A6 [2].

There is only one CYP2B enzyme in humans, CYP2B6. A second CYP2B gene, CYP2B7, was identified as a splice variant of CYP2B6 but is not transcribed into protein [254]. CYP2B6 is expressed mostly in the liver [15, 254]. In a panel of 19 human liver microsome samples, CYP2B6 protein expression showed a 100-fold interindividual variability [255]. CYP2B6 shows sex and ethnic differences in expression and activity [256]. CYP2B6 is involved in the metabolism of relatively few drugs. It has been shown to catalyze the 4-hydroxylation of cyclophosphamide, and the N-demethylation of benzphetamine, (S)-mephenytoin, and diazepam [2]. Moreover, CYP2B6 catalyzes the O-dealkylation of 7-benzyloxyresorufin, methoxychlor, and 7-ethoxycoumarin [253]. However, the activities are not specific to CYP2B6 as other CYP enzymes such as CYP2C9 and CYP3A4 also contribute to these reactions. In rats, members of the CYP2B subfamily include CYP2B1, CYP2B2, and CYP2B3 [396]. Hepatic CYP2B1 and CYP2B2 are highly inducible in the rat following exposure to phenobarbital [15, 257]. Unlike the rat, little is known about induction of CYP2B6 in humans. In cultured human hepatocytes, CYP2B6 expression was increased following treatment with rifampicin, dexamethasone, and phenobarbital [255].

The CYP2C subfamily consists of four genes in humans, namely, CYP2C8, CYP2C9, CYP2C18, and CYP2C19. The four CYP2C enzymes are >80% identical in terms of amino acid sequence [15]. All four CYP2C enzymes are expressed primarily in liver (see Table 18.8), with CYP2C9 typically present at a higher level than CYP2C8, CYP2C18, or CYP2C19. CYP2C9 and CYP2C19 exhibit genetic polymorphism (see Table 18.4), with two allelic variants described for CYP2C9 and five allelic variants described for CYP2C19. CYP2C enzymes are involved in the metabolism of several important drugs. For example, CYP2C8 catalyzes the 6α-hydroxylation of taxol and the 4-hydroxylation of retinol and all-*trans* retinoic acid. CYP2C9 catalyzes tolbutamide hydroxylation, tienilic acid hydroxylation, phenytoin 4′-hydroxylation, diclofenac 4′-hydroxylation, and (S)-warfarin 7-hydroxylation [2]. CYP2C19 preferentially catalyzes the hydroxylation of (S)-mephenytoin at the 4′-position, which serves as a marker activity for this enzyme. No specific reactions have been identified for CYP2C18, which is expressed in trace amounts in liver. Sulfaphenazole is a potent selective inhibitor of CYP2C9 [2]. Inhibitors of CYP2C8 and CYP2C19 are known but they are not very specific.

There is a single functional member of the CYP2D subfamily in humans. CYP2D6 is expressed primarily in liver. Low levels have also been detected in extrahepatic tissues. CYP2D6 is a highly polymorphic enzyme. More than 60 allelic variants, which affect the amount of expression of the enzyme and its catalytic activity, have been described (see Table 18.4). The polymorphisms affecting CYP2D6 have clinical relevance because this enzyme is involved in the metabolism of at least 100 different drugs (see Table 18.10). For example, CYP2D6 catalyzes the 4-hydroxylation of propranolol and debrisoquine, O-demethylation of dextromethorphan, 1′-hydroxylation of bufuralol, 5′-hydroxylation of propafenone, and hydroxylation of sparteine, all of which can be used as marker activities for this enzyme. Quinidine is a relatively selective inhibitor of CYP2D6 [2].

CYP2E1 is the only member of the CYP2E subfamily in humans. It is expressed constitutively in liver, lung, and kidney [2]. Relatively few drugs are metabolized by CYP2E1, but this enzyme catalyzes ethanol oxidation, N1- and N7-demethylation of caffeine, N-oxidation of acetaminophen, and chlorzoxazone 6-hydroxylation, which serves as a marker activity for CYP2E1. CYP2E1 can be induced by ethanol and isoniazid. 4-Methylpyrazole is a relatively selective inhibitor for CYP2E1 [2].

CYP2F and CYP2J are two minor subfamilies with only one functional gene in each. CYP2F1 is expressed primarily in human lung. It has been shown to catalyze the oxidation of ethoxycoumarin and propoxycoumarin, and of 4-ipomeanol and 3-methylindole, two lung toxicants [13]. CYP2J2 is expressed in liver and intestine. It has been shown to catalyze the hydroxylation of ebastine, a second-generation antihistamine [357].

Additional enzymes in the CYP2 family include CYP2S1, CYP2U1, and CYP2W1, but their function remains unknown, as substrates for these enzymes have not been identified [11].

18.4.4   CYP3 Family

CYP3A enzymes are the predominant CYP enzymes expressed in human liver and intestine [14, 154]. The human CYP3A subfamily consists of CYP3A4, CYP3A5, CYP3A7, and CYP3A43. CYP3A enzymes catalyze the biotransformation of a wide variety of xenobiotic compounds, as well as bile acids and steroids (Table 18.11). Indeed, CYP3A substrates represent diverse chemical structures including cyclosporin A, which is the largest CYP substrate known. The prominent role played by CYP3A enzymes in drug metabolism is highlighted by an estimate that CYP3A enzymes are responsible for the biotransformation of greater than 50% of all prescription medications [154].

CYP3A enzymes catalyze the N-dealkylation of alfentanil, benzphetamine, codeine, dextromethorphan, erythromycin, imipramine, and tamoxifen, hydroxylation of midazolam at the 1′-position, hydroxylation of alprazolam at the 4-position, and N-oxidation of dihydropyridines such as nifedipine [50]. A catalytic activity that is common to CYP3A enzymes in many mammalian species, and is often used as a marker activity, is the stereoselective hydroxylation of testosterone and cortisol at the 6β-position [15] (see Table 18.7). Inhibitors of CYP3A include the macrolide antibiotics, antifungal agents such as clotrimazole and ketoconazole, HIV protease inhibitors, particularly ritonavir, and gestodene [2].

CYP3A4 is the single most abundant CYP enzyme in human liver and small intestine [14, 154]. All human liver and small intestine samples appear to contain CYP3A4, but levels vary by 10-fold or more among individuals [14, 155]. In contrast, CYP3A5 is expressed at a lower level (approximately one-third or less) than

TABLE 18.11 Substrates for Human CYP3A4

	Category of Substrates	Examples of Substrates[a]
CYP3A4	Azole antifungals	Clotrimazole, fluconazole, itraconazole, ketoconazole, miconazole, voriconazole
	Bile acids	Chenodeoxycholic acid, cholic acid, deoxycholic acid, lithocholic acid, taurochenodeoxycholic acid
	Carcinogens	
	Mycotoxins	Aflatoxin B_1, aflatoxin G_1, ochratoxin A, sterigmatocystin
	Polycyclic aromatics	6-Aminochrysene, benzo[a]pyrene, benzo[a]pyrene-7,8-diol, DDB[a]P, DDB[b]F, DDMBA, 1,6-dinitropyrene, 1-ethylpyrene, 1-methylpyrene, naphthalene, nitropyrene, phenanthrene
	Various carcinogens	17β-Estradiol, MeIQ, methoxyaminoazobenzene, MOCA, NNK, NNN, senecionine, Tris-BP
	Chloroaromatics	1,2-Dichlorobenzene, 1,2,4-trichlorobenzene, 1,2,3,5-tetrachlorobenzene, pentachlorobenzene
	Coumarins	BFC
	Endogenous compounds	9,10-Epoxystearic acid, N-hydroxyarginine, leukotoxin, PGH_2
	Ergot alkaloids	Bromocriptine, dihydroergotamine
	Flavonoids	Apigenin, 7,8-benzoflavone, genistein, kaempferol, naringenin, tamarixetin
	Fluorescent probes	Dibenzylfluorescein
	Fungicides	Furametpyr, o-phenylphenol
	Hormones	$1\alpha,25$-Dihydroxyvitamin D_3
	Insect repellents	N,N-Diethyl-m-toluamide
	Macrolides	Clarithromycin, erythromycin, miocamycin, roxithromycin, sirolimus, tacrolimus, troleandomycin
	Mycotoxins, other toxins	Myristicin, territrems B and C
	Pesticides	Acetochlor, alachlor, aldrin, ametryne, atrazine, butachlor, carbofuran, chlorpyrifos, chlortoluron, diazinon, endosulfan, methoxychlor, parathion, terbutryne
	Retinoids	Retinal, all-trans-retinoic acid, 9-cis-retinoic acid
	Rifamycins and derivatives	Benzoxazinorifamycins, rifalazil, rifampicin
	Steroid hormones, steroids	Androstenedione, budesonide, corticosterone, cortisol, dehydroepiandrosterone, dexamethasone, DHEA, dutasteride, estrone, 17α-ethinylestradiol, finasteride, fluticasone, gestodene, levonorgestrel, liloprisitone, medroxyprogesterone, mestranol, methandienone, methylprednisolone, mifepristone, norethisterone, onapristone, prednisolone, prednisone, pregnenolone, progesterone, testosterone
	Terpenes	Eucalyptol, limonene

TABLE 18.11 *Continued*

Category of Substrates	Examples of Substrates[a]
Drugs	Acetaminophen, adinazolam, albendazole, alfentanil, alfuzosin, alpidem, alprazolam, ambroxol, aminopyrine, aminopyrine, amiodarone, amitriptyline, amlodipine, amprenavir, anastrozole, antipyrine, aprepitant, AQ4N, aripiprazole, arteether, artelinic acid, artemether, artemisinin, astemizole, atazanavir, atorvastatin, azelastine, azimilide, barnidipine, benzphetamine, bepridil, bezafibrate, bicalutamide, bisoprolol, bosentan, brinzolamide, bromoperidol, brotizolam, bupivacaine, buprenorphine, bupropion, buspirone, busulfan, capravirine, capsaicin, carbamazepine, carvedilol, cerivastatin, chloroquine, chlorpromazine, cibenzoline, cimetidine, ciprofibrate, cisapride, citalopram, clindamycin, clobazam, clofibrate, clomethiazole, clomipramine, clonazepam, clopidogrel, clozapine, cocaine, codeine, colchicine, cyclobenzaprine, cyclophosphamide, cyclosporine, dantrolene, dapsone, delavirdine, desipramine, desmethyladinazolam, dextromethorphan, diazepam, diclofenac, digitoxin, dihydralazine, dihydrocodeine, diltiazem, disopyramide, docetaxel, dolasetron, donepezil, dorzolamide, doxepin, doxorubicin, ebastine, ecabapide, efavirenz, eletriptan, ellipticine, enalapril, eplerenone, esomeprazole, eszopiclone, ethosuximide, ethylmorphine, etizolam, etoperidone, etoposide, etoricoxib, exemestane, ezlopitant, felbamate, felodipine, fenofibrate, fentanyl, flosequinan, flunitrazepam, flutamide, fluvastatin, galantamine, gallopamil, ganaxolone, gefitinib, gemfibrozil, gepirone, germander, glibenclamide, glyceryltrinitrate, granisetron, halofantrine, haloperidol, hydrocodone, hydromorphone, ifosfamide, imatinib, imipramine, imiquimod, indinavir, ipomeanol, irinotecan, isoniazid, isosorbide dinitrate, isradipine, ivermectin, karenitecin, ketamine, ketobemidone, lansoprazole, laquinimod, letrozole, lidocaine, lisofylline, lisuride, lonafarnib, loperamide, lopinavir, loratadine, losartan, lovastatin, lumefantrine, MBDB, MDA, MDE, MDMA, medifoxamine, mefloquine, meloxicam, methadone, mexazolam, mianserin, mibefradil, midazolam, mifepristone, mirtazapine, MMDX, modafinil, montelukast, mosapride, mycophenolic acid, nateglinide, navelbine, nefazodone, nefiracetam, nelfinavir, nevirapine, nicardipine, nifedipine, niludipine, nilvaldipine, nimodipine, nisoldipine, nitrendipine, noralfentanil,

nordiazepam, nortriptyline, norverapamil, omeprazole, ondansetron, orphenadrine, oxodipine, oxybutynin, paclitaxel, pantoprazole, perazine, perospirone, perphenazine, phencyclidine, phenprocoumon, pimozide, pioglitazone, piroxicam, pradefovir, pranidipine, pravastatin, praziquantel, primaquine, propafenone, proguanil, pyrilamine, quetiapine, quinidine, quinine, rabeprazole, raloxifene, ranolazine, reboxetine, repaglinide, resiquimod, risperidone, ritonavir, rofecoxib, ropinirole, ropivacaine, roquinimex, rupatadine, salmeterol, saquinavir, selegiline, seratrodast, sertindole, sertraline, sibutramine, sildenafil, simvastatin, sterinodole, sufentanil, sulfadiazine, sulfamethoxazole, sulfamidine, tafenoquine, tamoxifen, tamsulosin, targretin, tasosartan, tauromustine, tazofelone, temazepam, teniposide, tentoxin, terbinafine, terfenadine, terguride, THC, theophylline, thiamylal, thioTEPA, tiagabine, ticlopidine, tinidazole, tipranavir, tirilazad, tolmetin, tolterodine, toremifene, trazodone, triazolam, triazolone, trimethadione, trimethoprim, trofosfamide, troglitazone, tropisetron, valdecoxib, valspodar, vanoxerine, vardenafil, venlafaxine, verapamil, vesnarinone, vinblastine, vincristine, vindesine, vinorelbine, warfarin, yohimbine, zafirlukast, zaleplon, zatosetron, zidovudine, zileuton, ziprasidone, zopiclone, zolpidem, zomepirac, zonisamide, zotepine

[a]Abbreviations: AQ4N, 1,4-bis[[2-(dimethylamino-N-oxide)ethyl]amino]-5,8-dihydroxyanthracene-9,10-dione; BFC, 7-benzyloxy-4-trifluoromethylcoumarin; DDB[a]P, 7,8-dihydroxy-7,9-dihydrobenzo[a]pyrene; DDB[b]F, 9,10-dihydroxy-9,10-dihydrobenzo[b]fluoranthene; DDMBA, 3,4-dihydroxy-3,4-dihydro-7,12-dimethylbenz[a]anthracene; DHEA, dehydroepiandrosterone; MBDB, N-methylbenzodioxazolylbutanamine; MDA, 3,4-methylenedioxyamphetamine; MDE, 3,4-methylenedioxyethylamphetamine; MDMA, 3,4-methylenedioxymethamphetamine; MeIQ, 2-amino-3,5-dimethylimidazo[4,5-f]quinoline; MMDX, methoxymorpholinodoxorubicin; MOCA, 4,4′-methylene-bis(2-chloroaniline); NNK, 4-(methylnitrosamino)-1-(3-pyridyl)-1-butanone; NNN, nornitrosonicotine; PGH$_2$, prostaglandin H$_2$; THC, Δ^9-tetrahydrocannabinol; thioTEPA, triethylenethiophosphoramide; Tris-BP, tris-(2,3-dibromopropyl)phosphate.

Source: Compiled from Refs. 59, 118, 199, 212, 221, 238, 244, 247, and 258–344. A comprehensive listing of substrates for CYP3A enzymes can be found in book chapters [2, 15, 50, 53, 55], a review article [89], and websites [397, 398].

CYP3A4 and in only 10–30% of human liver and intestine samples [14, 155]. CYP3A5 has also been detected in human kidney [2]. The lack of CYP3A5 expression in most humans is thought to be due to a splice site mutation [345]. CYP3A7 is considered to be a fetal enzyme and accounts for 30–50% of total CYP content in fetal liver [345]. CYP3A7 is now recognized to be expressed in some adult livers [345]. CYP3A43 mRNA is expressed at low levels in the liver and at relatively high levels in the testis and prostate. In earlier studies, a fifth CYP3A enzyme, CYP3A3, was identified. This enzyme showed strong homology to CYP3A4. It is now believed that CYP3A3 is in fact an allelic variant of CYP3A4 [345]. Both CYP3A5 and CYP3A7 have similar substrate specificities as CYP3A4. The substrate specificity of CYP3A43 is unknown since only low levels of expression have been achieved in recombinant systems [345]. The human CYP3A enzymes can be induced by treatment with drugs such as phenobarbital, rifampicin, phenytoin, and troglitazone [50], and this induction can result in clinically relevant drug interactions.

In rats, the CYP3A subfamily includes CYP3A1, CYP3A2, CYP3A9, CYP3A18, and CYP3A62 [346, 396]. A sixth rat CYP3A enzyme, CYP3A23, has also been reported in the literature, but this is now believed to be an allelic variant of CYP3A1 [346, 347]. CYP3A2, CYP3A9, CYP3A18, and CYP3A62 display age- and sex-specific regulation and induction [348, 349]. For example, CYP3A2 is constitutively expressed in hepatic microsomes from immature rats of both sexes and mature male rats but not in adult female rats [348]. CYP3A18 is expressed predominantly in adult male rats, whereas CYP3A9 is expressed at higher levels in adult female rats than in male rats [350]. Dexamethasone treatment increases hepatic microsomal levels of CYP3A2 in immature rats and adult male but not adult female rats [348]. CYP3A1 is undetectable in hepatic microsomes from untreated rats of either sex but following administration of dexamethasone, hepatic levels of CYP3A1 are increased dramatically [348]. CYP3A1 can account for 30–37% of total CYP content in hepatic microsomes prepared from dexamethasone-treated immature and mature rats of both sexes. Expression of hepatic CYP3A9, CYP3A18, and CYP3A62 enzymes is also increased by administration of dexamethasone [346, 348]. Other inducers of rat CYP3A enzymes include phenobarbital, rifampicin, isosafrole, and pregnenolone 16α-carbonitrile [348].

18.4.5 CYP4 Family

Members of the CYP4 family generally metabolize endogenous fatty acid substrates such as lauric, palmitic, and arachidonic acids and their derivatives including prostaglandins, thromboxane, prostacyclin, and leukotrienes (Table 18.12). CYP4 enzymes play a minor role in the metabolism of drugs and other xenobiotics.

The CYP4A subfamily consists of CYP4A9 and CYP4A11. CYP4A11 is expressed in human liver and kidney. The expression and function of CYP4A9 is not known at present. CYP4A11 preferentially catalyzes the ω (terminal carbon) hydroxylation of fatty acids, although it can also catalyze hydroxylation at the ω-1 (penultimate carbon) position [2]. Hence the characteristic activity of CYP4A11 is hydroxylation of lauric acid at the 12-(ω) position (see Table 18.7). CYP4A enzymes in rats are inducible by peroxisomal proliferators such as clofibrate. Induction of CYP4A11 by clofibrate has also been reported in primary cultures of human hepatocytes [360].

TABLE 18.12   Substrates for Human CYP4 Enzymes

CYP	Category of Substrates	Examples of Substrates[a]
CYP4A11	Fatty acids, leukotrienes	Arachidonic acid, lauric acid, LTB_4, linoleic acid, palmitic acid, 9,10-epoxystearic acid, isoleukotoxin, leukotoxin
	Eicosanoic acids	15-HETE
	Prostaglandins	9,11-Epoxymethano-PGH_2, 11,9-epoxymethano-PGH_2, 9,11-diazo-15-deoxy-PGH_2
	Drugs	Artesunate, pentamidine
CYP4F2	Aromatic hydrocarbons	7-Ethoxycoumarin, p-nitroanisole
	Fatty acids, leukotrienes, lipoxins	Arachidonic acid, hydroxystearic acids, LTB_4, 6-*trans*-LTB_4, oleic acid, lipoxin A_4, 9,10-epoxystearic acid, isoleukotoxin, leukotoxin
	Eicosanoic acids	5,6-EET, 8,9-EET, 11,12-EET, 14,15-EET, 5-HETE, 8-HETE, 9-HETE, 11-HETE, 12-HETE, 15-HETE
CYP4F3B	Fatty acids, leukotrienes	Arachidonic acid, 9,10-dihydroxyoctadec-12-enoic acid, 12,13-dihydroxyoctadec-9-enoic acid, 9,10-dihydroxystearic acid, LTB_4, 9,10-epoxystearic acid, isoleukotoxin, leukotoxin
	Eicosanoic acids	5,6-DHET, 8,9-DHET, 11,12-DHET, 14,15-DHET, 5,6-EET, 8,9-EET, 11,12-EET, 14,15-EET
CYP4F11	Fatty acids, leukotrienes	Arachidonic acid, LTB_4
	Eicosanoic acids	8-HETE
	Drugs	Benzphetamine, chlorpromazine, erythromycin, ethylmorphine, imipramine, theophylline, verapamil
CYP4F12	Fatty acids, leukotrienes	Arachidonic acid, LTB_4
	Prostaglandins	11,9-Epoxymethano-PGH_2, 9,11-diazo-15-deoxy-PGH_2
	Drugs	Ebastine

[a]Abbreviations: DHET, dihydroxyeicosatrienoic acid; EET, epoxyeicosatrienoic acid; HETE, hydroxyeicosatetraenoic acid; LTB_4, leukotriene B_4; PGH_2, prostaglandin H_2.
Source: Compiled from Refs. 15, 29, 55, 89, and 351–361.

The human CYP4F subfamily consists of five genes, CYP4F2, CYP4F3, CYP4F8, CYP4F11, and CYP4F12 [358, 359]. CYP4F enzymes have been detected at the level of mRNA in numerous tissues in humans including leukocytes, liver, lung, kidney, intestine, heart, brain, and skin [358, 359]. CYP4F enzymes are involved in the oxidation of fatty acids, leukotrienes, and prostaglandins (Table 18.12).

18.4.6   Regulation of CYP Enzyme Expression

The expression of CYP genes in many species is highly regulated by age, hormonal factors including sex steroids, growth hormone, and thyroid hormones, diet and nutritional status, and disease states. Indeed, regulation of hepatic CYP enzymes is complex. Although the mechanisms and consequences of induction of CYP enzymes have been studied intensively, relatively little is known about the mechanisms by which CYP enzymes are regulated by physiological factors. In humans, CYP enzyme expression appears to be regulated mainly via induction by xenobiotics (i.e., drugs, environmental compounds including those present in cigarette smoke, dietary components, and ethanol) and possibly by hormones. CYP enzyme induction has consequences in terms of drug pharmacokinetics, accumulation, and toxicity.

Induction of CYP enzymes usually occurs at the level of transcription and results in *de novo* protein synthesis. There are several mechanisms that involve interactions with regulatory elements in the relevant CYP gene, by which CYP genes can be induced. Most commonly, inducers bind to a receptor protein, which then binds to regulatory elements in the DNA, and activates gene transcription and translation. Alternatively, the inducer can interact, either directly or indirectly, with a repressor protein that would normally be bound to the operator region of the CYP gene and repress its expression. Binding of the inducer would release the repressor and result in increased transcription of the structural region of the gene [15]. Specific xenobiotic receptor proteins have now been identified as being involved in gene induction by four distinct mechanisms [369, 370]. Inducing agents can bind to four different xenobiotic receptors, namely, the aryl hydrocarbon receptor (AhR), the constitutive androstane receptor (CAR), the pregnane X receptor (PXR), and the peroxisomal proliferator-activated receptor (PPAR). Typical inducers of human CYP enzymes are presented in Table 18.13.

The Ah receptor is a ligand-activated nuclear transcription factor that controls the expression of a battery of genes including CYP1A1, CYP1A2, and CYP1B1 [371, 372]. The AhR is ubiquitously expressed in most organs and is conserved across many species including mammals and invertebrates [181]. Once activated, the AhR translocates to the nucleus, where it forms a heterodimer with the aryl hydrocarbon nuclear translocator (ARNT) [373]. This heterodimer complex then binds to a

TABLE 18.13   Inducers of Human CYP Enzymes

CYP	Inducers[a]
CYP1A1	Chargrilled meat, omeprazole, PCBs, polycyclic aromatics (e.g., DMBA, MC), TCDD
CYP1A2	Chargrilled meat, cruciferous vegetables (e.g., broccoli, Brussels sprouts), hyperforin, omeprazole, PCBs, polycyclic aromatics, TCDD
CYP1B1	PCBs, polycyclic aromatics, TCDD
CYP2A6	Phenobarbital
CYP2B6	Nevirapine, phenobarbital, dexamethasone, troglitazone
CYP2C8	Rifampicin
CYP2C9	Hyperforin, phenobarbital, rifampicin
CYP2C19	Rifampicin, ritonavir
CYP2D6	Unknown
CYP2E1	Ethanol, isoniazid
CYP3A4	Bosentan, carbamazepine, cortisol, dexamethasone, efavirenz, felbamate, hyperforin, nevirapine, phenobarbital, phenytoin, primidone, rifampicin, rifapentin, sulfadimidine, topiramate, troglitazone
CYP4A11	Clofibrate

[a]Abbreviations: DMBA, 7,12-dimethylbenz[*a*]anthracene; MC, 3-methylcholanthrene; PCBs, polychlorinated biphenyls; TCDD, 2,3,7,8-tetrachlorodibenzo-*p*-dioxin.

Source: Compiled from Refs. 19, 26, 158, and 360–370. A comprehensive listing of CYP inducers can be found in book chapters [2, 15, 50, 55], a review article [89], and a website [398].

xenobiotic response element in the promoter region upstream of the CYP1A1 and CYP1A2 genes. Binding of the heterodimer complex to the xenobiotic response element results in recruitment of coregulatory proteins and relaxation of chromatin structure, which promotes transcription [181]. One of the most potent inducers of CYP1A expression is the highly toxic compound, TCDD. Other xenobiotic AhR ligands include 3-methylcholanthrene, indolo[2,3-*b*]carbazole, and coplanar PCBs [181] (Table 18.14). Endogenous AhR ligands include tryptamine, bilirubin, and indirubin [181].

Phenobarbital is a prototype agent for a variety of structurally unrelated inducers that elicit induction of CYP2B enzymes in a number of mammalian species. Induction of the CYP2B enzymes occurs mainly through the activation of CAR, a novel nuclear receptor. Following exposure to phenobarbital-type inducers, CAR translocates from the cytoplasm to the nucleus, where it binds and activates a phenobarbital-responsive element upstream of the CYP2B genes [374]. CAR, which is highly expressed in liver, is known to dimerize with the retinoid X receptor (RXR) and can constitutively activate its target genes even in the absence of inducers. Normally, endogenous androstane-like steroids bind to CAR and maintain it in an inactive state. The binding of phenobarbital-type inducers interferes with the binding of the inhibitory steroids so that receptor activity is derepressed and gene transcrip-

TABLE 18.14   Receptors and Xenobiotic Activators/Ligands of Human CYP Genes

Receptors[a]	Xenobiotic Activators/Ligands[a]	Regulated CYP Genes
AhR	Guanabenz, omeprazole, PCBs, polycyclic aromatics (e.g., benzo[*a*]pyrene, MC), TCDD, TCDF, thiabendazole	CYP1A1, CYP1A2, CYP1B1
CAR	CITCO, hyperforin, methoxychlor, phenobarbital, phenytoin, rifampicin	CYP2A6, CYP2B6, CYP2C8, CYP2C9, CYP2C19, CYP3A4
PPARα	Bezafibrate, clofibrate, fenofibrate, fenoprofen, flufenamic acid, gemfibrozil, herbicides, ibuprofen, indomethacin, phthalates, Wy-14,643	CYP4A11
PXR	Amprenavir, avasimibe, bosentan, carbamazepine, chlorpyrifos, CITCO, clotrimazole, cypermethrin, dexamethasone, DDT, dieldrin, efavirenz, endosulfan, endrin, etoposide, glibenclamide, hyperforin, lovastatin, mifepristone, methoxychlor, nelfinavir, nifedipine, nonylphenol, paclitaxel, phenobarbital, phenytoin, rifabutin, rifampicin, ritonavir, simvastatin, tamoxifen, TCPOBOP, topiramate, triclosan, troglitazone	CYP2A6, CYP2B6, CYP2C8, CYP2C9, CYP2C19, CYP3A4

[a]Abbreviations: AhR, aryl hydrocarbon receptor; CAR, constitutive androstane receptor; CITCO, 6-(4-chlorophenyl)imidazo[2,1-*b*][1,3]thiazole-5-carbaldehyde *O*-(3,4-dichlorobenzyl)oxime; DDT, dichlorodiphenyltrichloroethane; MC, 3-methylcholanthrene; PCBs, polychlorinated biphenyls; PPARα, peroxisome proliferator-activated receptor α; PXR, pregnane X receptor; TCDD, 2,3,7,8-tetrachlorodibenzo-*p*-dioxin; TCDF, 2,3,7,8-tetrachlorodibenzofuran; TCPOBOP, 1,4-bis[2-(3,5-dichloropyridyloxy)]benzene; Wy-14,643, [4-chloro-6-(2,3-xylidino)pyrimidynylthio]acetic acid.
Source: Compiled from Refs. 23, 26, 94, 154, 181, 366, and 369–395.

tion can proceed [369, 370]. CYP2B enzymes can be induced by a variety of anti-microbials, barbiturates, and pesticides. Some examples include clotrimazole, rifampicin, phenytoin, methoxychlor, and dichlorodiphenyltrichloroethane (DDT) [374, 375].

Another novel nuclear receptor, PXR (also known as PAR and SXR) [376], mediates induction of CYP3A genes in response to glucocorticoids such as dexamethasone and drugs such as rifampicin [28] (Table 18.14). CYP3A4 and CYP3A5 enzymes are inducible following administration of rifampicin although CYP3A5 is induced to a lesser extent than CYP3A4 [345]. Induction of the CYP3A subfamily occurs mainly through activation of PXR. PXR binds as a heterodimer with RXR to xenobiotic response elements in the proximal promoter regions of the CYP3A genes [154]. Induction of the CYP3A subfamily shows distinct species-specific differences. For example, rifampicin is a potent inducer of human CYP3A4 but is a weak inducer of rat CYP3A2 [154]. Studies have suggested that CAR may also be involved in transcriptional activation of the CYP3A genes since CAR can bind to xenobiotic response elements in the promoter region of the CYP3A genes [154]. Experimental evidence indicates that the glucocorticoid receptor may participate in the induction of CYP3A4, but the molecular mechanism is not clear [377].

The peroxisomal proliferator-activated receptor (PPAR) is highly expressed in liver and mediates peroxisome proliferation and induction of CYP4A enzymes [369] (Table 18.14).

18.5   CONCLUSION

Insight into the biotransformation of drugs by CYP and other drug-metabolizing enzymes is a prerequisite for the evaluation of drug safety and risk assessment. Moreover, comprehensive knowledge of the regulation and activity of CYP enzymes and an awareness of possible drug interactions is needed to avoid possible adverse effects associated with the common practice of prescribing several drugs simultaneously.

There are still many gaps in our knowledge of CYP enzymes. There is a practical need for better and more specific reagents to measure CYP enzyme activity and CYP enzyme levels in various tissues. For example, the ready availability of highly specific inhibitory antibodies and potent specific chemical inhibitors for each CYP enzyme would be highly desirable. This would allow investigators to identify the individual CYP enzymes involved in the metabolism of a particular drug and to quantify the enzymes in both hepatic and extrahepatic tissues. Also needed are highly selective and safe *in vivo* probes of CYP activity to allow investigators to estimate CYP levels in patients without the need to take liver biopsy samples. The large interindividual variability in CYP enzyme levels complicates drug therapy and efficacy. Expression profiling studies with larger banks of human tissues and human subjects are needed to discover the extent of variation of individual CYP protein levels, to delineate the causes of the variation, and to map distribution patterns of CYP enzymes within a population.

Recent advances are expanding our knowledge of the CYP enzymes and providing therapeutic benefits. For example, the development of CYP knockout mouse models is enabling investigators to explore the role and importance of CYP enzymes in normal physiology. Pharmacogenomic testing is also currently receiving much attention because of the increasing awareness of the benefits of incorporating pharmacogenomics into the selection of drug regimens. The selection of proper drug regimen and dose based on the patient's individual genetic makeup could eliminate the unpredictable response of drug treatment, which may arise because of genetic polymorphisms that affect drug metabolism, clearance, and tolerance. Lastly, computational models can be used to predict the metabolism of specific drugs by CYP enzymes, to "design out" unfavorable drug interactions, and to help guide the drug design process.

ACKNOWLEDGMENTS

Research in the authors' laboratory has been supported by grants from the Natural Sciences and Engineering Research Council of Canada, the Canadian Institutes of Health Research, and the Toxic Substances Research Initiative (Health Canada). The authors thank Dr. Ted Lakowski and Mr. Patrick Edwards for their highly valued input in the preparation of this chapter.

REFERENCES

1. Wrighton SA, Stevens JC. The human hepatic cytochromes P450 involved in drug metabolism. *Crit Rev Toxicol* 1992;22:1–21.
2. Parkinson A. Biotransformation of xenobiotics. In Klaasen CD, Ed. *Casarett and Doull's Toxicology: The Basic Science of Poisons*, 6th ed. New York: McGraw Hill; 2001, pp 133–224.
3. Peterson JA, Graham-Lorence SE. Bacterial P450s: structural similarities and functional differences. In *Ortiz de Montellano PR, Ed. Cytochrome P450: Structure, Mechanism, and Biochemistry*, 2nd ed. New York: Plenum Press; 1995, pp 151–180.
4. von Wachenfeldt C, Johnson EF. Structures of eukaryotic cytochrome P450 enzymes. In *Ortiz de Montellano PR, Ed. Cytochrome P450: Structure, Mechanism, and Biochemstry*, 2nd ed. New York: Plenum Press; 1995, pp 183–223.
5. Axelrod J. The enzymic demethylation of ephedrine. *J Pharmacol Exp Ther* 1955;114: 430–438.
6. Brodie B, Axelrod J, Cooper JR, Gaudette L, LaDu BN, Mitoma C, Udenfriend S. Detoxification of drugs and other foreign compounds by liver microsomes. *Science* 1955;121:603–604.
7. Klingenberg M. Pigments of rat liver microsomes. *Arch Biochem Biophys* 1958;75: 376–386.
8. Garfinkel D. Studies on pig liver microsomes. I. Enzymic and pigment composition of different microsomal fractions. *Arch Biochem Biophys* 1958;77:493–509.
9. Omura T, Sato R. The carbon monoxide-binding pigment of liver microsomes. *J Biol Chem* 1964;239:2370–2378.
10. Bandiera SM. Cytochrome P450 enzymes as biomarkers of PCB exposure and modulators of toxicity. In Robertson LW, Hansen LG, Eds. *PCBs: Recent Advances in Environmental Toxicology and Health Effects*. Lexington: University Press of Kentucky, 2001, pp 185–192.

11. Guengerich FP, Wu ZL, Bartleson CJ. Function of human cytochrome P450s: characterization of the orphans. *Biochem Biophys Res Commun* 2005;338:465–469.

12. Nelson DR, Kamataki T, Waxman DJ, Guengerich FP, Estabrook RW, Feyereisen R, Gonzalez FJ, Coon MJ, Gunsalus IC, Gotoh O, Okuda K, Nebert DW. The cytochrome P450 superfamily: update on new sequences, gene mapping, accession numbers, and nomenclature. *Pharmacogenetics* 1996;6:1–42.

13. Ding X, Kaminsky LS. Human extrahepatic cytochromes P450: function in xenobiotic metabolism and tissue-selective chemical toxicity in the respiratory and gastrointestinal tracts. *Annu Rev Pharmacol Toxicol* 2003;43:149–173.

14. Paine MF, Hart HL, Ludington SS, Haining RL, Rettie AE, Zeldin DC. The human intestinal cytochrome P450 "pie." *Drug Metab Dispos* 2006;34:880–886.

15. Lewis DFV. *Cytochromes P450: Structure, Function and Mechanism*. London: Taylor and Francis; 1996.

16. Bhamre S, Anandatheerathavarada HK, Shankar SK, Boyd MR, Ravindranath V. Purification of multiple forms of cytochrome P450 from a human brain and reconstitution of catalytic activities. *Arch Biochem Biophys* 1993;301:251–255.

17. Hellmold H, Rylander T, Magnusson M, Reihnér E, Warner M, Gustafsson J-Å. Characterization of cytochrome P450 enzymes in human breast tissue from reduction mammaplasties. *J Clin Endocrinol Metab* 1998;83:886–895.

18. Mason JI, Estabrook RW, Purvis JL. Testicular cytochrome P450 and iron–sulfur protein as related to steroid metabolism. *Ann NY Acad Sci* 1973;212:406–419.

19. Lee IP, Suzuki K, Mukhtar H, Bend JR. Hormonal regulation of cytochrome P-450-dependent monooxygenase activity and epoxide-metabolizing enzyme activities in testis of hypophysectomized rats. *Cancer Res* 1980;40:2486–2492.

20. Watanabe M, Abe T. Aryl hydrocarbon hydroxylase and its components in human lung microsomes. *Gann* 1981;72:806–810.

21. Denisov IG, Markis TM, Sligar SG, Schlichting I. Structure and chemistry of cytochrome P450. *Chem Rev* 2005;105:2254–2277.

22. Nebert DW, Adesnik M, Coon MJ, Estabrook RW, Gonzalez FJ, Guengerich FP, Gunsalus IC, Johnson EF, Kemper B, Levin W, Phillips IR, Satoh R, Waterman MR. The P450 gene superfamily: recommended nomenclature. *DNA* 1987;6:1–11.

23. Honkakoski P, Negishi M. Regulation of cytochrome P450 (CYP) genes by nuclear receptors. *Biochem J* 2000;347:321–337.

24. Okey AB. Enzyme induction in the cytochrome P-450 system. *Pharmacol Ther* 1990;45:241–298.

25. Miners JO, McKinnon RA. CYP1A. In Levy RH, Thummel KE, Trager WF, Hansten PD, Eichelbaum M, Eds. *Metabolic Drug Interactions*. Philadelphia: Lippincott Williams & Wilkins; 2000, pp 61–73.

26. Nebert DW, Dalton TP, Okey AB, Gonzalez FJ. Role of aryl hydrocarbon receptor-mediated induction of the CYP1 enzymes in environmental toxicity and cancer. *J Biol Chem* 2004;279:23847–23850.

27. Ryan DE, Levin W. Purification and characterization of hepatic microsomal cytochrome P450. *Pharmacol Ther* 1990;45:153–239.

28. Schuetz EG, Brimer C, Schuetz JD. Environmental xenobiotics and the antihormones cyproterone acetate and spironolactone use the nuclear hormone pregnenolone X receptor to activate the *CYP3A23* hormone response element. *Mol Pharmacol* 1998;54:1113–1117.

29. Hoch U, Zhang Z, Kroetz DL, Ortiz de Montellano PR. Structural determination of the substrate specificities and regioselectivities of the rat and human fatty acid ω-hydroxylases. *Arch Biochem Biophys* 2000;373:63–71.

30. Imaoka S, Ogawa H, Kimura S, Gonzalez FJ. Complete cDNA sequence and cDNA-directed expression of CYP4A11, a fatty acid omega-hydroxylase expressed in human kidney. *DNA Cell Biol* 1993;12:893–899.

31. Kharasch ED, Hankins DC, Thummel KE. Human kidney methoxyflurane and sevoflurane metabolism: intrarenal fluoride production as a possible mechanism of methoxyflurane nephrotoxicity. *Anesthesiology* 1995;82:689–699.

32. Hakkola J, Pasanen M, Hukkanen J, Pelkonen O, Mäenpää J, Edwards RJ, Boobis AR, Raunio H. Expression of xenobiotic-metabolizing cytochrome P450 forms in human full-term placenta. *Biochem Pharmacol* 1996;51:403–411.

33. Huang Z, Fasco MJ, Figge HL, Keyomarsi K, Kaminsky LS. Expression of cytochromes P450 in human breast tissue and tumors. *Drug Metab Dispos* 1996;24:899–905.

34. Zheng Y-M, Fisher MB, Yokotani N, Fujii-Kuriyama Y, Rettie AE. Identification of a meander region praline critical for heme binding to cytochrome P450: implications for the catalytic function of human CYP4B1. *Biochemistry* 1998;37:12847–12851.

35. Gervot L, Rochat B, Gautier JC, Bohnenstengel F, Kroemer H, de Berardinis V, Martin H, Beaune P, de Waziers I. Human CYP2B6: expression, inducibility and catalytic activities. *Pharmacogenetics* 1999;9:295–306.

36. Rylander T, Neve EPA, Ingelman-Sundberg M, Oscarson M. Identification and tissue distribution of the novel human cytochrome P450 2S1 (CYP2S1). *Biochem Biophys Res Commun* 2001;281:529–535.

37. Smith G, Wolf CR, Deeni YY, Dawe RS, Evans AT, Comrie MM, Ferguson J, Ibbotson SH. Cutaneous expression of cytochrome P450 CYP2S1: individuality in regulation by therapeutic agents for psoriasis and other skin diseases. *Lancet* 2003;361:1336–1343.

38. Miksys S, Tyndale RF. The unique regulation of brain cytochrome P450 2 (CYP2) family enzymes by drugs and genetics. *Drug Metab Rev* 2004;36:313–333.

39. Swanson HI. Cytochrome P450 expression in human keratinocytes: an aryl hydrocarbon receptor perspective. *Chem-Biol Interact* 2004;149:69–79.

40. Kinobe RT, Parkinson OT, Mitchell DJ, Gillam EMJ. P450 2C18 catalyzes the metabolic bioactivation of phenytoin. *Chem Res Toxicol* 2005;18:1868–1875.

41. Savas U, Hsu M-H, Griffin KJ, Bell DR, Johnson EF. Conditional regulation of the human CYP4X1 and CYP4Z1 genes. *Arch Biochem Biophys* 2005;436:377–385.

42. Chinta SJ, Kommaddi RP, Turman CM, Strobel HW, Ravindranath V. Constitutive expression and localization of cytochrome P-450 1A1 in rat and human brain: presence of a splice variant form in human brain. *J Neurochem* 2005;93:724–736.

43. Karlgren M, Miura S-I, Ingelman-Sundberg M. Novel extrahepatic cytochrome P450s. *Toxicol Appl Pharmacol* 2005;207:S57–S61.

44. Raimundo S, Fischer JU, Eichelbaum M, Griese, E-U, Schwab M, Zanger UM. Elucidation of the genetic basis of the common metaboliser phenotype for drug oxidation by CYP2D6. *Pharmacogenetics* 2000;20:577–581.

45. Brockmöller J, Kirchheiner J, Meisel C, Roots I. Pharmacogenetic diagnostics of cytochrome P450 polymorphisms in clinical drug development and in drug treatment. *Pharmacogenomics* 2000;1:125–152.

46. Zanger U, Eichelbaum M, CYP2D6. In Levy RH, Thummel KE, Tager WF, Hansten PD, Eichebaum M, Eds. *Metabolic Drug Interactions*. Philadelphia: Lippincott Williams & Wilkins; 2000, pp 87–94.

47. Guengerich FP, Liebler DC. Enzymatic activation of chemicals to toxic metabolites. *CRC Crit Rev Toxicol* 1985;14:259–262.

48. Conney AH. Induction of microsomal enzymes by foreign chemicals and carcinogenesis by polycyclic aromatic hydrocarbons: G.H.A. Clowes Memorial Lecture. *Cancer Res* 1982;42:4875–4917.

49. Guengerich FP. Reactions and significance of cytochrome P450 enzymes. *J Biol Chem* 1991;266:10019–10022.

50. Williams DA. Drug metabolism. In Williams DA, Lemke TL, Eds. *Foye's Principles of Medicinal Chemistry*, 5th ed. Baltimore: Lippincott Williams & Wilkins; 2002, pp 174–233.

51. Guengerich FP, Shimada T. Oxidation of toxic and carcinogenic chemicals by human cytochrome P-450 enzymes. *Chem Res Toxicol* 1991;4:391–407.

52. Gonzalez FJ, Gelboin HV. Role of human cytochromes P450 in the metabolic activation of chemical carcinogens and toxins. *Drug Metab Rev* 1994;26:165–183.

53. Guengerich FP, Human cytochrome P450 enzymes. In Ortiz de Montellano PR, Ed. *Cytochrome P450: Structure, Mechanism, and Biochemistry*, 2nd ed. New York: Plenum Press; 1995, pp 473–535.

54. Low LK, Metabolic changes of drugs and related organic compounds. In Delgado JN, Remers WA, Eds. *Textbook of Organic Medicinal and Pharmaceutical Chemistry*. Philadelphia: Lippincott Williams & Wilkins; 1998, pp 43–122.

55. Lewis DFV, *Guide to Cytochromes P450: Structure and Function*. London: Taylor and Francis; 2001.

56. Shimada T, Oda Y, Gillam EMJ, Guengerich FP, Inoue K. Metabolic activation of polycyclic aromatic hydrocarbons and other procarcinogens by cytochromes P450 1A1 and P450 1B1 allelic variants and other human cytochromes P450 in *Salmonella typhimurium* NM2009. *Drug Metab Dispos* 2001;29:1176–1182.

57. Patterson LH, Murray GI. Tumour cytochrome P450 and drug activation. *Curr Pharm Design* 2002;8:1335–1347.

58. Rooseboom M, Commandeur JNM, Vermeulen NPE. Enzyme-catalyzed activation of anticancer prodrugs. *Pharmacol Rev* 2004;56:53–102.

59. Vignati L, Turlizzi E, Monaci S, Grossi P, de Kanter R, Monshouwer M. An *in vitro* approach to detect metabolite toxicity due to CYP3A4-dependent bioactivation of xenobiotics. *Toxicology* 2005;216:154–167.

60. Hrycay EG, O'Brien PJ. Cytochrome P-450 as a microsomal peroxidase in steroid hydroperoxide reduction. *Arch Biochem Biophys*, 1972;153:480–494.

61. Hrycay EG, O'Brien PJ, van Lier JE, Kan G. Pregnene 17α-hydroperoxides as possible precursors of the adrenosteroid hormones. *Arch Biochem Biophys*, 1972;153:495–501.

62. Hrycay EG, Gustafsson J-Å, Ingelman-Sundberg M, Ernster L. The involvement of cytochrome P-450 in hepatic microsomal steroid hydroxylation reactions supported by sodium periodate, sodium chlorite, and organic hydroperoxides. *Eur J Biochem* 1976;61:43–52.

63. Hrycay EG, Bandiera SM. Spectral interactions of tetrachlorobiphenyls with hepatic microsomal cytochrome P450 enzymes. *Chem-Biol Interact* 2003;146:285–296.

64. Aoyama T, Yamano S, Guzelian PS, Gelboin HV, Gonzalez FJ. Five of 12 forms of Vaccinia virus-expressed human hepatic cytochrome P450 metabolically activate aflatoxin B_1. *Proc Natl Acad Sci USA* 1990;87:4790–4793.

65. Larrey D, Tinel M, Letteron P, Maurel P, Loeper J, Belghiti J, Pessayre D. Metabolic activation of the new tricyclic antidepressant tianeptine by human liver cytochrome P450. *Biochem Pharmacol* 1990;40:545–550.

66. Czerwinski M, McLemore TL, Philpot RM, Nhamburo PT, Korzekwa K, Gelboin HV, Gonzalez FJ. Metabolic activation of 4-ipomeanol by complementary DNA-expressed human cytochromes P-450: evidence for species-specific metabolism. *Cancer Res* 1991;51:4636–4638.

67. Tanimoto Y, Kaneko H, Ohkuma T, Oguri K, Yoshimura H. Site-selective oxidation of strychnine by phenobarbital inducible cytochrome P-450. *J Pharmacobio-Dynamics* 1991;14:161–169.

68. Shou M, Korzekwa KR, Krausz KW, Crespi CL, Gonzalez FJ, Gelboin HV. Regio- and stereo-selective metabolism of phenanthrene by twelve cDNA-expressed human, rodent, and rabbit cytochromes P-450. *Cancer Lett* 1994;83:305–313.

69. Rauschenbach R, Gieschen H, Husemann M, Salomon B, Hildebrand M. Stable expression of human cytochrome P450 3A4 in V79 cells and its application for metabolic profiling of ergot derivatives. *Eur J Pharmacol* 1995;293:183–190.

70. Caccia S, Metabolism of the newer antidepressants. *Clin Pharmacokinet* 1998;34: 281–302.

71. Daly JW. Thirty years of discovering arthropod alkaloids in amphibian skin. *J Nat Products* 1998;61:162–172.

72. Strolin-Benedetti M, Brogin G, Bani M, Oesch F, Hengstler JG. Association of cytochrome P450 induction with oxidative stress *in vivo* as evidenced by 3-hydroxylation of salicylate. *Xenobiotica* 1999;29:1171–1180.

73. Prior TI, Chue PS, Tibbo P, Baker GB. Drug metabolism and atypical antipsychotics. *Eur Neuropsychopharmacol* 1999;9:301–309.

74. Baker GB, Urichuk LJ, McKenna KF, Kennedy SH. Metabolism of monoamine oxidase inhibitors. *Cell Mol Neurobiol* 1999;19:411–426.

75. Rotzinger S, Bourin M, Akimoto Y, Coutts RT, Baker GB. Metabolism of some "second-" and "fourth-" generation antidepressants: iprindole, viloxazine, bupropion, mianserin, maprotiline, trazodone, nefazodone, and venlafaxine. *Cell Mol Neurobiol* 1999;19:427–442.

76. Chouinard G, Lefko-Singh K, Teboul E. Metabolism of anxiolytics and hypnotics: benzodiazepines, buspirone, zoplicone, and zolpidem. *Cell Mol Neurobiol* 1999;19: 533–552.

77. Lanza DL, Yost GS. Selective dehydrogenation/oxygenation of 3-methylindole by cytochrome P450 enzymes. *Drug Metab Dispos* 2001;29:950–953.

78. O'Neil MJ, Smith A, Heckelman PE, Budavari S. *The Merck Index: An Encyclopedia of Chemicals, Drugs, and Biologicals*, 13th ed. Whitehouse Station: Merck & Co; 2001.

79. Rogers JF, Nafziger AN, Bertino JS. Pharmacogenetics affects dosing, efficacy, and toxicity of cytochrome P450-metabolized drugs. *Am J Med* 2002;113:746–750.

80. Kelly P, Kahan BD. Metabolism of immunosuppressant drugs. *Curr Drug Metab* 2002;3:275–287.

81. Miyazawa M, Shindo M, Shimada T. Metabolism of (+)- and (−)-limonenes to respective carveols and perillyl alcohols by CYP2C9 and CYP2C19 in human liver microsomes. *Drug Metab Dispos* 2002;30:602–607.

82. Zhang W, Ramamoorthy Y, Tyndale RF, Glick SD, Maisonneuve IM, Kuehne ME, Sellers EM. Metabolism of 18-methoxycoronaridine, an ibogaine analog, to 18-hydroxycoronaridine by genetically variable CYP2C19. *Drug Metab Dispos* 2002;30:663–669.

83. Otake Y, Walle T. Oxidation of the flavonoids galangin and kaempferide by human liver microsomes and CYP1A1, CYP1A2, and CYP2C9. *Drug Metab Dispos* 2002;30: 103–105.

84. Tolleson WH, Doerge DR, Churchwell MI, Marques MM, Roberts DW. Metabolism of biochanin A and formononetin by human liver microsomes in vitro. *J Agric Food Chem* 2002;50:4783–4790.

85. Breinholt VM, Offord EA, Brouwer C, Nielsen SE, Brøsen K, Friedberg T. *In vitro* investigation of cytochrome P450-mediated metabolism of dietary flavonoids. *Food Chem Toxicol* 2002;40:609–616.

86. Hijazi Y, Boulieu R. Contribution of CYP3A4, CYP2B6, and CYP2C9 isoforms to N-demethylation of ketamine in human liver microsomes. *Drug Metab Dispos* 2002;30:853–858.

87. Canadian Pharmacists Association. *Compendium of Pharmaceuticals and Specialties.* Ottawa, Canada: Canadian Pharmacists Association, 2002.

88. Williams DA, Lemke TL, *Foye's Principles of Medicinal Chemistry*, 5th ed. Baltimore: Lippincott Williams & Wilkins, 2002.

89. Rendic S. Summary of information on human CYP enzymes: human P450 metabolism data. *Drug Metab Rev* 2002;34:83–448.

90. Jann MW, Shirley KL, Small GW. Clinical pharmacokinetics and pharmacodynamics of cholinesterase inhibitors. *Clin Pharmacokinet* 2002;41:719–739.

91. Smith JA, Newman RA, Hausheer FH, Madden T. Evaluation of *in vitro* drug interactions with karenitecin, a novel, highly lipophilic camptothecin derivative in phase II clinical development. *J Clin Pharmacol* 2003;43:1008–1014.

92. Reilly CA, Ehlhardt WJ, Jackson DA, Kulanthaivel P, Mutlib AE, Espina RJ, Moody DE, Crouch DJ, Yost GS. Metabolism of capsaicin by cytochrome P450 produces novel dehydrogenated metabolites and decreases cytotoxicity to lung and liver cells. *Chem Res Toxicol* 2003;16:336–349.

93. Li X-Q, Björkman A, Andersson TB, Gustafsson LL, Masimirembwa CM. Identification of human cytochrome P450s that metabolise anti-parasitic drugs and predictions of *in vivo* drug hepatic clearance from *in vitro* data. *Eur J Clin Pharmacol* 2003;59:429–442.

94. Chen G, Bunce NJ. Polybrominated diphenyl ethers as Ah receptor agonists and antagonists. *Toxicol Sci* 2003;76:310–320.

95. Breinholt VM, Rasmussen SE, Brøsen K, Friedberg TH. *In vitro* metabolism of genistein and tangeretin by human and murine cytochrome P450s. *Pharmacol Toxicol* 2003;93: 14–22.

96. Yun C-H, Lee HS, Lee H-Y, Yim S-K, Kim K-H, Kim E, Yea S-S, Guengerich FP. Roles of human liver cytochrome P450 3A4 and 1A2 enzymes in the oxidation of myristicin. *Toxicol Lett* 2003;137:143–150.

97. Paul LD, Springer D, Staack RF, Kraemer T, Maurer HH. Cytochrome P450 isoenzymes involved in rat liver microsomal metabolism of californine and protopine. *Eur J Pharmacol* 2004;485:69–79.

98. Neels HM, Sierens AC, Naelaerts K, Scharpé SL, Hatfield GM, Lambert WE. Therapeutic drug monitoring of old and newer anti-epileptic drugs. *Clin Chem Lab Med* 2004;42:1228–1255.

99. Slaughter D, Takenaga N, Lu P, Assang C, Walsh DJ, Arison BH, Cui D, Halpin RA, Geer LA, Vyas KP, Baillie TA. Metabolism of rofecoxib *in vitro* using human liver subcellular fractions. *Drug Metab Dispos* 2003;31:1398–1408.

100. Zhou S, Koh H-L, Gao Y, Gong Z-Y, Lee EJD. Herbal bioactivation: the good, the bad and the ugly. *Life Sci* 2004;74:935–968.

101. Naritomi Y, Terashita S, Kagayama A. Identification and relative contributions of human cytochrome P450 isoforms involved in the metabolism of glibenclamide and lansopra-

zole: evaluation of an approach based on the *in vitro* substrate disappearance rate. *Xenobiotica* 2004;34:415–427.

102. Ma X, Idle JR, Krausz KW, Gonzalez FJ. Metabolism of melatonin by human cytochromes P450. *Drug Metab Dispos* 2005;33:489–494.

103. Obach RS, Cox LM, Tremaine LM. Sertraline is metabolized by multiple cytochrome P450 enzymes, monamine oxidases, and glucuronyl transferases in human: an *in vitro* study. *Drug Metab Dispos* 2005;33:262–270.

104. Death AK, McGrath KCY, Handelsman DJ. Valproate is an anti-androgen and anti-progestin. *Steroids* 2005;70:946–953.

105. Hodgson E, Rose RL. Human metabolism and metabolic interactions of deployment-related chemicals. *Drug Metab Rev* 2005;1:1–39.

106. van Schaik RHN. Cancer treatment and pharmacogenetics of cytochrome P450 enzymes. *Invest New Drugs* 2005;23:513–522.

107. Mutch E, Williams FM. Diazinon, chlorpyrifos and parathion are metabolized by multiple cytochromes P450 in human liver. *Toxicology* 2006;224:22–32.

108. Jeurissen SMF, Bogaards JJP, Boersma MG, ter Horst JPF, Awad HM, Fiamegos YC, van Beek TA, Alink GM, Sudhölter EJR, Cnubben NHP, Rietjens IMCM. Human cytochrome P450 enzymes of importance for the bioactivation of methyleugenol to the proximate carcinogen 1′-hydroxymethyleugenol. *Chem Res Toxicol* 2006;19:111–116.

109. Chen C, Tu M-H. Transannular dioxygenation of 9,10-dimethyl-1,2-benzanthracene by cytochrome P-450 oxygenase of rat liver. *Biochem J* 1976;160:805–808.

110. Vaz ADN, Coon MJ. Hydrocarbon formation in the reductive cleavage of hydroperoxides by cytochrome P450. *Proc Natl Acad Sci USA* 1987;84:1172–1176.

111. Yang CS, Lu AYH, The diversity of substrates for cytochrome P450. In Guengerich FP, Ed. *Mammalian Cytochromes P450*. Boca Raton, FL; CRC Press, 1987, pp 1–17.

112. Koop DR. Oxidative and reductive metabolism by cytochrome P450 2E1. *Fed Am Soc Exp Biol J* 1992;6:724–730.

113. Nakasa H, Komiya M, Ohmori S, Rikihisa T, Kiuchi M, Kitada M. Characterization of human liver microsomal cytochrome P450 involved in the reductive metabolism of zonisamide. *Mol Pharmacol* 1993;44:216–221.

114. Chang TKH, Gonzalez FJ, Waxman DJ. Evaluation of triacetyloleandomycin, α-naphthoflavone and diethyldithiocarbamate as selective chemical probes for inhibition of human cytochromes P450. *Arch Biochem Biophys* 1994;311:437–442.

115. Veal GJ, Back DJ. Metabolism of zidovudine. *Gen Pharmacol* 1995;26:1469–1475.

116. Coon MJ, Vaz ADN, Bestervelt LL. Peroxidative reactions of diversozymes. *Fed Am Soc Exp Biol J* 1996;10:428–434.

117. Pan-Zhou X-R, Cretton-Scott E, Zhou X-J, Yang M-X, Lasker JM, Sommadossi J-P. Role of human liver P450s and cytochrome b_5 in the reductive metabolism of 3′-azido-3′-deoxythymidine (AZT) to 3′-amino-3′-deoxythymidine. *Biochem Pharmacol* 1998;55: 757–766.

118. Grace JM, Skanchy DJ, Aguilar AJ. Metabolism of artelinic acid to dihydroqinqhaosu by human liver cytochrome P4503A. *Xenobiotica* 1999;29:703–717.

119. Kudo S, Okumura H, Miyamoto G, Ishizaki T. Cytochrome P450 isoforms involved in carboxylic acid ester cleavage of Hantzsch pyridine ester of pranidipine. *Drug Metab Dispos* 1999;27:303–308.

120. Patterson LH, McKeown SR, Robson T, Gallagher R, Raleigh SM, Orr S. Antitumour prodrug development using cytochrome P450 (CYP) mediated activation. *Anti-Cancer Drug Design* 1999;14:473–486.

121. Guengerich FP. Common and uncommon cytochrome P450 reactions related to metabolism and chemical toxicity. *Chem Res Toxicol* 2001;14:611–650.

122. Kalgutkar AS, Nguyen HT, Vaz ADN, Doan A, Dalvie DK, McLeod DG, Murray JC. *In vitro* metabolism studies on the isoxazole ring scission in the anti-inflammatory agent leflunomide to its active α-cyanoenol metabolite A771726: mechanistic similarities with the cytochrome P450-catalyzed dehydration of aldoximes. *Drug Metab Dispos* 2003;31: 1240–1250.

123. Lesca P, Beaune P, Monsarrat B. Ellipticines and human liver microsomes: spectral interaction with cytochrome P-450 and hydroxylation. Inhibition of aryl hydrocarbon metabolism and mutagenicity. *Chem-Biol Interact* 1981;36:299–309.

124. Inaba T, Tyndale RE, Mahon WA. Quinidine: potent inhibition of sparteine and debrisoquine oxidation in vivo. *Br J Clin Pharmacol* 1986;22:199–200.

125. Tassaneeyakul W, Birkett DJ, Veronese ME, McManus ME, Tukey RH, Quattrochi LC, Gelboin HV, Miners JO. Specificity of substrate and inhibitor probes for human cytochromes P450 1A1 and 1A2. *J Pharmacol Exp Ther* 1993;265:401–407.

126. Brosen K, Skjelbo E, Rasmussen BB, Poulsen HE, Loft S. Fluvoxamine is a potent inhibitor of cytochrome P4501A2. *Biochem Pharmacol* 1993;45:1211–1214.

127. Kunze KL, Trager WF. Isoform-selective mechanism-based inhibition of human cytochrome P450 1A2 by furafylline. *Chem Res Toxicol* 1993;6:649–656.

128. Strobl GR, von Kruedener S, Stockigt J, Guengerich FP, Wolff T. Development of a pharmacophore for inhibition of human liver cytochrome P-450 2D6: molecular modeling and inhibition studies. *J Med Chem* 1993;36:1136–1145.

129. Mäenpää J, Juvonen R, Raunio H, Rautio A, Pelkonen O. Metabolic interactions of methoxsalen and coumarin in humans and mice. *Biochem Pharmacol* 1994;48:1363–1369.

130. Burke MD, Thompson S, Weaver RJ, Wolf CR, Mayer RT. Cytochrome P450 specificities of alkoxyresorufin *O*-dealkylation in human and rat liver. *Biochem Pharmacol* 1994;48:923–936.

131. López-Garcia MP, Dansette PM, Mansuy D. Thiophene derivatives as new mechanism-based inhibitors of cytochromes P-450: inactivation of yeast-expressed human liver cytochrome P-450 2C9 by tienilic acid. *Biochemistry* 1994;33:166–175.

132. Halpert JR, Guengerich FP, Bend JR, Correia MA. Contemporary issues in toxicology: selective inhibitors of cytochromes P450. *Toxicol Appl Pharmacol* 1994;125:163–175.

133. Baldwin SJ, Bloomer JC, Airton AD, Clarke SE, Chenery RJ. Ketoconazole and sulphaphenazole as the respective selective inhibitors of P450 3A and 2C9. *Xenobiotica* 1995;25:261–270.

134. Wienkers LC, Wurden CJ, Storch E, Kunze KL, Rettie AE, Trager WF. Formation of (*R*)-8-hydroxywarfarin in human liver microsomes. A new metabolic marker for the (*S*)-mephenytoin hydroxylase, P4502C19. *Drug Metab Dispos* 1996;24:610–614.

135. Roberts ES, Hopkins NE, Foroozesh M, Alworth WL, Halpert JR, Hollenberg PF. Inactivation of cytochrome P450s 2B1, 2B4, 2B6, and 2B11 by arylalkynes. *Drug Metab Dispos* 1997;25:1242–1248.

136. Moody GC, Griffin SJ, Mather AN, McGinnity DF, Riley RJ. Fully automated analysis of activities catalysed by the major human liver cytochrome P450 (CYP) enzymes: assessment of human CYP inhibition potential. *Xenobiotica* 1999;29:53–75.

137. Hasler JA, Estabrook R, Murray M, Pikuleva I, Waterman M, Capdevila J, Holla V, Helvig C, Falck JR, Farrell G, Kaminsky LS, Spivack SD, Boitier E, Beaune P. Human cytochromes P450. *Mol Aspects Med* 1999;20:1–137.

138. Chan WK, Delucchi AB. Resveratrol, a red wine constituent, is a mechanism-based inactivator of cytochrome P450 3A4. *Life Sci* 2000;67:3103–3112.

139. Rochat B, Morsman JM, Murray GI, Figg WD, McLeod HL. Human CYP1B1 and anti-cancer agent metabolism: mechanism for tumor-specific drug inactivation? *J Pharmacol Exp Ther* 2001;296:537–541.

140. Rae JM, Soukhova NV, Flockhart DA, Desta Z. Triethylenethiophosphoramide is a specific inhibitor of cytochrome P450 2B6: implications for cyclophosphamide metabolism. *Drug Metab Dispos* 2002;30:525–530.

141. Li X-Q, Björkman A, Andersson TB, Ridderström M, Masimirembwa CM. Amodiaquine clearance and its metabolism to *N*-desethylamodiaquine is mediated by CYP2C8: a new high affinity and turnover enzyme-specific probe substrate. *J Pharmacol Exp Ther* 2002;300:399–407.

142. Václavíková R, Horský S, Šimek P. Paclitaxel metabolism in rat and human liver microsomes is inhibited by phenolic antioxidants. *Naunyn Schmiedebergs Arch Pharmacol* 2003;368:200–209.

143. Turpeinen M, Nieminen R, Juntunen T, Taavitsainen P, Raunio H, Pelkonen O. Selective inhibition of CYP2B6-catalyzed bupropion hydroxylation in human liver microsomes in vitro. *Drug Metab Dispos* 2004;32:626–631.

144. Walsky RL, Obach RS. Validated assays for human cytochrome P450 activities. *Drug Metab Dispos* 2004;32:647–660.

145. Locuson, CW II, Suzuki H, Rettie AE, Jones JP. Charge and substituent effects on affinity and metabolism of benzbromarone-based CYP2C19 inhibitors. *J Med Chem* 2004;47:6768–6776.

146. Dutreix C, Peng B, Mehring G, Hayes M, Capdeville R, Pokorny R, Seiberling M. Pharmacokinetic interaction between ketoconazole and imatinib mesylate (Glivec) in healthy subjects. *Cancer Chemother Pharmacol* 2004;54:290–294.

147. Miyata N, Seki T, Tanaka Y, Omura T, Taniguchi K, Doi M, Bandou K, Kametani S, Sato M, Okuyama S, Cambj-Sapunar L, Harder DR, Roman RJ. Beneficial effects of a new 20-hydroxyeicosatetraenoic acid synthesis inhibitor, TS-011 [*N*-(3-chloro-4-morpholin-4-yl)phenyl-*N*-hydroxyimidoformamide], on hemorrhagic and ischemic stroke. *J Pharmacol Exp Ther* 2005;314:77–85.

148. Kim M-J, Kim H, Cha I-J, Park J-S, Shon J-H, Liu K-H, Shin J-G. High-throughput screening of inhibitory potential of nine cytochrome P450 enzymes *in vitro* using liquid chromatography/tandem mass spectrometry. *Rapid Commun Mass Spectrom* 2005;19:2651–2658.

149. Moon YJ, Wang X, Morris ME. Dietary flavonoids: effects on xenobiotic and carcinogen metabolism. *Toxicol In Vitro* 2006;20:187–210.

150. Guengerich FP. Enzymatic oxidations of xenobiotic chemicals. *CRC Crit Rev Biochem Mol Biol* 1990;25:97–153.

151. De Voss JJ, Sibbessen O, Zhang Z, Ortiz De Montellano PR. Substrate docking algorithms and prediction of the substrate specificity of cytochrome P450$_{cam}$ and its L244A mutant. *J Am Chem Soc* 1997;119:5480–5498.

152. Josephy PD, Mannervik B, Ortiz de Montellano PR. Cytochrome P450. In *Molecular Toxicology*. Oxford: Oxford University Press; 1997, pp 209–252.

153. Yasui H, Hayashi S, Sakurai H. Possible involvement of singlet oxygen species as multiple oxidants in P450 catalytic reactions. *Drug Metab Pharmacokinet* 2005;20:1–13.

154. Kliewer SA, Goodwin B, Willson TM. The nuclear pregnane X receptor: a key regulator of xenobiotic metabolism. *Endocr Rev* 2002;23:687–702.

155. Shimada T, Yamazaki H, Mimura M, Inui Y, Guengerich FP. Interindividual variations in human liver cytochrome P450 enzymes involved in the oxidation of drugs, carcinogens and toxic chemicals: studies with liver microsomes of 30 Japanese and 30 Caucasians. *J Pharmacol Exp Ther* 1994;270:414–423.

156. Edwards RJ, Adams DA, Watts PS, Davies DS, Boobis AR. Development of a comprehensive panel of antibodies against the major xenobiotic metabolizing forms of cytochrome P450 in humans. *Biochem Pharmacol* 1998;56:377–387.

157. Rodrigues AD. Integrated cytochrome P450 reaction phenotyping. *Biochem Pharmacol* 1999;57:465–480.

158. Chang TKH, Chen J, Pillay V, Ho J-Y, Bandiera SM. Real-time polymerase chain reaction analysis of CYP1B1 gene expression in human liver. *Toxicol Sci* 2003;71:11–19.

159. Nerurkar PV, Park SS, Thomas PE, Nims RW, Lubet RA. Methoxyresorufin and benzyloxyresorufin: substrates preferentially metabolized by cytochromes P4501A2 and 2B, respectively, in the rat and mouse. *Biochem Pharmacol* 1993;46:933–943.

160. Sesardic D, Cole KJ, Edwards RJ, Davies DS, Thomas PE, Levin W, Boobis AR. The inducibility and catalytic activity of cytochromes P450c (P450IA1) and P450d (P450IA2) in rat tissues. *Biochem Pharmacol* 1990;39:499–506.

161. Gu L, Gonzalez FJ, Kalow W, Tang BK. Biotransformation of caffeine, paraxanthine, theobromine and theophylline by cDNA-expressed human CYP1A2 and CYP2E1. *Pharmacogenetics* 1992;2:73–77.

162. Jayyosi Z, Villoutreix J, Ziegler JM, Batt AM, de Maack F, Siest G, Thomas PE. Identification of cytochrome P-450 isozymes involved in the hydroxylation of dantrolene by rat liver microsomes. *Drug Metab Dispos* 1993;21:939–945.

163. Shou M, Korzekwa KR, Crespi CL, Gonzalez FJ, Gelboin HV. The role of 12 cDNA-expressed human, rodent, and rabbit cytochromes P450 in the metabolism of benzo[*a*]pyrene and benzo[*a*]pyrene *trans*-7,8-dihydrodiol. *Mol Carcinog* 1994;10: 159–168.

164. Rodrigues AD, Kukulka MJ, Roberts EM, Ouellet D, Rodgers TR. [*O*-methyl ^{14}C]naproxen *O*-demethylase activity in human liver microsomes: evidence for the involvement of cytochrome P4501A2 and P4502C9/10. *Drug Metab Dispos* 1996;24:126–136.

165. Bloomer JC, Clarke SE, Chenery RJ. *In vitro* identification of the P450 enzymes responsible for the metabolism of ropinirole. *Drug Metab Dispos* 1997;25:840–844.

166. Shimada T, Gillam EMJ, Sutter TR, Strickland PT, Guengerich FP, Yamazaki H. Oxidation of xenobiotics by recombinant human cytochrome P450 1B1. *Drug Metab Dispos* 1997;29:617–622.

167. Lee SH, Slattery JT. Cytochrome P450 isozymes involved in lisofylline metabolism to pentoxifylline in human liver microsomes. *Drug Metab Dispos* 1997;25:1354–1358.

168. Sanderink G-J, Bournique B, Stevens J, Petry M, Martinet M. Involvement of human CYP1A isoenzymes in the metabolism and drug interactions of riluzole in vitro. *J Pharmacol Exp Ther* 1997;282:1465–1472.

169. Kinzig-Schippers M, Fuhr U, Zaigler M, Dammeyer J, Rüsing G, Labedzki A, Bulitta J, Sörgel F. Interaction of pefloxacin and enoxacin with the human cytochrome P450 enzyme CYP1A2. *Clin Pharmacol Ther* 1999;65:262–274.

170. Szotakova B, Wsol V, Skalova L, Kvasnickova E. Role of cytochrome P4501A in biotransformation of the potential anticancer drug oracin. *Exp Toxicol Pathol* 1999;51: 428–431.

171. Chen H, Howald WN, Juchau MR. Biosynthesis of all-*trans*-retinoic acid from all-*trans*-retinol: catalysis of all-*trans*-retinol oxidation by human P-450 cytochromes. *Drug Metab Dispos* 2000;28:315–322.

172. Hu M, Krausz K, Chen J, Ge X, Li J, Gelboin HL, Gonzalez FJ. Identification of CYP1A2 as the main isoform for the phase I hydroxylated metabolism of genistein and a prodrug converting enzyme of methylated isoflavones. *Drug Metab Dispos* 2003;31:924–931.

173. Granfors MT, Backman JT, Laitila J, Neuvonen PJ. Tizanidine is mainly metabolized by cytochrome P450 1A2 in vitro. *Br J Clin Pharmacol* 2003;57:349–353.

174. Peng W-X, Wang L-S, Li H-D, El-Aty AMA, Chen G-L, Zhou H-H. Evidence for the involvement of human liver microsomes CYP1A2 in the mono-hydroxylation of daidzein. *Clin Chim Acta* 2003;334:77–85.

175. Smith KS, Smith PL, Heady TN, Trugman JM, Harman WD, Macdonald TL. *In vitro* metabolism of tolcapone to reactive intermediates: relevance to tolcapone liver toxicity. *Chem Res Toxicol* 2003;16:123–128.

176. Piver B, Fer M, Vitrac X, Merillon J-M, Dreano Y, Berthou F, Lucas D. Involvement of cytochrome P450 1A2 in the biotransformation of *trans*-resveratrol in human liver microsomes. *Biochem Pharmacol* 2004;68:773–782.

177. Fuhr U, Kober S, Zaigler M, Mutschler E, Spahn-Langguth H. Rate-limiting biotransformation of triamterene is mediated by CYP1A2. *Int J Clin Pharmacol Ther* 2005;43:327–334.

178. Goda R, Nagai D, Akiyama Y, Nishikawa K, Ikemoto I, Aizawa Y, Nagata K, Yamazoe Y. Detection of a new *N*-oxidized metabolite of flutamide, *N*-[4-nitro-3-(trifluoromethyl)phenyl]hydroxylamine, in human liver microsomes and urine of prostate cancer patients. *Drug Metab Dispos* 2006;34:828–835.

179. Shimada T, Guengerich FP. Inhibition of human cytochrome P450 1A1-, 1A2-, and 1B1-mediated activation of procarcinogens to genotoxic metabolites by polycyclic aromatic hydrocarbons. *Chem Res Toxicol* 2006;19:288–294.

180. Stoilov I, Akarsu AN, Sarfarazi M. Identification of three different truncating mutations in the cytochrome P450 1B1 (CYP1B1) gene as the principal cause of primary congenital glaucoma (buphthalmos) in families linked to the GLC3A locus on chromosome 2p21. *Hum Mol Genet* 1997;6:641–647.

181. Fujii-Kuriyama Y, Mimura J. Molecular mechanisms of AhR functions in the regulation of *cytochrome P450* genes. *Biochem Biophys Res Commun* 2005;338:311–317.

182. Guengerich FP, Kim D-H, Iwasaki M. Role of human cytochrome P-450 IIE1 in the oxidation of many low molecular weight cancer suspects. *Chem Res Toxicol* 1991;4:168–179.

183. Narimatsu S, Kariya S, Isozaki S, Ohmori S, Kitada M, Hosokawa S, Masubuchi Y, Suzuki T. Involvement of CYP2D6 in oxidative metabolism of cinnarizine and flunarizine in human liver microsomes. *Biochem Biophys Res Commun* 1993;193:1262–1268.

184. Clement B, Jung F. *N*-hydroxylation of the antiprotozoal drug pentamidine catalyzed by rabbit liver cytochrome P-450 2C3 or human liver microsomes, microsomal retroreduction, and further oxidative transformation of the formed amidoximes: possible relationship to the biological oxidation of arginine to N^G-hydroxyarginine, citrulline, and nitric oxide. *Drug Metab Dispos* 1994;22:486–497.

185. Fischer V, Vickers AEM, Heitz F, Mahadevan S, Baldeck J-P, Minery P, Tynes R. The polymorphic cytochrome P-4502D6 is involved in the metabolism of both 5-hydroxytryptamine antagonists, tropisetron and ondansetron. *Drug Metab Dispos* 1994;22:269–274.

186. Miners JO, Rees DLP, Valente L, Veronese ME, Birkett DJ. Human hepatic cytochrome P450 2C9 catalyzes the rate-limiting pathway of torsemide metabolism. *J Pharmacol Exp Ther* 1995;272:1076–1081.

187. Yumibe N, Huie K, Chen K-J, Snow M, Clement RP, Cayen MN. Identification of human liver cytochrome P450 enzymes that metabolize the nonsedating antihistamine lorata-dine: formation of descarboethoxyloratadine by CYP3A4 and CYP2D6. *Biochem Pharmacol* 1996;51:165–172.

188. Tracy TS, Marra C, Wrighton SA, Gonzalez FJ, Korzekwa KR. Studies of flurbiprofen 4'-hydroxylation: additional evidence suggesting the sole involvement of cytochrome P450 2C9. *Biochem Pharmacol* 1996;52:1305–1309.

189. Ring BJ, Catlow J, Lindsay TJ, Gillespie T, Roskos LK, Cerimele BJ, Swanson SP, Hamman MA, Wrighton SA. Identification of the human cytochromes P450 responsible for the *in vitro* formation of the major oxidative metabolites of the antipsychotic agent olanzapine. *J Pharmacol Exp Ther* 1996;276:658–666.

190. Liu C, Zhuo X, Gonzalez FJ, Ding X. Baculovirus-mediated expression and characteriza-tion of rat CYP2A3 and human CYP2D6: role in metabolic activation of nasal toxicants. *Mol Pharmacol* 1996;50:781–788.

191. Kariya S, Isozaki S, Uchino K, Suzuki T, Narimatsu S. Oxidative metabolism of flunari-zine and cinnarizine by microsomes from β-lymphoblastoid cell lines expressing human cytochrome P450 enzymes. *Biol Pharm Bull* 1996;19:1511–1514.

192. Bonnabry P, Leemann T, Dayer P. Role of human liver microsomal CYP2C9 in the bio-transformation of lornoxicam. *Eur J Clin Pharmacol* 1996;49:305–308.

193. Sanwald P, David M, Dow J. Characterization of the cytochrome P450 enzymes involved in the *in vitro* metabolism of dolasetron. Comparison with other indole-containing 5-HT3 antagonists. *Drug Metab Dispos* 1996;24:602–609.

194. Ren S, Yang JS, Kalhorn TF, Slattery JT. Oxidation of cyclophosphamide to 4-hydroxy-cyclophosphamide and deschloroethylcyclophosphamide in human liver microsomes. *Cancer Res* 1997;57:4229–4235.

195. Kudo S, Uchida M, Odomi M. Metabolism of carteolol by cDNA-expressed human cytochrome P450. *Eur J Clin Pharmacol* 1997;52:479–485.

196. Chiba M, Xu X, Nishime JA, Balani SK, Lin JH. Hepatic microsomal metabolism of montelucast, a potent leukotriene D_4 receptor antagonist, in humans. *Drug Metab Dispos* 1997;25:1022–1031.

197. Kamimura H, Oishi S, Matsushima H, Watanabe T, Higuchi S, Hall M, Wood SG, Chasseaud LF. Identification of cytochrome P450 isozymes involved in metabolism of the α_1-adrenoceptor blocker tamsulosin in human liver microsomes. *Xenobiotica* 1998;28:909–922.

198. Hiroi T, Imaoka S, Funae Y. Dopamine formation from tyramine by CYP2D6. *Biochem Biophys Res Commun* 1998;249:838–843.

199. Chesne C, Guyomard C, Guillouzo A, Schmid J, Ludwig E, Sauter T. Metabolism of meloxicam in human liver involves cytochromes P4502C9 and 3A4. *Xenobiotica* 1998;28:1–13.

200. Ko J-W, Desta Z, Flockhart DA. Human *N*-demethylation of (*S*)-mephenytoin by cyto-chrome P450s 2C9 and 2B6. *Drug Metab Dispos* 1998;26:775–778.

201. Lasker JM, Wester MR, Aramsombatdee E, Raucy JL. Characterization of CYP2C19 and CYP2C9 from human liver: respective roles in microsomal tolbutamide, *S*-mephenytoin, and omeprazole hydroxylations. *Arch Biochem Biophys* 1998;353:16–28.

202. Gentile DM, Verhoeven CHJ, Shimada T, Back DJ. The role of CYP2C in the *in vitro* bioactivation of the contraceptive steroid desogestrel. *J Pharmacol Exp Ther* 1998;287:975–982.

203. Obach RS, Pablo J, Mash DC. Cytochrome P4502D6 catalyzes the *O*-demethylation of the psychoactive alkaloid ibogaine to 12-hydroxyibogamine. *Drug Metab Dispos* 1998;26:764–768.

204. Venkatakrishnan K, von Moltke LL, Greenblatt DJ. Relative quantities of catalytically active CYP 2C9 and 2C19 in human liver microsomes: application of the relative activity factor approach. *J Pharm Sci* 1998;87:845–853.

205. Coller JK, Somogyi AA, Bochner F. Comparison of (*S*)-mephenytoin and proguanil oxidation *in vitro*: contribution of several CYP isoforms. *Br J Clin Pharmacol* 1999;48: 158–167.

206. de Groot MJ, Ackland MJ, Horne VA, Alex AA, Jones BC. A novel approach to predicting P450 mediated drug metabolism. CYP2D6 catalyzed *N*-dealkylation reactions and qualitative metabolite predictions using a combined protein and pharmacophore model for CYP2D6. *J Med Chem* 1999;42:4062–4070.

207. Ekins S, Wrighton SA. The role of CYP2B6 in human xenobiotic metabolism. *Drug Metab Rev* 1999;31:719–754.

208. Kobayashi K, Abe S, Nakajima M, Shimada N, Tani M, Chiba K, Yamamoto T. Role of human CYP2B6 in *S*-mephobarbital *N*-demethylation. *Drug Metab Dispos* 1999;27: 1429–1433.

209. Bourrié M, Meunier V, Berger Y, Fabre G. Role of cytochrome P-4502C9 in irbesartan oxidation by human liver microsomes. *Drug Metab Dispos* 1999;27:288–296.

210. Bachus R, Bickel U, Thomsen T, Roots I, Kewitz H. The *O*-demethylation of the anti-dementia drug galanthamine is catalyzed by cytochrome P450 2D6. *Pharmacogenetics* 1999;9:661–668.

211. Chow T, Hiroi T, Imaoka S, Chiba K, Funae Y. Isoform-selective metabolism of mianserin by cytochrome P-450 2D. *Drug Metab Dispos* 1999;27:1200–1204.

212. Niwa T, Shiraga T, Mitani Y, Terakawa M, Tokuma Y, Kagayama A. Stereoselective metabolism of cibenzoline, an antiarrhythmic drug, by human and rat liver microsomes: possible involvement of CYP2D and CYP3A. *Drug Metab Dispos* 2000;28:1128–1134.

213. Gillam EMJ, Notley LM, Cai H, de Voss JJ, Guengerich FP. Oxidation of indole by cytochrome P450 enzymes. *Biochemistry* 2000;39:13817–13824.

214. Pelkonen O, Rautio A, Raunio H, Pasanen M. CYP2A6: a human coumarin 7-hydroxylase. *Toxicology* 2000;144:139–147.

215. Tang C, Shou M, Mei Q, Rushmore TH, Rodrigues AD. Major role of human liver microsomal cytochrome P450 2C9 (CYP2C9) in the oxidative metabolism of celecoxib, a novel cyclooxygenase-II inhibitor. *J Pharmacol Exp Ther* 2000;293:453–459.

216. Thijssen HH, Flinois J-P, Beaune PH. Cytochrome P4502C9 is the principal catalyst of racemic acenocoumarol hydroxylation reactions in human liver microsomes. *Drug Metab Dispos* 2000;28:1284–1290.

217. Scheen AJ. Pharma-clinics medication of the month. Nebivolol (Nobiten). *Rev Méd Liège* 2000;56:788–791.

218. Oda Y, Hamaoka N, Hiroi T, Imaoka S, Hase I, Tanaka K, Funae Y, Ishizaki T, Asada A. Involvement of human liver cytochrome P4502B6 in the metabolism of propofol. *Br J Clin Pharmacol* 2001;51:281–285.

219. Brachtendorf L, Jetter A, Beckurts KT, Hölscher AH, Fuhr U. Cytochrome P-450 enzymes contributing to demethylation of maprotiline in man. *Pharmacol Toxicol* 2002;90:144–149.

220. Desta Z, Wu GM, Morocho AM, Flockhart DA. The gastroprokinetic and antiemetic drug metoclopramide is a substrate and inhibitor of cytochrome P450 2D6. *Drug Metab Dispos* 2002;30:336–343.

221. Jacobson PA, Green K, Birnbaum A, Remmel RP. Cytochrome P450 isozymes 3A4 and 2B6 are involved in the *in vitro* metabolism of thiotepa to TEPA. *Cancer Chemother Pharmacol* 2002;49:461–467.

222. Matsumoto S, Hirama T, Matsubara T, Nagata K, Yamazoe Y. Involvement of CYP2J2 on the intestinal first-pass metabolism of antihistamine drug, astemizole. *Drug Metab Dispos* 2002;30:1240–1245.

223. Usmani KA, Rose RL, Goldstein JA, Taylor WG, Brimfield AA, Hodgson E. *In vitro* human metabolism and interactions of repellent *N, N*-diethyl-*m*-toluamide. *Drug Metab Dispos* 2002;30:289–294.

224. Marill J, Capron CC, Idres N, Chabot GG. Human cytochrome P450s involved in the metabolism of 9-*cis*- and 13-*cis*-retinoic acids. *Biochem Pharmacol* 2002;63:933–943.

225. Evans DC, O'Connor D, Lake BG, Evers R, Allen C, Hargreaves R. Eletriptan metabolism by human CYP450 enzymes and transport by human P-glycoprotein. *Drug Metab Dispos* 2003;31:861–869.

226. Skinner MH, Kuan H-Y, Pan A, Sathirakul K, Knadler MP, Gonzales CR, Yeo KP, Reddy S, Lim M, Ayan-Oshodi M, Wise SD. Duloxetine is both an inhibitor and a substrate of cytochrome P4502D6 in healthy volunteers. *Clin Pharmacol Ther* 2003;73:170–177.

227. Miyazawa M, Sugie A, Shimada T. Roles of human CYP2A6 and 2B6 and rat CYP2C11 and 2B1 in the 10-hydroxylation of (−)-verbenone by liver microsomes. *Drug Metab Dispos* 2003;31:1049–1053.

228. Kajita J, Fuse E, Kuwabara T, Kobayashi H. The contribution of cytochrome P450 to the metabolism of tegafur in human liver. *Drug Metab Pharmacokinet* 2003;18:303–309.

229. Ward BA, Gorski JC, Jones DR, Hall SD, Flockhart DA, Desta Z. The cytochrome P450 2B6 (CYP2B6) is the main catalyst of efavirenz primary and secondary metabolism: implication for HIV/AIDS therapy and utility of efavirenz as a substrate marker of CYP2B6 catalytic activity. *J Pharmacol Exp Ther* 2003;306:287–300.

230. Le Gal A, Dréano Y, Lucas D, Berthou F. Diversity of selective environmental substrates for human cytochrome P450 2A6: alkoxyethers, nicotine, coumarin, *N*-nitrosodiethylamine, and *N*-nitrosobenzylmethylamine. *Toxicol Lett* 2003;144:77–91.

231. Cheng JB, Motola DL, Mangelsdorf DJ, Russell DW. De-orphanization of cytochrome P450 2R1. *J Biol Chem* 2003;278:38084–38093.

232. Yu A-M, Idle JR, Krausz KW, Küpfer A, Gonzalez FJ. Contribution of individual cytochrome P450 isozymes to the *O*-demethylation of the psychotropic β-carboline alkaloids harmaline and harmine. *J Pharmacol Exp Ther* 2003;305:315–322.

233. Attar M, Dong D, Ling K-HJ, Tang-Liu DD-S. Cytochrome P450 2C8 and flavin-containing monooxygenases are involved in the metabolism of tazarotenic acid in humans. *Drug Metab Dispos* 2003;31:476–481.

234. Benetton SA, Borges VM, Chang TKH, McErlane KM. Role of individual human cytochrome P450 enzymes in the *in vitro* metabolism of hydromorphone. *Xenobiotica* 2004;34:335–344.

235. Wójcikowski J, Pichard-Garcia L, Maurel P, Daniel WA. The metabolism of the piperazine-type phenothiazine neuroleptic perazine by the human cytochrome P-450 isoenzymes. *Eur Neuropsychopharmacol* 2004;14:199–208.

236. Tougou K, Gotou H, Ohno Y, Nakamura A. Stereoselective glucuronidation and hydroxylation of etodolac by UGT1A9 and CYP2C9 in man. *Xenobiotica* 2004;34:449–461.

237. Giraud C, Tran A, Rey E, Vincent J, Tréluyer J-M, Pons G. *In vitro* characterization of clobazam metabolism by recombinant cytochrome P450 enzymes: importance of CYP2C19. *Drug Metab Dispos* 2004;32:1279–1286.

238. Ufer M, Svensson JO, Krausz KW, Gelboin HV, Rane A, Tybring G. Identification of cytochromes P_{450} 2C9 and 3A4 as the major catalysts of phenprocoumon hydroxylation *in vitro*. *Eur J Clin Pharmacol* 2004;60:173–182.

239. Hirani VN, Raucy JL, Lasker JM. Conversion of the HIV protease inhibitor nelfinavir to a bioactive metabolite by human liver CYP2C19. *Drug Metab Dispos* 2004;32: 1462–1467.

240. Akimoto M, Iida I, Itoga H, Miyata A, Kawahara S, Kohno Y. The *in vitro* metabolism of desglymidodrine, an active metabolite of prodrug midodrine, by human liver microsomes. *Eur J Drug Metab Pharmacokinet* 2004;29:179–186.

241. Maurer HH, Kraemer T, Springer D, Staack RF. Chemistry, pharmacology, toxicology, and hepatic metabolism of designer drugs of the amphetamine (ecstasy), piperazine, and pyrrolidinophenone types: a synopsis. *Ther Drug Monit* 2004;26:127–131.

242. Kubo M, Koue T, Inaba A, Takeda H, Maune H, Fukuda T, Azuma J. Influence of itraconazole co-administration and CYP2D6 genotype on the pharmacokinetics of the new antipsychotic Aripiprazole. *Drug Metab Pharmacokinet* 2005;20:55–64.

243. Winter HR, Unadkat JD. Identification of cytochrome P450 and arylamine *N*-acetyltransferase isoforms involved in sulfadiazine metabolism. *Drug Metab Dispos* 2004; 33:969–976.

244. Yasar Ü, Annas A, Svensson J-O, Lazorova L, Artursson P, Al-Shurbaji A. Ketobemidone is a substrate for cytochrome P4502C9 and 3A4, but not for P-glycoprotein. *Xenobiotica* 2005;35:785–796.

245. Bland TM, Haining RL, Tracy TS, Callery PS. CYP2C-catalyzed delta(9)-tetrahydrocannabinol metabolism: kinetics, pharmacogenetics and interaction with phenytoin. *Biochem Pharmacol* 2005;70:1096–1103.

246. Nakashima A, Kawashita H, Masuda N, Saxer C, Niina M, Nagae Y, Iwasaki K. Identification of cytochrome P450 forms involved in the 4-hydroxylation of valsartan, a potent and specific angiotensin II receptor antagonist, in human liver microsomes. *Xenobiotica* 2005;35:589–602.

247. Kajosaari LI, Laitila J, Neuvonen PJ, Backman JT. Metabolism of repaglinide by CYP2C8 and CYP3A4 *in vitro*: effect of fibrates and rifampicin. *Basic Clin Pharmacol Toxicol* 2005;97:249–256.

248. Obach RS, Cox LM, Tremaine LM. Sertraline is metabolized by multiple cytochrome P450 enzymes, monoamine oxidases, and glucuronyl transferases in human: an *in vitro* study. *Drug Metab Dispos* 2005;33:262–270.

249. Kimura M, Yamazaki H, Fujieda M, Kiyotani K, Honda G, Saruwatari J, Nakagawa K, Ishizaki T, Kamataki T. CYP2A6 is a principal enzyme involved in hydroxylation of 1,7-dimethylxanthine, a main caffeine metabolite, in humans. *Drug Metab Dispos* 2005;33:1361–1366.

250. Cederbaum AI. CYP2E1—biochemical and toxicological aspects and role in alcohol-induced liver injury. *Mt Sinai J Med* 2006;73:657–672.

251. Aiba I, Yamasaki T, Shinki T, Izumi S, Yamamoto K, Yamada S, Terato H, Ide H, Ohyama Y. Characterization of rat and human CYP2J enzymes as vitamin D 25-hydroxylases. *Steroids* 2006;71:849–856.

252. Casabar RCT, Wallace AD, Hodgson E, Rose RL. Metabolism of endosulfan-alpha by human liver microsomes as a simultaneous *in vitro* probe for CYP2B6 and CYP3A4. *Drug Metab Dispos* 2006;34:1779–1785.

253. Pritchard MP, Wolf CR. Other CYP: 2A6, 2B6, 4A. In Levy RH, Thummel KE, Trager WF, Hansten PD, Eichelbaum M, Eds. *Metabolic Drug Interactions*. Philadelphia: Lippincott Williams & Wilkins; 2000, pp 145–160.

254. Hanna IH, Reed JR, Guengerich FP, Hollenberg PF. Expression of human cytochrome P450 2B6 in *Escherichia coli*: characterization of catalytic activity and expression levels in human liver. *Arch Biochem Biophys* 2000;376:206–216.

255. Ekins S, Vandenbranden M, Ring BJ, Gillespie JS, Yang TJ, Gelboin HV, Wrighton SA. Further characterization of the expression in liver and catalytic activity of CYP2B6. *J Pharmacol Exp Ther* 1998;286:1253–1259.

256. Lamba V, Lamba J, Yasuda K, Strom S, Davila J, Hancock ML, Fackenthal JD, Rogan PK, Ring B, Wrighton SA, Schuetz EG. Hepatic CYP2B6 expression: gender and ethnic differences and relationship to CYP2B6 genotype and CAR (constitutive androstane receptor) expression. *J Pharmacol Exp Ther* 2003;307:906–922.

257. Souček P, Gut I. Cytochrome P-450 in rats: structures, functions, properties and relevant human forms. *Xenobiotica* 1992;22:83–103.

258. Sattler M, Guengerich FP, Yun C-H, Christians U, Sewing K-F. Cytochrome P-450 3A enzymes are responsible for biotransformation of FK506 and rapamycin in man and rat. *Drug Metab Dispos* 1992;20:753–761.

259. Ward S, Back DJ. Metabolism of gestodene in human liver cytosol and microsomes *in vitro*. *J Steroid Biochem Mol Biol* 1993;46:235–243.

260. Zhou-Pan X-R, Sérée E, Zhou X-J, Placidi M, Maurel P, Barra Y, Rahmani R. Involvement of human liver cytochrome P450 3A in vinblastine metabolism: drug interactions. *Cancer Res* 1993;53:5121–5126.

261. Zhou X-J, Zhou-Pan X-R, Gauthier T, Placidi M, Maurel P, Rahmani R. Human liver microsomal cytochrome P450 3A isozymes mediated vindesine biotransformation. Metabolic drug interactions. *Biochem Pharmacol* 1993;45:853–861.

262. Huskey S-EW, Dean DC, Miller RR, Rasmusson GH, Chiu S-HL. Identification of human cytochrome P450 isozymes responsible for the *in vitro* oxidative metabolism of finasteride. *Drug Metab Dispos* 1995;23:1126–1135.

263. Pichard L, Gillet G, Bonfils C, Domergue J, Thénot J-P, Maurel P. Oxidative metabolism of zolpidem by human liver cytochrome P450s. *Drug Metab Dispos* 1995;23:1253–1262.

264. Labroo RB, Thummel KE, Kunze KL, Podoll T, Trager WF, Kharasch ED. Catalytic role of cytochrome P4503A4 in multiple pathways of alfentanil metabolism. *Drug Metab Dispos* 1995;23:490–496.

265. Ono S, Hatanaka T, Miyazawa S, Tsutsui M, Aoyama T, Gonzalez FJ, Satoh T. Human liver microsomal diazepam metabolism using cDNA-expressed cytochrome P450s: role of CYP2B6, 2C19 and the 3A subfamily. *Xenobiotica* 1996;26:1155–1166.

266. Wienkers LC, Steenwyk RC, Sanders PE, Pearson PG. Biotransformation of tirilazad in human: 1. Cytochrome P450 3A-mediated hydroxylation of tirilazad mesylate in human liver microsomes. *J Pharmacol Exp Ther* 1996;277:982–990.

267. Kumar GN, Rodrigues AD, Buko AM, Denissen JF. Cytochrome P450-mediated metabolism of the HIV-protease inhibitor ritonavir (ABT-538) in human liver microsomes. *J Pharmacol Exp Ther* 1996;277:423–431.

268. Tateishi T, Krivoruk Y, Ueng YF, Wood AJ, Guengerich FP, Wood M. Identification of human liver cytochrome P-450 3A4 as the enzyme responsible for fentanyl and sufentanil *N*-dealkylation. *Anesth Analg* 1996;82:167–172.

269. Sanwald P, David M, Dow J. Characterization of the cytochrome P450 enzymes involved in the *in vitro* metabolism of dolasetron. Comparison with other indole-containing 5-HT3 antagonists. *Drug Metab Dispos* 1996;24:602–609.

270. Delaforge M, Andre F, Jaouen M, Dolgos H, Benech H, Gomis JM, Noel JP, Cavelier F, Verducci J, Aubagnac JL, Liebermann B. Metabolism of tentoxin by hepatic cytochrome P-450 3A isozymes. *Eur J Biochem* 1997;250:150–157.

271. Iatsimirskaia E, Tulebaev S, Storozhuk E, Utkin I, Smith D, Gerber N, Koudriakova T. Metabolism of rifabutin in human enterocyte and liver microsomes: kinetic parameters,

identification of enzyme systems, and drug interactions with macrolides and antifungal agents. *Clin Pharmacol Ther* 1997;61:554–562.

272. Surapaneni SS, Clay MP, Spangle LA, Paschal JW, Lindstrom TD. *In vitro* biotransformation and identification of human cytochrome P450 isozyme-dependent metabolism of tazofelone. *Drug Metab Dispos* 1997;25:1383–1388.

273. Prueksaritanont T, Gorham LM, Ma B, Liu L, Yu X, Zhao JJ, Slaughter DE, Arison BH, Vyas KP. *In vitro* metabolism of simvastatin in humans: identification of metabolizing enzymes and effect of the drug on hepatic P450s. *Drug Metab Dispos* 1997;25: 1191–1199.

274. Teramura T, Fukunaga Y, van Hoogdalem EJ, Watanabe T, Higuchi S. Examination of metabolic pathways and identification of human liver cytochrome P450 isozymes responsible for the metabolism of barnidipine, a calcium channel blocker. *Xenobiotica* 1997;27:885–900.

275. Butler AM, Murray M. Biotransformation of parathion in human liver: participation of CYP3A4 and its inactivation during microsomal parathion oxidation. *J Pharmacol Exp Ther* 1997;280:966–973.

276. von Moltke LL, Greenblatt DJ, Grassi JM, Granda BW, Fogelman SM, Harmatz JS, Kramer SJ, Fabre LF, Shader RI. Gepirone and 1-(2-pyrimidinyl)-piperazine *in vitro*: human cytochromes mediating transformation and cytochrome inhibitory effects. *Psychopharmacology* 1998;140:293–299.

277. Renwick AB, Mistry H, Ball SE, Walters DG, Kao J, Lake BG. Metabolism of zaleplon by human hepatic microsomal cytochrome P450 isoforms. *Xenobiotica* 1998;28:337–348.

278. Hashizume T, Mise M, Terauchi Y, O L, Fujii T, Miyazaki H, Inaba T. *N*-dealkylation and hydroxylation of ebastine by human liver cytochrome P450. *Drug Metab Dispos* 1998;26:566–571.

279. Yaich M, Popon M, Medard Y, Aigrain EJ. *In-vitro* cytochrome P450 dependent metabolism of oxybutynin to *N*-deethyloxybutynin in humans. *Pharmacogenetics* 1998;8:449–451.

280. Haaz MC, Rivory L, Riche C, Vernillet L, Robert J. Metabolism of irinotecan (CPT-11) by human hepatic microsomes: participation of cytochrome P-450 3A and drug interactions. *Cancer Res* 1998;58:468–472.

281. Zeng Z, Andrew NW, Arison BH, Luffer-Atlas D, Wang RW. Identification of cytochrome P4503A4 as the major enzyme responsible for the metabolism of ivermectin by human liver microsomes. *Xenobiotica* 1998;28:313–321.

282. Postlind H, Danielson A, Lindgren A, Andersson SHG. Tolterodine, a new muscarinic receptor antagonist, is metabolized by cytochromes P450 2D6 and 3A in human liver microsomes. *Drug Metab Dispos* 1998;26:289–293.

283. Baune B, Flinois JP, Furlan V, Gimenez F, Taburet AM, Becquemont L, Farinotti R. Halofantrine metabolism in microsomes in man: major role of CYP 3A4 and CYP 3A5. *J Pharm Pharmacol* 1999;51:419–426.

284. Becquemont L, Mouajjah S, Escaffre O, Beaune P, Funck-Brentano C, Jaillon P. Cytochrome P-450 3A4 and 2C8 are involved in zopiclone metabolism. *Drug Metab Dispos* 1999;27:1068–1073.

285. Salphati L, Benet LZ. Metabolism of digoxin and digoxigenin digitoxosides in rat liver microsomes: involvement of cytochrome P4503A. *Xenobiotica* 1999;29:171–185.

286. Nebbia C, Ceppa L, Dacasto M, Carletti M, Nachtmann C. Oxidative metabolism of monensin in rat liver microsomes and interactions with tiamulin and other

chemotherapeutic agents: evidence for the involvement of cytochrome P-450 3A sub-family. *Drug Metab Dispos* 1999;27:1039–1044.

287. Guengerich FP. Cytochrome P-450 3A4: regulation and role in drug metabolism. *Annu Rev Pharmacol Toxicol* 1999;39:1–17.

288. Suzuki A, Iida I, Tanaka F, Akimoto M, Fukushima K, Tani M, Ishizaki T, Chiba K. Identification of human cytochrome P-450 isoforms involved in metabolism of *R*(+)- and *S*(−)-gallopamil: utility of *in vitro* disappearance. *Drug Metab Dispos* 1999;27:1254–1259.

289. Shiraga T, Kaneko H, Iwasaki K, Tozuka Z, Suzuki A, Hata T. Identification of cytochrome P450 enzymes involved in the metabolism of zotepine, an antipsychotic drug, in human liver microsomes. *Xenobiotica* 1999;29:217–229.

290. Wienkers LC, Allievi C, Hauer MJ, Wynalda MA. Cytochrome P-450-mediated metabolism of the individual enantiomers of the antidepressant agent reboxetine in human liver microsomes. *Drug Metab Dispos* 1999;27:1334–1340.

291. May-Manke A, Kroemer H, Hempel G, Bohnenstengel F, Hohenlöchter B, Blaschke G, Boos J. Investigation of the major human hepatic cytochrome P450 involved in 4-hydroxylation and *N*-dechlorethylation of trofosfamide. *Cancer Chemother Pharmacol* 1999;44:327–334.

292. Zalma A, von Moltke LL, Granda BW, Harmatz JS, Shader RI, Greenblatt DJ. *In vitro* metabolism of trazodone by CYP3A: inhibition by ketoconazole and human immunodeficiency viral protease inhibitors. *Biol Psychiatry* 2000;47:655–661.

293. Gantenbein M, Attolini L, Bruguerolle B, Villard P-H, Puyoou F, Durand A, Lacarelle B, Hardwigsen J, Le-Treut Y-P. Oxidative metabolism of bupivacaine into pipecolylxylidine in humans is mainly catalyzed by CYP3A. *Drug Metab Dispos* 2000;28:383–385.

294. Kasahara M, Suzuki H, Komiya I. Studies on the cytochrome P450 (CYP)-mediated metabolic properties of miocamycin: evaluation of the possibility of a metabolic intermediate complex formation with CYP, and identification of the human CYP isoforms. *Drug Metab Dispos* 2000;28:409–417.

295. Prakash C, Kamel A, Cui D, Whalen RD, Miceli JJ, Tweedie D. Identification of the major human liver cytochrome P450 isoform(s) responsible for the formation of the primary metabolites of ziprasidone and prediction of possible drug interactions. *Br J Clin Pharmacol* 2000;49(Suppl 1):35S–42S.

296. Lefèvre G, Bindschedler M, Ezzet F, Schaeffer N, Meyer I, Thomsen MS. Pharmacokinetic interaction trial between co-artemether and mefloquine. *Eur J Pharm Sci* 2000;10:141–151.

297. Rawden HC, Kokwaro GO, Ward SA, Edwards G. Relative contribution of cytochromes P-450 and flavin-containing monooxygenases to the metabolism of albendazole by human liver microsomes. *Br J Clin Pharmacol* 2000;49:313–322.

298. Kobayashi K, Mimura N, Fujii H, Minami H, Sasaki Y, Shimada N, Chiba K. Role of human cytochrome P450 3A4 in metabolism of medroxyprogesterone acetate. *Clin Cancer Res* 2000;6:3297–3303.

299. Fitzpatrick JL, Ripp SL, Smith NB, Pierce WM Jr, Prough RA. Metabolism of DHEA by cytochromes P450 in rat and human liver microsomal fractions. *Arch Biochem Biophys* 2001;389:278–287.

300. Pearce RE, Gotschall RR, Kearns GL, Leeder JS. Cytochrome P450 involvement in the biotransformation of cisapride and racemic norcisapride *in vitro*: differential activity of individual human CYP3A isoforms. *Drug Metab Dispos* 2001;29:1548–1554.

301. Hyland R, Roe EGH, Jones BC, Smith DA. Identification of the cytochrome P450 enzymes involved in the *N*-demethylation of sildenafil. *Br J Clin Pharmacol* 2001; 51:239–248.

302. Igel M, Sudhop T, von Bergmann K. Metabolism and drug interactions of 3-hydroxy-3-methylglutaryl coenzyme A-reductase inhibitors (statins). *Eur J Clin Pharmacol* 2001;57:357–364.

303. Ishigami M, Honda T, Takasaki W, Ikeda T, Komai T, Ito K, Sugiyama Y. A comparison of the effects of 3-hydroxy-3-methylglutaryl-coenzyme A (HMG-CoA) reductase inhibitors on the CYP3A4-dependent oxidation of mexazolam *in vitro*. *Drug Metab Dispos* 2001;29:282–288.

304. Kassahun K, McIntosh IS, Shou M, Walsh DJ, Rodeheffer C, Slaughter DE, Geer LA, Halpin RA, Agrawal N, Rodrigues AD. Role of human liver cytochrome P4503A in the metabolism of etoricoxib, a novel cyclooxygenase-2 selective inhibitor. *Drug Metab Dispos* 2001;29:813–820.

305. Cherstniakova SA, Bi D, Fuller DR, Mojsiak JZ, Collins JM, Cantilena LR. Metabolism of vanoxerine, 1-[2-[bis(4-fluorophenyl)methoxy]ethyl]-4-(3-phenylpropyl) piperazine, by human cytochrome P450 enzymes. *Drug Metab Dispos* 2001;29:1216–1220.

306. Ibrahim A, Karim A, Feldman J, Kharasch E. The influence of parecoxib, a parenteral cyclooxygenase-2 specific inhibitor, on the pharmacokinetics and clinical effects of midazolam. *Anesth Analg* 2002;95:667–673.

307. Eagling VA, Wiltshire H, Whitcombe IW, Back DJ. CYP3A4-mediated hepatic metabolism of the HIV-1 protease inhibitor saquinavir *in vitro*. *Xenobiotica* 2002;32:1–17.

308. Yan Z, Caldwell GW, Wu WN, McKown LA, Rafferty B, Jones W, Masucci JA. *In vitro* identification of metabolic pathways and cytochrome P450 enzymes involved in the metabolism of etoperidone. *Xenobiotica* 2002;32:949–962.

309. Chen Q, Ngui JS, Doss GA, Wang RW, Cai X, DiNinno FP, Blizzard TA, Hammond ML, Stearns RA, Evans DC, Baillie TA, Tang W. Cytochrome P450 3A4-mediated bioactivation of raloxifene: irreversible enzyme inhibition and thiol adduct formation. *Chem Res Toxicol* 2002;15:907–914.

310. Cook CS, Berry LM, Kim DH, Burton EG, Hribar JD, Zhang L. Involvement of CYP3A in the metabolism of eplerenone in humans and dogs: differential metabolism by CYP3A4 and CYP3A5. *Drug Metab Dispos* 2002;30:1344–1351.

311. Guay DR. Clinical pharmacokinetics of drugs used to treat urge incontinence. *Clin Pharmacokinet* 2003;42:1243–1285.

312. Kim SY, Suzuki N, Laxmi YRS, Rieger R, Shibutani S. α-Hydroxylation of tamoxifen and toremifene by human and rat cytochrome P450 3A subfamily enzymes. *Chem Res Toxicol* 2003;16:1138–1144.

313. Tréluyer JM, Bowers G, Cazali N, Sonnier M, Rey E, Pons G, Cresteil T. Oxidative metabolism of amprenavir in the human liver. Effect of the CYP3A maturation. *Drug Metab Dispos* 2003;31:275–281.

314. Galetin A, Clarke SE, Houston JB. Multisite kinetic analysis of interactions between prototypical CYP3A4 subgroup substrates: midazolam, testosterone, and nifedipine. *Drug Metab Dispos* 2003;31:1108–1116.

315. Greenblatt DJ, von Molke LL, Giancarlo GM, Garteiz DA. Human cytochromes mediating gepirone biotransformation at low substrate concentrations. *Biopharm Drug Dispos* 2003;24:87–94.

316. Wynalda MA, Hutzler JM, Koets MD, Podoll T, Wienkers LC. *In vitro* metabolism of clindamycin in human liver and intestinal microsomes. *Drug Metab Dispos* 2003; 31:878–887.

317. Cockshott ID. Bicalutamide: clinical pharmacokinetics and metabolism. *Clin Pharmacokinet* 2004;43:855–878.

318. Dalvie DK, O'Connell TN. Characterization of novel dihydrothienopyridinium and thienopyridinium metabolites of ticlopidine *in vitro*: role of peroxidases, cytochromes P450, and monoamine oxidases. *Drug Metab Dispos* 2004;32:49–57.

319. Bu H-Z, Pool WF, Wu EY, Raber SR, Amantea MA, Shetty BV. Metabolism and excretion of capravirine, a new non-nucleoside reverse transcriptase inhibitor, alone and in combination with ritonavir in healthy volunteers. *Drug Metab Dispos* 2004;32:689–698.

320. Sanchez RI, Wang RW, Newton DJ, Bakhtiar R, Lu P, Chiu S-HL, Evans DC, Huskey S-EW. Cytochrome P450 3A4 is the major enzyme involved in the metabolism of the substance P receptor antagonist aprepitant. *Drug Metab Dispos* 2004;32:1287–1292.

321. Galetin A, Brown C, Hallifax D, Ito K, Houston JB. Utility of recombinant enzyme kinetics in prediction of human clearance: impact of variability, CYP3A5, and CYP2C19 on CYP3A4 probe substrates. *Drug Metab Dispos* 2004;32:1411–1420.

322. Berecz R, Dorado P, De La Rubia A, Caceres MC, Degrell I, Llerena A. The role of cytochrome P450 enzymes in the metabolism of risperidone and its clinical relevance for drug interactions. *Curr Drug Targets* 2004;5:573–579.

323. Ferrari A, Coccia CPR, Bertolini A, Sternieri E. Methadone—metabolism, pharmacokinetics and interactions. *Pharmacol Res* 2004;50:551–559.

324. Naritomi Y, Terashita S, Kagayama A. Identification and relative contributions of human cytochrome P450 isoforms involved in the metabolism of glibenclamide and lansoprazole: evaluation of an approach based on the *in vitro* substrate disappearance rate. *Xenobiotica* 2004;34:415–427.

325. Picard N, Cresteil T, Prémaud A, Marquet P. Characterization of a phase 1 metabolite of mycophenolic acid produced by CYP3A4/5. *Ther Drug Monit* 2004;26:600–608.

326. Usmani KA, Hodgson E, Rose RL. *In vitro* metabolism of carbofuran by human, mouse, and rat cytochrome P450 and interactions with chlorpyrifos, testosterone, and estradiol. *Chem-Biol Interact* 2004;150:221–232.

327. Kalgutkar AS, Vaz ADN, Lame ME, Henne KR, Soglia J, Zhao SX, Abramov YA, Lombardo F, Collin C, Hendsch ZS, Hop CECA. Bioactivation of the nontricyclic antidepressant nefazodone to a reactive quinine-imine species in human liver microsomes and recombinant cytochrome P450 3A4. *Drug Metab Dispos* 2005;33:243–253.

328. Zhu M, Zhao W, Jimenez H, Zhang D, Yeola S, Dai R, Vachharajani N, Mitroka J. Cytochrome P450 3A-mediated metabolism of buspirone in human liver microsomes. *Drug Metab Dispos* 2005;33:500–507.

329. Ghosal A, Chowdhury SK, Tong W, Hapangama N, Yuan Y, Su A-D, Zbaida S. Identification of human liver cytochrome P450 enzymes responsible for the metabolism of lonafarnib (Sarasar). *Drug Metab Dispos* 2005;34:628–635.

330. Picard N, Cresteil T, Djebli N, Marquet P. *In vitro* metabolism study of buprenorphine: evidence for new metabolic pathways. *Drug Metab Dispos* 2005;33:689–695.

331. Tuvesson H, Hallin I, Persson R, Sparre B, Gunnarsson PO, Seidegård J. Cytochrome P450 3A4 is the major enzyme responsible for the metabolism of laquinimod, a novel immunomodulator. *Drug Metab Dispos* 2005;33:866–872.

332. Duisken M, Sandner F, Blömeke B, Hollender J. Metabolism of 1,8-cineole by human cytochrome P450 enzymes: identification of a new hydroxylated metabolite. *Biochim Biophys Acta* 2005;1722:304–311.

333. Kitamura A, Mizuno Y, Natsui K, Yabuki M, Komuro S. Characterization of human cytochrome P450 enzymes involved in the *in vitro* metabolism of perospirone. *Biopharm Drug Dispos* 2005;26:59–65.

334. Le Tiec C, Barrail A, Goujard C, Taburet AM. Clinical pharmacokinetics and summary of efficacy and tolerability of atazanavir. *Clin Pharmacokinet* 2005;44:1035–1050.

335. Beulz-Riché D, Grudé P, Puozzo C, Sautel F, Filaquier C, Riché C, Ratanasavanh D. Characterization of human cytochrome P450 isoenzymes involved in the metabolism of vinorelbine. *Fundam Clin Pharmacol* 2005;19:545–553.

336. Tokairin T, Fukasawa T, Yasui-Furukori N, Aoshima T, Suzuki A, Inoue Y, Tateishi T, Otani K. Inhibition of the metabolism of brotizolam by erythromycin in humans: *in vivo* evidence for the involvement of CYP3A4 in brotizolam metabolism. *Br J Clin Pharmacol* 2005;60:172–175.

337. Kassahun K, Skordos K, McIntosh I, Slaughter D, Doss GA, Baillie TA, Yost GS. Zafirlukast metabolism by cytochrome P450 3A4 produces an electrophilic α,β-unsaturated iminium species that results in the selective mechanism-based inactivation of the enzyme. *Chem Res Toxicol* 2005;18:1427–1437.

338. Peng F-C, Chang C-C, Yang C-Y, Edwards RJ, Doehmer J. Territrems B and C metabolism in human liver microsomes: major role of CYP3A4 and CYP3A5. *Toxicology* 2006;218:172–185.

339. Xu Y, Hashizume T, Shuhart MC, Davis CL, Nelson WL, Sakaki T, Kalhorn TF, Watkins PB, Schuetz EG, Thummel KE. Intestinal and hepatic CYP3A4 catalyze hydroxylation of 1α,25-dihydroxyvitamin D_3: implications for drug-induced osteomalacia. *Mol Pharmacol* 2006;69:56–65.

340. Tanaka E, Nakamura T, Inomata S, Honda K. Effects of premedication medicines on the formation of the CYP3A4-dependent metabolite of ropivacaine, 2′, 6′-pipecoloxylidide, on human liver microsomes *in vitro*. *Basic Clin Pharmacol Toxicol* 2006;98: 181–183.

341. Chen Q, Doss GA, Tung EC, Liu W, Tang YS, Braun MP, Didolkar V, Strauss JR, Wang RW, Stearns RA, Evans DC, Baillie TA, Tang W. Evidence for the bioactivation of zomepirac and tolmetin by an oxidative pathway: identification of glutathione adducts *in vitro* in human liver microsomes and *in vivo* in rats. *Drug Metab Dispos* 2006;34:145–151.

342. Cho TM, Rose RL, Hodgson E. *In vitro* metabolism of naphthalene by human liver microsomal cytochrome P450 enzymes. *Drug Metab Dispos* 2006;34:176–183.

343. Lin C-C, Fang C, Benetton S, Xu G-F, Yeh L-T. Metabolic activation of pradefovir by CYP3A4 and its potential as an inhibitor or inducer. *Antimicrob Agents Chemother* 2006;50:2926–2931.

344. Najib J. Eszopiclone, a nonbenzodiazepine sedative-hypnotic agent for the treatment of transient and chronic insomnia. *Clin Ther* 2006;28:491–516.

345. Daly AK. Significance of the minor cytochrome P450 3A isoforms. *Clin Pharmacokinet* 2006;45:13–31.

346. Matsubara T, Kim HJ, Miyata M, Shimada M, Nagata K, Yamazoe Y. Isolation and characterization of a new major intestinal CYP3A form, CYP3A62, in the rat. *J Pharmacol Exp Ther* 2004;309:1282–1290.

347. Rekka E, Evdokimova E, Eeckhoudt S, Labar G, Calderon PB. Role of temperature on protein and mRNA cytochrome P450 3A (CYP3A) isozymes expression and midazolam oxidation by cultured rat precision-cut liver slices. *Biochem Pharmacol* 2002; 64:633–643.

348. Cooper KO, Reik LM, Jayyosi Z, Bandiera S, Kelley M, Ryan DE, Daniel R, McCluskey SA, Levin W, Thomas PE. Regulation of two members of the steroid-inducible cytochrome P450 subfamily (3A) in rats. *Arch Biochem Biophys* 1993;301:345–354.

349. Mahnke A, Strotkamp D, Roos PH, Hanstein WG, Chabot GG, Nef P. Expression and inducibility of cytochrome P450 3A9 (CYP3A9) and other members of the CYP3A subfamily in rat liver. *Arch Biochem Biophys* 1997;337:62–68.

350. Kawai M, Bandiera SM, Chang TKH, Bellward GD. Growth hormone regulation and developmental expression of rat hepatic CYP3A18, CYP3A9, and CYP3A2. *Biochem Pharmacol* 2000;59:1277–1287.

351. Castle PJ, Merdink JL, Okita JR, Wrighton SA, Okita RT. Human liver lauric acid hydroxylase activities. *Drug Metab Dispos* 1995;23:1037–1043.

352. Powell PK, Wolf I, Lasker JM. Identification of CYP4A11 as the major lauric acid omega-hydroxylase in human liver microsomes. *Arch Biochem Biophys* 1996;335: 219–226.

353. Jin R, Koop DR, Raucy JL, Lasker JM. Role of human CYP4F2 in hepatic catabolism of the proinflammatory agent leukotriene B4. *Arch Biochem Biophys* 1998;359:89–98.

354. Kikuta Y, Kusunose E, Kusunose M. Characterization of human liver leukotriene B₄ ω-hydroxylase P450 (CYP4F2). *J Biochem* 2000;127:1047–1052.

355. Bylund J, Bylund M, Oliw EH. cDNA cloning and expression of CYP4F12, a novel human cytochrome P450. *Biochem Biophys Res Commun* 2001;280:892–897.

356. Kikuta Y, Kusunose E, Kusunose M. Prostaglandin and leukotriene ω-hydroxylases. *Prostaglandins Other Lipid Mediators* 2002;68–69:345–362.

357. Hashizume T, Imaoka S, Mise M, Terauchi Y, Fujii T, Miyazaki H, Kamataki T, Funae Y. Involvement of CYP2J2 and CYP4F12 in the metabolism of ebastine in human intestinal microsomes. *J Pharmacol Exp Ther* 2002;300:298–304.

358. Kalsotra A, Turman CM, Kikuta Y, Strobel HW. Expression and characterization of human cytochrome P450 4F11: putative role in the metabolism of therapeutic drugs and eicosanoids. *Toxicol Appl Pharmacol* 2004;199:295–304.

359. Le Quéré V, Plée-Gauthier E, Potin P, Madec S. Human CYP4F3s are the main catalysts in the oxidation of fatty acid epoxides. *J Lipid Res* 2004;45:1446–1458.

360. Raucy JL, Lasker J, Ozaki K, Zoleta V. Regulation of CYP2E1 by ethanol and palmitic acid and CYP4A11 by clofibrate in primary cultures of human hepatocytes. *Toxicol Sci* 2004;79:233–241.

361. Kroetz DL, Xu F. Regulation and inhibition of arachidonic acid ω-hydroxylases and 20-HETE formation. *Annu Rev Pharmacol Toxicol* 2005;45:413–438.

362. Petersen KU. Omeprazole and the cytochrome P450 system. *Aliment Pharmacol Ther* 1995;9:1–9.

363. Probst-Hensch NM, Tannenbaum SR, Chan KK, Coetzee GA, Ross RK, Yu MC. Absence of the glutathione S-transferase M1 gene increases cytochrome P4501A2 activity among frequent consumers of cruciferous vegetables in a Caucasian population. *Cancer Epidemiol Biomarkers Prev* 1998;7:635–638.

364. Rae JM, Johnson MD, Lippman ME, Flockhart DA. Rifampin is a selective, pleiotropic inducer of drug metabolism genes in human hepatocytes: studies with cDNA and oligonucleotide expression arrays. *J Pharmacol Exp Ther* 2001;299:849–857.

365. Raucy JL. Regulation of CYP3A4 expression in human hepatocytes by pharmaceuticals and natural products. *Drug Metab Dispos* 2003;31:533–539.

366. Dingemanse J, van Giersbergen PLM. Clinical pharmacology of bosentan, a dual endothelin receptor antagonist. *Clin Pharmacokinet* 2004;43:1089–1115.

367. Komoroski BJ, Zhang S, Cai H, Hutzler JM, Frye R, Tracy TS, Strom SC, Lehmann T, Ang CYW, Cui YY, Venkataramanan R. Induction and inhibition of cytochromes P450 by the St. John's wort constituent hyperforin in human hepatocyte cultures. *Drug Metab Dispos* 2004;32:512–518.

368. Larsen JT, Brøsen K. Consumption of charcoal-broiled meat as an experimental tool for discerning CYP1A2-mediated drug metabolism *in vivo*. *Basic Clin Pharmacol Toxicol* 2005;97:141–148.

369. Waxman DJ. P450 gene induction by structurally diverse xenochemicals: central role of nuclear receptors CAR, PXR, and PPAR. *Arch Biochem Biophys* 1999;369:11–23.

370. Savas U, Griffin KJ, Johnson EF. Molecular mechanisms of cytochrome P-450 induction by xenobiotics: an expanded role for nuclear hormone receptors. *Mol Pharmacol* 1999;56:851–857.

371. Rowlands JC, Gustafsson, J-Å. Aryl hydrocarbon receptor-mediated signal transduction. *Crit Rev Toxicol* 1997;27:109–134.

372. Whitlock JP Jr. Induction of cytochrome P4501A1. *Annu Rev Pharmacol Toxicol* 1999;39:103–125.

373. Hankinson O. The aryl hydrocarbon receptor complex. *Annu Rev Pharmacol Toxicol* 1995;35:307–340.

374. Wang H, Negishi M. Transcriptional regulation of cytochrome P450 2B genes by nuclear receptors. *Curr Drug Metab* 2003;4:515–525.

375. Li HC, Dehal SS, Kupfer D. Induction of the hepatic CYP2B and CYP3A enzymes by the proestrogenic pesticide methoxychlor and by DDT in the rat. Effects on methoxychlor metabolism. *J Biochem Toxicol* 1995;10:51–61.

376. Blumberg B, Sabbagh W Jr, Bolado J Jr, van Meeter CM, Ong ES, Evans RM. SXR, a novel steroid and xenobiotics sensing nuclear receptor. *Genes Dev* 1998;12:3195–3205.

377. Burk O, Wojnowski L. Cytochrome P450 3A and their regulation. *Naunyn Schmiedebergs Arch Pharmacol* 2004;369:105–124.

378. Lehmann JM, Lenhard JM, Oliver BB, Ringgold GM, Kliewer SA. Peroxisome proliferator-activated receptors α and γ are activated by indomethacin and other non-steroidal anti-inflammatory drugs. *J Biol Chem* 1997;272:3406–3410.

379. Gonzalez FJ, Peters JM, Cattley RC. Mechanism of action of the nongenotoxic peroxisome proliferators: role of the peroxisome proliferator-activated receptor α. *J Natl Cancer Inst* 1998;90:1702–1709.

380. Moore LB, Parks DJ, Jones SA, Bledsoe RK, Consler TG, Stimmel JB, Goodwin B, Liddle C, Blanchard SG, Willson TM, Collins JL, Kliewer SA. Orphan nuclear receptors constitutive androstane receptor and pregnane X receptor share xenobiotic and steroid ligands. *J Biol Chem* 2000;275:15122–15127.

381. Staudinger JL, Goodwin B, Jones SA, Hawkins-Brown D, MacKenzie IK, LaTour A, Liu Y, Klaassen CD, Brown KK, Reinhard J, Willson TM, Koller BH, Kliewer SA. The nuclear receptor PXR is a lithocholic acid sensor that protects against liver toxicity. *Proc Natl Acad Sci USA* 2001;98:3369–3374.

382. Goodwin B, Moore LB, Stoltz CM, McKee DD, Kliewer SA. Regulation of the human *CYP2B6* gene by the nuclear pregnane X receptor. *Mol Pharmacol* 2001;60:427–431.

383. Ripp SL, Fitzpatrick JL, Peters JM, Prough RA. Induction of *CYP3A* expression by dehydroepiandrosterone: involvement of the pregnane X receptor. *Drug Metab Dispos* 2002;30:570–575.

384. Maglich JM, Stoltz CM, Goodwin B, Hawkins-Brown D, Moore JT, Kliewer SA. Nuclear pregnane X receptor and constitutive androstane receptor regulate overlapping but distinct sets of genes involved in xenobiotic detoxification. *Mol Pharmacol* 2002;62: 638–646.

385. Denison MS, Nagy SR. Activation of the aryl hydrocarbon receptor by structurally diverse exogenous and endogenous chemicals. *Annu Rev Pharmacol Toxicol* 2003;43: 309–334.

386. Handschin C, Meyer UA. Induction of drug metabolism: the role of nuclear receptors. *Pharmacol Rev* 2003;55:649–673.

387. Chen Y, Ferguson SS, Negishi M, Goldstein JA. Induction of human *CYP2C9* by rifampicin, hyperforin, and phenobarbital is mediated by the pregnane X receptor. *J Pharmacol Exp Ther* 2004;308:495–501.

388. Pascussi J-M, Gerbal-Chaloin S, Drocourst L, Assénat E, Larrey D, Pichard-Garcia L, Vilarem M-J, Maurel P. Cross-talk between xenobiotic detoxication and other signalling pathways: clinical and toxicological consequences. *Xenobiotica* 2004;34:633–664.

389. van Raalte DH, Li M, Pritchard PH, Wasan KM. Peroxisome proliferator-activated receptor (PPAR)-α: a pharmacological target with a promising future. *Pharm Res* 2004;21:1531–1538.

390. Chen Y, Kissling G, Negishi M, Goldstein JA. The nuclear receptors constitutive androstane receptor and pregnane X receptor cross-talk with hepatic nuclear factor 4α to synergistically activate the human *CYP2C9* promoter. *J Pharmacol Exp Ther* 2005;314:1125–1133.

391. Kretschmer XC, Baldwin WS. CAR and PXR: xenosensors of endocrine disrupters? *Chem-Biol Interact* 2005;155:111–128.

392. Tirona RG, Kim RB. Nuclear receptors and drug disposition gene regulation. *J Pharm Sci* 2005;94:1169–1186.

393. Ferguson SS, Chen Y, LeCluyse EL, Negishi M, Goldstein JA. Human *CYP2C8* is transcriptionally regulated by the nuclear receptors constitutive androstane receptor, pregnane X receptor, glucocorticoid receptor, and hepatic nuclear factor 4α. *Mol Pharmacol* 2005;68:747–757.

394. Chang TK, Waxman DJ. Synthetic drugs and natural products as modulators of constitutive androstane receptor (CAR) and pregnane X receptor (PXR). *Drug Metab Rev* 2006;38:51–73.

395. Itoh M, Nakajima M, Higashi E, Yoshida R, Nagata K, Yamazoe Y, Yokoi T. Induction of human CYP2A6 is mediated by the pregnane X receptor with peroxisome proliferator-activated receptor-γ coactivator 1α. *J Pharmacol Exp Ther* 2006;319:693–702.

396. Nelson D. Cytochrome P450 homepage, 18 July 2006. http://drnelson.utmem.edu/CytochromeP450.html.

397. Ragueneau-Majlessi I, Hachad H, Levy RH. M&T drug interaction database. 2004. http://didbase@u.washington.edu.

398. Flockhart D. Drug interactions. 29 August, 2006. http://www.drug-interactions.com.

19

METABOLISM KINETICS

CHARLES W. LOCUSON AND TIMOTHY S. TRACY
University of Minnesota, Minneapolis, Minnesota

Contents

19.1 INTRODUCTION

It is common to apply kinetic models to *in vitro* data in an attempt to determine parameters, such as intrinsic clearance, that can be used to make correlations to the *in vivo* situation. These estimations are generally predicated on the data following a hyperbolic profile such that the Michaelis–Menten equation can be applied. This

Preclinical Development Handbook: ADME and Biopharmaceutical Properties,
edited by Shayne Cox Gad
Copyright © 2008 John Wiley & Sons, Inc.

allows determination of V_m and K_m and thus the determination of intrinsic clearance. However, it is increasingly being recognized that, for many substrates, these "typical kinetic" conditions may not exist and "atypical kinetics" may be observed. Unfortunately, application of the Michaelis–Menten equation to these "atypical" situations results in misestimation of V_m and K_m and, subsequently, intrinsic clearance. Thus, it is important to understand the assumptions behind typical kinetics in drug metabolism reactions, the different types of atypical kinetic profiles that may also be observed, and what models and equations can be used to estimate kinetic parameters from each of these types of data.

19.2   TYPICAL KINETICS

19.2.1   Michaelis–Menten Equation and Its Use in Drug Metabolism

One of the most widely taught and used biochemical principles is embodied in an equation, which has remained the very foundation of enzymology for nearly a century. This equation allows quantitative descriptions of many enzyme-catalyzed reactions in terms of rate and concentration and therefore helps us describe the molecular workings of the cell. Enzymology has aided in the diagnoses of diseases as well as the development of therapies used to treat them, and at the heart of enzymology is the Michaelis–Menten equation:

$$v = \frac{V_m \cdot [S]}{K_m + [S]} \tag{19.1}$$

where reaction velocity, v, is described as a function of substrate concentration, [S], multiplied by a limiting rate, V_m (also known as V or V_{max} whose subscript is not to be confused with that of K_m), and divided by the sum of [S] and constant K_m, whose subscript refers to its name, the Michaelis constant.

Following up on the theory of A. J. Brown and V. Henri that enzymatic catalysis results from the formation of an intermediate enzyme–substrate complex, Michaelis and Menten reaffirmed Henri's basic assumption.[1] Mainly, the effect of substrate concentration on velocity could be described by an equilibrium between enzyme and substrate and that their complexation can lead to product.

$$E + S \underset{k_{-1}}{\overset{k_1}{\rightleftharpoons}} ES \overset{k_2}{\longrightarrow} E + P \tag{19.2}$$

Derivation of the rate equation for Eq. 19.2 based on the initial concentration of enzyme and substrate, and the definition of the substrate dissociation constant, K_S, gives

$$v = \frac{k_2 \cdot E_0 \cdot [S]}{K_S + [S]} \tag{19.3}$$

---

[1]The following details were compiled largely from Cornish-Bowden [6], and for further details, consultation of this book is highly recommended.

where E_0 is the initial enzyme concentration. By avoiding any assumption about equilibrium in the first step of Eq. 19.2 (i.e., substrate binding to enzyme), Briggs and Haldane actually made the final contribution to the Michaelis–Menten equation with their steady-state treatment. Their steady-state assumption was that the concentration of the enzyme–substrate intermediate would become constant soon after initiation of the reaction. Using the same scheme (Eq. 19.2), K_S in Eq. 19.3 is substituted with the Michaelis constant:

$$K_m = \frac{k_{-1} + k_2}{k_1} \tag{19.4}$$

using the steady-state assumption as shown in the derivation available in most biochemistry textbooks. This is probably the preferred treatment unless specific details regarding substrate binding are known that enable the use of K_S. Whether K_m or K_S is used, the form of the equation is the same:

$$v = \frac{k_{cat} \cdot E_0 \cdot [S]}{K_m + [S]} \tag{19.5}$$

with the substitution of k_2 for k_{cat} (the observed rate[2] of reaction) so that no assumption is made about the number of steps that occur between substrate binding and the chemistry described by $k_{cat} \times E_0$. In other words, k_2 in Eq. 19.2 does not reflect the rate of catalysis except for the simplest two-step mechanism such that k_{cat} is used to represent the observed rate of reaction if there are more than two steps, even if the true number of steps is not known. For the same reason K_m is often more complex than shown in Eq. 19.4. E_0 and k_{cat} are then multiplied to produce the parameter V_m to yield the familiar Eq. 19.1.

Equation 19.2 does not consider the reversibility of the k_2 step, which would result in the subtraction of the reverse rate in the numerator ($k_P \times E_0 \times [P]$) and a term that includes a K_m for product P in the denominator. Even so, the Michaelis–Menten equation in its commonest form (Eq. 19.1) adequately describes the kinetics of metabolism for many drugs by enzymes like the cytochromes P450. Ideally, the rate of reaction at each substrate concentration would follow the method of *initial rates*, meaning several measurements over a limited amount of time (i.e., less than a few minutes) are subjected to linear regression to determine a rate. This prevents excessive amounts of product from building up and reversibly (or irreversibly) inhibiting the enzyme, or undergoing significant reversal back to substrate. However, this is often not feasible if time-expensive methods like liquid-chromatography separation or even extraction into organic solvent are needed to measure metabolized drug. In addition, even an incubation carried out with recombinant P450 is

---

[2]k_{cat}, the *catalytic constant* or *turnover number*, describes the number of turnovers an enzyme can accomplish in a given unit of time. Determination of k_{cat} requires accurately estimating V_m, therefore requiring the use of a sufficient range of substrate concentration to ensure saturation, and knowledge of E_0 ($k_{cat} = V_m/E_0$). V_m is determined preferably by nonlinear regression (although certain linear plots have been used for estimates). The initial enzyme concentration, E_0 or E_{total}, is in the same concentration units as V_m (e.g., μM/time) so that the unit of k_{cat} is time^{-1}.

much more complex than most may realize. Using the steady-state treatment, a P450 incubation may be thought of as possessing a K_m not only for drug, but for oxygen, P450 oxidoreductase (which has a K_m for NADPH), and possibly any other partially rate-limiting steps required for catalysis. Fortunately, most of these variables are kept constant and/or saturating. Considering the number of variables in P450–drug incubations and some of the difficulties involved in analyzing the products of such reactions, the Michaelis–Menten equation nevertheless remains remarkably useful.

Therefore, although proper controls must be carried out (see below), triplicate end-point measurements and their analysis with the Michaelis–Menten equation are probably the most fundamental and useful experiments in drug metabolism.

19.2.2   The Case of Multiple Substrates

Cofactors are heavily relied upon by drug metabolizing enzymes. The UDP-glucuronosyltransferases (UGTs), glutathione S-transferases (GSTs), flavin mono-oxygenases (FMOs), sulfotransferases (more correctly, sulfonyltransferases), N-acetyltransferases (NATs), and thiopurine S-methyltransferase (TPMT) all utilize nucleotide-containing cofactors for oxygen activation (e.g., FMO) or for conjugation (e.g., all others). FMOs can remain poised for oxidation without drug substrate ever binding as long as saturating levels of NADPH are present. UGTs, on the other hand, require a ternary complex of enzyme and two substrates (UDP-glucuronic acid and the aglycone substrate to be conjugated) to form before catalysis can occur.

Unfortunately, the number of parameters in rate equations expands substantially when describing models involving additional reaction steps. For instance, take the example of the kinetic mechanism of UGT that generally occurs through the ordered binding of two cosubstrates [1]. If the reverse reaction is ignored and any amount of product formed during the course of the reaction is considered negligible, the rate equation requires concentration information and estimation of K_m values for both substrates:

$$v = \frac{V_m[A][B]}{K_{iA}K_{mB} + K_{mB}[A] + K_{mA}[B] + [A][B]} \tag{19.6}$$

where A and B represent the two substrates each with their own K_m (K_{mA} and K_{mB}) and K_{iA} is the dissociation constant for the EA complex. Even with the aforementioned assumption, a substantial number of data points would be needed to fit this rate equation due to the number of parameters involved. However, if substrate B is always present in saturating concentrations and care is taken to avoid the buildup of products, Eq. 19.6 *reduces eventually to the Michaelis–Menten equation* (Eq. 19.1). In fact, this experimental and analytical simplification is probably the standard and preferred method for determining V_m as well as the K_m for each substrate. With further analysis this method also has the benefit of revealing features of the kinetic mechanism such as whether substrate binding is random or ordered, or if the first substrate is turned over and leaves before the second substrate can be turned over (i.e., Ping-Pong mechanism) [2].

19.2.3 Use of the Michaelis–Menten Equation and Its Parameters

Most are familiar with the rectangular hyperbola that results from plotting reaction velocity (y-axis) versus substrate concentration (x-axis) and that these plotted data can be fit to the Michaelis–Menten equation using nonlinear regression (although the curve itself was never used by Michaelis and Menten and therefore is *not* called a Michaelis–Menten curve). Therefore, the parameters V_m and K_m, as best fit by the nonlinear version of the equation (Eq. 19.1), are reviewed.

At low [S], Eq. 19.1 demonstrates that velocity becomes proportional to [S]:

$$v \approx \frac{k_{cat} \cdot E_0 \cdot [S]}{K_m} = \frac{V \cdot [S]}{K_m} \tag{19.7}$$

The middle expression of Eq. 19.7 is important because a very useful parameter is obtained from the ratio of k_{cat}/K_m known as the *specificity constant*. k_{cat}/K_m (units of time^{-1} × concentration^{-1}) is an excellent evaluation of substrate specificity for an enzyme. Imagine two substrates for the same enzyme that can each be turned over without the other present. The substrate with the highest specificity constant will correctly predict that it will be turned over faster than the other substrate if both were present at any equimolar concentration. Even if one substrate has a larger k_{cat}, a substrate with a higher k_{cat}/K_m will be turned over faster if the two are compared at the same concentration.

Low substrate concentrations (i.e., much lower than K_m) are also relevant to *in vivo–in vitro* correlations. If the therapeutic dosage of a drug results in sub-K_m plasma concentrations (the most common situation), where kinetics are largely first order for the enzyme(s) metabolizing it, Eq. 19.7 can be defined as the intrinsic clearance ($CL_{int} = V_m/K_m$, units time^{-1}), which is the clearance of drug from a tissue via metabolism independent of blood flow, protein binding, and other restrictions. Although the units are different from that for k_{cat}/K_m, V_m/K_m is still a specificity constant and the comparison of CL_{int} values for different drugs with the same enzyme may prove useful in predicting the reduced CL_{int} for *each* drug involved in a drug–drug interaction or polypharmacy.

Next, when the substrate concentration is equal to K_m, K_m can be defined operationally as the *concentration of substrate where velocity equals* $\frac{1}{2}V_m$. Often, K_m in this sense is used as a measure of the affinity of substrate for enzyme as if they were in equilibrium (K_S); however, without additional information regarding rate constants, K_m should never be assumed to be anything more than an estimate of K_S with no guarantees attached. Finally, when substrate is said to be saturating so that every enzyme molecule is bound to substrate, K_m becomes negligible and $v \approx V_m$. In other words, the rate is limited by the amount of enzyme present, and hence, V_m is perhaps better described as a limiting rate rather than a maximum.

19.3 ATYPICAL KINETICS DISPLAYED BY DRUG METABOLIZING ENZYMES

Atypical kinetics is a term that has come to be used to describe any *in vitro* drug metabolism kinetics that do not fit the hyperbolic function seen when velocity is plotted versus substrate concentration. *Allosterism* is another term used frequently in the P450 literature that refers to the ability of a ligand (a.k.a. effector) other than the substrate being turned over to bind in a distinct, noncatalytic site on an enzyme and affect the rate of metabolism of the substrate. The effector can be a second (or third or fourth, etc.) substrate molecule binding to the same enzyme or it can be a molecule that is structurally dissimilar from the substrate. Several lines of evidence suggest that some of the allosteric sites in P450s 3A4 and 2C9 are really distinct sites within the same binding pocket that substrate occupies; however, we think allosterism is still a suitable term to define this phenomenon since the P450s most likely do not bind every substrate in the same orientation or subregion of their active sites anyway.

Much attention has been given to the atypical kinetics of P450s in drug metabolism, but it is becoming apparent that phase II enzymes and drug transporters may occasionally display atypical kinetics likely stemming from the simultaneous occupancy of a single protein by multiple ligand (in addition to the normal substrates, if there are multiple substrates required for catalysis). In fact, almost all of the theoretical mechanisms that could give rise to atypical kinetics are plausible with drug metabolizing enzymes whether it occurs via one substrate (*homotropic*) or combinations of substrate and effector (*heterotropic*). Using P450s as an example, it is completely reasonable to hypothesize atypical kinetics arise from effector binding that modifies P450–P450, P450–P450 reductase, or P450–cytochrome-b_5 interactions, where the site can be in the same binding pocket as substrate or remote and be either homotropic or heterotropic.

19.3.1 Sigmoidal Kinetics with a Single Substrate

Sigmoidicity in substrate–velocity plots usually brings to mind cooperativity, which is generally thought of as arising from multimeric enzymes, like the textbook example of hemoglobin. Here, the sites where substrate binds are equivalent on each enzyme so cooperativity, not allosterism (e.g., effect of BPG on O_2 binding by hemoglobin), is used to describe the kinetic phenomenon. Evidence, however, now suggests P450s may display homotropic activation (or homotropic cooperativity), where a monomeric enzyme displays sigmoidal kinetics (Fig. 19.1) presumably through substrate binding to both a catalytic site and an effector site [3–5]. In any case, a useful expression called the Hill equation (Eq. 19.8) is adequate for describing many cases of this type of kinetics with just a few parameters:

$$v = \frac{V_m[S]^n}{K^n + [S]^n} \qquad (19.8)$$

where V_m and K are analogous to the parameters in the Michaelis–Menten equation (but the parameter[3] K is *not* called the Michaelis constant) and n is the Hill coefficient. The Hill equation is empirical with respect to the parameter n because while

---

[3]It is not essential that K be to the power n except that since n is often not a whole integer, K as the substrate concentration that gives the half-maximal velocity will have the same units as [S], but not be directly relatable to it.

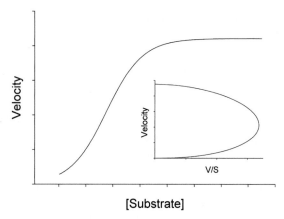

FIGURE 19.1 Graphical representation of a kinetic profile exhibiting sigmoidal (autoactivation) kinetics. Inset demonstrates the Eadie–Hofstee plot of a sigmoidal kinetic profile.

it measures relative cooperativity, it does not necessarily equal the number of binding sites for substrate because it is often not an integer. A more biochemically logical description of multiple binding sites is obtained with the use of the Adair equation (described in Cornish-Bowden [6]); however, the parameters of the Hill equation remain practical for most applications, including the study of drug metabolizing enzymes. For example, substrates (e.g., testosterone, carbamazepine, pyrene) that induce sigmoidal kinetics by CYP3A4 can all be meaningfully compared to each other using the Hill equation to determine which ones have the highest efficiency (V_m/K) and cooperativity (n).

When cooperativity is caused by an effector other than the target substrate in a monomeric enzyme (a.k.a. *heterotropic activation*) [7, 8], for instance, during inhibition screening, the Hill equation can still be used. Or, to better define the V_m and K_m parameters for substrate when it is known that the effector turnover rate is insignificant or much less than it is for substrate, Eq. 19.9 may prove useful by giving K_m and V_m in the absence or presence of effector (subscripts 1 and 2, respectively):

$$v = \frac{\dfrac{V_{m1}\cdot[S]}{K_{m1}} + \dfrac{V_{m2}\cdot[S]^2}{K_{m1}\cdot K_{m2}}}{1 + \dfrac{[S]}{K_{m1}} + \dfrac{[S]^2}{K_{m1}\cdot K_{m2}}} \qquad (19.9)$$

Equation 19.9, although working under the assumption of equilibrium, will also give the K_m and V_m of a substrate metabolized in two distinct subsites within the substrate binding pocket, each with different binding affinities and velocities. More complex rate equations have been developed for sigmoidal kinetics in drug metabolism and more rare mechanisms behind cooperativity can be found in Cornish-Bowden [6], and these sources should be consulted for a full description.

19.3.2 Biphasic Kinetics (Nonasymptotic)

As defined here, a biphasic kinetic profile does not follow saturation kinetics and has two distinct phases. (*Note that sigmoidal kinetics may also be biphasic but exhibits saturation.*) At low substrate concentrations, the kinetic profile exhibits curvature similar to that observed with hyperbolic kinetics; however, at high substrate concentrations, the velocity of the reaction continues to increase in a linear fashion (Fig. 19.2), as opposed to becoming asymptotic as would be expected with hyperbolic kinetics. This type of profile most commonly occurs when the metabolism of a substrate is carried out by more than one enzyme in a multienzyme system. However, when using a single, purified enzyme source, it is most likely the result of substrate binding in a productive orientation to more than one region within the active site, but these binding regions exhibit different affinities for the substrate and also differential turnover rates. In this case, a single enzyme behaves as if it were a multienzyme system. The enzyme thus exhibits a low K_m/low V_m component (responsible for the semihyperbolic nature of the profile) and another high K_m/high V_m component (producing the linear portion of the profile). In order to model this type of kinetic profile, one must use equations that describe the kinetics of one substrate interacting with two binding sites within the same enzyme species, such as Eq. 19.10.

$$v = \frac{(V_{m1} \cdot [S]) + (CL_{int} \cdot [S]^2)}{K_{m1} + [S]} \qquad (19.10)$$

The parameters V_{m1} and K_{m1} are estimated from data representing the curved portion of the plot at lower substrate concentrations and are the estimates of V_m and K_m for the low V_m, low K_m site, respectively. CL_{int} describes the linear portion of the plot exhibited at higher substrate concentrations and is the ratio of V_{max2}/K_{m2} (i.e., the high V_{max}, high K_m component of the profile). Because this upper portion of the plot is linear, one cannot estimate the actual V_m and K_m parameters for this portion of the profile since saturation is not achieved. Thus, CL_{int} is the slope (rate) for this linear portion of the kinetic profile.

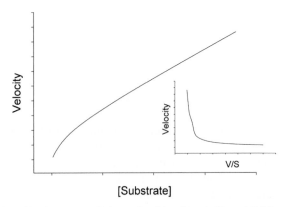

FIGURE 19.2 Graphical representation of a kinetic profile exhibiting biphasic kinetics. Inset demonstrates the Eadie–Hofstee plot of a biphasic kinetic profile.

19.3.3 Hyperbolic (Nonessential) Activation

The most straightforward kind of activation in terms of fitting K_m and V_m values to velocity versus [S] plots is probably hyperbolic activation. The name refers to the replot of K_m/V_m against reciprocal activator concentration, which is hyperbolic, not linear. (These plots for sigmoidal and biphasic kinetics are also not expected to be linear.) It is nonessential, because the effector is not necessary for catalysis to occur. While V_m and often K_m change for a substrate in the presence of an activating effector, the shape of the velocity vesus [S] curve remains a hyperbola. Therefore, the term hyperbolic activation has a more important meaning in drug metabolism kinetics because it can also refer to homo- or heterotropic activation that results in hyperbolic curves rather than sigmoidal or biphasic curves. As one might expect, changes in K_m and V_m can be fit at each activator concentration using the Michaelis–Menten equation. One of the best documented cases of this heterotropic activation is the activation of flurbiprofen (S) hydroxylation by the effector dapsone (B) in P450 2C9 and a mechanistic scheme has been proposed (Fig. 19.3). A graphical representation of the kinetic profile for this hyperbolic activation is shown in Fig. 19.4.

The equation (Eq. 19.11) for fitting multiple curves representing different activator concentrations has a manageable number of parameters including the usual K_m (which is assumed to be an estimate of K_S in this equilibrium model) and V_m for substrate in the absence of activator:

$$v = \frac{V_m \cdot [\text{S}]}{K_m \dfrac{1+[\text{B}]/K_B}{1+\beta[\text{B}]/\alpha K_B} + [\text{S}] \dfrac{1+[\text{B}]/\alpha K_B}{1+\beta[\text{B}]/\alpha K_B}} \tag{19.11}$$

where [B] is the concentration of activator, α is the factor by which K_S for substrate changes, and β can be thought of as the factor by which V_m changes (see Fig. 19.3 for further explanation of parameters).

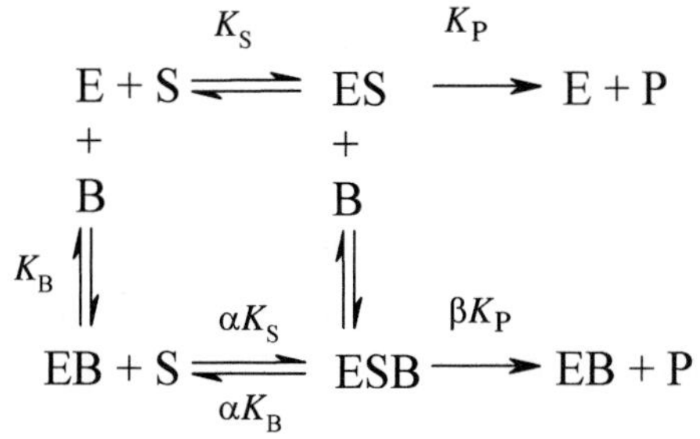

FIGURE 19.3 Kinetic mechanism for nonessential activation [2] demonstrates that the effector, B, is not essential for product formation. Furthermore, it can be seen that this scheme is flexible as α and β can be greater or less than unity. In the case of flurbiprofen, metabolism in the presence of effector dapsone results in a decrease in α, indicating an *increase* in affinity of P450 2C9 for flurbiprofen. This was further supported by equilibrium binding experiments. Parameter β was increased, indicating the velocity for oxidation of flurbiprofen has increased. Activation could also be achieved with $\alpha > 1$ but this would require higher substrate concentrations to be observed. Alternatively, if $\alpha < 1$, but $\beta < 1$, activation could result at low substrate concentrations and then result in inhibition at higher substrate concentrations.

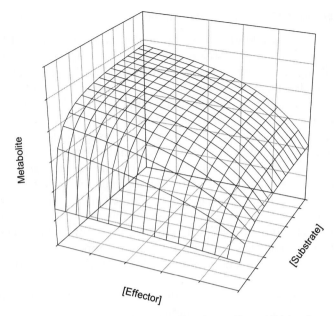

FIGURE 19.4 Graphical representation of a kinetic profile exhibiting heterotropic cooperativity (activation).

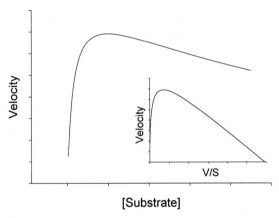

FIGURE 19.5 Graphical representation of a kinetic profile exhibiting substrate inhibition kinetics. Inset demonstrates the Eadie–Hofstee plot of a substrate inhibition kinetic profile.

19.3.4   Substrate Inhibition

In the case of substrate inhibition kinetics, as the concentration of substrate is increased, to determine V_m an inflection point in the velocity versus [S] curve occurs so that rather than plateau, the velocity starts to decrease and continues to do so as [S] is raised further (Fig. 19.5). Assuming the reactions were carried out appropriately (see Section 19.3.6), two likely scenarios arise when substrate inhibition is noted:

1. If the experiment is conducted with P450, the most likely cause is analogous to uncompetitive inhibition where two or more ligands (in this case, two substrate molecules) binding to the enzyme decrease its ability to catalyze substrate oxidation.
2. If the experiment is conducted with UGT, inhibition is likely the result of aglycone substrate binding right after a glucuronide conjugate is released from a previous round of catalysis, thereby trapping UDP and forming an inactive ternary complex. For many UGTs there appears to be a preference to bind UDP-glucuronic acid first, followed by aglycone, suggesting an ordered ternary complex mechanism.

In either case, K_m and V_m can be estimated via use of the appropriate equation. It should be noted, however, that the derived parameters (e.g., V_m and K_m) are not truly equivalent to the usual situation. Because V_m is never truly reached (or to simulate it unless the inhibition is very weak), the true K_m is also not discernible. In the past, researchers have incorrectly fit these types of data by either eliminating the points showing decreasing velocity or simply applying the Michaelis–Menten equation to the entire dataset. Lin and colleagues [9] have demonstrated the necessity to fit the entire dataset to the proper equation and the hazards of not doing so. For substrate inhibition occurring through promiscuous binding of a second substrate (case 1), the following rate equation (Eq. 19.12) is useful. It is derived from the uncompetitive inhibition model using an extra substrate molecule instead of inhibitor, therefore leading to a squared term in the denominator when multiplied out:

$$v = \frac{V_m[S]}{K_m + [S] + \dfrac{[S]^2}{K_{si}}} \tag{9.12}$$

However, in the course of kinetic analyses one may wish to gain additional information from the available kinetic data, allowing for estimation of additional kinetic parameters that may provide more insight into the processes taking place. Thus, more complicated equations for kinetic modeling of substrate inhibition kinetics have been derived (e.g., Eq. 19.13) that allow for the estimation of interaction factors and additional kinetic parameters.

$$v = \frac{V_m\left(\dfrac{1}{K_S} + \dfrac{\beta \cdot [S]}{\alpha K_i K_S}\right)}{\dfrac{1}{[S]} + \dfrac{1}{K_S} + \dfrac{1}{K_i} + \dfrac{[S]}{\alpha K_S K_i}} \tag{9.13}$$

In the case of Eq. 19.13, $K_S \approx K_m$, K_i is the dissociation constant of substrate binding to the inhibitory site, α is the factor by which the dissociation (K_S and K_i) of substrate at both sites changes when a second substrate is bound, and β is the factor by which V_m changes when a second substrate is bound. Because of the number of parameters being estimated in Eq. 19.13, modeling with this equation will generally require substantially more data points than required for Eq. 19.12.

For substrate inhibition mechanisms involving ordered ternary complex, such as the UGTs (case 2), Eq. 19.14 is applicable:

$$v = \frac{V_m[A][B]}{K_{iA}K_{mB} + K_{mB}[A] + K_{mA}[B] + [A][B]\left(1 + \frac{[B]}{K_{SiB}}\right)}$$ (19.14)

where K_{SiB} is *not* a dissocation constant.

19.3.5   Explanations for Atypical Kinetics in P450 Enzymes and Their Detection

Reports on the actual mechanism(s) behind the activation kinetics of drug metabolizing enzymes (mainly P450) are few compared to the kinetic models that have been devised to fit nonhyperbolic velocity data [10–12]. The approaches that have been taken to understand the interplay of substrate, effector, and enzyme are, however, diverse and include isotope effects, fluorescence spectroscopy [13], and nuclear magnetic resonance [14, 15] in addition to assays for distinct steps in the P450 catalytic cycle [16]. One of the most influential hypotheses behind the action of effectors that prompted the use of these varied techniques is that the effector binding site could be located in the active site with the substrate. Over the past few years evidence for simultaneous ligand binding to the same active site has now been provided for at least two microsomal enzymes, human CYP3A4 and CYP2C9 , and three bacterial enzymes, CYP102A1 (BM3) , CYP107A1 (eryF) [17], and CYP158A2 [18] as discussed below. Of course, allosterism can result from binding at remote sites or through protein–protein interactions.

Presence of Multiple Ligands Temporally Bound in the Same Active Site   In the case of 3A4, the substrate pyrene could be used to demonstrate multiple ligand binding to the same enzyme active site during catalysis. Pyrene induces a sigmoidal kinetic response with increasing concentrations, and its planarity, coupled with its multiring fused aromatic structure, gives it a large surface for intermolecular pyrene–pyrene pi-stacking (a.k.a. excimer formation). After showing binding of pyrene to 3A4 by visible difference spectrophotometry and changes in fluorescence of pyrene and the enzyme, differences in the excitation spectra (absorbance of monomer and excimer in the ground state) gave multiple indications that there are excimers in the presence of enzyme distinct from those that form in solution. Crystal structures of 3A4 do demonstrate active volumes sufficiently large enough (>1000 Å) for multiple ligands in their closed conformations [19]. Some investigators have even suggested triply occupied active sites [20], but defining the nature of atypical kinetics in terms of different subsites still remains a challenge due to the dependency on the structure of both substrate and effector.

Shortly after the 3A4/pyrene report, a series of isotope effect experiments with P450 BM3 suggested that multiple fatty acids could bind to the same enzyme active site simultaneously. This explained why the F87A mutant produced a different metabolic profile of hydroxylated products in the presence of laurate. Mutation of

F87 to alanine results in an increase in hydroxylation of the ω-1 position as laurate concentrations are raised. Since the alanine substitution gives a smaller side chain, and therefore more space, it is unclear why the ratio of metabolites would change unless the presence of a second substrate or the collapse of the enzyme constricts the available volume. This is where isotope effects appear to be capable of detecting multiple ligand binding without the need for fluorescent molecules. The theory is that given two enzyme-bound ligands in rapid equilibrium, mixing protio substrate (all hydrogens) and substrate substituted with deuteriums (the deuterium–carbon bond possesses a lower vibrational energy and requires more energy for abstraction) at the site of metabolism will favor metabolism of the nonlabeled substrate. Hence, a bias in the rate of labeled and un labeled substrate metabolism is produced and it favors the hydrogen-containing substrate (i.e., k_H/k_D ratio is greater than unity). In this case, the bias for ω-1 hydroxylation of palmitate was increased even more when deuterated laurate was added. Further validation of this technique is awaited for its use as a powerful tool with possibly untapped potential.

There are now crystal structures for two of the three major families of human microsomal P450s, 2 and 3 [21], but none have captured multiple ligands in the same pocket. However, crystallography has provided convincing electron density for multiple ligand binding in the same pocket for two bacterial enzymes. While not exactly a high throughput technology, even with the use of robotics, crystallography has generated structures that are invaluable for the predictive modeling of drug–drug interactions. P450 eryF in complex with two molecules of 9-aminophenanthrene and, more recently, P450 158A2 with two molecules of flaviolin have been reported. Both structures show one ligand above the heme with the second ligand lying above the first. Interestingly, both ligands are aromatic and planar, possibly owing some of their binding to each other. As of now, there are no examples with two different ligands bound, nor does a single structure indicate the order of their binding or the extent at which they move about inside the enzyme.

With the help of crystallography, nuclear magnetic resonance spectroscopy (NMR) has the capability to provide more details about the sequence and location of binding without the need for assigning every resonance. Yoon et al. [15] have reported on the use of protein NMR spectroscopy to study the binding of 9-aminophenanthrene to P450 eryF using enzyme expressed with ^{15}N-phenylalanine so that all phenylalanine residues would have detectable amide nitrogen nuclei. Titration of 9-aminophenanthrene to levels that are substoichiometric to enzyme altered the signal intensity for Phe residues that are different from those whose intensity changed in the presence of higher levels of 9-aminophenanthrene ([substrate] > [enzyme]). Further arguments regarding the time scale of on and off rates and their interpretation in terms of the mechanism of cooperative binding were also drawn from this study. Surely, the ability to distinguish two binding events at different locations inside the enzyme will greatly complement other analytical methods, and studies with human P450s will no doubt bring a more detailed understanding to drug–drug interactions induced by atypical kinetics.

An additional use of NMR involves the enhanced relaxation rate of substrate nuclei near the iron of the heme, which is paramagnetic in the ferric state [22]. Using P450 2C9, Hummel et al. [14] studied the proton relaxation times of the substrate flurbiprofen in the absence and presence of heteroactivator dapsone. Time-averaged distances of each substrate proton can be estimated by carrying out a T_1 relaxation experiment both with the ferric enzyme and the ferrous carbon monoxide complex, which is not paramagnetic. T_1 refers to the longitudinal relaxation and refers to the time it takes for the irradiated substrate protons to recess back to alignment with the magnetic field. The site of hydroxylation (4 -proton) was found to be closer to the iron of the heme group in the presence of heteroactivator, suggesting that its hyperbolic activation may result from increased collision frequency of substrate with the reactive iron-oxene or enhanced spin state conversion via heme dehydration.

Another dimension to the action of dapsone on flurbiprofen metabolism by P450 2C9 was provided by a study that compared the coupling of NADPH consumption to metabolite formation versus shunting to the side products superoxide, H_2O_2, and water. Catalytic coupling can be defined as the fraction of metabolite formed per NADPH consumed and is thus a measure of enzyme efficiency distinct from k_{cat}/K_m. In addition to increasing the rate of flurbiprofen metabolite formation, the effector dapsone was found to stimulate the consumption of NADPH, but decrease the formation of H_2O_2. Overall, the coupling of flurbiprofen metabolism was increased. Therefore, the distance of a substrate relative to the heme iron as altered by effectors appears to have multiple consequences as shown for P450 2C9. Possible effector-mediated changes in the position of substrate could displace the water that occupies the sixth coordination position of the iron to increase its reduction potential, keep the substrate closer to the active oxidant, and therefore decrease uncoupling of the catalytic cycle.

19.3.6   Artifactual Sources of Atypical Kinetics

During the conduct of *in vitro* drug metabolism experiments, it is prudent to be alert for the possible occurrence of atypical kinetics. However, the researcher must also be aware that there are several potential artifactual causes of atypical kinetic profiles that may lead to a misinterpretation of the data. Thus, extreme care must be taken to assure the validity of the results. The comments below address several of these potential sources of error and how to minimize their impact on the kinetic profiles observed.

One of the fundamental assumptions when conducting enzyme kinetic experiments is that the substrate (and effector concentration if drug–drug interactions are being studied) remains constant throughout the experiment. For substrates and effectors that exhibit substantial turnover, one must worry about substrate/effector depletion. This will result in constantly changing substrate/effector concentrations throughout the experiment and invalidate the assumption of steady state. Related to constantly changing (and decreasing) drug concentrations are potential sources of error when the actual substrate/effector concentration is lower than believed. This can occur if either compound undergoes substantial nonspecific binding to the incubation matrix (i.e., protein) or when the drug has very low solubility. In these cases, the free drug concentration (i.e., that available to interact with the enzyme) is substantially lower than believed, resulting in overestimates of kinetic parameters such as K_m, and K_i.

Although less of an issue in today's environment of widespread LC/MS/MS availability, insufficient analytical sensitivity to accurately and reproducibly quantitate metabolite production at the extreme low end of the substrate concentration–

velocity curve may result in erroneous assignment of the kinetic profile. This is most problematic in the case of sigmoidal kinetics, where inadequate sensitivity hinders determining the less steep slope during the initial portion of the curve. One must also be cautious when using multienzyme systems (e.g., human liver microsomes) for kinetic characterization since multiple enzymes are present. This is particularly problematic with respect to observations of biphasic kinetics, since more than one enzyme may be producing the metabolite. In this case, the kinetic phenomena observed are actually a hybrid of the concerted effects of multiple enzymes and result in *apparent* kinetic constants.

Finally, the kinetic profile observed may be affected by incubation conditions and preparation. Choice of buffer salt to be used in the incubation can result in differing kinetic profiles [23] and the presence of certain organic solvents (particularly at concentrations above 2%) have also been shown to activate enzyme kinetic processes [24]. Finally, the inclusion (or exclusion) of cytochrome-b_5 can result in different kinetic profiles observed [25]. Thus, one must pay particular attention to controls and conditions when making the assignment of atypical kinetic phenomena.

19.4 CONCLUSION

Proper estimation of kinetic parameters is critical to successful extrapolation of *in vitro* data to the *in vivo* situation. In addition to standard hyperbolic kinetics, sigmoidal (autoactivation), biphasic, substrate inhibition, and heterotropic activation have all been observed in the kinetic profiles of drug metabolism reactions. The most common hypothesis for the occurrence of these types of "atypical" kinetic profiles is based on data suggesting that two (or more) substrate molecules (or a substrate and effector molecule) bind within the enzyme active site simultaneously and alter the enzyme kinetics. The occurrence of these atypical kinetic profiles complicates the determination of *in vitro–in vivo* correlations and thus requires the use of more complex equations appropriate to the type of profile observed in order to properly estimate the kinetic parameters.

ACKNOWLEDGMENT

This work was supported in part by a grant from the National Institutes of Health (#GM 063215).

REFERENCES

1. Luukkanen L, Taskinen J, Kurkela M, Kostiainen R, Hirvonen J, Finel M. Kinetic characterization of the 1A subfamily of recombinant human UDP-glucuronosyltransferases. *Drug Metab Dispos* 2005;33:1017–1026.
2. Segel IH. *Rapid Equilibrium Bireactant and Terreactant Systems*. Hoboken, NJ: Wiley; 1975.

3. Shou M, Mei Q, Ettore MWJr, Dai R, Baillie TA, Rushmore TH. Sigmoidal kinetic model for two co-operative substrate-binding sites in a cytochrome P450 3A4 active site: an example of the metabolism of diazepam and its derivatives. *Biochem J* 1999;340(Pt 3):845–853.

4. Korzekwa KR, Krishnamachary N, Shou M, Ogai A, Parise RA, Rettie AE, Gonzalez FJ, Tracy TS. Evaluation of atypical cytochrome P450 kinetics with two-substrate models: evidence that multiple substrates can simultaneously bind to cytochrome P450 active sites. *Biochemistry* 1998;37:4137–4147.

5. Ueng YF, Kuwabara T, Chun YJ, Guengerich FP. Cooperativity in oxidations catalyzed by cytochrome P450 3A4. *Biochemistry* 1997;36:370–381.

6. Cornish-Bowden A. *Fundamentals of Enzyme Kinetics*. London: Portland Press; 2004.

7. Rock DA, Perkins BN, Wahlstrom J, Jones JP. A method for determining two substrates binding in the same active site of cytochrome P450BM3: an explanation of high energy omega product formation. *Arch Biochem Biophys* 2003;416:9–16.

8. Hutzler JM, Hauer MJ, Tracy TS. Dapsone activation of CYP2C9-mediated metabolism: evidence for activation of multiple substrates and a two-site model. *Drug Metab Dispos* 2001;29:1029–1034.

9. Lin Y, Lu P, Tang C, Mei Q, Sandig G, Rodrigues AD, Rushmore TH, Shou M. Substrate inhibition kinetics for cytochrome P450-catalyzed reactions. *Drug Metab Dispos* 2001;29:368–374.

10. Galetin A, Clarke SE, Houston JB. Quinidine and haloperidol as modifiers of CYP3A4 activity: multisite kinetic model approach. *Drug Metab Dispos* 2002;30:1512–1522.

11. Galetin A, Clarke SE, Houston JB. Multisite kinetic analysis of interactions between prototypical CYP3A4 subgroup substrates: midazolam, testosterone, and nifedipine. *Drug Metab Dispos* 2003;31:1108–1116.

12. Kenworthy KE, Clarke SE, Andrews J, Houston JB. Multisite kinetic models for CYP3A4: simultaneous activation and inhibition of diazepam and testosterone metabolism. *Drug Metab Dispos* 2001;29:1644–1651.

13. Dabrowski MJ, Schrag ML, Wienkers LC, Atkins WM. Pyrene–pyrene complexes at the active site of cytochrome P450 3A4: evidence for a multiple substrate binding site. *J Am Chem Soc* 2002;124:11866–11867.

14. Hummel MA, Gannett PM, Aguilar JS, Tracy TS. Effector-mediated alteration of substrate orientation in cytochrome P450 2C9. *Biochemistry* 2004;43:7207–7214.

15. Yoon MY, Campbell AP, Atkins WM. "Allosterism" in the elementary steps of the cytochrome P450 reaction cycle. *Drug Metab Rev* 2004;36:219–230.

16. Hutzler JM, Wienkers LC, Wahlstrom JL, Carlson TJ, Tracy TS. Activation of cytochrome P450 2C9-mediated metabolism: mechanistic evidence in support of kinetic observations. *Arch Biochem Biophys* 2003;410:16–24.

17. Cupp-Vickery J, Anderson R, Hatziris Z. Crystal structures of ligand complexes of P450eryF exhibiting homotropic cooperativity. *Proc Natl Acad Sci USA* 2002;97:3050–3055.

18. Zhao B, Guengerich FP, Bellamine A, Lamb DC, Izumikawa M, Lei L, Podust LM, Sundaramoorthy M, Kalaitzis JA, Reddy LM, Kelly SL, Moore BS, Stec D, Voehler M, Falck JR, Shimada T, Waterman MR. Binding of two flaviolin substrate molecules, oxidative coupling, and crystal structure of *Streptomyces coelicolor* A3(2) cytochrome P450 158A2. *J Biol Chem* 2005;280:11599–11607.

19. Scott EE, Halpert JR. Structures of cytochrome P450 3A4. *Trends Biochem Sci* 2005;30:5–7.

20. He YA, Roussel F, Halpert JR. Analysis of homotropic and heterotropic cooperativity of diazepam oxidation by CYP3A4 using site-directed mutagenesis and kinetic modeling. *Arch Biochem Biophys* 2003;409:92–101.

21. Johnson EF, Stout CD. Structural diversity of human xenobiotic-metabolizing cytochrome P450 monooxygenases. *Biochem Biophys Res Commun* 2005;338:331–336.

22. Yao H, Costache AD, Sem DS. Chemical proteomic tool for ligand mapping of CYP antitargets: an NMR-compatible 3D QSAR descriptor in the Heme-Based Coordinate System. *J Chem Inf Comput Sci* 2004;44:1456–1465.

23. Hutzler JM, Powers FJ, Wynalda MA, Wienkers LC. Effect of carbonate anion on cytochrome P450 2D6-mediated metabolism *in vitro*: the potential role of multiple oxygenating species. *Arch Biochem Biophys* 2003;417:165–175.

24. Hickman D, Wang JP, Wang Y, Unadkat JD. Evaluation of the selectivity of *in vitro* probes and suitability of organic solvents for the measurement of human cytochrome P450 monooxygenase activities. *Drug Metab Dispos* 1998;26:207–215.

25. Jushchyshyn MI, Hutzler JM, Schrag ML, Wienkers LC. Catalytic turnover of pyrene by CYP3A4: evidence that cytochrome b5 directly induces positive cooperativity. *Arch Biochem Biophys* 2005;438:21–28.

20

DRUG CLEARANCE

Sree D. Panuganti[1] and Craig K. Svensson[2]

[1]*Purdue University, West Lafayette, Indiana*
[2]*Osmetech Molecular Diagnostics, Pasadena, California*

Contents

20.1 INTRODUCTION

Drug discovery and development is a complex process involving various sequential stages broadly grouped as preclinical and clinical evaluation. Both phases require the characterization of the pharmacokinetics of the molecule being evaluated as a

Preclinical Development Handbook: ADME and Biopharmaceutical Properties,
edited by Shayne Cox Gad
Copyright © 2008 John Wiley & Sons, Inc.

potential drug candidate. In drug discovery and development, it is of particular interest to understand the pharmacokinetic behavior of potential drug candidates as early as possible in order to select the most promising compounds for further development while not wasting unnecessary resources on those compounds that will not prove to be viable for clinical use. While many pharmacokinetic processes contribute to the viability of drug candidates, clearance processes arguably have the greatest impact on determining whether or not a compound possesses the pharmacokinetic characteristics amenable to further development of the candidate. The clearance of a drug candidate is frequently the primary factor in determining the bioavailability, dosing frequency, duration of action, and viable routes of administration for the clinical use of the compound. Thus, the rate and routes of drug clearance can be critical in determining whether or not the development of a candidate compound should move forward. It is therefore imperative that development scientists possess an understanding of the determinants and characterization of drug clearance. Our objective in this chapter is to provide an overview of clearance concepts, ranging from a description of the routes by which drugs are cleared from the body to pathophysiological conditions that may alter these processes qualitatively and quantitatively. In subsequent chapters, authors will describe the importance of drug clearance in the overall context of pharmacokinetic analysis.

20.2   ROUTES OF DRUG ELIMINATION

Avoidance of accumulation of drugs subsequent to repeated exposure necessitates varied pathways for elimination of such compounds from the body. The rate of elimination will be a key determinant of the time for which critical body sites are exposed to effective concentrations of a drug. Hence, the duration of pharmacologic effect *in vivo* is generally determined by the rate of elimination. The routes of elimination are important in determining the likelihood of altered drug disposition in various disease states, as well as the potential for drug–drug interactions. Based on the anticipated patient population for a new chemical entity, it may be preferable to have a drug that is primarily eliminated by the liver, as opposed to the renal route, as the primary pathway of elimination. The importance of such factors in assessment of compounds under development makes it imperative that development scientists possess a good understanding of the potential pathways and means for quantifying drug elimination.

20.2.1   Potential Routes of Elimination

Mechanisms of drug elimination are largely determined by the physiochemical characteristics of the ingested compounds. Small water-soluble compounds are readily eliminated unchanged by the kidney, while large molecules and lipophilic agents must undergo biotransformation in the liver prior to being excreted by the kidney. While generally quantitatively minor, elimination by alternative routes may be of clinical/practical importance.

Renal Elimination   It may be argued that essentially all drugs are eliminated to some degree via the renal route. While large lipophilic molecules are not directly eliminated by the kidney, their biotransformation products (metabolites) are generally more water soluble and subject to renal elimination. This reality is important to recognize when considering the potential impact of renal disease on drug elimination. While the elimination of a lipophilic or large molecular weight parent compound may not be altered in the presence of renal disease, the elimination of its metabolites may be altered significantly. If those metabolites exhibit pharmacologic or toxicologic effects, renal disease may alter patient response, despite the lack of alterations in the disposition of the parent compound. As it represents one of the two most important pathways of drug elimination, renal elimination will be considered in further detail in a subsequent section.

Hepatic Elimination   The liver is an organ of critical importance for drug elimination. This is in part due to the fact that disease- and drug-induced alterations in metabolic capacity can have such a profound impact on the ability of the liver to metabolize drugs. It is, however, important to recognize that the liver also eliminates numerous drugs unchanged through its capacity for biliary excretion. As one of the two major organs for drug elimination (the other being the kidney), concepts of hepatic clearance are covered in further depth in a subsequent section.

Pulmonary Elimination   As the general population is aware of the use of ethanol measurements in exhaled breath to approximate blood ethanol concentrations, the ability to put pulmonary excretion of xenobiotics to practical use is obvious. While pulmonary elimination is a minor route for ethanol elimination, the constant ratio of alveolar to blood ethanol concentration permits extrapolation of the latter from the former. The number of compounds for which the pulmonary route is quantitatively significant in terms of the overall elimination of the drug is small and mostly limited to gaseous anesthetics. The ability to measure $^{13}CO_2$ or $^{14}CO_2$ in excreted breath has been utilized as an indirect means of measuring drug elimination for compounds that undergo oxidative metabolism in the liver. Several such tests are commercially available as a means of phenotyping the metabolic capacity of patients via specific cytochrome P450s (e.g., CYP3A4). These tests are dependent on the one-carbon oxidation that gives rise to CO_2, which is then excreted in exhaled breath.

Other Routes of Elimination   While also quantitatively minor, additional routes of elimination (e.g., tears, sweat, hair) may be of practical or clinical significance. For example, while the fraction of a dose of drug that is excreted in tears is quite small, it may have very important implications for patients. Rifampin is a compound that is eliminated in tears and is capable of staining contacts a yellow-orange color when worn by patients during therapy with this drug. Another pathway of elimination that is of minor quantitative importance is hair. However, measurement of drug concentration in hair permits assessment of drug exposure over a longer time period than possible with blood or urine. This fact is applied in the numerous commercially available kits to measure drugs of abuse in hair samples. Its noninvasive nature makes this means of exposure assessment attractive.

20.2.2   Characterization of Elimination

There are two primary ways in which drug elimination may be quantified. The first is through estimation of the *half-life* of a drug in some reference fluid (e.g., plasma).

The half-life represents the time required for 50% of the drug to be eliminated from the body. For drugs that are eliminated in a first-order fashion, this time is independent of dose or concentration. However, since many drugs are eliminated by processes that involve the direct interaction of drug with a macromolecule (e.g., an enzyme or transporter protein), large doses will result in saturation of enzymatic or transport process and give rise to altered half-lives (compared to that observed with lower doses). This is important to keep in mind in preclinical studies where large doses may be utilized. The importance of dose-dependent pharmacokinetics and the application in toxicokinetics is discussed in other chapters (see Chapters 31 and 36 in this volume).

The most useful parameter for quantifying drug elimination *in vivo* is *clearance*. Assessment of elimination using clearance is preferred over that of half-life, since the latter is a function of both clearance and distribution (see Chapters 31 and 36 in this volume). For this reason, half-life fails to provide insight into the mechanism of drug elimination and cannot be used to predict the likely impact of disease or drug interactions on drug elimination. Clearance is defined as *the volume of blood from which all of the drug would appear to be removed per unit time*. As such, it is expressed in terms of volume per unit time and may be related to real physiological volumes, such as hepatic blood flow or renal plasma flow.

An understanding of the concept of clearance can be gained by consideration of the perfusion of an isolated organ with blood containing drug (Fig. 20.1). The rate of drug entry into and out of the organ can be described as

$$\text{Rate in} = QC_a$$
$$\text{Rate out} = QC_v$$

where Q is the organ perfusion rate, C_a is the concentration of drug in arterial blood, and C_v is the concentration of drug in venous blood. Whenever $C_v < C_a$, elimination of drug occurs in the organ and it is referred to as a clearing organ. The rate of elimination can be determined as

$$\text{Rate of elimination} = QC_a - QC_v = Q(C_a - C_v)$$

A common means for describing the efficiency by which a single organ removes a drug from blood is the *extraction ratio (E)*, where

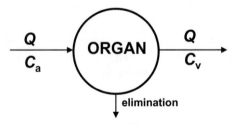

FIGURE 20.1   Schematic representation of a clearing organ. C_a designates arterial drug concentration, C_v is the venous drug concentration, and Q represents the blood flow to the organ. This schematic assumes that blood flow across the organ does not change significantly.

$$E = \frac{\text{Rate of elimination}}{\text{Rate of entry}}$$

$$E = \frac{Q(C_a - C_v)}{QC_a} = \frac{C_a - C_v}{C_a}$$

The clearance (CL) of the organ for a specific compound can be given as

$$CL = QE = Q\left(\frac{C_a - C_v}{C_a}\right)$$

The above equation reveals two potential extremes for CL. The first is when E →1, under which conditions $CL \sim Q$. Hence, for a drug that displays a high extraction ratio, the clearance is said to be *perfusion rate limited*; meaning that the rate-limiting step in the clearance is the delivery of drug to the clearing organ. Under such conditions, changes in organ perfusion rate will result in proportional changes in drug clearance. In contrast, when E is very low, changes in perfusion have little impact on drug clearance.

From the above equations, one can readily develop the means to calculate the total body clearance for a drug, CL_T, where

$$CL_T = \frac{\text{Elimination rate}}{\text{Concentration in blood}} = \frac{dX/dt}{C}$$

$$CL_T = \frac{\int_0^\infty (dX/dt)\,dt}{\int_0^\infty C\,dt}$$

where

$$\int_0^\infty \frac{dX}{dt}\,dt = \text{Total amount of drug eliminated}$$

and

$$\int_0^\infty C\,dt = AUC_0^\infty$$

where AUC is the area under the drug concentration versus time curve, X is the amount of drug in the body, and t is time. When the drug is administered intravenously, 100% of the drug enters the systemic circulation. Therefore, after intravenous administration, the total amount of drug ultimately eliminated is equal to the intravenous dose (D_{IV}). Hence,

$$CL_T = \frac{D_{IV}}{AUC_0^\infty}$$

From the above equation, it can be seen that the total clearance (sometimes also referred to as the *systemic* clearance) can readily be determined after intravenous

(IV) administration of a drug. The total clearance can be determined after non-intravenous routes of administration by accounting for the fraction of drug that reaches the systemic circulation (described in more detail in Chapter 36 in this volume).

An important principle related to the use and determination of organ-specific clearance is the additivity of clearance. Specifically, the total clearance is the sum of the individual organ clearance such that, for example,

$$\text{Total clearance} = \text{Renal clearance} + \text{Hepatic clearance}$$

This additivity arises from the fact that organs of elimination are fractionally perfused in parallel. An exception to this principle is pulmonary clearance, which arises as a result of the fact that the entire cardiac output traverses the pulmonary bed prior to being fractionally distributed to other organs of elimination (e.g., liver and kidney).

20.3   RENAL CLEARANCE

20.3.1   Basic Kidney Structure and Function

The most important functions of the kidney include regulation of body water content, mineral composition, and acidity. The kidney also plays an important role in the removal of endogenous metabolic waste products and xenobiotics and their metabolites from the body. Indeed, the major organ in mammals for the clearance of drugs and their metabolites is the kidney. Humans have two kidneys located in the upper rear region of the abdominal cavity. The functional units of kidney are called nephrons and each kidney is composed of over one million nephrons. Figure 20.2 illustrates different components of the nephron.

Each nephron consists of vascular and tubular components. The glomerulus is made up of a network of glomerular capillaries and Bowman's capsule, which is a

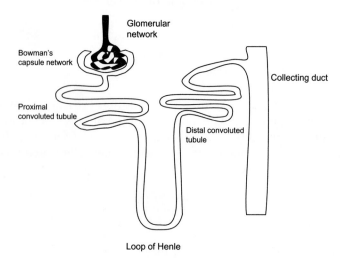

FIGURE 20.2   Components of the renal nephron.

thin double membrane that surrounds the glomerulus and functions as a filter. Blood is filtered at the glomerulus so that only protein-free filtrate is allowed to pass into the nephron. The resulting glomerular filtrate travels through the proximal convoluted tubule, where approximately 80% of the water is reabsorbed. The loop of Henle connects the proximal convoluted tubule to the distal convoluted tubule. A large collecting duct collects kidney filtrate from the distal convoluted tubules of each nephron and carries it to the bladder.

The kidney can be divided into two portions histologically: the outer renal cortex and the inner renal medulla. The renal cortex contains the glomeruli, proximal and distal convoluted tubules, the outer portion of the loop of Henle, and collecting ducts, whereas the renal medulla contains the lower ends of the loop of Henle and collecting ducts.

20.3.2 Mechanisms of Renal Clearance

The kidney excretes endogenous and xenobiotic compounds and their metabolites by three distinct mechanisms: glomerular filtration, tubular secretion, and tubular reabsorption. Glomerular filtration and tubular secretion remove drugs from the circulation, whereas tubular reabsorption can be considered as a redistribution mechanism by which drug moves from the inner tubule back into the circulation. While drugs may also be metabolized in the kidney, the quantitative contribution of this route is insignificant in terms of the overall clearance of drugs.

Glomerular Filtration   Glomerular filtration is a passive process. In this process drugs and other endogenous compounds of molecular weight less than 6 kDa are filtered effectively. Drug molecules that are bound to plasma proteins, such as albumin, will not be filtered. In other words, only unbound drug in plasma water is available for glomerular filtration. The glomerular filtration rate (GFR) can be determined using marker compounds that undergo filtration only (i.e., do not undergo secretion or reabsorption) and are not bound to plasma proteins. The renal clearance of such compounds is equal to the GFR. The most common marker compounds used to measure GFR are inulin (MW 5200) and creatinine (MW 131). The rate of filtration of a drug can be given as

$$\text{Rate of filtration} = GFR \times C_{\text{fup}}$$

where C_{fup} is the concentration of free (unbound) drug in plasma. Furthermore, since $C_{\text{fup}} = f_{\text{up}} \times C$,

$$\text{Rate of filtration} = f_{\text{up}} \times GFR \times C$$

If drug is only filtered and all of the drug filtered is excreted in the urine, the rate of drug excretion will be equal to the rate of filtration. Hence

$$CL_{\text{R}} = \frac{\text{Rate of excretion}}{\text{Plasma concentration}} = \frac{f_{\text{up}} \times GFR \times C}{C} = f_{\text{up}} \times GFR$$

Thus the renal clearance of a compound that is only filtered can be determined based on a knowledge of the protein binding and the GFR (as approximated by inulin or creatinine).

The glomerular filtration rate varies from individual to individual, but in healthy subjects ranges from 110 to 130 mL/min (~180 L/day). While single-point determinations of GFR are often used to estimate drug clearance, it should be recognized that GFR is subject to circadian variation. GFR is highest in the active phase (morning) and lowest in the inactive phase (evening), with an amplitude of variation of about 20–30% [1, 2].

Tubular Secretion   The kidney receives about 10–25% of the cardiac output, or about 700–1500 mL/min, assuming a cardiac output of 6000 mL/min [3], of which 60% will be the plasma flow. Approximately 18% of the effective plasma flow is filtered at the glomeruli. The remaining renal blood bathing the tubules permits access to the secretory processes in these tubules.

When the renal clearance of a drug exceeds $f_{up} \times GFR$, the drug must undergo active tubular secretion. There are two distinct systems involved in tubular secretion: one for organic anions (acids) and one for organic cation (bases). These systems are made up of multiple transporters. Both the anion and cation transport systems are located in the proximal convoluted tubule of the nephron. The most important transporters from a drug interaction perspective are the organic anion transporters. This process is thought to be localized primarily at the basolateral membrane of the proximal convoluted tubule. The transport of the organic anions across this membrane occurs through a three-step process (Fig. 20.3a).

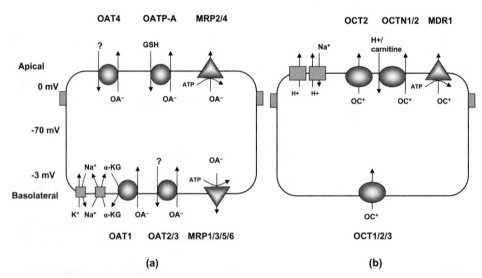

FIGURE 20.3   Functional and proposed models of organic anion (a) and cation (b) transporters in renal tubules. OA$^-$, organic anion; OAT, organic anion transporter; OATP, organic anion transporting polypeptide; OC$^+$, organic cation; OCT, OCTN, organic cation transporter; MRP, multidrug resistance associated protein; MDR, multidrug resistance P-glycoprotein. (Adapted from Ref. 19.)

The organic anion transport system (OAT1) is dependent on a cell membrane Na/K-ATPase that maintains the intracellular electrochemical gradient. Initially, ATP is hydrolyzed to drive the sodium pump. In the second step, the resulting Na^+ gradient drives α-ketogluterate (α-KG) cotransport across the basolateral membrane. The third step in this process is the exchange of α-KG with the organic anion (OA$^-$), as α-KG markedly stimulates the transport of organic anions. Once inside the proximal tubule cell, the organic acid is eliminated on the luminal side of the cell by a carrier-mediated transport system [4–6].

At present, it is difficult to predict whether a new drug candidate will interact with renal tubular secretion mechanisms based on structure–activity relationships alone. However, certain generalizations can be made based on transport studies using analogue compounds with different characteristics. In general, substrates with two negative charges will interact with anion transport systems, which are influenced by the molecular distance between the charges. Substances that interact with the organic anion transport system must have a hydrophobic area and two partial negative charges, a hydrophobic area and one negative ionic charge, or a large hydrophobic area and a partial negative charge [3].

Comparatively less is known about the organic cation transport system. This is partly due to the toxic side effects of the marker compounds on the cardiovascular system that could be used to study the transport process. As the organic anion transporters are responsible for the tubular secretion of organic acids, the organic cation transport systems are responsible for weak bases; often nitrogen-containing compounds that are ionized at physiological pH. Similar to anion transport, the organic cation transport also proceeds in three steps (Fig. 20.3b). In contrast to filtration, protein-bound toxicants are available for active transport. Binding to plasma proteins usually does not hinder tubular secretion of drugs because of the dynamic equilibrium that exists between free and bound drug. As free drug is removed and transported across the tubular epithelium, immediate dissociation of the drug–protein complex usually occurs [7, 8].

Since tubular secretion is an active process, there may be competitive inhibition of the secretion of one compound by coadministration of a second compound secreted via the same transporter. This can actually be taken advantage of clinically to prolong the systemic exposure to a drug readily secreted by the kidney. For example, probenecid inhibits the secretion of penicillin and coadministration of these two agents can be used to decrease the dose and frequency of penicillin that needs to be administered.

Tubular Reabsorption   When the $CL_R < f_{up} \times GFR$, it is apparent that a portion of the filtered drug must undergo reabsorption. Most of the filtrate that enters the renal tubules is reabsorbed, with urine output accounting for less than 1% of the filtrate fraction that enters the tubules. This creates a large concentration gradient across the tubule and plasma, representing a driving force for passive reabsorption of solutes back into the circulation. Small molecular weight substances that are sufficiently lipophilic and un-ionized will be reabsorbed. In contrast, compounds that have large molecular weight are polar or ionized will not be reabsorbed. As many drugs are either weak bases or acids, the pH of the glomerular filtrate can greatly influence the extent of tubular reabsorption. Even small changes in pH of filtrate, either because of diet or drugs, can result in significant variations in the percentage of drug reabsorbed or excreted. For example, the pK_a of phenobarbital (a weak acid) is 7.2 with an ionic strength equal to plasma. At a plasma pH of 7.4, the drug exists in ionized form and at pH values less than 7.2 the un-ionized form of the drug dominates and will be excreted. In the case of a drug overdose, it is possible to increase the excretion of some drugs by suitable adjustment of urine pH.

20.3.3   Determination of Renal Clearance and Mechanisms of Renal Clearance

General Model for Renal Clearance   The total renal clearance of a drug is the sum of all the renal elimination mechanisms involved in the elimination of that specific drug:

$$CL_R = CL_{Fil} + CL_{ATS} - CL_{TR}$$

where CL_{Fil} is the filtration clearance, CL_{ATS} is the active tubular secretion clearance, and CL_{TR} is the reabsorption clearance [3, 9]. As indicated previously, the filtration clearance of a drug is given as $f_{up} \times GFR$, while the active tubular secretion clearance can be described as

$$CL_{ATS} = \frac{Q_{RPF} f_{up} CL_{usint}}{Q_{RPF} + f_{up} CL_{usint}}$$

where Q_{RPF} is renal plasma flow and CL_{usint} is secretory clearance of unbound drug. Since the amount of drug reabsorbed represents a fraction of that which is filtered and secreted (F_{TR}), the renal clearance can be expressed as

$$CL_R = f_{up} GFR + \frac{Q_{RPF} f_{up} CL_{usint}}{Q_{RPF} + f_{up} CL_{usint}} - F_{TR} \left(f_{up} GFR + \frac{Q_{RPF} f_{up} CL_{usint}}{Q_{RPF} + f_{up} CL_{usint}} \right)$$

The above equation represents the complex relationship between plasma protein binding, renal plasma flow, glomerular filtration rate, and intrinsic secretory activity. More complex models that take into account urine flow, pH gradient, and transport saturation are needed to fully account for the many physiological variables governing renal clearance. While this complexity may leave the reader with the impression that determination and assessment of renal clearance is hopelessly complex, such is not the case. Simple measurement of renal clearance can provide valuable insight into mechanisms when compared with the renal clearance of marker compounds, as described in subsequent sections.

Determination of Renal Clearance from Urine and Plasma Concentrations   There are numerous methods available for calculation of renal clearance from measurements of plasma and urine drug concentrations. One common method is based on knowledge of the additivity of clearance. After a single intravenous dose of a drug, the fraction eliminated renally (f_R) is given as

$$f_R = \frac{Ae^{\infty}}{D_{IV}}$$

where Ae^{∞} is the total amount of drug excreted unchanged in urine. Determination of this value necessitates the collection of urine until all the drug has been eliminated from the body. If blood samples have also been obtained so that total clearance can be calculated as described previously, the renal clearance is determined as

$$CL_R = f_R \times CL_T$$

Alternatively, using the same data, one can calculate renal clearance from the relationship

$$CL_R = \frac{Ae^{\infty}}{AUC_0^{\infty}}$$

Renal clearance can also be calculated using excretion rate determinations rather than total drug excretion, where

$$CL_R = \frac{\Delta Ae/\Delta t}{C_{mid}}$$

C_{mid} represents the plasma concentration at the midpoint of the urine collection, ΔAe is the amount of drug excreted in urine unchanged over the collection interval, and Δt is the collection interval. As the renal clearance may vary somewhat between collection intervals, the best way to utilize this method is to determine the excretion rate over several different intervals. This can then be plotted against the midpoint concentration for each excretion rate. The result will provide a straight line with a slope equal to the renal clearance. Alternatively, if the drug is administered as a constant infusion until steady state is achieved,

$$CL_R = \frac{(\Delta Ae/\Delta t)_{ss}}{C_{ss}}$$

Assessment of Mechanism(s) of Renal Elimination from Renal Clearance Determinations   Renal clearance estimates are commonly used to determine the mechanism of renal elimination of compounds. If the renal clearance is approximately equal to $f_{up} \times$ GFR, filtration is the predominant mechanism. If renal clearance is less than $f_{up} \times GFR$, tubular reabsorption must occur, while a renal clearance greater than $f_{up} \times GFR$ indicates that tubular secretion is occurring in addition to filtration. Since renal clearance is the sum of all renal elimination mechanisms, a renal clearance equal to $f_{up} \times GFR$ does not rule out other mechanisms of renal elimination, as it is possible that secretion and reabsorption occur to an equal extent and thus negate one another.

As indicated previously, the most commonly used markers for estimating GFR are inulin and endogenous creatinine [1]. Inulin is one of the most accurate methods to estimate GFR. However, determination of inulin clearance is not practical for routine clinical use as it requires the infusion of an exogenous substance. In contrast, estimation of GFR via creatinine does not involve the administration of an additional substance.

Experimentally, concurrent determination of the renal clearance of a drug of interest and the clearance of inulin can be used to probe the mechanisms of renal elimination for the compound of interest. Once the renal clearance values are determined, the ratio of drug clearance to inulin clearance is determined, as shown in Table 20.1. Adjustments for plasma protein binding may need to be taken into account when using this method for elucidating the mechanisms of drug elimination.

As a means of more routine estimation of GFR, clearance of the endogenous marker creatinine can be determined by

$$CL_{cr} = \frac{U_{cr} \times V}{S_{cr}}$$

where U_{cr} is the urine creatinine concentration, V is the urine flow rate, and S_{cr} is the serum creatinine concentration sampled at the midpoint of the urinary collection period.

Creatinine clearance is often considered as an ideal method to assess GFR because (1) daily creatinine production is constant, (2) serum and urinary creatinine concentrations are easily measured in the laboratory, and (3) by making the urinary collection period sufficiently long, problems associated with short collection intervals can be avoided [10, 11]. Although the results obtained by creatinine clearance estimates correlate well with estimates of GFR, some deviation from GFR is to be expected, especially at very high and very low GFR values [12]. For most applications of GFR estimated through creatinine clearance, this deviation is insignificant. Creatinine clearance can also be estimated through use of S_{cr}, body weight, height, and sex. Such estimates are particularly useful for determining initial dosage regimens for drugs in a clinical setting.

A drug that is highly extracted by the kidney, meaning it undergoes extensive active tubular secretion, will exhibit a renal clearance that approximates renal plasma flow. A widely used model compound that exhibits these characteristics is p-aminohippuric acid (PAH). PAH has been widely used to determine the impact of interventions of renal plasma flow and to compare the renal clearance of a compound to the renal plasma flow in the same subjects.

TABLE 20.1 Use of Clearance Ratios to Determine Mechanisms of Renal Clearance

Clearance Ratio	Probable Mechanisms
$\dfrac{CL_{drug}}{CL_{inulin}} < 1$	Filtration and reabsorption
$\dfrac{CL_{drug}}{CL_{inulin}} = 1$	Filtration
$\dfrac{CL_{drug}}{CL_{inulin}} > 1$	Filtration and active tubular secretion

While a renal clearance less than $f_{up} \times GFR$ is indicative of tubular reabsorption, confirmation of this mechanism can be obtained by perturbations in urine flow and pH. As the concentration gradient is the driving force for reabsorption, increasing urine flow in the presence of reabsorptive mechanisms will result in an increase in the renal clearance. While pH manipulations may alter the renal tubular reabsorption of some drugs, drugs whose ionization does not change within the range of physiologically achievable urine pH (~5–8) will not exhibit an altered renal clearance despite changes in urine pH. Hence, the observation of pH-dependent renal clearance for ionizable compounds confirms the presence of tubular reabsorption, but such changes will not be expected for neutral compounds.

20.3.4 Factors Influencing Renal Clearance

Factors that influence the ability of the kidney to eliminate drugs may cause marked changes in the pharmacokinetics of some compounds. Such factors include age, disease, plasma protein binding, drug concentration or dose, and drug interactions at the site of elimination.

Age Many functions of the kidney are not fully developed at birth. As a result, some xenobiotics are eliminated more slowly in newborns than in adults. Similarly, the aging kidney exhibits reductions both in mass and in GFR. These changes may be associated with other age-related conditions, such as atherosclerosis and hypertension, which reduce renal blood flow. An age-dependent decline in the number of nephrons also occurs. The decline in GFR is in turn responsible for the reduced renal clearance of drugs that are normally removed by the kidney. With age the capacity to excrete acid load is diminished independent of decreased GFR. The diminished capacity of older subjects to excrete acid load could be due to an insufficient decrease in the tubular reabsorption.

Drug–Protein Binding The degree of plasma protein binding affects the filtration of drugs, as protein–xenobiotic complexes are too large to pass through the pores of the glomeruli. Whether or not changes in plasma protein binding alter renal clearance is dependent on the renal extraction ratio for the drug in question. For example, furosemide exhibits a low extraction ratio and its renal clearance changes proportionally to the free fraction of drug in plasma [13]. In contrast, the renal clearance of drugs that exhibit a high renal extraction ratio, and are therefore extensively secreted, is not significantly altered by changes in protein binding. Binding to plasma proteins usually does not hinder tubular secretion of drugs because of the rapid equilibrium that exists between free and bound drug. As free drug is removed and transported across the tubular epithelium, immediate dissociation of the drug–protein complex usually occurs—freeing more drug for secretion.

Concentration or Dose As tubular secretion involves the interaction of drug with transport carriers, which are limited in number, there is the potential for saturation of these membrane transport proteins as the dose or concentration of drug is increased. In the absence of saturation, the renal clearance of a drug will be independent of dose or concentration. However, when doses are administered that give rise to concentrations that saturate the transporters, the renal clearance will decrease.

Similarly, if the tubular reabsorption is by a carrier-mediated transport process (as is the case for ascorbic acid), increasing concentrations will saturate the carriers, resulting in an *increase* in the renal clearance (since the fraction reabsorbed will be reduced and more drug will be excreted in the urine). Such saturation has practical implications for the dosing of compounds that display saturation within the range of therapeutic concentrations. It is also important for the development scientist to keep the potential for such dose- or concentration-dependent changes in mind when utilizing high doses in preclinical studies.

A limited number of drugs exhibit concentration-dependent plasma protein binding at concentrations in the range achieved after therapeutic doses. An increase in the free fraction of a drug as the dose/concentration is increased will result in an increase in the filtration clearance (since this value is equal to $f_{up} \times GFR$). In this scenario, increasing the dose of a drug may fail to give rise to the expected increases in steady-state concentration since clearance is increased with dose. Several nonsteroidal anti-inflammatory drugs, such as naproxen, exhibit this type of dose/concentration-dependent changes in renal clearance.

Drug Interactions   The most well known drug–drug interactions that occur at the level of renal elimination are those in which one drug acts as a competitive inhibitor for another drug at a renal transport site. Competitive inhibitors will decrease the renal secretion of other substrates, but will not impact the filtration or extent of reabsorption that occurs passively. Such inhibition will result in a decrease in the clearance of a drug, which in turn increases the steady-state plasma concentration and results in a prolonged half-life of the drug.

Other sites of drug–drug interaction, though less common, can also affect the renal elimination of drugs. For example, antacids can alter urine pH and change the fraction of an ionizable drug that undergoes tubular reabsorption. Drugs that inhibit the renal metabolism of drugs represent another mechanism of potential interaction.

20.4   HEPATIC CLEARANCE

20.4.1   Basic Liver Structure and Function

The liver is the second largest organ in the body, weighing about 1.5 kg. The liver is located in the right upper quadrant of the abdomen, just below the diaphragm. Main functions of the liver include bile production, detoxification of waste products, storage of iron, vitamins, and trace elements, and the biotransformation of toxic compounds for excretion by the kidneys. Because of its location and ability to efficiently extract a wide variety of compounds from the portal circulation, the liver plays a central role in removing toxic materials before their entry into the systemic circulation. The extracting ability of the liver may result in a substantial decrease in the systemic availability of drugs after oral administration. In addition to its ability to biotransform a wide variety of toxicants, the liver may also directly excrete drugs and/or their metabolites into bile. Thus, the liver possesses two mechanisms for xenobiotic elimination—biotransformation and biliary excretion.

The liver is anatomically divided into two lobes, right and left. Each lobe is further divided into approximately one million lobules. These hepatic lobules are the functional units of the liver. The liver is composed of two types of epithelial cells: hepatocytes, which account for approximately 80% of the nuclear population, and cholangiocytes (epithelial cells that line intrahepatic bile ducts), which account for 3–5% of the liver cell population. A lobule is a hexagonal arrangement of plates of hepatocytes radiating outward from a central vein in the center. Roughly 75% of blood entering the liver arises from venous blood draining into the portal vein. Importantly, all of the venous blood returning from the small intestine, stomach, pancreas, and spleen converges into the portal vein, as does a portion of that which drains from the large intestine. The remaining 25% of the blood supply to the liver is arterial blood delivered through the hepatic artery (Fig. 20.4). The hepatic vascular system has several unique characteristics relative to other organs.

Terminal branches of the hepatic portal vein and hepatic artery empty together and mix as they enter sinusoids in the liver. Hence, the sinusoids are exposed to drug that originates from the gastrointestinal system as well as from the systemic circulation; and such exposure occurs simultaneously. This fact may have important implications in modeling hepatic clearance. The sinusoids are distensible vascular channels bounded circumferentially by hepatocytes. Blood flows through the sinusoids and empties into the central vein of each lobule. As blood flows through the sinusoids, nutrients and other endogenous and exogenous compounds are distributed into the hepatocytes. Hepatocytes are arranged in plates with their apical surfaces facing and surrounding the sinusoids. The basal faces of adjoining hepatocytes are welded together by junctional complexes to form canaliculi, the first channel in the biliary system. Hepatocytes secrete bile into the canaliculi, and those secretions flow antiparallel to the blood flow in sinusoids. At the ends of the

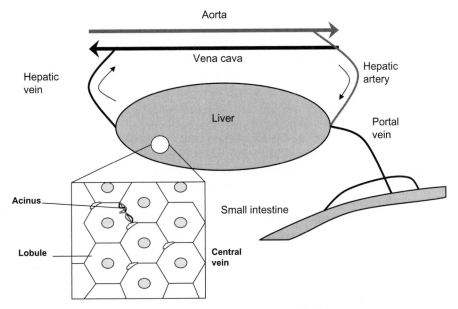

FIGURE 20.4 Hepatic vascular system and lobular structure.

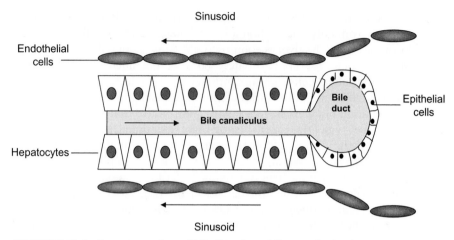

FIGURE 20.5   Representation of bile flow from bile canaliculus into the bile duct.

canaliculi, bile flows into bile ducts, which are true ducts lined with epithelial cells. Bile ducts thus begin in very close proximity to the terminal branches of the portal vein and hepatic artery.

Hepatocytes are the chief functional cells of the liver and perform a large number of metabolic, endocrine, and secretory functions. As mentioned previously, roughly 80% of the mass of the liver is hepatocytes. In three dimensions, hepatocytes are arranged in plates that are in membrane-to-membrane contact with one another. The cells are polygonal in shape and their sides are in contact either with sinusoids (sinusoidal face or apical face) or neighboring hepatocytes (basal faces). A portion of the basal faces of hepatocytes are modified, giving rise to bile canaliculi (Fig. 20.5). Bile originates as secretions from the basal surface of hepatocytes, which collect in canalicular channels. These secretions flow toward the periphery of lobules and into bile ductules and interlobular bile ducts, ultimately collecting in the hepatic duct outside the liver.

20.4.2   Mechanism of Drug Transport Across the Hepatocytes

The portal venous blood contains all of the products absorbed from the gastrointestinal (GI) tract, such as major and minor nutrients originating from ingested food, some endogenous substrates secreted into and reabsorbed from the GI tract, and drugs or other ingested xenobiotics. Drugs delivered to the liver via the portal vein or hepatic artery can be taken up by the hepatocytes and metabolized to more polar compounds. Drugs and their metabolites may then redistribute back into the sinusoids, from where they reach the systemic circulation. Alternatively, drugs or their metabolites may be secreted into the intestinal tract via the biliary system. These secreted compounds and their metabolites can be reabsorbed from the intestine or excreted through feces. Uptake of solutes from sinusoidal blood involves stepwise processes: transport, across the sinusoidal membrane, intrahepatocellular transport, and transport across the canalicular membrane.

Transport Across the Sinusoidal Membrane Once in the sinusoidal blood, drugs may be absorbed from the sinusoids by an active transport process or diffuse passively across the hepatocyte plasma membranes at the apical face. For drugs undergoing an active transport process, traversing the membrane involves several steps. The first is reversible binding of the drug to the membrane transport protein on the sinusoidal side of the cell membrane. Traversing the lipid bilayer itself could occur by a flip-flop process involving the hydrophilic region of the molecule. To aid this process, the carboxyl group of fatty acids becomes protonated by hydrogen bonding either with constituents in the membrane/water interface or constituents within the membrane itself. The uptake process is completed by dissociation of the drug at the cytosolic side of the cell membrane.

Specific plasma membrane transporters exist in the sinusoidal and canalicular membranes of hepatocytes (Fig. 20.6). These include Na^+-dependent and Na^+-independent anionic transporters, as well as cationic transporters. These plasma membrane transporters in humans include Na^+-taurocholate cotransporting polypeptide (NTCP), human organic anion transporting polypeptides (OATP1 and

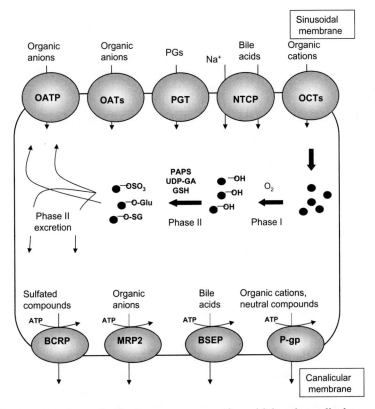

FIGURE 20.6 Uptake and efflux transporters on sinusoidal and canalicular membranes. OAT, organic anion transporter; OATP, organic anion transporting polypeptide; PGT, prostaglandin transporter; NTCP, Na^+-taurocholate cotransporting polypeptide; OCT, organic cation transporter; BCRP, breast cancer resistance protein; MRP, multidrug resistance associated protein; BSEP, bile salt export pump; P-gp, P-glycoprotein.

OATP2), prostaglandin transporter (PGT), and various organic cation transporters; including the organic cation transporter associated with uptake of hydrophilic aliphatic and certain aromatic cations (OCT1). These membrane transporters are involved in the transport of bile acids, organic anions, and organic cations.

Intrahepatocellular Transport   Intrahepatocellular drug transport may occur through several processes. These include cytoplasmic diffusion, protein mediated diffusion, cytoplasmic flow, vesicular transport, and drug transfer from intracellular membranes to intracellular proteins. Cytoplasmic diffusion and protein mediated diffusion of drugs are important in intracellular drug disposition. The transfer of solutes from the sinusoidal membrane to the canalicular membrane involves several different steps. These include lateral diffusion of the unbound ligand through the cytoplasm, lateral diffusion of the unbound ligand through membranes, vesicular transport, and transport by cytosolic binding proteins. It is also possible that transporters facilitate the uptake of some solutes by intrahepatic organelles such as lysosomes and mitochondria. Lipophilic basic drugs accumulate in the relatively acidic hepatic lysosomes as a result of the pH difference between lysosomes and the cytoplasm, but may also be due to binding to lipophilic substances and/or aggregation within lysosomes. The sequestration of cationic drugs in the liver also occurs by both slow and fast binding to proteins and membrane sites, as well as ion trapping into mitochondria and lysosomes. The accumulation of cationic lipophilic drugs in the liver, probably primarily due to trapping in mitochondria and lysosomes as well as binding, results in a slow elution and a low availability of cationic lipophilic drugs for excretion in the bile and enterohepatic transport.

Transport Across the Canalicular Membrane   Transport of solutes across the canalicular membrane into the bile occurs via active transport by several membrane proteins. Mechanistically, biliary elimination of anionic compounds, including glutathione *S*-conjugates, is mediated by multidrug resistance associated protein (MRP) transporter MRP2, whereas bile salts are excreted by a bile salt export pump (BSEP). MRP2 can recognize many kinds of organic anions and is responsible for the biliary excretion of many endogenous compounds and drugs. Also expressed in the canalicular membrane is P-glycoprotein, which mediates the biliary excretion of hydrophobic, mostly organic cationic and neutral metabolites. All of the canalicular membrane transport proteins are driven by ATP hydrolysis to transport a number of drug conjugates that undergo enterohepatic recycling, including glucuronide, sulfate, and glutathione conjugates. Figure 20.6 illustrates various sinusoidal and canalicular membrane transporters involved in the uptake and efflux of solutes.

Although hepatocytes lining the sinusoids are polarized (i.e., transport compounds from sinusoidal surface to canalicular surface), there is a possibility for back-transport into the sinusoids. For instance, certain multidrug resistance associated protein (MRP) transporters (MRP1, MRP3, and MRP6) exist at the sinusoidal surface of the membrane [14]. These active transporters can transport certain drugs and metabolites from hepatocytes back into sinusoids. In some cases there is preferential excretion of the solutes back into the sinusoids rather than into the bile, thus minimizing potential enterohepatic recycling. Other drug anion conjugates are also preferentially excreted into the sinusoids by a saturable transport mechanism.

In general, transporters such as MRP1 are present in the sinusoidal membrane only at very low levels in quiescent cells.

20.4.3 Role of Liver in First-Pass Metabolism

Although every tissue has some ability to metabolize drugs, the liver is the principal organ of drug metabolism. Other tissues that display considerable activity include the gastrointestinal tract, the lungs, the skin, and the kidneys. Drugs that are administered orally are absorbed from the gastrointestinal tract, carried via the hepatic portal vein to the liver. Many drugs are absorbed intact from the small intestine and transported to the liver, where they undergo extensive metabolism by the liver before the systemic organs are exposed to the drug. This removal of a drug by the liver, before the drug has become available in the systemic circulation, is called the *first-pass effect*. First-pass metabolism can occur in the gut and/or the liver, since the entire dose of the drug absorbed after oral administration must pass through these organs prior to reaching the systemic circulation. This process may greatly limit the bioavailability of orally administered drugs, such that alternative routes of administration must be employed to achieve therapeutically effective blood levels.

20.4.4 Biliary Clearance

Xenobiotic compounds excreted into bile are often divided into three classes on the basis of the ratio of their concentration in bile versus that in plasma. Class A substances have a ratio of nearly 1 and include sodium, potassium, glucose, mercury, thallium, cesium, and cobalt. Class B substances have a ratio of bile to plasma greater than 1. Class B substances include bile acids, bilirubin, sulfobromophthalein, lead, arsenic, manganese, and many other xenobiotics. Class C substances have a ratio below 1 (e.g., inulin, albumin, zinc, iron, gold, and chromium). Compounds rapidly excreted into bile are most likely to be found among class B substances.

The mechanism by which the body directs some compounds to the biliary excretion is as yet unclear. However, it is apparent that molecular weight of the compound is a key factor in determining biliary excretion. The molecular weight threshold for humans is estimated to be 500–600. Compounds with molecular weights less than this threshold are excreted primarily in the urine. This knowledge may be useful in drug design when one objective is to achieve a lead compound exhibiting primarily biliary excretion—which obviates the need for dosage adjustment in renal disease.

Drugs that undergo biliary secretion have the potential to be reabsorbed from the GI tract and exhibit enterohepatic recycling. Enterohepatic recycling prolongs the half-life of drugs primarily excreted in bile. Interruption of this cycling through the oral administration of nonabsorbable adsorbants (e.g., activated charcoal) may enhance the clearance of affected compounds. In addition, since the gallbladder empties episodically in humans, drugs that undergo significant enterohepatic recycling may exhibit discontinuous plasma concentrations (as a portion of the excreted dose is periodically reabsorbed, resulting in increases in the plasma concentration of drug).

20.4.5 Determination of Hepatic Clearance

Determination of the hepatic clearance (CL_H) of a compound is generally achieved through applying the principle of the additivity of clearance. In particular, the total and renal clearance are determined as described previously. If there is no evidence of nonrenal/nonhepatic elimination of the drug, the CL_H is given as

$$CL_H = CL_T - CL_R$$

This means of determination for hepatic clearance obviously requires numerous assumptions that must be validated experimentally. Hepatic clearance may also be estimated from *in vitro* data, taking into account protein binding and liver blood flow.

20.4.6 Models of Hepatic Clearance

Predicting the impact of pharmacological, physiological, and pathophysiological interventions on hepatic clearance necessitates the elucidation of the determinants of hepatic clearance such that a quantitative model can be developed. Among the various mathematical models proposed to describe hepatic clearance, the venous equilibrium model (also known as the well-stirred model) represents the simplest model that appears to provide reasonably robust predictive capacity [15, 16].

Venous Equilibrium Model of Hepatic Clearance   The venous equilibrium model assumes the liver to be represented as a single, homogeneous, well-stirred compartment, such that all metabolic enzymes in the liver are exposed to the same concentration of drug (Fig. 20.7). This model simplistically assumes that drug bathing the sinusoids is in equilibrium with that in hepatic venous blood (hence the name venous equilibrium). Such a model obviously does not account for various anatomical complexities present in the liver, such as its network of branching tubes each with a zonal distribution of enzymes. It is also physiologically naive to envision drug concentration as unchanging as blood traverses the sinusoidal bed. Nevertheless, despite the fact that experimental evidence suggests that the hepatic sinusoid is not

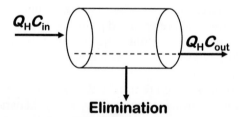

Elimination

FIGURE 20.7 Schematic of the venous equilibrium or well-stirred model of hepatic clearance. This model in essence envisions drug concentration dropping immediately upon entry into the hepatic sinusoids and not declining further as blood traverses across the sinusoidal bed. Hence the drug concentration bathing the sinusoids is viewed as being in equilibrium with the concentration in venous blood. Q_H, blood flow; C_{in}, concentration of drug in blood entering the liver; C_{out}, concentration of drug in venous blood exiting the liver. Dashed line represents the drug concentration in the sinusoids. (Adapted from Ref. 20.)

well stirred [17], the model has been found to provide good estimates of the impact of various changes on hepatic clearance and drug concentration. This model identifies three independent, noninteracting determinants of hepatic clearance: hepatic blood flow (Q_H), fraction of unbound drug in blood (f_{ub}), and the unbound intrinsic hepatic clearance (CL_{uint}) The CL_{uint} represents the ability of the liver to remove drug from blood in the absence of confounding factors (e.g., protein binding and blood flow) and is determined by the ability of the liver to metabolize or secrete (via biliary secretion) the drug. Accordingly, the hepatic clearance (CL_H) and hepatic extraction ratio (E_H) for the venous equilibrium model can be expressed as [15, 16, 18, 19]

$$CL_H = \frac{Q_H f_{ub} CL_{uint}}{Q_H + f_{ub} CL_{uint}}$$

$$E_H = \frac{f_{ub} CL_{uint}}{Q_H + f_{ub} CL_{uint}}$$

This model provides important insight into the impact of changes in blood flow, protein binding, and drug metabolism/transport on hepatic clearance—particularly at the extreme values of the unbound intrinsic hepatic clearance. For example, when $Q_H \gg f_{ub}CL_{uint}$, the value of CL_H will approach $f_{ub}CL_{uint}$ (i.e., $CL_H \approx f_{ub}CL_{uint}$). For such drugs, changes in hepatic clearance will be proportional to changes in protein binding or the unbound intrinsic clearance. Hence, coadministration of an enzyme inducer that increases the metabolism of such a drug will result in an increase in the hepatic clearance of the agent. Moreover, increases in the free fraction of drug will also result in proportional increases in the clearance of the drug. This indicates that the clearance of the drug is "restricted" to the free drug. Such drugs are therefore sometimes referred to as exhibiting restrictive clearance. Drugs in this category are also often classified as possessing a low intrinsic clearance. Agents that exhibit a hepatic extraction ratio < 0.3 can be viewed as possessing a low intrinsic clearance. Importantly, however, changes in hepatic blood flow will not alter the clearance of such drugs, provided the decrease is not sufficient to cause hypoxia and result in hepatocellular damage. Examples of drugs that fall into this category are diazepam, phenytoin, tolbutamide, and warfarin.

At the opposite extreme are those drugs for which $Q_H \ll f_{ub}CL_{uint}$, sometimes denoted as high intrinsic clearance drugs. Under these conditions, the value of CL_H will approach Q_H (i.e., $CL_H \approx Q_H$). Such drugs are referred to as exhibiting blood flow-dependent clearance (or perfusion rate limited), meaning that changes in blood flow result in proportional changes in clearance. Under these conditions, increases in enzyme or transport activity will not result in further increases in hepatic clearance, as drug is already being cleared as rapidly as it is delivered to the liver. Modest reductions in enzyme activity will also not result in significant alterations in drug clearance. However, if an inhibitor of metabolism or transport causes a magnitude of reduction such that the assumption that $Q_H \ll f_{ub}CL_{uint}$ is no longer true, coadministration of an inhibitor with a drug exhibiting a high intrinsic clearance may result in significant changes in drug clearance. Drugs with an extraction ratio > 0.7 are generally classified as exhibiting a high intrinsic clearance. Moreover, drug is removed so rapidly under these conditions that it is not restricted to free drug.

This model also provides important insight into factors that influence the systemic availability of drugs after oral administration. If a drug is completely absorbed after oral administration and is not metabolized by the gut, the fraction of drug that reaches the systemic circulation can be described as

$$F = 1 - E_H$$

Since

$$E_H = \frac{f_{ub}CL_{uint}}{Q_H + f_{ub}CL_{uint}}$$

F can be determined as

$$F = 1 - E_H$$

$$F = 1 - \frac{f_{ub}CL_{uint}}{Q_H + f_{ub}CL_{uint}}$$

$$F = \frac{Q_H}{Q_H + f_{ub}CL_{uint}}$$

The relationship given above indicates that when $Q_H \gg f_{ub}CL_{uint}$, $F \to 1$. Such drugs will not exhibit any significant first-pass effect during passage through the liver. Hence, coadministration of an enzyme inducer or inhibitor will not significantly alter the systemic availability of drugs with these characteristics. In contrast, when $Q_H \ll f_{ub}CL_{uint}$, $F \to 0$ and little of the drug will reach the systemic circulation after oral administration. Under these circumstances, changes in enzyme activity, as produced by inhibitors or inducers, may have profound effects on the systemic availability of drugs. Among the drugs that exhibit a high first-pass effect and low systemic availability are propranolol, verapamil, and nitroglycerin. Because of the high first-pass effect, oral doses of such drugs are substantially (sometimes an order of magnitude) greater than intravenous doses in order achieve the desired pharmacologic effect. In addition, there is generally much more inter- and intrapatient variability in the pharmacokinetics of drugs subject to extensive metabolism. As a consequence, one objective in lead optimization is often to utilize rationale drug design to eliminate first-pass metabolism.

This model of hepatic drug clearance also demonstrates the importance of understanding the role of first-pass metabolism in the interpretation of values of drug clearance obtained from the ratio of dose and area under the drug concentration versus time curve. This is most readily seen for a drug that is eliminated solely by hepatic metabolism and completely absorbed after oral administration. For such compounds, the hepatic clearance after intravenous administration can be determined as

$$CL_H = \frac{D_{IV}}{AUC_{IV}}$$

where D_{IV} is the intravenous dose and AUC_{IV} is the area under the drug concentration versus time curve for that dose. Similarly, the hepatic clearance after oral administration is given as

$$CL_H = \frac{F \times D_o}{AUC_o}$$

where F is the systemic availability, D_o is the oral dose, and AUC_o is the area under the drug concentration versus time curve after that dose. Remembering that

$$CL_H = \frac{Q_H f_{ub} CL_{uint}}{Q_H + f_{ub} CL_{uint}}$$

and

$$F = \frac{Q_H}{Q_H + f_{ub} CL_{uint}}$$

one can substitute these equalities for CL_H and F, yielding

$$\frac{Q_H f_{ub} CL_{uint}}{Q_H + f_{ub} CL_{uint}} = \frac{Q_H}{Q_H + f_{ub} CL_{uint}} \times \frac{D_o}{AUC_o}$$

This relationship simplifies to

$$f_{ub} CL_{uint} = \frac{D_o}{AUC_o}$$

Importantly, note that the ratio of oral dose to AUC does not provide the value for hepatic clearance, but rather $f_{ub}CL_{uint}$. When calculated in this fashion, this is referred to as the oral clearance (CL_o). For a low intrinsic clearance drug, this value will be essentially equal to the hepatic clearance. However, for a high intrinsic clearance drug, the value will be much higher than the hepatic clearance and will exceed the value for hepatic blood flow.

This relationship also provides a means by which the unbound intrinsic hepatic clearance and hepatic blood flow can be determined experimentally. If an intravenous dose of radiolabeled drug and an oral dose of "cold" drug are administered simultaneously, the hepatic and intrinsic clearances can be calculated from the above relationships. Once these values are determined, the blood flow can be calculated from the knowledge of these two parameters. While similar determinations can be made by administering nonradiolabeled drug by both routes on different days, simultaneous administration by both routes obviates the need to account for day to day variability in hepatic blood flow or enzyme activity.

Parallel Tube Model of Hepatic Clearance   The parallel tube model represents the liver sinusoids as identical parallel tubes. This model also assumes that metabolic

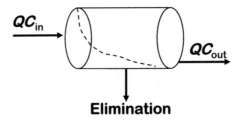

Elimination

FIGURE 20.8 Schematic representation of the parallel tube model of hepatic drug clearance. This model envisions the liver as being comprised of a series of parallel tubes (one of which is shown) with drug concentration declining as blood traverses through the sinusoidal space. See Fig. 20.7 for abbreviations. (Adapted from Ref. 20.)

enzymes are uniformly distributed along the sinusoid [20]. In this model, drug concentration is envisioned as declining exponentially as drug traverses the sinusoidal tube (Fig. 20.8). This leads to different equalities for extraction ratio, hepatic clearance, and systemic availability:

$$E = 1 - e^{-f_{ub}CL_{uint}/Q_H}$$
$$CL_H = Q_H(1 - e^{-f_{ub}CL_{uint}/Q_H})$$
$$F = e^{-f_{ub}CL_{uint}/Q_H}$$

The differences between the parallel tube and venous equilibrium models in prediction of the effect of changes in blood flow, enzyme activity, and protein binding are insignificant for drugs that exhibit a low intrinsic clearance (i.e., $E <$ 0.3). For intermediate drugs (i.e., $0.3 < E < 0.7$) the differences are also generally insignificant except with oral administration. The difference in model prediction is most clearly seen for drugs with high intrinsic clearance values. Using a variety of experimental models, most commonly the isolated perfused rat liver, numerous investigators have demonstrated substantial differences in the predictive capacity of these two models for such drugs. However, it should be noted that these differences are probably not of clinical significance for the overwhelming number of therapeutic agents. Therefore, the use of the most simplistic model provides important insight for the practical application of clearance concepts.

Other Models of Hepatic Clearance In addition to the two models described earlier, additional models of hepatic clearance have been proposed. The distributed model is a modification of the parallel tube model, where each tube has a distinct blood flow rate and metabolic capacity [19]. The dispersion model adds complexity via consideration of the transit time of the drug in the model. A series compartment model has also been proposed, which envisions the liver to be comprised of a series of well-stirred compartments. The review of Morgan and Smallwood [21] is recommend for readers interested in further consideration of various models of hepatic clearance.

20.5 EFFECT OF DISEASE ON DRUG CLEARANCE

From the foregoing discussion, it should be obvious that disease states that alter the functional capacity of organs of elimination may result in substantial changes in drug clearance. It is also important to recognize that the contribution of a given organ of elimination to the overall elimination of a drug may change dramatically in the face of significant pathology of another organ of elimination. Consider, for example, a drug that is eliminated 85% by the kidneys unchanged and 15% by hepatic metabolism. For such a drug, alteration of hepatic metabolism by administration of an enzyme inhibitor is unlikely to have a clinically significant impact on the disposition of the compound. In contrast, in the presence of renal disease such that hepatic metabolism becomes the predominant route of elimination, interaction with an enzyme inhibitor may be of substantial significance.

The impact of renal disease on the renal clearance of drugs has been the most widely studied disease-induced alteration of drug disposition. This is, in part, due to the ready ability to quantify kidney function via creatinine clearance. Hence, it has been possible to evaluate the impact of various degrees of functional deficit on the renal elimination of drugs. Renal diseases, mainly acute and chronic renal failure, are associated with nephron loss to varying degrees depending on the stage of the renal disease. Bricker's "intact nephron" hypothesis provides an explanation for the kidney's ability to compensate and preserve homeostasis despite a significant loss of nephron function in renal disease [22]. During renal failure, regardless of etiology, injury occurs to the nephrons in a progressive manner. Significant damage to groups of nephrons will eliminate them from contributing to the maintenance of normal renal function. The remaining intact nephrons will compensate by experiencing cellular hypertrophy. This growth process will enable them to accept larger blood volumes for clearance, thus contributing to maintenance of glomerulotubular balance and the excretion of greater solute levels, resulting in compensation. Thus, varieties of adaptations compensate for the decreased GFR and allow a new steady state of external balance to exist. However, in the process of adapting, a second component becomes disordered. The classic examples are the secondary hyperparathyroidism and uremic syndrome of chronic renal failure. Thus, renal diseases not only influence the overall elimination of drugs directly but also result in secondary abnormalities.

Progressive renal disease evolves to a multiorgan syndrome such that the disposition of drugs via nonrenal routes may be altered. For example, patients with renal disease may accumulate endogenous compounds that displace drugs from plasma protein binding sites. This has the potential to increase the hepatic clearance of low intrinsic clearance drugs. Furthermore, the accumulation of the endogenous products normally excreted in the kidney may impair the functional capacity of the liver, such that drug metabolism (and thus hepatic clearance) is impaired.

The kidney makes the major contribution to excretion of unchanged drug and also the excretion of metabolites. A range of physiological and pathophysiological states may influence the efficiency of renal clearance as described earlier. It is evident that renal drug clearance is altered to a clinically significant extent in a number of disease states. Even though the intact nephrons compensate for the decreased clearance by adaptation, they cannot completely reestablish the normal kidney function. For a drug, if the renal clearance contributes only 25–30% to overall clearance, the renal impairment may not influence the total body clearance significantly; while for the drugs that are predominantly cleared by the kidneys, total clearance is significantly affected by renal impairment. Therefore, drug removal by artificial means (renal replacement therapy) such as hemodialysis becomes essential in subjects with substantial loss of renal function. Similar to renal clearance, the extent to which the drug is affected by dialysis is determined primarily by physico-chemical characteristics such as molecular size, protein binding, volume of distribution, hydrophilicity, and plasma clearance of the drug. In addition, technical aspects of the dialysis procedure such as characteristics of dialysis membrane and dialysate flow rates may also determine the extent of drug removal [23, 24]. Drugs that are significantly cleared by the kidney often undergo substantial removal during dialysis and dosing adjustments are often required for such drugs. Only the unbound drug is available for filtration and drugs with high protein binding are poorly cleared by dialysis. The influence of renal diseases on protein binding of drugs is not well understood. It has been reported that low albumin levels are found in critically ill patients, which may increase the unbound fraction of many drugs with possible deleterious effects. These patients also often have increased levels of acid α-glycoprotein, which may increase protein binding of some drugs. Thus, the unbound fraction in healthy volunteers and in patients with renal impairment may differ substantially from the unbound fraction of drugs in critically ill patients receiving dialysis. Similarly, in critically ill patients the actual volume of distribution may differ significantly from that of healthy subjects, and it also exhibits great inter- and intraindividual variation [24, 25].

The ability of the liver to metabolize drugs depends on hepatic blood flow and enzyme activity, both of which can be affected by liver damage. Hepatic diseases can selectively modify the kinetics of drug metabolism in the liver [26]. Previous studies on the effects of hepatic disease have shown that cytochrome P450 (CYP) enzymes are more susceptible to hepatocellular injury than are NADPH-cytochrome P450 reductase or phase II enzymes, such as UDP-glucuronosyltrans-ferases involved in drug conjugation reactions. Patients with severe liver diseases such as cirrhosis or severe hepatitis with liver failure have significant impairment of CYP enzymes. Moreover, in patients with liver damage, expression of some CYP isoforms remains unaffected while other isoforms are significantly reduced. For instance, in liver cirrhosis expression of CYP1A2 and CYP3A4 is decreased, while in cirrhosis with cholestasis expression of CYP2C and CYP2E isoforms is reduced [27, 28]. Therefore, a thorough knowledge of the particular enzyme involved in the metabolism of a drug and the impact of hepatic damage on that enzyme is essential to provide a reasonable basis for dosage adjustment in patients with hepatic impairment. In addition, liver failure can influence the binding of a drug to plasma proteins. These changes can occur alone or in combination; when they coexist their effect on drug kinetics can be synergistic. The kinetics of drugs with a low hepatic extraction are sensitive to hepatic failure rather than to liver blood flow changes. While the kinetics of many drugs are altered by liver disease, quantifying the required dosing changes remains a challenge. At present, there is no satisfactory test that provides a quantitative measure of liver function, with which drug clearance is highly correlated.

Liver diseases may also impair the biliary excretion of drugs. Cholestasis is a hepatic abnormality in which there is stagnation of bile flow, which may arise from a physical obstruction of the biliary tree (extrahepatic cholestasis) or a decrease in the secretion of the bile by the hepatocytes (intrahepatic cholestasis). The impairment of biliary secretions may result in the accumulation of metabolites, such as glucuronide conjugates, that may be transported into blood. Under these conditions, the overall time that a compound remains in the body increases considerably. There are other clinical conditions in which the metabolism of drugs is altered, including heart failure and other liver diseases.

It is also important to recognize that chronic renal failure can significantly affect the disposition of both low and high hepatic extraction drugs, which are cleared predominantly by the liver. Renal diseases have also been suggested to affect biliary clearance through the accumulation of some P-glycoprotein substrates in the plasma, which may in turn inhibit the secretion of some drugs [9, 29].

REFERENCES

1. van Acker BA, Koomen GC, Koopman MG. Discrepancy between circadian rhythms of inulin and creatinine clearance. *J Lab Clin Med* 1992;120:400–410.

2. Koopman MG, Koomen GC, Krediet RT. Circadian rhythm of glomerular filtration rate in normal individuals. *Clin Sci* 1989;77:105–111.

3. Bonate PL, Reith K, Weir S. Drug interactions at the renal level: implications for drug development. *Clin Pharmacokinet* 1998;34:375–404.

4. Ullrich KJ, Rumrich G. Contraluminal transport systems in the proximal renal tubules involved in secretion of organic ions. *Am J Physiol* 1989;254:F453–F462.

5. Burkhardt G, Ullrich KJ. Organic anion transport across the contraluminal membrane KG dependence on sodium. *Kidney Int* 1989;36:370–377.

6. Lee W, Kim RB. Transporters and renal drug elimination. *Annu Rev Pharmacol Toxicol* 2004;44:137–166.

7. Rennick BR. Renal tubule transport of organic cations. *Am J Physiol* 1981;240: F83–F89.

8. Dorian C, Gattene VH II, Klaassen CD. Renal cadmium deposition and injury as a result of accumulation of cadmium-metallothionein (CdMT) by proximal concoluted tubules— a light microscope autoradiographic study with [109]CdMT. *Toxicol Appl Pharmacol* 1992;114:173–181.

9. Dreisbach AW, Lartora JJL. The effect of chronic renal failure on hepatic drug metabolism and drug disposition. *Semin Dialysis* 2003;16:45–50.

10. Rule AD, Larson TS, Bergstralh EJ, Slezak JM, Jacobsen SJ, Cosio FG. Using serum creatinine to estimate glomerular filtration rate: accuracy in good health and in chronic kidney disease. *Ann Intern Med* 2004;141:929–937.

11. Rule AD, Gussak HM, Pond GR, Bergstralh EJ, Stegall MD, Cosio FG, Larson, TS. Measured and estimated GFR in healthy potential kidney donors. *Am J Kidney Dis* 2004;43:112–119.

12. Branten AJ, Vervoort G, Wetzels JF. Serum creatinine is a poor marker of GFR in nephrotic syndrome. *Nephrol Dial Transplant* 2005;20:707–711.

13. Hall SD, Rowland M. Influence of fraction unbound upon the renal clearance of furosemide in the isolated perfused rat kidney. *J Pharmacol Exp Ther* 1985;232:263–268.

14. Chandra P, Brouwer KLR. The complexities of hepatic drug transport: current knowledge and emerging concepts. *Pharm Res* 2004;21:719–735.

15. Perrier D, Gibaldi M. Clearance and biological half-life as indices of intrinsic hepatic metabolism. *J Pharmacol Exp Ther* 1974;191:17–24.

16. Wilkinson GR, Shand DG. A physiological approach to hepatic drug clearance. *Clin Pharmacol Ther* 1975;18:377–390.

17. Weisiger RA, Mendel CM, Cavalieri RR. The hepatic sinusoid is not well-stirred: estimation of the degree of axial mixing by analysis of lobular concentration gradients formed during uptake of thyroxine by the perfused liver. *J Pharm Sci* 1986;75:263–268.

18. Ridgeway D, Tuszynski JA, Tam YK. Reassessing models of hepatic extraction. *J Biol Phys* 2003;29:1–21.

19. Ahmad AB, Bennette PN, Routland M. Models of hepatic drug clearance: discrimination between the well-stirred and parallel tube models. *J Pharm Pharmac* 1983;35:219–224.

20. Pang SK, Rowland M. Hepatic clearance of drugs I. Theoretical considerations of a "well-stirred" model and a "parallel tube" model. Influence of hepatic blood flow, plasma and blood cell binding and the hepatocellular enzymatic activity on hepatic drug clearance. *J Pharmacokinet Biopharm* 1977;5:625–653.

21. Morgan DJ, Smallwood RA. Clinical significance of pharmacokinetic models of hepatic elimination. *Clin Pharmacokinet* 1990;18:61–76.

22. Bricker NS. On the meaning of the intact nephron hypothesis. *Am J Med* 1969;46:1–11.

23. Hudson JQ, Comstock TJ, Feldman GM. Evaluation of an *in vitro* dialysis system to predict drug removal. *Nephrol Dial Transplant* 2004;19:400–405.

24. Driscoll DF, McMahon M, Blackburn GL, Bistrain BR. Phenytoin toxicity in a critically ill, hypoalbuminemic patient with normal serum drug concentrations. *Crit Care Med* 1988;16:1248–1249.

25. Brugge JF. Pharmacokinetics and drug dosing adjustments during continuous venovenous hemofiltration or hemodiafiltration in critically ill patients. *Acta Anesthesiol Scand* 2001;45:929–934.

26. Rodighiero V. Effects of liver disease on pharmacokinetics. An update. *Clin Pharmacokinet* 1999;37:399–431.

27. Blouin RA, Farrell GC, Ionnides C, Renton KW, Watlington CO. Impact of diseases on detoxication. *J Biochem Mol Toxicol* 1999;13:215–218.

28. George J, Murray M, Byth K, Farrell GC. Differential alterations of cytochrome P450 proteins in livers from patients with severe chronic liver disease. *Hepatology* 1995;21:120–128.

29. Nolin TD, Frye RF, Matzke GR. Hepatic drug metabolism and transport in patients with kidney disease. *Am J Kidney Dis* 2003;42:906–925.

21

IN VITRO METABOLISM IN PRECLINICAL DRUG DEVELOPMENT

OLAVI PELKONEN,[1] ARI TOLONEN,[1,2] MIIA TURPEINEN,[1] AND JOUKO UUSITALO[2]

[1]*University of Oulu, Oulu, Finland*
[2]*Novamass Analytical Ltd., Oulu, Finland*

Contents

Preclinical Development Handbook: ADME and Biopharmaceutical Properties,
edited by Shayne Cox Gad
Copyright © 2008 John Wiley & Sons, Inc.

21.1   INTRODUCTION

In drug therapy, some important questions concerning the efficient and safe use of a drug are the following: (1) What is the size of the dose? (2) How often should it be given? (3) Is there interference from other simultaneously used drugs or other chemicals? (4) Are there important idiosyncratic reactions due to a drug? (5) Are there important patient characteristics to be considered? [1]. The first two questions relate to basic pharmacokinetic characteristics of a drug, principally to its bioavailability and clearance. The third question relates to potential interactions. The fourth concerns the possibility of metabolism-related toxicities, and the fifth relates to endogenous, host-related and genetic features of an individual patient to whom a drug is administered. At the basic level, we need to know about the drug substance (1) its clearance and factors contributing to it, (2) major and minor, including potentially toxic, metabolites (i.e., metabolite profile), and (3) drug-metabolizing enzymes catalyzing (at least) rate-limiting routes, and their inhibition and induction and physiological and pathological behavior.

In this chapter, metabolism in preclinical drug development is the principal topic. However, before going into details, some more general concerns during drug discovery and development should be expressed. Drug development is the optimization of not a single feature but multiple features, even regarding metabolism and kinetics [2, 3]. Consequently, optimization is always a trade-off between several independent or interdependent features. Thus, there are no preset answers to the optimization problem; instead, it is a continuous cross-talk between various optimization tasks. It is therefore difficult to say that one *in vitro* test is more important than another, because the relative importance depends on the individual substance under study and its unique characteristics. However, this is not to say that we do not need a general strategy to study drug metabolism and pharmacokinetics by *in vitro* methods. We need a general strategy, but it has to be modified depending on the substance, its stage of development, and many other considerations.

In Table 21.1, an attempt has been made to put metabolism into a wider perspective in pharmacokinetic (PK) processes. Optimization of metabolic features in the context of pharmacokinetics is divided into characteristics, which should be pre-

TABLE 21.1 Metabolic Processes, Characteristics, and Factors that Should Be Predicted on the Basis of *In Vitro* Screening Assays or Assumed During the *In Vitro–In Vivo* Extrapolationa

PK Process	Characteristic	Factors	Assays
Systemic exposure			
Hepatic clearance	Hepatic blood flow	Protein binding permeability	Animals *in vivo*
	Hepatic metabolic clearance	CYP enzymes, phase II enzymes	*In vitro* and cell based (see text)
	Biliary clearance	Transporters	Liver perfusion
Bioavailability			
First-pass clearance	Intestinal clearance	Efflux transporters and intestinal metabolism	Caco-2
	Hepatic clearance	See above	
Interactions			
Metabolism	Inhibition	CYP enzymes	*In vitro* microsomes, recombinant CYPs or cell based
		Phase II enzymes	as above
	Induction		Hepatocytes, receptor-binding
Metabolic activation	Reactive metabolites, oxygen radicals, etc.	Producing enzymes	*In vitro* systems

aFor some illustrative examples concerning various PK aspects, see chapters in a book by Pelkonen et al. [6].

dicted on the basis of *in vitro* information, factors (i.e., biological phenomena or constituents mediating them), and assays or screens (i.e., systems available to measure a factor or a characteristic). Furthermore, an additional entry depicts metabolic activation, which is thought to be of importance for "idiosyncratic" reactions (see Section 21.5).

One more introductory note: the literature on subjects in this chapter is very large and making proper acknowledgments to all important contributions is impossible. Selection of references thus reflects our somewhat personal view, but hopefully contains the most useful ones, from which the reader can go further.

21.2   *IN VITRO* BIOLOGICAL SYSTEMS TO CATALYZE METABOLISM

The questions posed at the beginning of this chapter will be definitively and unequivocally answered during the clinical phase, including postmarketing pharmacovigilance, of drug development. However, this is too late from the early drug development point of view and thus, to avoid failures and withdrawals later on, the basic information for answering these questions should preferably be produced in the nonclinical phase of development. In the current paradigm of nonclinical drug development, *in vitro* screening systems are used for producing the appropriate answers through correlation and extrapolation, which actually are absolute requirements for the judicious use of *in vitro* studies to support drug development. Because of interspecies differences and extrapolation uncertainties, human-derived or humanized *in vitro* systems are preferably used. Important goals for using various human liver derived *in vitro* systems are the following: (1) to elucidate and determine principal metabolic routes of a new chemical entity (NCE) and to tentatively identify principal metabolites; (2) to identify phase I enzymes, especially cytochrome P450 (CYP), catalyzing the principal oxidation routes (primary metabolites) and phase II enzymes catalyzing the conjugated metabolites, and to gain some quantitative data on their significance for the overall metabolic fate of an NCE; and (3) to provide useful background information for characterizing potential interactions and physiological, genetic, and pathological factors affecting the kinetics and variability of an NCE in the *in vivo* situation.

21.2.1   Metabolic Competence of the *In Vitro* System

When screening potential drug candidates, one is faced with a question. How large or restricted should the set of enzymes be to cover a reasonable number of potential drug-metabolizing enzymes; that is, what is the optimal range of enzymes to be screened? In the end, each drug is an individual, with its characteristic physicochemical properties, metabolic reactions, metabolizing enzymes, kinetics, and so on. Regarding metabolism, thus far the main focus has been on CYP enzymes. This is natural, because the CYP enzyme superfamily is responsible for approximately 70–80% of the rate-limiting phase I metabolism of drugs [4]. However, there are a large number of other important enzymes participating in the metabolism of drugs. For example, should we routinely screen for various UGT or SULT enzymes and at which stage of the development? Table 21.2 gives an overview of drug-metabolizing enzymes, which should be considered when studying the metabolic competence of a given *in vitro* screening system [5, 6]. Although it is impossible to give unequivocal recommendations for how comprehensive metabolic competence should be employed in the *in vitro* test system, it is always useful to consider this matter and explicitly state objectives of the specific test and reasons for selecting the specific biological preparation, with a specified set of enzymes.

21.2.2   From Recombinants to Perfusions

Enzyme sources (i.e., biological preparations), are another concern. Most important possibilities are briefly described in Table 21.3, which presents an overview of current biological preparations for use as enzyme sources and some of their advantages and disadvantages. Liver microsomes have been the preferred source of enzymes for *in vitro* metabolism screening. Recombinant expressed enzymes have become more and more usable, because of easy availability and lack of variability. Isolated and/or cultured cells have a larger complement of enzymes in more natural cellular surroundings. These aspects have been very thoroughly covered recently [13, 14]. There are strong arguments in favor of using human primary hepatocytes [15], but obviously their availability for early and extensive screening is rather difficult. There are only a few studies in which several enzyme sources have been

TABLE 21.2 Drug–Metabolizing Enzymes (Preferably Human) that Should/Could/Might Be Included in the *In Vitro* Assays

Enzyme Classes/Enzymes	(Types of) Drugs Metabolized (Examples)	Sources Available	Need of Incorporation into *In Vitro* Systems
Cytochrome P450 enzymes (about 10–13 drug-metabolizing enzyme forms)	Practically 90% of all drug substances	Hepatocytes most versatile and comprehensive; other tissues and cell types selectively	Incorporation of P450-competent enzyme source is necessary for most purposes
An example: CYP1A1	Few pharmaceutics, principally polycyclic aromatic hydrocarbons and other carcinogens	Recombinant enzyme; mainly extrahepatic expression (e.g., placenta from smokers)	Induction usually required for expression; incorporation not necessary routinely
An example: CYP3A4	A majority, >50%, of all clinically used drugs	Hepatocytes, recombinant	Incorporation necessary for comprehensive screening
Flavin-monooxygenases (FMOs) (five forms)	Compounds with secondary and tertiary amines or sulfhydryl groups (chlorpromazine, desipramine, methimazole)	Hepatocytes most versatile and comprehensive	Incorporation comes automatically with hepatocytes; specific incorporation only in special circumstances
Prostaglandin H synthase	PAH-diols, aflatoxin B1, aromatic amines	Liver, kidney, bladder (microsomes)	Incorporation advisable for toxicity screening?
Alcohol/aldehyde dehydrogenases and oxidases	Various compounds with alcohol and aldehyde functions (ethanol)	Many tissues; cytosol	Some incorporation comes automatically with hepatocytes or hepatic homogenate; specific incorporation only in special circumstances
Monoamine oxidase	Selegiline, moclobemide	Many tissues; mitochondria	Incorporation advisable in specific situations

TABLE 21.2 *Continued*

Enzyme Classes/Enzymes	(Types of) Drugs Metabolized (Examples)	Sources Available	Need of Incorporation into *In Vitro* Systems
Esterases/hydrolases/peptidases	Compounds with cleavable ester/amide bond (procaine, succinylcholine, lidocaine)	Many tissues including blood and blood cells	At least some activity present when liver preparation is incorporated into the test system
Reductases	Many substances with azo, nitro, and carbonyl functions (chloramphenicol, naloxone); importance not well characterized	Present in hepatocytes (cytosol, some in microsomes)	Activity needs special circumstances; need of incorporation not adequately defined
UDP-glucuronosyltransferases (UGTs); glucuronide conjugation	Most drugs with suitable O-, S-, and N-functional groups (morphine, diazepam, paracetamol)	Hepatocytes most versatile and comprehensive (microsomes); subcellular systems need UDPGA	Incorporation of UGT-competent enzyme source is advisable for most purposes
Sulfotransferases (SULTs); sulfate conjugation	Phenols, alcohols, aromatic amines (paracetamol, methyldopa)	Hepatocytes most versatile and comprehensive (cytosol); subcellular systems need PAPS	Incorporation not adequately defined
GSH transferases (GSTs); glutathione conjugation	Epoxides, arene oxides, nitro groups, hydroxylamines (ethacrynic acid)	Hepatocytes most versatile and comprehensive (cytosol, microsomes)	Incorporation not adequately defined
Acyl-CoA glycinetransferase; amino acid conjugation	Acyl-CoA derivatives of carboxylic acids (salicylic acid)	Hepatocytes (mitochondria)	Incorporation advisable only in special cases
N-acetyltransferases (NATs); acylation	Amines (sulfonamides, isoniazid, clonazepam, dapsone)	Hepatocytes (cytosol)	Incorporation advisable only in special cases
Methyl transferases; methylation	Catecholamines, phenols, amines (L-dopa, thiouracil)	Various tissues (cytosol)	Incorporation advisable only in special cases

Sources: Adapted from Refs. 5 and 41.

TABLE 21.3 Comparison of *In Vitro* Enzyme Sources Used in Preclinical Research

Enzyme Sources	Availability	Advantages	Disadvantages
Liver homogenates [7]	Relatively good; commercially available	Contains basically all hepatic enzymes	Liver architecture lost; cofactor addition necessary
Microsomes [7]	Relatively good; transplantations or commercial sources	Contains most important rate-limiting enzymes; relatively inexpensive; easy storage	Contains only phase I enzymes and UGTs; requires strictly specific substrates or antibodies for individual DMEs; cofactor addition necessary
Recombinant CYP enzymes [8]	Commercially available	Can be utilized with HTS substrates; role of individual CYPs in the metabolism can be easily studied	The effect of only one enzyme at a time can be studied
Primary hepatocytes [9, 10, 15]	Difficult to obtain; relatively healthy tissue needed; commercially available	Contains the whole complement of DMEs cellularly integrated; induction effect of an NCE can be studied; cryopreservation possible	Requires specific techniques and well established procedures; levels of many DMEs decrease rapidly during cultivation
Liver slices [11]	Difficult to obtain; fresh tissue needed.	Contains the whole complement of DMEs and cell–cell connections; induction effect of an NCE can be studied; cryopreservation possible	Requires specific techniques and well established procedures; limited viability
Immortalized Cell lines [12]	Available at request; only a few adequately characterized cell lines exist	Nonlimited source of enzymes	Expression of most DMEs is poor; genotype/phenotype instability

Sources: Adapted from Refs. 5 and 41.

rigorously compared [16–18], but it seems that the currently used enzyme systems—recombinant enzymes, human liver microsomes and/or homogenates, liver slices, and hepatocytes—all give fairly reliable results, if their inherent restrictions are taken into consideration.

21.2.3 Current Types and Components of *In Vitro* Systems

During the development of an NCE, according to the current paradigm, several types of investigations are usually carried out, the earlier the better. The enzyme sources in these studies are usually human-derived systems. A summary of the major *in vitro* methods is provided in Table 21.4. The most important objectives of these studies are the elucidation of metabolic stability of an NCE, identification of metabolites and metabolic routes, and identification of CYP forms metabolizing an NCE. The following paragraphs summarize briefly these approaches. More details are given in subsequent sections.

1. The metabolic stability of an NCE determines its future as a drug candidate. By determining the time and concentration dependence of disappearance and/or metabolite formation *in vitro* in an appropriate system, its hepatic clearance *in vivo* can be predicted [23, 24].

2. Metabolite identification, at least at the tentative level, can be developed from incubations with human liver cells and other preparations, for example, homogenates or microsomes (see Section 21.4).

TABLE 21.4 *In Vitro* Studies for the Characterization of Metabolism and Metabolic Interactions of Potential Drugs[a]

In Vitro Test	Preparations	Parameters	Extrapolations
Metabolic stability	Microsomes, homogenates, cells, slices	Disappearance of the parent molecule or appearance of (main) metabolites	Intrinsic clearance, interindividual variability
Metabolite identification	Same as above	Tentative identification of metabolites, for example, by LC-TOF-MS and LC-MS-MS	Metabolic routes, qualitative (semiquantitative, if possible) metabolic chart
Identification of metabolizing enzymes	Microsomes with inhibitors or inhibitory antibodies; recombinant individual enzymes	Assignment and relative ability of enzymes to metabolize a compound	Prediction of effects of various genetic, environmental, and pathological factors; interindividual variability
Enzyme inhibition	Microsomes, recombinant enzymes	Inhibition of model activities by a substance	Potential drug–drug interactions
Enzyme induction	Cells, slices, permanent cell lines (if available), constructs	Induction of model activities (or mRNA); receptor binding (e.g., PXR or CAR)	Induction potential of a substance

[a]For some salient background data and examples, see Refs. 15 and 19–22.

3. After characterizing the metabolic stability and metabolic routes of an NCE, the *in vivo* prediction requires clarification of the enzymes that participate in the *in vitro* biotransformation of the NCE. After determining the initial velocity conditions and enzyme kinetic parameters for identified rate-limiting pathways, some of the main tools and approaches used in enzyme assignment are CYP selective chemical inhibitors and antibodies, cDNA expressed CYPs, correlation analysis, and measures of affinities of an NCE for CYPs (by inhibition).

Numerous compounds have been characterized for their inhibitory potency against different CYPs. Many of them are selective for the desired enzyme only at relatively low concentrations. Today, there are several commercial sources for CYP-specific inhibitory antibodies. Inhibitory antibodies raised specifically against a certain CYP form are a good tool in distinguishing between CYP forms.

cDNA expressed enzymes are convenient tools when a specific activity or a selective chemical inhibitor cannot be used in metabolic studies. Recombinant enzymes are used to ascertain the role of a certain CYP in the metabolism of an NCE. Still, the biotransformation of an NCE by a single CYP does not necessarily mean its participation in the reaction *in vivo*.

For correlation analysis, a well characterized bank of human liver samples is needed. In correlation analysis, the measured CYP-specific activities are correlated against the rate of the metabolic pathway of an NCE in every individual liver sample. Correlation analysis gives information about the possible extent of the contribution of certain CYPs to the reaction under study.

4. The effect of an NCE on characteristic CYP-selective activities is studied by coincubating series of dilutions of an NCE with a specific substrate. By comparing the effects of an NCE on the CYP-specific activities to the respective effects of diagnostic inhibitors, a tentative prediction of the *in vivo* situation can be made.

21.2.4 Measuring Induction Potential *In Vitro*

Induction of xenobiotic-metabolizing enzymes is an adaptive cellular response that usually leads to enhanced metabolism and termination of the pharmacological action of drugs. A majority of the drug-metabolizing CYP enzymes are inducible, including the most important CYP3A4. Induction of human CYP enzymes is difficult to study because there are no human liver cell lines that express the full complement of CYP enzymes or reproduce the induction observed *in vivo* [25]. Thus, there is increasing interest in the development of mechanism-based test systems for CYP induction, and proof of principle has been demonstrated for the nuclear receptors CAR, PXR, and PPARα. The main *in vitro* methods used are direct and indirect binding assays as well as cell-based reporter gene protocols [26, 27].

Because these systems are based ultimately on the inducer/receptor interaction, they cannot detect inducers that require *in vivo* transformation to active species or inducers that act via an alternative mechanism. For instance, dexamethasone may increase the expression of the PXR and CAR receptors and thus induce CYP enzymes or synergize with other inducers. Even though the mechanism-based induction screens may not detect every CYP inducer, they are still expected to be valuable as preliminary screens.

21.2.5   Species Considerations

Species differences in drug-metabolizing enzymes are large and more often than not unpredictable. Ortologous enzymes can be rather closely related in terms of sequence homology and still display large quantitative and qualitative differences toward potential substrates and inhibitors. A much cited example is concerned with mouse hepatic Cyp2a4 and Cyp2a5, which differ in only 11 amino acids and still there is an almost complete reversal of substrate specificity concerning testosterone and coumarin [28]. On the other hand, metabolic reaction of a given compound may be catalyzed by enzymes belonging to different subfamilies in different species (see examples in Ref. 29). Currently, it is practically impossible to predict species differences in metabolism. Thus, it is advisable to perform some comparative studies in the preclinical phase. For example, metabolic stability studies give at least a tentative view about differences in clearance rates between different species. Metabolite identification in hepatic preparations from different species may point to important considerations when trying to extrapolate results from *in vivo* animal studies to human risk assessment. The earlier these types of comparative studies are being performed, the better their results can be taken into consideration, for example, in the selection of appropriate species for certain types of toxicity studies.

21.3   ASSIGNMENT OF METABOLIZING ENZYMES

In terms of potential clinical consequences, the assignment of metabolizing enzymes is perhaps the most important single task in *in vitro* metabolic studies. For the identification of the CYP (or basically any other) enzyme responsible for the metabolite formation, a number of different and complementary approaches are used. The indirect method utilizes specific CYP enzyme inhibitors, which are each added in turn into the incubation with the study compound in the presence of liver microsomal preparation, and the formation of the metabolite is monitored quantitatively. The decreasing metabolite formation indicates that the CYP responsible for the metabolite formation is being inhibited. Different inhibitor concentrations can be used to calculate the IC_{50} value of the inhibitor toward the metabolite formation, but often only single inhibitor concentration (high enough for good inhibition of certain CYP but low enough to keep the inhibition CYP-selective) is used. The use of CYP-specific antibodies is carried out similarly to the inhibitors. Another often used and complementary method is the use of recombinant CYP enzymes, where the involvement of a certain CYP in the metabolite formation can be directly detected as a metabolite peak in LC-MS. In addition, CYP activity phenotyped liver preparations are used to reflect the formation of the metabolites. The increasing metabolite formation paralleling the increasing activity of a certain CYP enzyme in the different liver preparations suggests also a probable involvement of that selective CYP isoform in the biotransformation.

21.3.1   Affinity (Inhibition) Studies

Inhibition of CYP enzymes is the most common cause of drug–drug interactions and has led to the removal of several drugs from the market during the past few years [30, 31]. Thus, studying the inhibitory effect of NCEs is extremely important; an inhibitory profile would also give an idea about the affinity spectrum of the compound.

The most common method is to compare metabolite formation of the known CYP-selective biotransformation in a liver microsomal incubation with and without the study compound. The probe substrate in a biotransformation reaction is chosen so that its monitored metabolite is known to be formed specifically via one certain CYP enzyme. These studies are often carried out as a cocktail-type approach using a number of different CYP-specific probe substrates (3–10) simultaneously in the one incubation, and the formed metabolites are usually analyzed with a single LC/MS-MS method developed for the simultaneous analysis of all the different metabolites (see Ref. 32). The cocktail approach is especially good for the screening of possible CYP interactions of an NCE, as the one incubation and one LC/MS run give information of all studied CYP enzymes in a time-efficient manner. If high inhibition potential toward certain CYPs in a cocktail-type screening for an NCE is detected, then the more accurate IC_{50} values can be evaluated using single-probe metabolite reactions and also using metabolite spiked standard samples for more accurate quantitation in LC/MS.

21.3.2   Enzyme-Selective Substrates, Inhibitors, and Antibodies

Selection of model drugs and reactions is an important consideration in many *in vitro* testing systems. For example, recent surveys [33, 34] give lists of CYP-selective substrates and inhibitors and some potential alternatives for situations in which preferable probes cannot be used. A validation study of several CYP substrates has also been published [35]. Without going into extensive details here, one important consideration is clinical relevance: probe substances should preferably be clinically used drugs for which relatively good and comprehensive *in vivo* data is available [36]. This would make *in vitro–in vivo* extrapolations more reliable, because these probes could then be used as comparators for molecules under study. Table 21.5 compiles currently used substrates and biotransformations as well as inhibitors, which display at least some selectivity toward specific CYP enzymes.

In the metabolizing enzyme identification studies employing diagnostic inhibitors, the approach is essentially the same as in the CYP interaction studies, but the detected analytes are the metabolites of the studied compound, and the concentration of the diagnostic inhibitor in the incubation is varied. The use of diagnostic inhibitors has become rather routine in the early screening of promising candidate drugs.

21.3.3   Recombinant Enzymes

Isolated heterogeneous human CYP enzymes, expressed as single enzymes at a time from cDNA in bacterial, yeast, and mammalian cells, have been commercially avail-

TABLE 21.5   Summary of Human Hepatic Drug-Metabolizing CYP Enzymes and Their Selected Probe Substrates and Inhibitors Used in *In Vitro* and *In Vivo* Studies

CYP	Percentage (%) in Liver[a]	Substrate	Inhibitor	Other Characteristics
1A2	~10	Ethoxyresorufin Melatonin Caffeine Phenacetin	Furafylline Fluvoxamine	Inducible Polymorphic
2A6	~8	Coumarin Nicotine	Tranylcypromine	Inducible Polymorphic
2B6	~2	Bupropion Efavirenz Cyclophosphamide	Thio-Tepa Ticlopidine	Inducible Polymorphic
2C8	~5	Paclitaxel Amodiaquine Rosiglitazone	Montelukast Quercetin	Polymorphic
2C9	~20	S-warfarin Diclophenac Tolbutamide Losartan	Sulfaphenazole	Polymorphic Inducible
2C19	~2	Omeprazole S-mephenytoin Proguanil	Fluconazole	Polymorphic Inducible
2D6	~2	Dextromethorphan Debrisoquine Bufuralol Propranololol	Quinidine Paroxetine	Polymorphic
2E1	~15	Chlorzoxazone Ethanol	Pyridine Disulfiram	Inducible
3A4	~40	Midazolam Testosterone Simvastatin Nifedipine Erythromycin	Ketoconazole Itraconazole	Inducible

[a]Relative and absolute amounts of hepatic P450 proteins vary highly among people. Rounded values are based on a meta-analysis by Rowland Yeo et al. [45].

Sources: Data adapted from Refs. 37–44.

able for several years. Recombinant CYPs have been adopted as frontline tools in early drug development. These systems can be utilized to ascertain whether an NCE is a substrate for a particular CYP form and what metabolite is generated by that specific enzyme. Moreover, recombinant enzymes can be used as small-scale bioreactors to generate usable amounts of metabolic product [46–48]. They have been used also for clearance predictions and drug–drug interaction studies [49]. It should be kept in mind, however, that recombinant expressed enzymes are not in their natural microsomal environment and consequently there is a concern about the extent of applicability of the findings.

21.3.4   Enzyme Kinetic Characterization of Principal Metabolic Reactions

It is of importance to determine enzyme kinetic characteristics of at least the principal and rate-limiting reactions of a substance for scaling up and predicting *in vivo* kinetics of an NCE. If there is only one rate-limiting reaction catalyzed by a single enzyme, this investigation is easier, but if there are several reactions and multiple enzymes, the task is obviously more difficult and the prediction may become more imprecise. The importance of enzyme kinetic characterization becomes apparent in the extrapolation process: the first step in the scheme is determining "enzyme efficiency or enzyme intrinsic clearance," essentially reflecting V_{max}/K_m, which is then scaled to liver unit weight.

21.4   IDENTIFICATION AND QUANTIFICATION OF METABOLITES

Analytical tools are at the heart of metabolic studies during early drug development. Metabolism studies start with analyses of the parent compound in simple metabolic stability studies, in which the substrate loss is being determined, and continue to more complex structural analyses on the identification of major and minor metabolites produced by the catalysis of oxidative and conjugative enzymes, and ending with development of routine analytical methods for the identification of the respective enzymes and also addressing other drug interaction-related metabolism studies.

Although the measurement of the disappearance of an NCE in human liver preparations (i.e., "metabolic stability") sounds rather simple, it is actually a rather complicated undertaking, including the development of an assay for the parent compound, and contains a lot of caveats, starting with chemical stability and binding problems. However, if this assay is expanded with the identification of metabolites produced, it gives very useful information for drug development and for planning of subsequent experiments. With current mass spectrometry (MS) techniques and the use of liver preparations, microsomes, the S9 supernatant, or homogenate, fortified with all appropriate cofactors, a tentative understanding of metabolites and metabolic routes can be obtained. On this basis, educated guesses about the involvement of potential metabolizing enzymes can also be made. Current analytical repertoire makes it relatively easy to devise appropriate routine assays for measuring metabolism of a compound. Naturally, it depends on the results of the identification of principal metabolites for a compound, but if a compound is metabolized, a routine method has to be developed for the identification of metabolizing enzymes.

21.4.1   First Incubations—Tentative Identification of Metabolites

The approach used for elucidating the *in vitro* biotransformation of an NCE is dependent on the needed specificity of the data to be obtained [50]. For an NCE with no known metabolites or any information about metabolic behavior, the easiest and time-efficient way to identify the *in vitro* metabolites is to produce all oxidative and conjugative metabolites with a single incubation with cultured hepatocytes or liver homogenates that include all CYP enzymes, as well as the principal conjugative enzymes, at least UGT, SULT, GST, and NAT (Table 21.2). After incubating the drug substance with cultured hepatocytes or in liver homogenate together with the cofactors NADPH, UDPGA, GSH, and PAPS, needed for function of the enzymes, the metabolites formed are identified usually by liquid chromatography–mass spectrometry (LC/MS) techniques [51–53]. If some more specific information concerning the metabolism is needed, other types of liver preparations can be utilized, and the number of added cofactors can be varied. For example, if only phase I oxidative reactions need to be studied, liver microsomal fraction is used instead of the homogenate, as it contains all the oxidative CYP enzymes but lacks the GST and SULT enzymes. However, glucuronide conjugation may also occur with microsomal fraction, if cofactor UDPGA is used in incubation (for more detailed description, see Sections 21.1 and 21.2).

After the metabolite peak has been found from the chromatographic (LC/MS) data, the biotransformation can be identified according to the mass spectrum obtained for the metabolite. With modern LC/MS instruments equipped with atmospheric pressure ion sources, most commonly electrospray (ESI) [52, 53], usually only molecular ions are detected in the spectrum. This enables the elucidation of the shift in the molecular weight during the biotransformation from the substrate to metabolite. Some common shifts in molecular weights caused by metabolic reactions are given in the Table 21.6. Depending on the MS instrument type used, fragment ion MS data can also be obtained from the metabolite, enabling the elucidation of the biotransformation site in the substrate. With mass spectrometers capable of high resolution and good mass accuracy, accurate mass data from the metabolites

TABLE 21.6   Changes in Molecular Mass Due to the Most Common Metabolic Reactions

Biotransformation	Mass Change (u)	Charasteristic Fragmentation[a] (NL = Neutral Loss)
Dehydrogenation (oxidation)	−2	
Demethylation	−14	
Desethylation	−28	
Oxidative desulfuration	−32	
Hydrogenation (reduction)	+2	
Methylation	+14	
Hydroxylation	+16	
N/S-oxidation	+16	
Epoxidation	+16	
Acetylation	+42	
Sulfation	+80	−80 u (NL of SO_3)
Glucuronidation	+176	−176 u (NL of $C_6H_8O_6$)
Glutathionation	+305[b]	−129 u (NL of $C_5H_7NO_3$)
		−275 u (NL of $C_{10}H_{17}N_3O_6$, aryl-GSH)
Amino acid conjugation		
Glycine	+57	m/z 76 (Gly + H⁺), m/z 74 (Gly − H⁺)
Taurine	+107	m/z 126 (Tau + H⁺), m/z 124 (Tau − H⁺)

[a]The fragments of phase I metabolites are typically the same as for the substrate, or differ equally from the molecular weight.
[b]The glutathionation may lead to a number of different molecular mass changes; the addition of 305 u is the most simple case where glutathione replaces hydrogen atom in the substrate.

can be obtained, enabling differentiation in the biotransformation with a different molecular formula but the same nominal mass change, for example, distinquishing simultaneous demethylation and hydroxylation from hydrogenation, even though both reactions lead to an increase in molecular weight of two mass units. Additional H/D exchange studies can be conducted to distinguish different types of oxidations, for example, hydroxylation versus N-oxidation, giving the same mass shift but completely different biotransformation [54].

21.4.2 Absolute Structures—Reference Metabolites and NMR Studies

In some cases the data obtained by LC/MS methods as above does not give a clear enough picture about the structure of the formed metabolite, or the obtained tentative structure of the metabolite has to be elucidated in a more detailed manner. In these cases, the most simple and unambiguous approach is to synthesize the possible structures obtained for the metabolite (after LC/MS), and the LC/MS behavior of the synthesized compounds is compared with the unknown metabolite to confirm/ exclude the elucidated structure. This of course may take more time for the chemists to synthesize the desired structure(s). To reliably conclude that the synthesized compound and the metabolite have the exact same structure, more than one single chromatographic method (different columns, different eluent pH) should be used to verify the similar LC/MS behavior.

An alternative possibility is to isolate and purify the metabolite from the incubation matrix, and to elucidate the exact structure using nuclear magnetic resonance (NMR) methods [55, 56]. However, the sensitivity of the NMR is not even close to the level of mass spectrometric methods, and about 100 nanograms of sample has to be obtained from purification to be able to acquire definitive NMR data in sensible time (i.e., overnight), and orders of magnitude more for more insensitive two-dimensional NMR experiments. Fortunately, in many cases, the most sensitive simple NMR measurement (i.e., basic one-dimensional ^{1}H NMR) may already help in confirmation of the structure. Also online coupled LC/NMR instruments [57] are now available to avoid the purification step, but the chromatographic separation in these systems always suffers in comparison to more easily coupled LC/MS techniques.

21.4.3 Quantitative Studies

Besides the qualitative LC/MS studies in metabolite identification, quantitative data is also needed from a number of different studies with *in vitro* liver preparations. Among these, the most typical are the P450 enzyme interaction studies, direct drug–drug interaction studies, metabolizing CYP enzyme identification studies, and the estimation of metabolic stability (already mentioned). To save time, these analyses are often carried out semiquantitatively, that is, without spiked standard samples, and the results are reported as relative LC/MS peak areas of each detected compound in different samples, and these areas are expressed in percentages by comparing them to reference incubation samples (e.g., without an inhibitor or zero time incubation). In this stage of drug development, this sort of approach usually gives the accuracy needed, as the main purpose is to see if there are interactions or not, or to evaluate the general level of metabolic stability. Also, in this phase the metabolites themselves are usually not available to be used as external standards for quantitation (for creating a calibration curve), and so if any spiked standard samples are used, the metabolites are quantified as "substrate equivalents." This in turn may sometimes lead to large differences between the results obtained and the real metabolite concentrations, as the mass spectrometric response between the drug and its metabolite may vary a lot due to different ionization and fragmentation properties, especially if the biotransformation occurs in the same functional group of the compound where the ionization occurs in the ionization process of the LC/MS analysis.

The main issue in the analyses of early drug development is to have good specificity, to be sure to monitor the correct compound (metabolite), and to have good linearity of detection response, so that the relative peak areas, obtained without calibration curves created by spiked standard samples, are representative of the concentration differences in different samples. When the need for high sensitivity is added to the list of requirements, the usual analytical system of choice is LC/MS-MS with triple quadrupole mass spectrometers.

21.4.4 Requirements for Analytical Instrumentation

Although the range of modern analytical instrumentation commercially available for metabolism studies is very large, today's metabolism studies are carried out using high performance liquid chromatography coupled online with mass spectrometry (LC/MS), and additionally some other detector types, such as UV-diode array (DAD, PDA), fluorescence, or radioactive detectors, are used. The additional detectors are solely used for "detecting purposes"—not for identification of the compound but for its quantitation or detection if the mass spectrometric response of the analyte is poor. The fluorescence detector can be used as a very sensitive detector for certain types of fluorescing compounds if suitable excitation and emission wavelengths are chosen, and the radioactive detector can be used for screening and quantification of the metabolites of the radiolabeled substrate. However, these are rarely needed in *in vitro* studies; the LC/MS instruments can give many types of data from a single run, including detection and identification of the metabolites, and at least semiquantitative concentration estimates.

Generally, any kind of mass spectrometer with HPLC compatible ion source can be used in metabolite idenfication and quantitation, but unfortunately, none of the mass spectrometer types is the optimal instrument for all kinds of studies (qualitative vs. quantitative), and thus at least two different types of instrument are required if all the studies are to be conducted at a state-of-the-art level. The strengths and drawbacks of the most common types of mass spectrometer studies are given in Table 21.7. The table includes only the time-of-flight/QTOF [58, 59], ion trap [60, 61], and triple quadrupole [62, 63] type instruments, but recently a number of hybrid instruments containing features from many instrument types have been introduced by manufacturers. Of these new instrument types, most useful in the analysis of small drug-like molecules are the triple quadrupole/linear ion trap instrument, where the last quadrupole of a traditional triple quadrupole instrument is replaced by a linear ion trap to increase the full scan sensitivity [64], and the ion-trap-TOF instrument, where the collision cell of QTOF is replaced by an ion trap to enable MS^n

TABLE 21.7 Applicability of the Most Common Type Mass Spectrometers for *In Vitro* Drug Metabolism Studies (in LC/MS)

Parameters	Time-of-Flight (TOF-MS)	Ion Trap (IT-MS)	Triple Quadrupole (QQQ-MS)	Quadrupole-TOF (QTOF-MS)
Strengths	• High full scan sensitivity • High resolution for exact mass measurement • Very fast data acquisition (for HTS) • Easy to operate	• High full scan sensitivity • CID MS/MS and even MS^3 possibility	• Very high sensitivity for known analytes (MRM) • High linear range • High quality CID MS/MS, also with precursor ion and neutral loss scanning • Very fast data acquisition (in MRM mode)	• High full scan sensitivity • High resolution for exact mass measurement • Very fast data acquisition (for HTS) • CID MS/MS
Drawbacks	• Poor linear range • No real MS/MS possibility (only "in-source" MS/MS)	• Poor linear range • No exact mass possibility • No precursor ion or neutral loss scanning MS/MS • Slow scanning speed	• No exact mass possibility • Poor full scan sensitivity (for screening)	• Poor linear range • No precursor ion or neutral loss scanning MS/MS
Optimal use	Excellent for metabolite screening and identification of biotransformations	For metabolite screening and their tentative identifications; identification of biotransformation site	Excellent for quantitative analysis of known analytes; identification of biotransformation site; HTS applications	For metabolite screening; identification of biotransformations and their sites; HTS applications
Price	200,000–300,000 €	100,000–160,000 €	160,000–300,000 €	350,000–600,000 €

experiments with high resolution for fragment ions [65]. For higher mass resolution studies, mostly needed when working with biomolecules, the Orbitrap [66] and ion cyclotron resonance [67] mass spectrometers offer superior performance.

The basic rule of thumb is that the time-of-flight mass spectrometers are the instruments of choice for a screening type of analysis (biotransformation screening and tentative metabolite identification), whereas the triple quadrupole instruments are superior in quantitative work. For metabolite screening the instrument needed should have good sensitivity with wide scan range to detect all unexpected metabolites simultaneously; also, it should be able to give qualitative data for at least tentative identification of the metabolites. The time-of-flight instruments have all this, the qualitative data coming from easy operation, accurate mass measurements, and in-source fragment ion data.

21.5   ACTIVE/REACTIVE/TOXIC METABOLITES

It would be very useful to know whether metabolism is needed for the biological action (pharmacologic or toxicologic) of drugs. Metabolic activation, which may be pharmacologically useful (prodrug metabolism) or toxicologically adverse, is an established primary mechanism of action for many drugs and toxicants [68–71]. Especially during early drug development, a screening system able to detect the formation of reactive drug metabolites would provide crucial information for the development program. In toxicity risk assessment, a robust and validated screening system is urgently needed, because metabolism is often needed for tissue toxicity, immunotoxicity, genotoxicity, and/or carcinogenicity to be initiated. In Table 21.8,

TABLE 21.8   Potential *In Vitro* Screening Systems for Detecting the Formation of Reactive Metabolites

Type of Assay	Rationale	Example
Inhibition of drug metabolism	"Suicide" binding of a reactive metabolite with the enzyme	Tienilic acid
Formation of GSH conjugate	Binding of a reactive metabolite with GSH	Paracetamol
Covalent binding	Detection of bound reactive metabolite by radioactivity or by MS	Many carcinogens and mutagens
Lipid peroxidation	Detection of reactive oxygen species and/or peroxides by thiobarbituric acid reagent	Many halogenated substances
Target cell toxicity	Toxicity, for example, cell viability of metabolites produced either in the target cell itself or exogenously	Practically all substances are ultimately toxic to cells at high enough concentrations; mediation of toxicity by metabolism has to be incorporated into the test

several potential screening systems are summarized. Generally, the generation of short-lived reactive metabolites is relatively straightforward to observe in various *in vitro* systems, although, it has to be stressed, none of them are adequately validated [72]. Because reactive metabolites are usually short-lived and unstable, they cannot usually be detected as such, but only after binding to trapping agents, cellular macromolecules, or other cell components. However, it is difficult to predict whether the formation of metabolites capable of binding with trapping agents or macromolecules will ultimately result in serious toxicity *in vivo* [73].

During early drug development, assays for mechanism-based inhibition are perhaps more widely used than other assays for detecting reactive metabolites. Mechanism-based inhibition can occur via the formation of metabolite intermediate complexes or via the strong covalent binding of reactive intermediates to the protein or heme of the CYP. Mechanism-based inhibition is terminated by enzyme resynthesis and is therefore usually long-lasting [74, 75]. In some cases, the metabolic product inactivates the enzyme completely. This is referred to as suicide inhibition. The most important phenomenon of mechanism-based inhibition is the time-, concentration-, and NADPH-dependent enzyme inactivation [2, 74]. Classical mechanism-based inhibitors include furafylline (CYP1A2) [76, 77] and gestodene (CYP3A4) [78]. It is worth noting that many compounds display both mechanism-based and competitive modes of inhibition; one such example is ticlopidine [79].

Although the need to detect and identify reactive metabolites is widely recognized for drug development, there are large gaps in our knowledge and also uncertainties about which kinds of strategies to employ. Detecting reactive metabolites does not necessarily mean that tissue toxicity or immunotoxicity will ensue. Metabolic activation seems to be behind many immunotoxic manifestations, but unequivocal evidence has been difficult to produce [80, 81]. One of the more important problems has been the selectivity of binding of reactive intermediates. Previously, it was thought that binding of reactive metabolites with cellular macromolecules is essentially a nonselective process. Now it has become more and more apparent that the process is primarily a selective process and even slightly different reactive species display large differences in their binding targets [82]. Development of screening methods that would differentiate toxicologically significant reactive metabolites from inactive ones would be a significant advance. Interesting analyses for future developments in research on metabolic activation from the industrial perspective are provided by Evans et al. [83] and Baillie [73].

21.6   TESTING CONFIGURATIONS

With the advent of combinatorial chemistry and large libraries of chemicals, a need for high throughput screening (HTS) has become ever more pressing in the pharmaceutical industry. Most major drug companies make use of various HTS configurations for efficient screening. Regarding the metabolic properties of NCEs, screenings of metabolic stability and drug–drug interactions have advanced to a considerable extent [22]. Often, rather sophisticated detection systems based on fluorescence are used in HTS systems. In the following, MS detection techniques are described.

21.6.1   Sample Preparation

Because of relatively defined incubation conditions with liver preparations or hepatocytes, sample preparation for LC/MS can usually be kept very simple. Usually the
simple centrifugation of the incubation sample and careful pipetting of the supernatant into an HPLC autosampler vial is enough for an LC/MS compatible sample.
However, when performing quantitative analyses, even for relative peak areas
without external standards, the use of an internal standard is preferable. If long
sample lists are acquired (e.g., overnight from an autosampler), the high buffer and
salt concentrations together with other biomolecules or high concentration incubation media components may contaminate the mass spectrometer ion source, leading
to general decrease in the sensitivity level toward the end of the sample list. By
using an internal standard in the samples and using the relative peak area between
the analyte and the internal standard as a result, instead of a plain analyte peak
area, the effect of ion source contamination on the results can be avoided (as long
as the sensitivity level stays acceptable).

21.6.2   Single Enzyme/Activity Systems

Many *in vitro* metabolism studies—such as interaction studies with CYP-selective
inhibitors and antibodies, inhibition screens using studied NCEs with CYP-selective
substrates, and studies with recombinant enzymes—are relatively routine and robust
from the biochemical and analytical point of view, and there is a wide literature
background for using these tools in various *in vitro* settings. Detailed descriptions
of the methodological aspects of the more widely used CYP-selective substrates and
inhibitors can be found in recent articles [35] (see also Table 21.5).

21.6.3   Medium to High Throughput Systems

Thorough surveys of medium to high throughput systems for *in vitro* absorption,
distribution, metabolism, and excretion (ADME) have recently been published [84,
85]. When identifying the metabolizing or interacting CYP enzymes for larger
numbers of compounds, the use of recombinant CYP enzymes and diagnostic CYP
inhibitors are both suitable for HTS mode. With diagnostic CYP inhibitors, only one
inhibitor concentration is used, low enough to be specific for inhibition of the target
CYP but high enough for adequate inhibition if the study compound is metabolized
via the same CYP. In the HTS approach the LC/MS analysis time is a crucial factor,
and therefore very specific analytical methods for detecting only the monitored
metabolites in a very short time are needed. The study compounds may also be
incubated as mixtures of compounds, and the LC/MS method is adjusted to detect
all the desired metabolites from each compound in a single analysis, again increasing
the analytical challenge. However, the possible interaction with the simultaneously
incubated compounds may affect the results obtained; especially with recombinant
enzymes, the formation of monitored metabolite is a sign of the involvement of the
certain CYP enzyme in the metabolite formation.

   For fast screening of P450 inhibition, it is possible to employ a cocktail-type
analysis of known CYP-selective biotransformations in liver microsomal incubations. A number of assays for different CYP enzymes have been developed and

published [22]. The most simple cocktails contain only a few important CYP iso-forms, whereas the most complete assays contain all nine of the most important CYPs and also more than one probe reaction for some isoforms [32]. If a HTS for a large number of study compounds is needed, usually only one concentration per compound is needed to give a rough estimate of the level of interaction with each CYP. However, the development and use of the cocktail approach is much more challenging than the use of single-substrate incubations, as the substrate concentrations have to be optimized so as not to cause any interactions between each other; also the reliable LC/MS analysis of many chemically different metabolites with a single run is quite challenging. If very high throughput is needed, the studied compounds may be delivered into the incubations as cocktails of several compounds, and the go or no-go decision is then given to all of the compounds tested together. However, this approach contains a risk of losing good lead candidates, as only one potent inhibitor in the mixture of simultaneously tested compounds may lead to wasting the other, noninhibiting, compounds.

21.6.4   Analytical Considerations

From the analytical point of view, the issues covered in Section 21.4 are all valid here as well. The quantitative analyses in these studies are usually carried out as relative LC/MS peak areas, without any spiked calibration standard samples. The excellent linear range and specificity of triple quadrupole mass spectrometers makes them the best choice for LC/MS instrumentation, enabling very sensitive detection of the low metabolite concentrations. Also, when detecting metabolites from several compounds incubated simultaneously in the same well/vessel, the triple quadrupole instruments provide the most specific detection for each analyte. Even structural analogues with the same molecular weight and the same retention times can still be separated, as long as the compounds have different fragmentation pathways in the collision-induced dissociation. However, with HTS applications and constantly changing analytes, the time-of-flight mass spectrometers (or ion trap instruments) may offer a good alternative for instrumentation, as the excellent sensitivity for acquiring data over a high mass range enables the detection of all different analytes, without the need to adjust the detection parameters before the analysis, as is the case with triple quadrupole instruments. Therefore, with LC/TOF-MS and LC/QTOF-MS, the same generic method may be used for a large set of completely different compounds in HTS applications [86]. With QTOF, the MS/MS option in data acquisition is available. However, if the application is for P450 inhibition screening, where detected compounds remain the same all the time, the triple quadrupole mass spectrometer is the best possible instrument for the analysis.

When the aim in analyses is to produce as much data as possible from a single LC/MS run, many software packages can control the data acquisition with so-called data-dependent operations [87], which may be particularly useful with MS/MS instruments, as the detection of high abundance ions with the certain m/z in the spectrum of a high abundance ion may trigger some other type of data acquisition using this ion as a precursor mass—such as product ion scanning and selected reaction monitoring. This way, both qualitative and quantitative data can be acquired simultaneously. If the molecular weights of the studied metabolites are known before analysis, the same acquisition functions can of course be set manually, which usually provides better quality data.

21.7 PRIORITIES OF *IN VITRO* METABOLISM STUDIES AND *IN VITRO–IN VIVO* EXTRAPOLATION

One of the important questions concerning the starter *in vitro* test of metabolism is: Which one is best as a first test? Because each molecule is rather unique in terms of metabolism and kinetics, we would need a rather comprehensive test, which should cover as many salient features of a compound as possible. But this requirement is contradictory to simplicity, rapidity, and economy, which are needed for early testing.

There is no fixed single strategy for performing metabolic studies during early drug development. Rather, major drug companies employ their own slightly variable schemes. Table 21.9 presents one possible strategy of metabolism studies in early drug development, which is described below. Whatever strategy is adopted, assessment of metabolic stability is very important to perform early on in the drug development program, because it determines, despite many caveats inherent in current testing systems, to a large extent the usefulness of the molecule and gives an important value for *in vitro–in vivo* extrapolation.

21.7.1 Priorities of *In Vitro* Metabolism Studies

Determination of basic physicochemical properties is the prerequisite for every subsequent property determination. When developing adequate analytical methods for NCEs, it is important to know solubility, pK_a, lipophilicity, and also chemical

TABLE 21.9 Example of a Rough Priority Scheme for *In Vitro* Studies Related to Metabolic Properties of an NCE

Properties of an NCE	Remarks
Solubility, lipophilicity, pK_a, chemical stability, possible inpurities, plasma protein binding (free fraction)	These data are absolutely required before metabolism studies to prevent unpleasant surprises; free fraction (plasma protein binding) needed for proper extrapolation
Metabolic stability in microsomes/homogenates or hepatocytes	A crucial piece of information for the extrapolation of hepatic clearance
Metabolite identification in microsomes, homogenates, or hepatocytes	Human hepatocytes are an enzyme source of choice if available
Inhibitory interactions in human liver microsomes	Also help pinpoint enzymes with affinity toward the studied compound
Identification of metabolizing CYPs	Primarily employed: diagnostic inhibitors, recombinant enzymes, correlation analysis (if a liver bank is available)
Induction of drug metabolism	Preferably in human hepatocytes if available
Metabolic stability and identification of metabolites in animal liver preparations	To search for appropriate species for certain toxicity studies

stability. A cost-effective approach is to integrate method development, simple degradation study, and physicochemical property characterization together with plasma protein binding and nonspecific binding. It is feasible to start *in vitro* metabolism and permeation studies after the physicochemical, degradation, and binding properties of an NCE are already known. It is easier to incubate, to analyze, and most importantly to predict the *in vivo* situation, if possible interfering problems are dealt with before starting the metabolism experiments.

Metabolism data using human liver preparations are irreplaceable if the drug candidates are intended for human use. Since a rat is not human, it is not feasible to start metabolism studies with rat or any other animal liver preparations; their time is later, when animal models for toxicological studies are selected. A good practice is to start metabolism studies with human and several obvious animal models, but resources might be wasted if the compound is rejected. The first human *in vitro* metabolism studies should be conducted with a system involving all the possible drug-metabolizing enzymes and cofactors for the enzymes. High initial concentrations of parent compound should be used and all the possible (predicted and unpredicted, major and minor) metabolites should be identified. Special attention needs to be addressed to those metabolites potentially associated with toxicity, such as acyl glucuronides, epoxides, glutathione pathway metabolites, and hydroxyl amines, because their presence indicates a need for lead optimization. This primary metabolism screen for tentative metabolic stability and metabolite identification could best be conducted with a LC-TOF-MS or LC-QTOF-MS instrument. The preferred liver preparation would be human liver homogenate (pool of several individuals) due to its relatively easy access compared to hepatocytes. A permanent hepatocyte-like cell line would be highly desirable, but no such cell line has yet been found or developed.

For the compounds that survive the primary metabolism screen, several second tier studies are needed. First, kinetic metabolic stability and metabolite formation studies are needed for proper *in vivo* prediction. This is usually done in human liver microsomes, unless the metabolites found in the primary screen indicate homogenate, S9, or cytosol has to be used, with several time points, concentrations, and replicates. Second, rate-limiting CYP enzymes, or other enzymes if indicated by primary screen, should be identified to assess potential drug–drug interactions and also kinetic aspects. Human liver microsomal incubations of an NCE together with CYP-specific inhibitors or antibodies give a clear indication of which CYP enzymes are involved. If the picture is completed by incubations with recombinant CYP enzymes and both tests point to the same CYP enzyme, an involvement of a certain CYP enzyme in a particular biotransformation can be relatively reliably confirmed. Third, a microsomal study to be conducted at this stage is CYP enzyme inhibition screen. A simple cocktail approach with one concentration of NCE aiming at "% activity inhibited" will usually do the trick. If something risky is observed, more thorough investigations including mechanistic studies should be done.

In the third round and for the molecules that remain, one should study CYP induction in human hepatocytes. Once the hepatocytes are employed, it will be cost efficient to study the other metabolic properties on hepatocytes also: confirmation of the previous investigations in microsomes/homogenates/S9. Thus, one should again study metabolic stability, metabolite identification, CYP inhibition and induction, and metabolizing CYP enzymes. A good add-on would be a study of accumulation of the parent and metabolites in hepatocyte cells, because this information may be crucial for the interpretation of *in vitro–in vivo* extrapolation.

Finally, the rat (or mouse or dog or monkey) becomes relevant. If the candidate drug passes the *in vitro* tests with human preparations, a multispecies metabolism study would be appropriate to find out the most relevant species for toxicological investigations. Special attention should be given to the metabolites formed—not metabolic stability—as every relevant human metabolite should be found from the toxicological species.

21.7.2 *In Vitro–In Vivo* Extrapolation

Metabolic clearance (intrinsic clearance, CL_{int}) is an important determinant for extrapolation purposes. CL_{int} is a direct measure of the efficacy of an enzyme to metabolize a substrate. Knowing that the drug concentrations in *in vivo* situations are usually far below their K_m values (i.e., under linear velocity conditions), CL_{int} is equal to the ratio of V_{max}/K_m [88, 89]. When the contribution of multiple enzymes to the metabolism is assumed, the net *in vitro* CL_{int} in the whole study system can be expressed as the sum of each metabolic pathway [89, 90].

Several elements limit the reliability of predicting CL_{int} on the basis of *in vitro* studies. The most important factor to be taken into account is the nonspecific binding of the substrate to the microsomal protein fraction. Generally, for drugs with high protein binding affinity, underestimations with CL_{int} can occur if protein binding is taken into account. However, inclusion of both microsomal and plasma protein binding usually results in good agreement between extrapolated and actual clearance values [91, 92].

Altered hepatic blood flow may have an impact on the accuracy of the *in vitro–in vivo* extrapolation. On the basis of their hepatic clearances, drugs can be classified either as low clearance or high clearance compounds. In the first case, the hepatic blood flow has a minor effect on the total clearance of the drug (enzyme-limited clearance), whereas in the latter case, changes in the hepatic blood flow will have a drastic effect on the total clearance of the drug (flow-limited clearance). However, the clinical outcome is hard to predict, as conditions affecting portal blood flow usually involve concurrent complications [2, 93].

In general, *in vitro–in vivo* extrapolations are performed with two objectives in mind: prediction of the intrinsic clearance (CL_{int}) of an NCE and prediction of potential drug–drug interactions. Other pharmacokinetic parameters, such as plasma half-life, volume of distribution, and oral bioavailability, have also to be considered for the estimation of *in vivo* kinetics on the basis of *in vitro* studies. Many *in vivo* factors affect the results of extrapolation. One of these is the binding to plasma and tissue proteins and, ultimately, the distribution volume of the drug. Details of various models and equations can be found in recent reviews [94, 95].

21.8 VALIDATION OF *IN VITRO* SYSTEMS

The main purpose of *in vitro* tests used in preclinical departments of drug companies is to aid drug development, not registration. Naturally, companies are interested in the precision and accuracy of *in vitro* tests, but there is no requirement of formal validation. Consequently, validation is done primarily in-house. If the results of the tests are being used in regulatory applications, then a certain amount of validation—even if not formal—is required. FDA, EMEA, and authorities in Japan have all published some guidelines under which circumstances of *in vitro* drug interaction results can be used to support marketing authorization. The current view is that prediction of drug–drug interactions on the basis of *in vitro* studies is most advanced from the validation and reliability points of view [1, 96–98].

In vitro systems are generally useful in identifying compounds with severe potential liabilities, such as metabolic instability, very high affinity to a principal metabolizing enzyme, or metabolism by a polymorphic enzyme (e.g., CYP2D6). Whether false positives in these respects are rare or common, is not known. Also, the frequency of false negatives is not known. Discussions with company scientists about their unpublished data have led to a view that the predictive power of various *in vitro* tests tends to weaken when the number and structural variability of tested substances increase. There is no consensus about what is the acceptable frequency of false positives or negatives, or more precisely, what are the acceptable tolerances for findings. The only remedy for these uncertainties is validation according to the established principles [99].

21.9 CONCLUSION

Metabolism is a major determinant governing both pharmacokinetics and clinical response of the majority of drugs and a great deal of effort is now directed at assessing key metabolic parameters in the early stages of drug development. Several *in vitro* methods are now available for determination of metabolic features, often yielding data that reasonably well predict *in vivo* behavior of the studied drug molecules [1]. Further development and refining of these methods will provide us with methods having increased precision and robustness, allowing for highly reliable analysis and prediction of metabolic features. In addition, analogous methodology will be employed on predicting absorption, organ uptake, and efflux mediated by various transporter systems, plasma protein binding, and cellular determinants of intrinsic clearance. As an outcome of this development, we are already witnessing a diminishing number of drug candidates being withdrawn from clinical studies (or the market) due to major kinetic problems, such as strong metabolism induction or interaction potential.

An important consideration concerns the integration of results from various *in vitro* tests. Pharmacokinetics is actually an integrated whole, and different pieces are valuable only in the context of the whole. Development of modeling and simulation tools, for example, physiologically based pharmacokinetic models, will aid in incorporation of the results from *in vitro* studies into realistic models and in understanding genetic, physiological, and pathological factors affecting the behavior of an NCE when a substance is administered for the first time to a human being. Although much has already been done, there is still a need for reliable and robust pharmacokinetic models that would incorporate various factors and processes affecting the fate of a molecule. With the help of these *in silico* models, information from *in vitro* tests becomes continuously integrated into the database.

The use of human-derived biological systems seems rather natural, because we are interested primarily in human metabolism and kinetics. Human hepatocyte assay is regarded as the gold standard for metabolic screening, but there are several problems in this approach. There is an urgent need to develop a renewable, immortal hepatocyte-like permanent cellular model, which would express all the necessary enzymes and transporters at the level resembling *in vivo* hepatocyte. One promising candidate is a recently developed hepatic cell line, HepaRG, which expressed most enzymes and transporters at a relatively high level [100, 101].

An important drawback, at least in some academic laboratories that work to develop *in vitro* techniques to measure drug metabolism, is the absolute necessity of expensive mass spectrometric techniques for analytical work. However, we feel that rational and productive research on *in vitro* drug metabolism tests is not possible without up-to-date analytical techniques. Analytical chemistry is at the heart of early drug development.

REFERENCES

1. Pelkonen O, Raunio H. *In vitro* screening of drug metabolism during drug development: Can we trust the predictions? *Expert Opin Drug Metab Toxicol* 2005;1:49–60.
2. Lin JH, Lu AYH. Role of pharmacokinetics and metabolism in drug discovery and development. *Pharmacol Rev* 1997;49:403–449.
3. Van de Waterbeemd H, Gifford E. ADMET *in silico* modelling: towards prediction paradise? *Nat Rev Drug Dev* 2003;2:192–203.
4. Guengerich FP, Rendic S. Human cytochrome P450 enzymes (human CYPs): human cytochrome P450 enzymes, a status report summarizing their reactions, substrates, inducers, and inhibitors—1st update. *Drug Metab Rev* 2002;34:1–450.
5. Coecke S, Ahr H, Blaauboer BJ, Bremer S, Casati S, Castell J, Combes R, Corvi R, Crespi CL, Cunningham ML, Elaut G, Eletti B, Freidig A, Gennari A, Ghersi-Egea JF, Guillouzo A, Hartung T, Hoet P, Ingelman-Sundberg M, Munn S, Janssens W, Ladstetter B, Leahy D, Long A, Meneguz A, Monshouwer M, Morath S, Nagelkerke F, Pelkonen O, Ponti J, Prieto P, Richert L, Sabbioni E, Schaack B, Steiling W, Testai E, Vericat JA, Worth A. Metabolism: a bottleneck in *in vitro* toxicological test development. The Report and Recommendations of ECVAM Workshop 54. *Altern Lab Anim* 2006;34:49–84.
6. Pelkonen O, Baumann A, Reichel A. *Pharmacokinetic Challenges in Drug Discovery*. Ernst Schering Research Foundation Workshop 37. Berlin: Springer; 2002.
7. Kremers P. Liver microsomes: a convenient tool for metabolism studies but.... In Boobis AR, Kremers P, Pelkonen O, Pithan K, Eds. *European Symposium on the Prediction of Drug Metabolism in Man: Progress and Problems*. Office for Official Publications of the European Communities; 1999, pp 38–52.
8. Rodrigues AD. Integrated cytochrome P450 reaction phenotyping: attempting to bridge the gap between cDNA-expressed cytochromes P450 and native human liver microsomes. *Biochem Pharmacol* 1999;57:465–480.
9. Guillouzo A. Acquisition and use of human *in vitro* liver preparations. *Cell Biol Toxicol* 1995;11:141–145.
10. Guillouzo A, Morel F, Fardel O, Meunier B. Use of human hepatocyte cultures for drug metabolism studies. *Toxicology* 1993;82:209–219.

11. Ferrero JL, Brendel K. Liver slices as a model in drug metabolism. *Adv Pharmacol* 1997;43:131–169.

12. Allen DD, Caviedes R, Cardenas AM, Shimahara T, Segura-Aguilar J, Caviedes PA. Cell lines as *in vitro* models for drug screening and toxicity studies. *Drug Dev Ind Pharm* 2005;31:757–768.

13. Brandon EFA, Raap CD, Meijerman I, Beijnen JH, Schellens JHM. An update on *in vitro* test methods in human hepatic drug biotransformation research: pros and cons. *Toxicol Appl Pharmacol* 2003;189:233–246.

14. Plant N. Strategies for using *in vitro* screens in drug metabolism. *DDT* 2004;9:328–336.

15. Gomez-Lechon MJ, Donato MT, Castell JV, Jover R. Human hepatocytes in primary culture: the choice to investigate drug metabolism in man. *Curr Drug Metab* 2004;5:443–462.

16. Andersson TB, Sjöberg H, Hoffmann K-J, Boobis AR, Watts P, Edwards RJ, Lake BG, Price RJ, Renwick AB, Gómez-Lechón MJ, Castell JV, Ingelman-Sundberg M, Hidestrand M, Goldfarb PS, Lewis DFV, Corcos L, Guillouzo A, Taavitsainen P, Pelkonen O. An assessment of human liver-derived *in vitro* systems to predict the *in vivo* metabolism and clearance of almokalant. *Drug Metab Dispos* 2001;29:712–720.

17. Salonen JS, Nyman L, Boobis AR, Edwards RJ, Watts P, Lake BG, Price RJ, Renwick AB, Gómez-Lechón MJ, Castell JV, Ingelman-Sundberg M, Hidestrand M, Guillouzo A, Corcos L, Goldfarb PS, Lewis DFV, Taavitsainen P, Pelkonen O. Comparative studies on the CYP-associated metabolism and interaction potential of selegiline between human liver-derived *in vitro* systems. *Drug Metab Dispos* 2003;31:1093–1102.

18. Pelkonen O, Myllynen P, Taavitsainen P, Boobis AR, Watts P, Lake BG, Price RJ, Renwick AB, Gómez-Lechón MJ, Castell JV, Ingelman-Sundberg M, Hidestrand M, Guillouzo A, Corcos L, Goldfarb PS, Lewis DFV. Carbamazepine: a "blind" assessment of CYP-associated metabolism and interactions in human liver-derived *in vitro* systems. *Xenobiotica* 2001;31:321–343.

19. Thompson TN. Early ADME in support of drug discovery: the role of metabolic stability studies. *Curr Drug Metab* 2000;1:215–241.

20. Gebhardt R, Hengstler JG, Muller D, Glockner R, Buenning P, Laube B, Schmelzer E, Ullrich M, Utesch D, Hewitt N, Ringel M, Hilz BR, Bader A, Langsch A, Koose T, Burger HJ, Maas J, Oesch F. New hepatocyte *in vitro* systems for drug metabolism: metabolic capacity and recommendations for application in basic research and drug development, standard operation procedures. *Drug Metab Rev* 2003;35:145–213.

21. Masimirembwa CM, Bredberg U, Andersson TB. Metabolic stability for drug discovery and development: pharmacokinetic and biochemical challenges. *Clin Pharmacokinet* 2003;42:515–528.

22. Ansede JH, Thakker DR. High-throughput screening for stability and inhibitory activity of compounds toward cytochrome P450-mediated metabolism. *J Pharm Sci* 2004;93: 239–255.

23. Obach RS, Baxter JG, Liston TE, Silber BM, Jones BC, MacIntyre F, Rance DJ, Wastall P. The prediction of human pharmacokinetic parameters from preclinical and *in vitro* metabolism data. *J Pharmacol Exp Ther* 1999;283:46–58.

24. Clarke SE, Jeffrey P. Utility of metabolic stability screening: comparison of *in vitro* and *in vivo* clearance. *Xenobiotica* 2001;31:591–598.

25. Pelkonen O, Hukkanen J, Honkakoski P, Hakkola J, Viitala P, Raunio H. *In vitro* screening of cytochrome P450 induction potential. In Pelkonen O, Baumann A, Reichel A, Eds. *Pharmacokinetics Challenges in Drug Discovery*. Ernst Schering Research Foundation Workshop 37. Berlin: Springer Verlag; 2002, pp 105–137.

26. Honkakoski P, Negishi M. Regulation of cytochrome P450 (CYP) genes by nuclear receptors. *Biochem J* 2000;347:321–337.

27. Honkakoski P. Nuclear receptors CAR and PXR in metabolism and elimination of drugs. *Curr Pharmacogenomics* 2003;1:75–85.

28. Lindberg RL, Negishi M. Alteration of mouse cytochrome P450coh substrate specificity by mutation of a single amino-acid residue. *Nature* 1989;339:632–634.

29. Pelkonen O, Breimer DD. Role of environmental factors in the pharmacokinetics of drugs: considerations with respect to animal models, P-450 enzymes, and probe drugs. In Welling PG, Balant LP, Eds. *Handbook of Experimental Pharmacology*, Volume 110. Berlin: Springer-Verlag; 1994, pp 289–332.

30. Friedman MA, Woodcock J, Lumpkin MM, Shuren JE, Hass AE, Thompson LJ. The safety of newly approved medicines: do recent market removals mean there is a problem? *JAMA* 1999;281:1728–1734.

31. Lasser KE, Allen PD, Woolhandler SJ, Himmelstein DU, Wolfe SM, Bor DH. Timing of new black box warnings and withdrawals for prescription medications. *JAMA* 2002; 287:2215–2220.

32. Turpeinen M, Uusitalo J, Jalonen J, Pelkonen O. Multiple P450 substrates in a single run: rapid and comprehensive *in vitro* interaction assay. *Eur J Pharm Sci* 2005;24:123–132.

33. Tucker GT, Houston JB, Huang S-M. EUFEPS Conference Report. Optimising drug development: strategies to assess drug metabolism/transporter interaction potential—towards a consensus. *Eur J Pharm Sci* 2001;13:417–428.

34. Yuan R, Madani S, Wei X-X, Reynolds K, Huang S-M. Evaluation of cytochrome P450 probe substrates commonly used by the pharmaceutical industry to study *in vitro* drug interactions. *Drug Metab Dispos* 2002;30:1311–1319.

35. Walsky RL, Obach RS. Validated assays for human cytochrome P450 activities. *Drug Metab Dispos* 2004;32:647–660.

36. Streetman DS, Bertino JS Jr, Nafziger AN. Phenotyping of drug-metabolizing enzymes in adults: a review of *in-vivo* cytochrome P450 phenotyping probes. *Pharmacogenetics* 2000;10:187–216.

37. Bertz RJ, Granneman GR. Use of *in vitro* and *in vivo* data to estimate the likelihood of metabolic pharmacokinetic interactions. *Clin Pharmacokinet* 1997;32:210–258.

38. Kremers P. *In vitro* tests for predicting drug–drug interactions: the need for validated procedures. *Pharmacol Toxicol* 2002;91:209–217.

39. Pelkonen O, Maenpaa J, Taavitsainen P, Rautio A, Raunio H. Inhibition and induction of human cytochrome P450 (CYP) enzymes. *Xenobiotica* 1998;28:1203–1253.

40. Pelkonen O. Human CYPs: *in vivo* and clinical aspects. *Drug Metab Rev* 2000; 34:37–46.

41. Pelkonen O, Turpeinen M, Uusitalo J, Rautio A, Raunio H. Prediction of drug metabolism and interactions on the basis of *in vitro* investigations. *Basic Clin Pharmacol Toxicol* 2005;96:167–175.

42. Lewis DF. Human cytochromes P450 associated with the phase 1 metabolism of drugs and other xenobiotics: a compilation of substrates and inhibitors of the CYP1, CYP2 and CYP3 families. *Curr Med Chem* 2003;10:1955–1972.

43. Ingelman-Sundberg M. Pharmacogenetics of cytochrome *P*450 and its applications in drug therapy: the past, present and future. *Trends Pharmacol Sci* 2004;25:193–200.

44. Totah RA, Rettie AE. Cytochrome P450 2C8: substrates, inhibitors, pharmacogenetics, and clinical relevance. *Clin Pharm Ther* 2005;77:341–352.

45. Rowland Yeo K, Rostami-Hodjegan A, Tucker GT. Abundance of cytochromes P450 in human liver: a meta analysis. *Br J Clin Pharmacol* 2004;57:687–688.

46. Friedberg T, Henderson CJ, Pritchard MP, Wolf CR. *In vivo* and *in vitro* recombinant DNA technology as a powerful tool in drug development. In Woolf TF, Ed. *Handbook of Drug Metabolism*. New York: Marcel Dekker; 1999, pp 322–362.

47. Moody GC, Griffin SJ, Mather AN, McGinnity DF, Riley RJ. Fully automated analysis of activities catalysed by the major human liver cytochrome P450 (CYP) enzymes: assessment of human CYP inhibition potential. *Xenobiotica* 1999;29:53–75.

48. McGinnity DF, Riley RJ. Predicting drug pharmacokinetics in humans from *in vitro* metabolism studies. *Biochem Soc Trans* 2001;29(Pt 2):135–139.

49. Galetin A, Brown C, Hallifax D, Ito K, Houston JB. Utility of recombinant enzyme kinetics in prediction of human clearance: impact of variability, CYP3A5, and CYP2C19 on CYP3A4 probe substrates. *Drug Metab Dispos* 2004;32:1411–1420.

50. Nassar A-EF, Talaat RE. Strategies for dealing with metabolite elucidation in drug discovery and development. *DDT* 2004;9:317–327.

51. Kostiainen R, Kotiaho T, Kuuranne T, Auriola S. Liquid chromatography/atmospheric pressure ionization–mass spectrometry in drug metabolism studies. *J Mass Spectrom* 2003;38:357–372.

52. Cole MJ, Janiszewski JS, Fouda HG. Electrospray mass spectrometry in contemporary drug metabolism and pharmacokinetics. In Pramanik BN, Ganguly AK, Gross ML, Eds. *Applled Electrospray Mass Spectrometry*. New York: Marcel Dekker; 2002, pp 211–249.

53. Lee MS, Kerns EH. LC/MS applications in drug development. *Mass Spectrom Rev* 1999;18:187–279.

54. Tolonen A, Turpeinen M, Uusitalo J, Pelkonen O. A simple method for differentiation of monoisotropic drug metabolites with hydrogen–deuterium exchange LC/MS. *Eur J Pharm Sci* 2005;25:155–162.

55. Pellecchia M, Sem DS, Wutrich K. NMR in drug discovery. *Nat Rev Drug Discov* 2002;1:211–219.

56. Keifer PA. NMR spectroscopy in drug discovery: tools for combinatorial chemistry, natural products, and metabolism research. *Prog Drug Res* 2000;55:137–211.

57. Corcoral O, Spraul M. LC-NMR-MS in drug discovery. *Drug Discov Today* 2003;8:624–631.

58. Zhang N, Fountain ST, Bi H, Rossi DT. Quantification and rapid metabolite identification in drug discovery using API time-of-flight LC/MS. *Anal Chem* 2000;72:800–806.

59. Plumb RS, Stumpf CL, Granger JH, Castro-Perez J, Haselden JN, Dear GJ. Use of liquid chromatography/time-of-flight mass spectrometry and multivariate statistical analysis shows promise for the detection of drug metabolites in biological fluids. *Rapid Commun Mass Spectrom* 2003;17:2632–2638.

60. March RE, Todd JFJ, Eds. *Practical Aspects of Ion Trap Mass Spectrometry*. Boca Raton, FL: CRC Press; 1995.

61. Kantharaj E, Tuytelaars A, Proost PEA, Ongel Z, van Assouw HP, Gilissen RAHJ. Simultaneous measurement of drug metabolic stability and identification of metabolites using ion-trap mass spectrometry. *Rapid Commun Mass Spectrom* 2003;17:2661–2668.

62. Brewer E, Henion J. Atmospheric pressure ionization LC/MS/MS techniques for drug disposition studies. *J Pharm Sci* 1998;87:395–402.

63. Xu X, Veals J, Korfmacher WA. Comparison of conventional and enhanced mass resolution triple-quadrupole mass spectrometers for discovery bioanalytical applications. *Rapid Commun Mass Spectrom* 2003;17:832–837.

64. Hopfgartner G, Varesio E, Tschappat V, Grivet C, Bourgogne E, Leuthold LA. Triple quadrupole linear ion trap mass spectrometer for the analysis of small molecules and macromolecules. *J Mass Spectrom* 2004;39:845–855.

65. Collings BA, Campbell JM, Mao D, Douglas DJ. A combined linear ion trap time-of-flight system with improved performance and MS^n capabilities. *Rapid Commun Mass Spectrom* 2001;15:1777–1795.

66. Hu Q, Noll RJ, Li H, Makarov A, Hardman M, Cooks RG. The Orbitrap: a new mass spectrometer. *J Mass Spectrom* 2005;40:430–443.

67. Marshall AG, Hendrickson CL, Jackson GS. Fourier transform ion cyclotron resonance mass spectrometry: a primer. *Mass Spectrom Rev* 1998;17:1–35.

68. Park BK, Kitteringham NR, Maggs JL, Pirmohamed M, Williams DP. The role of metabolic activation in drug-induced hepatotoxicity. *Annu Rev Pharmacol Toxicol* 2005; 45:177–202.

69. Walgren JL, Mitchell MD, Thompson DC. Role of metabolism in drug-induced idiosyncratic hepatotoxicity. *Crit Rev Toxicol* 2005;35:325–361.

70. Zhou S, Chan E, Duan W, Huang M, Chen Y-Z. Drug bioactivation, covalent binding to target proteins and toxicity relevance. *Drug Metab Rev* 2005;1:41–213.

71. Kaplowitz N. Idiosyncratic drug hepatotoxicity. *Nat Rev Drug Discov* 2005;4:489–499.

72. Baillie TA, Cayen MN, Fouda H, Gerson RJ, Green JD, Grossman SJ, Klunk LJ, LeBlanc B, Perkins DG, Shipley LA. Contemporary issues in toxicology. Drug metabolites in safety testing. *Toxicol Appl Pharmacol* 2002;182:188–196.

73. Baillie TA. Future of toxicology—metabolic activation and drug design: challenges and opportunities in chemical toxicology. *Chem Res Toxicol* 2006;19:889–893.

74. Halpert JR. Structural basis of selective cytochrome P450 inhibition. *Annu Rev Pharmacol Toxicol* 1995;35:29–53.

75. Kent UM, Juschyshyn MI, Hollenberg PF. Mechanism-based inactivators as probes of cytochrome P450 structure and function. *Curr Drug Metab* 2001;2:215–243.

76. Sesardic D, Boobis AR, Murray BP, Murray S, Segura J, de la Torre R, Davies DS. Furafylline is a potent and selective inhibitor of cytochrome P450IA2 in man. *Br J Clin Pharmacol* 1990;29:651–663.

77. Kunze KL, Trager WF. Isoform-selective mechanism-based inhibition of human cytochrome P450 1A2 by furafylline. *Chem Res Toxicol* 1993;6:649–656.

78. Back DJ, Houlgrave R, Tjia JF, Ward S, Orme ML. Effect of the progestogens, gestodene, 3-keto desogestrel, levonorgestrel, norethisterone and norgestimate on the oxidation of ethinyloestradiol and other substrates by human liver microsomes. *J Steroid Biochem Mol Biol* 1991;38:219–225.

79. Turpeinen M, Nieminen R, Juntunen T, Taavitsainen P, Raunio H, Pelkonen O. Selective inhibition of CYP2B6-catalyzed bupropion hydroxylation in human liver microsomes *in vitro*. *Drug Metab Dispos* 2004;36:626–631.

80. Uetrecht J. Screening for the potential of a drug candidate to cause idiosyncratic drug reactions. *DDT* 2003;8:832–837.

81. Williams DP, Park BK. Idiosyncratic toxicity: the role of toxicophores and bioactivation. *DDT* 2003;8:1044–1050.

82. Dennehy MK, Richards KAM, Wernke GR, Shyr GR, Liebler DC. Cytosolic and nuclear protein targets of thiol-reactive electrophiles. *Chem Res Toxicol* 2006;19:20–29.

83. Evans DC, Watt AP, Nicoll-Griffith DA, Baillie TA. Drug–protein covalent adducts: an industry perspective on minimizing the potential for drug bioactivation in drug discovery and development. *Chem Res Toxicol* 2004;17:3–16.

84. van de Waterbeemd H. High-throughput and *in silico* techniques in drug metabolism and pharmacokinetics. *Curr Opin Drug Discov Dev* 2002;5:33–43.

85. Wunberg T, Hendrix M, Hillisch A, Lobell M, Meier H, Schmeck C, Wild H, Hinzen B. Improving the hit-to-lead process: data-driven assessment of drug-like and lead-like screening hits. *Drug Discov Today* 2006;11:175–180.

86. Castro-Perez J, Plumb R, Granger JH, Beattie I, Joncour K, Wright A. Increasing throughput and information content for *in vitro* drug metabolism experiments using ultra-performance liquid chromatography coupled to a quadrupole time-of-flight mass spectrometer. *Rapid Commun Mass Spectrom* 2005;19:843–848.

87. Lopez LL, Yu X, Cui D, Davis MR. Identification of drug metabolites in biological matrices by intelligent automated liquid chromatography/tandem mass spectrometry. *Rapid Commun Mass Spectrom* 1999;12:1756–1760.

88. Houston JB. Utility of *in vitro* drug metabolism data in predicting *in vivo* metabolic clearance. *Biochem Pharmacol* 1994;47:1469–1479.

89. Iwatsubo T, Hirota N, Ooie T, Suzuki H, Shimada N, Chiba K, Ishizaki T, Green CE, Tyson CA, Sugiyama Y. Prediction of *in vivo* drug metabolism in the human liver from *in vitro* metabolism data. *Pharmacol Ther* 1997;73:147–171.

90. Ito K, Iwatsubo T, Kanamitsu S, Nakajima Y, Sugiyama Y. Quantitative prediction of *in vivo* drug clearance and drug interactions from *in vitro* data on metabolism, together with binding and transport. *Annu Rev Pharmacol Toxicol* 1998;38:461–499.

91. Obach RS. Prediction of human clearance of twenty-nine drugs from hepatic microsomal intrinsic clearance data: an examination of *in vitro* half-life approach and nonspecific binding to microsomes. *Drug Metab Dispos* 1999;27:1350–1359.

92. Obach RS. The prediction of human clearance from hepatic microsomal metabolism data. *Curr Opin Drug Discov Dev* 2001;4:36–44.

93. Rowland M, Tozer TN. *Clinical Pharmacokinetics: Concepts and Applications*, 3rd ed. Philadelphia: Lippincott Williams & Wilkins; 1994.

94. Houston JB, Galetin A. Progress towards prediction of human pharmacokinetic parameters fron *in vitro* technologies. *Drug Metab Rev* 2003;35:393–415.

95. Shiran MR, Proctor NJ, Howgate EM, Rowland-Yeo K, Tucker GT, Rostami-Hodjegan A. Prediction of metabolic drug clearance in humans: *in vitro–in vivo* extrapolation vs allometric scaling. *Xenobiotica* 2006;36:567–580.

96. Bjornsson TD, Callaghan JT, Einolf HJ, Fischer V, Gan L, Grimm S, Kao J, King SP, Miwa G, Ni L, Kumar G, McLeod J, Obach RS, Roberts S, Roe A, Shah A, Snikeris F, Sullivan JT, Tweedie D, Vega JM, Walsh J, Wrighton SA. The conduct of *in vitro* and *in vivo* drug–drug interaction studies: a Pharmaceutical Research and Manufacturers of America (PhRMA) perspective. *Drug Metab Dispos* 2003;31:815–832.

97. Ito K, Brown HS, Houston JB. Database analyses for the prediction of *in vivo* drug–drug interactions from *in vitro* data. *Br J Clin Pharmacol* 2004;57:473–486.

98. Obach RS, Walsky RL, Venkatakrishnan K, Gaman EA, Houston JB, Tremaine LM. The utility of *in vitro* cytochrome P450 inhibition data in the prediction of drug–drug interactions. *J Pharmacol Exp Ther* 2006;316:336–348.

99. Hartung T, Bremer S, Casati S, Coecke S, Corvi R, Fortaner S, Gribaldo L, Halder M, Hoffmann S, Roi AJ, Prieto P, Sabbioni E, Scott L, Worth A, Zuang V. A modular approach to the ECVAM principles on test validity. *Altern Lab Anim* 2004;32: 467–472.

100. Aninat C, Piton A, Glaise D, Le Charpentier T, Langouet S, Morel F, Guguen-Guillouzo C, Guillouzo A. Expression of cytochromes P450, conjugating enzymes and nuclear receptors in human hepatoma HepaRG cells. *Drug Metab Dispos* 2006;34:75–83.

101. Le Vee M, Jigorel E, Glaise D, Gripon P, Guguen-Guillouzo C, Fardel O. Functional expression of sinusoidal and canalicular hepatic drug transporters in the differentiated human hepatoma HepaRG cell line. *Eur J Pharm Sci* 2006;28:109–117.

22

UTILIZATION OF *IN VITRO* CYTOCHROME P450 INHIBITION DATA FOR PROJECTING CLINICAL DRUG–DRUG INTERACTIONS

JANE R. KENNY, DERMOT F. MCGINNITY, KEN GRIME, AND ROBERT J. RILEY

AstraZeneca R&D Charnwood, Loughborough, United Kingdom

Contents

Preclinical Development Handbook: ADME and Biopharmaceutical Properties, edited by Shayne Cox Gad
Copyright © 2008 John Wiley & Sons, Inc.

22.1 INTRODUCTION

Adverse drug reactions (ADRs) are recognized as a significant cause of hospitalizations and up to 2.8% of hospital admissions may be a consequence of drug–drug interactions (DDIs) [1, 2]. The possibility of DDIs presents whenever two or more drugs are administered simultaneously; an ever more likely occurrence in an aging population often exposed to polypharmacy [3]. Moreover, it has been estimated that >90% of ADRs are also associated with dose-dependent pharmacokinetic/pharmacodynamic (PK/PD) events, which are one of the top five causes of death in the United States, resulting in over 100, 000 deaths each year [1, 2, 4]. While this is alarming, it is noteworthy that of the drugs associated with preventable drug-related hospital admissions, only four drug groups account for more than 50% of ADRs [5]. Indeed, drug concentration-dependent pharmacological reactions (classified as type A adverse reactions) account for approximately 75% of all ADRs and in principle should be preventable [6]. Such statistics highlight the need for improved mechanistic understanding and clear risk avoidance strategies, both during the drug discovery/development process and in the clinic.

DDIs may occur at the metabolic level with impact on drug clearance at the site of gastrointestinal absorption, on plasma or tissue binding, by inhibition or induction of hepatic drug metabolizing enzymes, and on carrier mediated transport (including renal and hepatic uptake and biliary efflux) [7]. All these interactions may induce changes in the PK profiles of the drugs involved, resulting in altered PD response or promotion of a toxicological effect not associated with the primary pharmacology [8, 9]. Several clinically relevant and severe DDI cases, such as those resulting in the withdrawal of terfenadine and cerivastatin [10], have increased the focus on metabolism-based interactions, particularly those involving cytochrome P450 (CYP) enzymes. Indeed, CYP inhibition is reported to account for as much as half of all reported DDIs [11]. These metabolic interactions can occur whenever the metabolism of one "victim" drug is inhibited by the presence of another "perpetrator" drug. The resultant decrease in clearance of the victim drug leads to increased systemic concentrations that are pronounced if the inhibited pathway is the major route of elimination. Several CYP mediated DDIs have resulted in severe clinical reactions and fatalities in extreme cases [10, 12], so real emphasis is placed on the prediction and hence avoidance of DDIs in drug discovery [7, 13–15]. Indeed, there has been substantial academic and industrial effort directed toward the accurate prediction of DDIs with the aim of reducing their impact in the clinic by designing out such interactions.

DDIs as a potential source or contributor to drug attrition, either directly or indirectly, has contributed to the industry focus on this area. In the late 1980s poor drug metabolism and pharmacokinetics (DMPK) properties and toxicity were predominantly responsible for the discontinued development of new chemical entities (NCEs) during late stage clinical trials [16, 17]. In response to this, and to increase competitive advantage (e.g., by avoiding product interaction labels), the pharmaceutical industry has increasingly aligned DMPK to the early drug discovery phase. The failure of NCEs at a late stage is a cost the pharmaceutical industry can ill afford; it is estimated that the total preapproval costs for a new drug are in excess of 800 million U.S. dollars [18]. The industry has responded to both the clinical and economic factors by front-loading DDI screens early in the discovery phase to predict the risk of DDI for NCEs. High throughput automated assays to evaluate the impact of CYP inhibition are now common as early as the hit identification stage [19]. Increased importance is placed on evaluation of the risk for NCEs participating in DDIs, as a victim and/or perpetrator of such interactions. However, despite the focus that DDIs and potentially associated ADRs have received over the last two decades, it was recently reported that there has been little reduction in their clinical impact [6, 17], although with a drug development time in excess of ten years it is perhaps too early to identify the impact of such DDI screens on these clinical statistics.

In the following sections several examples of DDIs are introduced to demonstrate the clinical consequences of CYP inhibition. The kinetics of reversible and irreversible inhibition are presented along with discussion of *in vitro* methodology. Accurate *in vitro* kinetic data is an absolute prerequisite for *in vitro–in vivo* extrapolation (IVIVE), and the current literature models for predicting clinical inhibition are presented. Overall, this chapter aims to summarize the current knowledge base and the complexities of CYP inhibition and to provide a guide for embarking on prediction of clinical DDIs with particular emphasis on the drug discovery setting.

22.2 CYTOCHROME P450 AND ITS ROLE IN DRUG–DRUG INTERACTIONS

The CYP family of enzymes are the primary facilitators of oxidative biotransformation in the liver and are responsible for the metabolism, at least in part, of the majority of human drugs [20]. These heme-containing enzymes are primarily situated in the lipid bilayer of the endoplasmic reticulum of hepatocytes, but are also located in extrahepatic tissues, including the gastrointestinal tract (GIT), kidney, and lung [21]. Fifty-seven different human CYP enzymes have been identified [22] and of these, 23 human isoforms are from the CYP1, CYP2, and CYP3 families that are recognized as important in xenobiotic metabolism [23]. However, it has been estimated that approximately 90% of human drug oxidations can be attributed to just five CYPs, namely, CYP1A2, CYP2C9, CYP2C19, CYP2D6, and CYP3A4/5 [24, 25]. CYP3A4 is the most abundant of these and can constitute up to 50% of total hepatic CYP content [26]. This enzyme is also the most prolific, with approximately 60% of all oxidative biotransformations being attributed to CYP3A4 [27]. The CYP family metabolize a very broad range of substrates, from endogenous steroids and vitamins to small drug molecules of all charge types [28]. For example, CYP3A4 metabolizes large lipophilic molecules including testosterone, erythromycin, and cyclosporine as well as smaller molecules like midazolam and nifedipine. CYP2C9 favors medium sized acidic or neutral molecules such as diclofenac and tienilic acid; CYP2D6 favors basic, lipophilic molecules such as dextromethorphan and metoprolol, while CYP1A2 has affinity for neutral planar molecules such as theophylline and phenacetin [28]. Since CYPs are the major enzyme family in xenobiotic/drug metabolism, they retain a central role in the mediation of clinically relevant DDIs.

22.2.1 Clinical Consequences of Cytochrome P450 Mediated Drug–Drug Interactions

There is a wealth of literature around CYP mediated DDIs. The most documented DDIs resulting in severe clinical adverse reactions are listed in Table 22.1. In the following section examples of drugs as either victims or perpetrators of DDIs will be presented with specific cases exemplifying (1) reversible and irreversible inhibition at the major CYPs and (2) the role of intestinal metabolism and enzyme polymorphisms within the patient population.

The antihistamine terfenadine, a victim of DDI, was withdrawn because of patient fatality following coadministration with ketoconazole [10]. Competitive inhibition of CYP3A4-dependent terfenadine methyl-hydroxylation by ketoconazole resulted in up to a 40-fold increase in the area under the plasma concentration–time curve (*AUC*) of terfenadine. This increased concentration manifested itself clinically as QT prolongation and torsades de pointes [37]. Other victims of DDI are simvastatin and lovastatin. Both are 3-hydroxy-3-methylglutaryl coenzyme A (HMG-CoA) reductase inhibitors, which although exceedingly well tolerated, incur a small risk of myopathy or potentially fatal rhabdomyolysis, particularly when coadministered with medications that increase their systemic exposure [44]. These statins both have a substantial CYP3A4 component to their metabolism, and large (hepatic and intestinal) first-pass metabolism makes them particularly susceptible to interactions via CYP3A4 inhibition. Intestinal metabolism may be effectively abolished in the presence of a potent oral CYP3A4 inhibitor, resulting in an increase in plasma concentration of up to threefold for drugs such as cyclosporine, midazolam, lovastatin, and simvastatin [44–46]. This was elegantly confirmed in clinical studies where midazolam was administered either via the oral or intravenous route alongside the CYP3A4 inhibitors itraconazole and fluconazole [46]. Following an intravenous dose the *AUC* of midazolam was increased 3.5-fold in the presence of itraconazole; however, the *AUC* increased sevenfold when midazolam was administered orally [46]. Clearly, for drugs with a high hepatic extraction, the impact of metabolic inhibition will give rise to large changes in oral exposure, compounded by any effect of inhibition on intestinal metabolism.

Another statin, cerivastatin, was anticipated to have less potential for CYP3A4 mediated DDIs than the other statins due to the additional role of CYP2C8 in its metabolism [47]. Prior to launch it was thought that cerivastatin would provide a safer alternative to simvastatin and lovastatin due to its alternative metabolic pathway. Indeed, interaction studies with erythromycin and itraconazole, two potent inhibitors of CYP3A4, have shown little impact on cerivastatin plasma levels [48–50]. However, coadministration with gemfibrozil increases the *AUC* of cerivastatin about sixfold [33]. This is assumed to be due to inhibition of CYP2C8 by gemfibrozil and its glucuronide metabolite. Interestingly, the glucuronide metabolite demonstrates a 20-fold increase in inhibitory potency at CYP2C8 over its parent (IC_{50} of 80 µM and 4 µM for gemfibrozil and its glucuronide metabolite, respectively [51]) and is actively concentrated in the liver [51, 52]. It is also worth noting that gemfibrozil also inhibits the OATP1B1-mediated hepatic uptake of statins and that this mechanism could well have contributed to this and indeed other gemfibrozil–statin interactions [52, 53]. During cerivastatin monotherapy, the incidence rate of rhabdomyolysis was 10–100 times higher than with the other statins and gemfibrozil

TABLE 22.1 Examples of Marketed Drugs Involved in Clinically Significant Drug–Drug Interactions

Predominant CYP Isoform	Victim Drug	Perpetrator Drug	Maximum Clinical AUC Increase of Victim Drug	Clinical Consequences	References
CYP1A2	Theophylline	Ciprofloxacin	Variable	Theophylline toxicity	29
	Tizanidine	Ciprofloxacin	10-fold	Excess hypotensive and sedative effects	30
CYP2C8	Tacrine	Fluvoxamine	~sixfold	Hepatotoxicity	31, 32
	Cerivastatin[a]	Gemfibrozil	sixfold	Rhabdomylosis	33
CYP2C9	Tolbutamide	Sulfaphenazole	5.3-fold	Hypoglycemia	34
	Warfarin	Fluconazole	50% decrease in clearance	Enhanced hypoprothrombinemic effect	35
CYP2D6	Desipramine	Fluoxetine	~sixfold		31
	Metoprolol	Mibefradil[a]	4–5-fold	Effect on cardioselectivity	36
CYP3A4	Terfenadine[a]	Ketoconazole	~40-fold	Torsades des pointes	2, 10, 37, 38
	Lovastatin	Itraconazole	~20-fold	Rhabdomylosis	39, 40
	Simvastatin	Mibefradil[a]	5–10-fold	Rhabdomylosis	41
	Midazolam	Erythromycin	threefold	Excess sedation	42
	Cisapride[a]	Erythromycin	Variable	QT prolongation	12, 43

[a]Withdrawn from the market between 1990 and 2001.

greatly increased this risk; the number of rhabdomyolysis cases reported to the U.S. Food and Drug Administration with the gemfibrozil–cerivastatin combination was 533 [53]. As a result, cerivastatin was voluntarily withdrawn from the market in 2003.

Adverse events can be manifest without particularly large changes in the *AUC* of the victim drug. In epileptic patients stabilized on carbamazepine therapy, addition of the antidepressant agent viloxazine has resulted in side effects of carbamazepine intoxication (fatigue, dizziness, and ataxia). This is associated with an *AUC* elevation of carbamazepine (approximately twofold) and carbamazepine 10,11-epoxide (approximately 1.3-fold) [54]. The most likely mechanism for this interaction is CYP3A4 inhibition by viloxazine [55]. This example shows how a modest elevation can be detrimental if the therapeutic window of the victim drug is narrow; in this case resulting in an exaggerated pharmacological effect.

Mibefradil, a novel calcium antagonist for the treatment of hypertension and angina and a perpetrator of DDI, was voluntarily withdrawn from the market in 1997, less than a year after its launch [36]. Several severe adverse reactions were observed during mibefradil therapy in combination with various drugs including simvastatin and lovastatin [36, 41]. During its development, mibefradil had been identified as having inhibitory effects on CYP3A4 and CYP2D6, consequently coadministration was contraindicated with terfenadine and metoprolol (a CYP2D6 substrate) and the labeling carried a list of drugs that might require dose adjustment. When mibefradil was withdrawn, an additional complication arose; life-threatening reactions occurred if therapy was replaced with β-blockers or calcium channel antagonists within 5 days of discontinuing mibefradil therapy [36]. This was attributed to the long elimination half-life of mibefradil, but subsequently, it has been observed that mibefradil is a time-dependent inhibitor of CYP3A4 [56, 57] and also inhibits P-gp *in vitro* (K_i of 1.6 μM [58]). The time-dependent nature of its CYP3A4 inhibition could explain the long "wash-out" period of mibefradil mediated inhibition. There are suggestions in the literature that some of the severe interactions observed with mibefradil could have been predicted from the *in vitro* and *in vivo* data available at the time [36, 45, 59].

The extent of DDIs can vary substantially within the population due to variability in enzyme expression. This variation is observed in the ciprofloxacin–theophylline interaction and has implications for the severity of the clinical outcome. The inhibitory effect of ciprofloxacin at CYP1A2 can result in varying changes in theophylline levels across a patient population. In sensitive patients, theophylline clearance can decrease significantly, increasing the risk of theophylline related toxicity [29, 60]. In another case, ciprofloxacin inhibits the CYP1A2 mediated metabolism of tizanidine, resulting in AUC increases of up to 10-fold, dangerously escalating its hypotensive and sedative effects [30]. CYP1A2 is the primary clearance mechanism for both theophylline and tizanidine [61, 62], and there is considerable interindividual variability in the *in vivo* metabolic activity of CYP1A2 (demonstrated by caffeine clearance [63]); therefore, inhibition results in significant changes in plasma levels in sensitive patients only.

As is the case for all polymorphic CYPs, the CYP2D6 related DDIs are complicated by the genetic polymorphisms observed for this enzyme (between 5% and 10% of the Caucasian population are CYP2D6 poor metabolizers). Investigation of potential DDIs observed via CYP2D6 inhibition may be confounded by the presence of individuals with the poor metabolizer phenotype within the study group [64]. It is evident that poor metabolizers are unlikely to suffer DDIs through CYP2D6 inhibition and therefore will not display the same magnitude of interaction predicted from *in vitro* studies [6]. CYP2D6 is inhibited by antipsychotic drugs and the propensity for interactions is increased for this patient population as psychopharmacologic medications are often taken for long periods of time and commonly coprescribed with other medications [65]. For example, the CYP2D6 inhibitor fluoxetine has been demonstrated to substantially increase the plasma levels of desipramine (between four- and sixfold) [31].

The clinical interactions presented here highlight the need to assess an NCE's involvement in potential DDIs from *both* perspectives of inhibition, either as a victim drug where metabolism is altered by a coadministered inhibitor or as the perpetrator of DDI. The cases also highlight the importance of fully defining the elimination and metabolic profile of an NCE: reaction phenotyping can lend greater understanding to potential interactions as can an understanding of the target patient population and likely coadministered drugs.

22.2.2   Mechanisms of Cytochrome P450 Inhibition

There are different mechanisms through which CYP inhibition may occur, all of which are a function of the metabolic capacity of the enzyme. In nearly all cases of clinically relevant *reversible* inhibition, the perpetrator is a substrate competing for the same CYP mediated metabolism. Simple Michaelis–Menten kinetics often satisfactorily describes CYP metabolism *in vitro*, provided that the enzyme and substrate are in thermodynamic equilibrium.

Enzyme Kinetics   In the reaction scheme shown in Fig. 22.1, a steady-state equilibrium is assumed to be reached (the ES complex rapidly reaches a constant value such that $d[ES]/dt = 0$). This assumption is key to the derivation of the Michaelis–Menten equation, which underpins not only prediction of metabolic clearance from *in vitro* data but also prediction of DDIs (since the prediction of DDI magnitude from *in vitro* data always starts with a modification of the Michaelis–Menten equation). The reason that the investigator needs to be aware of this is that experimental conditions are important in making this assumption. For $d[ES]/dt = 0$, the reverse reaction rate should be negligible and the formation of the [ES] complex should not significantly alter the substrate concentration [S]. In other words, the substrate concentration should greatly exceed the enzyme concentration and the substrate concentration should not be significantly depleted during the incubation (less than 20% metabolism). To this end, it is noteworthy that in a typical human liver microsome (HLM) preparation, CYP3A4 concentration may be as much as $0.25\,\mu M$ when the incubation contains $1\,mg/mL$ HLM.

Equations 22.1 and 22.2 are the Michaelis–Menten equation (22.1) and its rearrangement (22.2), where v is the observed rate of metabolite formation, V_{max} is the maximum rate of this metabolite formation, K_m is the Michaelis–Menten constant representing the enzyme:substrate affinity and is the concentration that supports half the maximum rate of metabolite formation, and [S] is the substrate concentration at the enzyme active site. The derivation of these equations is shown in Appendix A.

$$E + S \underset{k_{-1}}{\overset{k_{+1}}{\rightleftharpoons}} ES \overset{k_2}{\longrightarrow} E + P$$

FIGURE 22.1   Schematic representing Michaelis–Menten kinetics, where E is enzyme, S is substrate, k_{+1} is the association rate constant describing ES formation from E + S, k_{-1} is the dissociation rate constant from ES to E + S, ES is substrate-bound enzyme, P is the product of enzyme, and k_2 is the dissociation rate constant from ES to E + P.

$$v = \frac{V_{max} \cdot [S]}{K_m + [S]} \tag{22.1}$$

$$= \frac{V_{max}}{1 + K_m/[S]} \tag{22.2}$$

Only simple one-site binding can be accurately described by hyperbolic Michaelis–Menten kinetics but there is substantial literature evidence that atypical kinetics and multisite binding exist for the CYP enzymes. This is most clear for CYP3A4 [66] but is also observed for CYP2C9 [67, 68]. Positive or negative cooperative effects, where a bound substrate molecule influences the binding of a second molecule, have implications in terms of probe substrate selection and make full kinetic characterizations complex. It must be noted, however, that while cooperativity is clearly demonstrable *in vitro*, there is little evidence of its influence *in vivo* [69, 70]. Only simple one-site models of inhibition will be discussed here and detailed explanation of atypical (or sigmoidal) kinetics in inhibition can be found elsewhere in the scientific literature [14, 66, 71–73].

Reversible Inhibition   Having explained the basis of simple CYP kinetics, the details of inhibition can be described. Reversible CYP inhibition can be categorized into three main forms: competitive, noncompetitive, and uncompetitive. Figure 22.2 describes each type of inhibition and the rate equations associated with them are presented below. In competitive inhibition the substrate and inhibitor compete for the same binding site within the enzyme; inhibition therefore decreases as the enzyme becomes saturated with substrate. Competitive inhibitors interfere with substrate binding so as to raise K_m by a factor of $[I]/K_i$ without affecting V_{max} (i.e., the affinity of the substrate for the enzyme, K_m, is decreased by a factor dependent in magnitude on the ratio of inhibitor concentration and the affinity of the inhibitor for the enzyme, K_i (Eq. 22.3)):

$$v = \frac{V_{max} \cdot [S]}{K_m(1 + [I]/K_i) + [S]} \tag{22.3}$$

It is common to relate the potency of competitive inhibition to IC_{50} (the concentration of inhibitor for which the reaction rate is suppressed by 50%). Equation 22.4 is derived from Eq. 22.3 when v becomes $v/2$ and I becomes IC_{50}.

$$IC_{50} = K_i(1 + [S]/K_m) \tag{22.4}$$

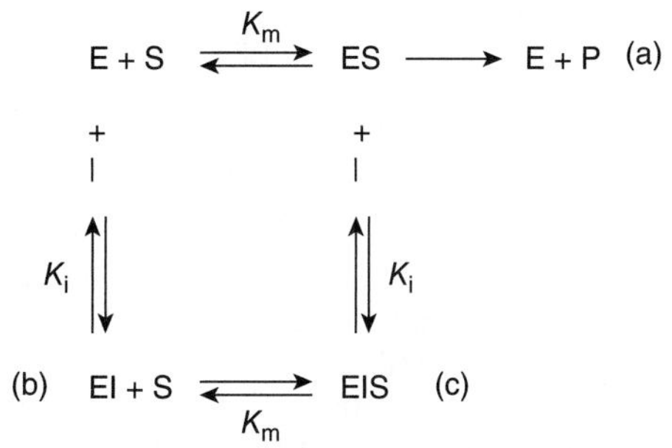

$$E + S \underset{}{\overset{K_m}{\rightleftarrows}} ES \longrightarrow E + P \quad (a)$$

$$+ \qquad\qquad +$$
$$| \qquad\qquad\quad |$$

$$K_i \updownarrow \qquad\qquad \updownarrow K_i$$

$$(b) \quad EI + S \underset{K_m}{\overset{}{\rightleftarrows}} EIS \quad (c)$$

FIGURE 22.2 Schematic of competitive inhibition, representing Michaelis–Menten kinetics. Pathway (a), competitive inhibition; pathway (b), uncompetitive inhibition; pathway (c), noncompetitive inhibition. E is enzyme, S is substrate, ES is substrate-bound enzyme, P is the product of enzyme and substrate, I is inhibitor, EI is inhibitor-bound enzyme, EIS is inhibitor- and substrate-bound enzyme, K_m is the Michaelis–Menten constant, and K_i is the inhibition constant. Note that K_m can be described as $(k_2 + k_{-1}/k_{+1})$—see Appendix A. However, if it is assumed that rapid formation of the ES complex occurs when the enzyme and substrate are mixed; $k_{+1} \gg k_2$ and K_m can be described as k_{-1}/k_{+1}.

In noncompetitive inhibition the inhibitor binds at a site distinct from the substrate binding site and can interact with either the substrate-free or the substrate-bound form of the enzyme. It is assumed that the inhibitor binds to both states of the enzyme with the same affinity and so the degree of inhibition is independent of substrate concentration. The binding affinity (K_m) is unaffected but the inhibitor acts to remove active enzyme and consequently the maximal reaction velocity (V_{max}) is decreased. The metabolic rate of noncompetitive inhibition is described by

$$v = \frac{V_{max}/(1+[I]/K_i)\cdot[S]}{K_m + [S]} \quad (22.5)$$

The substrate-independent nature of inhibition is further demonstrated by the IC_{50}, which is equivalent to the inhibitor constant $K_i(IC_{50} = K_i)$, derived from Eq. 22.5 when v becomes $v/2$ and $[I]$ becomes IC_{50}.

In uncompetitive inhibition (which is extremely rare for CYP metabolism [71]), only the substrate-bound form of the enzyme is open to inhibitor binding; the inhibitor cannot bind to free enzyme and so the degree of inhibition will increase with substrate concentration. The metabolic rate in the presence of an uncompetitive inhibitor can be described by Eq. 22.6 and the corresponding IC_{50} by Eq. 22.7:

$$v = \frac{V_{max}/(1+[I]/K_i)\cdot[S]}{K_m(1+[I]/K_i)+[S]} \quad (22.6)$$

$$IC_{50} = K_i(1 + K_m/[S]) \quad (22.7)$$

Mechanism-Based Inhibition Irreversible inhibition or mechanism-based inactivation is an unusual occurrence with most enzymes. It is, however, observed in reactions catalyzed by CYP in somewhat higher frequency [74]. In contrast with

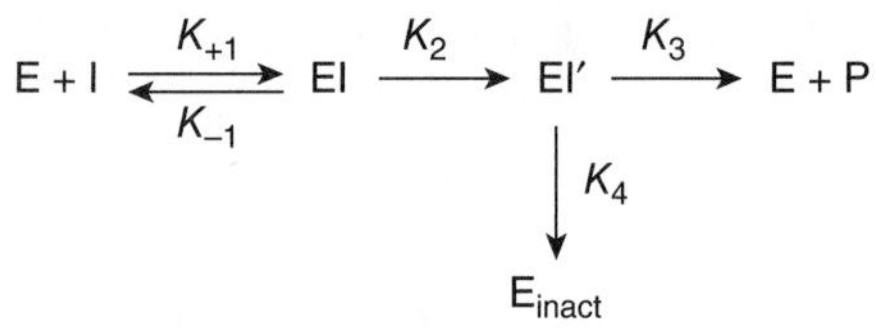

FIGURE 22.3 Schematic of mechanism-based inhibition, where E is enzyme, I is inhibitor, EI is inhibitor-bound enzyme, EI′ is the initial complex formed between metabolic intermediate and enzyme, P is the product of enzyme and inhibitor complex that escapes reactive binding in the active site, $E_{inactive}$ is the inactive enzyme with irreversibly bound metabolic intermediate, k_{+1} is the association rate constant for E + I forming EI, k_2 is the association rate constant for EI forming EI′, k_3 is the dissociation rate constant for EI′ to E + P, and k_4 is the rate constant from EI′ to E_{inact}.

reversible inhibition, the effects of mechanism-based inhibition (MBI) are more profound after multiple dosing and the recovery period, typically several days, is independent of continued exposure to the drug [75, 76]. This MBI transpires when a CYP is quasi-irreversibly or irreversibly inhibited by reactive intermediates formed during the metabolic process. The inhibitory intermediates may form covalently bound adducts to the CYP heme or apoprotein; alternatively, they may form a metabolic inhibitory complex (MIC) in the active site. This MBI is characterized by NADPH-, concentration-, and time-dependent inactivation. Additionally, the inactivation rate is diminished in the presence of a competing substrate, enzyme activity is not restored by dialysis or filtration (as inhibitor is covalently bound), and *de novo* synthesis of protein is required to recover metabolic activity [77]. Figure 22.3 shows a schematic representation of this inhibition [78] and the inhibition for the initial rate of enzyme deactivation can be described as follows.

From Fig. 22.3 it can be seen that the change in concentration over time of inhibitor-bound enzyme, [EI], the initial complex formed between metabolic intermediate and enzyme, [EI′], and the inactive enzyme with irreversibly bound metabolic intermediate, [E_{inact}], respectively can be expressed as

$$d[EI]/dt = k_{+1}[I]\cdot[E] - (k_{-1} + k_2)[EI] \tag{22.8}$$

$$d[EI′]/dt = k_2[EI] - (k_3 + k_4)[EI′] \tag{22.9}$$

$$d[E_{inact}]/dt = k_4[EI′] \tag{22.10}$$

where [E] is the concentration of the unbound active enzyme and [I] is the concentration of the mechanism-based inhibitor.

The parameters k_{inact} (the maximal inactivation rate constant) and K_I (the inhibitor concentration that supports half the maximal rate of inactivation) are described by Eqs. 22.11 and 22.12, respectively, using the association constants shown in Fig. 22.3.

$$k_{inact} = k_2 k_4 / (k_2 + k_3 + k_4) \tag{22.11}$$

$$K_I = \frac{(k_3 + k_4)(k_{-1} + k_2)}{(k_2 + k_3 + k_4)k_1} \tag{22.12}$$

The apparent inactivation rate constant of the enzyme, k_{obs}, is described by

$$k_{obs} = \frac{k_{inact}[I]}{[I] + K_I} \qquad (22.13)$$

The derivation of these equations is included in Appendix B to show the mathematical assumptions that must be made to allow such parameters to be defined experimentally.

The partition ratio (r) is a useful additional parameter to k_{inact} and K_I. It is defined as the number of moles of reactive metabolite escaping the enzyme without inactivating it (product) per number of moles of reactive metabolite inactivating the enzyme (trapped product) ($r = k_3/k_4$; Fig. 22.3). As the partition ratio approaches 0, inhibition is more efficient; for every cycle of the enzyme and substrate that results in product, a cycle also results in inactivated enzyme. For a potent inhibitor, the reactive species is less likely to escape the active site without adduct formation. While the partition ratio may be helpful in ranking compounds in order of inhibitory efficiency (as is the k_{inact}/K_I ratio), any use beyond this is limited.

22.3 ASSESSMENT OF CYTOCHROME P450 INHIBITION *IN VITRO*

Over the last decade there have been tremendous advances in the understanding of both the theoretical and technical aspects of generating *in vitro* kinetic data to engender predictions of DDIs [7, 11, 13, 21, 71, 79, 80]. The advantages of using *in vitro* assays to study inhibition include allowing inexpensive and rapid assessment of inhibition potential and consequent evaluation of DDI risk, facilitating detailed kinetic analysis of drugs known to cause DDIs in the clinic, and helping to further develop our understanding of these interactions and ultimately striving toward the avoidance of DDIs for NCEs. However, despite the undoubted usefulness of *in vitro* models, there are limitations, primarily due to the fact that, to date, there is no consensus toward a model that quantitatively predicts interactions in humans from *in vitro* data. Indeed, there is no single method for generating *in vitro* data. Despite the lack of consensus, there are some fundamentally common elements to the existing methodologies and these form the basis of the remainder of this chapter. Prior to modeling data, accurate *in vitro* assessments must be made. There are many parameters to consider when embarking on inhibition studies to generate good *in vitro* data, the key elements of which are discussed here.

22.3.1 Enzyme Systems

Historically, the majority of inhibition studies have been conducted using subcellular fractions of liver. Clear species differences exist in hepatic enzyme content and function [81]. In most cases a homolog of the human enzyme is present in the preclinical species. For example, CYP3A1 and CYP3A2 are the major 3A isoforms in the rat and share substrate crossover to human CYP3A4 and CYP3A5. Likewise CYP2C11 in rodent liver is homologous to CYP2C9 in humans. However, the species-specific isoforms of CYP1A, CYP2C, CYP2D, and CYP3A do show appreciable interspecies differences in terms of catalytic activity [81]. While laboratory species can be a useful tool for investigating pharmacokinetic species differences and for providing confidence in IVIVE, clinical DDI potential must be investigated *in vitro* using human derived tissues and/or enzymes because of such species differences.

Human liver microsomes (HLMs) are prepared from liver homogenates by differential ultracentrifugation, first removing the cytosolic (S9) fraction, then with further ultracentrifugation collecting the subcellular fraction, which includes membrane-bound enzymes [82]. The utility of HLMs is clear; they can be isolated from a relatively small amount of human liver, can be stored almost indefinitely at −80 °C, contain functional CYPs (and other enzymes such as UDP-glucuronosyltransferases and flavin monooxygenases), and can be used as a single donor or pooled to provide a representation of enzyme expression in the population. However, due to the presence of multiple CYP isoforms with overlapping substrate selectivity, kinetic investigations must be thorough and carefully planned as inhibitors may be substrates for more than one CYP isoform. Consequently, for CYP inhibition studies using HLMs, the use of selective probe reactions is paramount and often relies on careful adjustment of substrate concentration to ensure selectivity.

In the last decade, the use of recombinant human CYP (rCYP) proteins, expressed in yeast, baculovirus-infected insect cells, or *Escherichia coli*, has become widespread and indeed now forms the backbone of screening efforts in the pharmaceutical industry. There are considerable advantages to using a single rCYP enzyme in an assay as it allows manipulation of substrates and inhibitors without the complications of enzyme selectivity. A notable example of this is CYP3A5, which has broad substrate crossover with CYP3A4, making it difficult to characterize reactions that are specific to or of equal affinity at CYP3A5 with respect to CYP3A4 [83]. A sometimes-perceived disadvantage of rCYP is the increased enzyme activity per unit of membrane protein compared to that of HLM. However, the high CYP expression levels give rise to low incubational protein content and low non-specific substrate and inhibitor binding, resulting in more accurate estimations of unbound K_{+1} values. Finally, the utility of rCYP in reaction phenotyping and inhibition studies has been well validated [84–86] and the versatility of rCYPs lends them to enhanced throughput screening.

Isolated human hepatocytes are an alternative *in vitro* tool and can be used to add refinement to data generated using subcellular fractions, as the impact of drug transporter activity on K_i, accounting for intracellular free drug concentrations, can be investigated. As whole cells, hepatocytes express not only all membrane-bound enzymes but also hepatic cytosolic enzymes; moreover, they contain the necessary cofactors. Under the correct conditions, human hepatocytes retain some functionality for many days, express the transcriptional machinery to regulate enzymes, and contain functional proteins for active drug transport across membranes [87]. The utility of hepatocytes for investigation of metabolic stability [88–90] and DDIs mediated by CYP induction [87, 91, 92] is well established. More recently, hepatocytes have been used to describe the impact of reversible [68, 93, 94] and time-dependent CYP inhibition *in vitro* [95, 96]. Primary hepatocytes in culture provide the closest *in vitro* model to human liver and may offer advantages when predicting clinical DDI. Metabolites of one pathway may lead to inhibition of another; this phenomenon is indiscernible using single rCYPs and exemplifies the usefulness of hepatocytes [97].

There is little published comparative data of inhibition constants generated in rCYPs and human hepatocytes. Data generated in this laboratory demonstrates $IC_{50,apparent}$ values generated in human hepatocytes, using probe substrates specific to the CYP isoform, were systematically higher than those determined using the respective rCYP [68]. This was predominantly the result of greater nonspecific binding in hepatocytes compared to rCYPs, as for the majority of compounds tested there was a good concordance between the respective $IC_{50,unbound}$ values (Fig. 22.4a).

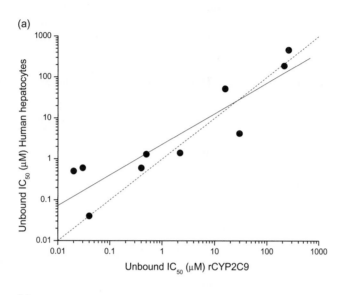

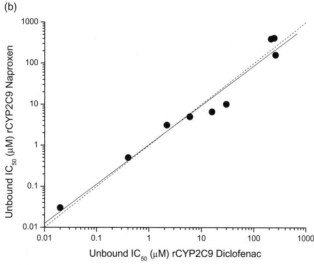

FIGURE 22.4 (a) Relationship between $IC_{50,unbound}$ for CYP2C9 in human hepatocytes and rCYPs. The dotted line is unity. The solid line indicates linear regression of the data ($r^2 = 0.88$, $p < 0.0001$) (b) $IC_{50,unbound}$ comparisons using naproxen and diclofenac as substrates for rCYP2C9. The dotted line is unity. The solid line indicates linear regression of the data ($r^2 = 0.77$, $p < 0.002$). (Part (b) from Ref. 68.)

It can be speculated that the impact of hepatic transporters may explain some discrepancies in $IC_{50,unbound}$ between rCYP and hepatocytes as compound can be actively effluxed from or taken up into the hepatocyte, altering the concentration of drug exposed to the enzyme [97]. Additionally, the impact of time-dependent CYP inhibition in primary cultures of human hepatocytes has been evaluated, again using a cocktail of CYP substrates, which allows the maximum amount of data to be extracted from this limited resource [95]. K_I and k_{inact} values were estimated from nonlinear regression analysis and compared with values obtained from rCYPs and HLMs (Table 22.2). The values generated are also comparable to several literature reports of K_I and k_{inact} estimates using rCYP and HLMs and the results from our laboratory using rCYP, HLMs, and human hepatocytes were consistent with these

TABLE 22.2   Kinetic Parameters of Time-Dependent Inhibitors in Different *In Vitro* Matrices

Compound	CYP Isoform	Enzyme Source	K_I (µM)	k_{inact} (min^{-1})	Reference
Tienilic acid	CYP2C9	rCYP2C9	2	0.19	95
		rCYP2C9 (2C10)	4	0.20	99
		Human hepatocytes	2	0.05	95
AZ1	CYP2C9	rCYP2C9	30	0.02	95
		Human hepatocytes	19	0.02	95
Fluoxetine	CYP2C19	rCYP2C19	0.4	0.5	95
		HLM	8[a] (0.8)	0.03	95
		Human hepatocytes	0.2	0.04	95
	CYP3A4	rCYP3A4	2	0.03	95
		HLM	5[a] (0.5)	0.01	95
		HLM	5[a]	0.02	100
		Human hepatocytes	1	0.01	95
Erythromycin	CYP3A4	rCYP3A4	9	0.12	98
		rCYP3A4	5	0.12	101
		HLM	16[a]	0.07	102
		HLM	82[a]	0.07	103
		HLM	13[a]	0.02	104
		HLM	10[a]	0.08	105
		HLM	11[a]	0.05	106
		HLM	15[a]	0.07	96
		Human hepatocytes	11	0.07	95
Troleandomycin	CYP3A4	rCYP3A4	0.3	0.12	98
		rCYP3A4	0.2	0.15	101
		HLMs	2[a]	0.03	96
		Human hepatocytes	0.4	0.05	95

[a]Apparent K_I values. All other values are *unbound* K_I estimates.

Source: From Ref. 95.

reports. Indeed, the CYP3A4-dependent K_I and k_{inact} values in human hepatocytes are comparable to values determined in rCYP3A4 and HLMs (Table 22.2) when corrected for nonspecific binding in the incubation.

Finally, an element of interlaboratory variability can be expected for different tissue preparations. However, an interlaboratory comparison found the rank order of five HLM preparations was conserved across five laboratories, all using different methodologies, despite differences in absolute values (based on protein content, CYP content, and activity) [107]. Irrespective of the enzyme system used, there are some common factors that must be considered for all *in vitro* inhibition incubations. The assay must be designed such that linear initial rate conditions for the reaction under investigation are assured. To make certain of this, preliminary experiments will be required to ensure product formation is linear with respect to both time and enzyme (protein) concentration [72]. Additionally, protein concentration should be kept as low as reasonably possible to reduce the impact of nonspecific binding [108]. As discussed with respect to hepatocytes and rCYPs, the fraction unbound in the incubation (f_{uinc}) can have a pronounced effect on the apparent K_i, K_I, and IC_{50} determined (Fig. 22.5). This is especially the case for lipophilic inhibitors such as ketoconazole, for which the apparent IC_{50} can vary between 0.005 and 0.3 μM [109]. It is important that such drug binding terms be incorporated by default when making IVIVE to improve the accuracy of *in vitro* data [88], and the importance of considering the fraction unbound in an *in vitro* incubation (f_{uinc}) when relating *in vitro* and *in vivo* data was proposed many years ago by Gillette (1963). The term itself can readily be determined and indeed predicted with accuracy from physiochemical properties [88, 110, 111]. Another important factor is the amount of solvent vehicle, which must be minimized ideally to 1% (or less) of the final incubation volume, as activation or inhibition of CYP activity can be manifest through solvent effects alone (Fig. 22.6). Acetonitrile appears the most favored solvent, having minimal inhibitory effects, despite it being able to activate CYP1A2; although DMSO is commonly used to ensure adequate NCE solubility, it can result in inhibition of metabolism, especially for basic CYP3A4 substrates [88, 112]. Solvent effects

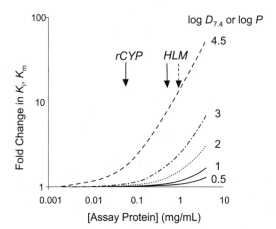

FIGURE 22.5 Simulated effects of microsomal or hepatocyte concentration on K_i or K_m as a function of log P or log $D_{7.4}$-dependent nonspecific binding. (From Ref. 88.)

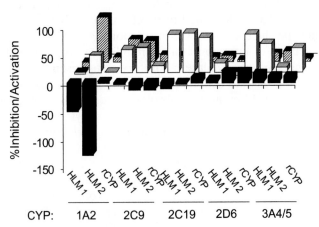

FIGURE 22.6   Overview of potential effects of commonly used organic solvents (1%, v/v) on CYP activities with recombinant proteins and HLMs (solid bars = acetonitrile, open bars = DMSO, hatched bars = methanol). (From Ref. 112.)

can also be selective for probe and enzyme source [113], so it is advisable to check the effects of an alternative solvent for key studies.

22.3.2   Probe Substrate Selection

An important component of *in vitro* inhibition study design is the selection of appropriate probe substrates. Nonselective probes in HLM or human hepatocyte assays can result in hybrid inhibition measurements where multiple enzymes (with varying sensitivity to the inhibitor) can contribute to the reaction under investigation [14]. To avoid such complications, a selective marker substrate is required for each CYP isoform being assessed. These probes should meet the following criteria: possess high affinity for the specific enzyme; be metabolized to a specific product metabolite; provide the ability to detect the product separately from the substrate (using the analytical system of choice); and, finally, the turnover of the probe substrate should be optimized in each enzyme system and be linear with respect to time resulting in less than 20% loss of parent compound to maintain constant reaction velocity throughout the experiment [106, 114]. Industry representatives and regulatory bodies have made recommendations for preferred probe substrates for each CYP isoform (Table 22.3), many of which have the additional benefit of being clinically relevant [117, 120]. These substrates have been rigorously validated for human CYPs [115] and the usefulness and caveats associated with them are well documented [14].

An advantage to the availability of highly selective probes is that, coupled with the improved analytical sensitivity afforded by advances in detection systems such as LC/MS-MS, a cassette of substrates can be used to evaluate the inhibitory potential of a compound upon multiple CYP isoforms in a single incubation. The usefulness of cassette assays derives from increasing the throughput of inhibition screening, although they do require careful optimization and validation to ensure selectivity is maintained [116, 118, 121].

TABLE 22.3 Specific Probe Substrate Reactions for Individual CYP Enzymes

CYP	Substrate	Reaction	Analytical Method	Comments[a]	References
CYP1A2	Phenacetin[b]	O-deethylation	LC/MS-MS	High specificity at <100 μM ($K_m \approx$ 50 μM)	115, 116
	Ethoxyresorufin (EROD)	O-deethylation	Fluorescence	$K_m \approx$ 0.2 μM; not clinically relevant	117
CYP2A6	Caffeine	N3-demethylation	UV-HPL	Low affinity $K_m \approx$ 600 μM	117
	Coumarin	7-Hydroxylation	LC/MS-MS Fluorescence	High specificity $K_m \approx$ 0.5 μM	115, 117
CYP2B6	Bupropion[b]	Hydroxylation	LC/MS-MS	High specificity $K_m \approx$ 90 μM	115, 118
	S-Mephenytoin	N-demethylation	LC/MS-MS	Not CYP2B6 specific $K_m \approx$ 2000 μM (CYP2C9 high affinity $K_m \approx$ 150 μM)	14
CYP2C8	Amodiaquine[b]	N-deethylation	LC/MS-MS	High specificity $K_m \approx$ 2 μM	115, 118
CYP2C9	Diclofenac[b]	4'-Hydroxylation	LC/MS-MS	Good specificity $K_m \approx$ 2 μM (some CYP2C19 $K_m \approx$ 80 μM)	115, 116
	Tolbutamide	Hydroxylation	LC/MS-MS Radiometric	$K_m \approx$ 200 μM (some CYP2C19 $K_m \approx$ 500 μM)	115, 119
CYP2C19	S-Mephenytoin[b]	4'-Hydroxylation	LC/MS-MS	High specificity $K_m \approx$ 40 μM	115, 116
CYP2D6	Bufuralol[b]	1-Hydroxylation	LC/MS-MS	High affinity component for CYP2D6 $K_m \approx$ 5 μM (CYP2C19 and CYP2C9 at high concentrations)	116
	Dextromethorphan	O-demethylation	LC/MS-MS	Questionable specificity $K_m \approx$ 700 μM	115
CYP2E1	Chlorzoxazone	7-Hydroxylation	LC/MS-MS		115, 117
CYP3A4	Midazolam[b]	1'-Hydroxylation	LC/MS-MS	High specificity benzodiazepine $K_m \approx$ 3 μM	56, 115, 116
	Testosterone	6β-Hydroxylation	UV-HPLC Radiometric	High specificity steroid $K_m \approx$ 50 μM	56, 115, 117
	Nifedipine	Oxidations	UV-HPLC	High specificity dihydropyridine $K_m \approx$ 50 μM	87

[a]Comments from Ref. 14.
[b]Primary Substrate used in this laboratory.

An additional aspect to be considered for *in vitro* assays is that CYP inhibition can be substrate dependent, particularly for CYP3A4 [122]. CYP3A4 is thought to bind substrates and inhibitors in multiple modes and/or binding sites [66, 123]. As a result, inhibitory interactions observed with one probe substrate may not be representative of those observed with other substrates [19]. This is due to the cooperative nature of substrate–inhibitor interactions within the active site [124]. Kenworthy et al. [122] classified 10 CYP3A4 substrates into three distinct groups: a benzodiazepine group (including diazepam, midazolam, triazolam, and dextromethorphan), a large molecular weight group (including testosterone, erythromycin, and cyclosporine), and finally nifedipine and benzyloxyresorufin (BROD), which fit in neither of the previous groups and are distinct from each other. These substrate groups were classified according to analysis of their behavior as probe reactions for the effect of 34 compounds on CYP3A4 mediated metabolism, with different inhibitor profiles being observed with different substrate groups. For example, the IC_{50} for inhibition of CYP3A4 mediated nifedipine oxidation by haloperidol was $0.1\,\mu M$, while for dextromethorphan N-demethylation it was $>100\,\mu M$ [122]. It is postulated that haloperidol is able to inhibit CYP3A4 by binding at more than one site, with the effect being dependent on the substrate, reflecting the cooperative nature of CYP3A4.

There is also increasing evidence that similar multisite kinetics and substrate-dependent interactions are observed for CYP2C9 *in vitro* [67–69]. Therefore, while there is little evidence of auto-/heteroactivation *in vivo* in humans [69, 70, 125], it is good practice to evaluate the inhibitory potential of NCEs against CYP3A4 and CYP2C9 using at least two structurally dissimilar probe substrates, to afford a better predictive quality to the *in vitro* data as *in vivo* effects can be substrate dependent. In our laboratory, routine screens are conducted with drug-like probes for both CYP3A4 (midazolam) and CYP2C9 (diclofenac); for key compounds, a second and potentially a third probe is used to fully evaluate inhibition of these isoforms, for example, erythromycin and naproxen for CYP3A4 and CYP2C9, respectively. Figure 22.4b shows the effect of using either diclofenac or naproxen as probe substrate to measure the IC_{50} for a range of compounds demonstrating CYP2C9 inhibition. On average, it was found that the $IC_{50,apparent}$ generated in an assay using naproxen as a substrate could be approximately 1.5-fold times that using diclofenac. This could be corrected from a consideration of $IC_{50,unbound}$ [68] (see Fig. 22.4b).

22.3.3   Analysis Methods

Several analytical methods are available for determining the impact of inhibition on a probe substrate. The selection of an analytical endpoint depends on the probe under investigation, the availability of the detection system, and the throughput required. LC/MS-MS is probably the system of choice for the pharmaceutical industry due to the selectivity and sensitivity it affords [115, 126]. This, combined with the fact that LC/MS-MS is the backbone of analysis within DMPK laboratories and therefore readily available, has driven its increased use in CYP inhibition assays. There are several LC/MS-MS methods that enable routine analysis of metabolites generated in microsomal and rCYP incubations, and importantly LC/MS-MS facilitates the use of clinically relevant probes. Additionally, the sensitivity afforded by LC/MS-MS has allowed multiple reaction monitoring of substrate cassettes, facilitating the investigation of test inhibitors for multiple CYP isoforms [20, 116, 121]. In our laboratory we routinely screen for CYP inhibition using a substrate cassette and a rCYP cocktail; the details of this and other assays used are shown in Table 22.4.

An alternative to LC/MS-MS is HPLC-radioflow. This allows separation of metabolites of ^{14}C or ^{3}H labeled probe substrates. It is, however, a time-consuming technique requiring meticulous optimization of conditions and long run times, and LC/MS-MS is a more rapid alternative [115, 116, 118, 126]. A higher throughput radiometric endpoint assay is available and is flexible, sensitive, robust, and free from analytical interference [119, 127]. This laboratory uses a range of automated assays with [*O*- or *N*-methyl-^{14}C]-substrates, which liberate [^{14}C]-formaldehyde as the product of enzyme-specific oxidative demethylation [119]. However, the extra considerations involved with the use of radioactivity, such as the highly regulated disposal of isotopes and additional safety requirements, does constrain their use perhaps to second substrate selection.

Fluorometric assays are commonly used for CYP inhibition studies, especially in early drug discovery, as their speed and cost advantages lend them to enhanced throughput (compared to detailed manual assays) or true HTS (miniaturized assays employing robotics to utilize 96-, 384-, or 1536-well plate formats with rapid endpoints). Indeed, they are widely used throughout the pharmaceutical industry. Fluorescent-based assays are very amenable to multiwell plate assays; but despite their utility in rapidly generating large sets of inhibition data there are drawbacks. There can be fluorescent interference from the test compound or its product and issues with fluorescent quenching as well as lack of probe molecule specificity for an individual CYP [20]. The nonselective nature of fluorescent probes can, of course, be overcome by the use of single rCYPs. A potential concern for these assays is the non-drug-like qualities of most fluorescent probes, particularly in terms of clinically relevant CYP interactions. A detailed study evaluating inhibition data generated using fluorescent probes compared to that of conventional drug probes suggested that in general only a weak correlation between the two endpoints existed, with both endpoints not detecting inhibition by a significant number of compounds [19, 88]. Cohen et al. [19] suggest that concerns over fluorogenic probes not resembling drug molecules are unfounded and that it is the architecture of the CYP active site, permitting binding of structurally diverse molecules, that underlies interprobe differences in IC_{50} values, be they fluorescent or not. In our laboratory, fluorometric assays have been widely replaced by LC/MS-MS-based assays but are still used as an alternative substrate assay to cross-check inhibition data for CYP3A4 and CYP2C9, as it is prudent to assess inhibition in detailed studies using multiple probes and alternative endpoints as least for these enzymes.

Finally, luminescence-based CYP selective probes have recently become commercially available, such as those used in the Promega P450-Glo™ assays. These assays provide a luminescent method for measuring CYP activity from recombinant and native sources. A conventional CYP reaction is performed by incubating the CYP with a luminogenic CYP substrate and NADPH regeneration system. The substrates in the P450-Glo assays are derivatives of beetle luciferin ((4*S*)-4,5-dihydro-2-(6-hydroxybenzothiazolyl)-4-thiazolecarboxylic acid) and are substrates for CYP but not luciferase. The derivatives are converted by CYP to a luciferin product that is detected in a second reaction with a luciferin detection reagent. The amount of light produced in the second reaction is directly proportional to the activity of the CYP (http://www.promega.com). Such assays lend themselves to true

TABLE 22.4 Assay Conditions Used for IC$_{50}$ Generation in the Authors' Laboratory Utilizing Fluorescent or Radiometric Endpoints and a Single rCYP Isoform and LC/MS-MS Endpoint with a Cocktail of rCYPs and Cassette of Substrates[a]

Isoform	Substrate	Final [Substrate] (µM)	[CYP] (pmol/mL)	Incubation Time (min)	Endpoint	Vehicle (1% v/v)	Inhibitor (IC$_{50}$; µM)
CYP1A2	Ethoxyresorufin	0.7	17	15	λ_{ex} 530 nm; λ_{em} 590 nm	DMSO	Fluvoxamine (0.17)
CYP2C9	7-Methoxy-4-(trifluoromethyl)coumarin	50	50	20	λ_{ex} 410 nm; λ_{em} 535 nm	DMSO	Sulfaphenazole (0.3)
CYP2C19	7-Methoxy-4-(trifluoromethyl)coumarin	50	57	20	λ_{ex} 405 nm; λ_{em} 535 nm	MeCN	Omeprazole (3)
CYP2D6	3-[2-(N,N-diethyl-N-methylammonium)ethyl]-7-methoxy-4-methlycoumarin	10	56	15	λ_{ex} 530 nm; λ_{em} 590 nm	DMSO	Quinidine (0.060)
CYP3A4	7-Benzyloxy-4-(trifluoromethyl)coumarin	10	9	15	λ_{ex} 405 nm; λ_{em} 535 nm	MeOH /MeCN	Ketoconazole (0.007)
CYP2C9	Naproxen	109	70	15	Liquid scintillation counting	DMSO	Sufaphenazole (0.45)
CYP2C19	Diazepam	21	40	15	Liquid scintillation counting	DMSO	Omeprazole (3)
CYP2D6	Dextromethorphan	5	20	15	Liquid scintillation counting	DMSO	Quinidine (0.025)
CYP3A4	Erythromycin	19	25	10	Liquid scintillation counting	DMSO	Ketoconazole (0.035)
5 CYP cocktail	1A2–Phenacetin	26	15	10	LC/MS-MS	DMSO	α-Naphthoflavone(0.014)
	2C9–Diclofenac	2	5				Sulfaphenazole (0.26)
	2C19–S-mephenytoin	31	3				Tranylcypromine (3.60)
	2D6–Bufurolol	9	5				Quinidine (0.018)
	3A4–Midazolam	3	5				Ketoconazole (0.0036)
			Total 33				
3 CYP cocktail	2B6–Bupropion	20	18	10	LC/MS-MS	DMSO	Ticlopidine (0.55)
	2C8–Amodiaquine	2	1				Quercetin (5.12)
	3A5–Midazolam	2	5				Ketoconazole (0.17)
			Total 24				

[a]See Refs. 116, 118, and 119. Data is mean *n* > 50.

TABLE 22.5   Some Considerations in the Selection of CYP Assay Endpoints

Consideration	Assay Type			
	Radiolabeled	Fluorescent	LC/MS-MS	Luminescent
Cost	++	+++	+	++
Throughput	+	+++	++	HTS
Accessibility	++	++	+	++
Interference	+++	+	++	+
Health and safety	+	+++	+++	+++
Published information	++	+++	+++	+
Marketed drug substrates	++	—	+++	—

HTS capabilities, providing quick readouts on multiple well plates. Table 22.5 shows a comparison of LC/MS-MS, fluorometric, radiometric, and luminescent endpoints to aid consideration of assay choice.

Using fluorescent or luminescent assays for enhanced/HTS and rapid generation of IC_{50} data may be invaluable for the development of structure–activity relationships (SARs) for the different CYPs [69, 128]. The utility of high throughput CYP inhibition screens has allowed generation of large datasets, facilitating development of statistical *in silico* approaches. To this end, quantitative *in silico* models now exist for prominent CYPs, often based on physical-chemical properties alone. These models can classify compounds as "noninhibitors" with reasonable accuracy (~80% of compounds were classified correctly for CYP3A4 and CYP2D6 [128]) and can guide medicinal chemistry away from CYP interactions at early stages of drug discovery programs [128, 129]. In theory, these *in silico* models allow predictions of inhibitory potency to be made even before a compound has been synthesized [129].

22.4   GENERATION OF *IN VITRO* CYTOCHROME P450 INHIBITION DATA

Fundamentally, *in vitro* kinetic data must be accurate, meaningful, and relevant. As discussed previously, all assays should be preoptimized for time and protein linearity to ensure the reaction proceeds under linear conditions. The objective is to determine K_i for predicting the likelihood and extent of DDIs. Experimentally, this is achieved by either defining the IC_{50} or by directly determining a K_i. From Eqs. 22.4 and 22.7, it is clear that if $[S] = K_m$, the K_i can be estimated to within twofold from an accurate IC_{50} determination. This may well be less than the error in determining K_i by an extensive (and laborious) fully inhibited Michaelis–Menten study. Furthermore, the mechanism of inhibition must be defined and, if irreversible, generation of K_I and k_{inact} is required for accurate assessment of DDIs.

When generating *in vitro* inhibition data, particularly when evaluating the propensity of NCEs to behave as CYP inhibitors, it is important to include the appropriate positive controls. To this end, known inhibitors should be included in any incubations as markers, and it has been suggested that K_i or IC_{50} values generated for these standard inhibitors should fall within threefold of the median literature value for an assay to be deemed acceptable [130].

22.4.1 Reversible Inhibition (IC$_{50}$ and K_i)

An IC$_{50}$ is generated using a single concentration of substrate. Inhibitor concentrations should cover at least two log units (e.g., 0, 0.1, 0.3, 1, 3, 10 μM) to ensure a range of measurements from negligible to virtually complete inhibition. The percentage of total enzyme activity remaining (from control incubations) is plotted against log inhibitor concentration [I] to generate an IC$_{50}$ curve. Plotting log [I] results in more accurate confidence intervals when using nonlinear regression, as the data is equally spaced on a log axis, allowing symmetrical confidence intervals to be calculated. In the authors' laboratory, an automated assay to determine IC$_{50}$ is adopted; K_i is estimated to be half the IC$_{50}$ (as [S] = K_m). The automated assay utilizes a pool of recombinant CYPs (CYP1A2, CYP2C9, CYP2C19, CYP2D6, and CYP3A4) to minimize nonspecific binding in the incubation, at protein concentrations and incubation times designed to ensure the selective metabolism of a substrate cassette at concentrations equivalent to the K_m (phenacetin, diclofenac, *S*-mephenytoin, bufuralol, and midazolam, respectively). LC/MS-MS analysis of specific metabolite formation allows comparison of peak area in the presence of increasing concentration of test inhibitor against a DMSO control. Recently, an additional assay was developed for CYP2B6, CYP2C8, and CYP3A5 due to the emerging importance of these enzymes [118]. This second automated assay again uses a pool of rCYPs and a substrate cassette of bupropion, amodiaquine, and midazolam, respectively. Table 22.4 shows the reaction conditions for these assays.

An alternative approach is to experimentally define the inhibition constant K_i. To do this accurately, the inhibitor concentration should span a range around the suspected K_i (based on a prior IC$_{50}$ estimation) using at least five concentrations, for example, $0K_i$, $0.3K_i$, K_i, $3K_i$, and $10K_i$. Typically, 8–10 substrate concentrations should be used to investigate each concentration of inhibitor and these should span from $K_m/3$ to $3K_m$. The range of substrate concentration needs to be expanded for increased inhibitor concentrations, since the K_m shifts up when the substrate's metabolism is competitively inhibited. K_i determinations therefore require large numbers of incubations, as all parts of the velocity–substrate concentration profile need to be defined for each inhibitor concentration. Accurate determinations of any one of the parameters (K_m, V_{max}, K_i) depends on accurate determination of all three.

Once generated, the data can be visually inspected for the mechanism of inhibition; this is commonly achieved using two types of graphical representation—the Eadie–Hofstee plot (v against v/[S]) and the Dixon plot ($1/v$ against [I]). The type of inhibition can be determined from the shape of the linearized data and examples of these plots for each type of reversible inhibition are shown in Fig. 22.7. Kinetic parameters should never be determined from linear transforms such as these as doing so generally leads to inaccurate estimation of K_i (the two-dimensional nature of the data fit does not fully describe the effect of changing inhibitor concentrations on different concentrations of substrate). The plots are solely for the purpose of aiding interpretation of the inhibition type. Consequently, nonlinear regression software is an absolute requirement to facilitate iterative modeling of changing sub-

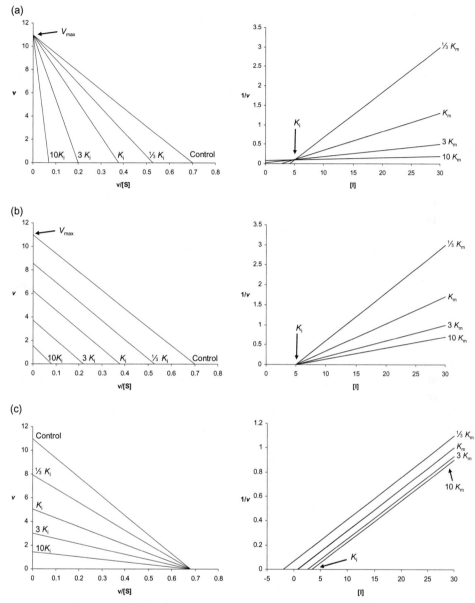

FIGURE 22.7   Graphical representation of inhibition plots: Eadie–Hofstee plots (v against v/[S] on the left) and Dixon plots ($1/v$ against [I] on the right) for (a) competitive inhibition, (b) noncompetitive inhibition, (c) and uncompetitive inhibition.

strate and inhibitor concentrations, fitting the untransformed data to the appropriate rate equation (for competitive, noncompetitive, or uncompetitive inhibition, Eqs. 22.3, 22.5, and 22.6, respectively). In practice, this means nonlinear regression modeling of all the substrate concentration, velocity, and inhibitor concentration data simultaneously using the equation for competitive inhibition (Eq. 22.3). The data should be weighted by $1/y$, to compensate for unequal experimental variance in the different experimental points. (Velocity–substrate concentration plots tend to have a constant relative error associated such that the residual—the difference between predicted and observed velocity—will be larger at higher reaction velocities. This is true because the error is the same at low and high velocities, giving rise to larger standard deviations from the mean observed velocity at higher velocities.) The same dataset should then be reanalyzed using the equation for noncompetitive inhibition (Eq. 22.5). The two mathematical models can then be discriminated by evaluation of "goodness-of-fit" criteria. For a full explanation, see Mannervik [131]. Generally, goodness-of-fit criteria (e.g., Akaike values) and accuracy of parameter estimates (standard deviation and coefficient of variance) should be compared for both models and the most appropriate model (type of inhibition) chosen.

22.4.2   Mechanism-Based Inhibition (K_I, k_{inact}, and IC_{50})

True irreversible inhibition or mechanism-based inhibition (MBI) of CYPs can only be defined according to the criteria detailed previously and may be established by mechanistic studies such as dialysis of the inhibited CYP or spectral shifts in absorbance [100]. MBI is not readily detected in standard *in vitro* assay formats. Time-dependent inhibition (TDI) is a collective term for a change in potency of CYP inhibitors during an *in vitro* incubation or dosing period *in vivo*. Such changes usually result in an increase in inhibitory potency; potential mechanisms include the formation of more inhibitory metabolites and MBI. In the following assays, it is the time-, concentration-, and/or NADPH-dependent nature of the inhibition under investigation.

In essence, an assay to detect TDI involves a preincubation step, where enzyme is incubated with and without NADPH and in the presence of varying inhibitor concentrations. This reaction is allowed to proceed over a predetermined time course, before dilution of the reaction mixture into a second incubation that includes a probe substrate to assess the degree of enzyme inactivation [77]. To accurately define the inhibitory constants of TDI, the conditions governing the two separate incubations must be carefully chosen. A useful critical evaluation of experimental design, methodology, and data analysis for TDI protocols in published literature highlighted not only the variation between laboratories but the subsequent impact on the predicted effects of TDI *in vivo* if the *in vitro* kinetic parameters are incorrectly defined [79].

The experimental design of a TDI assay must adhere to the same conditions as those for reversible inhibition (linear enzyme reactions, etc.) and protocols have to be adjusted to correctly define the kinetics of different inhibitors. These adjustments are dependent on the potency of the inhibitor under investigation, as potent inhibitors require considerably shorter preincubation times than weaker inhibitors [75, 79]. To this end, the time course of the pre-incubation must be such that the inhibition at each concentration of inhibitor is linear with respect to time—at least over the initial preincubation period. Allowing the preincubation reaction to proceed over a large time course with multiple dilution points into the second assay (0, 0.5, 1, 2, 3, 5, 10, 20, and 30 min) should gauge this; however, this is not necessarily practical due to the large reaction volume required in the preincubation to sustain multiple dilution points. In practice, two separate assays may have to be conducted: an initial assessment where preincubation occurs over an intermediate time course (such as 5, 10, and 20 min), and a second assay where times are adjusted for more accurate definition of the inhibition profile (based on inspection of the data generated in the initial assessment). In addition to this, it is vital to ensure all the CYP inactivation occurs in this preincubation, to allow accurate measurement of inhibited enzyme with respect to incubation time, without concurrent inhibition and probe substrate metabolism in the second incubation. To this end, the dilution of the preincubation reaction mixture into the second incubation should be as large as possible (in general, 10–50-fold) while still guaranteeing analytical sensitivity for the probe substrate metabolite. Additionally, the concentration of CYP selective substrate in the final incubation should be high relative to its K_m (in general, 5–10-fold), again to minimize further CYP inactivation after the preincubation step, and the final incubation time should be minimized. Finally, since the enzyme can undergo some inactivation in the absence of inhibitor, the enzyme activity remaining following each preincubation time point should be determined by comparison to control (enzyme incubated without inhibitor). In the authors' laboratory, two automated assays with an LC/MS-MS endpoint are used to assess TDI potential [98] and have been modified to allow detection of weaker time-dependent inhibitors [75]. An initial screen generates an IC_{50} value using HLMs and a cassette of CYP specific probe substrates. A single inhibitor concentration is tested using a single preincubation time of 30 min and a 20-fold dilution. If inhibition is detected in this IC_{50} assay, a second assay is then used to generate values for K_I and k_{inact} from rCYPs. This assay adheres to the strict criteria detailed earlier in order to accurately define the kinetic parameters. Five preincubation times (up to 23 min) are used with six inhibitor concentrations and a dilution factor of 20-fold. There is a good correlation between k_{inact}/K_I ratio (a measure of inhibitory efficiency) generated in rCYP and the IC_{50} from the HLM assay, thus allowing NCE evaluation from a reasonable throughput assay [98] (see Fig. 22.8).

The analysis of data generated in TDI assays must be carefully conducted. First, the natural log of the percent control activity remaining is plotted against time. The slope of the linear portion for each inhibitor concentration is equivalent to the inactivation rate constant, k (or k_{obs}). Graphical representations of these plots are shown in Fig. 22.9. Using nonlinear regression, this data can be fitted to Eq. 22.13 to estimate k_{inact} and K_I. A common fault is to use linear Kitz–Wilson plots rather than nonlinear regression, as two-dimensional fitting of the data cannot yield accurate estimations for k_{inact} and K_I. [79]. It is also worth noting that if all the CYP inactivation occurs in the preincubation step, the point where the log-linear fits of each inhibitor concentration cross the y axis (time = 0) represents the reversible inhibition component. However, if the dilution of the preincubation is not sufficient, considerable reversible inhibition may occur during the second incubation, making data interpretation more problematic [98].

Finally, an additional utility of a TDI screen in drug discovery may be as a "flag" for reactive metabolite formation. Electrophilic species are often generated during CYP MBI and there is a high chance that these may escape from the CYP active site and react elsewhere in the body, either via detoxification processes (glutathione deactivation) or more worryingly via reaction with proteins or nucleic acids. It is not at all surprising that the same chemical groups implicated in reactive metabolite formation are also known to inhibit CYPs irreversibly [75]. Perhaps linked to this,

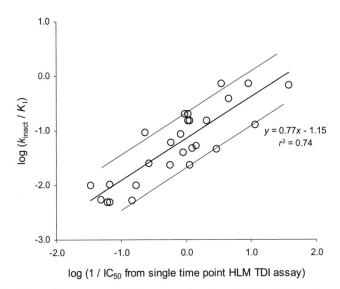

$$y = 0.77x - 1.15$$
$$r^2 = 0.74$$

log (1 / IC$_{50}$ from single time point HLM TDI assay)

FIGURE 22.8   Plot of log unbound IC$_{50}$ against log (k_{inact}/K_I) for 28 time-dependent inhibitors of CYP3A4. IC$_{50}$ values were generated using the automated single time point, single inhibitor concentration human liver microsomal time-dependent inhibition screen [98]. These values were adjusted for incubational binding to give unbound IC$_{50}$ values (according to the mathematical model of Austin et al. [111]). K_I and k_{inact} were estimated using the 3 time point, 6 inhibitor concentration, recombinant CYP automated time-dependent inhibition assay. The solid line is the line of best fit, with dashed lines representing threefold deviation from the line. (From Ref. 98.)

it is found that many drugs exhibiting TDI are also associated with adverse drug reactions (e.g., erythromycin, diclofenac, tacrine, valproic acid, halothane, suprofen, ticlopidine, tienilic acid, isoniazid, zileuton) [132, 133]. Using TDI screening, alongside cold trapping and/or radiolabeled binding studies, may be advantageous in minimizing the potential for reactive metabolite formation as early as possible in a drug discovery screening cascade.

22.5   *IN VITRO–IN VIVO* EXTRAPOLATION OF CYTOCHROME P450 BASED DRUG–DRUG INTERACTIONS

The clinical implications of DDIs and the importance of generating accurate *in vitro* data have been discussed; from this it follows that IVIVE requires careful data handling using the approach outlined below to generate predictions of clinical impact. Over the last 10–15 years, predicting the extent of DDI in a semiquantitative way has been the subject of many publications and the most effective models are presented here.

22.5.1   Approach for Reversible Inhibitors

If the metabolism of a drug is reversibly inhibited, the magnitude of the effect will be $1 + [I]/K_i$ (sometimes termed the inhibition index, I_i), provided that the concen-

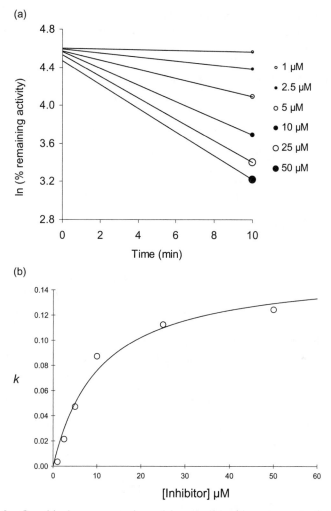

FIGURE 22.9 Graphical representation of irreversible (time-dependent) inhibition. (a) Inhibition of control activity against time for increasing inhibitor concentration; and (b) nonlinear regression of k against inhibitor concentration giving k_{inact} of $0.16\,min^{-1}$ and K_I of $10.6\,\mu M$ (circles are observed data points and line is predicted data fit).

tration of substrate undergoing inhibition is well below its K_m value and that it is eliminated by the single pathway being inhibited [134]. This is because the magnitude of effect is dependent not only on how much affinity the inhibitor has for the enzyme (K_i) but also on the concentration of inhibitor available. For competitive inhibition, the K_m of the victim drug will be increased to $K_m + K_m\,[I]/K_i$ (or $K_m(1 + [I]/K_i)$) and therefore the intrinsic clearance (CL_{int}) (as $CL_{int} = V_{max}/K_m$) will be decreased to $V_{max}/(K_m(1 + [I]/K_i)$ or $CL_{int}/(1 + [I]/K_i)$.

For an IV administered victim drug, the following is true:

$$CL = Dose/AUC \tag{22.14}$$

$$CL/CL' = AUC'/AUC \tag{22.15}$$

where CL is the *in vivo* clearance in the absence and CL' in the presence of inhibitor, respectively, and AUC is area under the plasma–concentration time curve in the absence and AUC' in the presence of inhibitor', respectively.

$$\frac{AUC'}{AUC} = \frac{Q_h \cdot CL_{int} \cdot f_{ub}}{Q_h + CL_{int} \cdot f_{ub}} \cdot \frac{Q_h + CL'_{int} \cdot f_{ub} \cdot 1/I_i}{Q_h \cdot CL'_{int} \cdot f_{ub} \cdot I_i} \tag{22.16}$$

$$= \frac{Q_h^2 \cdot CL_{int} \cdot f_{ub} + Q_h^2 \cdot CL_{int} \cdot f_{ub} \cdot 1/I_i \cdot CL_{int} \cdot f_{ub}}{Q_h^2 \cdot f_{ub} \cdot CL_{int} \cdot 1/I_i + Q_h^2 \cdot f_{ub} \cdot CL_{int} \cdot f_{ub} \cdot CL_{int} \cdot 1/I_i} \tag{22.17}$$

$$= \frac{Q_h + (f_{ub} \cdot CL_{int})/I_i}{Q_h/I_i + (f_{ub} \cdot CL_{int})/I_i} \tag{22.18}$$

$$\frac{AUC'}{AUC} = \frac{Q_h \cdot I_i + f_{ub} \cdot CL_{int}}{Q_h + f_{ub} \cdot CL_{int}} \tag{22.19}$$

where Q_h is hepatic blood flow and I_i is the inhibition index $1 + [I]/K_i$. If $f_{ub} \cdot CL_{int} \ll Q_h$, there is a high inhibitory effect and the AUC ratio approximates to I_i $(1 + [I]/K_i)$. If $f_{ub} \cdot CL_{int} \gg Q_h$, there is little effect since the AUC ratio approximates to 1.

For an orally administered victim drug, the fraction escaping hepatic first-pass extraction in the presence (F') or absence (F) of inhibitor is

$$\frac{F'}{F} = \frac{1 - CL'_h/Q_h}{1 - CL_h/Q_h} \tag{22.20}$$

Rearranging the well stirred model [135],

$$CL_{int} = \frac{CL_h}{f_{ub}(1 - CL_h/Q_h)} \tag{22.21}$$

$$= \frac{CL_h}{F \cdot f_{ub}} \tag{22.22}$$

It follows that

$$F = \frac{CL_h}{CL_{int} \cdot f_{ub}} \tag{22.23}$$

Therefore,

$$F = \frac{CL_{int} \cdot f_{ub} \cdot Q_h}{CL_{int} \cdot f_{ub} + Q_h} \cdot \frac{1}{CL_{int} \cdot f_{ub}} \tag{22.24}$$

$$= \frac{Q_h}{CL_{int} \cdot f_{ub} + Q_h} \tag{22.25}$$

Putting this back into Eq. 22.20, we find

$$\frac{F'}{F} = \frac{Q_h}{CL_{int} \cdot f_{ub}/I_i + Q_h} \cdot \frac{CL_{int} \cdot f_{ub} + Q_h}{Q_h} \tag{22.26}$$

$$\frac{F'}{F} = \frac{CL_{int} \cdot f_{ub} + Q_h}{(CL_{int} \cdot f_{ub}/I_i) + Q_h} \tag{22.27}$$

So, when $f_{ub} \cdot CL_{int} \ll Q_h$, there is little inhibitor effect since the ratio of the fraction escaping first pass is approximately 1. When $f_{ub} \cdot CL_{int} \gg Q_h$, the ratio of the fraction escaping first pass in the presence and absence of inhibitor approximates to $1 + [I]/K_i$.

It is recognized as a "rule of thumb" that inhibitors with $[I]/K_i < 0.1$ represent a low DDI risk, those with $[I]/K_i$ between 0.1 and 1 are moderate risk, and those with $[I]/K_i > 1$ are high risk. The relationship between the AUC ratio and $[I]/K_i$ ratio is depicted in Fig. 22.10 and is the most simple model of CYP inhibition [80, 130, 136, 137]. A more detailed approach, that is, the fundamental basis of most IVIVE for CYP inhibition, expands on the inhibition index $(1 + [I]/K_i)$ by including the relative metabolic contribution (*fm*) of each inhibited CYP to the *in vivo* metabolism of the substrate under investigation:

$$\frac{AUC'}{AUC} = \frac{1}{\dfrac{fm_{CYP}}{1+[I]/K_i} + (1 - fm_{CYP})} \tag{22.28}$$

The impact of *fm* on the magnitude of inhibition can be visualized in Fig. 22.11 [56, 68, 138]. From this plot it is clear that *fm* > 0.5 is required for inhibition to generate significant increases in AUC and that predictions are very sensitive to the *fm* used when it approaches 1. Within a population, *fm* will vary and individuals most at risk

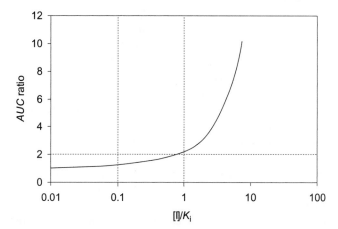

FIGURE 22.10 Qualitative zoning of the prediction of the magnitude and risk of drug–drug interactions mediated by reversible inhibition (AUC ratio) using $[I]/K_i$ ratio. Low risk, <0.1; medium risk, 0.1–1; high risk, >1.

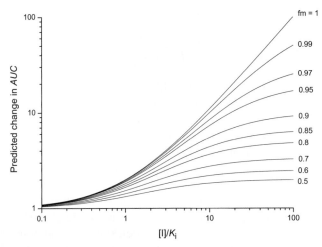

FIGURE 22.11   Simulation of predicted change in *AUC* as a function of $[I]/K_i$ with different *fm* values. The simulation is based on Eq. 22.28, where *fm* is the fraction of substrate clearance mediated by the inhibited metabolic pathway. (Adapted from Ref. 98.)

of DDI will be those with the highest *fm*. The model can be expanded further to include inhibition of multiple CYP isoforms and the effect of each contribution to overall clearance of the victim drug and other routes of elimination need to be considered [136, 138].

The choice of which [I] to use in these predictions has been a source of much debate in the literature [7, 13, 80, 88, 139, 140]. Classical pharmacology states that only the unbound fraction of a drug is able to cross membranes and interact with a target protein; from this it follows that a drug associated with proteins in the plasma or tissue is unavailable for interaction. It follows that the use of unbound drug concentrations and inhibition constants should be the starting point in IVIVE and doing so can give good predictions when other relevant factors are included [88]. Changes in the unbound fraction of a drug in the blood (f_{ub}) is in itself a potential mechanism of DDI; f_{ub} is increased when one drug is displaced by other drugs at the site of plasma protein binding. These interactions rarely cause serious clinical problems [7, 141]. However, despite the rationale for using corrections of unbound drug concentrations to predict clearance [108, 142], the use of drug binding terms in predictive IVIVE models remains controversial [13, 88, 97, 139].

Across the spectrum of literature on the subject, inconsistencies in the use of drug binding terms and the choice of *in vivo* inhibitor concentration may have clouded the general understanding and inadvertently reduced confidence in IVIVE for anything other than *qualitative* DDI predictions (average steady plasma concentration, $[I]_{av}$, peak steady-state plasma concentration, $[I]_{max}$, maximum hepatic input concentration $[I]_{in}$; see Table 22.6) [7, 13, 80, 144]. The suggestion that total blood concentrations can be used with unbound *in vitro* K_i values to achieve good predictivity is less than helpful, since it leaves the reader potentially unsure as to the impact of blood binding *in vivo*. Binding to blood components may not reach equilibrium during the short time period in the portal vein, leading to a greater free-drug concentration than may be predicted and underestimation of DDI [136]. However,

TABLE 22.6 Choice of *In Vivo* Inhibitor Concentration Advocated in the Literature in Recent Years

Which [I]	K_i Adjusted for f_{uinc}?	Equation	Author Comments	References
Maximum *unbound* hepatic input concentration, $[I]_{in}$, where [I] is $[I] \cdot f_{ub}$	No	$[I]_{av} = \dfrac{D/\tau}{CL/F}$ $[I]_{in} = [I]_{av} + \dfrac{k_a \cdot F_a \cdot D}{Q_h}$	The incidence of false-negative predictions was largest using $[I_{av}]$ for unbound drug concentration and smallest using $[I_{in}]$ for total drug concentration for each of the CYP enzymes. The use of $[I_{in}]$ is recommended because true negatives can be identified and, in contrast to the use of other [I] values, false negatives eliminated.	137
Maximum *total* hepatic input concentration, $[I]_{in}$	No	$[I]_{in} = [I]_{av} + \dfrac{k_a \cdot F_a \cdot D}{Q_h}$	True negatives can be identified and, in contrast to the use of other values for [I], false negatives are eliminated. True positives are also predicted well and, although the incidence of false-positive predictions is quite high, the use of hepatic input concentration is recommended.	80
Maximum *total* hepatic input concentration $[I]_{in}$	No	$[I]_{in} = [I]_{av} + \dfrac{k_a \cdot F_a \cdot D}{Q_h}$	The use of $[I]_{in}$ incorporating both fm_{CYP} and refined k_a values resulted in the most successful prediction overall.	143
Average *total* steady plasma concentration, $[I]_{av}$, or maximum *total* hepatic input concentration, $[I]_{in}$	Yes	$[I]_{in} = [I]_{av} + \dfrac{k_a \cdot F_a \cdot D}{Q_h}$ $[I]_{av} = \dfrac{D/\tau}{CL/F}$	Either the average systemic plasma concentration after repeated oral administration ($[I]_{av}$) or the maximum hepatic input concentration ($[I]_{in}$)	56
Average *total* steady plasma concentration, $[I]_{av}$	Yes	$[I]_{av} = \dfrac{D/\tau}{CL/F}$	The use of $[I]_{av}$ as the [I] surrogate generated the most successful predictions as judged by several criteria. Using $[I]_{av}$ incorporation of either plasma protein binding of inhibitor or gut wall CYP3A4 inhibition did not result in a general improvement of DDI predictions.	13
Maximum *unbound* hepatic input concentration, $[I]_{in,u}$, where [I] is $[I] \cdot f_{ub}$	Yes ([protein] low so f_{uinc} assumed negligible)	$[I]_{in} = [I]_{av} + \dfrac{k_a \cdot F_a \cdot D}{Q_h}$	The use of estimated unbound hepatic inlet C_{max} during the absorptive phase yielded the most accurate predictions of the magnitudes of DDI.	139

the "free-drug" theory should be regarded as the default situation and if successful predictions cannot be made, the reason(s) should be sought.

Equation 22.29 shows the maximum hepatic input of inhibitor (the sum of the contribution from the systemic circulation and the absorption phase; $[I]_{in}$) calculated using the absorption rate constant (k_a), the fraction absorbed (F_a), and dose [7].

$$[I]_{in} = [I]_{av} + (k_a \cdot F_a \cdot \text{Dose})/Q_h) \qquad (22.29)$$

Often it is assumed that the rate of absorption is instantaneous (approaching $0.1\,\text{min}^{-1}$); however, changes in k_a can account for marked differences in $[I]_{in}$ and the value chosen should be carefully considered [143].

In the authors' laboratory, good predictions have been made using unbound maximum hepatic concentration $[I]_{in,u}$ along with correction of K_i for binding in the incubation (f_{uinc}) [88]. Using a published dataset of clinical DDIs [80], an 84% success rate was achieved for prediction of DDI at CYP3A4 and a 91% success rate predicting CYP2D6 interactions (Fig. 22.12) [88]. There were some noticeable outliers in the dataset, however; these highlighted that subtle changes in some parameters (e.g., plasma protein values for a highly bound drug) can result in large discrepancies in calculated unbound concentration and that measured *AUC* changes for drugs with low oral bioavailability are subject to large errors. Additionally, it was apparent that the impact of the $[I]/K_i$ estimate on *AUC* change becomes small once fm_{CYP} falls below 0.85 (Fig. 22.11) [88]. The clinical dataset is substantially smaller for CYP2C9 than for CYP3A4 and CYP2D6, but it was found that using $[I]_{in,u}$ and $K_{i,u}$ to predict changes in *AUC* resulted in 14 correct assignations and 1 false negative [68]. However, the desire to avoid false negatives in a drug discovery screening

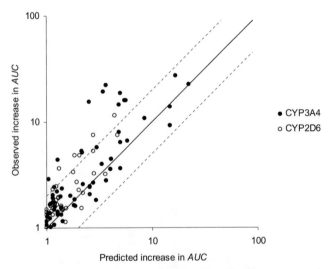

FIGURE 22.12   Observed and predicated *AUC* values for CYP3A4 and CYP2D6 DDIs. The square box represents twofold increase in *AUC*, the solid line is unity and the dashed lines are twofold errors in either direction. (Adapted from Ref. 88.)

cascade perhaps explains the popularity for using *total* concentration terms for [I], despite the decreased accuracy in absolute prediction afforded by doing so.

The multifaceted nature of CYP inhibition *in vivo* requires a great deal of understanding for accurate prediction, and the reasons behind the lack of a unifying model can be appreciated. As the IVIVE field progresses, it is anticipated that prediction accuracy will increase as there is profound interest and utility in such models within the pharmaceutical industry and considerable academic effort being made toward this goal. The ultimate aim is an integrated approach toward CYP inhibition prediction, which encompasses the role of all CYP isoforms and is underpinned by sound pharmacokinetic principles.

22.5.2   Approach for Mechanism-Based Inhibitors

Two models are currently presented in the literature and they rely on some key parameters for accurate predictions of DDI [7, 100]. As for reversible inhibition, the relevant concentration of inhibitor at the target CYP and the fraction of substrate clearance affected by inhibiting the enzyme are fundamental. In addition to this, predictions of MBI also employ the *in vivo* rate of enzyme synthesis (k_{synth}) and of degradation (k_{degrad}), and the *in vitro* inactivation kinetic parameters (K_I and k_{inact}). Where the currently available models differ is in the complexity of predicting the effect of changing inhibitor concentration over a dosing interval and the impact of this on the overall amount of inactivated CYP.

A model first presented by Hall and co-workers and subsequently expanded by the same group [100, 145, 146] is used most widely. This model assumes that the rates of enzyme synthesis and degradation are unaffected by enzyme inactivation and rely on the steady-state concentration of active enzyme being proportional to the ratio of the rate of synthesis and the rate of degradation. In the presence of inhibitor, the rate of degradation is then the sum of the *in vivo* degradation rate constant (k_{degrad}) and the rate constant describing the drug-induced inactivation (λ), where

$$\lambda = ([I] \cdot k_{inact}/[I] + K_I) \tag{22.30}$$

The model including inactivation of intestinal CYP and the fraction of drug metabolized by the inhibited pathway in the absence of the inhibitor is given in by

$$\frac{AUC}{AUC'} = \frac{F'}{F} \cdot \left(1 + \frac{fm}{([I] \cdot k_{inact})/(k_{degrad} \cdot (K_I + 1))} + (1 - fm) \right)^{-1} \tag{22.31}$$

This model has been shown to predict well for verapamil [145] and other mechanism-based inhibitors [147]. The accuracy of prediction is dependent on the k_{degrad} used, especially for substrates undergoing substantial ($fm > 0.9$) metabolism by the inhibited enzyme [56].

As with reversible CYP inhibition, a nonlinear regression model encompassing the various parameters predicting changing inhibitor and substrate concentrations affords the most sophisticated approach. To that end, an elegant model was proposed by Ito et al. [7], which predicts the effect of macrolide antibiotics on CYP3A4 [104]. A real advantage of this model is that it allows visualization of the plasma concentration–time profiles for the affected substrate and the inhibitor, and more importantly the change in active enzyme concentration over time. This model encompasses not only k_{inact} and K_I and the rate of resynthesis of active enzyme but also the changing concentration of the inhibitor as a function of its own disposition. Three compartments are represented: portal vein, liver, and systemic blood. The rate of change of inhibitor over time is modeled in each compartment with and without coadministered drug and a final compartment describes inactivation of hepatic CYP (Fig. 22.13). The use of this model requires nonlinear regression in a seven-compartment model which, while possible, is not necessarily practicable. Consequently, in the authors' laboratory, an analogous model has been written and implemented using a Microsoft Excel spreadsheet format [75], allowing simple manipulation and interrogation of this complex model.

Alongside the validation of this model presented by Ito et al. [104], where the interaction between erythromycin and clarithromycin with midazolam in humans was accurately predicted, the isolated perfused rat liver model (IPRL) has been used to demonstrate the effect of known mechanism-based inhibitors and NCEs [148]. Using the IPRL allowed ready validation of the predicted impact of TDI *in vivo*. It provides a bridge between the *in vitro* effect and *in vivo* impact for compounds with existing clinical data and NCEs, using pre-clinical species to bring confidence to predicted effect in humans. An adapted five-compartment model was used to fit the data and the *ex vivo* effects, although modest, were well predicted. The interplay between inhibitory potency and pharmacokinetic parameters was demonstrated; a less potent inhibitor with longer PK duration can impact hepatic CYPs to the same extent as a much more potent inhibitor with short duration. This was confirmed for troleandomycin and erythromycin in the IPRL; troleandomycin was found to be over 100-fold more efficient at inhibiting CYP3A2 than erythromycin *in vitro*, yet in the IPRL only a two fold increase over the effect of erythromycin was observed, reflecting the clinical situation for these drugs [149, 150]. This point was further confirmed by a study in cultured human hepatocytes performed in the authors' laboratory [95], where a compound that is a relatively weak time-dependent inhibitor of CYP2C9 was observed to have a dramatic impact on CYP2C9 activity over a prolonged culture period due to the large unbound concentration in the incubation combined with its metabolic stability. However, when the *in vivo* effect was modeled using predicted human PK parameters and dose, only a 5% decrease in *in vivo* CYP2C9 activity was predicted (Fig. 22.14).

22.5.3 Key Concepts

The literature regarding IVIVE of pharmacokinetics and drug interactions is vast, not only in terms of predicting human pharmacokinetic parameters but also the impact of potential DDIs and the correct use of *in vitro* data to engender the most accurate prediction of clinical DDIs. A summary of the underlying key concepts not already covered for CYP mediated DDIs is presented here.

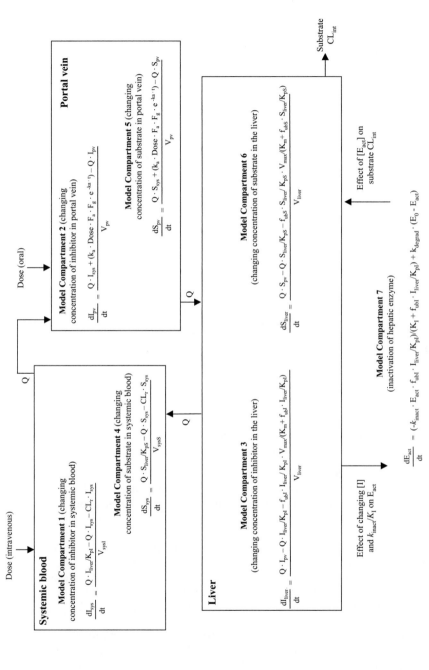

FIGURE 22.13 Model present by Ito et al. [7] for predicting effect of TDI. Seven compartments are described representing the changing inhibitor concentration in systemic blood (compartment 1), the changing inhibitor concentration in the portal vein following an oral dose (compartment 2), the changing inhibitor concentration in the liver (compartment 3), the changing substrate concentration in systemic blood (compartment 4), the changing substrate concentration in the portal vein following an oral dose (compartment 5), the changing substrate concentration in the liver (compartment 6), and the inactivation of hepatic enzyme (compartment 7), where I and S are the concentrations of inhibitor and substrate, respectively; I_{sys}, S_{sys} and I_{liver}, S_{liver} are the concentration in the systemic circulation and liver; V_{sysI}, V_{sysS} represent the volumes of distribution in the central compartment; K_{pI}, K_{pS} are the liver-to-blood concentration ratios; f_{ubS}, f_{ubI} are the fraction unbound in blood; I_{pv}, S_{pv} represent the concentrations in the portal vein; V_{pv} represents the volume of the portal vein; Q is blood flow, CL_r represents renal clearance; k_a is the absorption rate constant; F_a is fraction absorbed from an oral dose; and F_g represents the intestinal availability.

809

In the figure:

Systemic blood

Model Compartment 1 (changing concentration of inhibitor in systemic blood)

$$\frac{dI_{sys}}{dt} = \frac{Q \cdot I_{liver}/K_{pI} - Q \cdot I_{sys} - CL_r \cdot I_{sys}}{V_{sysI}}$$

Model Compartment 4 (changing concentration of substrate in systemic blood)

$$\frac{dS_{sys}}{dt} = \frac{Q \cdot S_{liver}/K_{pS} - Q \cdot S_{sys} - CL_r \cdot S_{sys}}{V_{sysS}}$$

Portal vein

Model Compartment 2 (changing concentration of inhibitor in portal vein)

$$\frac{dI_{pv}}{dt} = \frac{Q \cdot I_{sys} + (k_a \cdot Dose \cdot F_a \cdot F_g \cdot e^{-k_a t}) - Q \cdot I_{pv}}{V_{pv}}$$

Model Compartment 5 (changing concentration of substrate in portal vein)

$$\frac{dS_{pv}}{dt} = \frac{Q \cdot S_{sys} + (k_a \cdot Dose \cdot F_a \cdot F_g \cdot e^{-k_a t}) - Q \cdot S_{pv}}{V_{pv}}$$

Liver

Model Compartment 3 (changing concentration of inhibitor in the liver)

$$\frac{dI_{liver}}{dt} = \frac{Q \cdot I_{pv} - Q \cdot I_{liver}/K_{pI} - f_{ubI} \cdot I_{liver}/K_{pI} \cdot V_{max}/(K_m + f_{ubI} \cdot I_{liver}/K_{pI})}{V_{liver}}$$

Model Compartment 6 (changing concentration of substrate in the liver)

$$\frac{dS_{liver}}{dt} = \frac{Q \cdot S_{pv} - Q \cdot S_{liver}/K_{pS} - f_{ubS} \cdot S_{liver}/K_{pS} \cdot V_{max}/(K_m + f_{ubS} \cdot S_{liver}/K_{pS})}{V_{liver}}$$

Model Compartment 7 (inactivation of hepatic enzyme)

$$\frac{dE_{act}}{dt} = -(k_{inact} \cdot E_{act} \cdot f_{ubI} \cdot I_{liver}/K_{pI})/(K_I + f_{ubI} \cdot I_{liver}/K_{pI}) + k_{degrad} \cdot (E_0 - E_{act})$$

Effect of changing [I] and k_{inact}/K_I on E_{act}

Effect of [E_{act}] on substrate CL_{int}

Dose (intravenous)

Dose (oral)

Substrate CL_{int}

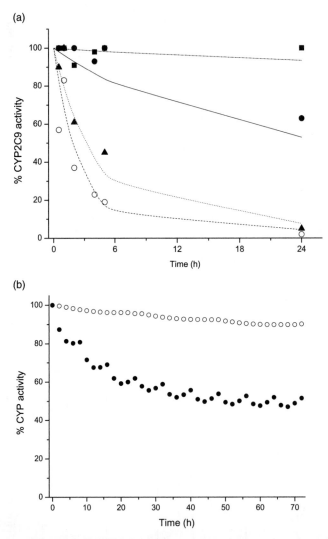

FIGURE 22.14 Effect of CYP2C9 inhibition observed *in vitro* and predicted *in vivo*. (a) CYP2C9 activity in cultured human hepatocytes after incubation with AZ1: CYP2C9-dependent diclofenac 4′-hydroxylation after incubation with AZ1 was determined after incubation with 0.1 μM (solid squares), 1 μM (solid circles), 5 μM (solid triangles), and 10 μM (open circles) AZ1. The dash-dot, solid, dotted, and dashed lines indicate nonlinear regression of the 0.1, 1, 5, and 10 μM AZ1 data, respectively. (b) Simulated profiles of CYP activity in human liver after oral dosing with AZ1 and erythromycin, respectively, using the methodology of Ito et al. [104]: CYP2C9 activity in human liver was simulated after oral dosing with AZ1 (70 mg every 24 h for 72 h open circles) and CYP3A4 activity in human liver after oral dosing with erythromycin (500 mg every 8 h for 72 h closed circles) (From Ref. 95.).

Making quantitative predictions of *in vivo* DDI using *in vitro* data requires consideration not only of inhibitor K_i (or K_I and k_{inact} for mechanism-based inhibition), but also f_{uinc}, $f_{u,b}$, CL, volume, fm_{CYP}, dose, and k_a. Use of such factors has resulted in relatively accurate predictions of DDI for reasonably large datasets [75, 88, 139, 147], with some exceptions (possibly compounds with an active component to their hepatic uptake/efflux—clearly there is more to learn in this area). For detailed predictions of individual DDIs, computer-modeling software should be used to simulate not only the impact of the scenarios detailed earlier, but also the changing drug concentrations with time as a result of the individual PK parameters; this allows a detailed interrogation of the interaction. If a worst-case scenario is to be provided, the maximum unbound inhibitor concentration at the enzyme site should be used. For this, knowledge of the extent to which the inhibitor concentrates in the hepatocyte is important (if no information is available, 10× the maximum unbound blood concentration has been proposed [7]). Additionally, assuming that elimination of substrate is by a single hepatic CYP predicts a worse-case scenario for the inhibited pathway *in vivo*. These approaches are of utility in a discovery setting when selecting compounds for further progression, but it can be appreciated that it generally leads to an overestimation of the inhibitory effect, especially when combined with the assumption of complete and instantaneous absorption of the inhibitor from an oral dose.

Refinement and improved predictivity is afforded by including the contribution of the inhibited CYP to the total clearance of the substrate (fm_{CYP}) and more realistic estimations of the fraction and rate of absorption for the inhibitor, essentially by estimating not only the concentration of inhibitor in the liver more accurately but also its impact on the metabolic pathway of the substrate. Information on the *in vivo* fm_{CYP} for specific substrates can be found in the literature [68, 138, 151]. As demonstrated by the clinical cases of DDI presented previously, CYP inhibition has greatest impact when a substrate is predominantly cleared by the inhibited pathway; consequently, multiple pathways for drug elimination reduce the chance of clinically significant DDI. However, consideration must be given to the target patient population as, for example, renal impairment can dramatically affect the elimination pathway of a drug.

Recently, an *in vitro* approach aimed at overcoming the difficulty of assessing inhibitor concentration at the enzyme was presented [152]. It involves using human hepatocytes suspended in human plasma to generate K_i without the need for correction for free concentration at the active site (with the caveat that active transport in hepatocytes *in vitro* may not fully represent that *in vivo*). Using this method, the authors claim accurate prediction of several clinically relevant CYP DDIs by including the CYP phenotypic metabolism for each substrate. This method requires a large range of inhibitor concentrations in the *in vitro* incubations and relies heavily on acute analytical sensitivity. A limitation of this and other methods utilizing fm_{CYP} is the level of understanding required for each substrate under investigation (optimal concentration range for determining K_i and an accurate estimation of the contribution of different CYPs to the substrates' *in vivo* metabolism). This method is one approach to minimizing the difficulty of predicting [I] at the active site.

Other points of consideration for IVIVE of DDI include using appropriate substrate–inhibitor combinations *in vitro* so the *in vivo* interaction is correctly assessed; this further emphasizes the importance of using clinically relevant probe substrates in the *in vitro* determinations. Consideration must also be given to the metabolites of an inhibitor, which can often have a significant inhibitory effect in their own right. If they persist in the systemic circulation or are actively concentrated in the liver, their influence can lead to underprediction of the magnitude of the interaction if they are discounted.

There are several pharmacokinetic parameters to be considered for both substrate and inhibitor when making predictions of DDIs. These considerations essentially require estimating levels of drug within the body, be it in the circulating plasma, liver, portal vein, or gastrointestinal tract. Dose and clearance are the primary determinants for these parameters. For drugs in preclinical development, accurate prediction of the relative impact of DDI relies on reasonable assessment of dose level, frequency, and route. It follows that by minimizing dose the potential of DDI will also be minimized. The route of administration of the victim drug must also be considered. A compound with high (intestinal and hepatic) first-pass extraction will behave very differently in the presence of an inhibitor when administered orally as opposed to intravenously. For a drug with a high extraction ratio, the C_{max} will be significantly increased in the presence of an inhibitor but the elimination half-life will be quite similar in the presence and absence of inhibitor. Conversely, for a compound with a low extraction ratio, the same inhibitor will have limited effect on C_{max} following an oral dose but the elimination half-life may be considerably larger; this will also be the case following an IV dose [130].

Predictions of CYP inhibition made in isolation of other contributing factors, albeit sometimes unknown, may only result in an approximation of *in vivo* effect. The ultimate goal is to be able to predict *in vivo* disposition by encompassing not only multiple mechanisms of CYP (and indeed other enzyme) inhibition but also the potential inductive capacity and transporter interactions for the compound under evaluation. Many drugs exhibit numerous interactive attributes, one such example is the antiviral protease inhibitor ritonavir. *In vitro* ritonavir has been demonstrated to induce CYP3A4 expression through activation of the Pregnane X receptor [153]; it is also a potent mechanism-based inhibitor of CYP3A4 [154] and a substrate and inducer of the P-glycoprotein transporter [155]. Despite accurate *in vitro* assessment of its inhibitory capacity, predictions of the *in vivo* effect of ritonavir are often erroneous due to varying contribution of all these factors and also are dependent on the time course of drug exposure. Initially, ritonavir exerts an inhibitory effect on CYP3A4 mediated metabolism *in vivo* but with prolonged exposure the inductive capacity of the drug predominates. For example, short-term low-dose administration of ritonavir produces a large and significant impairment of triazolam clearance and enhancement of clinical effects [156] with the *AUC* of triazolam increasing from 13.6 to 553 ng/mL·h following 1 day of ritonavir treatment but following 10 days of treatment falling to 287 ng/mL·h [157]. Accurate prediction of such situations becomes difficult. A unifying model allowing all factors to be encompassed, although complex, would be beneficial.

As discussed, a comprehensive, integrated, and systematic approach is required for IVIVE of CYP mediated DDIs. To this end there exists Simcyp® (http://www.simcyp.com), a population-based prediction software tool that offers such an evaluation for CYP mediated DDIs. This software incorporates physiological, genetic, and epidemiological information, which, together with *in vitro* data, facilitates the modeling and simulation of the time course and fate of drugs in representative virtual patient populations. Simcyp uses information from routine *in vitro* studies generated in most drug discovery departments and with this information predicts individual pharmacokinetic parameters (such as F_{abs}, CL, and V_{ss}) and simulates CYP mediated drug interactions and the likely associated population variability. This allows prediction of outcomes in relevant patient populations, identifying those individuals at most risk from a DDI, not just a single value in an average individual. The software has the potential to simulate the effect of combined CYP induction and inhibition and can also be applied to DDIs involving time-dependent inhibition. Simcyp may assist in the evaluation and optimization of candidate drugs, in the estimation of early human doses and exposures in the clinic, and the prioritization and planning of suitable *in vitro* and clinical interaction studies in the development phase. Tools such as Simcyp are attracting a lot of interest in the pharmaceutical industry and may facilitate a more aligned strategy and as such are worthy of further investment and validation.

22.5.4   FDA Guidelines

The FDA defines a significant DDI as a two fold (or more) increase in the *AUC* of the substrate drug in the presence of an inhibitor. The two fold threshold is given as inter-individual variation and polymorphisms in CYP expression within the population could account for changes less than this [158]. If a risk of DDI is predicted from *in vitro* data, a clinical study evaluating the risk and a thorough investigation of the mechanism of CYP inhibition (along with understanding of the potential coadministered drugs in the target patient population) may make it possible to launch a candidate drug, providing it carries a product label stating possible risk of DDI. For example, if a drug has been determined to be a "strong" inhibitor of CYP3A, a warning about an interaction with "sensitive CYP3A substrates" and CYP3A substrates with narrow therapeutic range may be required [158].

The FDA has released guidance documents, which reflect current thinking in the field specifically aimed at industry evaluating metabolism-based drug interactions; *Guidance for Industry: Drug Metabolism/Drug Interaction Studies in the Drug Development Process—Studies in Vitro*; and *Guidance for Industry: In Vivo Drug Metabolism/Drug Interaction Studies—Study Design, Data Analysis and Recommendations for Dosing and Labelling* [159]. The *in vitro* studies guide, as well as providing a summary of drug metabolism and relevant concepts, describes *in vitro* techniques for evaluating the potential of metabolism-based interactions, the correlation of *in vitro* and *in vivo* findings, and the timing of *in vitro* studies and subsequent product labeling. It defines the goals of evaluating *in vitro* drug metabolism as: (1) to identify all of the major metabolic pathways that affect the test drug and its metabolites, including the specific enzymes responsible for elimination and the intermediates formed; and (2) to explore and anticipate the effects of the test drug on the metabolism of other drugs and the effects of other drugs on its metabolism.

22.6   CONCLUSION

Undoubtedly, using *in vitro* data to make accurate predictions of clinical DDIs involving inhibition of CYP is possible providing that there is understanding of the various processes involved. The availability of clinical data is central to building predictive models and is required for feedback on their accuracy and further iteration of these algorithms. Misinterpretation of the risk of CYP inhibition can be costly both in terms of patient safety and pharmaceutical resources; in a drug discovery setting predicting the worst-case scenario is a prudent approach.

In brief, CYP inhibition may/can result in serious clinical adverse reactions, the prediction of which is a maturing science. Accurate predictions are possible and the pitfalls and progress in using *in vitro* inhibition data to project clinical drug–drug interactions have been presented. Clearly, accurate predictions start with the production of high quality *in vitro* data, require rational examination of the kinetics of inhibition, and, finally, require the application of sound pharmacokinetic theory. The approaches discussed here should guide the researcher in implementing this best practice.

REFERENCES

1. Pirmohamed M, James S, Meakin S, Green C, Scott AK, Walley TJ, Farrar K, Park BK, Breckenridge AM. Adverse drug reactions as cause of admission to hospital: prospective analysis of 18,820 patients. *Br Med J* 2004;329(7456):15–19.

2. Lazarou J, Pomeranz BH, Corey PN. Incidence of adverse drug reactions in hospitalised patients. *JAMA* 1998;279(15):1200–1205.

3. Frankfort SV, Tulner LR, van Campen JPCM, Koks CHW, Beijnen JH. Evaluation of pharmacotherapy in geriatric patients after performing complete geriatric assessment at a diagnostic day clinic. *Clin Drug Invest* 2006;26(3):169–174.

4. Jankel C, Fitterman LK. Epidemiology of drug–drug interactions as a cause of hospital admissions. *Drug Safety* 1993;9:51–59.

5. Howard RL, Avery AJ, Slavenburg S, Royal S, Pipe G, Lucassen P, Pirmohamed M. Which drugs cause preventable admissions to hospital? A systematic review. *Br J Clin Pharmacol* 2007;63(2):136–147.

6. Shah RR. Mechanistic basis of adverse drug reactions: the perils of inappropriate dose schedules. *Expert Opin Drug Safety* 2005;4(1):103–128.

7. Ito K, Iwatsubo T, Kanamutsu S, Ueda K, Suzuki H, Sugiyama Y. Prediction of pharmacokinetic alterations caused by drug–drug interactions: metabolic interaction in the liver. *Pharmacol Rev* 1998;50(3):387–411.

8. Kumar V, Wahlstrom JL, Rock DA, Warren CJ, Gorman LA, Tracy TS. CYP2C9 inhibition: impact of probe selection and pharmacogenetics on *in vitro* inhibition profiles. *Drug Metab Dispos* 2006;34(12):1966–1075.

9. Shou M. Prediction of pharmacokinetics and drug–drug interactions from *in vitro* metabolic data. *Curr Opin Drug Discov Dev* 2005;8(1):66–77.

10. Zimmermann M, Duruz H, Guinand O, Broccard O, Levy P, Lacatis D, Bloch A. Torsades de pointes after treatment with terfenadine and ketoconazole. *Eur Heart J* 1992; 13(7):1002–1003.

11. Backmann KA, Lewis JD. Predicting inhibitory drug–drug interactions and evaluating interaction reports using inhibition constants. *Ann Pharmacother* 2005;39:1064–1072.

12. Wysowsk DK, Bacsanyi J. Cisapride and fatal arrhythmia. *N Engl J Med* 1996; 335(4):290–291.

13. Brown HS, Galetin A, Halifax D, Houston JB. Prediction of *in vivo* drug–drug interactions from *in vitro* data: factors affecting prototypic drug–drug interactions involving CYP2C9, CYP2D6 and CYP3A4. *Clin Pharmacokinet* 2006;45(10):1035–1050.

14. Venkatakrishnan K, von Moltke LL, Obach RS, Greenblatt DJ. Drug metabolism and drug interactions: application and clinical value of *in vitro* models. *Curr Drug Metab* 2003;4:423–459.

15. Lin JH, Lu AYH. Interindividual variability in inhibition and induction of cytochrome P450 enzymes. *Annu Rev Pharmacol Toxicol* 2001;41:535–567.

16. Prentis RA, Lis Y, Walker SR. Pharmaceutical innovation by the seven UK-owned pharmaceutical companies (1964–1985). *Br J Clin Pharmacol* 1988;25:387–396.

17. Schuster D, Laggner C, Langer T. Why drugs fail—a study on side effects in new chemical entities. *Curr Pharm Des* 2005;11:3545–3559.

18. DiMasi JA, Hansen RW, Grabowski HG. The price of innovation: new estimates of drug development costs. *J Health Econ* 2003;22:151–185.

19. Cohen LH, Remley MJ, Raunig D, Vaz ADN. *In vitro* drug interactions of cytochrome P450: an evaluation of fluorogenic to conventional substrates. *Drug Metab Dispos* 2003;31:1005–1015.

20. Wienkers LC, Heath TG. Predicting *in vivo* drug interactions from *in vitro* drug discovery data. *Nat Rev (Drug Disco)* 2005;4:825–833.

21. Donato MT, Gomez-Lechón MJ. Inhibition of P450 enzymes: an *in vitro* approach. *Curr Enzyme Inhib* 2006;2:281–304.

22. Lewis DFV. 57 varieties: the human cytochromes P450. *Pharmacogenomics* 2004; 5(3):305–318.

23. Girault I, Rougier N, Chesné C, Lideraue R, Beaune P, Biéche I, De Waziers I. Simultaneous measurement of 23 isoforms from the human cytochrome P450 families 1 to 3 by quantitative reverse transcriptase-polymerase chain reaction. *Drug Metab Dispos* 2005;33:1803–1810.

24. Tanaka E. Clinically important pharmacokinetic drug–drug interactions: role of cytochrome P450 enzymes. *J Clin Pharm Ther* 1998;23:403–416.

25. Bertz RJ, Granneman GR. Use of *in vitro* and *in vivo* data to estimate the likelihood of metabolic pharmacokinetic interactions. *Clin Pharmacokin* 1997;32(3):210–258.

26. Shimada T, Yamazaki H, Mimura M, Yukiharu I, Guengerich FP. Interindividual variations in human liver cytochrome P450 enzymes involved in oxidation of drugs, carcinogens and toxic chemicals; studies with liver microsomes of 30 Japanese and 30 Caucasians. *J Pharmacol Exp Ther* 1994;270:414–423.

27. Dresser GK, Spence JD, Bailey DG. Pharmacokinetic–pharmacodynamic consequences and clinical relevance of cytochrome P450 inhibition. *Clin Pharmacokinet* 2000; 38(1):41–57.

28. Lewis JD, Bachmann KA. Cytochrome P450 enzymes and drug–drug interactions: an update on the superfamily. *J Pharm Technol* 2006;22:22–31.

29. Batty KT, Davis TME, Ilett KF, Dusci LJ, Langton SR. The effect of ciprofloxacin on theophylline pharmacokinetics in healthy subjects. *Br J Clin Pharmacol* 1995; 39(3):305–311.

30. Granfors MT, Backman JT, Neuvonen M, Neuvonen PJ. Ciprofloxacin greatly increases concentrations and hypotensive effect of tizanidine by inhibiting its cytochrome P450 1A2-mediated presystemic metabolism. *Clin Pharmacol Ther* 2004;76(6):598–606.

31. Hemeryck A, Belpaire FM. Selective serotonin reuptake inhibitors and cytochrome P-450 mediated drug–drug interactions: an update. *Curr Drug Metab* 2002;3:13–37.

32. Becquemont L, Bot MA, Le Riche C, Beaune P. Influence of fluvoxamine on tacrine metabolism *in vitro*: potential implication for hepatotoxicity *in vivo*. *Fundam Clin Pharmacol* 1996;10(2):156–157.

33. Backman JT, Kyrklund C, Neuvonen M, Neuvonen PJ. Gemfibrozil greatly increases plasma concentrations of cerivastatin. *Clin Pharmacol Ther* 2002;72:685–691.

34. Veronese ME, Miners JO, Randles D, Gregov D, Birkett DJ. Validation of the tolbutamide metabolic ratio for population screening with use of sulfaphenazole to produce model phenotypic poor metabolizers. *Clin Pharmacol Ther* 1990;47:403–411.

35. Crussell-Porter LL, Rindone JP, Ford MA, Jaskar DW. Low-dose fluconazole therapy potentiates the hypoprothrombinemic response of warfarin sodium. *Arch Intern Med* 1993;153(1):102–104.

36. Krayenbühl JC, Vozeh S, Kondo-Oestreicher M, Dayer P. Drug–drug interactions of new active substances: mibefradil example. *Eur J Clin Pharmacol* 1999;55:559–565.

37. Boxenbaum H. Cytochrome P450 3A4 *in vivo* ketoconazole competitive inhibition: determination of K_i and dangers associated with high clearance drugs in general. *J Pharm Pharm Sci* 1999;2(2):47–52.

38. Honig PK, Woosley RL, Zamani K, Conner DP, Cantilena LR, Jr. Changes in the pharmacokinetics and electrocardiograph pharmacodynamics of terfenadine with concomitant administration of erythromycin. *Clin Pharmacol Ther* 1992;52(3):231–238.

39. Ishigam M, Uchiyama M, Kondo T, Iwabuchi H, Inoue SI, Takasaki W, Ikeda T, Komai T, Ito K, Sugiyama Y. Inhibition of *in vitro* metabolism of simvastatin by itraconazole in humans and prediction of *in vivo* drug–drug interactions. *Pharm Res* 2001;18(5):622–631.

40. Corpier CL, Jones PH, Suki WN, Lederer ED, Quinones MA, Schmidt SW, Young JB. Rhabdomyolysis and renal injury with lovastatin use. Report of two cases in cardiac transplant recipients. *JAMA* 1998;260(2):239–241.

41. Schmassmann-Suhijar D, Bullingham R, Gasser R, Schmutz J, Haefeli WE. Rhabdomyolysis due to interaction of simvastatin with mibefradil [letter]. *Lancet* 1998;351:1929–1930.

42. Kantola T, Kivisto KT, Neuvonen PJ. Erythromycin and verapamil considerably increase serum simvastatin and simvastatin acid concentrations. *Clin Pharmacol Ther* 1998;64(2):177–182.

43. Michalets EL, Williams CR. Drug interactions with cisapride: clinical implications. *Clin Pharmacokinet* 2000;39(1):49–75.

44. Jacobsen W, Kirchner G, Hallensleben K, Mancinelli L, Deters M, Hackbarth I, Baner K, Benet LZ, Sewing K, Christians U. Small intestinal metabolism of the 3-hydroxy-3-methylglutaryl-coenzyme A reductase inhibitor lovastatin and comparison with pravastatin. *J Pharmacol Exp Ther* 1999;291(1):131–139.

45. Spoendlin M, Peters J, Welker H, Bock A, Thiel G. Pharmacokinetic interaction between oral cyclosporin and mibefradil in stabilized post-renal-transplant patients. *Nephrol Dial Transplant* 1998;13:1787–1791.

46. Olkkola KT, Ahonen J, Neuvonen PJ. The effect of the systemic antimycotics, itraconazole and fluconazole, on the pharmacokinetics and pharmacodynamics of intravenous and oral midazolam. *Anesth Analg* 1996;82(3):511–516.

47. Muck W. Rational assessment of the interaction profile of cerivastatin supports its low propensity for drug interactions. *Drugs* 1998;56(1s):15–23.

48. Muck W, Ochmann K, Rohde G, Unger S, Kuhlmann J. Influence of erythromycin pre- and co-treatment on single-dose pharmacokinetics of the HMG-CoA reductase inhibitor cerivastatin. *Eur J Clin Pharmacol* 1998;53:469–473.

49. Kantola T, Kivisto KT, Neuvonen PJ. Effect of itraconazole on cerivastatin pharmacokinetics. *Eur J Clin Pharmacol* 1999;54:851–855.

50. Mazzu AL, Lasseter KC, Shamblen EC, Agarwal V, Lettieri J, Sundaresen P. Itraconazole alters the pharmacokinetics of atorvastatin to a greater extent than either cerivastatin or pravastatin. *Clin Pharmacol Ther* 2000;68:391–400.

51. Shitara Y, Sugiyama Y. Pharmacokinetic and pharmacodynamic alterations of 3-hydroxy-3-methylglutaryl coenzyme A (HMG-CoA) reductase inhibitors: drug–drug interactions and interindividual differences in transporter and metabolic enzyme functions. *Pharmacol Ther* 2006;112(1):71–105.

52. Shitara Y, Hirano M, Sato H, Sugiyama Y. Gemfibrozil and its glucuronide inhibit the organic anion transporting polypeptide 2 (OATP2/OATP1B1:SLC21A6)-mediated hepatic uptake and CYP2C8-mediated metabolism of cerivastatin: analysis of the mechanism of the clinically relevant drug–drug interaction between cerivastatin and gemfibrozil. *J Pharmacol Exp Ther* 2004;311:228–236.

53. Neuvonen PJ, Mikko Niemi M, Backman JT. Drug interactions with lipid-lowering drugs: mechanisms and clinical relevance. *Clin Pharmacol Ther* 2006;80(6):565–581.

54. Pisani F, Narbone MC, Fazio A, Crisafulli P, Primerano G, D'Agostino AA, Oteri G, Di Perri R. Increased serum carbamazepine levels by viloxazine in epileptic patients. *Epilepsia* 1986;25:482–285.

55. Rotzinger S, Bourin M, Akimoto Y, Coutts RT, Bake GB. Metabolism of some "second"– and "fourth"–generation antidepressants: iprindole, viloxazine, bupropion, mianserin, maprotiline, trazodone, nefazodone, and venlafaxine. *Cell Mol Neurobiol* 1999;19(4):427–442.

56. Galetin A, Ito K, Halifax D, Houston JB. CYP3A4 substrate selection and substitution in the prediction of potential drug–drug interactions. *J Pharmacol Exp Ther* 2005;314(1):180–190.

57. Prueksaritanont T, Ma B, Tang C, Meng Y, Assang C, Lu P, Reider PJ, Lin JH, Baillie TA. Metabolic interactions between mibefradil and HMG-CoA reductase inhibitors: an *in vitro* investigation with human liver preparations. *Br J Clin Pharmacol* 1999;47(3):291–298.

58. Wandel C, Kim RB, Guengerich PF, Wood AJJ. Mibefradil is a P-glycoprotein substrate and a potent inhibitor of P-glycoprotein and CYP3A4 *in vitro*. *Drug Metab Dispos* 2000;28:895–898.

59. Reynolds KS. Drug interactions: regulatory perspective. In Piscitelle S, Rodvold K, Eds. *Drug Interactions in Infectious Diseases*, 2nd eds. Totowa, NJ: Humana Press; 2005.

60. Venkatakrishnan K, von Moltke LL, Greenblatt DJ. Effects of the antifungal agents on oxidative drug metabolism: clinical relevance. *Clin Pharmacokinet* 2000;8(2):111–180.

61. Granfors MT, Backman JT, Jouko L, Neuvonen PJ. Tizanidine is mainly metabolized by cytochrome P450 1A2 *in vitro*. *Br J Clin Pharmacol* 2004;57(3):349–353.

62. Ha HR, Chen J, Freiburghaus AU, Follath F. Metabolism of theophylline by cDNA-expressed human cytochromes P-450. *Br J Clin Pharmacol* 1995;39(3):321–326.

63. Ilett KF, Castleden WM, Vandongen YK, Stacey MC, Butler MA, Kadlubar FF. Acetylation phenotype and cytochrome P450IA2 phenotype are unlikely to be associated with peripheral arterial disease. *Clin Pharmacol Ther* 1993;54(3):317–322.

64. Dorado P, Berecz R, Penas-Lledo EM, Caceres MC, Llerena A. Clinical implications of CYP2D6 genetic polymorphism during treatment with antipsychotic drugs. *Curr Drug Targets* 2006;7(12):1671–1680.

65. Preskorn SH, Harvey AT. Cytochrome P450 enzymes and psychopharmacology. In Bloom FE, Kupfer DJ, Eds. *Psychopharmacology—The Fourth Generation of Progress*, 4threv ed. Philadelphia: Raven Press; 1995.

66. Kenworthy KE, Clarke SE, Andrews J, Houston JB. Multisite kinetic models for CYP3A4: simultaneous activation and inhibition of diazepam and testosterone metabolism. *Drug Metab Dispos* 2001;29(12):1644–1651.

67. Hutzler JM, Hauer MJ, Tracy TS. Dapsone activation of CYP2C9-mediated metabolism: evidence for activation of multiple substrates and a two-site model. *Drug Metab Dispos* 2001;29(7):1029–1034.

68. McGinnity DF, Tucker J, Trigg S, Riley RJ. Prediction of CYP2C9-mediated drug–drug interactions: a comparison using data from recombinant enzymes and human hepatocytes. *Drug Metab Dispos* 2005;33(11):1700–1707.

69. Egnell A-C, Eriksson C, Albertson N, Houston B, Boyer S. Generation and evaluation of a CYP2C9 heteroactivation pharmacophore. *J Pharmacol Exp Ther* 2003;307:878–887.

70. Egnell A-C, Houston B, Boyer S. *In vivo* CYP3A4 heteroactivation is a possible mechanism for the drug interaction between felbamate and carbamazepine. *J Pharmacol Exp Ther* 2003;305(3):1251–1262.

71. Zhang Z, Wong YN. Enzyme kinetics for clinically relevant CYP inhibition. *Curr Drug Metab* 2005;6:241–257.

72. Tracy TS, Hummell MA. Modelling kinetic data from *in vitro* drug metabolising enzyme experiments. *Drug Metab Rev* 2004;26(2):231–242.

73. Houston JB, Kenworthy KE, Galetin A. Typical and atypical enzyme kinetics. In Lee JS, Obach RS, Fisher MB, Eds. *Drug Metabolising Enzymes, Cytochrome P450 and Other Enzymes in Drug Discovery and Development*. New York: Marcel Dekker; 2003, pp 211–254.

74. Hollenberg PF. Characteristics and common properties of inhibitors, inducers, and activators of CYP enzymes. *Drug Metab Rev* 2002;34(1–2):17–35.

75. Riley RJ, Grime K, Weaver R. Time-dependent CYP inhibition. *Expert Opin Drug Metab Toxicol* 2007;3(1):51–66.

76. Zhou S, Yung Chan S, Cher Goh B, Chan E, Duan W, Huang M, McLeod HL. Mechanism-based inhibition of cytochrome P450 3A4 by therapeutic drugs. *Clin Pharmacokinet* 2005;44(3):279–304.

77. Silverman RB. Mechanism-based enzyme inactivation. In *Chemistry and Enzymology*, Vol 1. Boca Raton, FL: CRC Press; 1988, pp 3–30.

78. Waley SG. Kinetics of suicide substrates: practical procedures for determining parameters. *Biochem J* 1985;227:843–849.

79. Ghanbari F, Rowland-Yeo K, Bloomer JC, Clarke SE, Lennard MS, Tucker GT, Rostami-Hodjegan A. A critical evaluation of the experimental design of studies of mechanism-based enzyme inhibition, with implications for *in vitro–in vivo* extrapolation. *Curr Drug Metab* 2006;7:315–334.

80. Ito K, Brown HS, Houston JB. Database analyses for the prediction of *in vivo* drug–drug interactions from *in vitro* data. *Br J Clin Pharmacol* 2004;57(4):473–486.

81. Martignoni M, Groothuis GMM, de Kanter R. Species differences between mouse, rat, dog, monkey and human CYP-mediated drug metabolism, inhibition and induction. *Expert Opin Drug Metab Toxicol* 2006;2(6):875–894.

82. Gill HJ, Tingle MD, Park BK. N-Hydroxylation of dapsone by multiple enzymes of cytochrome P450: implications for inhibition of hemotoxicity. *Br J Clin Pharmacol* 1995;40(6):531–538.

83. Soars MG, Grime K, Riely RJ. Comparative analysis of substrate and inhibitor interactions with CYP3A4 and CYP3A5. *Xenobiotica* 2006;36(4):287–299.

84. Tang W, Wang WW, Lu AYH. Utility of recombinant cytochrome P450 enzymes: a drug metabolism perspective. *Curr Drug Metab* 2005;6:503–517.

85. Proctor NJ, Tucker GT, Rostami-Hodjegan A. Predicting drug clearance from recombinantly expressed CYPs: intersystem extrapolation factors. *Xenobiotica* 2004;34(2):151–178.

86. McGinnity DF, Riley RJ. Predicting drug pharmacokinetics in humans from *in vitro* metabolism studies. *Biochem Soc Transact* 2001;29(2):135–139.

87. Gomez-Lechón MJ, Donato MT, Castell JV, Jover R. Human hepatocytes in primary culture: the choice to investigated drug metabolism in man. *Curr Drug Metab* 2004;5:443–462.

88. Grime K, Riley RJ. The impact of *in vitro* binding on *in vitro–in vivo* extrapolations, projections of metabolic clearance and clinical drug–drug interactions. *Curr Drug Metab* 2006;7(3):251–264.

89. Griffin SJ, Houston JB. Comparison of fresh and cryopreserved rat hepatocyte suspensions for the prediction of *in vitro* intrinsic clearance. *Drug Metab Dispos* 2004;32:552–558.

90. Houston JB, Carlile DJ. Prediction of hepatic clearance from microsomes, hepatocytes and liver slices. *Drug Metab Rev* 1997;29:891–922.

91. Dickins M. Induction of cytochromes P450. *Curr Top Med Chem* 2004;4(16): 1745–1766.

92. LeCluyse EL. Human hepatocyte culture systems for the *in vitro* evaluation of cytochrome P450 expression and regulation. *Eur J Pharm Sci* 2001;13(4):343–368.

93. Oleson FB, Berman CL, Li AP. An evaluation of the P450 inhibition and induction potential of daptomycin in primary human hepatocytes. *Chem Biol Interact* 2004; 150:137–147.

94. Li AP, Lu C, Brent JA, Pham C, Fackett A, Ruegg CE, Silber PM. Cryopreserved human hepatocytes: characterization of drug-metabolizing enzyme activities and applications in higher throughput screening assays for hepatotoxicity, metabolic stability, and drug–drug interaction potential. *Chem Biol Interact* 1999;121:17–35.

95. McGinnity DF, Berry AJ, Kenny JR, Grime K, Riley RJ. Evaluation of time-dependent cytochrome P450 inhibition using cultured human hepatocytes. *Drug Metab Dispos* 2006;34:1291–1300.

96. Zhao P, Kunze KL, Lee CA. Evaluation of time-dependent inactivation of CYP3A in cryopreserved human hepatocytes. *Drug Metab Dispos* 2005;33:853–861.

97. Soars MG, McGinnity DF, Grime K, Riely RJ. The pivotal role of hepatocytes in drug discovery. *Chem-Biol Interact* 2007;168(1):2–15.

98. Atkinson A, Kenny JR, Grime K. Automated assessment of time-dependent inhibition of human cytochrome P450 enzymes using liquid chromatography-tandem mass spectrometry analysis. *Drug Metab Dispos* 2005;33:1637–1647.

99. Lopez-Garcia MP, Dansette PM, Mansuy D. Thiophene derivatives as new mechanism-based inhibitors of cytochromes P-450: inactivation of yeast-expressed human liver cytochrome P-450 2C9 by tienilic acid. *Biochemistry* 1994;33(1):166–175.

100. Mayhew BS, Jones DR, Hall SD. An *in vitro* model for predicting *in vivo* inhibition of cytochrome P450 3A4 by metabolic intermediate complex formation. *Drug Metab Dispos* 2000;28:1031–1037.

101. Chan WK, Delucchi AB. Resveratrol, a red wine constituent, is a mechanism-based inactivator of cytochrome P450 3A4. *Life Sci* 2000;67(25):3103–3112.

102. Kanamitsu S, Ito K, Green CE, Tyson CA, Shimada N, Sugiyama Y. Prediction of *in vivo* interaction between triazolam and erythromycin based on *in vitro* studies using human liver microsomes and recombinant human CYP3A4. *Pharm Res* 2000;17(4):419–426.

103. Yamano K, Yamamoto K, Katashima M, Kotaki H, Takedomi S, Matsuo H, Ohtani H, Sawada Y, Iga T. Prediction of midazolam-CYP3A inhibitors interaction in the human liver from *in vivo/in vitro* absorption, distribution, and metabolism data. *Drug Metab Dispos* 2001;29(4):443–452.

104. Ito K, Ogihara K, Kanamitsu S, Itoh T. Prediction of the *in vivo* interaction between midazolam and macrolides based on *in vitro* studies using human liver microsomes. *Drug Metab Dispos* 2003;31(7):945–954.

105. Dai R, Wei X, Luo G, Sinz M, Marathe P. Metabolism-dependent P450 3A4 inactivation with multiple substrates. Abstract from 12th North American ISSX Meeting, Providence, RI. *Drug Metab Rev* 2003;35:341.

106. McConn DJ, Zhao Z. Integrating *in vitro* kinetic data from compounds exhibiting induction, reversible inhibition and mechanism-based inactivation: *in vitro* study design. *Curr Drug Metab* 2004;5:141–146.

107. Boobis AR, McKillop D, Robinson DT, Adams DA, McCormick DJ. Interlaboratory comparison of the assessment of P450 activities in human hepatic microsomal samples. *Xenobiotica* 1998;28(5):493–506.

108. Obach RS. Prediction of human clearance of twenty-nine drugs from hepatic microsomal intrinsic clearance data: an examination of *in vitro* half-life approach and nonspecific binding to microsomes. *Drug Metab Dispos* 1999;27:1350–1359.

109. Riley RJ. The potential pharmacological and toxicological impact of P450 screening. *Curr Opin Drug Discov Dev* 2001;4:45–54.

110. Austin RP, Barton P, Mohmed S, Riley RJ. The binding of drugs to hepatocytes and its relationship to physicochemical properties. *Drug Metab Dispos* 2005;33(3):419–425.

111. Austin RP, Barton P, Cockroft SL, Wenlock MC, Riley RJ. The influence of nonspecific microsomal binding on apparent intrinsic clearance, and its prediction from physicochemical properties. *Drug Metab Dispos* 2002;30(12):1497–1503.

112. Riley RJ, Grime K. Metabolic screening *in vitro*: metabolic stability, CYP inhibition and induction. *Drug Discov Today* 2004;1(4):365–372.

113. Tang C, Shou M, Rodrigues AD. Substrate-dependent effect of acetronitrile on human liver microsomal cytochrome P450 2C9 (CYP2C9) activity. *Drug Metab Dispos* 2000;28:567–572.

114. Baranczewski P, Stanczak A, Sundberg K, Svensson R, Wallin A, Jansson J, Garberg P, Postlind H. Introduction to *in vitro* estimation of metabolic stability and drug interactions of new chemical entities in drug discovery and development. *Pharmacol Rep* 2006;58:453–472.

115. Walsky RL, Obach RS. Validated assays for human cytochrome P450 activities. *Drug Metab Dispos* 2004;32:647–660.

116. Weaver R, Grime K, Beatie IG, Riley RJ. Cytochrome P450 inhibition using recombinant proteins and mass spectrometry/multiple reaction monitoring technology in a cassette incubation. *Drug Metab Dispos* 2003;31:955–966.

117. Tucker GT, Houston JB, Huang S. Optimising drug development: strategies to assess drug metabolism/transport interaction potential—towards a consensus. *Pharm Res* 2001;18(8):1071–1080.

118. O'Donnell CJ, Grime K, Courtney P, Slee D, Riley RJ. The development of a cocktail CYP2B6, CYP2C8 and CYP3A5 inhibition assay and a preliminary assessment of utiliy in a drug discovery setting. *Drug Metab Dispos* 2007;35(3):381–385.

119. Moody GC, Griffin SJ, Mather AN, McGinnity DF, Riley RJ. Fully automated analysis of activities catalysed by the major human liver cytochrome P450 (CYP) enzymes: assessment of human CYP inhibition potential. *Xenobiotica* 1999;29(1):53–75.

120. US Food and Drug Administration, Center for Drug Evaluation and Research website. Drug Development And Drug Interactions information page. http://www.fda.gov/cder/drug/drugInteractions/.

121. Bu H-Z, Magis L, Knuth K, Teitelbaum P. High-throughput cytochrome P450 (CYP) inhibition screening via a cassette probe-dosing strategy. VI. Simultaneous evaluation of inhibition potential of drugs on human hepatic isozymes CYP2A6, 3A4, 2C9, 2D6 and 2E1. *Rapid Commun Mass Spectrom* 2001;15(10):741–748.

122. Kenworthy KE, Bloomer JC, Clarke SE, Houston JB. CYP3A4 drug interactions: correlation of 10 *in vitro* probe substrates. *Br J Clin Pharmacol* 1999;48(5):716–727.

123. Shou M, Lin Y, Lu P, Tang C, Mei Q, Cui D, Tang W, Ngui JS, Lin CC, Singh R, Wong BK, Yergey JA, Lin JH, Pearson PG, Baillie TA, Rodrigues AD, Rushmore TH. Enzyme kinetics of cytochrome P450-mediated reactions. *Curr Drug Metab* 2001;2(1):17–36.

124. Ueng YF, Kuwabara T, Chun YJ, Guengerich FP. Cooperativity in oxidations catalyzed by cytochrome P450 3A4. *Biochemistry* 1997;36(2):370–381.

125. Zhang Z, Li Y, Shou M, Zhang Y, Ngui JS, Stearns RA, Evans DC, Baillie TA, Tang W. Influence of different recombinant systems on the cooperativity exhibited by cytochrome P4503A4. *Xenobiotica* 2004;34(5):473–486.

126. Janiszewski JS, Rogers KJ, Whalen KM, Cole MJ, Liston TE, Duchosiav E, Fouda HG. A high-capacity LC-MS system for the bioanalysis of samples generated from plate based metabolic screening. *Anal Chem* 2001;73(7):1495–1501.

127. DiMarco A, Marcucci I, Verdirame M, Perez J, Sanchez M, Pelaez F, Chaudhary A, Laufer R. Development and validation of a high throughput radiometric CYP3A4 inhibition assay using tritiated testosterone. *Drug Metab Dispos* 2005;33:349–358.

128. Jensen BF, Vind C, Padkjr SB, Brockhoff PB, Refsgaard HHF. *In silico* prediction of cytochrome P450 2D6 and 3A4 inhibition using Gaussian kernel weighted k-nearest neighbor and extended connectivity fingerprints, including structural fragment analysis of inhibitors versus noninhibitors. *J Med Chem* 2007;50(3):501–511.

129. Refsgaard HHF, Jensen BF, Christensen IT, Hagen N, Brockhoff PB. *In silico* prediction of cytochrome P450 inhibitors. *Drug Dev Res* 2006;67:417–429.

130. Bachmann KA. Inhibition constants, inhibitor concentrations and the prediction of inhibitory drug drug interactions: pitfalls, progress and promise. *Curr Drug Metab* 2006;7:1–14.

131. Mannervik B. Regression analysis in design and analysis. In Purich DL, Ed. *Contemporary Enzyme Kinetics and Mechanism*, 2nd ed. San Diego, CA: Academic Press; 1996.

132. Kalgutkar AS, Gardner I, Obach RS, Shaffer CL, Callegari E, Henne KR, Mutlib AE, Dalvie DK, Lee JS, Nakai Y, O'Donnell JP, Boer J, Harriman SP. A comprehensive listing of bioactivation pathways of organic functional groups. *Curr Drug Metab* 2005; 6(3):161–225.

133. Li AP. A review of the common properties of drugs with idiosyncratic hepatotoxicity and the "multiple determinant hypothesis" for the manifestation of idiosyncratic drug toxicity. *Chem Biol Interact* 2002;142(1–2):7–23.

134. Segel IH. Simple inhibition systems. In *Enzyme Kinetics: Behaviour and Analysis of Rapid Equilibrium and Steady-State Enzyme Systems*. Hoboken, NJ: Wiley; 1975.

135. Wilkinson GR, Shand DG. A physiological approach to hepatic drug clearance. *Clin Pharmacol Ther* 1975;18:377–390.

136. Rostami-Hodjegan A, Tucker G. *In silico* simulations to assess the *in vivo* consequences of *in vitro* metabolic drug–drug interactions. *Drug Discov Today* 2004;1(4):441–448.

137. Houston JB, Galetin A. Progress towards prediction of human pharmacokinetic parameters from *in vitro* technologies. *Drug Metab Rev* 2003;35(4):393–415.

138. Ito K, Halifax D, Obach RS, Houston JB. Impact of parallel pathways of drug elimination and multiple cytochrome P450 involvement on drug–drug interactions: CYP2D6 paradigm. *Drug Metab Dispos* 2005;33(6):837–844.

139. Obach RS, Walsky RL, Venkatakrishnan K, Gaman EA, Houston JB, Termaine LM. The utility of *in vitro* cytochrome P450 inhibition data in the prediction of drug–drug interactions. *J Pharmacol Exp Ther* 2006;316:336–348.

140. Kato M, Tachibana T, Ito K, Sugiyama Y. Evaluation of methods for predicting drug–drug interactions by Monte Carlo simulation. *Drug Metab Pharmacokinet* 2003;18(2):121–127.

141. Rowland M, Tozer TN. Interacting drugs. In Rowland M, Tozer TN, Eds. *Clinical Pharmacokinetics: Concepts and Applications*. Philadelphia: Williams & Wilkins; 1995, pp 267–289.

142. Riley RJ, McGinnity DF, Austin RP. A unified model for predicting human hepatic, metabolic clearance from *in vitro* intrinsic clearance data in hepatocytes and microsomes. *Drug Metab Dispos* 2005;33(9):1304–1311.

143. Brown HS, Ito K, Galetin A, Houston JB. Prediction of *in vivo* drug–drug interactions from *in vitro* data: impact of incorporating parallel pathways of drug elimination and inhibitor absorption rate constant. *Br J Clin Pharmacol* 2005;60(5):508–518.

144. Blanchard N, Richert L, Coassolo P, Lave T. Qualitative and quantitative assessment of drug–drug interaction potential in man, based on K_i, IC_{50} and inhibitor concentration. *Curr Drug Metab* 2006;5(2):147–156.

145. Wang YH, Jones DR, Hall SD. Prediction of cytochrome P450 3A inhibition by verapamil enantiomers and their metabolites. *Drug Metab Dispos* 2004;32(2):259–266.

146. Ernest CS, Hall SD, Jones DR. Mechanism-based inactivation of CYP3A by HIV protease inhibitors. *J Pharmacol Exp Ther* 2005;312(2):583–591.

147. Obach RS, Walsky RL, Venkatakrishnan K. Mechanism based inactivation of human cytochrome P450 enzymes and the prediction of drug–drug interactions. *Drug Metab Dispos* 2007;35(2):246–255.

148. Kenny JR, Grime K. Pharmacokinetic consequences of time-dependent inhibition using the isolated perfused rat liver model. *Xenobiotica* 2006;36(5):351–365.

149. Warot D, Bergougnan L, Lamiable D, Berlin I, Bensimon G, Danjou P, Puech AJ. TroleandomycIn–triazolam interaction in healthy volunteers: pharmacokinetic and psychometric evaluation. *Eur J Clin Pharmacol* 1987;32:389–393.

150. Phillips JP, Antal EJ, Smith RB. A pharmacokinetic drug interaction between erythromycin and triazolam. *J Clin Psychopharmacol* 1986;6:297–299.

151. Galetin A, Burt H, Gibbons L, Houston JB. Prediction of time-dependent CYP3A4 drug–drug interactions: impact of enzyme degradation, parallel elimination pathways, and intestinal inhibition. *Drug Metab Dispos* 2006;34(1):166–175.

152. Lu C, Miwa GT, Prakash SR, Gan L, Balani SK. A novel method for the prediction of drug–drug interactions in humans based on *in vitro* CYP phenotypic data. *Drug Metab Dispos* 2007;35(1):79–85.

153. Luo G, Cunningham M, Kim S, Burn T, Lin J, Sinz M, Hamilton G, Rizzo C, Jolley S, Gilbert D, Downey A, Mudra D, Graham R, Carroll K, Xie J, Madan A, Parkinson A, Christ D, Selling B, Lecluyse E, Gan L. CYP3A4 induction by drugs: correlation between a pregnane X receptor reporter gene assay and CYP3A4 expression in human hepatocytes. *Drug Metab Dispos* 2002;30(7):795–804.

154. von Moltke LL, Durol ALB, Duan SX, Greenblatt DJ. Potent mechanism-based inhibition of human CYP3A *in vitro* by amprenavir and ritonavir: comparison with ketoconazole. *Eur J Clin Pharmacol* 2000;56(3):259–261.

155. Perloff MD, Stoermer E, von Moltke LL, Greenblatt DJ. Rapid assessment of P-glyco-protein inhibition and induction *in vitro*. *Pharm Res* 2003;20(8):1177–1183.

156. Greenblatt DJ, von Moltke LL, Harmatz JS, Durol ALB, Daily JP, Graf JA, Mertzanis P, Hoffman JL, Shader RI. Differential impairment of triazolam and zolpidem clearance by ritonavir. *J Acquir Immune Defic Syndr Hum Retrovirol* 2000;24(2):129–136.

157. Culm-Merdek KE, von Moltke LL, Gan L, Horan KA, Reynolds R, Harmatz JS, Court MH, Greenblatt DJ. Effect of extended exposure to grapefruit juice on cytochrome P450 3A activity in humans: comparison with ritonavir. *Clin Pharmacol Ther* 2006;79(3):243–254.

158. US Food and Drug Administration, Center for Drug Evaluation and Research website. http://www.fda.gov/CDER.

159. US Food and Drug Administration, Center for Drug Evaluation and Research website. Guidance web page. http://www.fda.gov/CDER/guidance.

APPENDIX A

From Fig. 22.1 it can be seen that

$$d[ES]/dt = k_1 \cdot [E] \cdot [S] - k_{-1} \cdot [ES] - k_2 \cdot [ES] \tag{A.1}$$

But at steady state, $d[ES]/dt = 0$; therefore,

$$k_1 \cdot [E] \cdot [S] = k_{-1} \cdot [ES] + k_2 \cdot [ES] \tag{A.2}$$

The total enzyme concentration is

$$[E]_0 = [E] + [ES] \tag{A.3}$$

and the total substrate concentration is

$$[S]_0 = [S] + [ES] \tag{A.4}$$

and therefore

$$[E] = [E]_0 - [ES] \tag{A.5}$$

and

$$[S] = [S]_0 - [ES] \tag{A.6}$$

Therefore, substituting Eqs. A.5 and A.6 into Eq. A.2 gives

$$k_1 \cdot [S]([E]_0 - [ES]) = (k_{-1} + k_2) \cdot [ES] \tag{A.7}$$

Dividing through by [ES] gives

$$\frac{k_1 \cdot [E]_0 \cdot [S]}{[ES]} - k_1 \cdot [S] = k_{-1} + k_2 \tag{A.8}$$

and therefore

$$k_{-1} + k_2 + k_1 \cdot [S] = k_1 \cdot \frac{[E]_0 \cdot [S]}{[ES]} \tag{A.9}$$

and

$$[ES] = \frac{k_1 \cdot [E]_0 \cdot [S]}{k_1 \cdot [S] + k_{-1} + k_2} \tag{A.10}$$

Dividing through by k_1 gives

$$[ES] = \frac{[E]_0 \cdot [S]}{[S] + (k_{-1} + k_2/k_1)} \tag{A.11}$$

since from the reaction scheme in Fig. 22.1 the overall dissociation rate constant for enzyme–substrate complex, $[ES] = (k_{-1} + k_2)/k_1$. This is referred to as the Michaelis–Menten constant K_m. Therefore, Eq. A.11 becomes

$$[ES] = \frac{[E]_0 \cdot [S]}{[S] + K_m} \tag{A.12}$$

Referring again to the reaction scheme in Fig. 22.1, the rate of reaction, v, or product formation, $d[P]/dt = k_2 \cdot [ES]$. Substituting this into Eq. A.12 gives

$$\frac{d[P]}{dt} = v = \frac{k_2 \cdot [E]_0 \cdot [S]}{[S] + K_m} \tag{A.13}$$

where $[S] \gg K_m$ and v tends to $k_2 \cdot [E]_0$ such that the maximal reaction rate can be described as $V_{max} = k_2 \cdot [E]_0$. Equation A.13 therefore becomes

$$v = \frac{V_{max} \cdot [S]}{K_m + [S]} \tag{A.14}$$

$$= \frac{V_{max}}{1 + K_m/[S]} \tag{A.15}$$

APPENDIX B

$$d[EI]/dt = k_{+1} \cdot [I] \cdot [E] - (k_{-1} + k_2) \cdot [EI] \tag{B.1}$$

$$d[EI']/dt = k_2 \cdot [EI] - (k_3 + k_4) \cdot [EI'] \tag{B.2}$$

$$d[E_{inact}]/dt = k_4 \cdot [EI'] \tag{B.3}$$

The *initial* rate of enzyme degradation, v_{inact}, is described by Eq. B.1, where k_{obs} is the apparent inactivation rate constant of the enzyme

$$v_{\text{inact}} = d[\text{E}_{\text{inact}}]/dt = k_4 \cdot [\text{EI}'] = k_{\text{obs}} \cdot [\text{E}]_0 \qquad (\text{B.4})$$

It is assumed that $[\text{E}_{\text{inact}}]$ is negligible before $[\text{EI}']$ reaches steady state; therefore, the total enzyme concentration, $[\text{E}]_0$, remains the same whether it is free, in complex with inhibitor, $[\text{EI}]$, or inactivated $[\text{EI}']$:

$$[\text{E}]_0 = [\text{E}] + [\text{EI}] + [\text{EI}'] \qquad (\text{B.5})$$

Referring to Fig. 22.3, when the levels of the inhibitor-bound enzyme are at steady state, $d[\text{EI}]/dt = 0$,

$$k_1 \cdot [\text{E}] \cdot [\text{I}] = (k_{-1} + k_2) \cdot [\text{EI}] \qquad (\text{B.6})$$

therefore,

$$[\text{EI}] = \frac{k_1 \cdot [\text{E}] \cdot [\text{I}]}{k_{-1} + k_2} \qquad (\text{B.7})$$

and when the levels of the initial complex formed between metabolic intermediate and enzyme are at steady state, $d[\text{EI}']/dt = 0$,

$$k_2 \cdot [\text{EI}] = (k_3 + k_4) \cdot [\text{EI}'] \qquad (\text{B.8})$$

therefore,

$$[\text{EI}'] = \frac{k_2 \cdot [\text{EI}]}{k_3 + k_4} \qquad (\text{B.9})$$

Substituting Eq. B.4 into Eq. B.6 gives

$$[\text{EI}'] = \frac{k_2 \cdot k_1 \cdot [\text{I}] \cdot [\text{E}]}{(k_3 + k_4) \cdot (k_{-1} + k_2)} \qquad (\text{B.10})$$

Substituting Eqs. B.8 and B.9 into Eq. B.5 gives

$$[\text{E}]_0 = [\text{E}] + \frac{k_1 \cdot [\text{I}] \cdot [\text{E}]}{(k_{-1} + k_2)} + \frac{k_2 \cdot k_1 \cdot [\text{I}] \cdot [\text{E}]}{(k_3 + k_4) \cdot (k_{-1} + k_2)} \qquad (\text{B.11})$$

To simplify Eq. B.11, the common denominator $(k_3 + k_4) \cdot (k_{-1} + k_2)$ is used:

$$[\text{E}]_0 = \frac{(k_3 + k_4) \cdot (k_{-1} + k_2)}{(k_3 + k_4) \cdot (k_{-1} + k_2)} \cdot [\text{E}] + \frac{(k_3 + k_4) \cdot k_1 \cdot [\text{I}] \cdot [\text{E}]}{(k_3 + k_4) \cdot (k_{-1} + k_2)} + \frac{k_2 \cdot k_1 \cdot [\text{I}] \cdot [\text{E}]}{(k_3 + k_4) \cdot (k_{-1} + k_2)} \qquad (\text{B.12})$$

$$= [E] \cdot \frac{(k_3 + k_4) \cdot (k_{-1} + k_2) + (k_3 + k_4) \cdot k_1 \cdot [I] + k_2 \cdot k_1 \cdot [I]}{(k_3 + k_4) \cdot (k_{-1} + k_2)} \tag{B.13}$$

Therefore,

$$[E] = \frac{(k_3 + k_4) \cdot (k_{-1} + k_2) \cdot [E]_0}{k_2 \cdot k_1 \cdot [I] + (k_3 + k_4) \cdot k_1 \cdot [I] + (k_3 + k_4) \cdot (k_{-1} + k_2)} \tag{B.14}$$

Substituting Eq. B.13 into Eq. B.10 gives

$$[EI'] = \frac{k_2 \cdot k_1 \cdot [I] \cdot [E]}{(k_3 + k_4) \cdot (k_{-1} + k_2)} \cdot \frac{(k_3 + k_4) \cdot (k_{-1} + k_2) \cdot [E]_0}{k_2 \cdot k_1 \cdot [I] + (k_3 + k_4) \cdot k_1 \cdot [I] + (k_3 + k_4) \cdot (k_{-1} + k_2)} \tag{B.15}$$

$$= \frac{k_2 \cdot k_1 \cdot [I] \cdot [E]_0}{k_2 \cdot k_1 \cdot [I] + (k_3 + k_4) \cdot k_1 \cdot [I] + (k_3 + k_4) \cdot (k_{-1} + k_2)} \tag{B.16}$$

Dividing through by k_1 gives

$$[EI'] = \frac{k_2 \cdot [I] \cdot [E]_0}{k_2 \cdot [I] + (k_3 + k_4) \cdot [I] + ((k_3 + k_4) \cdot (k_{-1} + k_2)/k_1)} \tag{B.17}$$

Then dividing through by $(k_2 + k_3 + k_4)$ gives

$$[EI'] = \frac{(k_2/(k_2 + k_3 + k_4)) \cdot [I] \cdot [E]_0}{[I] + \dfrac{(k_3 + k_4) \cdot (k_{-1} + k_2)}{(k_2 + k_3 + k_4) \cdot k_1}} \tag{B.18}$$

From Eq. B.18, we have

$$k_4 \cdot [EI'] = \frac{(k_2 \cdot k_4/(k_2 + k_3 + k_4)) \cdot [I] \cdot [E]_0}{[I] + \dfrac{(k_3 + k_4) \cdot (k_{-1} + k_2)}{(k_2 + k_3 + k_4) \cdot k_1}} \tag{B.19}$$

Substituting Eq. B.17 into Eq. B.3 gives

$$k_{obs} = \frac{(k_2 \cdot k_4/(k_2 + k_3 + k_4)) \cdot [I]}{[I] + \dfrac{(k_3 + k_4) \cdot (k_{-1} + k_2)}{(k_2 + k_3 + k_4) \cdot k_1}} \tag{B.20}$$

$$k_{obs} = \frac{k_{inact} \cdot [I]}{[I] + K_I} \tag{B.21}$$

where k_{inact} is the maximal inactivation rate constant and K_I is the inhibitor concentration that supports half the maximal rate of inactivation and, referring to Fig. 22.3, can be described by

$$k_{\text{inact}} = k_2 \cdot k_4 / (k_2 + k_3 + k_4) \tag{B.22}$$

$$K_I = \frac{(k_3 + k_4) \cdot (k_{-1} + k_2)}{(k_2 + k_3 + k_4) \cdot k_1} \tag{B.23}$$

23

IN VIVO METABOLISM IN PRECLINICAL DRUG DEVELOPMENT

SEVIM ROLLAS

Marmara University, Istanbul, Turkey

Contents

23.1 INTRODUCTION

Drug biotransformation plays an important role in the absorption, distribution, metabolism, excretion, and toxicology (ADMET) properties. Undesirable ADMET properties are the cause of many drug development failures [1–3]. Many toxic side effects (carcinogenicity, tissue necrosis, apoptosis, hypersensitivity, teratogenicity) of

Preclinical Development Handbook: ADME and Biopharmaceutical Properties,
edited by Shayne Cox Gad
Copyright © 2008 John Wiley & Sons, Inc.

drugs are directly attributable to the formation of chemically reactive metabolites [4–6]. The liver is a major site for the metabolism of xenobiotics (drugs and other exogenous compounds) and endogenous compounds. Other tissues such as kidney, lungs, adrenals, placenta, brain, intestinal mucosa, and skin have some degree of drug-metabolizing capability. Drug metabolism reactions have been divided into two main classes, phase I (functionalization) includes oxidation, reduction, and enzymatic hydrolysis reactions and phase II (conjugation) includes glucuronidation, sulfation, acetylation, methylation, amino acid and glutation conjugation, and mercapturic acid formation reactions. In phase I reactions, the cytochrome P450 (CYP) enzymes are responsible for oxidative biotransformation of many organic compounds [7]. Other drug-metabolizing enzymes, flavin-containing monooxygenase, monoamine oxidase, epoxide hydrolase, UDP-glucuronosyltransferase, glutation *S*-transferase, sulfotransferase, methyltransferase, and *N*-acetyltransferase may also be important when the drug is primarily metabolized by a non-P450 enzyme [8]. Glucuronidation is a well known major drug-metabolizing reaction (pathway) in humans and changes the structure of the parent drug, and thus its chemical and biological reactivity.

Individual differences in drug biotransformation exist. Some people metabolize a drug rapidly so that therapeutically effective blood and tissue levels are not achieved; others metabolize the same drug slowly so that toxicity results. Most CYP enzymes that belong to the CYP 1, 2, or 3 families are polymorphic [9]; so it may be difficult to predict a clinical response to a particular dose of a drug. Genetic polymorphisms have played an important role in these differences [10].

Metabolites can be obtained from plasma, urine, and bile after administration of compounds to laboratory animals and are used in preclinical *in vivo* studies as a reference standard [11–13]. The synthesis of metabolites is mostly done with parent compounds or is performed by total synthesis [14]. In addition, microbial methods can be used to obtain metabolites. The last two methods are very important for active metabolite synthesis.

Prodrug approches are very valuable in drug development. The goal of prodrug development is to solve specific pharmaceutical or pharmacological problems. The prodrug itself is inactive and is converted to the active drug *in vivo*. Early screening of their *in vitro* and/or *in vivo* plasma stability provides vital information for a stability profile of prodrug candidates [15, 16].

The application of well established preclinical *in vitro* and *in vivo* methodologies, such as gas chromatography–mass spectrometry (GC-MS) and liquid chromatography–mass spectrometry (LC-MS), is essential for drug discovery. Sensitive and specific analytical methods—for example liquid chromatography–high resolution nuclear magnetic resonance spectrometry [17, 18], LC-MS/MS (tandem mass spectrometry) [19–22], liquid chromatography–nuclear magnetic resonance/mass spectrometry (LC-NMR/MS) [23], and quadrupole time-of-flight mass spectrometry [24]—provide the identification and quantitation of metabolites. In general, this chapter is devoted to the preclinical *in vivo* metabolism of drug candidates. In the first part of this chapter, isolation, identification, synthesis, protein binding, and preclinical experimental studies are discussed, while in the following parts, *in vivo* metabolism of prodrugs, acyl glucuronides, and the role of active metabolites are covered.

23.2 *IN VIVO* METABOLISM OF DRUG CANDIDATES

In preclinical drug discovery, investigation of the *in vitro, in vivo* metabolism and toxicity screening of a drug candidate together play a very important role in the drug's success before entering into clinical use [25]. Rapid metabolism is one of the most important problems in achieving therapeutic drug levels [26]. Liver microsomal incubation has routinely been carried out by pharmaceutical companies to survey the metabolisim of potential drugs. Phase I and phase II drug-metabolizing enzymes affect the overall therapeutic and toxicity profiles of a drug. Several *in vitro* models, such as isolated perfused livers, liver tissue slices, freshly isolated hepatocytes in suspension, primary hepatocyte cultures, cell lines, microsomes, mitochondria, and expression systems, in particular, have been developed to profile human metabolism [1]. *In silico* (computational) techniques are tools that are used to predict the metabolic profiles of drugs that are in the design phase, but there is still insufficient data on the efficacy of *in silico* techniques. That is why *in vivo* metabolism studies should be performed on pharmacophore groups for an *in silico* database. *In vivo* metabolism is still being studied for conventional drugs in humans or animals for the detection of unknown metabolites [27–31]. During drug development, *in vivo* drug absorption, metabolic fate, and hepatic first-pass metabolism studies generally are performed in rats, dogs, and/or monkeys [32–34]. Indeed, the results of *in vitro* metabolism may not be the same as results of *in vivo* metabolism in animals and humans. Reliable human tests should be carried out. Human hepatocytes are used to model biotransformation in the human liver to predict human clearance [35–37]. Dog hepatocytes have also been used. However, the most successful results have been provided using human hepatocytes [38, 39]. Investigating the stereoselective metabolism of optical isomers of drugs is crucial in distinguishing their pharmacokinetic behaviors. The formation of sulfone, hydroxy, and 5-*O*-demethyl metabolites from *S*- and *R*-omeprazole using liver microsomes has been reported [40]. The metabolism of the optical isomers of omeprazole exhibits a significant stereoselectivity. Current strategies in high throughput chemistry are focused on high quality lead compounds [41]. Therefore animal testing is the most important step for lead identification and *in vitro–in vivo* correlation. The preclinical evaluation of selected lead compounds is represented in Fig. 23.1.

23.2.1 Isolation and Identification of Metabolites

Metabolite isolation and identification are important processes in discovery and development of new drugs. In many cases, the isolation and identification of metabolites are diffucult because of the low concentration or instability of these compounds in biological matrix. Therefore metabolites are synthesized and characterized by spectroscopic methods. The drug metabolism methodologies may be divided into isolation technologies (e.g., extraction, fractioning, chromatography) and chemical characterization (by means of spectroscopic techniques). For *in vivo* characterization of metabolites, biological samples are collected and it is determined what extraction methods (e.g., preparative solid phase extraction, solid phase extraction, liquid–liquid extraction, or protein precipitation (deproteination)) are necessary for analysis of the samples. Several studies reported use of extraction processes [13, 14,

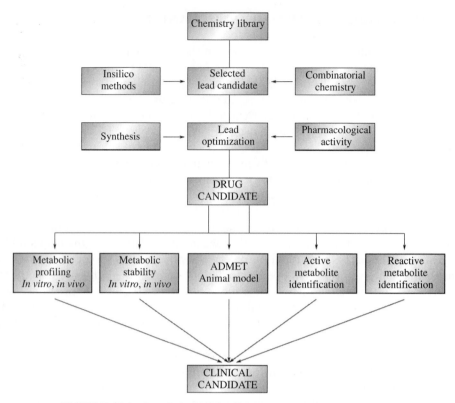

FIGURE 23.1   Preclinical evaluation of selected lead candidates.

19, 34, 42–46]. Recently, the use of turbulent flow chromatography with online solid phase extraction and column switching for sample preparation has been reported by Ong et al. [47]. Development of an analytical methodology suitable for accurate determination of both drug and metabolite in biological fluids is an advantange for the examination of the metabolic profile of a drug. The well known technique of liquid chromatography–tandem mass spectrometry (LC-MS/MS), can provide information for the identification for drug metabolites [25, 48]. High resolution nuclear magnetic resonance (NMR) spectroscopy is widely used for structure elucidation of organic compounds and their metabolites in biological samples [49–51]. The most high throughput analytical method for substrate and metabolite analysis is liquid chromatography with parallel NMR and mass spectrometry (LC-NMR/MS) [23, 49]. Timm and colleagues [42] reported another method for the analysis of oral platelet aggregation inhibitor, a double protected prodrug, and its metabolites by using HPLC—column switching combined with turbo ion spray single quadrupole mass spectrometry after precipitation of plasma protein by 0.5 M perchloric acid. Deproteination is a suitable method for sample preparation. Acetonitrile, methanol, perchloric acid, and trichloroacetic acid are used as deproteination agents [52–56]. Hydrophilic glucuronide conjugates may be hydrolyzed by β-glucuronidase in acetate buffer [28, 29, 57] or by acid or alkali [46, 58, 59] before being analyzed. In recent years, ultra performance liquid chromatography (UPLC) [60] has been used

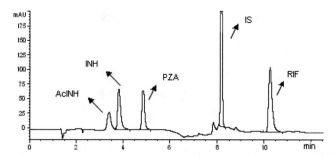

FIGURE 23.2   HPLC chromatogram of AcINH (acetylisoniazide), INH (isoniazide), PZA (pyrazinamide), IS (internal standard), and RIF (rifampin). Pore size is 4 μm Pore 3.9 × 150 mm long Nova-Pak C_{18} column. Signals were monitored by diode array detector. Gradient elution was used.

for drug and metabolite identification in biological fluids [61, 62]. Johnson and Plump [62] reported human metabolism of acetaminophen using UPLC with quadrupole time-of-flight mass analysis. Dear et al. [52] also reported a new approach by using UPLC for *in vivo* metabolite identification. These novel fast and successful methods may be applied to preclinical *in vivo* metabolite identification of drug candidates.

Metabolites alter the quantity of drug during pharmacokinetic or drug monitoring studies if an efficient separation is not provided. In our study on the monitoring of isoniazide, pyrazinamide, and rifampicin, for the separation of isoniazid and its major metabolite acetylisoniazid, we developed an HPLC analysis method represented in Fig. 23.2 for the drug monitoring study [55].

23.2.2 Synthesis of Metabolites

Metabolite identification and synthesis are important processes in the development of new lead candidates for drug metabolite profiling, pharmacokinetic studies (interference of metabolite), pharmacological activity testing (for active metabolite), metabolite quantification, CYP identification, and toxicity testing. Therefore a synthesis of methods are needed to obtain authentic metabolites. The synthesis of metabolites that are not easily obtained by chemistry methods may be produced by microbial biotransformation of the drugs. Chemical synthesis [14, 63] and microbial methods [64–66] are reported in the literature. Sulfadimethoxine *N*-glucuronide was prepared by Bridges et al. [67] starting from sodium sulfadimethoxine and methyl 2,3,4-tri-*O*-acetyl-1-bromoglucuronate. Ketotifen [68] and soraprazam [69] glucuronides have also been prepared synthetically. The N-oxide metabolite of the model compound *N*-benzyl-*N*-methylaniline was prepared by oxidizing with hydrogen peroxide [70]. Sulfinpyrazone sulfide metabolite was prepared by He et al. [71] by the reduction of sulfinpyrazone with iron powder. The hydroxamic acid metabolites are usually obtained from molecules containing an ester functional group [72].

The use of microbial models is a suitable method to produce a sufficient quantity of metabolites [73, 74]. Most bacterial species have P450 enzymes [75]. Enantiomeri-

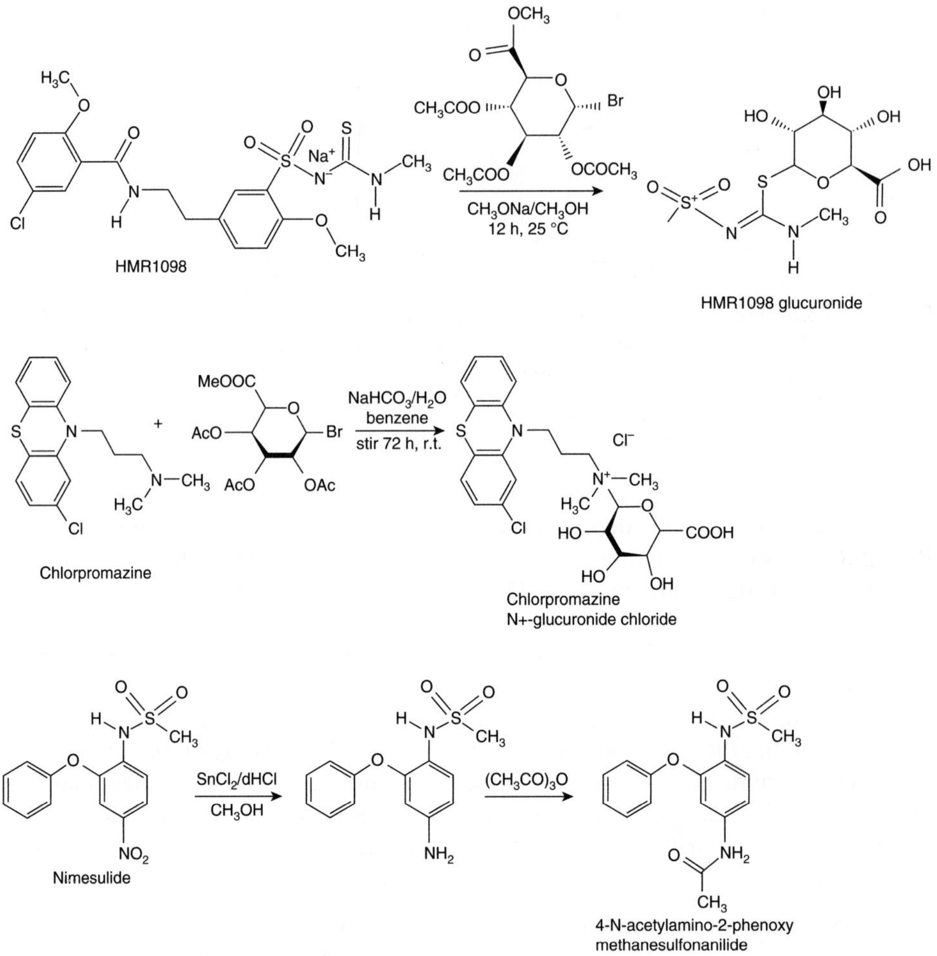

FIGURE 23.3   Examples for synthesis of some metabolites.

cally pure sulfoxides may be synthesized by biocatalytic methods using microorganisms or isolated enzymes. Ricci et al. [76] prepared aromatic sulfoxides from sulfides employing Basidiomycetes. Zhang et al. [77] reported biotransformation of amitriptyline by the filamentous fungus *Cunninghamella elegans*. The amitriptyline N-oxide metabolite that is produced from fungus can also be obtained by the oxidation of amitriptyline with 3-chloroperoxybenzoic acid to compare with the microbial product. The biosynthesis of drug glucuronides may be performed using suitable animal microsomes to obtain glucuronide metabolites [78]. The synthesis route of some metabolites is shown in Fig. 23.3 [20, 79, 80].

23.2.3   Protein Binding of Metabolites

Most drugs and/or their metabolites bind to plasma proteins and other blood components such as red blood cells [81–84]. Generally, free drug molecules can arrive

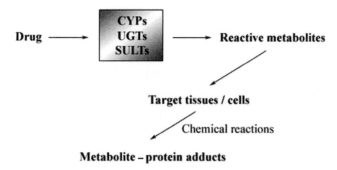

FIGURE 23.4 Formation of metabolite–protein adducts of drugs.

at the site of action. They are distributed into tissues for direct binding to tissue proteins [85]. Binding of a drug to plasma protein influences the drug's ADME processes. Yamazaki and Kanaoka [86] have developed a computational method that can provide precise and useful prediction of plasma protein binding for new drug candidates. However, preclinically, the *in vivo* studies must also be performed on drug candidates. The binding of drugs and/or their metabolites to plasma and tissue proteins is reversible. In some cases, they may covalently bind to plasma and tissue proteins, resulting of drug–protein or metabolite–protein adducts [87–89]. In most cases, the covalent binding by drugs is via their reactive metabolites [90–93]. Covalent binding to tissue proteins has been demonstrated for several metabolites such as acetaminophen–quinoneimine metabolite [94], carbamazepine–10,11-epoxide metabolite [95], furosemide–epoxide metabolite [88], ibuprofen–glucuronide metabolite [96], clozapine–nitrenium ion derived from clozapine N-oxide metabolite [97], and valproic acid–4-ene metabolite [98]. Formation of metabolite–protein adducts of drugs is represented in Fig. 23.4.

23.2.4 Preclinical Experimental Studies

The application of human-based preclinical *in vitro* hepatic metabolism (hepatocyte or liver microsome) is a must for the evaluation of drug metabolism and the selection of drug candidates with a probability of clinical success. However, *in vitro* metabolic stability and metabolite profiling studies should be correlated with *in vivo* experiments with relevant laboratory animal species for prediction of *in vivo* human drug properties [99]. Sample preparation is the most important element in *in vivo* metabolism studies. Conventional solid phase extraction is performed with a C_{18} cartridge [82, 100, 101]. Recently, Oasis HLB (hydrophilic–lipophilic balance), MCX (mixed mode, cation-exchange), and MAX (mixed mode, anion-exchange) cartridges have been developed to prepare samples [102–104]. Cleanup of the samples by means of solid phase extraction is shown Fig. 23.5.

Examples of *in vivo* metabolism studies are given next. The metabolite profile of 5-(2-ethyl-2*H*-tetrazol-5-yl)-1-methyl-1,2,3,6-tetrahydropyridine (Lu 25-109), a muscarine agonist, has been reported in mice, rats, dogs, and humans in plasma and

HLB, MCX, MAX
Oasis cartridge 1cc/30mg

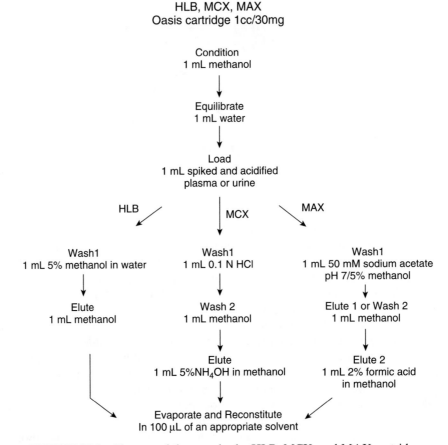

Condition
1 mL methanol

Equilibrate
1 mL water

Load
1 mL spiked and acidified
plasma or urine

HLB   MCX   MAX

| Wash1 | Wash1 | Wash1 |
| 1 mL 5% methanol in water | 1 mL 0.1 N HCl | 1 mL 50 mM sodium acetate pH 7/5% methanol |

| Elute | Wash 2 | Elute 1 or Wash 2 |
| 1 mL methanol | 1 mL methanol | 1 mL methanol |

Elute
1 mL 5%NH₄OH in methanol

Elute 2
1 mL 2% formic acid
in methanol

Evaporate and Reconstitute
In 100 µL of an appropriate solvent

FIGURE 23.5   Cleanup of the samples by HLB, MCX, and MAX cartridges.

urine after oral administration of [¹⁴C]Lu 25-109. The *N*-deethyl metabolite is a major metabolite in human plasma. The formation of a pyridine derivative has only been shown in rats [105].

The myocardial binding of the high potency antipsychotic benzisoxazol derivative risperidone and its active metabolite, 9-hydroxyrisperidone, was studied by using equilibrium dialysis *in vitro* and using intraperitoneal administration *in vivo* on plasma and tissue samples of guinea pig by Titier et al [106]. Risperidone and its metabolite concentrations have been determined by the HPLC method with UV detection. The plasma protein and tissue binding of 9-hydroxyrisperidone was lower than that of the more lipophilic risperidone. This method can be applied for other drugs and for therapeutic drug monitoring [106].

In our laboratory, *in vivo* metabolic pathway selected model compounds—1,2,4-triazole-3-thiones [82, 107], hydrazide [108], thiourea derivative [109], azo compounds [110, 111], and quinazolinone [112] and pyridazine [113] rings compounds—were investigated in rats (Fig. 23.6). The potential metabolites of substrate, which cannot be provided, were synthesized. Unknown metabolites were

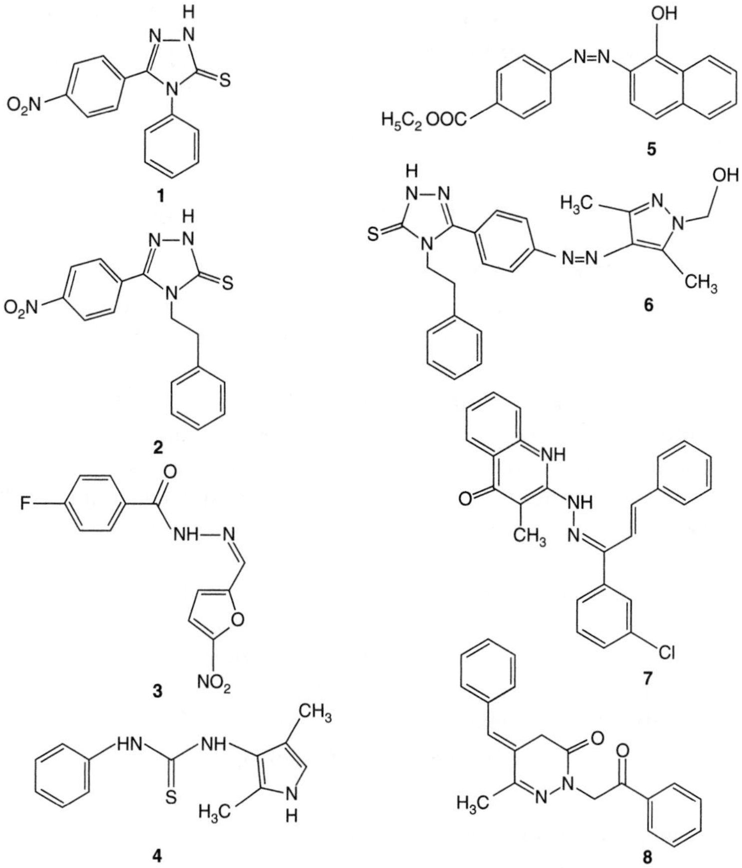

FIGURE 23.6 Examples of model compounds investigated for their *in vivo* meta-bolism: (**1**) 5-(4-nitrophenyl)-4-phenyl-2,4-dihydro-3*H*-1,2,4-triazole-3-thione [82]; (**2**) 5-(4-nitrophe-nyl)-4-(2-phenylethyl)-2,4-dihydro-3*H*-1,2,4-triazole-3-thione [107]; (**3**) 4-fluorobenzoic acid [(5-nitro-2-furanyl)methylene]hydrazide [108]; (**4**) *N*-phenyl-*N'*-(3,5-dimethyl-pyrazole-4-yl)thiourea [109]; (**5**) ethyl 4-[(2-hydroxy-1-naphthyl)azo]benzoate [110]; (**6**) 4-phenylethyl-5-[4-(1-(2-hydroxy-ethyl)-3,5-dimethyl-4-pyrazolylazo)-phenyl]-2,4-dihydro-3*H*-1,2,4-triazole-3-thione[111];(**7**)2-[1'-phenyl-3'-(3-chlorophenyl)-2'-propenylyden]hydrazino-3-methyl-4(3*H*)-quinazolinone [112]; (**8**) 3-oxo-5-benzylidene-6-methyl-(4*H*)-2-(benzoylmethyl)pyridazine [113].

collected during HPLC studies for mass analysis. Desulfurization reaction did not occur in the 1,2,4-triazole-3-thiones model compounds. Their oxygen analogues were synthesized and used as a reference standard in these studies. Examples of model compounds investigated for their *in vivo* metabolism are shown in Fig. 23.6.

4-Fluorobenzoic acid [(5-nitro-2-furanyl)methylene]hydrazide (substrate) is active against *Staphylococcus aureus* ATCC 29213 (MIC value 3.25 µg/mL) [114]. It was administered intraperitoneally in doses of 50 or 100 mg/kg. Blood samples were collected after administration. The substrate and its potential metabolites were synthesized and separated using HPLC [108]. The substrate and its potential metab-olites were not detected in plasma. After plasma proteins were denatured, 4-

fluorobenzoic acid (1.5 h) was detected. However, it rapidly metabolizes via a hydrolytic reaction in rats and shows poor metabolic stability *in vivo.*

23.3   *IN VIVO* METABOLISM OF PRODRUGS

Drug activation has been known since the identification of prontosil as a bioreductive prodrug of sulfanylamide. The aim of prodrug development is to solve specific pharmaceutical or pharmacological problems. Various drugs with groups that can be modified by chemical reactions can be converted into prodrugs. They can be synthesized to improve drug stability and absorption, to reduce diverse effects, to extend the duration of action, to increase water solubility or other desirable properties, and to allow site-specific delivery [115]. Generally, synthetic or natural compounds with therapeutic potential as bioactive agents contain alcohol, phenol, ester, thioether, amino, or nitro groups in their structure. In the synthesis of prodrugs, mainly esters, amides, ethers, phosphamides, hydroxamic acids, imines, N-oxides, Mannich bases, azo groups, glycosides, peptides, salts, polymers, and complexes from the parent drug are obtained. The anti-inflammatory drug sulindac is a prodrug and its two active metabolites—sulindac sulfide and sulindac sulfone—result from reduction and oxidation, respectively [116]. This type of prodrug is called a *bioprecursor.* Examples of other bioprecursors are diazepam, primidone, and clofibrate. Quantitative prediction of the effect of a prodrug's enzymatic catalysis *in vivo* is diffucult due to the variety and complexity of enzyme systems [117]. The conversion of a prodrug into a parent drug is represented schematically in Fig. 23.7.

23.3.1   Ester and Amide Prodrugs

Esterification and amidation are two important reactions for the synthesis of prodrugs. Many drugs contain free carboxylic acid and/or an amine group. Chandrasekaran et al. [118] reported that the nonsteroidal anti-inflammatory drug indomethacin conjugated with triethylene glycol at the carboxylic acid to obtain its ester and amide prodrugs. Sriram et al. [119] synthesized the amino acid ester prodrug of stavudine for the effective treatment of HIV/AIDS. Wu et al. [120] synthesized lipophilic metronidazol esters using enzymes as catalyst. The best enzymatic transesterfication is provided by *Candida antarctica* lipase acrylic resin.

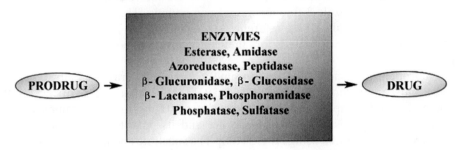

FIGURE 23.7   Conversion of prodrug to parent drug.

23.3.2 Other Prodrugs

Generally, prodrugs are designed for dealing with problems like rapid metabolism or poor absorption or reducing diverse effects seen with conventional drugs. In recent years, tumor-activated prodrug (TAP) strategies have become a very important approach in cancer therapy [121]. These prodrugs can be selectively activated in tumor tissue. The aromatic and aliphatic N-oxides, quinones, aromatic nitro groups, and cobalt complexes are the most important structures in developing hypoxia-selective TAPs [122]. Monoclonal antibody–enzyme conjugates (antibody-directed enzyme prodrugs) have recently been developed and rituximab, cetuximab, and trastuzumab are being used in the clinical setting [123,124]. β-Lactamase-dependent prodrugs have also been developed for antibody-directed enzyme therapy [125].

Another class of prodrugs is the dendritic prodrugs, which can improve drug delivery and solubility: thus decreasing dosages and prolonging drug release [126–128]. Najlah et al. [129] reported that the design, synthesis, and characterization of polyamidoamine (PAMAM) dendrimer-based prodrugs are described by selecting as the model compound naproxen, a poorly water-soluble drug. Propranolol-G_3 PAMAM dendrimer conjugates were also synthesized to increase propranolol solubility [130]. Salamonczyk [131] prepared phosphorus-based dendrimers of acyclovir.

23.3.3 Metabolic Stability of Prodrugs

The metabolic stability of a drug candidate in liver microsomes of different animal species is determined in order to assess the potential of this drug to form undesired, potentially toxic, or pharmacologically inactive/active metabolites. In the determination of metabolic stability, *in vitro* models were widely used in order to investigate the metabolic fate of drug candidates. Liver microsomes and S9 (cytosolic and mitochondrial) fractions as drug-metabolizing enzyme sources are used for metabolic stability studies [132]. Di et al. [133] have suggested a single time-point microsomal stability assay and incubation time of 15 min for metabolic stability profiling at the early stage of drug discovery. The duration and/or the intensity of action of most drugs are determined by their rate of metabolism by hepatic enzymes [134]. The metabolic stability procedure involves the following [15, 16, 135]:

- Preparation of buffers
- Preparation of stock solution of test compound (in DMSO or water)
- Incubation (at 37 °C)
- Sample preparation
- Determination of loss of parent compound (using LC-MS, LC-MS/MS)

Screening of plasma stability of the prodrugs is very important for rapid conversion in plasma [136]. However, *in vitro* hydrolysis rates of prodrugs of ester or amide must be correlated with *in vivo* hydrolysis rates [137]. Lai and Khojasteh-Bakht [138] reported a new method for prodrug stability—an automated online liquid chromatographic–mass spectrometric method.

23.4   ACYL GLUCURONIDES

Glucuronidation reaction represents the major route for elimination and detoxification of drugs. The biosynthesis of glucuronides is catalyzed by the uridine diphosphate glucuronosyltransferases, which are localized in hepatic endoplasmic reticulum. However, the glucuronidation of some drugs has been observed in human kidney microsomes [135]. Seventeen human UDP-glucuronosyltransferases have been identified to date [139]. The mechanism of glucuronidation is a nucleophilic substitution reaction and the resulting glucuronide has the 1β-glycosidic configuration.

The rate of glucuronidation is dependent on the nucleophilic character of the substrate and enzyme concentration. The most systematic investigations were initiated in the 1930s by R. T. Williams and collaborators [140, 141]. Acyl glucuronide metabolites of carboxylic acid may be hydrolyzed under physiological conditions. Therefore the glucuronides produced can potentially interfere with the pharmacokinetics of the parent drug. In this case, early pharmacokinetic study is important in animal models to regulate dosing and duration of action.

On the other hand, glucuronide conjugates are capable of cellular injury (e.g., hepatotoxicity, carcinogenesis) by facilitating the formation of reactive electrophilic intermediates and their transport into target tissues [87]. Acyl glucuronides are chemically unstable in aqueous solution and undergo the intramolecular acyl migration. The acyl group may migrate to the C-2, C-3, or C-4 position of the glucuronic acid from the 1β position [142]. In addition, unstable acyl glucuronides have also been shown to form covalent adducts with proteins under *in vivo* conditions. The existence of genetic polymorphism in the rate of drug acylation has important consequences in drug therapy. Chen et al. [143] developed a rapid *in vitro* method for the assessment of the stability of acyl glucuronides. Many nonsteroidal anti-inflammatory drugs, such as diclofenac, diflunisal, zomepirac, and naproxen, and other drugs, such as valproic acid, citalopram, and furosemide, which bear the carboxylic functional group, have been metabolized to form acy lglucuronides [49, 144, 145].

23.5   ROLE OF ACTIVE METABOLITES IN PRECLINICAL DRUG DEVELOPMENT

Drugs can metabolize inactive, reactive, or pharmacologically active molecules [146, 147]. Fura et al. [148] and Guengerich et al. [149] define an active metabolite as the active metabolic product possessing the same pharmacological activity as the parent drug. Pharmacologically active metabolites should be recognized at the drug discovery stage, because the potential contribution of an active metabolite to total activity is an important factor for pharmacokinetic properties of a drug candidate. Therefore active metabolite kinetics should be studied in animal models. Klein et al. [150] reported a population pharmacokinetic model for irinotecan and two of its metabolites, SN-38 and SN-38 glucuronide. The active metabolite 7-hydroxycamptothecin (SN-38) is 300–1000 times more potent than its parent molecule irinotecan. Therefore it is important to develop dosing strategies for irinotecan. Mak and Weglicki [151] reported on the antioxidant properties of 4-hydroxypropranolol, a major metabolite of propranolol. It is four- to eightfold more potent than vitamin E. As a result, 4-hydroxypropranolol may contribute to the cardiovascular therapeutic benefits of propranolol because of its endothelial cytoprotective efficacy against cell injury.

Active metabolites play a role as lead candidates during lead optimization [148, 152]. For example, ezetimibe was found during the lead optimization phase [152]. During drug development, it is sometimes impossible to characterize the pharmacological activity of active metabolites because of the difficulties in their synthesis by common methods. They may be more active than their respective parent molecules. However, a number of active metabolites have been marketed as drugs: for example, acetaminophen, cetirizine, imipramine, desloratadine, fexofenadine, mesoridazone, nortriptyline, and oxazepam [148].

Metabolism of the antifungal drug itraconazole (ITZ) involves both phase I (oxidative) and phase II (conjugative) pathways. One of these metabolites, hydroxy-itraconazole (OH-ITZ), possesses antifungal activity similar to that of ITZ [153]. Therefore, the pharmacokinetic behavior of ITZ may be affected by its active metabolites. Gasparro et al. [154] reported that the active metabolite *R*-desmethyl-deprenyl of *R*-deprenyl has been shown to be more active than R-deprenyl. Ciclesonide, an inhaled corticosteroid with prolonged anti-inflammatory activity, is being developed for the treatment of asthma. Nave et al. [155] reported ciclesonide is converted to an active metabolite, desisobutyryl-ciclesonide, which undergoes reversible fatty acid conjugation in *in vitro* studies. Cannell et al. [144] demostrated that nonsteroidal anti-inflammatory drugs (diflunisal, zomepirac, and diclofenac), acyl glucuronides, and their rearrangement isomers had antiproliferative activity on human adenocarcinoma HT-29 cells in culture.

In conclusion, active metabolites may:

- Alter pharmacokinetic properties of parent compounds.
- Cause enzyme induction or inhibition.
- Alter pharmacokinetics of drugs when used together.
- Show different pharmacological activity.
- Be toxic.

23.6 CURRENT APPROACHES FOR EVALUATING PRECLINICAL *IN VIVO* METABOLISM

Metabolism is one of the most important steps in ADMET studies. Metabolites affect pharmacokinetic results [156]. *In vivo* pharmacokinetic behavior involves permeability, metabolic stability, inhibition, and induction of CYP isoenzymes and plasma protein binding. A new approach may be the use of ultra performance liquid chromatography [52], online hyphenated LC-NMR/MS [48], and an integrated high capacity solid phase extraction–MS/MS system [157] for *in vivo* metabolite identification in the future. Metabolism is also one of the most complicated of the pharmacokinetic properties. Genetic, environmental, and physiological factors may affect drug metabolism. Computational approaches for predicting CYP-related metabolism is very important for the evaulation of a successful new drug [158]. Therefore, CYP inhibitors, CYP inducers, CYP regioselectivity, and CYP substrates have been studied for the development of a reliable predictive model.

Computational or virtual ADME [2, 26, 159–162] and metabolism models derived from past *in vitro* and *in vivo* data have been developed to contribute to new drug discovery in the pharmaceutical industry [163, 164]. Klopman et al. [165] evaluated a computer model for prediction of intestinal absorption in humans. This model may be applied to particularly active metabolites. Recent studies have shown that one of the current trends will be drug-induced autoimmunity. Idiosyncratic drug reactions that do not occur in most patients are an important clinical problem [166]. Most of these reactions appear to be immune-mediated reactions. It is nessesary to develop new animal models, in addition to the present models, for preclinical studies. However, the newest approaches of drug discovery may be the mechanism-based, the function-based, and the physiology-based approaches [167].

23.7 CONCLUSION

In the last few years, much effort in drug discovery and development has focused on defining the metabolic profile, toxicity, stereoselective metabolism, and pharmacokinetics of new drug candidates. Understanding the role of drug–metabolizing enzymes in drug metabolism is an important area of research for human toxicology testing. *In vitro* and *in vivo* models have been used as part of high throughput screening programs to characterize lead identification, drug metabolic profiling, metabolic stability, drug permeability, drug solubility, and drug safety. *In vitro* studies generally provide a valuable insight into a drug's metabolic profile in humans; however, sometimes there are discrepancies between *in vitro* results and *in vivo* findings. In the future, the use of *in silico* predictive models and ultra developed analysis techniques for preclinical *in vivo* studies will be an essential requirement for the discovery and development of successful new drugs.

REFERENCES

1. Sivaraman A, Leach JK, Townsend S, Iida T, Hogan BJ, Stolz DB, Fry R, Samson LD, Tannenbaum SR, Griffith LG. A microscale *in vitro* physiological model of the liver: predictive screens for drug metabolism and enzyme induction. *Curr Drug Metabolism* 2005;6:569–591.
2. Bugrim A, Nikolskaya T, Nikolsky Y. Early prediction of drug metabolism and toxicity: systems biology approach and modeling. *Drug Discov Today* 2004;9:127–135.
3. Ekins S, Ring BJ, Grace J, McRobie-Belle DJ, Wrighton SA. Present and future *in vitro* approaches for drug metabolism. *Pharmacol Toxicol Methods* 2000;44:313–324.
4. Wells PG, Kim PM, Laposa RR, Nicol CJ, Parman T, Winn LM. Oxidative damage in chemical teratogenesis. *Mutat Res* 1997;396:65–78.
5. Williams DP. Toxicophores: investigations in drug safety. *Toxicology* 2006;226:1–11.
6. Park KB, Dalton-Brown E, Hirst C, Williams DP. Selection of new chemical entities with decreased potential for adverse drug reactions. *Eur J Pharmacol* 2006;549:1–8.
7. Rendic S. Summary of information on human CYP enzymes: human P450 metabolism data. *Drug Metab Rev* 2002;34:438–448.
8. Lu AYH, Wang RW, Lin JH. Cytochrome P450 *in vitro* reaction phenotyping: a re-evaluation of approaches used for P450 isoform identification. *Drug Metab Dispos* 2003;31:345–350.

9. Agundez JAG. Cytochrome P450 gene polymorphism and cancer. *Curr Drug Metab* 2004;5:211–224.

10. Dorne JLCM, Walton K, Renwick AG. Human variability in xenobiotic metabolism and pathway-related uncertainty factors for chemical risk assessment: a review. *Food Chem Toxicol* 2005;43:203–216.

11. Williams RT. Studies in detoxification 13. The biosynthesis of aminophenyl- and sulphonamidoaminophenyl- glucuronides in the rabbit and their action on haemoglobin *in vitro*. *Biochem J* 1943;37:329–333.

12. Turgeon J, Pare JRJ, Lalande M, Grech-Belanger O, Belanger PM. Isolation and structural characterization by spectroscopic methods of two glucuronide metabolites of mexiletine after N-oxidation and deamination. *Drug Metab Dispos* 1992;20:762–769.

13. Sidelman UG, Christiansen E, Krogh L, Cornett C, Tjornelund J, Hansen SH. Prufication and ^{1}H NMR spectroscopic characterization of phase II metabolites of tolfenamic acid. *Drug Metab Dispos* 1997;25:725–731.

14. Lantz RJ, Gillespie TA, Rash TJ, Kuo F, Skinner M, Kuan HY, Knadler MP. Metabolism, excretion, and pharmacokinetics of duloxetine in healthy human subjects. *Drug Metab Dispos* 2003;31:1142–1150.

15. Di L, Kerns EH, Hong Y, Chen H. Develoment and application of high throughput plasma stability assay for drug discovery. *Int J Pharm* 2005;297:110–119.

16. Kerns EH, Di L. Pharmaceutical profiling in drug discovery. *Drug Discov Today* 2003; 8:316–323.

17. Mutlib AE, Chen H, Nemeth GA, Markwalder JA, Seitz SP, Gan LS, Christ DD. Identification and characterization of efavirenz metabolites by liquid chromatography/mass spectrometry and high field NMR: species differences in the metabolism of efavirenz. *Drug Metab Dispos* 1999;27:1319–1333.

18. Zhang KE, Hee B, Lee CA, Liang B, Potts BCM. Liquid chromatography–mass spectrometry and liquid chromatography–NMR characterization of *in vitro* metabolites of a potent and irreversible peptidomimetic inhibitor or rhinovirus 3C protease. *Drug Metab Dispos* 2001;29:729–734.

19. Bramer SL, Tata PNV, Vengurlekar SS, Brisson JH. Method for the quantitative analysis of cilostazol using LC/MS/MS. *J Pharm Biomed Anal* 2001;26:637–650.

20. Kucukguzel SG, Kucukguzel I, Oral B, Sezen S, Rollas S. Detection of nimesulide metabolites in rat plasma and hepatic subcellular fractions by HPLC-UV/DAD and LC-MS/MS studies. *Eur J Drug Metab Pharmacokinet* 2005;30:127–134.

21. Lampinen-Salomonsson M, Beckman E, Bondesson U, Hedeland M. Detection of altrenogest and its metabolites in post administration horse urine using liquid chromatography tandem mass spectrometry—increased sensitivity by chemical derivatization of glucuronic acid conjugate. *J Chromatogr B* 2006;833:245–256.

22. Guo L, Qi M, Jin X, Wang P, Zhao H. Determination of active metabolite of prulifloxacin in human plasma by liquid chromatography–tandem mass spectrometry. *J Chromatogr B* 2006;832:280–285.

23. Corcoran O, Spraul M. LC-NMR-MS in drug discovery. *Drug Discov Today* 2003; 8:624–631.

24. Ishigai M, Langridge JI, Bordoli RS. A new approach for dynamics of enzyme-catalyzed glutation conjugation by electrospray quadrupole/time–of-flight mass spectrometry. *Anal Biochem* 2001;298:83–92.

25. Lee M-Y, Dordick JS. High-throughput human metabolism and toxicity analysis. *Curr Opin Biotechnol* 2006;17:1–9.

26. Tarbit MH, Berman J. High-throughput approaches for evaluating absorption, distribution, metabolism and excretion properties of lead compounds. *Curr Opin Chem Biol* 1998;2:411–416.

27. Schaber G, Wiatr G, Wachsmuth H, Dachtler M, Albert K, Gaertner I, Breyer-Pfaff U. Isolation and identification of clozapine metabolites in patient urine. *Drug Metab Dispos* 2001;29:923–931.

28. Strickmann DB, Blaschke G. Isolation of an unknown metabolite of non-steroidal anti-inflammatory drug etodolac and its identification as 5-hydroxy etodolac. *J Pharm Biomed Anal* 2001;25:977–984.

29. Desmoulin F, Gilard V, Martino R, Malet-Martino M. Isolation of an unknown metabolite of capecitabine, an oral 5-fluorouracil prodrug, and its identification by nuclear magnetic resonance and liquid chromatography–tandem mass spectrometry as a glucuroconjugate of 5′-deoxy-5-fluorocytidine, namely 2′-(β-D-glucuronic acid)-5′-deoxy-5-fluorocytidine. *J Chromatogr B* 2003;792:323–332.

30. Walles M, Thum T, Levsen K, Borlak J. Metabolism of verapamil: 24 new phase I and phase II metabolites identified in cell cultures of rat hepatocytes by liquid chromatography–tandem mass spectrometry. *J Chromatogr B* 2003;798:265–274.

31. Aresta A, Carbonara T, Palmisano F, Zambonin CG. Profiling urinary metabolites of naproxen by liquid chromatography–electrospray mass spectrometry. *J Pharm Biomed Anal* 2006;41:1312–1316.

32. Bertrand M, Jackson P, Walther B. Rapid assessment of drug metabolism in the drug discovery process. *Eur J Pharm Sci* 2000;11(Suppl 2):S61–S62.

33. Ward KW, Smith BR. A comprehensive quantitative and qualitative evaluation of extrapolation of intravenous pharmacokinetic parameters from rat, dog and monkey to humans. I. Clearance. *Drug Metab Dispos* 2004;32:603–611.

34. Mattiuz EL, Ponsler GD, Barbuch RJ, Wood PG, Mullen JH, Shugert RL, Li Q, Wheeler WJ, Kuo F, Conrad PC, Sauer J-M. Disposition and metabolic fate of atomoxetine hydrocloride: pharmacokinetics, metabolism, and excretion in the Fischer 344 rats and beagle dog. *Drug Metab Dispos* 2003;31:88–97.

35. Wilkening S, Stahl F, Bader A. Comparison of primary human hepatocytes and hepatoma cell line HEPG2 with regard to their biotransformation properties. *Drug Metab Dispos* 2003;31:1035–1042.

36. Naritomi Y, Terashita S, Kagayama A, Sugiyama Y. Utility of hepatocytes in predicting drug metabolism: comparison of hepatic intrinsic clearance in rats and humans *in vivo* and *in vitro*. *Drug Metab Dispos* 2003;31:580–588.

37. Soars MG, Burchell B, Riley RJ. *In vitro* analysis of human drug glucoronidation and prediction of *in vivo* metabolic clearance. *J Pharmacol Exp Ther* 2001;301:382–390.

38. McGinnity DF, Soars MG, Urbanowicz RA, Riley RJ. Evaluation of fresh and cryopreserved hepatocytes as *in vitro* drug metabolism tools for the prediction of metabolic clearance. *Drug Metab Dispos* 2004;32:1247–1253.

39. Iwatsubo T, Hirota N, Ooide T, Suzuki H, Shimada N, Chiba K, Ishizaki T, Green CE, Tyson CA, Sugiyama Y. Prediction of *in vivo* drug metabolism in the human liver from *in vitro* metabolism data. *Pharmacol Ther* 1997;73:147–171.

40. Abelo A, Anderson TB, Antonsson M, Naudot AK, Skanberg I, Weidolf L. Stereoselective metabolism of omeprazole by human cytochrome P450 enzymes. *Drug Metab Dispos* 2000;28:966–972.

41. Steinmeyer A. The hit-to-lead process at Schering AG: strategic aspects. *ChemMedChem* 2006;1:31–36.

42. Timm U, Birnböck H, Erdin R, Hopfgartner G., Zumbrunnen R. Determination of oral platelet aggregation inhibitor Sibrafiban® in rat, dog and human plasma utilising

HPLC–column switching with turbo ion spray single quadrupole mass spectrometry. *J Pharm Biomed Anal* 1999;21:151–163.

43. Wang XJ, Jin YX, Ying JY, Zeng S, Yao TW. Determination of rutin deca(H-) sulfate sodium in rat plasma using ion-pairing liquid chromatography after ion-pairing solid-phase extraction. *J Chromatogr B* 2006;833:231–235.

44. Wang PG, Wei JS, Kim G, Chang M, El-Shourbagy T. Validation and application of a high-performance liquid chromatography–tandem mass spectrometric method for simultaneous quantification of lopinavir and ritonavir in human plasma using semi-automated 96-well liquid–liquid extraction. *J Chromatogr A* 2006;1130:302–307.

45. Dumasia MC. *In vivo* biotransformation of metoprolol in the horse and on-column esterification of the aminocarboxylic acid metabolite by alcohols during solid phase extraction using mixed mode columns. *J Pharm Biomed Anal* 2006;40:75–81.

46. Oruc EE, Kocyigit-Kaymakcioglu B, Yilmaz-Demircan F, Gurbuz Y, Kalaca S, Kucukguzel SG, Ulgen M, Rollas S. An high performance liquid chromatographic method for the quantification of cotinine in the urine of preschool children. *Pharmazie* 2006; 61:823–827.

47. Ong VS, Cook KL, Kosara CM, Brubaker WF. Quantitative bioanalysis: an integrated approach for drug discovery and development. *Int J Mass Spectrom* 2004;238:139–152.

48. Constanzer ML, Chavez-Eng CM, Fu I, Woolf EJ, Matuszewski BK. Determination of dextromethorphan and its metabolite dextrorphan in human urine using high performance liquid chromatography with atmospheric pressure chemical ionization tandem mass spectrometry: a study of selectivity of a tandem mass spectrometric assay. *J Chromatogr B* 2005;816:297–308.

49. Yang Z. Online hyphenated liquid chromatography–nuclear magnetic resonance spectroscopy–mass-spectrometry for drug metabolite and nature product analysis. *J Pharm Biomed Anal* 2006;40:516–527.

50. Sidelmann UG, Bjornsdottir I, Shockcor JC, Hansen SH, Lindon JC, Nicholson JK. Directly coupled HPLC-NMR and HPLC-MS approaches for the rapid characterisation of drug metabolites in urine: application to the human metabolism of naproxen. *J Pharm Biomed Anal* 2001;24:569–579.

51. Vanderhoeven SJ, Lindon JC, Troke J, Nicholson JK, Wilson ID. NMR spectroscopic studies of the transacylation reactivity 1-β-*O*-acyl glucuronide. *J Pharm Biomed Anal* 2006;41:1002–1006.

52. Dear GJ, Patel N, Kelly PJ, Webber L, Yung M. TopCount coupled to ultra-performance liquid chromatography for the profiling of radiolabeled drug metabolites in complex biological samples. *J Chromatogr B* 2006;844:96–103.

53. Gemesi LI, Kapas M, Szeberenyi SZ. Application of LC-MS analysis to the characterisation of the *in vitro* and *in vivo* metabolite profiles of RGH-1756 in the rat. *J Pharm Biomed Anal* 2001;24:877–885.

54. Mohri K, Okoda K, Benet LZ. Stereoselective metabolism of benoxaprofen in rats. Biliary excretion of benoxaprofen taurine conjugate and glucuronide. *Drug Metab Dispos* 1998;26:332–337.

55. Unsalan S, Sancar M, Bekce B, Clark PM, Karagoz T, Izzettin FV, Rollas S. Therapeutic monitoring of isoniazid, pyrazinamide and rifampicin in tuberculosis patients using LC. *Chromatographia* 2005;61:595–598.

56. Nobilis M, Vybiralova Z, Sladkova K, Lisa M, Holcapek M, Kvetina J. High-performance liquid-chromatographic determination of 5-aminosalicylic acid and its metabolites in bood plasma. *J Chromatogr A* 2006;1119:299–308.

57. Zhang JY, Yuan JJ, Wang YF, Roy H, Bible JR, Breau AP. Pharmacokinetics and metabolism of a COX-2 inhibitor, valdecoxib in mice. *Drug Metab Dispos* 2003;31:491–501.

58. Kamata T, Nishikawa M, Katagi M, Tsuchihashi H. Optimized glucuronide hydrolysis for the detection of psilocin in human urine samples. *J Chromatogr B* 2003; 796:421–427.

59. Groff M, Riffel K, Song H, Lo M-W. Stabilization and determination of a PPAR agonist in human urine using automated 96-well liquid–liquid extraction and liquid chromatography/tandem mass spectrometry. *J Chromatogr B* 2006;842:122–130.

60. Wren SAC. Peak capacity in gradient ultra performance liquid chromatography (UPLC). *J Pharm Biomed Anal* 2005;38:337–343.

61. Li R, Dong L, Huang J. Ultra performance liquid chromatography–tandem mass spectrometry for the determination of epirubicin in human plasma. *Anal Chim Acta* 2005;546:167–173.

62. Johnson KA, Plumb R. Investigation of the human metabolism of acetaminophen using UPLC and exact mass oa-TOF MS. *J Pharm Biomed Anal* 2005;39:805–810.

63. Yu W, Dener JM, Dickman DA, Grothaus P, Ling Y, Liu L, Havel C, Malesky K, Mahajan T, O'Brain C, Shelton EJ, Sperandio D, Tong Z, Yee R, Mordenti JJ. Identification of metabolites of the tryptase inhibitor CRA-9249: observation of a metabolite derived from an unexpected hydroxylation pathway. *Bioorg Med Chem Lett* 2006;16:4053–4058.

64. Funhoff EG, Salzmann J, Bauer U, Witholt B, Blein JB. Hydroxylation and epoxidation reactions catalyzed by CYP153 enzymes. *Enzyme Microbial Technol* 2007;40:806–812.

65. Medici R, Lewkowicz ES, Iribarren AM. Microbial synthesis of 2,6-diaminopurine nucleosides. *J Mol Catal B: Enzymatic* 2006;39:40–44.

66. Keppler AF, Porto ALM, Schoenlein-Crusius IH, Comasseto JV, Andrade LH. Enzymatic evaluation of different *Aspergillus* strains by biotransformation of cyclic ketones. *Enzyme Microbial Technol* 2005;36:967–975.

67. Bridges JW, Kibby MR, Williams RT. The structure of the glucuronide of sulphadimethoxine formed in man. *Biochem J* 1965;96:829–836.

68. Mey U, Wachsmuth H, Breyer-Pfaff U. Conjugation of the enantiomers of ketotifen to four isomeric quarternary ammonium glucuronides in humans *in vivo* and in liver microsomes. *Drug Metab Dispos* 1999;27:1281–1292.

69. Senn-Bilfinger J, Ferguson JR, Holmes MA, Lumbard KW, Huber R, Zech K, Hummel RP, Zimmermann PJ. Glucuronide conjugates of Soraprazan (BY359), a new potassium-competitive acid blocker (P-CAB) for the treatment of acid-related diseases. *Tetrahedron Lett* 2006;47:3321–3323.

70. Kucukguzel I, Ulgen M, Gorrod JW. *In vitro* hepatic metabolism of *N*-benzyl-*N*-methylaniline. *Il Farmaco* 1999;54:331–337.

71. He M, Rettie AE, Neal J, Trager WF. Metabolism of sulfinpyrazone sulfide and sulfinpyrazone by human liver microsomes and cDNA-expressed cytochrome p450s. *Drug Metab Dispos* 2001;29:701–711.

72. Mshvidobadze EV, Vasilevsky SF, Elguero J. A new route to pyrazolo[3,4-c] and [4,3-c]pyridinones via heterocyclization of *vic*-substituted hydroxamic acids of acetylenylpyrazoles. *Tetrahedron* 2004;60:11875–11878.

73. Duhart BT, Zhang JD, Deck J, Freeman JP, Cerniglia CE. Biotransformation of protriptyline by filamentous fungi and yeasts. *Xenobiotica* 1999;29:733–746.

74. Li L, Liu R, Ye M, Hu X, Wang Q, Bi K, Guo D. Microbial, metabolism of evodiamine by *Penicillium janthinellum* and its application for metabolite identification in rat urine. *Enzyme Microbial Technol* 2006;39:561–567.

75. Lewis DFV, Wiseman A. A selective review of bacterial forms of cytochrome P450 enzymes. *Enzyme Microbial Technol* 2005;36:377–384.

76. Ricci LC, Commasseto JV, Andrabe LH, Capelari M, Cass QB, Porto ALM. Biotransformations of aryl alkyl sulfides by whole cells of white-rot Basidiomycetes. *Enzyme Microbial Technol* 2005;36:937–946.

77. Zhang D, Evans FE, Freeman JP, Duhart B Jr, Cerniglia CE. Biotransformation of amitriptyline by Cunninghamella elegans. *Drug Metab Dispos* 1995;23:1417–1425.

78. Soars MG, Mattiuz ED, Jackson DA, Kulanthaivel P, Ehlhardt WJ, Wrighton SA. Biosynthesis of drug glucuronides for use as authentic standards. *J Pharmacol Toxicol Methods* 2002;47:161–168.

79. Ethell BT, Riedel J, Englert H, Jantz H, Oekonomopulos R, Burchell B. Glucuronidation of HMR-1098 in human microsomes: evidence for the involvement of UGT1A1 in the formation of *S*-glucuronides. *Drug Metab Dispos* 2003;31:1027–1034.

80. Luo H, Hawes EM., McKay G, Midha KK. Synthesis and charecterization of quaternary ammonium-linked glucuronide metabolites of drugs with an aliphatic tertiary amine group. *J Pharm Sci* 1992;81:1079–1083.

81. Tonn GR, Kerr CR, Axelson JE. *In vitro* protein binding of propafenone and 5-hydroxy-propafenone in serum, in solutions of isolated serum proteins, and to red blood cells. *J Pharm Sci* 1992;81:1098–1103.

82. Oruc EE, Rollas S, Kabasakal L, Uysal MK. The *in vivo* metabolism of 5-(4-nitrophenyl)-4-phenyl-2,4-dihydro-3*H*-1,2,4-triazole-3-thione in rats. *Drug Metab Drug Interact* 1999;15:127–140.

83. Degelman CJ, Ebner T, Ludwig E, Happich S, Schildberg FW, Koebe HG. Protein binding capacity *in vitro* changes metabolism of substrates and influences the predictability of metabolic patways *in vivo*. *Toxicol In Vitro* 2004;18:835–840.

84. Acharya MR, Sparreboom A, Sausville EA, Conley BA, Doroshow JH, Venitz J, Figg WD. Interspecies differences in plasma protein binding of MS-275, a novel histon deacetylase inhibitor. *Cancer Chemother Pharmacol* 2006;57:275–281.

85. Yang XX, Hu ZP, Chan SY, Zhou SF. Monitoring drug–protein interaction. *Clin Chim Acta* 2006;365:9–29.

86. Yamazaki K, Kanaoka M. Computational prediction of the plasma protein-binding present in diverse pharmaceutical compounds. *J Pharm Sci* 2004;93:1480–1494.

87. Bailey MJ, Dickinson RG. Acyl glucuronide reactivity in perspective: biological consequences. *Chem-Biol Interact* 2003;145:117–137.

88. Park K, Williams DP, Naisbitt DJ, Kitteringham NR, Pirmohamed M. Investigation of toxic metabolites during drug development. *Toxicol Appl Pharmacol* 2005;207:425–434.

89. Day SH, Mao A, White R, Schulz-Utermoehl T, Miller R, Beconi MG. A semi-automated method measuring the potential for protein covalent binding in drug discovery. *J Pharmacol Toxicol Methods* 2005;52:278–285.

90. Dahms M, Spahn-Langguth H. Covalent binding of acidic drugs via reactive intermediates: detection of benoxaprofen and flunoxaprofen protein adducts in biological material. *Pharmazie* 1996;51:874–881.

91. Dong JQ, Liu J, Smith PC. Role of benoxaprofen acyl glucuronides in covalent binding to rat plasma and liver proteins in vivo. *Biochem Pharmacol* 2005;70:937–948.

92. Grillo MP, Benet LZ. Studies on the reactivity of clofibryl-*S*-acyl CoA thioester with glutathione *in vitro*. *Drug Metab Dispos* 2002;30:55–62.

93. Fan PW, Bolton JL. Bioactivation of tamoxifen to metabolite E quinone methide: reaction with glutathione and DNA. *Drug Metab Dispos* 2001;29:891–896.

94. Muldrew KL, James LP, Coop L, McCullough SS, Hendrickson HP, Hinson JA, Mayeux PR. Determination of acetaminophen–protein in mouse liver and serum and human

serum after hepatotoxic doses of acetaminophen using high-performance liquid chromatography with electrochemical detection. *Drug Metab Dispos* 2002;30:446–451.

95. Bu HZ, Kang P, Deese AJ, Zhao P, Pool WF. Human *in vitro* glutathione and protein adducts of carbamazepine-10,11-epoxide, a stable and pharmacologically active metabolite of carbamazepine. *Drug Metab Dispos* 2005;33:1920–1924.

96. Castillo M, Lam YW, Dooley MA, Stahl E, Smith PC. Disposition and covalent binding of ibuprofen and its acyl glucuronide in the elderly. *Clin Pharmacol Ther* 1995; 57:636–644.

97. Williams DP, Pirmohamed M, Naisbitt DJ, Maggs JL, Park BK. Neutrophil cytotoxicity of the chemically reactive metabolite(s) of clozapine: possible role in agranulocytosis. *J Pharmacol Exp Ther* 1997;283:1375–1382.

98. Sadeque AJM, Fisher MB, Korzekwa KR, Gonzales FJ, Rettie AE. Human CYP2C9 and CYP2A6 mediate formation of the hepatotoxin 4-ene-valproic acid. *J Pharmacol Exp Ther* 1997;283:698–703.

99. Li AP. Preclinical *in vitro* screening assays for drug-like properties. *Drug Discov Today* 2003;2:179–185.

100. Flores JR, Nevado JJB, Salcedo AMC, Diaz MPC. Non-aqueous capillary zone electrophoresis method for the analysis of paroxetine, tamoxifen and their main metabolites in urine. *Anal Chim Acta* 2004;512:287–295.

101. Meng QH, Gauthier D. Simultaneous analysis of citalopram and desmethylcitalopram by liquid chromatography with fluorescence detection after solid-phase extraction. *Clin Biochem* 2005;38:282–285.

102. Francois-Bouchard M, Simonin G, Bossant M-J, Boursier-Neyret C. Simultaneous determination of ivabradine and its metabolites in human plasma by liquid chromatography–tandem mass spectrometry. *J Chromatogr B* 2000;745:261–269.

103. Djabarouti S, Boselli E, Allaouchiche B, Ba B, Nguyen AT, Gordien JB, Bernadou JM, Saux MC, Breilh D. Determination of levofloxacin in plasma, bronchoalveolar lavage and bone tissues by high-performance liquid chromatography with ultraviolet detection using a fully automated extraction method. *J Chromatogr B* 2004;799:165–172.

104. Rizzo M, Ventrice D, Sarro VD, Gitto R, Caruso R, Chimirri A. SPE-HPLC determination of new tetrahydroisoquinoline derivatives in rat plasma. *J Chromatogr B* 2005;821: 15–21.

105. Christensen EB, Andersen JB, Pedersen H, Jensen KG, Dalgaard L. Metabolites of [^{14}C]-5(2-ethyl-2*H*-tetrazol-5-yl)-1-methyl-1,2,3,6-tetrahydropyridine in mice, rats, dogs, and humans. *Drug Metab Dispos* 1999;27:1341–1349.

106. Titier K, Deridet E, Moore N. *In vivo* and *in vitro* myocardial binding of risperidone and 9-hydroxyrisperidone. *Toxicol Appl Pharmacol* 2002;180:145–149.

107. Oruc EE, Kabasakal L, Rollas S. The *in vivo* metabolism of 5-(4-nitrophenyl)-4-(2-phenylethyl)-2,4-dihydro-3*H*-1,2,4-triazole-3-thione in rats. *Eur J Drug Metab Pharmacokinet* 2003;28:113–118.

108. Gulerman NN, Oruc EE, Kartal F, Rollas S. *In vivo* metabolism of 4-fluorobenzoic acid [(5-nitro-2-furanyl)methylene]hydrazide in rats. *Eur J Drug Metab Pharmacokinet* 2000;25:103–108.

109. Kocyigit-Kaymakcioglu B, Rollas S, Kartal-Aricioglu F. *In vivo* metabolism of *N*-phenyl-*N*′-(3,5-dimethylpyrazole-4-yl)thiourea in rats. *Eur J Drug Metab Pharmacokinet* 2003;28(4):273–278.

110. Bekce B, Sener G, Oktav M, Ulgen M, Rollas S. *In vitro* and *in vivo* metabolism of ethyl 4-[(2-hydroxy-1-naphthyl)azo]benzoate. *Eur J Drug Metab Pharmacokinet* 2005; 30:91–97.

111. Kaymakcioglu BK, Oruc EE, Unsalan S, Kabasakal LEE, Rollas S. High-pressure liquid chromatographic analysis for identification of *in vitro* and *in vivo* metabolites of 4-phenethyl-5-[4-(1-(2-hydroxyethyl)3,5-dimethyl-4-pyrazolylazo)phenyl]-2,4-dihydro-3*H*-1,2,4-triazole-3-thione in rats. *J Chromatogr B* 2006;831:184–189.

112. Kaymakcioglu BK, Aktan Y, Suzen S, Gokhan N, Koyuncuoglu S, Erol K, Yesilada A, Rollas S. *In vivo* metabolism of 2-[1'-phenyl-3'-(3-chlorophenyl)-2'-propenylyden] hydrazino-3-methyl-4(3*H*)-quinazolinone in rats. *Eur J Drug Metab Pharmacokinet* 2005;3:255–260.

113. Oruc EE, Unsal O, Balkan A, Ozkanli F, Goren MZ, Terzioglu MZ, Rollas S. The *in vivo* metabolism of 3-oxo-5-benzylidene-6-methyl-(4*H*)-2-(benzoylmethyl)pyridazine in rats. *Eur J Drug Metabol Pharmacokinet* 2006;31:21–25.

114. Rollas S, Gulerman N, Erdeniz H. Synthesis and antimicrobial activity of some new hydrazones of 4-fluorobenzoic acid hydrazide and 3-acethyl-2,5-disubstitute-1,3,4-oxadiazolines. *Il Farmaco* 2002;57:171–174.

115. Sincula AA, Yalkowsky SH. Rationale for design of biologically reversible drug derivatives. Prodrugs. *J Pharm Sci* 1975;64:181–210.

116. Chen Y-L, Jong Y-J, Wu S-M. Capillary electrophoresis field-amplified sample stacking and electroosmotic flow suppressant for analysis of sulindac and its two metabolites in plasma. *J Chromatogr A* 2006;1119:176–182.

117. Testa B. Prodrug research: futile or fertile? *Biochem Pharmacol* 2004;68:2097–2106.

118. Chandrasekaran S, Al-Ghananeem AM, Riggs RM, Crooks PA. Synthesis and stability of two indomethacin prodrugs. *Bioorg Med Chem Lett* 2006;16:1874–1879.

119. Sriram D, Yogeeswari P, Srichakravarthy N, Bal TR. Synthesis of stavudine amino acid ester prodrugs with broad-spectrum chemotherapeutic properties for the effective treatment of HIV/AIDS. *Bioorg Med Chem Lett* 2004;14:1085–1087.

120. Wu Q, Wang M, Chen ZC, Lu DS, Lin XF. Enzymatic synthesis of metronidazole esters and their monosaccharide ester derivatives. *Enzyme Microbial Technol* 2006;39:1258–1263.

121. Chari RVJ. Targeted delivery of chemotherapeutics: tumor-activated prodrug therapy. *Adv Drug Delivery Rev* 1998;31:89–104.

122. Denny WA. Prodrug strategies in cancer therapy. *Eur J Med Chem* 2001;36:577–595.

123. Senter PD, Springer CJ. Selective activation of anticancer prodrugs by monoclonal antibody-enzyme conjugates. *Adv Drug Delivery Rev* 2001;53:247–264.

124. Baselga J. Epidermal growth factor receptor pathway inhibitors. *Update Cancer Ther* 2006;I:299–310.

125. Smyth TP, O'Donnell ME, O'Connor MJ, Ledger JO. β-Lactamase-dependent prodrugs—recent developments. *Tetrahedron* 2000;56:5699–5707.

126. Tang S, June SM, Howell BA, Chai M. Synthesis of salicylate dendritic prodrugs. *Tetrahedron Lett* 2006;47:7671–7675.

127. Li X, Wu Q, Lv D-S, Lin X-F. Controllable synthesis of polymerizable ester and amide prodrugs of acyclovir by enzyme in organic solvent. *Bioorg Med Chem* 2006;14:3377–3382.

128. Chandrasekar D, Sistla R, Ahmad FJ, Khar RK, Dwan PV. The development of folate–PAMAM dendrimer conjugates for targeted delivery of anti-arthritics and their pharmacokinetics and biodistribution in arthritic rats. *Biomaterials* 2006;28:504–512.

129. Najlah M, Freeman S, Attwood D, Emanuele DA. Synthesis, characterization and stability of dendrimer prodrugs. *Int J Pharm* 2006;308:175–182.

130. Emanuele AD, Jevprasesphant R, Penny J, Attwood D. The use of a dendrimer–propranolol prodrug to bypass efflux transporters and enhance oral bioavailability. *J Controlled Release* 2004;95:447–453.

131. Salamonczyk GM. Acyclovir terminated thiophosphate dendrimers. *Tetrahedron Lett* 2003;44:7449–7453.

132. Ansede JH, Thakker DR. High-throughput screening for stability and inhibitory activity of compounds toward cytochrome P450-mediated metabolism. *J Pharm Sci* 2004; 93:239–255.

133. Di L, Kerns EH, Gao N, Li SQ, Huang Y, Bourassa JL, Huryn DM. Experimental design on single-time point high-throughput microsomal stability assay. *J Pharm Sci* 2004;93:1537–1544.

134. Mandagere AK, Thompson TN, Hwang KK. Graphical model for estimating oral bio-availability of drugs in humans and other species from their Caco-2 permeability and *in vitro* liver enzyme metabolic stability rates. *J Med Chem* 2002;45:304–311.

135. Soars MG, Riley RJ, Findlay KAB, Coffey MJ, Riley RJ, Burchell B. Evidence for significant differences in microsomal drug glucuronidation by canine and human liver and kidney. *Drug Metab Dispos* 2001;29:121–126.

136. Di L, Kerns EH, Li SQ, Petusky SL. High throughput microsomal stability assay for insoluble compounds. *Int J Pharm* 2006;317:54–60.

137. Lorenzi PL, Landowski CP, Song X, Borysko KZ, Breitenbach JM, Kim JS, Hilfinger JM, Townsend LB, Drach JC, Amidon GL. Amino acid ester prodrugs of 2-bromo-5,6-dichloro-1-(beta-dribofuranosyl)benzimidazole enhance metabolic stability *in vitro* and *in vivo*. *J Pharmacol Exp Ther* 2005;314:883–890.

138. Lai F, Khojasteh-Bakht SC. Automated online liquid chromatographic/mass spectrometric metabolic study for prodrug stability. *J Chromatogr B* 2005;814:225–232.

139. Miners JO, Knights KM, Houston JB, Mackenzie PI. *In vitro–in vivo* correlation for drugs and others eliminated by glucuronidation in humans: pitfalls and promises. *Biochem Pharmacol* 2006;71:1531–1539.

140. Pryde JP, Williams RT. The biochemistry and physiology of glucuronic acid I. The structure of glucuronic acid of animal origin. *Biochem J* 1933;27:1197–1204.

141. Williams RT. Studies in detoxication II. (a) The conjugation of isomeric 3-menthanols with glucuronic acid and the asymmetric conjugation of *dl*-menthol and *dl*-isomenthol in the rabbit. (b) *d*-Isomenthylglucuronide, a new conjugated glucuronic acid. *Biochem J* 1938;32:1849–1855.

142. Ebner T, Heinzel G, Prox A, Beschke K, Wachsmuth H. Disposition and chemical stability of telmisartan 1-*O*-acylglucuronide. *Drug Metab Dispos* 1999;27:1143–1149.

143. Chen Z, Holt TG, Pivnichny JV, Leung K. A simple *in vitro* model to study the stability of acylglucuronides. *J Pharmacol Toxicol Methods* 2006;55:91–95.

144. Cannell GR, Vesey DA, Dickinson RG. Inhibition of proliferation of HT-29 colon adenocarcinoma cell by carboxylate NSAIDs and their acyl glucuronides. *Life Sci* 2001;70:37–48.

145. Shipkova M, Wieland E. Glucuronidation in therapeutic drug monitoring. *Clin Chim Acta* 2005;358:2–23.

146. Gad SC. Active drug metabolites in drug development. *Curr Opin Pharmacol* 2003; 3:98–100.

147. Fura A. Role of pharmacologically active metabolites in drug discovery and development. *Drug Discov Today* 2006;11:133–142.

148. Fura A, Shu YZ, Zhu M, Hanson RL, Roongta V. Discovering drugs through biological transformation: role of pharmacologically active metabolites in drug discovery. *J Med Chem* 2004;47:4339–4351.

149. Guengerich FP. Cytochrome P450s and other enzymes in drug metabolism and toxicity. *AAPS J* 2006;8:101–111.

150. Klein CE, Gupta E, Reid JM, Atherton PJ, Sloan JA, Pitot HC, Ratain MJ, Kastrissios H. Population pharmacokinetic model for irinotecan and two of its metabolites, SN-38 and SN-38 glucuronide. *Clin Pharmacol Ther* 2002;72:638–647.

151. Mak IT, Weglicki WB. Potent antioxidant properties of 4-hydroxyl-propranolol. *J Pharmacol Exp Ther* 2004;303:85–90.

152. Davis HR. Ezetimibe: first in a new class of cholesterol absorption inhibitors. *Int Cong Ser* 2004;1262:243–246.

153. Wong JW, Nisar U-R, Yuen KH. Liquid chromatographic method for the determination of plasma itraconazole and its hydroxy metabolite in pharmacokinetic/bioavailability studies. *J Chromatogr B* 2003;798:355–360.

154. Gasparro DM, Almeida DRP, Fülöp F. *Ab initio* multi-dimensional conformational analysis of *R*-(–)-desmethyldeprenyl: a potent neuroprotective metabolite of *R*-(–)-deprenyl. *J Mol Structure THEOCHEM* 2005;725:75–83.

155. Nave R, Meyer W, Fuhst R, Zech K. Formation of fatty acid conjugates of ciclesonide active metabolite in the rat lung after 4-week inhalation of ciclesonide. *Pulm Pharmacol Ther* 2005;18:390–396.

156. Eddershaw PJ, Beresford AP, Bayliss MK. ADME/PK as part of a rational approach to drug discovery. *Drug Discov Today* 2000;5:409–414.

157. Kerns EH, Kleintop T, Little D, Tobien T, Mallis L, Di L, Hu M, Hong Y, McConnell OJ. Integrated high capacity solid phase extraction–MS/MS system for pharmaceutical profiling in drug discovery. *J Pharm Biomed Anal* 2004;34:1–9.

158. Crivori P, Poggesi I. Computational approaches for predicting CYP-related metabolism properties in the screening of new drugs. *Eur J Med Chem* 2006;41:795–808.

159. Lipinski CA. Drug-like properties and the causes of poor solubility and poor permeability. *J Pharmacol Toxicol Methods* 2000;44:235–249.

160. Dickins M, Waterbeemd H. Simulation models for drug disposition and drug interactions. *Drug Discov Today Biosilico* 2004;2:38–45.

161. Davis AM, Riley RJ. Predictive ADMET studies, the challenges and The opportunities. *Curr Opin Chem Biol* 2004;8:378–386.

162. Huisinga W, Telgmann R, Wulkow M. The virtual laboratory to pharmacokinetics: design principles and concepts. *Drug Discov Today* 2006;11:800–805.

163. Ekins S, Waller CL, Swaan PW, Cruciani G, Wrighton SA, Wikel JH. Progress in predicting human ADME parameters *in silico*. *J Pharmacol Toxicol Methods* 2000;44:251–272.

164. Ekins S, Nikolsky Y, Nikolskaya T. Techniques: application of systems biology to absorption, distribution, metabolism, excretion and toxicity. *Trends Pharmacol Sci* 2005; 26(4):202–209.

165. Klopman G, Stefan L, Saiakhov RD. A computer model for the prediction of intestinal absorption in humans. *Eur J Pharm Sci* 2002;17:253–263.

166. Uetrecht J. Curreent trends in drug-induced autoimmunity. *Autoimmun Rev* 2005;4: 309–314.

167. Sams-Dodd F. Drug discovery. Selecting the optimal approach. *Drug Discov Today* 2006;11:465–472.

24

IN VITRO EVALUATION OF METABOLIC DRUG–DRUG INTERACTIONS: SCIENTIFIC CONCEPTS AND PRACTICAL CONSIDERATIONS

ALBERT P. LI

In Vitro ADMET Laboratories Inc., Columbia, Maryland

Contents

Preclinical Development Handbook: ADME and Biopharmaceutical Properties,
edited by Shayne Cox Gad
Copyright © 2008 John Wiley & Sons, Inc.

24.1   INTRODUCTION

Simultaneous coadministration of multiple drugs to a patient is highly probable. A patient may be coadministered multiple drugs to allow effective treatment of a single disease (e.g., cancer, HIV infection) or multiple disease or disease symptoms. It is now known that drug–drug interactions may have serious, sometimes fatal, consequences. Serious drug–drug interactions have led to the necessity of a drug manufacturer to withdraw or limit the use of marketed drugs. Examples of fatal drug–drug interactions are shown in Table 24.1. As illustrated by the examples in Table 24.1, a major mechanism of adverse drug–drug interactions is the inhibition of the metabolism of a drug by a coadministered drug, thereby elevating the systemic burden of the affected drug to a toxic level.

Besides toxicity, loss of efficacy can also result from drug–drug interactions. In this case, the metabolic clearance of a drug is accelerated due to the inducing effects of a coadministered drug on drug metabolism. A well known example is the occurrence of breakthrough bleeding and contraceptive failures in women taking oral contraceptives who were coadministered the enzyme inducer rifampin [7]. Examples of drug–drug interactions leading to the loss of efficacy are shown in Table 24.2.

Estimation of drug–drug interaction potential is therefore an essential element of drug development. Screening for drug–drug interaction in early phases of drug development allows the avoidance of the development of drug candidates with high potential for adverse drug interactions. Estimation of drug–drug interaction potential is a regulatory requirement—it is required for New Drug Applications (NDAs) to the U.S. FDA [11]. In this chapter, the scientific principles, technologies, and experimental approaches for the preclinical evaluation of drug–drug interactions are reviewed.

24.2   MECHANISMS OF ADVERSE DRUG–DRUG INTERACTIONS

Adverse effects in a patient due to coadministration of multiple drugs can be due to pharmacological or pharmacokinetic drug–drug interactions defined as follows:

Pharmacological Interactions.   Adverse effects that occur due to combined pharmacological activities, leading to exaggerated pharmacological effects. An example of pharmacological interaction is the serious, sometimes fatal, drop in blood pressure due to coadministration of nitroglycerin and Sildenafil [12].

TABLE 24.1   Drugs that Have Been Withdrawn from the Market Due to Fatal Interactions with Coadministered Drugs

Drug–Drug Interaction	Mechanism of Interactions	References
Terfenadine–ketoconazole interaction, leading to fatal arrhythmia (torsades de pointes). Terfenadine was withdrawn from the market in January 1997 and replaced by a safer alternative drug (fexofenadine), which is the active metabolite of terfenadine.	Terfenadine is metabolized mainly by CYP3A4 and has been found to interact with CYP3A4 inhibitors (e.g., ketoconazole), leading to elevation of plasma terfenadine level that reached cardiotoxic levels.	1–3; www.fda.gov/bbs/ topics/answers/ ans00853.html
Mibefradil interaction with multiple drugs, leading to serious adverse effects. Mibefradil interactions with statins has led to rhabdomyolysis. Mibefradil was withdrawn from the market in June 1998, less than a year after it was introduced to the market in August 1997.	Mibefradil is a potent CYP3A4 inhibitor known to elevate the plasma levels of over 25 coadministered drugs to toxic levels. Statins, especially simvastatin and cerivastatin, are known to cause rhabdomyolysis.	4; www.fda.gov/bbs/topics/ answers/ans00876.html
Sorivudine–5-fluorouracil (5-FU) interaction, leading to severe or fatal gastrointestinal and bone marrow toxicities. Soruvidine was withdrawn from the market in 1993.	Sorivudine inhibits dihydropyrimidine dehydrogenase, an enzyme pathway responsible for fluoropyrimidine metabolism.	5
Gemfibrozil–cerivastatin interaction, leading to rhabdomyolysis. Cerivastatin was withdrawn from the market in August 2001.	Inhibition of cerivastatin metabolism by gemfibrozil, apparently due to CYP2C8 inhibitory effects of gemfibrozil.	6; www.fda.gov/medwatch/ safety/2001/Baycol2. html

Pharmacokinetic Interactions. Adverse effects that occur due to altered body burden of a drug as a result of a coadministered drug that can occur because of the ability of one drug to alter the absorption, distribution, metabolism, and excretion (ADME properties) of the coadministered drug. Of the ADME properties, drug metabolism represents the most important and prevalent mechanism for pharmacokinetic interactions.

24.3   DRUG METABOLISM

All drugs administered to a patient are subject to biotransformation. Orally administered drugs are first subjected to metabolism by the intestinal epithelium and, upon

TABLE 24.2   Drug–Drug Interactions Leading to Loss of Efficacy

Drug–Drug Interaction	Mechanism	References
Oral contraceptive–rifampin interactions, leading to breakthrough bleeding and contraceptive failure	Rifampin accelerates the metabolism of the estrogenic component (e.g., 17 α-ethinylestradiol) of oral contraceptives via induction of the metabolizing enzymes (CYP3A4 and estrogen sulfotransferases)	7, 8
Cyclosporin–rifampin interaction, leading to rejection of transplanted organs	Rifampin induces CYP3A, leading to accelerated metabolic clearance of cyclosporine to nonimmunosuppressive level	9
St. John's wort (SJW) interactions with prescribed drugs, leading to loss of efficacy	SJW (*Hypericum perforatum*) is an herbal medicine found to contain ingredients that can induce CYP3A4, CYP2C9, CYP1A2, and various transporters, leading to clinically observed accelerated metabolic clearance and/or loss of efficacy of a large number of drugs including warfarin, phenprocoumon, cyclosporine, HIV protease inhibitors, theophylline, digoxin, and oral contraceptives. The incidents with SJW illustrate the importance of the evaluation of potential drug–drug interaction of herbal medicines.	10

absorption into the portal circulation, are metabolized by the liver before entering the systemic circulation. While multiple tissues have certain degrees of biotransformation capacity, it is generally accepted that hepatic metabolism represent the most important aspect of drug metabolism.

Drug metabolism can be classified into the following major categories:

Phase I Oxidation. This generally is described as the addition of an oxygen atom (e.g., as a hydroxyl moiety) to the parent molecule. Phase I oxidation is carried out by multiple enzyme pathways, including the various isoforms of the cytochrome P450 (CYP) family and the non-P450 biotransformation enzymes such as flavin-containing monooxygenase (FMO) and monamine oxidase (MAO).

Phase II Conjugation. Phase II conjugation represents enzyme reactions that lead to the addition of a highly water-soluble molecule to the chemical that is being metabolized, leading to highly water-soluble "conjugates" that allow efficient excretion. Examples of phase II enzymes are UDP-glucuronosyl transferase (UGT), sulfotransferase (ST), and glutathione-*S*-transferase (GST). Conjugation reactions often occur with the hydroxyl moiety of the parent structure or with the oxidative metabolites.

The major drug-metabolizing enzymes and subcellular locations are summarized in Table 24.3.

TABLE 24.3 Major Pathways for Drug Metabolism, Enzymes, Subcellular Locations, and *In Vitro* Experimental System Containing the Enzymes[a]

Major Classification	Enzyme	Subcellular Location	Representative *In Vitro* Experimental System
Phase I oxidation	Cytochrome P450 mixed function monooxygenases	Endoplasmic reticulum	Microsomes, S9, hepatocytes
	Monoamine oxidase	Mitochondria	Hepatocytes
	Flavin-containing monooxygenase	Endoplasmic reticulum	Microsomes, S9, hepatocytes
	Alchohol/aldehyde dehydrogenase	Cytosol	S9, hepatocytes
	Esterases	Cytosol and endoplasmic reticulum	Microsomes, S9, hepatocytes
Phase II conjugation	UDP-dependent glucuronyl transferase	Endoplasmic reticulum	Microsomes, S9, hepatocytes
	Phenol sulfotransferases; estrogen sulfotransferase	Cytosol	S9, hepatocytes
	N-acetyl transferase	Endoplasmic reticulum	Microsomes, S9, hepatocytes
	Soluble glutathione-S-transferases (GST)	Cytosol	S9, hepatocytes
	Membrane-bound GST	Endoplasmic retuculum	Microsomes, S9, hepatocytes

[a]These enzymes are grouped into phase I oxidation and phase II conjugation enzymes, although it is now believed that such classification may not be possible for all drug-metabolizing enzymes. Representative *in vitro* experimental systems containing these enzymes are shown to guide the selection of the most relevant approach for specific enzyme pathways. It is apparent that intact hepatocytes represent the most complete *in vitro* system for drug metabolism studies as they contain all the key hepatic drug-metabolizing enzyme pathways.

24.4 CYP ISOFORMS

Cytochrome P450-dependent monooxygenases (CYP) are the drug-metabolizing enzymes often involved in metabolic drug–drug interactions. The CYP family is represented by a large number of isoforms, each having selectivity for certain chemical structures. The major hepatic human CYP isoforms are CYP1A2, CYP2A6, CYP2B6, CYP2C8, CYP2C9, CYP2C19, CYP2D6, CYP2E1, and CYP3A4. Of these isoforms, the CYP3A isoforms are the most important in drug metabolism. CYP3A isoforms (CYP3A4 and CYP3A5) collectively represent the most abundant hepatic CYP isoforms (approximately 26%), followed by CYP2C isoforms (approximately 17%). In terms of the isoforms involved in drug metabolism, CYP3 isoforms are known to be involved in the metabolism of the most number of drugs (approximately 33%), followed by CYP2C isoforms (approximately 25%) [13].

P450 isoforms are known to have specific substrates, inhibitors, and inducers (Table 24.4).

TABLE 24.4   Major Human P450 Isoforms[a] Involved in Drug Metabolism

CYP Isoform	Substrate	Inhibitor	Inducer
CYP1A2	Phenytoin	Furafylline	Omeprazole
CYP2A6	Coumarin	Tranylcypromine	Rifampin
CYP2B6	Bupropion	Ticlopidine	Rifampin
CYP2C8	Taxol	Quercetin	Rifampin
CYP2C9	Tolbutamide	Sulfaphenazole	Rifampin
CYP2C19	S-mephenytoin	Omeprazole	Rifampin
CYP2D6	Dextromethorphan	Quinidine	None
CYP2E1	Chlorzoxazone	Diethyldithiocarbamate	Ethanol
CYP3A4	Testosterone	Ketoconazole	Rifampin

[a]The individual isoforms and examples of isoform-specific substrates, inhibitors, and inducers are shown.

24.5   HUMAN *IN VITRO* EXPERIMENTAL SYSTEMS FOR DRUG METABOLISM

Substantial species–species differences occur in drug metabolism pathways, especially for CYP isoforms. Because of the species–species differences, human *in vitro* hepatic experimental systems rather than nonhuman animals are viewed as the most relevant to the evaluation of xenobiotic properties, including human drug metabolism and metabolism-based drug–drug interactions [14–17]. The following are the commonly used *in vitro* experimental systems for the evaluation of metabolism-based drug–drug interactions.

24.5.1   Hepatocytes

Hepatocytes are the parenchymal cells of the liver, which are responsible for hepatic biotransformation of xenobiotics. Isolated hepatocytes represent the most physiologically relevant experimental system for drug metabolism studies as they contain all the major hepatic drug-metabolizing enzyme pathways that are not physically disrupted such as cell free fractions. Furthermore, the drug-metabolizing enzymes and cofactors in the hepatocytes are present at physiological concentrations. Freshly isolated hepatocytes and cryopreserved hepatocytes are generally believed to represent the most complete *in vitro* system for the evaluation of hepatic drug metabolism [18].

In the past, the use of human hepatocytes has been severely limited by their availability, as studies would be performed only if human livers were available for hepatocyte isolation. Furthermore, hepatocyte isolation from human livers is not a technology available to most drug metabolism laboratories. This limitation has been overcome in the past decade due to the advancements in the procurement of human livers for research, and the commercial availability of isolated human hepatocytes. The application of human hepatocytes in drug metabolism studies is also greatly aided by the successful cryopreservation of human hepatocytes to retain drug metabolism activities [8, 19, 20]. Recently, the usefulness of cryopreserved human hepatocytes was further extended through the development of technologies to cryopreserve human hepatocytes to retain their ability to be cultured as attached cultures (plateable cryopreserved hepatocytes), which can be used for longer term

TABLE 24.5   Viability and Plateability (Ability of Hepatocytes to Be Cultured as Monolayer Cultures) of the Various Lots of Cryopreserved Human Hepatocytes[a]

Lot	Yield (cells/vial)	Viability (trypan blue)	Plating	Confluency
HU4003	4.5×106	86%	Yes	100%
HU4001	6.0×106	80%	No	20%
HU4004	6.0×106	80%	No	30%
HU4000	7.2×106	93%	Yes	100%
HU4013	7.3×106	92%	Yes	75%
HU4016	6.2×106	81%	Yes	100%
HU4021	5.4×106	89%	Yes	70%
HU4022	5.5×106	91%	Yes	80%
HU4026	5.85×106	91%	No	10%
HU4027	5.9×106	92%	No	30%
HU4028	3.2×106	83%	Yes	50%
HU4023	2.1×106	89%	No	20%
HU4029	6.0×106	90%	Yes	80%

[a]Hepatocytes manufactured by APSciences Inc. in partnership with CellzDirect Inc.

studies such as enzyme induction studies [21]. Examples of the viability and plateability of cryopreserved human hepatocytes prepared in our laboratory are shown in Table 24.5.

24.5.2   Liver Postmitochondrial Supernatant (PMS)

Liver PMS is prepared by first homogenizing the liver, and then centrifuging the homogenate at a speed of either $9000g$ or $10,000g$ to generate the supernatants S9 or S10, respectively. Liver PMS contains both cytosolic and microsomal drug-metabolizing enzymes but lacks mitochondrial enzymes.

24.5.3   Human Liver Microsomes

Liver microsomes are the $100,000g$ pellet for the PMS. Microsome preparation procedures in general involve the homogenization of the liver, dilution of the homogenate with approximately 4 volumes of sample weight with a buffer (e.g., 0.1 M Tris-HCl, pH 7.4, 0.1 M KCl, 1.0 mM EDTA, 1.0 mM PMSF [22]) followed by centrifugation at $9000–14,000g$ to remove nonmicrosomal membranes, and then at $100,000–138,000g$ to pellet the microsomes [23]. Microsomes contain the smooth endoplasmic reticulum, which is the site of the major phase I oxidation pathway, the P450 isoforms, and esterases, as well as a major conjugating pathway, UGT.

24.5.4   Recombinant P450 Isoforms (rCYP)

These are microsomes derived from organisms transfected with genes for individual human P450 isoforms (e.g., bacteria, yeast, mammalian cells) [24–26] and therefore contain only one specific human isoform. The major human P450 isoforms involved in drug metabolism are available commercially as rCYP. This experimental system is widely used to evaluate the drug-metabolizing activities of individual P450 isoforms [15, 16].

TABLE 24.6   Comparison of the Key *In Vitro* Drug-Metabolizing Experimental Systems: Liver Microsomes (Microsomes), Liver Postmitochondrial Supernatant (S9), Liver Cytosol (Cytosol), and Hepatocytes and Their Major Drug-Metabolizing Enzymes[a]

In Vitro System	P450	MAO	UGT	ST	GST
Microsomes	+	−	+[b]	−	+[c]
S9	+	−	+[b]	+[b]	+
Cytosol	−	−	−[b]	+[b]	+[d]
Hepatocytes	+	+	+	+	+

[a]P450, cytochrome P450; MAO, monoamine oxidase; UGT, UDP-glucuronosyl transferase; ST, sulfotransferase; GST, glutathione-*S*-transferase.
[b]Activity of this drug-metabolizing enzyme requires the addition of specific cofactors, for instance, UDP-glucuronic acid (UDPGA) for UGT activity, and 3′-phosphoadenosine 5′-phosphosulfate (PAPS) for ST activity.
[c]Membrane-bound GST but not the soluble GST is found in the microsomes.
[d]Soluble GST but not membrane-bound GST are found in the cytosol.

24.5.5   Cytosol

The supernatant after the $100,000\,g$ centrifugation for microsome preparation is the cytosol, which is practically devoid of all membrane associated enzymes. *N*-acetyl transferases, sulfotransferases, and dehydrogenases are examples of cytosolic enzymes. While drug–drug interaction studies are mainly studied using liver microsomes, there are cases of drug–drug interactions involving phase II pathways that can be studied using liver cytosol [27].

A comparison of the different *in vitro* experimental systems and their drug-metabolizing enzymes are shown in Table 24.6.

24.6   MECHANISMS OF METABOLIC DRUG–DRUG INTERACTIONS

Metabolic drug–drug interaction results from the alteration of the metabolic clearance of one drug by a coadministered drug. There are two major pathways of metabolic drug–drug interactions:

Inhibitory Drug–Drug Interaction. When one drug inhibits the drug metabolism enzyme responsible for the metabolism of a coadministered drug, the result is a decreased metabolic clearance of the affected drug, resulting in a higher than desired systemic burden. For drugs with a narrow therapeutic index, this may lead to serious toxicological concerns. Most fatal drug–drug interactions are due to inhibitory drug–drug interactions.

Inductive Drug–Drug Interactions. Drug–drug interactions can also be a result of the acceleration of the metabolism of a drug by a coadministered drug. Acceleration of metabolism is usually due to the induction of the gene expression, leading to higher rates of protein synthesis and therefore higher cellular content of the induced drug–metabolizing enzyme and a higher rate of metabolism of the substrates of the induced enzyme. Inductive drug–drug interactions can lead to a higher metabolic clearance of the affected drug, leading to a decrease in plasma concentration and loss of efficacy. Inductive drug–drug interactions can also lead to a higher systemic burden of metabolites, which, if toxic, may lead to safety concerns.

24.7   MECHANISM-BASED APPROACH FOR THE EVALUATION OF DRUG–DRUG INTERACTION POTENTIAL

Due to the realization that it is physically impossible to evaluate empirically the possible interaction between one drug and all marketed drugs, and that most drug-metabolizing enzyme pathways are well defined, a mechanism-based approach is used for the evaluation of drug–drug interaction potential of a new drug or drug candidate [15, 16, 28]. This mechanism-based approach is now also recommended by the U.S. FDA (www.fda.gov/cber/gdlns/interactstud.htm). The approach consists of the following major studies.

Metabolic Phenotyping. Metabolic phenotyping is defined as the identification of the major pathways involved in the metabolism of the drug in question. The reasoning is that if the pathways are known, one can estimate potential interaction of the drug in question with known inhibitors or inducers of the pathway.

Evaluation of Inhibitory Potential for Drug-Metabolizing Enzymes. The ability of the drug in question to inhibit the activities of known pathways for drug metabolism is evaluated. If a drug is an inhibitor of a drug-metabolizing enzyme pathway, it will have the potential to cause inhibitory drug interactions with coadministered drugs that are substrates of the inhibited pathway.

Induction Potential for Drug-Metabolizing Enzymes. The ability of the drug in question to induce drug-metabolizing enzyme activities is evaluated. If the drug in question is an inducer of a specific pathway, it will have the potential to cause inductive drug interactions with coadministered drugs that are substrates of the induced pathway.

24.8   EXPERIMENTAL APPROACHES FOR THE *IN VITRO* EVALUATION OF DRUG–DRUG INTERACTION POTENTIAL

Because of the known species–species differences in drug metabolism, it is now believed that *in vitro*, human-based, experimental systems are more appropriate than nonhuman animal models for the evaluation of drug–drug interactions. *In vitro* positive findings are usually confirmed with *in vivo* clinical studies. The typical preclinical studies for drug–drug interactions [15, 16, 28] (www.fda.gov/cber/gdlns/interactstud.htm) are described next.

24.8.1   Study 1: Metabolic Phenotyping 1—Metabolite Identification

The objective of this study is to identify the major metabolites of the drug in question. For this study, the drug in question is incubated with an appropriate *in vitro* metabolic system to allow the formation of metabolites [15, 16]. Metabolites are then identified using analytical chemical approaches. The *in vitro* experimental system of choice is human hepatocytes, with high performance liquid chromatography/mass spectrometry (HPLC/MS) or tandem mass spectrometry (HPLC/MS/MS) as the most convenient analytical tool to identify the metabolites.

The metabolites are generally identified as metabolites of phase I oxidation or phase II conjugation. If phase I oxidation is concluded as the major pathway for the oxidative metabolism of the drug, Experiment 2 will be performed to evaluate which of the several oxidative pathways are involved. Phase II conjugation pathways can generally be identified by the identity of the metabolite and subsequent experiments to further identify the pathways may not be necessary. For instance, if the metabolite is a glucuronide, UGT can be identified as the enzyme involved.

A typical experimental design is as follows:

- *In vitro System.* Cryopreserved human hepatocytes pooled from two donors (male, female).

  Three drug concentrations: 1, 10, and 100 μM.

  Hepatocyte concentration: 0.5–1.0 million hepatocytes per mL.

  Three incubation times: 1, 2, and 4 hours (suspension culture); up to 24 hours (attached culture).

  Incubation in 24 well plates at 37 °C.

  Organic solvent (e.g., acetonitrile) to terminate reaction and to extract medium and intracellular metabolites.

  Stored frozen until analysis.

- *Analytical Chemistry.* HPLC-MS/MS.

  Quantification of disappearance of parent chemical in all samples.

  Identification of metabolites from 100 μM samples.

  Detection of metabolites in 1 and 10 μM samples.

24.8.2   Study 2: Metabolic Phenotyping 2—Identification of Major Metabolic Pathways

If oxidative metabolites are found to be the major metabolites, it is necessary to evaluate which major oxidative pathways are involved in the metabolism. This is performed via the use of liver microsomes and experimental conditions that would inhibit a specific pathway. The major pathways and experimental conditions are shown in Table 24.7.

As P450 pathways are considered the most important for metabolic drug–drug interactions, the study with the general P450 inhibitor, 1-aminobenzotriazole (ABT)

TABLE 24.7   Experimental Conditions to Reduce the Activity of the Major Drug-Metabolizing Enzyme Pathways (P450 Isoforms (CYP), Flavin-Containing Monooxygenases (FMOs), and Monoamine Oxidase (MAO)) Using the *In Vitro* Experimental Systems for Drug Metabolism (Liver Microsomes (Microsomes), Postmitochondrial Supernatant (S9), and Hepatocytes)

In Vitro System	Condition	Inactivated Pathway(s)
Microsomes	NADH omission	CYP, FMO
Microsomes or hepatocytes	1-Aminobenzotriazole treatment	CYP
Microsomes	Heat (45 °C) inactivation	FMO
S9	Pargyline treatment	MAO

Source: Adapted from http://www.fda.gov/cder/guidance/6695dft.pdf.

is the one that should be performed. ABT is known to inhibit all eight human P450 isoforms involved in drug metabolism [29]. Inhibition of metabolism of a test article by ABT would indicate that the test article is metabolized by the P450 pathway. A typical study with ABT is as follows:

- Human liver microsomes (0.5 mg protein/mL).
- Experiment 1: Evaluation of experimental conditions for the accurate quantification of metabolic clearance.
    - Incubation with three concentrations of test article (e.g., 0.1, 1, 10 μM) and three incubation times (e.g., 15, 30, and 60 minutes).
    - Quantification of test article disappearance.
- Experiment 2: Reaction phenotyping.
    - Incubation with one concentration of the test article at one incubation time (chosen from Experiment 1) in the presence and absence of three concentrations of ABT (100, 200, and 500 μM).
    - Quantification of test article disappearance and evaluation of the effects of ABT treatment.

24.8.3 Study 3: Metabolic Phenotyping 3—Identification of P450 Isoform Pathways (P450 Phenotyping)

If ABT is found to inhibit the metabolism of the drug or drug candidate in Study 2, P450 metabolism is ascertained. The next step is to identify which P450 isoforms are involved in the metabolism, a process termed P450 phenotyping [30, 31]. There are several major approaches for this study.

Liver Microsome and Isoform-Selective Inhibitors   In this experiment, the test article is incubated with human liver microsomes in the presence and absence of individual selective inhibitors for the eight major CYP isoforms. The ability of an inhibitor to inhibit metabolism of the test article would indicate that the pathway inhibited by the inhibitor is involved in metabolism. For instance, if ketoconazole, a potent CYP3A4 inhibitor, is found to inhibit the metabolism of the test article, then CYP3A4 is concluded to be involved in the metabolism of the test article. It is also a common practice to assign the degree of involvement by the maximum percent inhibition. For instance, if the maximum inhibition, expressed as percentages of the total metabolism in the absence of inhibitor, by sulfaphenazole (CYP2C9 inhibitor) and ketoconazole (CYP3A4 inhibitor) are 20% and 80%, respectively, it can be concluded that the CYP2C9 is involved in 20% and CYP3A4 in 80% of the metabolism of the test article. It is important to realize that the inhibitors are isoform selective rather than isoform specific, so data interpretation must be performed carefully to avoid an inaccurate assignment of enzyme pathways [31]. It is always prudent to confirm the results of this study with results using a different approach (e.g., using rCYP).

Incubation with Individual rCYPs   In this experiment, individual rCYP isoforms are used to evaluate which P450 isoforms are involved in the metabolism [30]. The test article is incubated with each rCYP and its disappearance quantified. A rCYP that leads to the disappearance of the test article would indicate that the isoform is involved in the metabolism of the test article. For instance, if rCYP2C19 incubation leads to the disappearance of the test article, then CYP2C19 is concluded to be involved in the metabolic clearance of the test article. It is important to realize that these studies are performed with a single P450 isoform and therefore lack competing enzyme pathways. Metabolism by a rCYP isoform may not be relevant *in vivo* because of higher affinity pathways.

Correlation Study with Human Liver Microsomes   In this experiment, the test article is incubated with multiple lots of human liver microsomes that have been previously characterized for the activities of the individual CYP isoforms [32]. The rate of metabolic clearance of the test article is then plotted against the CYP activities of the different lots of microsomes. A linear correlation between activity and rate of disappearance for a specific CYP would indicate that this pathway is involved in the metabolism of the test article. This study requires the evaluation of at least 10 liver microsome lots with well-distributed gradations of activities.

Liver Microsome/Inhibitor Study Design   In general, studies with liver microsomes are believed to be more relevant than studies with rCYP, as studies with individual rCYP does not allow competition in metabolism for isoforms with different affinities for the substrate and therefore may overemphasize the participation of low affinity pathways. It is important to use substrate concentrations similar to expected plasma concentrations. An artifactually high concentration would cause the substrate to be metabolized similarly by high and low affinity enzyme pathways [33]. Using liver microsomes with physiologically relevant substrate concentrations should provide the best results. A typical liver microsome experiment with inhibitors is as follows.

- Human liver microsomes (0.5 mg/mL).
- Experiment 1: Metabolic stability study.
    Incubation with three concentrations of test article (e.g., 0.1, 1, 10 µM) and three incubation times (e.g., 15, 30, and 60 minutes).
    Quantification of test article disappearance.
- Experiment 2: Reaction phenotyping.
    Incubation with one concentration of the test article at one incubation time (chosen from Experiment 1) in the presence and absence of isoform-specific inhibitors.
    Quantification of test article disappearance.

The isoform-specific inhibitors suggested by the U.S. FDA are shown in Table 24.8.

Evaluation of CYP Isoform Contributions Using Both Liver Microsomes and rCYP Isoforms   It is also possible to calculate the relative contribution of individual isoforms using data from both liver microsomes and rCYP isoforms using the following approach [34, 35]:

TABLE 24.8   Preferred and Acceptable P450 Isoform-Specific Inhibitors Suggested by U.S. FDA in the September 2006 Draft Guidance Document for Drug–Drug Interaction Evaluation and Preferred Inhibitors Used in the *In Vitro* ADMET Laboratories (IVAL)

CYP	FDA Preferred Inhibitor	FDA Acceptable Inhibitor	IVAL Preferred Inhibitor
1A2	Furafylline	α-Napthoflavone	Furafylline
2A6	Tranylcypromine, methoxsalen	Pilocarpine, tryptamine	Tranylcypromine
2B6		Ticlopidine, sertraline	Ticlopidine
2C8	Quercetin	Trimethoprim, gemfibrozil, rosiglitazone	Quercetin
2C9	Sulfaphenazole	Fluconazole	Sulfaphenazole
2C19		Ticlopidine	Omeprazole
2D6	Quinidine		Quinidine
2E1		Diethyldithiocarbamate	Diethyldithiocarbamate
3A4/5	Ketoconazole, itraconazole	Troleandomycin, verapamil	Ketoconazole

- The relative activity factor for individual isoforms (using isoform-specific substrates) is calculated first. This is necessary as each lot of liver microsomes would have different relative amounts of each P450 isoform. V_{max} and K_m values are determined for each isoform using isoform-specific substrates for both liver microsomes and rCYP isoforms. The relative activity factor (RAF) is calculated using the following equation:

$$RAF = \frac{(V_{max}/K_m \text{ of CYP in microsomes})}{V_{max}/K_m \text{ of rCYP}}$$

- Contribution of a specific CYP isoform to the metabolism of a test article is then calculated using the following equation:

$$\text{Contribution of CYP}(\%) = RAF \times \frac{V(\text{rCYP})}{V(\text{microsomes})}$$

24.8.4   Study 4: CYP Inhibitory Potential

The objective of this study is to evaluate if the drug or drug candidate in question is an inhibitor of a specific P450 isoform. This study can be performed with rCYP, human liver microsomes, and human hepatocytes.

rCYP Studies   rCYP studies represent the most convenient and rapid study for the evaluation of CYP inhibitory potential. As the study involves substrates that form metabolites that can be quantified by fluorescence, the laborious and time-consuming HPLC or LC/MS sample analysis is not required. For this reason, most drug development laboratories perform rCYP inhibition assays as a screen for P450 inhibitory potential of their drug candidates. The study involves the incubation of individual rCYP isoforms with the test article at various concentrations (e.g., seven concentrations plus solvent control) in triplicate, and a substrate that can be metabolized by the specific isoform. As the reaction contains only one isoform, isoform-specific substrates are not required to be used. The requirement is that the substrate generates metabolites that can be measured by a plate reader with the capability to quantify florescence.

Liver Microsome Studies Liver microsomes represent the most appropriate experimental system for the evaluation of the interaction of a drug with P450 isoforms. For the evaluation of CYP inhibitory potential, the test article is incubated with liver microsomes in the presence of individual isoform-specific substrates. The isoform-specific substrates and the metabolites quantified are shown in Table 24.9.

Human Hepatocyte Studies rCYP and human liver microsomes are cell-free systems, allowing direct interaction of the test article with the P450 isoforms. *In vivo*, the inhibitor is initially absorbed into the systemic circulation and then interacts with the enzymes after penetration through the hepatocyte plasma membrane. Once inside the cytoplasm, the inhibitor may be metabolized by phase I and/or phase II metabolism and/or actively transported out of the hepatocytes, for instance, via bile excretion. Furthermore, there may be transporters present to actively uptake the inhibitor. The result is that the intracellular concentration of the inhibitor may be substantially different from the plasma concentration. Results with rCYP and human liver microsomes may not be useful to estimate *in vivo* inhibitory effects based on plasma concentrations if the intracellular concentration of the inhibitor is not known.

The use of intact human hepatocytes may allow a more accurate extrapolation of *in vitro* results to *in vivo*. The study is performed using intact human hepatocytes incubated with isoform-specific substrate and the test article. The intact plasma membrane and the presence of all hepatic metabolic pathways and cofactors allow distribution and metabolism of the test article. The resulting inhibitory effect there-

TABLE 24.9   P450 Isoform-Specific Substrates and Their Respective Metabolites[a]

CYP	Substrate	Metabolite
1A2	Phenacetin	Acetaminophen
	Ethoxyresorufin	Resorufin
2A6	Coumarin	7-OH-coumarin
2B6	Bupropion	Hydroxypropion
2C8	Taxol	6-α-Hydroxypaclitaxel
2C9	Tolbutamide	4'-Hydroxytolbutamide
2C19	*S*-Mephenytoin	4-OH-mephenytoin
2D6	Dextromethorphan	Dextrophan
2E1	Chlorzoxazone	6-Hydroxychlorzoxazone
3A4/5	Testosterone	6-β-Hydroxytestosterone

[a]These substrates are used in *in vitro* experimental systems such as liver microsomes, liver S9, or hepatocytes in which multiple isoforms are expressed.

fore should be physiologically more relevant to the *in vivo* situation than results with cell-free systems.

It is recommended that inhibition studies with intact hepatocytes be performed if inhibitory effects of a drug or drug candidate have been observed with rCYP or liver microsomes to allow a more accurate prediction of the extent of *in vivo* inhibitory effects. Time-dependent inhibition of P450 can also be studied using intact human hepatocytes [36]. One precaution with the use of intact hepatocytes is to concurrently measure cytotoxicity. As dead hepatocytes are not active in drug metabolism, without cytotoxicity information, cytotoxic drug concentrations could be interpreted as inhibitory concentrations.

A recent advancement is to use intact hepatocytes suspended in whole human plasma for inhibition studies to allow correction for plasma protein binding [37]. As drugs *in vivo* are always in contact with 100% human blood, this is conceptually sound and therefore deserves further investigation on its general applicability. One disturbing finding in our laboratory is that testosterone, a compound that is readily metabolized *in vivo*, is not metabolized by intact human hepatocytes in whole plasma (A. P. Li, unpublished).

IC$_{50}$, K$_i$, K$_{inact}$ and [I]/K$_i$ Determinations   Enzyme inhibition data are often presented as IC$_{50}$, the concentration of the inhibitor to cause 50% inhibition at one chosen substrate concentration; K_i, the inhibition constant (dissociation constant from the inhibitor–enzyme complex) determined by enzyme kinetic analysis (e.g., Dixon plot); and K_{inact}, the time-dependent inhibition constant for mechanism-based inhibitors. IC$_{50}$ values can be estimated from the study described earlier. A positive inhibition, defined as dose-dependent inhibition, with the inhibited activity lower than 50% of that of the negative control, will require further experimentation to define K_i for a better evaluation of *in vivo* inhibitory potential. Furthermore, study to determine K_{inact} may be performed to evaluate if the inhibitor acts via covalent binding to the active site of the enzyme, leading to time-dependent irreversible inhibition.

IC$_{50}$ is generally determined by plotting the log of the relative activity (activity in the presence of the inhibitor as a percentage of the activity of the negative solvent control), and then estimating the concentration yielding 50% relative activity using linear regression analysis. IC$_{50}$ can also be calculated from the relationship between inhibitor concentrations and percent control activity with the aid of a nonlinear regression program such as SCIENTIST (Micromath, Salt Lake City, UT) [38].

K_i can be determined using a Dixon plot with the reciprocal of the activity as the *y*-axis and inhibitor concentration as the *x*-axis. Results with at least two substrate concentrations below V_{max} are plotted, with K_i calculated as the negative of the *x*-intercept [39]. K_i can also be estimated with the aid of nonlinear regression analysis software such as SYSTAT (SPPS, Inc., Chicago, IL) [40].

Most P450 inhibitors act via reversible (competitive or noncompetitive) mechanisms and their inhibitory potential can be estimated from their IC$_{50}$ or K_i values. Some inhibitors are "mechanism-based" or "time-dependent" inhibitors, which can cause irreversible inhibition due to the formation of reactive metabolites by the CYP isoform, leading to covalent binding to the active site and thereby causing irreversible inhibition of the affected enzyme molecule [41]. Irreversible inhibitors therefore will have prolonged inhibition of the enzyme even after clearance of the drug in question. K_{inact} is a measure of the potency of such "mechanism-based" inhibitors.

K_{inact} can be determined using the following approach [42]:

1. Plot the relative activity (activity in the presence of the inhibitor as a percentage of the activity of the solvent or negative control) versus time and determine the slope at each inhibitor concentration.
2. Plot (1/slope) versus (1/inhibitor concentration) (Kitz–Wilson plot). K_{inact} is calculated as the reciprocal of the y-intercept, and K_i as the negative of the reciprocal of the x-intercept.

$[I]/K_i$, the ratio of the anticipated or known steady-state plasma drug concentration to K_i, is generally used to determine the likelihood of clinical drug–drug interactions [43, 44]. A general rule of thumb suggested by the U.S. FDA (http://www.fda.gov/cder/guidance/6695dft.pdf) is as follows:

- $[I]/K_i < 0.1$: Unlikely to cause *in vivo* drug–drug interactions.
- $[I]K_i = 1$: Possible to cause *in vivo* drug–drug interactions.
- $[I]/K_i > 1$: Likely to cause *in vivo* drug–drug interactions.

K_i is estimated by an experiment with varying inhibitor and substrate concentrations. A typical K_i study is as follows:

- *In vitro* experimental system: rCYP, human liver microsomes or hepatocytes.
- Inhibitor concentrations: Five (ideally yielding 10–90% inhibition of activity).
- Substrate concentrations: Minimum of two for the Dixon plot; three is recommended.
- Timepoint: one (within the linear time course) if time course is known; multiple (e.g., 5, 10, and 15 minutes) if time course under the experimental conditions has not been established.
- K_i is determined by a Dixon plot, plotting the reciprocal of activity versus inhibitor concentration. The negative of the x-coordinate value corresponding to the intercept of the plots for the low and high substrate concentrations is the K_i.

For mechanism-based inhibitors, K_{inact} is estimated by an experiment with varying inhibitor concentration and preincubation time. A typical K_{inact} study is as follows:

- *In vitro* experimental system: rCYP, human liver microsomes or hepatocytes.
- Preincubation time (preincubation of enzyme with inhibitor): Five values (e.g., 5, 10, 15, 20, 30 minutes).
- Inhibitor concentration: Five (ideally yielding 10–90% inhibition of activity).
- Substrate concentration: one.

- Substrate incubation time: one (within the linear time course) if time course is known; multiple (e.g., 5, 10, and 15 minutes) if time course under the experimental conditions has not been established.
- K_{inact} is determined by the following approach:

    Plot activity as a percentage of the solvent control versus time.

    Estimate the first-order inactivation constants at each inhibitor concentration by multiplying the slope of the linear regression analysis by 2.303.

    Determine $t_{1/2}$ of the inactivation reaction as $0.693/k$.

    Plot the Kitz–Wilson plot of $t_{1/2}$ versus the reciprocal of the inhibitor concentration and estimate K_{inact} as the y-intercept, and K_i as the reciprocal of the x-intercept.

24.8.5   Study 5: Enzyme Induction Potential

Enzyme induction is a major mechanism for drug–drug interactions. Induction of a drug-metabolizing enzyme by one drug would lead to the enhanced metabolism of coadministered drugs that are substrates of the induced enzyme.

Experimental evaluation of enzyme induction involves the treatment of human hepatocytes for several days with the test article followed by evaluation of enzyme activities using P450 isoform-specific substrates [45, 46]. As freshly isolated hepatocytes possess endogenous activities, which may be the result of inducers present in the donor's systemic circulation, the isolated hepatocytes are cultured for 2–3 days to allow the P450 enzyme activities to return to a basal level. Testing for induction potential is initiated by treatment of the cultured hepatocytes for 2–3 days to allow full expression of the induced enzyme. Induction is generally evaluated by measuring enzyme activity, as activity represents the most relevant endpoint for drug–drug interaction. Both freshly isolated and plateable cryopreserved human hepatocytes can be used for the induction study [21, 47, 48].

As of this writing, all known inducers of P450 isoforms *in vivo* are inducers *in vitro* [21]. The known human P450 inducers are shown in Table 24.10.

TABLE 24.10   Clinically Demonstrated Human Enzyme Inducers and Their Respective *In Vitro* Induction Results as Well as Their Association with Severe Hepatotoxicity

In Vivo Enzyme Inducer	*In Vitro* Human Hepatocyte Induction Finding	Severe Clinical Hepatotoxicity
Carbamazepine	+	+
Dexamethasone	+	−
Isoniazid	+	+
Omeprazole	+	+
Phenobarbital	+	+
Phenytoin	+	+
Rifampin	+	+
Rifapentine	+	−
Rifabutin	+	−
Troglitazone	+	+
St. John's wort	+	+

The typical experimental procedures for an enzyme induction study are as follows:

- Day 0: Plate human hepatocytes (freshly isolated or plateable cryopreserved human hepatocytes).
- Day 1: Refresh medium.
- Day 2: Refresh medium.
- Day 3: Change medium to that containing test article, solvent control, or positive controls.

  Minimum of three test article concentrations, with the high concentration at least one order of magnitude greater than expected plasma concentration.

  If plasma concentration not known, evaluate concentrations ranging over at least two orders of magnitude (e.g., 1, 10, 100 µM).
- Day 4: Refresh treatment medium.
- Day 5: Refresh treatment medium.
- Day 6: Measure activity (*in situ* incubation with isoform-specific substrates).

The isoform-specific substrates described earlier for CYP inhibition studies are generally used for enzyme induction studies.

The known CYP inducers are now known to induce either CYP1A and/or CYP3A, with inducers of other inducible isoforms such as CYP2A6, CYP2C9, and CYP2C19 found also to be CYP3A inducers. For general enzyme induction evaluation for drug–drug interaction, it may be adequate to simply screen for CYP1A and CYP3A induction. If CYP3A induction is observed, then investigations into CYP2A6, CYP2C9, and CYP2C19 induction are warranted.

The two most common confounding factors for P450 induction studies are as follows:

1. *Inducers that Are Also Inhibitors.* The co-occurrence of P450 inhibition and induction (i. e., the compound is both an inhibitor and inducer) can confound induction results. Ritonavir is an example of a CYP3A4 inducer [49] that is also a potent CYP3A4 inhibitor [50]. The inhibitory effects can overcome any induction effects using activity as an endpoint. For the evaluation of enzyme induction potential of inhibitors, Western blotting for the amount of enzyme proteins would be most appropriate. Studies with mRNA expression would provide data to distinguish between induction of gene expression or protein stabilization as mechanisms. As in the case of ritonavir, induction effects persist after the clearance of the drug from the systemic circulation, leading to enhanced clearance of drugs that are substrates of the induced pathways. It is important to define the induction potential of a drug even if it is found to be an enzyme inhibitor.

2. *Cytotoxic Compounds.* Induction effects can be masked by the decrease of cell viability, as most induction assays quantify substrate metabolism *in situ* (in the same cell culture plate in which the cells are cultured) and assume that there is no change in cell number. Cytotoxicity evaluation therefore should always be performed concurrently with induction studies. In the presence of cytotoxicity, activity should be corrected by the viability for comparison with negative control activity to assess induction potential.

A compound is concluded to be an inducer if reproducible, statistically significant, and dose-dependent induction effects are observed. U.S. FDA recommends the use of the criterion of "40% or higher of the activity of positive controls" as a positive response (www.fda.gov/cber/gdlns/interactstud.htm).

24.8.6 Study 6: *In Vitro* Empirical Drug–Drug Interactions

The physiological significance of the findings based on the mechanistic approach may be substantiated by *in vitro* drug–drug interactions between frequently coadministered drugs that are likely to have interaction with the drug in question [28]. This is particularly important if the drug in question is either a CYP3A4 substrate or a CYP3A4 inhibitor. As CYP3A4 is now known to have different affinities for different substrates and inhibitors [51], the interaction potential for a drug and a particular coadministered drug may be substantially different from that estimated by using a surrogate substrate of CYP3A4.

This study can be performed with liver microsomes or hepatocytes. The use of hepatocytes probably would allow the development of data more relevant to humans *in vivo*.

24.9 DATA INTERPRETATION

The studies described previously allow one to develop data for the estimation of drug–drug interaction potential of the drug or drug candidate in question. Accurate prediction of *in vivo* effects is possible only through thorough and scientifically sound interpretation of the data. While every novel chemical structure will provide a unique set of data and therefore requires individualized data interpretation and/or further experimentation, the following guidelines can be used to aid the evaluation of the data generated.

24.9.1 Pathway Evaluation

Possible outcomes of a study are as follows:

1. The test article is not metabolized by liver microsomes or hepatocytes. This is indicated by the lack of metabolite formation and lack of parent disappearance in Studies 1 and 2. Hepatic metabolism is not involved in the metabolic clearance of the compound. There should be no concern with coadministered drugs that can alter drug-metabolizing enzyme activities.
2. The test article is metabolized but not metabolized by P450 isoforms. As P450-related drug–drug interactions are the most prevalent, non-P450 drug–drug interactions should be considered on a case-by-case basis. For instance, MAO interaction may be important if the drug in question may be coadministered with known MAO substrates or inhibitors. UGT substrates, for instance, may have drug interactions with UGT inhibitory drugs such as probenecid.
3. The test article is metabolized by a single P450 isoform. This represents the easiest data to interpret, albeit not a good scenario for a drug candidate. A drug that is metabolized predominantly by a single P450 isoform will very likely have drug–drug interactions with inhibitors of the isoform. The known cases of serious drug–drug interactions often involve a single P450 pathway,

with CYP3A4 being the most prominent. Drugs that have been withdrawn due to fatal drug–drug interactions are often CYP3A4 substrates or potent CYP3A4 inhibitors. Because of the role of CYP2C8 in the metabolism of statins, which are widely prescribed to combat hypercholesterolemia, CYP2C8 has become the second-most important isoform for drug–drug interactions. Cerivastatin, a CYP2C8 substrate, was withdrawn from the market in August 2001 after reports of fatal interactions with the CYP2C8 inhibitor gemfibrozil [52].

4. The test article is metabolized by multiple P450 isoforms. This is generally interpreted that the test article may not have serious interactions with a specific inhibitor of one of the P450 isoforms, as the metabolic clearance can be carried out by the unaffected pathways. However, there are examples of drugs that have been found to be metabolized by multiple pathways but later were found in clinical or postmarketing studies to have interactions with potent inhibitors of a specific pathway. An example is the antifungal terbinafine, which has been characterized using human liver microsomes and rCYP isoforms to be metabolized by multiple P450 isoforms: CYP1A2, CYP2C8, CYP2C9. CYP2C19, CYP2D6, and CYP3A4, leading to the conclusion that "the potential for terbinafine interaction with other drugs is predicted to be insignificant" [53]. In the same study, as terbinafine was a competitive inhibitor of CYP2D6, it was concluded that it would have interactions with CYP2D6 substrates. *In vivo* studies confirmed the CYP2D6 inhibitory effects as predicted by *in vitro* studies; however, it was also observed clinically that rifampin, a CYP3A4 inducer, caused a 100% increase in terbinafine clearance (www.fda. gov/medwatch/safety/2004/jan_PI/Lamasil_PI.pdf). One possible explanation of this is that, upon CYP3A4 induction, the total metabolism of terbinafine is greatly enhanced due to the high capacity of CYP3A4 for this substrate. It is therefore important to realize that if a drug is metabolized by multiple isoforms, it may still have significant drug interactions with inducers of isoforms with high capacity for the metabolism of the drug.

24.9.2 P450 Inhibition

The outcomes of P450 inhibition studies may include the following:

1. No inhibition is observed. If no inhibitory effects are observed with rCYP, microsomes, and hepatocytes, the substance in question is considered not to have the potential to cause inhibitory metabolic drug–drug interactions *in vivo*. As of now, there are no examples of *in vivo* enzyme inhibitors that are not inhibitors *in vitro*.

2. Significant inhibition is observed. A practical definition of significant inhibition is that the test article is found to cause dose-dependent and >50% inhibition of one or more P450 isoforms at the concentrations evaluated. The conclusion is that the test article is a potent inhibitor. As described earlier, the physiological significance is determined by the $[I]/K_i$ value, with any $[I]/K_i$ value of 0.1 or higher as possible or likely to cause *in vivo* drug–drug interactions. It is recommended that $[I]/K_i$ values obtained from cell-free systems (microsomes and rCYP) are confirmed with intact hepatocytes to aid an accurate prediction

of *in vivo* effects. If the results with hepatocytes are also determined to be significant, *in vivo* studies will need to be performed to estimate human *in vivo* drug–drug interaction potential.

3. No time-dependent inhibition is observed. The inhibitor is not a mechanism-based inhibitor.

4. Time-dependent inhibition is observed. The inhibitor is a time-dependent inhibitor. *In vivo* studies will need to be performed to further define its drug–drug interaction potential.

5. Additional safety concern. A time-dependent inhibitor may need to be further studied to define its hepatotoxic potential, as a number of time-dependent P450 inhibitors are found to cause idiosyncratic hepatotoxicity.

24.9.3 P450 Induction

The following outcomes may be observed:

1. No induction is observed. The substance evaluated is not an enzyme inducer if P450 inhibitory and cytotoxic potential are eliminated as confounding factors.

2. Induction is observed. The substance evaluated is observed to cause dose-dependent and physiologically significant induction (e.g., induced activity greater than twofold the negative control activity). If the doses found to be positive are within clinical plasma concentrations (e.g., within 10× of plasma C_{max}), *in vivo* studies may be needed to further define the test article's *in vivo* enzyme induction and the subsequent drug–drug interaction potential.

3. Additional safety concern. Enzyme inducers may need to be further evaluated for their hepatotoxic potential, as a large number of enzyme-inducing drugs are found to cause severe hepatotoxicity.

24.10   CONCLUSION

Drug–drug interactions can have serious adverse consequences and therefore should be evaluated accurately before a new drug is introduced to the human population. Due to the scientific advances in the understanding of key human drug-metabolizing pathways, and the availability of human *in vitro* systems for drug metabolism studies, human drug–drug interaction evaluations, especially drug metabolism-related interactions, can be performed rapidly and efficiently. A scientific, mechanism-based approach to evaluate drug–drug interactions remains the most appropriate approach:

1. Understanding of the major drug-metabolizing pathways in the metabolism of the drug or drug candidate in question will allow assessment of its potential interactions with existing drugs that are inhibitors or inducers of the pathways involved.

2. A careful and exhaustive evaluation of the inhibitory potential of the drug or drug candidate in question toward the major human drug metabolism enzymes

will allow assessment of its potential to cause interactions with existing drugs that are substrates of the inhibited enzymes.

3. Evaluation of induction potential of the drug or drug candidate in question for the inducible human drug-metabolizing enzymes will allow assessment of potential interactions with drugs that are substrates of the induced enzymes.

This approach is mainly applied toward P450 isoforms but can also be applied to non-P450 drug-metabolizing enzyme pathways. The next wave of major advances in drug–drug interactions is anticipated to be approaches for the evaluation of the interactions between drugs and drug transporters.

The success achieved with the scientific-based approaches in the evaluation of drug–drug interactions is a result of the extensive scientific research in the identification and characterization of drug-metabolizing enzymes, the definition of the mechanisms of metabolism-based drug–drug interactions, and the development, characterization, and intelligent application of the human-based *in vitro* experimental models for drug metabolism. Similar approaches should be adopted for the evaluation of other major adverse drug effects (e.g., idiosyncratic drug toxicity), which so far have eluded the routine drug safety evaluation approaches. It is through an open mind—a willingness to venture toward the development of a hypothesis, the testing of a hypothesis, and the development and adoption of approaches to investigate a problem based on the best science—that the field of drug safety evaluation can move forward.

REFERENCES

1. Vazquez E, Whitfield L. Seldane warnings. *Posit Aware* 1997;8:12.
2. Carlson AM, Morris LS. Coprescription of terfenadine and erythromycin or ketoconazole: an assessment of potential harm. *J Am Pharm Assoc (Wash)* 1996;NS36:263–269.
3. Von Moltke LL, Greenblatt DJ, Duan SX, Harmatz JS, Wright CE, Shader RI. Inhibition of terfenadine metabolism *in vitro* by azole antifungal agents and by selective serotonin reuptake inhibitor antidepressants: relations to pharmacokinetic interactions *in vivo*. *J Clin Psychopharmacol* 1996;16:104–112.
4. Omar MA, Wilson JP. FDA adverse event reports on statin associated rhabdomyolysis. *Ann Pharmacother* 2002;36:288–295.
5. Diasio RB. Sorivudine and 5-fluorouracil; a clinically significant drug–drug interaction due to inhibition of dihydropyrimidine dehydrogenase. *Br J Clin Pharmacol* 1998;46: 1–4.
6. Ozdemir O, Boran M, Gokce V, Uzun Y, Kocak B, Korkmaz S. A case with severe rhabdomyolysis and renal failure associated with cerivastatin–gemfibrozil combination therapy—a case report. *Angiology* 2000;51:695–697.
7. Zhang H, Cui D, Wang B, Han YH, Balimane P, Yang Z, Sinz M, Rodriqus AD. Pharmacokinetic drug interactions involving 17alpha-ethinylestradiol: a new look at an old drug. *Clin Pharmacokinet* 2007;46:133–157.
8. Li AP, Hartman NR, Lu C, Collins JM, Strong JM. Effects of cytochrome P450 inducers on 17 alpha-ethinyloestradiol (EE2) conjugation by primary human hepatocytes. *Br J Clin Pharmacol* 1999;48:733–742.
9. Capone D, Aiello C, Santoro GA, Gentile A, Stanziale P, D'Alessandro R, Imperatore P, Basile V. Drug interaction between cyclosporine and two antimicrobial agents, josamycin

and rifampicin, in organ-transplanted patients. *Int J Clin Pharmacol Res* 1996;16: 73–76.

10. Henderson L, Yue QY, Berqquist C, Gerden B, Arlett P. St. John's wort (*Hypericum perforatum*): drug interactions and clinical outcomes. *Br J Clin Pharmacol* 2002;54: 349–356.

11. Huang SM, Lesko LJ, Williams RL. Assessment of the quality and quantity of drug–drug interaction studies in recent NDA submissions: study design and data analysis issues. *J Clin Pharmacol* 1999;39:1006–1014.

12. Schalcher C, Schad K, Brunner-La Rocca HP, Schindler R, Oechslin E, Scharf C, Suetsch G, Bertel O, Kiowski W. Interaction of sildenafil with cAMP-mediated vasodilation *in vivo*. *Hypertension* 2003;40:763–767.

13. Guengerich FP. Cytochrome P450s and other enzymes in drug metabolism and toxicity. *AAPS J* 2006;8:E101–E111.

14. Li AP, Maurel P, Gomez-Lechon MJ, Cheng LC, Jurima-Romet M. Applications of primary human hepatocytes in the evaluation of P450 induction. *Chem Biol Interact* 1997;107:5–16.

15. Li AP. Screening for human ADME/Tox drug properties in drug discovery. *Drug Discov Today* 2001;6:357–366.

16. Li AP. *In vitro* approaches to evaluate ADMET drug properties. *Curr Top Med Chem* 2004;4:701–706.

17. MacGregor JT, Collins JM, Sugiyama Y, Tyson CA, Dean J, Smith L, Andersen M, Curren RD, Houston JB, Kadlubar FF, Kedderis GL, Krishnan K, Li AP, Parchment PE, Thummel K, Tomaszewski JE, Ulrich R, Vickers AE, Wrighton SA. *In vitro* human tissue models in risk assessment: report of a consensus-building workshop. *Toxicol Sci* 2001;59:17–36.

18. Hewitt NJ, Lechon MJ, Houston JB, Hallifax D, Brown HS, Maurel P, Kenna JG, Gustavsson L, Lohmann C, Skonberg C, Huillouzo A, Tuschi G, Li AP, Elcluyse E, Groothuis GM, Hengstler JG. Primary hepatocytes: current understanding of the regulation of metabolic enzymes and transporter proteins, and pharmaceutical practice for the use of hepatocytes in metabolism, enzyme induction, transporter, clearance, and hepatoxicity studies. *Drug Metab Rev* 2007;39:159–234.

19. Li AP, Gorycki PD, Hengstler JG, Kedderis GL, Koebe HG, Rahmani R, de Sousas G, Silva JM, Skett P. Present status of the application of cryopreserved hepatocytes in the evaluation of xenobiotics: consensus of an international expert panel. *Chem Biol Interact* 1999;121:117–123.

20. Li AP, Lu C, Brent JA, Pham C, Fackett A, Ruegg CE, Silber PM. Cryopreserved human hepatocytes: characterization of drug-metabolizing enzyme activities and applications in higher throughput screening assays for hepatotoxicity, metabolic stability, and drug–drug interaction potential. *Chem Biol Interact* 1999;121:17–35.

21. Li AP. Human hepatocytes: isolation, cryopreservation and applications in drug development. *Chem Biol Interact* 2007;168:16–29.

22. Raucy J, Lasker JM. Isolation of P450 enzymes from human livers. *Methods Enzymol* 1991;206:577–594.

23. Nelson AC, Huang W, Moody DE. Human liver microsome preparation: impact on the kinetics of L-α-acetylmethadol (LAAM) *N*-demethylation and dextromethorphan *O*-demethylation. *Drug Metab Dispos* 2001;29:319–325.

24. Barnes HJ, Arlotto MP, Waterman MR. Expression and enzymatic activity of recombinant cytochrome P450 17-alpha-hydroxylase in *Escherichia coli*. *Proc Natl Acad Sci USA* 1991;88:5597–5601.

25. Friedberg T, Pritchard MP, Bandera M, Hanlon SP, Yao D, McLaughlin LA, Ding S, Burhell B, Wolf CR. Merits and limitations of recombinant models for the study of human

P450-mediated drug metabolism and toxicity—an intralaboratory comparison. *Drug Metab Rev* 1999;31:523–544.

26. Donato MT, Jimenez N, Castell JV, Gomez-Lechon J. Fluorescence-based assays for screening nine cytochrome P450 (P450) activities in intact cells expressing individual human P450 enzymes. *Drug Metab Dispos* 2004;32:699–706.

27. Vtric F, Haefeli WE, Drewe, J, Krahenbuhl S, Wenk M. Interaction of ibuprofen and probenecid with metabolizing enzyme phenotyping procedures using caffeine as the probe drug. *Br J Clin Pharmacol* 2003;55:191–198.

28. Li AP. Scientific basis of drug-drug interactions: mechanism and preclinical evaluation. *Drug Inf J* 1998;32:657–664.

29. Emoto C, Murase S, Sawada Y, Jones BC, Iwasaki K. *In vitro* inhibitory effects of 1-aminobenzotriazole on drug oxidations catalyzed by human cytochrome P450 enzymes: a comparison with SKF-525A and ketoconazole. *Drug Metab Pharmacokinet* 2003;18:287–295.

30. Rodriques AD. Integrated cytochrome P450 reaction phenotyping: attempting to bridge the gap between cDNA-expressed cytochromes P450 and native human liver microsomes. *Biochem Pharmacol* 1999;57:465–480.

31. Lu AYH, Wang RW, Lin JH. Commentary: Cytochrome P450 *in vitro* reaction phenotyping: a re-evaluation of approaches for P450 isoform identification. *Drug Metab Dispos* 2003;31:345–350.

32. Ring BJ, Gillespie JS, Eckstein JA, Wrighton SA. Identification of human cytochromes P450 responsible for atomozetine metabolism. *Drug Metab Dispos* 2002;30:319–323.

33. Renwick AB, Surry D, Price RJ, Lake BG, Evans DC. Metabolism of 7-benzyloxy-4-trifluoromethylcoumarin by human hepatic cytochrome P450 isoforms. *Xenobiotica* 2004;30:955–969.

34. Crespi CL. Xenobiotic-metabolizing human cells as tools for pharmacological and toxicological research. *Adv Drug Res* 1995;26:179–235.

35. Uttamsingh V, Lu C, Miwa G, Gan LS. Relative contributions of the five major human cytochromes P450, 1A2, 2C9, 2C19, 2D6, and 3A4, to the hepatic metabolism of the proteasome inhibitor bortezomib. *Drug Metab Dispos* 2005;33:1723–1728.

36. McGinnity DF, Berry AJ, Kenny JR, Grime K, Riley RJ. Evaluation of time-dependent cytochrome P450 inhibition using cultured human hepatocytes. *Drug Metab Dispos* 2006;34:1291–1300.

37. Lu C, Miwa GT, Prakash SR, Gan LS, Balani SK. A novel model for the prediction of drug–drug interactions in humans based on *in vitro* cytochrome p450 phenotypic data. *Drug Metab Dispos* 2007;35:79–85.

38. Chiba M, Jin L, Neway W, Vacca JP, Tata JR, Chapman K, Lin JH. *Drug Metab Dispos* 2001;29:1–3.

39. Kim JY, Baek M, Lee S, Kim SO, Dong MS, Kim BR, Kim DH. Characterization of the selectivity and mechanism of cytochrome P450 inhibition by dimethyl-4,4'-dimethoxy-5,6,5',6'-dimethylenedioxybiphenyl-2,2'-dicarboxylate. *Drug Metab Dispos* 2001;29:1555–1560.

40. Wen X, Wang JS, Backman JT, Kivisto KT, Neuvonen PJ. Gemfibrozil as an inhibitor of human cytochrome P450 2C9. *Drug Metab Dispos* 2001;29:1359–1361.

41. Walsh CT. Suicide substrates, mechanism-based enzyme inactivators: recent developments. *Annu Rev Biochem* 1984;53:493–535.

42. Madeira M, Levine M, Chang TKH, Mirfazaelian A, Bellward G. The effect of cimetidine on dextromethorphan *O*-demethylase activity of human liver microsomes and recombinant CYP2D6. *Drug Metab Dispos* 2004;32:460–467.

43. Brown HS, Galetin A, Hallifax D, Houston B. Prediction of *in vivo* drug–drug interactions from *in vivo* data: factors affecting prototypic drug–drug interactions involving CYP2C9, CYP2D6 and CYP3A4. *Clin Pharmacokinet* 2006;45:1035–1050.

44. Kato M, Tachibana T, Ito K, Sugiyama Y. Evaluation of methods for predicting drug–drug interactions by Monte Carlo simulation. *Drug Metab Pharmacokinet* 2003;18:121–127.

45. Li AP, Rasmussen A, Xu L, Kaminski DL. Rifampicin induction of lidocaine metabolism in cultured human hepatocytes. *J Pharmacol Exp Ther* 1995;274:673–677.

46. Li AP. Primary hepatocyte cultures as an *in vitro* experimental model for the evaluation of pharmacokinetic drug–drug interactions. *Adv Pharmacol* 1997;43:103–130.

47. Roymans D, Van Looveren C, Leone A, Parker JB, McMillan M, Johnson MD, Koganti A, Gilissen R, Silber P, Mannens G, Meuldermans W. Determination of cytochrome P450 1A2 and P450 3A4 induction in cryopreserved human hepatocytes. *Biochem Pharmacol* 2004;67:427–437.

48. Roymans D, Annaert P, Van Houdt J, Weygers A, Noukens J, Sensenhauser C, Silva J, van Looveren C, Hendrickx J, Mannens G, Meuldermans W. Expression and induction potential of cytohromes P450 in human cryopreserved hepatocytes. *Drug Metab Dispos* 2005;33:1004–1016.

49. Hariparsad N, Nallani S, Sane RS, Buckley DJ, Buckley AR, Desai PB. Induction of CYP3A4 by efavirenz in primary human hepatocytes: comparison with rifampin and phenobarbital. *J Clin Pharmaol* 2004;44:1273–1281.

50. Lillibridge JH, Liang BH, Kerr BM, Webber S, Quart B, Shetty BV, Lee CA. Characterization of the selectivity and mechanism of human cytochrome P450 inhibition by the human immunodeficiency virus–protease inhibitor nelfinavir mesylate. *Drug Metab Dispos* 1998;26:609–616.

51. Wang RW, Newton DJ, Liu N, Atkins WM, Lu AYH. Human cytochrome P-450 3A4: *in vitro* drug–drug interaction patterns are substrate-dependent. *Drug Metab Dispos* 2000;28:360–366.

52. Backman JT, Kyrklund C, Neuvonen M, Neuvonen PJ. Gemfibrozil greatly increases plasma concentrations of cerivastatin. *Clin Pharmaol Ther* 2002;72:685–691.

53. Vickers AE, Sinclair JR, Zollinger M, Heitz F, Glanzel U, Johanson L, Fischer V. Multiple cytochrome P450s involved in the metabolism of terbinafine suggest a limited potential for drug–drug interactions. *Drug Metab Dispos* 1999;27:1029–1038.

25

MECHANISMS AND CONSEQUENCES OF DRUG–DRUG INTERACTIONS

DORA FARKAS, RICHARD I. SHADER, LISA L. VON MOLTKE, AND DAVID J. GREENBLATT

Tufts University School of Medicine, Boston, Massachusetts

Contents

Preclinical Development Handbook: ADME and Biopharmaceutical Properties,
edited by Shayne Cox Gad
Copyright © 2008 John Wiley & Sons, Inc.

25.1 PRINCIPLES OF DRUG–DRUG INTERACTIONS

25.1.1 Introduction

Understanding the mechanisms and consequences of drug–drug interactions is essential for the development of new pharmaceuticals and for the design of multidrug regimens. Drug interactions occur when one drug (the "perpetrator") changes the pharmacokinetic and/or the pharmacodynamic actions of another drug (the "victim"). This interaction can lead to changes in the clearance of the victim drug, which can influence its efficacy and safety. For drugs with narrow therapeutic indices, such as warfarin, digoxin, and theophylline, small changes in plasma concentrations can lead to toxicity.

Even after drugs undergo rigorous safety and efficacy testing during clinical trials, they can be withdrawn from the market due to the unanticipated possibility of toxic interactions with other drugs. For example, in the late 1990s the U.S. FDA recommended the withdrawal of the antihistamine terfenadine after it was discovered that its coadministration with the antifungal ketoconazole was associated with cardiac toxicity, which in a few instances was fatal. Terfenadine has been replaced by its metabolite, fexofenadine, which has similar efficacy but no known cardiac toxicity [1].

Drug–drug interactions are especially a concern for patients taking several drugs concurrently, such as the elderly and patients with serious medical diseases such as cancer or HIV. It is estimated that almost 40% of the elderly take five or more drugs simultaneously [2] and that 90% of them also use over-the-counter (OTC) medications, some of which may also contribute to drug interactions [3]. For example, the H_2 receptor antagonist cimetidine inhibits several cytochrome P450s and interacts with the CYP1A2 substrate theophylline [4]. Elderly patients are also thought to be 3–10 times more likely than younger patients to be susceptible to adverse drug–drug interactions due to changes in hepatic and renal clearance [5, 6]. In addition, with the increasing use of complementary alternative medicines such as herbal supplements, the probability of drug–drug interactions is increased. For example, it is estimated that over 50% of cancer patients take herbal remedies, even though there is evidence for adverse drug interactions with several herbs such as kava-kava, *Ginkgo biloba*, ginseng, and echinacea [6, 7].

Drug–drug interactions are not limited to prescription drugs, OTC drugs, and herbal remedies. Other substances such as foods, beverages, and excipients in drug tablets can enhance or inhibit the disposition of drugs. Grapefruit juice, for example, is an inhibitor of CYP3A, which is responsible for metabolizing an estimated 50% of prescription drugs. Further clinical trials demonstrated that grapefruit juice only inhibits intestinal CYP3A, and therefore, it is only expected to influence the pharmacokinetics of drugs that undergo significant enteric CYP3A metabolism [8], such as short half-life benzodiazepines [9]. More recent evidence suggests that certain other fruit juices also have the potential to inhibit CYP3A. For example, Seville orange juice was shown to inhibit enteric metabolism of felodipine [10] to a similar extent as grapefruit juice. In addition, *in vitro* and animal studies suggest that pomegranate juice is also a significant inhibitor of CYP3A [11, 12].

Interestingly, certain tablet excipients also influence absorption and bioavailability. For example, the cremophores EL and RH 40, which enhance lipid solubility, have been shown to increase the oral bioavailability of saquinavir and digoxin, respectively [13–15]. However, other excipients such as Tween 80 and HS15 can adversely affect the disposition of drugs by inhibiting the drug transporter P-glycoprotein (also known as ABCB1 and MDR1) and increasing intracellular levels of P-glycoprotein substrates such as the chemotherapy agent daunorubicin [15].

Drug–drug interactions can occur through four mechanisms of drug disposition, collectively known as ADME—*a*bsorption, *d*istribution, *m*etabolism, and *e*limination. Absorption of a drug across a lipid bilayer is influenced by several factors, including physicochemical properties of the drug, such as solubility, lipophilicity, the pH of the environment, gastric emptying rate, gastrointestinal motility, and bile secretion. Antacids such as H_2 receptor antagonists can inhibit the absorption of certain drugs, such as ketoconazole, which need an acidic environment, and the anxiolytic drug clorazepate, which needs an acidic environment to be converted to its metabolite, desmethyldiazepam [16]. Furthermore, multivalent cations, such as calcium, magnesium, zinc, iron, and aluminum, which form chemical complexes, can inhibit the absorption of the antibiotics tetracycline and ciprofloxacin [17, 18]. Thus, the consumption of milk or nutritional supplements containing these minerals is contraindicated with tetracycline. Gastrointestinal motility is also impaired by the anticholinergic effects of marijuana or enhanced by the gastrokinetic agent metoclopramide. A decrease (or increase) in gastrointestinal motility can increase (or decrease) the exposure of the intestine to drugs and may result in toxicity [17].

It was previously believed that when a drug is displaced from its plasma protein binding site by another drug, the victim drug's unbound concentration will increase, leading to increased efficacy or possibly toxicity [19]. There are actually very few cases where displacement from plasma protein causes clinically significant interactions [20, 21]. Exceptions include drugs with high extraction and narrow therapeutic indices. For example, extensively albumin-bound compounds may theoretically displace a drug such as warfarin; however, this effect is only transient and rarely of clinical importance [22, 23]. Some interactions were previously attributed primarily to displacement but were found to be a result of inhibition of clearance. Phenylbutazone, for example, inhibits the metabolism of warfarin [24, 25], while sulfonamides reduce the clearance of tolbutamide [26, 27].

Altered metabolism (including phase I and phase II) is the most common reason for drug interactions since many metabolic enzymes can be inhibited or induced by drugs. Inhibition and induction of transporter proteins, particularly P-glycoprotein, is also a clinically significant pathway for drug–drug interactions and will be discussed in more detail in the following sections.

Clearly, it is impossible for the prescribing physician to remember all potential drug interactions. However, an understanding of the principles of drug–drug interactions can aid in the design of a safe multidrug regimen. New analytical techniques and modeling tools combined with knowledge databases are enabling researchers to make better predictions of possible drug interactions. The goals of this chapter are to discuss (1) the common mechanisms of drug–drug interactions, (2) different experimental systems and modeling tools used to investigate possible drug interactions, and (3) pharmacokinetic principles of drug interactions. In Sections 25.2 and 25.3, we illustrate clinically significant drug–drug and drug–herb interactions in two different case studies.

25.1.2   Mechanisms of Drug–Drug Interactions

Metabolic Interactions   While there are several possible mechanisms for drug interactions, most of the interactions occur through alterations of hepatic or enteric drug metabolism. Metabolic interactions occur when a perpetrator drug inhibits or induces the activity of a drug-metabolizing enzyme, resulting in either decreased or increased metabolism of a victim drug. Most of the known drug interactions involve the cytochrome P450s (phase I metabolism); however, interactions may also involve phase II enzymes such as the UDP glucuronidases [28, 29]. Table 25.1 provides selected examples of some common prescription drugs that are inhibitors or inducers of the cytochrome P450s and the transporter P-glycoprotein. According to most studies, CYP2D6 is not an easily inducible enzyme. However, there are some studies that suggest that CYP2D6 might be induced by phenobarbital [30] and carbamazepine [31].

The cytochrome P450s implicated in most drug–drug interactions are CYP1A2, CYP2B6, CYP2C8, CYP2C9, CYP2C19, CYP2D6, and CYP3A4. The CYP3A family, particularly CYP3A4, is considered to be exceptionally important, since it mediates the clearance of many common prescription medications [29, 32]. Many prescription drugs, such as the antifungals ketoconazole and fluconazole, the macrolide antibiotic clarithromycin, and the antidepressant fluoxetine, are potent inhibitors of CYP3A and can lead to significant drug interactions. As mentioned previously, the antihistamine terfenadine was withdrawn from the market after it was discovered that coadministration with ketoconazole could lead to cardiac toxicity. The toxicity resulted from the accumulation of excess terfenadine in the bloodstream, since the CYP3A-mediated metabolism of terfenadine was inhibited by ketoconazole [33]. Antifungal agents also interact with other classes of metabolic enzymes. It is thought that fluconazole and miconazole can interact with the metabolism of warfarin, possibly by inhibiting CYP2C9 [6, 34]. However, not all CYP450 inhibitors lead to clinically significant interactions. For example, the antibiotics azithromycin and dirithromycin are weak CYP3A inhibitors and have not been observed to cause toxic drug–drug interactions [35–37].

Selective serotonin reuptake inhibitors (SSRIs) are also known to interact with most of the major cytochrome P450s. CYP1A2 is inhibited by fluvoxamine and to a lesser extent by citalopram, and CYP2D6 is known to be inhibited significantly by fluoxetine and paroxetine, and to a lesser extent by sertraline and citalopram. Many antineoplastic and antiretroviral drugs also interact with the CYP450s, which can be potentially dangerous when several of these drugs are coadministered. The anticancer drug paclitaxel, frequently used to treat breast and ovarian cancers, has been reported to cause toxicity when coadministered with CYP3A inhibitors such as the antiretrovirals delavirdine and saquinavir. Paclitaxel was also found to interact with the chemotherapeutic agent valspodar, possibly through the inhibition of P-glycoprotein by valspodar [6, 38].

Complicating clinical practice is the interindividual variability due to genetic differences in the drug metabolism enzymes [6]. Genetic differences in drug metabolism were first suggested in the 1950s. Hughes et al. [39] reported significant interindividual variability in the acetylation of isoniazid and observed that "slow acetylators" were more likely to experience toxicity from the drug [40]. In the years following this discovery, many epidemiological studies were carried out to confirm

TABLE 25.1 Prescription Drugs as Inducers and Inhibitors of the Major Cytochrome P450s and P-Glycoprotein

CYP1A2	CYP2B6	CYP2C9	CYP2C19	CYP2D6	CYP2E1	CYP3A4	P-Glycoprotein
Inducer(s)							
Omeprazole	Rifampin	Rifampin	Rifampin	None known	Isoniazid	Carbamazepine Dexamethasone Rifampin Phenytoin	Rifampin
Inhibitors							
Fluvoxamine Cimetidine	Ketoconazole Clopidogrel	Sulfaphenzole Fluvoxamine Fluconazole Miconazole	Fluoxetine Fluvoxamine	Fluoxetine Quinidine Methadone Paroxetine	Disulfiram	Clotrimazole Itraconazole Ketoconazole Miconazole Ritonazir Nefazodone	Verapamil Doxorubicin Clarithromycin Ritonavir Omeprazole

Source: Adapted from Refs. 15, 32, 43, 46, and 144.

883

interindividual differences in drug metabolism. For example, the cytochrome P450s CYP2D6 and CYP2C9 have significant genetic polymorphisms and they also metabolize an estimated 25% [41] and 16% [42] of prescription drugs, respectively. CYP2D6, in particular, has at least 80 allelic variants, resulting in a range from poor to ultrarapid metabolizers, and it is also inhibited by drugs such as fluoxetine and methadone [43]. CYP2C9 has five alleles with varying prevalences among different ethnic groups. Genetic variations in CYP2C9 are also a concern, since CYP2C9 is responsible for metabolizing substrates with narrow therapeutic indices such as warfarin and phenytoin [44].

Some of the most significant drug–drug interactions are due to mechanism-based, or irreversible, inhibition. In this case, the drug binds to the enzyme and can modify the heme, protein, or the complex through covalent binding and inactivate it irreversibly [45]. Mechanism-based inhibitors include paroxetine (CYP2D6) [28], tamoxifen, erythromycin, and fluoxetine (CYP3A4). The CYP3A inhibitor in grapefruit juice, 6′, 7′-dihydroxybergamottin, is also a mechanism-based inhibitor. In clinical trials where midazolam was used as a CYP3A probe, a 10 oz glass of white grapefruit juice led to approximately a 65% increase in midazolam's area under the curve (AUC). Subsequent administration of midazolam demonstrated that complete recovery of CYP3A takes about 3 days [8].

Although less investigated, drug–drug interactions also occur through enzyme induction. Induction is a much slower process than inhibition since it involves transcriptional activation of genes. CYP1A2 clearance is increased by cruciferous vegetables, charcoal-broiled beef, cigarette smoke, and omeprazole. The antibacterial rifampin is an inducer of CYP2C9, CYP2C19 and CYP3A4. CYP3A4 can be induced by a variety of compounds including barbiturates, glucocorticoids, phenytoin, carbamazepine, and St. John's wort [46]. Induction of cytochrome P450s typically occurs through the nuclear receptors primarily AhR, CAR, and PXR. In addition to interindividual differences among the cytochrome P450s, there are also differences in nuclear receptors [47, 48] and in their regulatory proteins [49, 50]. Chang et al. [51] measured the mRNAs of CYP2B6, CAR, and PXR in 12 human liver samples. They found a 240-fold interindividual variability among samples in CAR mRNA levels, and a 278-fold variability in the mRNA levels of CYP2B6. The variability in PXR was about 27-fold and it also correlated well with the variabilities in CYP2B6 and CAR [50]. Individual differences in drug disposition could also be due to genetic variations in drug transporters. In fact, there is recent evidence to suggest that interindividual variability in the metabolism of phenytoin and fexofenadine could be attributed to genetic differences in the transporter P-glycoprotein [52, 53].

Interactions Through Nonneuronal Efflux Transporters   Transporters are ubiquitously located throughout the body and play an important role in the disposition of drugs, particularly in the liver, the intestine, and the kidneys. While some transporters can interfere with the delivery of drugs inside the cells, they are essential for maintaining a physiologic barrier at several locations, such as the blood–brain barrier [54], testes, and placenta [15]. Transporters include both uptake and efflux proteins and have been classified into several families, including the ATP-binding cassette transporters (ABCs), the organic anion transporting polypeptides (OATPs), organic anion transporters (OATs), and the organic cation transporters (OCTs). Inhibition or induction of transporters can lead to increased or decreased drug concentration inside the cells, and therefore a better understanding of these transporters is essential for rational drug design and pharmacokinetic modeling.

The ABC family is further subdivided into several subfamilies such as ABCA, ABCB, and ABCC. The most widely recognized transporter is the multidrug resistance protein, MDR1, also known as ABCB1 or P-glycoprotein [55], and in this chapter we use P-glycoprotein as the model for demonstrating the importance of drug–drug interactions through transporters.

Some drugs such as the immunosuppressant cyclosporin A are interesting in that they are both substrates and inhibitors of P-glycoprotein [15]. For example, it has been shown *in vitro* that cyclosporin A inhibited transport of the cardiac drug digoxin, yet digoxin did not inhibit transport of cyclosporin A [56]. P-glycoprotein is especially critical in maintaining the intactness of the blood–brain barrier and cyclosporin A has led to the accumulation of vinblastine in the brain of mice [57]. In P-glycoprotein knockout mice, a normally harmless dose of the opiate loperamide (used as an antidiarrheal in humans) was lethal as the drug gained entry into the central nervous system [58, 59]. In rats, cyclosporine inhibited P-glycoprotein in other organs such as the testes, where it led to the accumulation of doxorubicin [60]. Cardiac toxicity in rats was also caused by another inhibitor of P-glycoprotein, verapamil, which increased the cardiac levels of the chemotherapeutic agent idarubicin [61].

While the presence of P-glycoprotein is associated with drug efflux from cells, it is important to point out that not all substrates of P-glycoprotein have poor bioavailability. Digoxin, in particular, has an oral bioavailability of 50–85% [62, 63]. Ritonavir, another P-glycoprotein substrate, has a bioavailability of 60% [63, 64]. The reason for the high bioavailability of these drugs is that bioavailability is also influenced by influx processes, which might outweigh the effects of the efflux transporters for some drugs. In addition, similar to enzymes, P-glycoprotein efflux is a saturable process. The K_m for many P-glycoprotein substrates, such as digoxin, verapamil, and indinavir, have been determined and the values are in the micromolar range. Thus, in theory, when the plasma concentration of the drug is significantly higher than its K_m value, the drug might be expected to have high bioavailability [62, 63].

Inhibition of P-glycoprotein can occur through multiple mechanisms and can be classified as competitive inhibition, noncompetitive inhibition, or cooperative stimulation. Inhibition can occur if the inhibitor occupies an active binding site or if it inhibits the ATP hydrolysis process that is necessary for efflux. Verapamil inhibits P-glycoprotein by occupying an active binding site, vanadate interacts with ATP hydrolysis, while cyclosporine inhibits P-glycoprotein through both mechanisms [63, 65]. Cooperative inhibition occurs when two inhibitors act together to inhibit P-glycoprotein. P-glycoprotein is thought to have at least two binding sites, and sometimes inhibitors bind to both sites, leading to synergism between the two binding sites to inhibit P-glycoprotein [66]. Inhibitors that were found to act at both sites included vinblastine, tamoxifen, and quinidine [67]. Modeling inhibition can be quite complex, because in addition to the multiple binding sites on P-glycoprotein, there are also allosteric interactions when multiple binding sites are occupied.

Induction of P-glycoprotein has also been observed in response to common P450 inducers such as 3-methylcholanthrene [68] and dexamethasone [69]. Certain cytotoxic agents such as adriamycin, daunomycin, and mitoxantrone have also been found to induce P-glycoprotein in rodent cells [70]. There is now data to suggest that induction of P-glycoprotein may occur through multiple mechanisms including PXR. Thus, species differences in P-glycoprotein induction are probably due in part to differences in the activation of species-specific PXR [63]. However, even within the same organism, P-glycoprotein is not necessarily induced to the same extent in every tissue, and the time until maximum induction can also vary significantly. Jette et al. [71] compared induction of P-glycoprotein by 10 mg/kg/day cyclosporine A in various organs in the rat. Whereas P-glycoprotein increased by more than 250% in the stomach, it only increased 69% in the lungs [63]. Furthermore, maximal response was observed after only 5 days in the heart, while it took 15 days for maximal response in the spleen and testes.

Pharmacoenhancement or Augmentatics   In the previous sections we have discussed examples of adverse drug–drug interactions. However, the pharmacokinetics of HIV combination protease inhibitors demonstrate the principles of pharmacoenhancement, where the "perpetrator" drug actually improves the effectiveness of the "victim" drug. In this section we illustrate the principles of pharmacoenhancement by discussing the pharmacokinetics of HIV protease inhibitors.

Protease inhibitors (PIs), introduced in the mid-1990s, are now standard therapy for HIV. However, in spite of their effectiveness, there is poor patient compliance, leading to treatment failure within 1 year in 40–60% of cases [72, 73]. Reasons for poor patient compliance include unpleasant side effects, the need for frequent dosing, and food- or fluid-dependent administration regimens. Poor patient compliance allows the viral load to get very high and can lead to resistance to the treatment. Combination PIs, where multiple drugs are combined within one formulation, are more effective in suppressing viral replication by increasing the overall exposure to the boosted drug. In addition, clinical trials have suggested better patient compliance because of fewer food restrictions, simpler dosing regimen, as well as lower interindividual variabilities.

Many PIs are combined with ritonavir as the "perpetrator" drug. Ritonavir, which is usually prescribed as 600 mg twice a day, is generally not well tolerated since it can lead to nausea, diarrhea, and other unpleasant side effects. However, a 100 mg dose of ritonavir has been shown to boost the effectiveness of several other PIs [72]. All approved HIV PIs are predominantly metabolized by CYP3A4, and they are all substrates for P-glycoprotein. Of all PIs, ritonavir is the most potent inhibitor of both CYP3A4 and P-glycoprotein [74]. The combination PI consisting of 400 mg of lopinavir and 100 mg of ritonavir has been shown to be well tolerated and effective [75] and is now a marketed drug as a twice-a-day prescription. The FDA has now approved other once-a-day regimens such as amprenavir and atazanavir for patients who are treatment-experienced. The effectiveness of administering lopinavir/saquinavir once-a-day is being currently evaluated [76]. Other drugs boosted by ritonavir include indinavir, amprenavir, saquinavir, lopinavir, atanazavir, and nelfinavir. Other PIs, such as efivarenz and nevirapine, are inducers of CYP3A4; thus, their inclusion in a treatment regimen might require an increase in the dose of other drugs [74].

The specific type of pharmacoenhancement with ritonavir depends on the individual PIs. The effects will be either (1) to increase C_{max}, C_{min}, and AUC and modestly increase $t_{1/2}$ (primarily C_{max} boosting) or (2) to increase $t_{1/2}$ and C_{min} and modestly increase AUC (primarily $t_{1/2}$ boosting). An increase in C_{min} is associated with higher efficacy and an increase in C_{max} also leads to higher drug exposure but could also result in toxicity unless the drug is well tolerated. A boosting of C_{max}, C_{min}, and AUC (the first type of effect) is observed with lopinavir and saquinavir, which have high first-pass metabolism. Indinavir and amprenavir have short half-lives and ritonavir primarily increases the $t_{1/2}$ and C_{min} and modestly increases AUC for these drugs (the second effect). It is also fortunate that the AUC and the C_{max} are not significantly boosted since an increase in the C_{max} for these drugs has been associated with adverse side effects [77].

Double-boosted PIs are also gaining popularity, especially in treatment-experienced patients. The advantages of this type of treatment are that (1) the levels of several different PIs are increased simulataneously and they are effective against viruses that might have resistance against one particular drug, and (2) addition of a second booster might further enhance the pharmacokinetic properties of the treatment. For example, addition of saquinavir to an atazanavir/ritonavir combination was reported to increase the C_{max} of atazanavir more than just adding ritonavir. The AUCs of atazanavir and saquinavir also increased compared to single-boosted regimens [78, 79].

While ritonavir seems to be effective in combination PIs, not all patients can tolerate it due to its adverse side effects. Another booster drug is the nonnucleoside reverse transcriptase inhibitor delavirdine, which has been shown to increase the half-life, AUC, and C_{max} of nelfinavir. Nelfinavir is metabolized partially by CYP2D6, which is missing in 7% of Caucasians and 1% of Asians [74]. Other individuals are ultrarapid CYP2D6 metabolizers and need higher doses to reach therapeutic drug concentrations. Thus, interindividual variability in drug-metabolizing phenotype also needs to be taken into consideration when prescribing the specific combination PI therapy.

25.1.3   Methods and Systems for Analyzing Drug–Drug Interactions

In Vitro Systems   Several systems are available for studying drug–drug interactions and the choice of system depends on the predicted type of interaction. Clearly, the most relevant system is the human body; however, clinical trials are expensive and only a few compounds can be tested per trial. Furthermore, species differences may limit the usefulness of animal experiments. *In vitro* and *in silico* (computational) studies can be useful in eliminating unlikely drug–drug interactions and determining the probable interactions that could be further investigated in clinical or animal studies. Microsomes are frequently used for inhibition studies because they are inexpensive and allow for simulataneous monitoring of several enzymes including the cytochrome P450s, the flavin monooxygenases, and the UDP-glucuronosyltransferases.

Induction studies are carried out in hepatocytes, since the cellular machinery is necessary for upregulating the transcription of genes. However, primary hepatocytes are known to rapidly lose metabolic functions after isolation; thus, special media and culture conditions are necessary for maintaining them. The main challenge regarding hepatocyte culture is that most factors stimulate either regeneration or differentiation but not both [40]. Long-term cultures of hepatocytes usually require a mitogenic compound, such as epidermal growth factor (EGF), which stimulates DNA synthesis. However, it has been shown that EGF leads to a downregulation of the metabolic enzymes, specifically CYP1A, CYP2B [80, 81], CYP2C11 [82], and CP3A [83]. Cell density also influences cell proliferation and metabolism. A low cell density increases cell proliferation but reduces the expression and inducibility of metabolic enzymes [84]. Culturing hepatocytes on structural matrix proteins, such as collagen, fibronectin, and laminin, has been found to maintain cell morphology and metabolic functions better than plating them on plastic. Culturing hepatocytes in a sandwich configuration is even more suitable for maintaining metabolically active cells. The most common matrices for sandwich cultures are collagen type I and Matrigel, an extract derived from the basement membrane of the Engelbreth–Holm–Sworm mouse sarcoma [85]. Both collagen–collagen and collagen–Matrigel sandwiches have been shown to maintain morphology and albumin secretion for several weeks [86], and they are also inducible for both CYP1A2 and CYP3A4 in systems with human hepatocytes [87].

In addition to optimizing cell culture parameters, special cell lines have been engineered that constitutively express cytochrome P450s and are also inducible for specific enzymes such as CYP3A4. For example, the DPX-3A4 cell line, which contains a luciferase-linked PXR promoter, has been shown to be inducible by a number of compounds such as rifampin, ginseng, and kava-kava [88]. Other cell lines such as the Fa2N-4 are inducible for multiple enzymes, including CYP1A2, CYP2C9, CYP3A4, and UGT1A and the MDR1 transporter [89]. The WIF-B9 cell line, which is a fusion of rat hepatoma and human fibroblasts, has been shown to constitutively express both human and rat cytochrome P450s [90].

For transporter studies involving P-glycoprotein, the human intestinally derived Caco-2 cell line is the most frequently used. The Madin–Darby canine kidney (MDCK) cells are also frequently tested since they require shorter culture period (3–5 days) and have high levels of P-glycoprotein expression [91, 92]. The two main issues with using cells lines for transporter studies are (1) the influence of passage number on the expression of P-glycoprotein and (2) expression of other transporter proteins. In particular, Caco-2 cells typically express the breast cancer resistance protein (BCRP) and the multidrug resistance-associated protein 2 (MRP2) [93–95].

Pharmacokinetic studies can also be carried out in more physiologic *in vitro* systems such as a bioartificial liver. The main challenge with such systems is designing conditions that can maintain hepatocytes long enough for the studies. Cell lines are easier to maintain than primary hepatocytes, but they usually do not express drug-metabolizing enzymes. Several new cell lines have been developed for this purpose such as a pig hepatocyte cell line and a couple of human-derived lines. The pig hepatocytes have been shown to express most of the cytochrome P450s as well as glutathione *S*-transferase and UDP-glucuronosyltransferase [96]. A HepG2-derived cell line was also found to express CYP3A4 at even higher levels than primary human hepatocytes [97]. Furthermore, a human hepatocellular carcinoma cell line has been engineered to be inducible for CYP3A4. This cell line, FLC-5, was cultured in a radial-flow bioreactor and shown to be inducible for CYP3A4 via PXR activation [98]. Thus, the development of these cell lines is a promising step in designing physiologically based perfused bioreactors for drug metabolism and drug interaction studies.

Computational Modeling and Data Processing Tools   Computational (or *in silico*) tools are also used widely in the pharmaceutical industry to evaluate possible metabolism and toxicity pathways for new drugs. While it is not possible to completely characterize most compounds *in silico*, a lot of the technology is already in place and incorporation of new data could lead to more reliable tools in the near future [99]. Quantitative structure–activity relationship (QSAR) models have been compiled for over 2000 compounds to determine possible substrates for the CYP450s [100]. Although many other pathways and endogenous factors influence the pharmacokinetics of drugs, these models can aid in modeling the binding potential of drugs to enzymes. Structure–activity models have been developed for the major cytochrome P450s, including CYP3A4, CYP2D6, and CYP2C9, and results from these models have shown over 90% correlation with experimental data [101]. More in-depth QSAR models have been built for individual P450s, such as CYP2C9, to examine interactions of the enzyme with a variety of potential inhibitors and also to determine the effect of mutations on enzyme activity [102]. Special computer-based models have also been developed for the prediction of drug–drug interactions, which incorporate all known data on drug metabolism enzymes. One example is Q-DIPS (quantitative drug interactions prediction system), which correctly predicted a potent inhibition of CYP3A4 by ketoconazole, and a weaker inhibition by fluconazole [103]. QSAR models have also been developed for drug transporters, especially P-glycoprotein. These models have identified several potential modulators of transporters in order to overcome drug resistance to many chemotherapeutic compounds [104, 105]. Thus, these models can be useful for discovering new compounds that could enter the drug pipelines; however, the development process of new drugs still relies heavily on *in vitro* and *in vivo* experimentation.

Another challenge of drug development is integration of all known data about a certain enzyme or the affected molecular pathway affected. Integration of data has become especially time consuming with the high throughput methods of genomics, proteomics, and metabonomics, which generate vast amounts of data. The goal of systems biology is to combine experimentally generated data with modeling tools in order to discover potential drug interactions and new therapeutic targets. Although many models have been developed, they are far from being complete, since only 15% of the human genome has known function. Nevertheless, these knowledge databases combined with high throughput screening have become useful for modeling ADME/Tox, discovering potential drug interactions and for visualizing the biological processes influenced by drugs [106].

25.1.4 Pharmacokinetic Principles of Drug–Drug Interactions

Kinetics Pharmacokinetic modeling is an essential tool for understanding drug disposition and for designing safe and effective treatment regimens. The simplest approach assumes linear, first-order Michaelis–Menten kinetics. This type of kinetics is described by

$$v = \frac{V_{max}[S]}{K_M + [S]}$$

where v is the reaction velocity, $[S]$ is the substrate concentration, and K_M is the substrate concentration at which the reaction velocity reaches half of the maximal velocity, V_{max}. When $[S] \ll K_M$ the reaction displays linear kinetics; thus, the rate is directly proportional to the substrate concentration. When $[S]$ get close to K_M

the enzyme starts becoming saturated and eventually the velocity, v, reaches its maximum, V_{max}.

If a drug is metabolized by more than one enzyme, the velocity of the reaction is the sum of the individual rates:

$$v = \frac{V_{max(1)}[S]}{K_{M(1)}+[S]} + \frac{V_{max(2)}[S]}{K_{M(2)}+[S]}$$

In this case each enzyme reaction has its own V_{max} and K_M, denoted by the appropriate subscripts. In order to recognize such a phenomenon, the data needs to be viewed on an Eadie–Hofstee plot (v vs. $v/[S]$), which will illustrate the biphasic characteristic of the reaction [28].

Inhibition and induction occur through different mechanisms and there are different mathematical models and *in vitro* tools for studying them. Inhibition is primarily a chemical phenomenon involving a reversible or irreversible binding of the inhibitor to the enzyme. For this reason inhibition is usually concentration dependent and is usually quantified by the inhibition constant K_i or the 50% inhibitory concentration, the IC_{50}. Inhibition can be competitive, noncompetitive, or uncompetitive. In competitive inhibition, the inhibitor binds to the active pocket of the enzyme and blocks the binding of the substrate. In noncompetitive inhibition, the inhibitor and the substrate bind independently to different sites, and in uncompetitive inhibition, the inhibitor binds to the substrate–enzyme complex and renders the complex inactive. In all three cases, the inhibitor interferes with the reaction velocity and the Michaelis–Menten kinetics are then modified accordingly [46].

For competitive inhibition,

$$v = \frac{V_{max}[S]}{[S]+K_M(1+[I]/K_i)}$$

For noncompetitive inhibition,

$$v = \frac{V_{max}[S]}{(1+[I]/K_i)(K_M+[S])}$$

For uncompetitive inhibition,

$$v = \frac{V_{max}[S]}{[S]+K_M+[I][S]/K_i}$$

The mechanism of inhibition can be determined from plotting experimental data. Figure 25.1 shows the plots of $1/v$, the reciprocal of the velocity, versus [I], the inhibitor concentration, for the three types of inhibition (also known as Dixon plots) [107]. Note that [I] and $1/v$ will be positive for all experimental data and the diagrammed intersection points can only be determined by extrapolating the lines. When the mechanism is competitive, the lines will intersect at the point where $[I] = -K_i$ and $1/v = 1/V_{max}$, and when it is noncompetitive the intersection point is at $[I] = -K_i$ and $1/v = 0$. In uncompetitive inhibition, the slopes are independent of [S] and hence

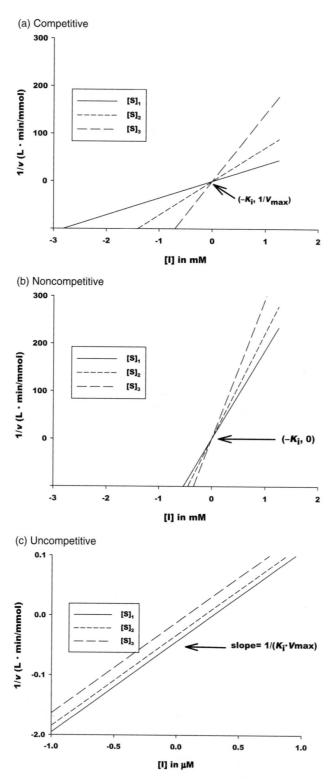

FIGURE 25.1 Relationship between concentration of inhibitor, [I], and the reciprocal of velocity ($1/v$) at different substrate concentrations for (a) competitive, (b) uncompetitive, and (c) noncompetitive inhibition with the following parameters: $K_m = 4.7 \times 10^{-5}\,$M; $V_{max} = 22\,\mu$Mol/(L·min); $K_i = 3 \times 10^{-4}\,$M. The three substrate concentrations were $[S]_1 = 2 \times 10^{-4}\,$M, $[S]_2 = 1 \times 10^{-4}\,$M, and $[S]_3 = 5 \times 10^{-5}\,$M.

TABLE 25.2   Pharmacokinetic Changes Due to Drug–Drug Interactions

Mechanism of Interaction	Change in Systemic Exposure	Theoretical Change in Exposure[a]
Competitive Inhibition	Increased	$\dfrac{AUC_i}{AUC} = 1 + \dfrac{[I]}{K_i}$
Noncompetitive inhibition	Increased	$\dfrac{AUC_i}{AUC} = 1 + \dfrac{[I]}{K_i}$
Uncompetitive inhibition	Increased	$\dfrac{AUC_i}{AUC} = 1 + \left(\dfrac{[I]}{K_i}\right)\left(\dfrac{[S]}{[S] + K_M}\right)$
Mechanism-based inhibition (irreversible inactivation)	Increased	$\dfrac{AUC_i}{AUC} = \dfrac{V_{max}}{V_{max(inhibited)}}$
Induction	Decreased	$\dfrac{AUC_i}{AUC} = \dfrac{V_{max}}{V_{max(inhibited)}}$

[a] AUC_i denotes the area under the curve after administration of the inhibitor. These equations assume that $[S] \ll K_M$.
Source: Adapted from Ref. 28.

the lines will be parallel [107]. Table 25.2 summarizes the changes in systemic exposure during different drug interaction scenarios [28].

Determining the type of inhibition mechanism and calculation of the inhibition constant, K_i, is very labor intensive, since the reaction velocity needs to be determined at several different inhibitor and substrate concentrations. Before determining the type of inhibition, it is helpful to investigate whether the inhibition is mechanism based, in which the case the inhibitor would irreversibly inactivate the enzyme. In this case, the inhibitor is preincubated with the enzyme for some time period before addition of the substrate. This preincubation allows the inhibitor to bind to the enzyme, and if the mechanism is irreversible, the reaction should proceed significantly slower than without preincubation.

Calculation of the IC_{50} is useful for determining whether the inhibitor is likely to have an *in vivo* significance. The IC_{50} can be determined by plotting the percentage of control (uninhibited) reaction velocity (R) versus the inhibitor concentration [I], at a constant substrate concentration. The resulting sigmoidal curve can be modeled with nonlinear regression and described with the following equation:

$$R = 100\left(1 - \frac{E_{max}C^A}{C^A + IC^A}\right)$$

where E_{max} is the maximum fractional inhibition, C is the concentration of the inhibitor, IC is the concentration that results in a reaction velocity of $50(2 - E_{max})$, which is the velocity at half the maximal inhibition, and A is an exponent relating the sigmoidal shape of the curve. The true IC_{50}, producing a velocity that is 50% of the control value, is calculated as [108]

$$IC_{50} = \frac{IC}{(2E_{max}-1)^{1/A}}$$

Using this approach, the calculation of IC_{50} is model independent, since its value does not depend on the biochemical mechanism of inhibition (competitive vs. non-competitive vs. uncompetitive). Lower IC_{50} values indicate greater inhibitory potency and IC_{50} will always be greater than or equal to K_i, the inhibition constant. If the mechanism of inhibition is "noncompetitive," they are equal [109]. If the mechanism of inhibition is reversible (competitive or noncompetitive), the preincubation process will not affect inhibitory potency, or may actually decrease inhibitory potency (higher IC_{50}) due to metabolic consumption of inhibitor in the microsomal system. If the inhibition is irreversible, the preincubation will increase inhibitory potency (lower IC_{50}).

Many metabolic enzymes obey atypical or nonlinear enzyme kinetics. CYP3A4 exhibits a sigmoidal saturation curve due to the existence of multiple binding sites on which substrates can bind cooperatively [110]. The v versus [S] plot is described by the following equation:

$$v = \frac{V_{max}[S]^n}{S_{50}^n + [S]^n}$$

in which n refers to a Hill coefficient (which has to be greater than 1.0), and S_{50} is the substrate concentration at which the velocity is half of V_{max} [28].

Another possible complication in modeling drug–drug interactions is the possibility of concurrent inhibition and induction. Ritonavir is an example, since it is an inhibitor of CYP3A, but long-term administration induces the enzyme through the PXR receptor [111]. St. John's wort was found to produce the same effect; certain components of it are potent inhibitors of CYP3A, yet St. John's wort also activates CYP3A through PXR [112]. Inhibition and induction can be distinguished from each other since they occur on different time scales. Inhibition is an immediate phenomenon and can be studied in microsomes, which do not have the cellular machinery for inducing enzymes. Induction is a time-consuming process, where transcription alone can take 4–6 hours; however, in clinical trials it could take days to see any inductive effects, especially if inhibition is competing with induction. For example, in a trial where ritonavir and alprazolam were coadministered, there was a small decrease in the plasma concentration of alprazolam after 12 days, suggesting that induction was overcoming inhibition [28].

Besides metabolism, efflux transport is also a form of clearance and modeling of transporter systems is useful for determining the most important parameters in this process. Several computational models have been developed to study transporters. Jang et al. [113] modeled the P-glycoprotein-mediated efflux of the anticancer drug paclitaxel. The P-glycoprotein-mediated efflux rate can described as

$$\text{P-gp – efflux rate} = \frac{J_{max} \cdot C_{max}}{K_{M,P\text{-gp}} + C_{free,c}}$$

In this equation, which is analogous to the Michaelis–Menten model, J_{max} is the maximum efflux rate per cell, $K_{M,P\text{-gp}}$ is the dissociation constant of the efflux process, and $C_{free,c}$ is the free drug concentration inside the cells [114]. The concentration of the drug is then modeled using mass balance equations, which describe the amount of paclitaxel inside and outside the cells as a function of time. Using this approach, it was determined that the most important factor influencing the transport process is the extracellular drug concentration, followed by intracellular binding capacity and binding affinity, and finally P-glycoprotein expression. Furthermore, it was also shown that, similar to enzyme kinetics, P-glycoprotein efflux is a saturable process [115]. Pharmacokinetic modeling can also be used to determine which transport process is most relevant for a certain drug and what the rate constants are for a particular process [116].

In Vitro/In Vivo Scaling   Clearance is an important parameter for *in vitro/in vivo* scaling, particularly in drug–drug interaction studies. *In vitro* studies are usually conducted in liver microsomes and several assumptions need to be made for scaling. First, one must assume that liver metabolism is the major route of clearance and that oxidative metabolism is much more significant than other forms of metabolism such as conjugation, hydrolysis, and reduction. Second, one must also assume that the rates of metabolism *in vivo* will be similar to those *in vitro*. The scaling factor is usually a function of the microsomal protein per gram liver and the weight of the liver in comparison to body weight. Livers are usually assumed to have 45–50 mg microsomes/gram liver. If one is to scale up from hepatocyte experiments, 120,000,000 hepatocytes/gram liver could be used as a scaling factor [28, 117]. If one is scaling up from hepatocyte experiments, it is not necessary to assume that oxidative metabolism is dominant since hepatocytes are capable of carrying out the other forms of biotransformation.

One of the challenges of scaling *in vitro* to *in vivo* is estimating the inhibitor concentration, [I]. In a microsomal incubation, [I] can be calculated directly from the experimental conditions. However, *in vivo* it is not clear what the proper [I] is, since the inhibitor concentration at the site of metabolism cannot be calculated from the administered dose. Some estimates of [I] include total inhibitor concentration in the plasma, unbound concentration in the plasma, or concentration at the target organ such as the intrahepatic concentration. So far, no general estimate has been found to correlate *in vitro* [I] to an *in vivo* [I] in every specific case. Complicating factors include intestinal metabolism, transporters, and flow-dependent clearance. In general, the larger the IC_{50} values, the less potent the inhibitor and the less likely that a clinically significant interaction will occur. Conversely, small IC_{50} values usually indicate a high likelihood of a clinical interaction. Large IC_{50} values are considered to be those higher than 100 μM, while small ones are usually less than 1 μM. The challenge is to interpret "intermediate" values of IC_{50}. Calculating $[I]/K_i$ can also be helpful in determining the likelihood of an *in vivo* interaction. The larger the ratio the more likely the possibility of an interaction. If the ratio is less than 0.5, the interaction is unlikely; but if $[I]/K_i$ is higher than 5, a clinically significant interaction is probable [109, 118].

25.1.5   Conclusions

Drug–drug interactions can occur through multiple pathways, where the perpetrator drug can influence the absorption, distribution, metabolism, and elimination of the victim drug. Based on empirical data, the most common interactions occur through the inhibition or induction of the cytochrome P450s and the efflux transporter P-glycoprotein. Clinically significant drug interactions can lead to an increase in systemic blood concentrations (possibly causing toxicity), or a decrease in the plasma concentrations (corresponding to lack of efficacy). The success of combination HIV protease inhibitors illustrates the principle of pharmacoenhancement, where the combined formulation of two drugs is designed such that one drug improves the efficacy of the second drug. This improvement usually occurs by increasing the AUC, C_{max}, or the half-life of the boosted drug, thus increasing the overall systemic exposure to the compound. In this section we have also discussed the pharmacokinetic principles of drug–drug interactions as well as the challenges associated with predicting *in vivo* interactions from *in vitro* data. It is clear that it is currently very difficult to make clinically significant predictions based on *in vitro* data, even with the use of mathematical modeling. In Case Study A, we discuss the pharmacokinetics of benzodiazepines, particularly triazolam. We show several aspects of drug interactions with benzodiazepines, including *in vitro* and *in vivo* studies, prediction of clinical interactions, differences between males and females and different age groups, and also pharmacokinetic/pharmacodynamic integration. As is clear from the discussion so far, over-the-counter preparations (including herbal supplements) and foods can significantly contribute to drug–drug interactions. In Case Study B, we review the most commonly used herbs, mechanisms of drug interactions, and reports of clinically significant adverse events.

25.2   CASE STUDY A: DRUG–DRUG INTERACTIONS WITH TRIAZOLAM AND OTHER BENZODIAZEPINES

25.2.1   Introduction

Among the most commonly prescribed benzodiazepines are triazolam, midazolam, lorazepam, diazepam, and alprazolam. Triazolam, a short half-life triazolobenzodiazepine, is now one of the accepted clinical probes for monitoring CYP3A activity in human studies as it is metabolized primarily by CYP3A [119]. Since triazolam is a hypnotic, it has also been useful for pharmacodynamic experiments. The purpose of this case study is to review the series of *in vitro* and *in vivo* experiments that explored the pharmacokinetics and pharmacodynamics of triazolam and related benzodiazepines in the presence of other drugs, particularly CYP3A inhibitors. This case study also discusses (1) contributions from different CYP3A isoforms, (2) hepatic versus intestinal CYP3A, (3) effects of benzodiazepines in young versus elderly individuals, and (4) pharmacokinetic/pharmacodynamic integration.

25.2.2   Metabolic Interactions

Triazolam is metabolized primarily by CYP3A4 and it forms the α-hydroxy and 4-hydroxy metabolites [120]. These compounds have less activity than triazolam and are further conjugated to the glucuronide metabolites [121]. Triazolam metabolism is known to be inhibited by several classes of CYP3A inhibitors such as macrolide antibiotics [122], azole antifungal agents [123], and some SSRI antidepressants [124].

On the other hand, drugs that induce CYP3A would be expected to impair the effectiveness of triazolam. Coadministration of rifampin, an inducer of CYP3A4, greatly reduces the pharmacodynamic effects of triazolam [125]. Coadministration of triazolam with ritonavir poses an interesting clinical dilemma because ritonavir has been shown to concurrently induce and inhibit CYP3A [126]. During short-term administration, ritonavir inhibits the clearance the triazolam, but during long-term dosage the net effect of the coadministration is not easily predicted [111].

25.2.3   *In Vitro* Studies

The metabolism of triazolam was examined *in vitro* in human liver microsomes in the presence of several CYP3A inhibitors including ketoconazole, erythromycin, and several types of SSRIs in order to assess the likelihood of a clinical interaction [33]. Without inhibition, the V_{max} and K_M values for the formation of the 4-OH metabolite were 10.3 nM/min/mg of protein and 304 μM. For the α-OH pathways, these values were 2.4 nM/min/mg and 74 μM, respectively [124]. However, the V_{max}/K_M ratios were the same for both metabolites, suggesting that each pathway contributes equally to clearance.

Ketoconazole was found to be the most potent inhibitor with a K_i of 0.006 μM for the α-OH metabolite and 0.023 for the 4-OH metabolite. The weakest inhibitor was erythromycin with K_i values of 36.6 μM and 111 μM for the α-OH and 4-OH pathways, respectively. Several SSRIs were also inhibitors of CYP3A, including fluoxetine, norfluoxetine, and sertraline.

The metabolism of midazolam was also examined *in vitro* in the presence of SSRIs and azole antifungal agents [127]. Midazolam also forms the α-OH and 4-OH metabolites, and without inhibition the formation of the α-OH metabolite was a higher affinity process ($K_M = 3.3$ μM) than the formation of the 4-OH metabolite ($K_M = 57$ μM). Based on the V_{max}/K_M ratios, it was estimated that α-OH accounted for 95% of intrinsic clearance. Competitive inhibition constants (K_i) versus the formation of the α-OH metabolite for the antifungal agents ketoconazole, itraconazole, and fluconazole were 0.0037 μM, 0.27 μM, and 1.27 μM, respectively. The K_i values for the α-OH pathway for fluoxetine and its metabolite norfluoxetine were 11.5 μM and 1.44 μM, respectively, which was consistent with previous clinical findings, which suggested that fluoxetine impairs the clearance of CYP3A substrates. Furthermore, these results suggest that most of the inhibition is due to the metabolite norfluoxetine rather than the parent compound fluoxetine.

The CYP3A family is thought to consist of at least three isoforms—CYP3A4, CYP3A5, and CYP3A7. While CYP3A4 is considered to be the dominant isoform, CYP3A5 has been detected in 10–25% of adult livers [128] and CYP3A7 is thought to be present in up to 50% of adult livers, particularly from African-Americans [129–131]. The metabolism of both triazolam and midazolam, as well as testosterone and nifedipine, was examined in human liver microsomes and recombinant CYP3A4 and CYP3A5 to investigate the contribution of each isoform in the metabolism of these drugs [132]. Overall, CYP3A4 contributed more than CYP3A5 in the metabolism of all the compounds. Ketoconazole significantly inhibited metabolism in microsomes and recombinant CYP3A4. The inhibition for CYP3A5 was 5–19-fold less than for CYP3A4 for all substrates, suggesting that CYP3A5 might not be as significant as CYP3A4 in drug interactions with ketoconazole. Although there seems to be a significant interindividual variability in CYP3A5 content, with some samples having up to 25% as much CYP3A5 as CYP3A4, the overall net contribution is probably dominated by CYP3A4.

25.2.4 Pharmacokinetic Clinical Studies

It is important to note that clinically significant drug–drug interactions are not very common and, most frequently, coadministration of two drugs results in no change in the pharmacokinetic or pharmacodynamic profile of either drug. Occasionally, there is a change in the kinetic profile but it is only rarely large enough to be clinically significant [133].

Inhibition of triazolam metabolism by ketoconazole was confirmed in clinical trials where a 200 mg dose of ketoconazole reduced the oral clearance of 0.125 mg triazolam ninefold and prolonged half-life fourfold [124]. This degree of inhibition was correctly predicted by an *in vitro–in vivo* scaling model, which assumed competitive inhibition:

$$\text{Fractional decrement} = \frac{I}{I + K_i(1 + S/K_M)}$$

If S is much less than K_M, this equation can be approximated as

$$\text{Fractional decrement} = \frac{I}{I + K_i}$$

This equation holds true in the case of noncompetitive inhibition regardless of the substrate concentration [124].

Triazolam is a relatively high extraction drug, metabolized primarily by CYP3A4, with oral bioavailability around 50%. The plasma levels of high extraction drugs are expected to be influenced significantly when combined with inhibitors of the key metabolic enzymes. Figure 25.2 shows the pharmacokinetic and pharmacodynamic profiles of triazolam when the drug was coadministered with ketoconazole. After coadministration, there was a 10-fold decrease in the clearance of triazolam, which was accompanied by a drop in the pharmacodynamic marker, the digit-symbol-substitution test (DSST). On the other hand, alprazolam is a low extraction drug (also metabolized by CYP3A4) with a bioavailability of 90%. After coadministration with ketoconazole, its clearance was only reduced threefold, in contrast to the 10-fold decrease observed with triazolam [134].

The expression of hepatic and intestinal CYP3A are influenced by different environmental factors and thus their contributions to the metabolism of drugs need to be distinguished. For example, 6,7-dihydroxybergamottin, a component in grapefruit juice, primarily inhibits intestinal CYP3A and is thus only expected to interfere with drugs whose metabolism is primarily carried out by enteric CYP3A. In order to distinguish between the contributions of hepatic and intestinal metabolism, a drug is usually administered in two separate trials: once orally, when the drug undergoes both hepatic and intestinal metabolism, and then intravenously when the contribution from intestinal metabolism is considered negligible. Midazolam is also one

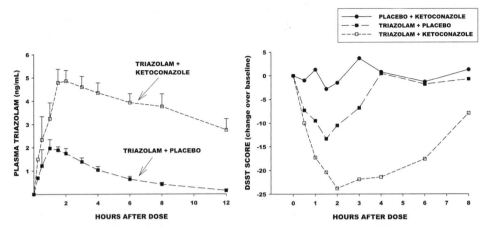

FIGURE 25.2   Pharmacokinetic and pharmacodynamic interactions between triazolam and ketoconazole. Healthy male volunteers received 0.25 mg triazolam and 200 mg ketoconazole or placebos orally. The diagram on the left shows the mean (+SE) plasma concentration of triazolam (ng/mL) with and without ketoconazole. The diagram on the right illustrates the results of the digit-symbol-substitution test (DSST) under the three conditions listed [134].

of the accepted CYP3A clinical probes and its metabolism was studied in the presence of ketoconazole to determine contributions from intestinal and hepatic CYP3A [129]. After ketoconazole administration the AUC of intravenous midazolam increased fivefold, whereas after oral administration it increased 16-fold. The bioavailability of the intestinal component also increased more significantly than the hepatic component after ketoconazole therapy. These results suggest that intestinal CYP3A contributes significantly to midazolam clearance after oral dosage. Interestingly, females had a higher clearance of midazolam than males. Most other studies with benzodiazepines found no statistically significant difference between males and females, although females in general have higher clearances than males, possibly because females have increased enteric CYP3A [135]. However, the sample size in this study was small (three females and six males), thus larger studies would be needed to confirm a difference.

On the other hand, the clearance of CYP3A substrates is found to decrease with age, particularly in men, possibly due to decreases in hepatic and renal clearance [136]. A clinical trial with triazolam showed that elderly women (over 60 years of age) had a small increase in AUC and a decrease in clearance compared with younger women (20–36 years of age) but these differences were not statistically significant. However, in elderly men the AUC values were 75% higher and clearances were 28% lower than in younger men (Fig. 25.3) [137]. These findings concur with previous research, which suggested that age-related decrease in clearance of CYP3A substrates might be more significant in men.

25.2.5   Pharmacokinetic/Pharmacodynamic Integration

The goal of pharmacokinetic/pharmacodynamic (PK/PD) studies is to correlate changes in the plasma levels of drugs with observed pharmacodynamic effects. In

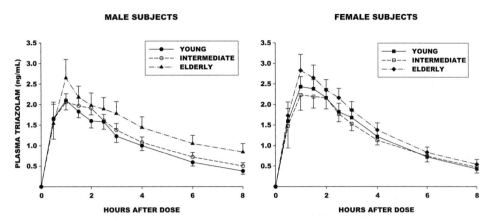

FIGURE 25.3   Mean (±SE) plasma triazolam levels (ng/mL) for male and female volunteers in different age groups after administration of 0.25 mg triazolam. The age groups were young (20–36 years old), intermediate (40–56 years old), and elderly (60–75 years old) [137].

the previous section we discussed that the pharmacokinetics of triazolam were more affected than the pharmacokinetics of alprazolam. Pharmacodynamic studies consisting of electroencephalographic (EEG) beta activity and the digit-symbol-substitution test (DDST) also showed a similar pattern. For alprazolam, ketoconazole increased EEG and DSST by factors of 1.35 and 2.29, respectively, whereas these numbers increased by factors of 2.51 and 4.33, respectively, for triazolam [134]. Thus, the consequences of coadministering a high extraction compound such as triazolam with a CYP3A inhibitor could be clinically more important than administering the CYP3A inhibitor with a low extraction drug such as alprazolam.

The pharmacodynamics of triazolam in elderly volunteers followed a pattern similar to the pharmacokinetics. Probably due to decreased clearance, elderly subjects experienced more pronounced pharmacodynamic effects such as sedation and impairment of motor coordination [137–139]. For example, the values for percent decrement in the DSST after triazolam administration were −5.9 ± 1.9 and −8.6 ± 1.9 in young and elderly women, respectively (Fig. 25.4) [137]. These values in young and elderly men were −5.4 ± 2 and −11.4 ± 2, respectively. It was of note that self-rated sedation actually decreased in elderly subjects after triazolam administration despite an increase in the observer-rated sedation and a decrease in the percent beta amplitude. It is possible that elderly subjects were not aware of their sedation or their reporting did not match with their true sedation levels. Thus, prescribing benzodiazepines for the elderly could be a concern if they are not fully aware of their sedation or cannot report the effects of these drugs.

Another concern with an elderly population is the increase in the likelihood of drug interactions within multidrug regimens. Steroid hormones, such as progesterone, have been known to exert effects on the central nervous system [140]. Thus, the pharmacodynamic interaction between triazolam and progesterone has been investigated in postmenopausal women, since this population previously was likely to be concurrently taking both drugs [141]. In a randomized trial, one group received intravenous triazolam plus oral progesterone (300 mg) or intravenous triazolam plus oral placebo. The pharmacokinetic parameters such as AUC were similar between

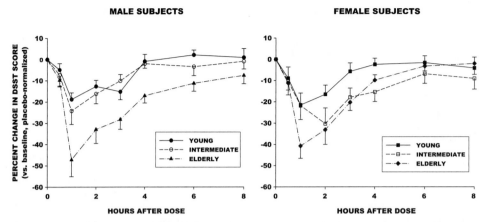

FIGURE 25.4   Percent change (±SE) in digit-symbol-substitution test (DSST) scores for male and female volunteers in different age groups after administration of 0.25 mg triazolam. The age groups were young (20–36 years old), intermediate (40–56 years old), and elderly (60–75 years old) [137].

both groups but pharmacodynamic testing showed that progesterone potentiated the sedative effects of triazolam, suggesting that women taking progesterone might have an increased sensitivity to triazolam or other benzodiazepines. The pharmaco-dynamic effects of progesterone are attributed to a metabolite 3α-hydroxy-5α-dihydroprogesterone, which modulates the GABA receptor complex and regulates brain excitability [141, 142].

Pharmacodynamic effects are influenced not only by plasma levels but also by the concentration of drug in the brain and the binding of the drug to its receptor. Interestingly, the pharmacodynamic effects of triazolam in the presence of ketocon-azole are less potent than expected based on plasma levels. Thus, the effects of ketoconazole on triazolam receptor binding were investigated in mice who received 50 mg/kg ketoconazole and 0.1–0.3 mg/kg of triazolam [143]. Ketoconazole was found in the brains at 31% of the plasma levels and its coadministration also increased triazolam levels in the brain compared to controls. *In vitro* binding studies also demonstrated that ketoconazole inhibits triazolam displacement of [³H]flunitrazepam binding by 36–89% depending on ketoconazole concentration. Thus, these data suggest that, in addition to inhibiting CYP3A metabolism, keto-conazole also interferes with triazolam binding in the brain and could impair its pharmacodynamic effects.

The efflux transporter P-glycoprotein, or MDR1, has been shown to be involved in drug disposition in many organs including the liver, kidney, intestines, and brain. As an efflux transporter, MDR1 can limit the transport of drugs into epithelial cells and enhance the excretion of drugs from hepatocytes and renal tubules [144]. The role of P-glycoprotein is especially critical in the blood–brain barrier, where the endothelial cells lining the blood vessels are joined so closely together that only lipophilic drugs can enter via passive diffusion [63]. Since triazolam needs to cross the blood–brain barrier to reach its receptor, one of the questions is whether efflux transport by P-glycoprotein influences the disposition of triazolam in the brain. The effect of P-glycoprotein on triazolam distribution was investigated by comparing brain levels of ketoconazole and triazolam in P-glycoprotein-deficient mice and matched controls [145]. Interestingly, triazolam levels were the same in both mouse types, but P-glycoprotein-deficient mice had higher levels of ketoconazole. Coadministration of the two drugs did not alter their levels in the brain. Thus, while triazolam is not a P-glycoprotein substrate in the blood–brain barrier, ketoconazole may be transported by P-glycoprotein.

25.2.6   Conclusions

We have discussed the methods for investigating different aspects of drug–drug interactions. An initial estimate of clinical significance comes from *in vitro* studies with microsomes, which can be later confirmed with clinical trials. In order to differentiate between enteric and hepatic metabolism it is necessary to administer a drug in clinical trials orally and intravenously and compare the clearances from each administration. *In vitro* studies have also shown that, among the CYP3A isoforms, CYP3A4 is probably an important contributor to the metabolism of benzodiazepines. It is also important to specify the study population in clinical trials. As we have shown, there are significant differences between age groups, both in terms of clearance of benzodiazepines and in their pharmacodynamic responses to the drugs. The elderly seem particularly susceptible to the sedative effects of benzodiazepines. This effect may be partially due to lower hepatic clearance. However, the concentration–effect relationship was also more pronounced in the elderly, suggesting that the same concentration produces a more significant effect than in younger volunteers. While a substantial difference between males and females could not be consistently demonstrated in benzodiazepine trials, CYP3A is known to be influenced by the hormonal environment. Thus, sex differences should also be considered as variables in human studies.

25.3   CASE STUDY B: DRUG INTERACTIONS WITH HERBS AND NATURAL FOOD PRODUCTS

25.3.1   Introduction

The consumption of herbal supplements is increasing among both adults and children. Although estimates of the percentage of adults using herbals varies depending on survey methods (ranging from 12% to over 50%), the sales of herbals have been increasing about 25% a year with the approximate yearly sales now being over 4 billion dollars [146]. Herbal usage has become especially common among chronically ill patients, including cancer and HIV patients, who are on multidrug regimens and have an increased risk of drug–herbal interactions. There have also been reports of as many as 45% of adults giving their children herbal supplements as well as 45% of pregnant women consuming herbals [147, 148].

Increased consumption of herbals is a concern for drug manufacturers since the FDA requires proper labeling of pharmaceuticals regarding possible adverse interactions. For example, the consumption of grapefruit juice is contraindicated on the labeling of several drugs, such as lovastatin, atorvastatin, and cyclosporine. Grapefruit juice is also reported to interact with other pharmaceuticals including calcium channel antagonists, sedatives, and HIV protease inhibitors [149]. The FDA is very aware of clinically significant interactions with herbs and natural food products. In February of 2000 the FDA issued a warning after clinical trials showed a substantial decrease in the plasma levels of indinavir when combined with St. John's wort. The FDA also warned against coadministration of St. John's wort with all other nonnucleoside reverse transcriptase protease, inhibitors, such as nevirapine [147, 150].

While herbs consist of chemical compounds just like pharmaceuticals, it is challenging to conduct a systematic investigation of potential herb–drug interactions because (1) herbs are regulated differently than pharmaceuticals, (2) they consist of several (sometimes over 100) active ingredients, and (3) there are many different preparations and batch-to-batch variations. Many reports of herb–drug interactions originate primarily from case studies rather than controlled trial studies, therefore cause–effect relationships are difficult to prove [151]. In this section we discuss the regulation of herbal products, mechanisms of drug–herb interactions, and clinically significant adverse events.

25.3.2 Regulation of Herbal Supplements

Herbs are considered dietary supplements and are regulated in the United States by the Dietary Supplement Health and Education Act of 1994. This legislation is significantly more lenient than European and Japanese regulations, which treat herbal products the same way as pharmaceuticals [152]. Herbal product manufacturers are allowed to make claims on the function of herbs without proof regarding safety and efficacy; however, they must also state that these statements have not been evaluated by the FDA. Under the Dietary Supplement Health and Education Act, the herb manufacturers are responsible for monitoring the safety of herbal products [153] but the safety guidelines are not well established. Surprisingly, according to surveys almost 60% of adults believe that herbs need approval before being sold [152]. However, manufacturers of herbal and dietary supplements do not need to report adverse events to the FDA, and the FDA needs to prove that supplements are unsafe before they can be removed from the market [154].

Commercially available herbal preparations vary substantially in their compositions and frequently their labeling does not reflect their true compositions. Thin-layer chromatographic analysis of 59 commercial echinacea preparations showed that the labeling was consistent with the content in only 31 samples and 6 samples contained no echinacea at all [155]. Another study with ginseng products showed that there was a 15–200-fold variation in the concentration of ginsenosides and eleutherosides, which are considered the biologically active ingredients [146, 156].

The most commonly used herbs in the United States are echninacea, garlic, *Ginkgo biloba*, saw palmetto, ginseng, grape seed extract, green tea, St. John's wort, bilberry, and aloe [146]. In order to illustrate the major concepts regarding herbal and food–drug interactions, this case study discusses primarily St. John's wort, *Ginkgo biloba*, garlic, and echinacea.

25.3.3 Influence of Herbal Constituents on Drug Metabolism *In Vitro*

Herbs are complex mixtures of chemicals such as flavonoids, polyphenols, alkaloids, triterpenoids, and anthraquinones—all of which have been shown to modulate CYP450 activity *in vitro* [157]. As will be discussed, multiple components may induce or inhibit an enzyme, but frequently they do not lead to clinically significant interactions.

Hyperforin and hypericin are the two components in St. John's wort believed to be responsible for the antidepressant effects. However, the inhibition and induction capacities of St. John's wort are attributed primarily to hyperforin [158]. *In vitro* studies with cDNA-expressed cytochrome P450 enzyme systems showed that hyperforin is a significant inhibitor of CYP1A2, CYP2C9, CYP2C19, and CYP3A4 with IC_{50} values of 3.87, 0.01, 0.02, and 4.20 μM, respectively. In general, potent inhibitors are considered those with IC_{50} values less than 10 μM [159], although clinically significant interactions are expected when the IC_{50} values are less than 1 μM. Hyperforin also induces intestinal P-glycoprotein in isolated cells [160] and volunteers [161]. This effect is also thought to be mediated by the binding of hyperforin to the pregnane X receptor (PXR) inducing CYP2B6, CYP3A4, and P-glycoprotein [147, 162, 163]. Other herbal inhibitors of P-glycoprotein include ginsenosides, piperine, sylmarin, and catechins from green tea [164].

Consumption of garlic is thought to be beneficial for many health conditions including atherosclerosis and peptic ulcer disease and as a chemopreventative agent for gastric tumors [165]. However, extracts from garlic, in particular, the volatile components, diallyl sulfide, dipropyl sulfide, and dipropyl disulfide, have been shown to interact with a number of CYP450s *in vitro* [166, 167]. CYP2C9, CYP2C19, CYP3A4, CYP3A5, CYP3A7, and CYP2E1 were shown to be inhibited, whereas CYP1A2, CYP2B, and CYP3A were induced [168–170]. Interestingly, garlic seemed to have little effect on CYP2D6 activity (less than 10% inhibition). In the study by Foster et al. [169], modulation of CYP450 was compared across several garlic preparations, specifically garlic oil, odorless garlic preparations, freeze-dried garlic tablets, and three types of garlic bulbs (common, elephant, and Chinese). CYP3A4 was significantly inhibited by all of the products and in the case of the tablets inhibition was over 95%. Inhibition of three CYP3A isoforms (CYP3A4, CYP3A5, CYP3A7) was also compared by the three types of garlic bulbs. All of the isoforms were inhibited, but CYP3A4 was affected the most with inhibition ranging from almost 40% to over 58%. Interestingly, these garlic preparations had little effect on P-glycoprotein compared with verapamil, the positive control [169].

An investigation of 29 constituents of *Ginkgo biloba* revealed inhibitory potential for all of the five major cytochrome P450s (CYP1A2, CYP2C9, CYP2C19, CYP2D6, and CYP3A) in human liver microsomes [171]. Quercetin and amentoflavone inhibited three or more isoforms and nine constituents inhibited CYP3A. The mean IC_{50} values ranged from 0.035 to over 100 μM, although most of the values were between 1 and 30 μM. In cDNA-expressed cytochrome P450 enzyme systems (CYP1A2, CYP2C9, CYP2C19, CYP2D6, and CYP3A4), ginkgolic acids I and II inhibited CYP1A2, CYP2C9, CYP2C19, CYP2D6, and CYP3A4 with the IC_{50} values being 4–5 μM for CYP1A2 and CYP2C19, around 2 μM for CYP2C9, 7–11 μM for CYP2D6, and 6–7 for CYP3A4 [159]. Interestingly, *Ginkgo biloba* increased clearance of the calcium channel blocker nicardipine in rats, suggesting induction of CYP3A2 [172]. Overall, *Ginkgo biloba* increased the expression of CYP2B1/2 and CYP3A1/2 in rats but did not affect CYP1A1/2, CYP2C11, or CYP4A1 [172, 173].

While *Ginkgo biloba* modulated CYP3A *in vitro* and in animal studies, there are few controlled clinical case studies suggesting herb–drug interactions through enzyme modulation by *Ginkgo biloba* [166, 174]. It must be noted that the absence of evidence for clinically significant CYP3A4 inhibition in humans does not necessarily mean that such an interaction could not occur. *In vitro* studies have demonstrated potent inhibition of this enzyme and conflicting findings on *Ginkgo biloba* in clinical trials could be due to variations in *Ginkgo biloba* preparations [175].

25.3.4 Clinically Significant Drug Interactions

While many of these investigations have been successful at identifying drug-inducing or drug-inhibiting components, many *in vitro* studies did not correctly predict clinically significant interactions [166]. As mentioned in Case Study A, clinically significant drug interactions are relatively rare and occur primarily when the therapeutic index is very narrow or if the perpetrator is a very significant modulator of a metabolic enzyme. Table 25.3 shows representative examples of clinically significant drug–herb interactions.

Warfarin, an example of a drug with a narrow therapeutic index, is metabolized almost exclusively by CYP2C9 [176]. In a small clinical study, American ginseng has been shown to cause a slight but statistically significant decrease in the AUC of warfarin as well as the INR (International Normalized Ratio, a number used to characterize blood clotting) of patients, suggesting that ginseng could decrease the efficacy of warfarin. *Ginkgo biloba* contains several inhibitors of CYP2C9, the most potent being amentoflavone with an IC_{50} around $0.035\,\mu M$ [171]. Several anectodal case reports suggested potentiation of warfarin coagulation by *Ginkgo biloba*; this phenomenon could not be demonstrated in controlled clinical trials [22, 177].

Herb–drug interactions are a particular concern for the elderly since they (1) are usually on multidrug regimens, increasing the likelihood of interactions, and (2) have decreased hepatic and renal clearance compared to a younger population [178]. Clinical studies with hyperforin in healthy elderly volunteers (60–76 years) showed a 140% induction of CYP3A4 compared to a 98% induction in young volunteers, despite the fact that the young volunteers were administered 2.5 times the dose of the elderly. Interestingly, the serum concentrations were also similar (42.6 ng/mL in

TABLE 25.3 Clinically Significant Interactions Between Herbs and Prescription Drugs

Herb/Food Product	Clinical Interaction	Potential Mechanism
St. John's wort	Digoxin [181]	Induction of P-gp
	Simvastatin [182], alprazolam, midazolam [180, 185]	Induction of CYP3A4
	Amitriptyline [183], indinavir [186], nevirapine [187]	Induction of CYP3A4 and P-gp
	Buspirone [184]	Inhibition of serotonin reuptake
Echinacea	Midazolam [188]	Induction of CYP3A4
	Caffeine [188]	Induction CYP 1A2
Garlic	Ritonavir [191], saquinavir [192]	Induction of transporter, not necessarily P-gp [169]
	Warfarin [195]	Enhancement of anticoagulation
Ginko biloba	Aspirin, warfarin [196], ibupofen [197], rofecoxib [147, 198]	Enhancement of anticoagulation

young vs. 51.2 ng/mL in old) [179]. This data suggests that the elderly are particularly susceptible to the inductive effects of hyperforin on CYP3A4 activity.

The antidepressant effect of St. John's wort has been confirmed in clinical trials [164] and is attributed partially to hyperforin, which inhibits the uptake of neurotransmitters in synapses. However, St. John's wort has been linked to many clinically significant and even potentially fatal drug interactions. Long-term (2 weeks) St. John's wort administration has been shown to induce both intestinal and hepatic CYP3A4 [147, 180]. St. John's wort has been reported to interact with protease inhibitors, oral contraceptives, and anticoagulants, as well as cyclosporine, digoxin, amitryptiline, and theophylline. Effects of these interactions included organ rejection (with cyclosporine), unplanned pregnancies and intermenstrual bleeding (with contraceptives), and decreases in the efficacies of antiretrovirals and anticoagulants [158].

In a clinical study, St. John's wort was also shown to decrease plasma levels of digoxin, probably through the induction of P-glycoprotein [181]. Clinical studies also reported decreased plasma concentration of simvastatin but not pravastatin when combined with St. John's wort [182]. Due to hyperforin's ability to inhibit the reuptake of brain neurotransmitters, such as serotonin, St. John's wort can also interact with antidepressants and anxiolytic drugs. In clinical studies, St. John's wort decreased the plasma and urine concentrations of the tricyclic antidepressant amitriptyline, presumably through the induction of P-glycoprotein and CYP3A4 [183]. In a reported case study, a patient experienced serotonin syndrome after combining St. John's wort with the anxiolytic drug buspirone, which is a 5-HT1 receptor agonist [184]. In multiple clinical studies, the plasma levels of the CYP3A4 probes alprazolam and midazolam were decreased after treatment with St. John's wort [180, 185]. The plasma concentrations of the antiretroviral drugs indinavir [186] and nevirapine [187] were also reduced when the drugs were combined with St. John's wort. Such an interaction could have serious implications, including reduced treatment efficacy and drug resistance [147].

Echinacea represents 10% of the U.S. herb market and is commonly used for immune system stimulation [155]. Echinacea is also known to modulate CYP3A4 and in human studies it was observed to induce hepatic CYP3A4 but inhibit intestinal CYP3A4 [188]. Specifically, echinacea increased the systemic but not the oral clearance of midazolam by 34%. Increase in systemic clearance is probably due to induction of CYP3A4 (since in this case the contribution of intestinal CYP3A4 is considered negligible) whereas with oral clearance, hepatic induction might be counteracted with intestinal inhibition of CYP3A4. Echinacea also reduced the oral clearance of caffeine (CYP1A2 substrate) and tolbutamide (CYP2C9 substrate), although the latter increase was not statistically significant. The clearance of the CYP2D6 substrate dextromethorphan was not affected. Thus, echinacea would be expected to interact with drugs that are substrates for CYP1A2 and CYP3A4 [188].

Garlic has been cultivated for over 5000 years as a culinary and medicinal herb and it was one of the best-selling herbs in 2002 [175, 189]. In clinical studies garlic did not influence the clearance of caffeine, dextromethorphan, and the CYP3A4 substrate alprazolam [190]. While these clinical studies suggest that garlic does not affect CYP3A4, garlic has been shown to decrease the AUC of ritonavir [191] and saquinavir [192]. Thus, the interaction may occur through a transporter, but not necessarily P-glycoprotein [169]. Garlic did not influence the metabolism of acetaminophen [193], but it did enhance the anticoagulant effects of warfarin, leading to an increase in clotting time [194, 195].

In vitro studies reported that *Ginkgo biloba* is an inhibitor of CYP1A2, CYP2C9, CYP2C19, CYP2D6, and CYP3A4 [171]. Furthermore, several case studies have suggested that this interaction could be of clinical importance; however, this has not been confirmed by clinical studies. In case studies *Ginkgo biloba* has been reported to lead to increased bleeding in patients taking nonsteroidal anti-inflammatory drugs such as aspirin[196], ibuprofen [197], and the cyclo-oxygenase-2 inhibitor rofecoxib [147, 198], and in one case the combination of *Ginkgo biloba* and ibuprofen led to intracerebral bleeding and death [197]. While in a case study *Ginkgo biloba* has been reported to increase the anticoagulant effect of warfarin [196], a randomized clinical trial showed that recommended doses of *Ginkgo biloba* did not affect the pharmacokinetics or pharmacodynamics of warfarin [199].

25.3.5 Conclusions

In vitro and clinical studies have clearly demonstrated the potential for serious and possibly fatal interactions between herbal supplements and prescription medications. In general, the public views these supplements as natural and safe, and more than half of adults believe that herbals need to be approved before reaching the market. With the FDA becoming increasingly aware of herb–drug interactions and requiring proper labeling (as in the case of grapefruit juice), drug developers need to consider the possibility of coadministration with herbal supplements. While it would be impossible to examine all the possible herb–drug interactions, the *in vitro* effects of most commonly used herbs have been examined. Thus, based on metabolic studies, one could predict which herbs a drug might interact with.

St. John's wort is of particular concern, due to its potent induction of both CYP3A4 and P-glycoprotein. Clinical studies have confirmed that this herb can lead to potent interactions with several prescription drugs such as digoxin, antidepressants, benzodiazepines, and antiretrovirals. In the case of cyclosporine, an interaction could lead to organ rejection and be fatal. Other herbs such as echinacea, garlic, and *Ginkgo biloba* have also been reported to interact with prescription drugs. While these are some of the most commonly used herbs, they are not the only ones suspected of drug interactions. Other herbs such as kava-kava, ginger, ginseng, and green tea have also been reported to lead to adverse effects when coadministered with certain prescription drugs, and further clinical studies are necessary to the assess the effects of these herbs on medications [147].

ACKNOWLEDGMENTS

Supported by Grants AT-003540, AG-017880, and AI-058784 from the United States Department of Health and Human Services.

REFERENCES

1. Pratt C, Brown AM, Rampe D, Mason J, Russell T, Reynolds R, Ahlbrandt R. Cardiovascular safety of fexofenadine HCl. *Clin and Exp Allergy* 1999;29(Suppl 3): 212–216.

2. Jorgensen T, Johansson S, Kennerfalk A, Wallander MA, Svardsudd K. Prescription drug use, diagnoses, and healthcare utilization among the elderly. *Ann Pharmacother* 2001;35:1004–1009.

3. Hanlon JT, Fillenbaum GG, Ruby CM, Gray S, Bohannon A. Epidemiology of over-the-counter drug use in community dwelling elderly: United States perspective. *Drugs Aging* 2001;18:123–131.

4. Nix DE, Di Cicco RA, Miller AK, Boyle DA, Boike SC, Zariffa N, Jorkasky DK, Schentag JJ. The effect of low-dose cimetidine (200 mg twice daily) on the pharmacokinetics of theophylline. *J Clin Pharmacol* 1999;39:855–865.

5. Anantharaju A, Feller A, Chedid A. Aging liver. A review. *Gerontology* 2002;48: 343–353.

6. Blower P, de Wit R, Goodin S, Aapro M. Drug–drug interactions in oncology: Why are they important and can they be minimized? *Crit Rev Oncol/Hematol* 2005;55:117–142.

7. Werneke U, Earl J, Seydel C, Horn O, Crichton P, Fannon D. Potential health risks of complementary alternative medicines in cancer patients. *Br J Cancer* 2004;90:408–413.

8. Greenblatt DJ, von Moltke LL, Harmatz JS, Chen G, Weemhoff JL, Jen C, Kelley CJ, LeDuc BW, Zinny MA. Time course of recovery of cytochrome P450 3A function after single doses of grapefruit juice. *Clin Pharmacol Ther* 2003;74:121–129.

9. Greenblatt DJ, Patki KC, von Moltke LL, Shader RI. Drug interactions with grapefruit juice: an update. *J Clin Psychopharmacol* 2001;21:357–359.

10. Malhotra S, Bailey DG, Paine MF, Watkins PB. Seville orange juice–felodipine interaction: comparison with dilute grapefruit juice and involvement of furocoumarins. *Clin Pharmacol Ther* 2001;69:14–23.

11. Hidaka M, Okumura M, Fujita K, Ogikubo T, Yamasaki K, Iwakiri T, Setoguchi N, Arimori K. Effects of pomegranate juice on human cytochrome P450 3A (CYP3A) and carbamazepine pharmacokinetics in rats. *Drug Metab Dispos* 2005;33:644–648.

12. Hidaka M, Fujita K, Ogikubo T, Yamasaki K, Iwakiri T, Okumura M, Kodama H, Arimori K. Potent inhibition by star fruit of human cytochrome P450 3A (CYP3A) activity. *Drug Metab Dispos* 2004;32:581–583.

13. Martin-Facklam M, Burhenne J, Ding R, Fricker R, Mikus G, Walter-Sack I, Haefeli WE. Dose-dependent increase of saquinavir bioavailability by the pharmaceutic aid Cremophor EL. *Br J Clin Pharmacol* 2002;53:576–581.

14. Tayrouz Y, Ding R, Burhenne J, Riedel KD, Weiss J, Hoppe-Tichy T, Haefeli WE, Mikus G. Pharmacokinetic and pharmaceutic interaction between digoxin and Cremophor RH40. *Clin Pharmacol Ther* 2003;73:397–405.

15. Balayssac D, Authier N, Cayre A, Coudore F. Does inhibition of P-glycoprotein lead to drug–drug interactions? *Toxicol Lett* 2005;156:319–329.

16. Ochs HR, Steinhaus E, Locniskar A, Knüchel M, Greenblatt DJ. Desmethyldiazepam kinetics after intravenous, intramuscular, and oral administration of clorazepate dipotassium. *Klin Wochenschrift* 1982;60:411–415.

17. Venkatakrishnan K, Shader RI, Greenblatt DJ. Concepts and mechanisms of drug disposition and drug interactions. In Ciraulo DA, Shader RI, Greenblatt DJ, Creelman W, Eds. *Drug Interactions in Psychiatry*. Philadelphia: Lippincott Williams & Wilkins; 2005, pp 1–46.

18. Kato R, Ueno K, Imano H, Kawai M, Kuwahara S, Tsuchishita Y, Yonezawa E, Tanaka K. Impairment of ciprofloxacin absorption by calcium polycarbophil. *J Clin Pharmacol* 2002;42:806–811.

19. Greenblatt DJ, Sellers EM, Koch-Weser J. Importance of protein binding for the interpretation of serum or plasma drug concentrations. *J Clin Pharmacol* 1982;22:259–263.

20. MacKichan JJ. Protein binding drug displacement interactions fact or fiction? *Clin Pharmacokinet* 1989;16:65–73.

21. Sansom LN, Evans AM. What is the true clinical significance of plasma protein binding displacement interactions? *Drug Safety* 1995;12:227–233.

22. Greenblatt DJ, von Moltke LL. Interaction of warfarin with drugs, natural substances, and foods. *J Clin Pharmacol* 2005;45:127–132.

23. Benet LZ, Hoener BA. Changes in plasma protein binding have little clinical relevance. *Clin Pharmacol Ther* 2002;71:115–121.

24. O'Reilly RA, Trager WF, Motley CH, Howald W. Stereoselective interaction of phenyl-butazone with [^{12}C/^{13}C]warfarin pseudoracemates in man. *J Clin Invest* 1980;65: 746–753.

25. Banfield C, O'Reilly R, Chan E, Rowland M. Phenylbutazone–warfarin interaction in man: further stereochemical and metabolic considerations. *Br J Clin Pharmacol* 1983;16:669–675.

26. Rolan PE. Plasma protein binding displacement interactions—why are they still regarded as clinically important? *Br J Clin Pharmacol* 1994;37:125–128.

27. Hansen JM, Christensen LK. Drug interactions with oral sulphonylurea hypoglycaemic drugs. *Drugs* 1977;13:24–34.

28. Venkatakrishnan K, von Moltke LL, Obach RS, Greenblatt DJ. Drug metabolism and drug interactions: application and clinical value of *in vitro* models. *Curr Drug Metab* 2003;4:423–459.

29. Williams JA, Hyland R, Jones BC, Smith DA, Hurst S, Goosen TC, Peterkin V, Koup JR, Ball SE. Drug–drug interactions for UDP-glucuronosyltransferase substrates: a pharma-cokinetic explanation for typically observed low exposure (AUC$_i$/AUC) ratios. *Drug Metab Dispos Biol Fate Chem* 2004;32:1201–1208.

30. Spina E, Avenoso A, Campo GM, Caputi AP, Perucca E. Phenobarbital induces the 2-hydroxylation of desipramine. *Ther Drug Monitor* 1996;18:60–64.

31. Ono S, Mihara K, Suzuki A, Kondo T, Yasui-Furukori N, Furukori H, de Vries R, Kaneko S. Significant pharmacokinetic interaction between risperidone and carbamazepine: its relationship with CYP2D6 genotypes. *Psychopharmacology (Berl)* 2002;162:50–54.

32. Parkinson A. Biotransformation of xenobiotics. In Klaassen C, Ed. *Casarett & Doull's Toxicology*. New York: McGraw-Hill; 1996, pp 113–186.

33. von Moltke LL, Greenblatt DJ, Duan SX, Harmatz JS, Shader RI. *In vitro* prediction of the terfenadine–ketoconazole pharmacokinetic interaction. *J Clin Pharmacol* 1994;34: 1222–1227.

34. Holbrook AM, Pereira JA, Labiris R, McDonald H, Douketis JD, Crowther M, Wells PS. Systematic overview of warfarin and its drug and food interactions. *Arch Intern Med* 2005;165:1095–1106.

35. Thummel KE, Wilkinson GR. *In vitro* and *in vivo* drug interactions involving human CYP3A. *Annu Rev Pharmacol Toxicol* 1998;38:389–430.

36. Baciewicz AM, and Baciewicz FA Jr. Ketoconazole and fluconazole drug interactions. *Arch Intern Med* 1993;153:1970–1976.

37. Gillum JG, Israel DS, Polk RE. Pharmacokinetic drug interactions with antimicrobial agents. *Clin Pharmacokinet* 1993;25:450–482.

38. Advani R, Fisher GA, Lum BL, Hausdorff J, Halsey J, Litchman M, Sikic BI. A phase I trial of doxorubicin, paclitaxel, and valspodar (PSC 833), a modulator of multidrug resistance. *Clin Cancer Res* 2001;7:1221–1229.

39. Hughes H, Biehl J, Jones A, Schmidt L. Metabolism of isoniazid in man as related to the occurence of peripheral neuritis. *Am Rev Tuberculosis* 1954;70:266–273.

40. Farkas D, Tannenbaum SR. *In vitro* methods to study chemically-induced hepatotoxicity: a literature review. *Curr Drug Metab* 2005;6:111–125.

41. Davis MP, Homsi J. The importance of cytochrome P450 monooxygenase CYP2D6 in palliative medicine. *Support Care Cancer* 2001;9:442–451.

42. Schwarz UI. Clinical relevance of genetic polymorphisms in the human CYP2C9 gene. *Eur J Clin Invest* 2003;33 (Suppl 2):23–30.

43. Ingelman-Sundberg M. Genetic polymorphisms of cytochrome P450 2D6 (CYP2D6): clinical consequences, evolutionary aspects and functional diversity. *Pharmacogenomics J* 2005;5:6–13.

44. Rettie AE, Jones JP. Clinical and toxicological relevance of CYP2C9: drug–drug interactions and pharmacogenetics. *Annu Rev Pharmacol Toxicol* 2005;45:477–494.

45. Zhou S, Chan E, Lim LY, Boelsterli UA, Li SC, Wang J, Zhang Q, Huang M, Xu A. Therapeutic drugs that behave as mechanism-based inhibitors of cytochrome P450 3A4. *Curr Drug Metab* 2004;5:415–442.

46. Alfaro CA, Piscitelli SC. Drug interactions. In Atkinson AJ, Daniels CE, Dedrick RL, Grudzinskas CV, Markey SP. eds. *Principles of Clinical Pharmacoglogy*. Boston: Academic Press; 2001, pp 167–180.

47. Ma Q, Lu AY. Origins of individual variability in P4501A induction. *Chem Res Toxicol* 2003;16:249–260.

48. Hustert E, Zibat A, Presecan-Siedel E, Eiselt R, Mueller R, Fuss C, Brehm I, Brinkmann U, Eichelbaum M, Wojnowski L, Burk O. Natural protein variants of pregnane X receptor with altered transactivation activity toward CYP3A4. *Drug Metab Dispos Biol Fate Chem* 2001;29:1454–1459.

49. Cao H, Hegele RA. Human aryl hydrocarbon receptor nuclear translocator gene (ARNT) D/N511 polymorphism. *J Hum Genet* 2000;45:92–93.

50. Tang C, Lin JH, Lu AY. Metabolism-based drug–drug interactions: what determines individual variability in cytochrome P450 induction? *Drug Metab Dispos Biol Fate Chem* 2005;33:603–613.

51. Chang TK, Bandiera SM, Chen J. Constitutive androstane receptor and pregnane X receptor gene expression in human liver: interindividual variability and correlation with CYP2B6 mRNA levels. *Drug Metab Dispos Biol Fate Chem* 2003;31:7–10.

52. Kerb R, Aynacioglu AS, Brockmöller J, Schlagenhaufer R, Bauer S, Szekeres T, Hamwi A, Fritzer-Szekeres M, Baumgartner C, Ongen HZ, Guzelbey P, Roots I, Brinkmann U. The predictive value of MDR1, CYP2C9, and CYP2C19 polymorphisms for phenytoin plasma levels. *Pharmacogenomics J* 2001;1:204–210.

53. Kim RB, Leake BF, Choo EF, Dresser GK, Kubba SV, Schwarz UI, Taylor A, Xie HG, McKinsey J, Zhou S, Lan LB, Schuetz JD, Schuetz EG, Wilkinson GR. Identification of functionally variant MDR1 alleles among European Americans and African Americans. *Clin Pharmacol Ther* 2001;70:189–199.

54. Begley DJ. ABC transporters and the blood–brain barrier. *Curr Pharm Design* 2004;10:1295–1312.

55. Chandra P, Brouwer KL. The complexities of hepatic drug transport: current knowledge and emerging concepts. *Pharm Res* 2004;21:719–735.

56. Okamura N, Hirai M, Tanigawara Y, Tanaka K, Yasuhara M, Ueda K, Komano T, Hori R. Digoxin–cyclosporin A interaction: modulation of the multidrug transporter P-glycoprotein in the kidney. *J Pharmacol Exp Ther* 1993;266:1614–1619.

57. Saito T, Zhang ZJ, Tokuriki M, Ohtsubo T, Shibamori Y, Yamamoto T, Saito H. Cyclosporin A inhibits the extrusion pump function of P-glycoprotein in the inner ear of mice treated with vinblastine and doxorubicin. *Brain Res* 2001;901:265–270.

58. Sadeque AJ, Wandel C, He H, Shah S, Wood AJ. Increased drug delivery to the brain by P-glycoprotein inhibition. *Clin Pharmacol Ther* 2000;68:231–237.

59. Schinkel AH, Wagenaar E, Mol CA, van Deemter L. P-glycoprotein in the blood–brain barrier of mice influences the brain penetration and pharmacological activity of many drugs. *J Clin Invest* 1996;97:2517–2524.

60. Hughes CS, Vaden SL, Manaugh CA, Price GS, Hudson LC. Modulation of doxorubicin concentration by cyclosporin A in brain and testicular barrier tissues expressing P-glycoprotein in rats. *J Neuro-Oncol* 1998;37:45–54.

61. Kang W, Weiss M. Influence of P-glycoprotein modulators on cardiac uptake, metabolism, and effects of idarubicin. *Pharm Res* 2001;18:1535–1541.

62. Kramer WG, Reuning RH. Use of area under the curve to estimate absolute bioavailability of digoxin. *J Pharm Sci* 1978;67:141–142.

63. Lin JH. Drug–drug interaction mediated by inhibition and induction of P-glycoprotein. *Adv Drug Deliv Rev* 2003;55:53–81.

64. Lin JH. Human immunodeficiency virus protease inhibitors. From drug design to clinical studies. *Adv Drug Deliv Rev* 1997;27:215–233.

65. Szabo K, Welker E, Bakos E, Müller M, Roninson I, Varadi A, Sarkadi B. Drug-stimulated nucleotide trapping in the human multidrug transporter MDR1. Cooperation of the nucleotide binding domains. *J Biol Chem* 1998;273:10132–10138.

66. Shapiro AB, Ling V. Positively cooperative sites for drug transport by P-glycoprotein with distinct drug specificities. *Eur J Biochem* 1997;250:130–137.

67. Ayesh S, Shao YM, Stein WD. Co-operative, competitive and non-competitive interactions between modulators of P-glycoprotein. *Biochim Biophys Acta* 1996;1316:8–18.

68. Fardel O, Lecureur V, Corlu A, Guillouzo A. P-glycoprotein induction in rat liver epithelial cells in response to acute 3-methylcholanthrene treatment. *Biochem Pharmacol* 1996;51:1427–1436.

69. Fardel O, Morel F, Guillouzo A. P-glycoprotein expression in human, mouse, hamster and rat hepatocytes in primary culture. *Carcinogenesis* 1993;14:781–783.

70. Chin KV, Chauhan SS, Pastan I, Gottesman MM. Regulation of mdr RNA levels in response to cytotoxic drugs in rodent cells. *Cell Growth Differ* 1990;1:361–365.

71. Jette L, Beaulieu E, Leclerc JM, Beliveau R. Cyclosporin A treatment induces over-expression of P-glycoprotein in the kidney and other tissues. *Am J Physiol* 1996; 270:F756–F765.

72. Boffito M, Maitland D, Samarasinghe Y, Pozniak A. The pharmacokinetics of HIV protease inhibitor combinations. *Curr Opin Infect Dis* 2005;18:1–7.

73. van Heeswijk RP, Veldkamp A, Mulder JW, Meenhorst PL, Lange JM, Beijnen JH, Hoetelmans RM. Combination of protease inhibitors for the treatment of HIV-1-infected patients: a review of pharmacokinetics and clinical experience. *Antiviral Ther* 2001;6:201–229.

74. Moyle G. Use of HIV protease inhibitors as pharmacoenhancers. *AIDS Reader* 2001;11:87–98.

75. Cvetkovic RS, Goa KL. Lopinavir/ritonavir: a review of its use in the management of HIV infection. *Drugs* 2003;63:769–802.

76. Scott JD. Simplifying the treatment of HIV infection with ritonavir-boosted protease inhibitors in antiretroviral-experienced patients. *Am J Health-System Pharm* 2005; 62:809–815.

77. Moyle GJ, Back D. Principles and practice of HIV-protease inhibitor pharmacoenhancement. *HIV Med* 2001;2:105–113.

78. Kashuba AD. Drug-drug interactions and the pharmacotherapy of HIV infection. *Topics HIV Med* 2005;13:64–69.

79. von Hentig NH, Mueller A, Haberl A. The ATSAQ-1 cohort study; pharmakinetic interactions of atazanavir (ATV) and saquinavir (SAQ) in a ritonavir (RTV) boosted protease inhibitor regimen. *XV International AIDS Conference*; 2004.

80. de Smet K, Loyer P, Gilot D, Vercruysse A, Rogiers V, Guguen-Guillouzo C. Effects of epidermal growth factor on CYP inducibility by xenobiotics, DNA replication, and caspase activations in collagen I gel sandwich cultures of rat hepatocytes. *Biochem Pharmacol* 2001;61:1293–1303.

81. de Smet K, Beken S, Depreter M, Roels F, Vercruysse A, Rogiers V. Effect of epidermal growth factor in collagen gel cultures of rat hepatocytes. *Toxicol in Vitro* 1999;13: 579–585.

82. Ching KZ, Tenney KA, Chen J, Morgan ET. Suppression of constitutive cytochrome P450 gene expression by epidermal growth factor receptor ligands in cultured rat hepatocytes. *Drug Metab Dispos Biol Fate Chem* 1996;24:542–546.

83. Greuet J, Pichard L, Ourlin JC, Bonfils C, Domergue J, Le Treut P, Maurel P. Effect of cell density and epidermal growth factor on the inducible expression of CYP3A and CYP1A genes in human hepatocytes in primary culture. *Hepatology* 1997;25:1166–1175.

84. LeCluyse EL. Human hepatocyte culture systems for the *in vitro* evaluation of cytochrome P450 expression and regulation. *Eur J Pharm Sci* 2001;13:343–368.

85. Moghe PV, Coger RN, Toner M, Yarmush ML. Cell–cell interactiOns are essential for MaIntenance of hepatocyte FunctiOn In collagen gel but not On Matrigel. *Biotechnol Bioeng* 1997;56:706–711.

86. Moghe PV, Berthiaume F, Ezzell RM, Toner M, Tompkins RG, Yarmush ML. Culture matrix configuration and composition in the maintenance of hepatocyte polarity and function. *Biomaterials* 1996;17:373–385.

87. LeCluyse E, Madan A, Hamilton G, Carroll K, DeHaan R, Parkinson A. Expression and regulation of cytochrome P450 enzymes in primary cultures of human hepatocytes. *J Biochem Mol Toxicol* 2000;14:177–188.

88. Raucy JL. Regulation of CYP3A4 expression in human hepatocytes by pharmaceuticals and natural products. *Drug Metab Dispos* 2003;31:533–539.

89. Mills JB, Rose KA, Sadagopan N, Sahi J, de Morais SM. Induction of drug metabolism enzymes and MDR1 using a novel human hepatocyte cell line. *J Pharmacol Exp Ther* 2004;309:303–309.

90. Biagini CP, Bender V, Borde F, Boissel E, Bonnet MC, Masson MT, Cassio D, Chevalier S. Cytochrome P450 expression-induction profile and chemically mediated alterations of the WIF-B9 cell line. *Biol Cell* 2005;98:23–32.

91. Polli JW, Wring SA, Humphreys JE, Huang L, Morgan JB, Webster LO, Serabjit-Singh CS. Rational use of *in vitro* P-glycoprotein assays in drug discovery. *J Pharmacol Exp Ther* 2001;299:620–628.

92. Tang F, Horie K, Borchardt RT. Are MDCK cells transfected with the human MRP2 gene a good model of the human intestinal mucosa? *Pharm Res* 2002;19:773–779.

93. Taub ME, Podila L, Ely D, Almeida I. Functional assessment of multiple P-glycoprotein (P-gp) probe substrates: influence of cell line and modulator concentration on P-gp activity. *Drug Metab Dispos Biol Fate Chem* 2005;33:1679–1687.

94. Taipalensuu J, Tornblom H, Lindberg G, Einarsson C, Sjoqvist F, Melhus H, Garberg P, Sjostrom B, Lundgren B, Artursson P. Correlation of gene expression of ten drug efflux proteins of the ATP-binding cassette transporter family in normal human jejunum and

in human intestinal epithelial Caco-2 cell monolayers. *J Pharmacol Exp Ther* 2001;299: 164–170.

95. Prime-Chapman HM, Fearn RA, Cooper AE, Moore V, Hirst BH. Differential multidrug resistance-associated protein 1 through 6 isoform expression and function in human intestinal epithelial Caco-2 cells. *J Pharmacol Exp Ther* 2004;311:476–484.

96. Donato MT, Castell JV, Gomez-Lechon MJ. Characterization of drug metabolizing activities in pig hepatocytes for use in bioartificial liver devices: comparison with other hepatic cellular models. *J Hepatol* 1999;31:542–549.

97. Omasa T, Kim K, Hiramatsu S, Katakura Y, Kishimoto M, Enosawa S, Ohtake H. Construction and evaluation of drug-metabolizing cell line for bioartificial liver support system. *Biotechnol Prog* 2005;21:161–167.

98. Iwahori T, Matsuura T, Maehashi H, Sugo K, Saito M, Hosokawa M, Chiba K, Masaki T, Aizaki H, Ohkawa K, Suzuki T. CYP3A4 inducible model for *in vitro* analysis of human drug metabolism using a bioartificial liver. *Hepatology* 2003;37:665–673.

99. Bugrim A, Nikolskaya T, Nikolsky Y. Early prediction of drug metabolism and toxicity: systems biology approach and modeling. *Drug Discov Today* 2004;9:127–135.

100. Korolev D, Balakin KV, Nikolsky Y, Kirillov E, Ivanenkov YA, Savchuk NP, Ivashchenko AA, Nikolskaya T. Modeling of human cytochrome P450-mediated drug metabolism using unsupervised machine learning approach. *J Med Chem* 2003;46:3631–3643.

101. Manga N, Duffy JC, Rowe PH, Cronin MT. Structure-based methods for the prediction of the dominant P450 enzyme in human drug biotransformation: consideration of CYP3A4, CYP2C9, CYP2D6. *SAR QSAR Environ Res* 2005;16:43–61.

102. Jones JP, He M, Trager WF, Rettie AE. Three-dimensional quantitative structure–activity relationship for inhibitors of cytochrome P4502C9. *Drug Metab Dispos Biol Fate Chem* 1996;24:1–6.

103. Bonnabry P, Sievering J, Leemann T, Dayer P. Quantitative drug interactions prediction system (Q-DIPS): a computer-based prediction and management support system for drug metabolism interactions. *Eur J Clin Pharmacol* 1999;55:341–347.

104. Langer T, Eder M, Hoffmann RD, Chiba P, Ecker GF. Lead identification for modulators of multidrug resistance based on *in silico* screening with a pharmacophoric feature model. *Arch Pharm (Weinheim)* 2004;337:317–327.

105. Rebitzer S, Annibali D, Kopp S, Eder M, Langer T, Chiba P, Ecker GF, Noe CR. *In silico* screening with benzofurane- and benzopyrane-type MDR-modulators. *Farmaco* 2003; 58:185–191.

106. Ekins S, Nikolsky Y, Nikolskaya T. Techniques: application of systems biology to absorption, distribution, metabolism, excretion and toxicity. *Trends Pharmacol Sci* 2005; 26:202–209.

107. Segel I. Enzymes. *Biochemical Calculations*. Hoboken, NJ: John Wiley & Sons, 1976; pp 208–323.

108. von Moltke LL, Greenblatt DJ, Grassi JM, Granda BW, Duan SX, Fogelman SM, Daily JP, Harmatz JS, Shader RI. Protease inhibitors as inhibitors of human cytochromes P450: high risk associated with ritonavir. *J Clin Pharmacol* 1998;38:106–111.

109. von Moltke LL, Greenblatt DJ, Schmider J, Wright CE, Harmatz JS, Shader RI. *In vitro* approaches to predicting drug interactions *in vivo*. *Biochem Pharmacol* 1998; 55:113–122.

110. Shou M, Mei Q, Ettore MW Jr, Dai R, Baillie TA, Rushmore TH. Sigmoidal kinetic model for two co-operative substrate-binding sites in a cytochrome P450 3A4 active site: an example of the metabolism of diazepam and its derivatives. *Biochem J* 1999;340 (Pt 3):845–853.

111. Greenblatt DJ, von Moltke LL, Daily JP, Harmatz JS, Shader RI. Extensive impairment of triazolam and alprazolam clearance by short-term low-dose ritonavir: the clinical dilemma of concurrent inhibition and induction. *J Clin Psychopharmacol* 1999;19: 293–296.

112. Obach RS. Inhibition of human cytochrome P450 enzymes by constituents of St. John's wort, an herbal preparation used in the treatment of depression. *J Pharmacol Exp Ther* 2000;294:88–95.

113. Jang SH, Wientjes MG, Au JL. Kinetics of P-glycoprotein-mediated efflux of paclitaxel. *J Pharmacol Exp Ther* 2001;298:1236–1242.

114. Hunter J, Jepson MA, Tsuruo T, Simmons NL, Hirst BH. Functional expression of P-glycoprotein in apical membranes of human intestinal Caco-2 cells. Kinetics of vinblastine secretion and interaction with modulators. *J Biol Chem* 1993;268:14991–14997.

115. Jang SH, Wientjes MG, Au JL. Interdependent effect of P-glycoprotein-mediated drug efflux and intracellular drug binding on intracellular paclitaxel pharmacokinetics: application of computational modeling. *J Pharmacol Exp Ther* 2003;304:773–780.

116. Hoffmaster KA, Zamek-Gliszczynski MJ, Pollack GM, Brouwer KL. Multiple transport systems mediate the hepatic uptake and biliary excretion of the metabolically stable opioid peptide [D-penicillamine2,5]enkephalin. *Drug Metab and Dispos Biol Fate Chem* 2005;33:287–293.

117. Zahlten RN, Stratman FW. The isolation of hormone-sensitive rat hepatocytes by a modified enzymatic technique. *Arch Biochem Biophys* 1974;163:600–608.

118. Bertz RJ, Granneman GR. Use of *in vitro* and *in vivo* data to estimate the likelihood of metabolic pharmacokinetic interactions. *Clin Pharmacokinet* 1997;32:210–258.

119. Greenblatt DJ, von Moltke LL, Harmatz JS, Durol AL, Daily JP, Graf JA, Mertzanis P, Hoffman JL, Shader RI. Differential impairment of triazolam and zolpidem clearance by ritonavir. *J Acquir Immune Defic Syndr* 2000;24:129–136.

120. Kronbach T, Mathys D, Umeno M, Gonzalez FJ, Meyer UA. Oxidation of midazolam and triazolam by human liver cytochrome P450IIIA4. *Mol Pharmacol* 1989;36:89–96.

121. Eberts FS Jr, Philopoulos Y, Reineke LM, Vliek RW. Triazolam disposition. *Clin Pharmacol Ther* 1981;29:81–93.

122. Phillips JP, Antal EJ, Smith RB. A pharmacokinetic drug interaction between erythromycin and triazolam. *J Clin Psychopharmacol* 1986;6:297–299.

123. Varhe A, Olkkola KT, Neuvonen PJ. Oral triazolam is potentially hazardous to patients receiving systemic antimycotics ketoconazole or itraconazole. *Clin Pharmacol Ther* 1994;56:601–607.

124. von Moltke LL, Greenblatt DJ, Harmatz JS, Duan SX, Harrel LM, Cotreau-Bibbo MM, Pritchard GA, Wright CE, Shader RI. Triazolam biotransformation by human liver microsomes *in vitro*: effects of metabolic inhibitors and clinical confirmation of a predicted interaction with ketoconazole. *J Pharmacol Exp Ther* 1996;276:370–379.

125. Villikka K, Kivistö KT, Backman JT, Olkkola KT, Neuvonen PJ. Triazolam is ineffective in patients taking rifampin. *Clin Pharmacol Ther* 1997;61:8–14.

126. Hsu A, Granneman GR, Bertz RJ. Ritonavir. Clinical pharmacokinetics and interactions with other anti-HIV agents. *Clin Pharmacokinet* 1998;35:275–291.

127. von Moltke LL, Greenblatt DJ, Schmider J, Duan SX, Wright CE, Harmatz JS, Shader RI. Midazolam hydroxylation by human liver microsomes *in vitro*: inhibition by fluoxetine, norfluoxetine, and by azole antifungal agents. *J Clin Pharmacol* 1996;36:783–791.

128. Wrighton SA, Ring BJ, Watkins PB, Vandenbranden M. Identification of a polymorphically expressed member of the human cytochrome P-450III family. *Mol Pharmacol* 1989;36:97–105.

129. Tsunoda SM, Velez RL, von Moltke LL, Greenblatt DJ. Differentiation of intestinal and hepatic cytochrome P450 3A activity with use of midazolam as an *in vivo* probe: effect of ketoconazole. *Clin Pharmacol Ther* 1999;66:461–471.

130. Schuetz JD, Beach DL, Guzelian PS. Selective expression of cytochrome P450 CYP3A mRNAs in embryonic and adult human liver. *Pharmacogenetics* 1994;4:11–20.

131. Kuehl P, Zhang J, Lin Y, Lamba J, Assem M, Schuetz J, Watkins PB, Daly A, Wrighton SA, Hall SD, Maurel P, Relling M, Brimer C, Yasuda K, Venkataramanan R, Strom S, Thummel K, Boguski MS, Schuetz E. Sequence diversity in CYP3A promoters and characterization of the genetic basis of polymorphic CYP3A5 expression. *Nat Genet* 2001;27:383–391.

132. Patki KC, von Moltke LL, Greenblatt DJ. *In vitro* metabolism of midazolam, triazolam, nifedipine, and testosterone by human liver microsomes and recombinant cytochromes p450: role of CYP3A4 and CYP3A5. *Drug Metab Dispos Biol Fate Chem* 2003; 31:938–944.

133. Greenblatt DJ, von Moltke LL. Drug–drug interactions: clinical perspective. In Rodrigues AD, ed. *Drug–Drug Interactions*. New York: Marcel Dekker; 2002, pp 565–584.

134. Greenblatt DJ, Wright CE, Von Moltke LL, Harmatz JS, Ehrenberg BL, Harrel LM, Corbett K, Counihan M, Tobias S, Shader RI. Ketoconazole inhibition of triazolam and alprazolam clearance: differential kinetic and dynamic consequences. *Clin Pharmacol Ther* 1998;64:237–247.

135. Gorski JC, Jones DR, Haehner-Daniels BD, Hamman MA, O'Mara EM Jr, Hall SD. The contribution of intestinal and hepatic CYP3A to the interaction between midazolam and clarithromycin. *Clin Pharmacol Ther* 1998;64:133–143.

136. Cotreau MM, von Moltke LL, Greenblatt DJ. The influence of age and sex on the clearance of cytochrome P450 3A substrates. *Clin Pharmacokinet* 2005;44:33–60.

137. Greenblatt DJ, Harmatz JS, von Moltke LL, Wright CE, Shader RI. Age and gender effects on the pharmacokinetics and pharmacodynamics of triazolam, a cytochrome P450 3A substrate. *Clin Pharmacol Ther* 2004;76:467–479.

138. Greenblatt DJ, Divoll M, Abernethy DR, Moschitto LJ, Smith RB, Shader RI. Reduced clearance of triazolam in old age: relation to antipyrine oxidizing capacity. *Br J Clin Pharmacol* 1983;15:303–309.

139. Greenblatt DJ, Harmatz JS, Shapiro L, Engelhardt N, Gouthro TA, Shader RI. Sensitivity to triazolam in the elderly. *N Engl J Med* 1991;324:1691–1698.

140. Callachan H, Cottrell GA, Hather NY, Lambert JJ, Nooney JM, Peters JA. Modulation of the GABAA receptor by progesterone metabolites. *Proc R Soc London Ser B Biol Sci* 1987;231:359–369.

141. McAuley JW, Reynolds IJ, Kroboth FJ, Smith RB, Kroboth PD. Orally administered progesterone enhances sensitivity to triazolam in postmenopausal women. *J Clin Psychopharmacol* 1995;15:3–11.

142. McAuley JW, Kroboth PD, Stiff DD, Reynolds IJ. Modulation of [^{3}H]flunitrazepam binding by natural and synthetic progestational agents. *Pharmacol Biochem Behav* 1993;45:77–83.

143. Fahey JM, Pritchard GA, von Moltke LL, Pratt JS, Grassi JM, Shader RI, Greenblatt DJ. Effects of ketoconazole on triazolam pharmacokinetics, pharmacodynamics and benzodiazepine receptor binding in mice. *J Pharmacol Exp Ther* 1998;285:271–276.

144. Lin JH, Yamazaki M. Role of P-glycoprotein in pharmacokinetics: clinical implications. *Clin Pharmacokinet* 2003;42:59–98.

145. von Moltke LL, Granda BW, Grassi JM, Perloff MD, Vishnuvardhan D, Greenblatt DJ. Interaction of triazolam and ketoconazole in P-glycoprotein-deficient mice. *Drug Metab Dispos Biol Fate Chem* 2004;32:800–804.

146. Bent S, Ko R. Commonly used herbal medicines in the United States: a review. *Am J Med* 2004;116:478–485.

147. Izzo AA. Herb–drug interactions: an overview of the clinical evidence. *Fundam Clin Pharmacol* 2005;19:1–16.

148. Ernst E. Are herbal medicines effective? *Int J Clin Pharmacol Ther* 2004;42:157–159.

149. Greenblatt DJ, Patki KC, von Moltke LL, Shader RI. Drug interactions with grapefruit juice: an update. *J Clin Psychopharmacol* 2001;21:357–359.

150. James, JS. St. John's Warning: Do Not Combine with Protease Inhibitors, NNRTI's. http://www.aids.org/atn/a-337-02.html. 2005.

151. Fugh-Berman A, Ernst E. Herb–drug interactions: review and assessment of report reliability. *Br J Clin Pharmacol* 2001;52:587–595.

152. Lewis JD, Strom BL. Balancing safety of dietary supplements with the free market. *Ann Intern Med* 2002;136:616–618.

153. Dietary Supplement Health Education Act of 1994. http://www.fda.gov/opacom/laws/dshea.html.

154. Dietary Supplements: Questions Answers. US Food Drug Aministration; Center for Food Safety Applied Nutrition; 2001. http://www.cfsan.fda.gov/~dms/ds-faq.html.

155. Gilroy CM, Steiner JF, Byers T, Shapiro H, Georgian W. Echinacea and truth in labeling. *Arch Intern Med* 2003;163:699–704.

156. Harkey MR, Henderson GL, Gershwin ME, Stern JS, Hackman RM. Variability in commercial ginseng products: an analysis of 25 preparations. *Am J Clin Nutr* 2001;73:1101–1106.

157. Zhou S, Gao Y, Jiang W, Huang M, Xu A, Paxton JW. Interactions of herbs with cytochrome P450. *Drug Metab Rev* 2003;35:35–98.

158. Ioannides C. Pharmacokinetic interactions between herbal remedies and medicinal drugs. *Xenobiotica* 2002;32:451–478.

159. Zou L, Harkey MR, Henderson GL. Effects of herbal components on cDNA-expressed cytochrome P450 enzyme catalytic activity. *Life Sci* 2002;71:1579–1589.

160. Perloff MD, von Moltke LL, Stormer E, Shader RI, Greenblatt DJ. Saint John's wort: an *in vitro* analysis of P-glycoprotein induction due to extended exposure. *Br J Pharmacol* 2001;134:1601–1608.

161. Dresser GK, Schwarz UI, Wilkinson GR, Kim RB. Coordinate induction of both cytochrome P4503A and MDR1 by St John's wort in healthy subjects. *Clin Pharmacol Ther* 2003;73:41–50.

162. Moore LB, Goodwin B, Jones SA, Wisely GB, Serabjit-Singh CJ, Willson TM, Collins JL, Kliewer SA. St. John's wort induces hepatic drug metabolism through activation of the pregnane X receptor. *Proc Nat Acad Sci USA* 2000;97:7500–7502.

163. Wentworth JM, Agostini M, Love J, Schwabe JW, Chatterjee VK. St John's wort, a herbal antidepressant, activates the steroid X receptor. *J Endocrinol* 2000;166:R11–R16.

164. Zhou S, Lim LY, Chowbay B. Herbal modulation of P-glycoprotein. *Drug Metab Rev* 2004;36:57–104.

165. Levi F, Pasche C, La Vecchia C, Lucchini F, Franceschi S. Food groups and colorectal cancer risk. *Br J Cancer* 1999;79:1283–1287.

166. Delgoda R, Westlake AC. Herbal interactions involving cytochrome P450 enzymes: a mini review. *Toxicol Rev* 2004;23:239–249.

167. Guyonnet D, Belloir C, Suschetet M, Siess MH, Le Bon AM. Liver subcellular fractions from rats treated by organosulfur compounds from Allium modulate mutagen activation. *Mutat Res* 2000;466:17–26.

168. Wu CC, Sheen LY, Chen HW, Kuo WW, Tsai SJ, Lii CK. Differential effects of garlic oil and its three major organosulfur components on the hepatic detoxification system in rats. *J Agric Food Chem* 2002;50:378–383.

169. Foster BC, Foster MS, Vandenhoek S, Krantis A, Budzinski JW, Arnason JT, Gallicano KD, Choudri S. An *in vitro* evaluation of human cytochrome P450 3A4 and P-glycoprotein inhibition by garlic. *J Pharm Pharm Sci* 2001;4:176–184.

170. Chen HW, Tsai CW, Yang JJ, Liu CT, Kuo WW, Lii CK. The combined effects of garlic oil and fish oil on the hepatic antioxidant and drug-metabolizing enzymes of rats. *Br J Nutr* 2003;89:189–200.

171. von Moltke LL, Weemhoff JL, Bedir E, Khan IA, Harmatz JS, Goldman P, Greenblatt DJ. Inhibition of human cytochromes P450 by components of *Ginkgo biloba*. *J Pharm Pharmacol* 2004;56:1039–1044.

172. Shinozuka K, Umegaki K, Kubota Y, Tanaka N, Mizuno H, Yamauchi J, Nakamura K, Kunitomo M. Feeding of *Ginkgo biloba* extract (GBE) enhances gene expression of hepatic cytochrome P-450 and attenuates the hypotensive effect of nicardipine in rats. *Life Sci* 2002;70:2783–2792.

173. Ginkgo. In LaGow B, Ed. *PDR for Herbal Medicine*. Montvale, NJ: Thomson PDR; 2004, pp. 368–378.

174. Gurley BJ, Gardner SF, Hubbard MA, Williams DK, Gentry WB, Cui Y, Ang CY. Cytochrome P450 phenotypic ratios for predicting herb-drug interactions in humans. *Clin Pharmacol Ther* 2002;72:276–287.

175. Sparreboom A, Cox MC, Acharya MR, Figg WD. Herbal remedies in the United States: potential adverse interactions with anticancer agents. *J Clin Oncol* 2004;22:2489–2503.

176. Yamazaki H, Shimada T. Human liver cytochrome P450 enzymes involved in the 7-hydroxylation of *R*- and *S*-warfarin enantiomers. *Biochem Pharmacol* 1997;54:1195–1203.

177. Engelsen J, Nielsen JD, Winther K. Effect of coenzyme Q10 and *Ginkgo biloba* on warfarin dosage in stable, long-term warfarin treated outpatients. A randomised, double blind, placebo-crossover trial. *Thromb Haemost* 2002;87:1075–1076.

178. Cotreau MM, von Moltke LL, Greenblatt DJ. The influence of age and sex on the clearance of cytochrome P450 3A substrates. *Clin Pharmacokinet* 2005;44:33–60.

179. Gurley BJ, Gardner SF, Hubbard MA, Williams DK, Gentry WB, Cui Y, Ang CY. Clinical assessment of effects of botanical supplementation on cytochrome P450 phenotypes in the elderly: St John's wort, garlic oil, Panax ginseng and *Ginkgo biloba*. *Drugs Agin* 2005;22:525–539.

180. Markowitz JS, Donovan JL, DeVane CL, Taylor RM, Ruan Y, Wang JS, Chavin KD. Effect of St John's wort on drug metabolism by induction of cytochrome P450 3A4 enzyme. *JAMA* 2003;290:1500–1504.

181. Jöhne A, Brockmöller J, Bauer S, Maurer A, Langheinrich M, Roots I. Pharmacokinetic interaction of digoxin with an herbal extract from St. John's wort (*Hypericum perforatum*). *Clin Pharmacol Ther* 1999;66:338–345.

182. Sugimoto K, Ohmori M, Tsuruoka S, Nishiki K, Kawaguchi A, Harada K, Arakawa M, Sakamoto K, Masada M, Miyamori I, Fujimura A. Different effects of St. John's wort on the pharmacokinetics of simvastatin and pravastatin. *Clin Pharmacol Ther* 2001;70:518–524.

183. Jöhne A, Schmider J, Brockmöller J, Stadelmann AM, Störmer E, Bauer S, Scholler G, Langheinrich M, Roots I. Decreased plasma levels of amitriptyline and its metabolites on comedication with an extract from St. John's wort (*Hypericum perforatum*). *J Clin Psychopharmacol* 2002;22:46–54.

184. Dannawi M. Possible serotonin syndrome after combination of buspirone and St John's wort. *J Psychopharmacol* 2002;16:401.

185. Wang Z, Gorski JC, Hamman MA, Huang SM, Lesko LJ, Hall SD. The effects of St John's wort (*Hypericum perforatum*) on human cytochrome P450 activity. *Clin Pharmacol Ther* 2001;70:317–326.

186. Piscitelli SC, Burstein AH, Chaitt D, Alfaro RM, Falloon J. Indinavir concentrations and St John's wort. *Lancet* 2000;355:547–548.

187. de Maat MM, Hoetelmans RM, Matht RA, van Gorp EC, Meenhorst PL, Mulder JW, Beijnen JH. Drug interaction between St John's wort and nevirapine. *AIDS* 2001;15:420–421.

188. Gorski JC, Huang SM, Pinto A, Hamman MA, Hilligoss JK, Zaheer NA, Desai M, Miller M, Hall SD. The effect of Echinacea (*Echinacea purpurea* root) on cytochrome P450 activity *in vivo*. *Clin Pharmacol Ther* 2004;75:89–100.

189. Blumenthal M. Herbs continue slide in mainstream market: sales down 14 percent. *HerbalGram* 2003;58:71.

190. Markowitz JS, DeVane CL, Chavin KD, Taylor RM, Ruan Y, Donovan JL. Effects of garlic (*Allium sativum* L.) supplementation on cytochrome P450 2D6 and 3A4 activity in healthy volunteers. *Clin Pharmacol Ther* 2003;74:170–177.

191. Gallicano K, Foster B, Choudhri S. Effect of short-term administration of garlic supplements on single-dose ritonavir pharmacokinetics in healthy volunteers. *Br J Clin Pharmacol* 2003;55:199–202.

192. Piscitelli SC, Burstein AH, Welden N, Gallicano KD, Falloon J. The effect of garlic supplements on the pharmacokinetics of saquinavir. *Clin Infect Dis* 2002;34:234–238.

193. Gwilt PR, Lear CL, Tempero MA, Birt DD, Grandjean AC, Ruddon RW, Nagel DL. The effect of garlic extract on human metabolism of acetaminophen. *Cancer Epidemiol Biomarkers Prev* 1994;3:155–160.

194. Hu Z, Yang X, Ho PC, Chan SY, Heng PW, Chan E, Duan W, Koh HL, Zhou S. Herb–drug interactions: a literature review. *Drug* 2005;65:1239–1282.

195. Evans V. Herbs and the brain: friend or foe? The effects of ginkgo and garlic on warfarin use. *J Neurosci Nurs* 2000;32:229–232.

196. Matthews MK Jr. Association of *Ginkgo biloba* with intracerebral hemorrhage. *Neurology* 1998;50:1933–1934.

197. Meisel C, Jöhne A, Roots I. Fatal intracerebral mass bleeding associated with *Ginkgo biloba* and ibuprofen. *Atherosclerosis* 2003;167:367.

198. Hoffman T. Ginkgo, Vioxx and excessive bleeding—possible drug–herb interactions: case report. *Hawaii Med J* 2001;60:290.

199. Jiang X, Williams KM, Liauw WS, Ammit AJ, Roufogalis BD, Duke CC, Day RO, McLachlan AJ. Effect of ginkgo and ginger on the pharmacokinetics and pharmacodynamics of warfarin in healthy subjects. *Br J Clin Pharmacol* 2005;59:425–432.

26

SPECIES COMPARISON OF METABOLISM IN MICROSOMES AND HEPATOCYTES

Niels Krebsfaenger

Schwarz Biosciences, Monheim, Germany

Contents

26.1   INTRODUCTION AND GENERAL ASPECTS

Species differences in metabolism may have significant impact on pharmacokinetics and toxicity of drugs. Therefore detailed knowledge of comparative metabolism across species is key for species selection in preclinical safety testing and interpretation of any animal data in respect to relevance for humans.

From the safety perspective, the primary concern is to identify any unique or major human metabolites. Early identification will allow for timely assessment of

Preclinical Development Handbook: ADME and Biopharmaceutical Properties,
edited by Shayne Cox Gad
Copyright © 2008 John Wiley & Sons, Inc.

potential safety issues in the development process and thereby reduce the risk for subjects included in clinical trials as well as for possible delays in the development process.

Since in early drug development animal and human *in vivo* metabolism data are usually lacking, *in vitro* species comparisons provide useful information to support a preliminary species selection for preclinical safety testing and interpretation of animal data.

26.1.1   Relevance of Liver Preparations for Metabolism Studies *In Vitro*

The liver is the major organ for biotransformation of xenobiotics including drugs. The majority of xenobiotic metabolizing enzymes (XMEs) are expressed in the liver and usually their abundance is higher than in other organs or tissues. Several standard methods have been established to investigate hepatic metabolism *in vitro* and there is comprehensive knowledge of their potential and limitations. Therefore, liver preparations such as tissue slices, hepatocytes, or microsomes are valuable and accepted tools for comparative studies on drug metabolism across species *in vitro* (see Section 26.1.5). As orally administered drugs enter first the liver via the portal vein before being distributed in the systemic circulation, and metabolism may have substantial impact on the toxicity of xenobiotics (see Chapter 28 in this volume), hepatotoxicity is a general concern in drug development (see Section 26.1.3). Therefore, toxicity testing in hepatocytes along with metabolism studies may provide additional useful information in early drug development.

However, it should be kept in mind that the liver is not the only metabolically competent organ. For example, cytochrome P450 (CYP) 3A4 is also expressed at high levels in the gut and may substantially contribute to metabolism of drugs even before they enter the liver. CYP1A1 expression is significantly induced in the lung by smoking but there is no such enzymatic activity in the liver, and several prodrugs are cleaved by plasma esterases. Accordingly, *in vitro* metabolism data based on liver preparations alone are not always fully predictive for the situation *in vivo*. Therefore, additional testing using, for example, pulmonary, intestinal, or kidney (microsomal) preparations may be appropriate in specific cases.

26.1.2   Liver Microsomes Versus Hepatocytes

Liver microsomes and primary hepatocytes are the most common *in vitro* systems to assess species differences in metabolism *in vitro*. However, they differ in many respects (Table 26.1).

Microsomes are subcellular membrane fractions obtained by differential centrifugation (see Section 26.2.1), which contain primarily the membrane-bound (smooth endoplasmic reticulum) phase I XMEs (CYPs). Liver microsomes of various species are commercially available (see Section 26.2.3) and are standard for screening of metabolic stability, CYP profiling, and inhibition (see Chapter 21 in this volume). Besides CYP-dependent metabolism, flavin-containing monooxygenase (FMO) and uridine diphosphoglucuronosyltransferase (UGT) metabolism can also be investigated in microsomes if the appropriate cofactors are added to the incubation (i.e., $FADH_2$ or UDP-glucuronic acid, respectively). Epoxide hydrolase

TABLE 26.1 Comparative Characteristics and Properties of Liver Microsomes and Primary Hepatocytes

Characteristic	Liver Microsomes	Primary Hepatocytes	
		Cryopreserved	Freshly Isolated
Metabolic competence	Phase I (CYPs, EH) No transporters High enzyme activities FMOs and UGTs (if supplemented with specific cofactors) Carboxylesterases (depending on preparation method)	Phases I and II Transporters Low enzyme activities	Phases I and II Transporters Low to intermediate enzyme activities
Cofactors	To be supplemented	Intrinsic	Intrinsic
Batch characterization	Usually precharacterized (enzyme activities, protein content, genotyping)	Usually precharacterized (enzyme activities, inducibility, viability, genotyping)	Limited precharacterization (characterization usually in parallel to experiment)
Incubation time (type)	Up to 1 hour (subcellular suspension)	Up to 2–4 hours (suspension) Days—weeks (plated[a])	Up to 2–4 hours (suspension) Days—weeks (plated)
Toxicity testing	Not possible	Limited	Various parameters possible
Species available[b]	Many	Many	Some
Availability	Excellent	Good	Unpredictable
Costs	Less expensive	Expensive	Most expensive

[a]Plating of cryopreserved hepatocytes is not possible with all species.
[b]See Table 26.6.

(EH) and—depending on the preparation method—carboxylesterase activity may also be maintained. Enzyme activities are comparably high and compensate for the limited incubation time due to enzyme degradation over time.

The major limitation of liver microsomes is the lack of phase II metabolic competence. Predictions for compounds that are readily conjugated may therefore be misleading. For example, compounds with free amino, carboxy, or hydroxy functions may be acetylated, glucuronidated, or sulfated without prior functionalization. Microsomal incubations may therefore overestimate the metabolic stability of such compounds. Similarly, the comparison of metabolic profiles over species is evidently limited if phase II metabolism is involved in biotransformation.

Primary hepatocytes overcome the obstacle of lacking phase II metabolism and provide the advantages of a "living" cellular test system such as intrinsic formation of cofactors, regeneration of XMEs (though not constant over time), and the possibility to implement the assessment of liver function and toxicological parameters (see Section 26.1.3). Hepatocytes allow also for investigation of XME induction. In addition, test substance concentrations at the enzyme are expected to be closer to the physiological situation compared to noncellular microsomal incubations due to the preserved natural orientation for linked enzymes and intact cellular and subcellular compartmentation as well as presence of transporters (see Chapter 12 in this volume). Overall, primary hepatocytes provide a much more physiological test situation. Freshly isolated primary hepatocytes and some batches of plateable cryopreserved hepatocytes can be cultured for up to weeks ahead, maintaining hepatocyte properties and forming organ-like structures (e.g., polarity, junctional complexes, bile canaliculi, and glycogen particles) [1, 2], although nonparenchymal cells are usually underrepresented.

The major limitations of primary hepatocytes are the high interbatch variability and lower enzyme activities, which may further decrease significantly during prolonged incubation. Also, primary hepatocytes are considerably more expensive than liver microsomes. Another drawback with freshly isolated primary hepatocytes as compared to cryopreserved hepatocytes and microsomes is the limited availability and lack of precharacterization; that is, the batch characteristics usually are only determined in parallel with the actual experiment.

26.1.3 Toxicity Testing in Primary Hepatocyte Metabolism Studies

During the last decade liver toxicity has been one of the most frequent reasons for pharmacovigilance safety reports and the withdrawal from the market of an approved medicinal product [3].

Accumulation of the parent drug itself or its metabolites in the liver (see Chapter 13 in this volume) and formation of reactive metabolites[1] are potential cause for concern. Even at therapeutic dose levels, drugs may affect expression of XMEs (induction or inhibition) and increase production of reactive metabolites. Therefore, the use of metabolically competent and potentially inducible hepatocytes is recommended as an *in vitro* tool for the early detection and mechanistic investigation of potential hepatotoxicity [3]. The concomitant assessment of liver function and toxicological parameters within comparative metabolism studies in hepatocytes offers the chance to link potential hepatotoxicity with critical metabolite(s) and identify possible species differences early on. This may help to interpret *in vivo* findings and their relevance for humans (Fig. 26.1). However, it should be stressed that cultured hepatocytes clearly do not represent the complex *in vivo* situation and important mechanisms of liver toxicity such as those mediated via an immunological cascade or idiosyncratic reactions are not represented.

Many of the standard clinical chemistry parameters for liver injury measured in plasma samples in *in vivo* studies can also be assessed in the supernatant of hepatocyte cultures *in vitro* (Table 26.2). *In vivo*, increases in the levels of alanine aminotransferase (ALT) and aspartate aminotransferase (AST) in serum, in combination with increased bilirubin levels, are actually considered to be the most

---

[1]Potential structural alerts for hepatotoxicity are furans, quinones, epoxides, thiophenes, carboxylic acids, phenoxyl radicals, phenols, acyl halides, acyl glucuronides, aniline radicals, and aromatic and hydroxy amines.

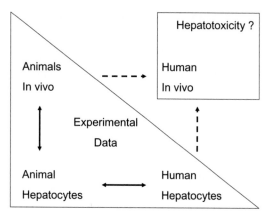

FIGURE 26.1 Prediction of human hepatotoxicity. Combining human *in vitro*, animal *in vitro*, and animal *in vivo* data improves the prediction of human hepatotoxicity *in vivo*. Human hepatocytes can provide the "missing link" for species extrapolation while animal *in vivo* data "test" the relevance of the respective *in vitro* data.

TABLE 26.2 Examples for Liver Function and Toxicological Parameters in Hepatocytes

Parameter	Correlation/Function	Assessment
Cell morphology and general appearance	General cell viability, necrotic or apoptotic cells, extra- or intracellular precipitates, etc.	Microscopical "in-life" examination of cells in culture well
Albumin secretion	Synthesis competence	Clinical chemistry of supernatant
ALT	Hepatocellular damage	Clinical chemistry of supernatant
AST	Hepatocellular damage	Clinical chemistry of supernatant
LDH	Hepatocellular damage	Clinical chemistry of supernatant
γ-GT	Hepatobiliary damage	Clinical chemistry of supernatant
aP	Hepatobiliary damage	Clinical chemistry of supernatant
GLDH	Mitochondrial damage	Clinical chemistry of supernatant
Lactate	Mitochondrial damage	Clinical chemistry of supernatant
ATP	Mitochondrial damage	Terminal intracellular detection
GSH	Redox status	Terminal intracellular detection
Trypan blue exclusion	Membrane integrity	Terminal staining of cells in well
Neutral red uptake	Membrane integrity	Terminal staining of cells in well
MTT reduction	Mitochondrial activity	Terminal staining of cells in well
XTT reduction	Mitochondrial activity	Terminal staining of cells in well
Sulforhodamine B staining	Protein content	Terminal staining of cells in well
Hoechst 33258 staining	DNA content	Terminal sampling of cells/DNA
Expression profiling	mRNA (or protein) levels	Terminal sampling of cells/mRNA

relevant signal of liver toxicity, and an increase of ALT activity in the range of two- to fourfold and higher compared to concurrent control average or individual pre-treatment values should raise concern as an indication of potential hepatic injury [3]. ALT is considered a more specific and sensitive indicator of hepatocellular injury than AST.

TABLE 26.3 General Rules on Interspecies Differences in DMPK

Species	DMPK Characteristics
Human	Polymorphisms (e.g., CYP2C9, CYP2C19, CYP2D6, NAT1, NAT2)
Dog	Low acetylation, high capacity for deacetylation; different absorption due to higher pH in gastrointestinal tract than in humans (consider use of synthetic gastric fluid to mimic human situation)
Rat	Often gender differences that are not observed in other species; abundant tetrahydrofolate (protects, e.g., against methanol ocular damage)
Rabbit	Low sulfation
(Mini)Pig	Low sulfation; gastrointestinal conditions similar to humans
Cat	Low glucuronidation; high sulfation

In addition, in cultured hepatocytes conventional cytotoxicity staining or expression profiling can be terminally performed (Table 26.2). Toxicogenomic data may support the elucidation of hepatotoxic mechanisms or interspecies differences and the development of appropriate biomarkers for liver toxicity.

26.1.4 Species Characteristics and Differences in Metabolism

As pointed out earlier, the knowledge of qualitative and quantitative interspecies differences in metabolism is key in species selection for preclinical safety studies and interpretation of any animal data.

Although there are some "general rules" on species differences in drug metabolism and pharmacokinetics (DMPK) (Table 26.3) like a decreasing rate of metabolism with an increasing size of organism, that is, mouse > rat > dog > human (see Chapter 29 in this volume for allometric scaling), which is also reflected *in vitro*, experimental testing of individual compounds is *conditio sine qua non* as there are also numerous more subtle but often decisive distinctions and the metabolic fate of a new chemical entity (NCE) cannot be reliably predicted today. The complexity of interspecies differences in the XME pattern is probably best exemplified by the many species differences in CYP isoforms [4]. Similarly, several species differences in isoforms have been identified for the major phase II XMEs: UGTs [5], sulfotransferases (SULTs) [6], *N*-acetyltransferases (NATs) [7], and glutathione *S*-transferases (GSTs) [8]. Information on typical phase I and II XME activities in liver preparations of different species is available on the websites of commercial vendors (Table 26.4) or, for example, in Refs. 9 and 10 (see Section 26.2.1).

For example, species comparison of 7-ethoxycoumarin (7-EC) phase I and II metabolism *in vitro*, which is typically used for (pre)characterization of human and animal hepatocytes (Table 26.5), suggests that human metabolism is best represented in cynomolgus monkeys with respect to the metabolite profile (glucuronidated metabolite (7-HCG) > sulfated metabolite (7-HCS) > O-deethylated metabolite (7-HC)); however, rats would be the more appropriate model with respect to the rate of metabolism (monkey ≈ rabbit ≈ dog > rat > human) [10].

26.1.5 Regulatory and Strategic Aspects

The importance of species comparisons in metabolism for safety assessment of NCEs and their metabolite(s) during drug development is reflected in several

TABLE 26.4   Examples of Commercial Sources for Liver Preparations and/or Specialized CROs for *In Vitro* Metabolism Studies (Status August 2006)

CRO/Vendor	Website @ www.	Comment[a]
BD Biosciences	bdbiosciences.com (gentest.com)	M, cH, fH, Services
GenPharmTox BioTech AG	genpharmtox.com	Services
In Vitro Technologies, Inc.	invitrotech.com	M, cH, fH, Services
tebu-bio	tebu-bio.com	M, cH, Services
XenoTech, LLC	xenotechllc.com	M, cH, fH, Services

[a]M, microsomes; cH, cryopreserved hepatocytes; fH, freshly isolated hepatocytes.

TABLE 26.5   Typical Marker Reactions for (Pre)Characterization of Human and Animal Liver Microsomes and Hepatocytes

XME	Marker Reaction
Phase I	
CYP(s)	7-Ethoxycoumarin O-deethylation (formation of 7-hydroxycoumarin)
Human isoenzyme	
CYP1A2	Phenacetin O-deethylation
CYP2A6	Coumarin 7-hydroxylation
CYP2B6	*S*-mephenytoin N-demethylation
CYP2C8	Taxol 6-hydroxylation
CYP2C9	Diclofenac 4′-hydroxylation
CYP2C19	*S*-mephenytoin 4′-hydroxylation
CYP2D6	Bufuralol 1′-hydroxylation
CYP2E1	Chlorzoxazone 6-hydroxylation
CYP3A4/5	Testosterone 6β-hydroxylation
Phase II	
UGT(s)	7-Hydroxycoumarin glucuronidation
SULT(s)	7-Hydroxycoumarin sulfation
GST(s)	1-Chloro-2,4-dinitro-benzene glutathione conjugation
NAT1 (human)	*p*-Aminobenzoic acid N-acetylation
NAT2 (human)	Sulfamethazine N-acetylation

regulatory guidance documents (status August 2006; see Chapter 37 in this volume):

- ICH M3, 1997: *Guidance for Industry on Nonclinical Safety Studies for the Conduct of Human Clinical Trials for Pharmaceuticals* [11].
- EMEA, 2000: *Note for Guidance on Repeated Dose Toxicity* [12].
- FDA/CDER, 2005: *Draft Guidance for Industry on Safety Testing of Drug Metabolites* [13].
- FDA/CDER, 1997: *Guidance for Industry: Drug Metabolism/Drug Interaction Studies in the Drug Development Process: Studies In Vitro* [14].

According to ICH M3, "exposure data in animals should be evaluated prior to human clinical trials. Further information on ADME[2] in animals should be made available to compare human and animal metabolic pathways. Appropriate information should usually be available by the time the Phase I (Human Pharmacology) studies have been completed."

The EMEA *Note for Guidance on Repeated Dose Toxicity* emphasizes the importance of comparative metabolism data for species selection in preclinical safety studies: "Within the usual spectrum of laboratory animals used for toxicity testing, the species should be chosen based on their similarity to humans with regard to pharmacokinetic profile including biotransformation. Exposure to the main human metabolite(s)[3] should be ensured. If this can not be achieved in toxicity studies with the parent compound, specific studies with the metabolite(s) should be considered."

And the FDA/CDER *Draft Guidance for Industry on Safety Testing of Drug Metabolites* encourages that "attempts be made to identify as early as possible during the drug development process differences in drug metabolism in animals used in nonclinical safety assessments compared to humans. It is especially important to identify metabolites that may be unique to humans."

Although the ultimate confirmation and justification on species selection can only be made after animal and human *in vivo* metabolite profiles are available (see Chapters 23 and 27 in this volume), this is, not before Clinical Phase I, *in vitro* species comparisons including human material provide an important—and the only—possibility to rationalize the species selection for pre-IND safety studies; usually on genotoxicity and repeated dose toxicity in one rodent and one nonrodent animal species [11] (see Chapter 37 in this volume). They further offer the possibility to compare human and several standard laboratory and potentially also nonstandard animal species in a relatively efficient approach. In addition, though obviously preferable, in contrast to *in vivo* studies, radiolabeled test substance is often not necessarily required to obtain at least qualitatively comparable metabolite profiles and "identify" the major metabolite(s) if state-of-the-art analytical equipment, usually HPLC/MS,[4] is available (see Chapter 27 in this volume).

While the early identification of unique or major metabolites will allow for timely assessment of potential safety issues, the discovery of unique or major human metabolites late in drug development can cause development delays and could have possible implications for marketing approval.

Accordingly, sponsors are encouraged by regulators "to conduct *in vitro* studies to identify and characterize unique human or major metabolites early in drug development" [13]. Liver preparations such as microsomes, hepatocytes, or tissue slices are considered appropriate for this purpose. This approach is also regarded as the "best practice" in the U.S. pharmaceutical industry [15, 16].

In vitro metabolism studies are not classical safety studies and regulatory agencies in the Unites States, Europe, and Japan therefore do not require compliance

---

[2]ADME: absorption, distribution, metabolism, excretion.
[3]The FDA/CDER *Draft Guidance for Industry on Safety Testing of Drug Metabolites* defines major metabolites primarily as those identified in human plasma that account for greater than 10% of drug-related material (administered dose or systemic exposure, whichever is less).
[4]HPLC, high performance liquid chromatography; MS, mass spectrometry.

with "Good Laboratory Practice" (GLP) regulations. However, testing under GLP may be considered since this may add to quality and improved processing and documentation, especially if studies are outsourced to contract research organizations (CROs), and there appears to be increasing interest in GLP compliance by regulators also for safety-related studies.

26.2 MATERIALS, METHODS, AND TECHNICAL ASPECTS

26.2.1 Preparation and Characterization of Liver Microsomes and Hepatocytes

Preparation of Liver Microsomes   The generalized procedure for preparation of (liver) microsomes by differential centrifugation is shown in Fig. 26.2. Tissue samples are homogenized and centrifuged at a lower force (e.g., 9000 g) to form a premicrosomal pellet containing cell debris, nuclei, peroxisomes, lysosomes, and mitochondria. The resulting postmitochondrial supernatant is subsequently centrifuged at a higher force (e.g., 138,000 g) to precipitate the microsomes. The cytosolic supernatant may directly be used in metabolism studies; the microsomal pellet is resuspended in buffer and is ready for direct use or storage below −70 °C until use.

A more detailed description of the procedure is given in Ref. 17. The assessment of different protocols [18–24] shows that there are a number of methodological variables such as the number of strokes used to homogenize the liver samples (four to eight), the centrifugation parameters (9000 g for 20 min to 18,000 g for 10 min in the first step and 100,000–143,000 g for 60–90 min in the second step), compositions of the homogenization and final suspension buffers (EDTA, potassium chloride,

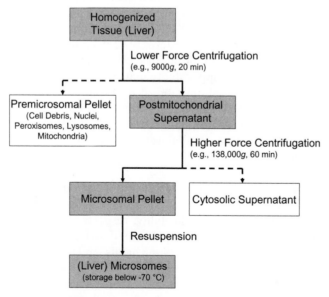

FIGURE 26.2 Preparation of (liver) microsomes. The generalized differential centrifugation procedure for preparation of microsomes is shown. For more detailed information (e.g., on tissue homogenization, buffer composition, repetition of steps), please refer to the references as given in the text.

glycerol, sucrose), and repetition of steps for more thorough extraction. Relative volumes, concentrations, and dilutions of the samples also differ. These variables may significantly affect the recovery and specific activities of microsomal components but do not appear to affect enzyme kinetics [17].

Preparation of Freshly Isolated Hepatocytes   There are two principal methods for isolation of primary hepatocytes: (1) *in situ* liver perfusion in anesthetized animals and (2) perfusion of human or animal liver samples after liver resection.

For the first method, the animal is anesthetized and the liver is perfused *in situ* via the vena portae with EGTA[5]/washing buffer to remove blood and prevent clotting of the capillaries. Subsequently, perfusion is continued with collagenase buffer to dissociate the cells from their matrix. After perfusion the liver is removed from the animal, the liver capsula is removed, and the cells are dissociated carefully in suspension buffer. The liver cell suspension is filtered and the filtrate is gently centrifuged for sedimentation of the hepatocytes. The cell pellet is washed in suspension buffer, centrifuged again, and resuspended in suspension buffer.

For the second method, the resected liver tissue is immediately transferred into ice-cold suspension buffer for storage and transport up to some hours until further processing. Liver samples are perfused with EGTA/washing buffer to remove blood and prevent clotting of the capillaries. Perfusion is performed by (several) blunt-end cannulae inserted into vessels of the cut surface. Thereafter, perfusion is continued with collagenase buffer to dissociate the cells from their matrix. The tissue is transferred into a large Petri dish with suspension buffer and the liver cells are gently scraped out with a spatula. The liver cell suspension is filtered and the filtrate is gently centrifuged for sedimentation of the hepatocytes. The cell pellet is washed in suspension buffer, centrifuged again, and resuspended in suspension buffer.

Detailed procedures for the isolation of primary rat and human hepatocytes by these methods are described in Ref. 9. Like with the preparation of microsomes, multiple variations of the general procedures have been described [25–31]. In principle, both methods are suitable for different species such as mouse, rat, rabbit, dog, minipig, or monkey. However, applicability may be limited by size of the organ or tissue sample or due to practical limitations; for example, human and sometimes animal livers may not be available for perfusion *in situ* but only after resection.

The freshly isolated primary hepatocytes may be used directly in suspension [9, 32], culture plated on collagen-coated wells (Fig. 26.3) [1, 26, 27, 29, 33], or cryopreserved and precharacterized for later use [9, 32, 34, 35].

(Pre)characterization of Liver Preparations   Microsomes and cryopreserved hepatocytes are usually precharacterized for XME activities and total protein and CYP content or cell viability and inducibility, respectively. Liver preparations of individual human donors are usually supplemented with information on the respective donor, such as age, gender, race, smoking habits, and premedication, and sometimes are also genotyped for polymorphic XMEs such as CYP2C9, CYP2C19, CYP2D6, NAT1, or NAT2. This enables one to select batches of preferred characteristics for the intended type of study and compound under investigation (Section 26.2.3).

---

[5]EGTA, ethylene glycol bis(β-aminoethyl-ether)-*N,N,N',N'*-tetraacetic acid.

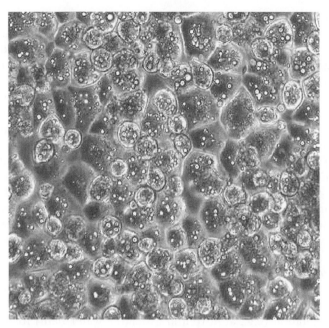

FIGURE 26.3   Light microscopical picture of plated primary human hepatocytes in culture. (Courtesy of GenPharmTox BioTech AG, Martinsried, Germany.)

If freshly isolated primary hepatocytes are directly employed after isolation, precharacterization is usually limited to cell viability and donor information but further indepth characterization (e.g., for enzyme activities) may only be performed concomitant to the actual experiment.

Typical marker reactions for (pre)characterization of human and animal liver microsomes and hepatocytes are listed in Table 26.5. A more comprehensive list of preferred and acceptable substrates, inhibitors, and inducers for *in vitro* experiments and the respective concentration ranges is given on the FDA website *Drug Development and Drug Interactions: Table of Substrates, Inhibitors and Inducers* at http://www.fda.gov/cder/drug/drugInteractions/tableSubstrates.htm#major.   Information on typical marker substrate activities for phase I and II XMEs in liver preparations of different species are available on the websites of commercial vendors (Table 26.4) or, for example, in Refs. 9 and 10.

26.2.2   Experimental Study Design

In the following, the principal experimental study designs for investigating metabolic stabilities and metabolite profiles of NCEs in liver microsomes, hepatocyte suspensions, and cultured hepatocytes are described. Depending on the test item properties and intended purpose of the study (e.g., for screening or a development project), manifold variations may be advisable, which cannot be discussed in detail here. However, some general points to consider will be highlighted later in the subsection "Points to Consider."

Metabolic Stability and Metabolite Profile in Liver Microsomes   An aliquot of test item stock solution(s) is added to the prewarmed reaction mix(es) including liver microsomes of the desired species, incubation buffer, and NADPH or a NADPH regenerating system and is incubated at 37 °C for different time intervals (usually 10–60 min). The reaction is terminated by addition of organic solvent (e.g., ice-chilled acetonitrile or methanol) and kept cool during sample preparation. In many cases, after centrifugation of the precipitated microsomal components, the supernatant can be directly submitted to HPLC-UV/VIS,[6] -FLD, -RD, and/or -MS analysis.

The loss of parent compound and/or formation of metabolite(s) is calculated compared to a zero time point control, a control without test item, and/or a control without NADPH to correct for chemical degradation, non-CYP-dependent metabolism, and artifact peaks. From this the rate of metabolism (i.e., metabolic half-life, intrinsic clearance, or simply percentage of test compound metabolized/remaining after a certain time) and/or qualitative information on the metabolite profile (i.e., minor, intermediate, major abundance of phase I metabolites) is derived.

Metabolic Stability and Metabolite Profile in Hepatocyte Suspensions   An aliquot of test item stock solution(s) is added to the prewarmed reaction mix(es) including hepatocytes of the desired species and incubation buffer and is incubated at 37 °C under slight agitation (e.g., at 40 rpm in a shaking water bath) for different time intervals (usually 15–120 min, maximum 4 hours). The reaction is terminated by addition of organic solvent (e.g., ice-chilled acetonitrile or methanol) and kept cool during sample preparation. In many cases, after centrifugation of the precipitated hepatocytes and other components, the supernatant can be directly submitted to analysis. The loss of parent compound and/or formation of metabolite(s) is calculated compared to a zero time point control and/or a control with heat-inactivated hepatocytes to correct for chemical degradation and artifact peaks. From this the rate of metabolism and/or qualitative information on the phase I and II metabolite profile is derived.

Metabolic Stability and Metabolite Profile in Cultured Hepatocytes   An aliquot of test item stock solution(s) is added to the preincubated hepatocyte culture (attachment phase of at least 4 hours, for long-term cultures often overnight) including hepatocytes of the desired species and incubation buffer and is incubated at 37 °C and 5% CO_2 for different time intervals (usually 2–24 hours, maximum several days). The reaction is terminated by addition of organic solvent (e.g., ice-chilled acetonitrile or methanol) and/or removal of the supernatant and kept cool during sample preparation. In many cases, after centrifugation of the precipitated hepatocytes and other components, the supernatant can be directly submitted to analysis.

The loss of parent compound and/or formation of metabolite(s) is calculated compared to a zero time point control and/or a control with heat-inactivated hepatocytes to correct for chemical degradation and artifact peaks. From this the rate of metabolism and/or qualitative information on the metabolite profile is derived.

As discussed in Section 26.1.3, it should be noted that cultured hepatocytes in addition allow for the concomitant assessment of several liver function and

---

[6]HPLC, high performance liquid chromatography; UV/VIS, ultraviolet/visible light detector; FLD, fluorescence detector; RD, radiometric detection; MS, mass spectrometry.

toxicological parameters, thereby offering the chance to link potential hepatotoxicity with critical metabolite(s) and identify possible species differences early in drug development.

Points to Consider   Low solubility of the test item in aqueous buffer at physiological pH is often a challenge in *in vitro* drug metabolism studies. Precipitation in the incubation mix is difficult to note due to the turbidity of the suspension; light microscopy with cultured hepatocytes may sometimes reveal precipitates, but in general solubility may already be limited before any precipitate is visible. The situation is even complicated by potentially solubilizing effects of lipids and proteins within the incubation.

Usually, stock solutions of the test item in organic solvent such as dimethyl sulfoxide, acetonitrile, ethanol, or methanol are prepared to enhance solubility for the serial dilution as well as within the actual incubation. If the high concentration stock solution was prepared in solvent, serial dilutions should also be prepared with solvent—not medium—to assure correct concentrations of the lower concentration stock solutions (i.e., to prevent precipitation during the serial dilution). Usually, final concentrations of up to 1% organic solvent are employed and tolerated by (sub)cellular test systems. However, it should be noted that different solvents interact with different XMEs even at considerably lower concentrations [36]. Another aspect linked with test item solubility is the recovery rate, which, if possible, may be worthwhile examining for proper interpretation of *in vitro* metabolism data.

Test item concentrations generally vary between 0.1 and 100 μM. In most cases, in early development the actual concentration in plasma or liver *in vivo* is not known but will usually be within this range. For determination of the rate of metabolism, lower concentrations of 0.1 or 1 μM are recommended in order not to overload the test system, while higher test item concentrations of 10 or 100 μM will facilitate detection of (minor) metabolites due to a higher absolute amount of metabolism. It should, however, be noted that metabolite profiles (*in vitro* and *in vivo*!) may differ for very high versus very low test item concentrations due to other sets of XMEs being preferred; for example, UGTs are low affinity but high capacity enzymes while SULTs show high affinity but low capacity. Appropriate test system concentrations, buffer composition, and detailed incubation/cultivation procedures may be derived from the commercial vendor's information (Section 26.2.3) or the referenced literature.

Incubation times are generally limited by loss of enzyme activity to about 1 or 2 hours for microsomes and hepatocyte suspensions, respectively. If minor metabolism is observed, incubation times may be extended (for up to 4 hours in suspension cultures) or cultured hepatocytes should be used, enabling incubation for up to several days. Chemical stability of the test item under the incubation conditions should also be considered.

For examination of metabolite profiles (see Chapter 27 in this volume), the use of a radiolabeled test item is obviously preferable as drug-related peaks are easier to differentiate from background and artifacts; metabolites can—at least approximately—easily be quantified and recovery can be assessed. However, metabolite profiles can also be derived from cold test substance if appropriate detection is possible, for example, by UV/VIS or FLD for absorbing compounds or by full-scan or targeted mass detection. In each case, it should be carefully considered which kind of metabolites would be detected—or missed—with the respective analytical method given its limitations and the structure and properties of the test compound (see Chapter 27 in this volume).

26.2.3   Commercial Suppliers and CROs

There are a number of commercial sources for liver preparations and/or CROs for outsourcing *in vitro* metabolism studies (Table 26.4). Standard species for which microsomes and hepatocytes are available are listed in Table 26.6. Preparations from other species are sometimes also available as "custom preparations," however, usually at substantially higher costs and sometimes unacceptable timelines.

When purchasing liver preparations, besides precharacterization data, quality, price, and a well established shipment procedure should be considered. Especially when liver preparations of "critical" species such as minipig (agricultural species) or monkey (strict animal welfare legislation) are purchased from vendors abroad, customs may delay delivery and biomaterials may degrade if not maintained appropriately. Therefore, especially in the case of freshly isolated hepatocytes, although there are elaborate shipment procedures established nowadays, it may be preferable to choose a local supplier in order to ensure the best possible quality and prompt delivery.

While some milligrams of test substance per species should usually be sufficient, it is difficult to give even a general rule on costs and timelines for outsourcing studies on species comparisons/metabolite profiles due to the many different possible study designs (number of replicates, time points, controls, etc.) and analytical methods (cold versus radiolabeled test substance, metabolite profile "scan" versus metabolite identification, etc.).

TABLE 26.6   Standard Species[a] for Which Microsomes and Hepatocytes Are Commercially Available at the Vendors Listed in Table 26.4 (Status August 2006)

Species	Strain	Liver Microsomes	Cryopreserved Hepatocytes	Freshly Isolated Hepatocytes
Human	Individual donor	+	+	+
	Pooled	+	+	
Monkey	Cynomolgus	+	+	+
	Rhesus	+	+	
	Marmoset	+	+	
Minipig	Goettingen	+	+	
	Yucatan	+		
	Sinclair	+		
Dog	Beagle	+	+	+
Rabbit	New Zealand White	+	+	
Guinea pig	Dunkin–Hartley	+	+	
Hamster	Golden Syrian	+		
Rat	Sprague–Dawley	+	+	+
	Wistar Han	+	+	
	Fischer 344	+		
Mouse	CD-1	+	+	+
	B6C3F1	+		

[a]Additional species may be available as "custom preparations."

26.3   CONCLUSION

Species differences in metabolism may have significant impact on pharmacokinetics and toxicity of drugs. Therefore detailed knowledge of comparative metabolism across species is key for species selection in preclinical safety testing and interpretation of any animal data in respect to relevance for humans. Although there are some "general rules" on species differences in drug metabolism and pharmacokinetics, experimental testing of individual compounds is *conditio sine qua non*, as there are also numerous more subtle but often decisive distinctions and the metabolic fate of an NCE cannot be reliably predicted today.

Liver preparations such as tissue slices, hepatocytes, or microsomes are valuable and accepted tools for comparative studies on drug metabolism across species *in vitro*. While liver microsomes of various species are easily commercially available and are standard for screening of metabolic stability, CYP profiling, and inhibition, freshly isolated or cryopreserved hepatocytes in suspension represent a well established, commercially readily available, and easy-to-handle *in vitro* system that generally correctly predicts interspecies differences in phase I and II metabolism of NCEs. If longer incubation periods are required (i.e., if the rate of metabolism is low or minor metabolites are to be assessed), hepatocyte culture systems may be used. Such systems allow in addition for the concomitant assessment of liver function and toxicological parameters within comparative metabolism studies and thereby offer the chance to link potential hepatotoxicity with critical metabolite(s) and identify possible species differences early on. This may help to interpret *in vivo* findings and their relevance for humans.

Although all *in vitro* systems have their inherent limitations and the ultimate confirmation and justification on species selection can only be made after animal and human *in vivo* metabolite profiles are available, *in vitro* species comparisons including human material provide an important—and the only—possibility to rationalize the species selection for early *in vivo* safety studies, and they further offer the possibility to compare human and several standard laboratory and potentially also nonstandard animal species in a relatively efficient approach.

REFERENCES

1. Koebe HG, Pahernik S, Eyer P, Schildberg FW. Collagen gel immobilization: a useful cell culture technique for long-term metabolic studies on human hepatocytes. *Xenobiotica* 1994;24(2):95–107.

2. Yamamoto N, Wu J, Zhang Y, Catana AM, Cai H, Strom S, Novikoff PM, Zern MA. An optimal culture condition maintains human hepatocyte phenotype after long-term culture. *Hepatol Res* 2006;35:169–177.

3. EMEA. *Guideline on Detection of Early Signal of Drug-Induced Hepatotoxicity in Non-Clinical Studies.* EMEA/CHMP/SWP/150115/2006.

4. Nelson DR, Koymans L, Kamataki T, Stegeman JJ, Feyereisen R, Waxman DJ, Waterman MR, Gotoh O, Coon MJ, Estabrook RW, Gunsalus IC, Nebert DW. P450 superfamily: update on new sequences, gene mapping, accession numbers and nomenclature. *Pharmacogenetics* 1996;6(1):1–42.

5. Mackenzie PI, Bock WK, Burchell B, Guillemette C, Ikushiro S, Iyanagi T, Miners JO, Owens IS, Nebert DW. Nomenclature update for the mammalian UDP glycosyltransferase (UGT) gene superfamily. *Pharmacogenetic Genomics* 2005;15(10):677–685.

6. Blanchard RL, Freimuth RR, Buck J, Weinshilboum RM, Coughtrie MW. A proposed nomenclature system for the cytosolic sulfotransferase (SULT) superfamily. *Pharmacogenetics* 2004;14(3):199–211.

7. Vatsis KP, Weber WW, Bell DA, Dupret J-M, Evans DA, Grant DM, Hein DW, Lin HJ, Meyer UA, Relling MV, Sim E, Suzuki T, Yamazoe Y. Nomenclature for *N*-acetyltransferases. *Pharmacogenetics* 1995;5(1):1–17.

8. Mannervik B, Board PG, Hayes JD, Listowsky I, Pearson WR. Nomenclature for mammalian soluble glutathione transferases. *Methods Enzymol* 2005;401:1–8.

9. Gebhardt R, Hengstler JG, Müller D, Glöckner R, Buenning P, Laube B, Schmelzer E, Ullrich M, Utesch D, Hewitt N, Ringel M, Reder-Hilz B, Bader A, Langsch A, Koose T, Burger H-J, Maas J, Oesch F. New hepatocyte *in vitro* systems for drug metabolism: metabolic capacity and recommendations for application in basic research and drug development, standard operation procedures. *Drug Metab Rev* 2003;35(2&3):145–213.

10. Li AP, Lu C, Brent JA, Pham C, Fackett A, Ruegg CE, Silber PM. Cryopreserved human hepatocytes: characterization of drug-metabolizing enzyme activities and applications in higher throughput screening assays for hepatotoxicity, metabolic stability, and drug-drug interaction potential. *Chem Biol Interact* 1999;121(1):17–35.

11. ICH M3. *Guidance for Industry on Nonclinical Safety Studies for the Conduct of Human Clinical Trials for Pharmaceuticals*; 1997.

12. EMEA. *Note for Guidance on Repeated Dose Toxicity*; 2000. EMEA/CPMP/SWP/1042/99 corr.

13. FDA/CDER. *Draft Guidance for Industry on Safety Testing of Drug Metabolites*; 2005.

14. FDA/CDER. *Guidance for Industry: Drug Metabolism/Drug Interaction Studies in the Drug Development Process: Studies In Vitro*; 1997.

15. Baillie TA, Cayen MN, Fouda H, Gerson RJ, Green JD, Grossman SJ, Klunk LJ, LeBlanc B, Perkins DG, Shipley LA. Drug metabolites in safety testing. *Toxicol Appl Pharmacol* 2002;182:188–196.

16. Hastings KL, El-Hage J, Jacobs A, Leighton J, Morse D, Osterberg R. Drug metabolites in safety testing. *Toxicol Appl Pharmacol* 2003;190(1):91–92.

17. Nelson AC, Huang W, Moody DE. Variables in human liver microsome preparation: impact on the kinetics of L-α-acetylmethadol (LAAM) N-demethylation and dextromethorphan O-demethylation. *Drug Metab Dispos* 2001;29(3):319–325.

18. Boobis AR, Brodie MJ, Kahn GC, Fletcher DR, Saunders JH, Davies DS. Monooxygenase activity of human liver in microsomal fractions of needle biopsy specimens. *Br J Clin Pharmacol* 1980;9:11–19.

19. Raucy J, Lasker JM. Isolation of P450 enzymes from human livers. *Methods Enzymol* 1991;206:577–594.

20. Kharasch ED, Thummel KE. Identification of cytochrome P450 2E1 as the predominant enzyme catalyzing human liver microsomal defluorination of sevoflurane, isoflurane, and methoxyflurane. *Anesthesiology* 1993;79:795–807.

21. Guengerich FP. In Hayes A, Ed. *Analysis and Characterization of Enzymes in Principles and Methods of Toxicology*. New York: Raven Press; 1994, pp 1259–1313.

22. Rodrigues AD, Kukulka MJ, Surber BW, Thomas SB, Uchic JT, Rotert GA, Michel G, Thome-Kromer B, Machinist JM. Measurement of liver microsomal cytochrome P450 (CYP2D6) activity using [O-methyl-^{14}C]dextromethorphan. *Anal Biochem* 1994;219: 309–320.

23. de Duve C. Tissue fractionation past and present. *J Cell Biol* 1971;50:20d–55d.

24. Papac DI, Franklin MR. N-benzylimidazole, a high magnitude inducer of rat hepatic cytochrome P-450 exhibiting both polycyclic aromatic hydrocarbon- and phenobarbital-type induction of phase I and phase II drug-metabolizing enzymes. *Drug Metab Dispos* 1988;16:259–264.

25. DeLeve LD. Cellular target of cyclophosphamide toxicity in the murine liver: role of glutathione and site of metabolic activation. *Hepatology* 1996;24(4):830–837.

26. Hengstler JG, Utesch D, Steinberg P, Ringel M, Swales N, Biefang K, Platt KL, Diener B, Boettger T, Fischer T, Oesch F. Cryopreserved primary hepatocytes as an *in vitro* model for the evaluation of drug metabolism and enzyme induction. *Drug Metab Rev* 2000;32:81–118.

27. Li AP, Roque AP, Beck DJ, Kaminski DL. Isolation and culturing of hepatocytes from human livers. *Methods Cell Sci* 1992;14(3):139–145.

28. Moldeus P, Hogberg J, Orrenius S. Isolation and use of liver cells. *Methods Enzymol* 1978;51:60–70.

29. Ryan CM, Carter EA, Jenkins RL, Sterling LM, Yarmush ML, Malt RA, Tompkins RG. Isolation and long-term culture of human hepatocytes. *Surgery* 1993;113:48–54.

30. Seglen PO. Preparation of isolated rat liver cells. *Methods Cell Biol* 1976;13:29–83.

31. Steffan AM, Gendrault JL, McCuskey RS, McCuskey PA, Kirn A. Phagocytosis, an unrecognized property of murine endothelial liver cells. *Hepatology* 1986;6(5):830–836.

32. Elaut G, Papeleu P, Vinken M, Henkens T, Snykers S, Vanhaecke T, Rogiers V. Hepatocytes in suspension. *Methods Mol Biol* 2006;320:255–263.

33. Dunn JC, Yarmush ML, Koebe HG, Tompkins RG. Hepatocyte function and extracellular matrix geometry: long-term culture in a sandwich configuration. *FASEB J* 1989;3(2):174–177. Erratum in: *FASEB J* 1989;3(7):1873.

34. Loretz LJ, Li AP, Flye MW, Wilson AG. Optimization of cryopreservation procedures for rat and human hepatocytes. *Xenobiotica* 1989;19(5):489–498.

35. Gomez-Lechon MJ, Lahoz A, Jimenez N, Castell VJ, Donato MT. Cryopreservation of rat, dog and human hepatocytes: influence of preculture and cryoprotectants on recovery, cytochrome P450 activities and induction upon thawing. *Xenobiotica* 2006;36(6): 457–472.

36. Busby WF Jr, Ackermann JM, Crespi CL. Effect of methanol, ethanol, dimethyl sulfoxide, and acetonitrile on *in vitro* activities of cDNA-expressed human cytochromes P-450. *Drug Metab Dispos* 1999;27(2):246–249.

27

METABOLITE PROFILING AND STRUCTURAL IDENTIFICATION

MEHRAN F. MOGHADDAM

Celgene, San Diego, California

Contents

27.1 INTRODUCTION

In the pharmaceutical and agrichemical arena, transformation of a compound into its metabolite(s) via *in vivo* or *in vitro* biochemical reactions is referred to as biotransformation reactions. Metabolite profiling refers to the process of identifying

Preclinical Development Handbook: ADME and Biopharmaceutical Properties,
edited by Shayne Cox Gad
Copyright © 2008 John Wiley & Sons, Inc.

all drug related metabolites generated through biotransformation reactions in animals or in *in vitro* systems. In animals, this process may result in the presence of metabolites in the circulation and in any and all tissues as well as the excreta, collectively referred to as animal matrices. In general, biotransformation reactions deactivate/detoxify xenobiotics and render them more water soluble and hence more amendable to excretion (Fig. 27.1a). This leads to clearance of drugs from the body. However, there are clear examples of bioactivation of compounds after biotransformation, which may lead to generation of pharmacologically or toxicologically active metabolites. As depicted in Fig. 27.1b, biotransformation can be beneficial in timely degradation of drugs so they do not accumulate in the body and exert their effects continuously. Also, generation of pharmacologically active metabolites can be viewed as a beneficial aspect of biotransformation. At the same time, the process of biotransformation can have deleterious effects on drug action when it results in rapid clearance of a drug or transforms it into toxic metabolites.

The goal of the ensuing discussion is to provide readers unfamiliar with the field of drug metabolite identification and profiling with an overall knowledge of the concepts involved and to enable them to understand the literature in this area of science.

27.2   WHY IS METABOLITE PROFILING IMPORTANT?

Metabolite profiling should be conducted as early in the process of drug discovery and development as possible for several reasons.

27.2.1   Biotransformation-Assisted Drug Design and Discovery

By identifying metabolite(s) of a compound in *in vitro* systems early in the discovery process, one may uncover the metabolic "weak spots" on a molecule. Medicinal chemists should be informed as soon as metabolites have been identified in order to stabilize "weak spots" on the experimental molecules via chemical modifications. This allows medicinal chemists to engender metabolic stability into and lower metabolic clearance of the chemical series of interest in a timely fashion [1]. Additionally, metabolites with chemical features capable of generating adverse effects should be pointed out to guide chemists to eliminate progenitors to such moieties.

27.2.2   Discovery of Pharmacologically Active Metabolites

In some instances, biotransformation of a drug can lead to a pharmacologically active metabolite (Fig. 27.1a). Although one may envision a more extensive definition, the literature defines a pharmacologically active metabolite as a metabolite with activity against the same pharmacological target as the parent drug [2, 3]. An example of a published pharmacologically active metabolite is Clarinex™ (desloratadine), which is a metabolite of Claritin™ (loratadine) with a 10-fold

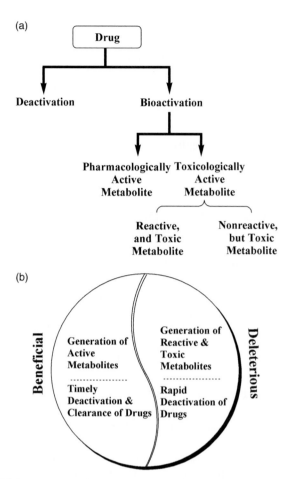

FIGURE 27.1   (a) Drug metabolism results in deactivation or bioactivation of a drug. Bioactivation of a drug leads to formation of either pharmacologically or toxicologically active metabolites. Toxic metabolites may or may not be chemically reactive in nature. (b) Drug metabolism is a process that can be viewed as beneficial or deleterious depending on the outcome. It may be beneficial if it generates pharmacologically active metabolites and degrades the drug slowly. However, it will be viewed as a deleterious process if it generates reactive metabolites and/or results in rapid clearance of drugs.

increase in its potency, longer half-life, and greater exposure [2]. Other examples include 6-*O*-glucuronide of morphine with higher levels of exposure and lower incidences of side effects, Allegra™ (fexofenadine) with no cardiac side effects as opposed to terfenadine, its parent drug, and Zyrtec™ (cetirizine) with a higher affinity for H1 receptor and a lack of distribution to brain (therefore nonsedative) as opposed to its parent drug, Atarax™ (hydroxyzine).

Early knowledge of the metabolic profile of a compound allows one to monitor it in plasma during pharmacokinetic (PK) and efficacy studies. In the discovery setting, this establishes the relevance of metabolites generated *in vitro* to *in vivo* findings and potentially uncovers pharmacologically active metabolites. Knowledge of active metabolites can assist in establishment of better PK/PD (pharmacokinetic/pharmacodynamic) correlations. Determination of the extent of contribution of an active metabolite to the efficacy of a drug is needed for more accurate dose selection in the clinic. Furthermore, pharmacologically active metabolites can be synthesized and tested as potential drugs themselves [3].

27.2.3 Detection of Toxicologically Active Metabolites

Early identification of metabolites may assist in safety assessment of molecules in the discovery process. From a regulatory and safety perspective, it is critical to demonstrate that all human metabolites are present in animal species tested in toxicology studies. This could be partially assessed by conducting *in vitro* studies with hepatocytes, S9 fractions, or microsomes from human and preclinical species, as discussed later.

In 2002, a group of scientists from the pharmaceutical industry proposed a guideline, "metabolites in safety testing" or "MIST," for assessing the safety of metabolites [4]. It was primarily proposed that human metabolites present in circulation at 25% or more of the total drug related material should be considered for testing. In 2005, in order to address this issue, the U.S. Food and Drug Administration (FDA) put forth a draft guidance (http://www.fda.gov/cder/guidance/6366dft.pdf). This document makes recommendations on when and how to identify, characterize, and evaluate major metabolites or metabolites unique to humans for safety. Unique metabolites are defined as metabolites that occur in humans only, and therefore have not been adequately tested for safety in preclinical species in toxicology testing. Major metabolites are defined as those identified in human plasma that account for greater than 10% of the drug related material (administered dose or systemic exposure, whichever is less), which again were not present in the preclinical species at significant amounts. The FDA recommends that attempts be made to identify any major metabolites or metabolites unique to humans, as early as possible so these molecules can be synthesized and properly tested for safety in a timely manner. It is warned that discovery of major metabolites or metabolites unique to humans late in the development process can cause delays and have possible implications for marketing approval of new drugs.

Although a cutoff point of 10% of circulating drug related material is used by the FDA, the Environmental Protection Agency (EPA) regards the threshold for metabolite identification and toxicological testing at 5% [5]. There are clear examples of metabolites circulating at levels below 10%, which have been reported to cause toxicity. Therefore it has been stated by the FDA that the issue of safety concerns should be handled on a case-by-case basis regardless of how a "major metabolite" is defined [5].

Some examples cited by the FDA include felbamate, cyclophosphamide, and acetaminophen. Felbamate, used for the treatment of epilepsy, has been associated with aplastic anemia and hepatotoxicity, both attributed to a reactive metabolite, atropaldehyde [6]. Atropaldehyde is found as a mercapturic acid urinary metabolite (~2% of felbamate concentration in urine) and mercapturic alcohol (~13% of felbamate concentration in urine). Cyclophosphamide is not directly cytotoxic. However, it is metabolized to several toxic metabolites, one of which, 4-

hydroxycyclophosphamide, represented about 8% of total plasma exposure [7]. Acetaminophen liver toxicity is attributed to *N*-acetyl-*p*-benzoquinonimine (NAPQI), detected in urine as thioether metabolites. The thioethers constitute approximately 9% of a therapeutic dose of acetaminophen [8]. Figure 27.2 shows the decision tree presented by the FDA regarding metabolite testing for safety. It is important to note that reactive metabolites often are too reactive to remain in the matrix. This makes their detection in circulation difficult and they may only be observed as conjugates in excreta or not detected at all (bound residues in tissues). Reactive metabolites have been implicated in idiosyncratic reactions as well. This is a subject worthy of a lengthy discussion; however, it is not the focus of this chapter so the reader is referred to a recent review article on this subject [9]. In brief, more than 10% of acute liver failures from consumption of drugs are due to idiosyncratic reactions. Liver failure is now a leading cause of drug failure in the clinic. Remarkably, most routine animal toxicology testing fails to predict this problem in humans. In fact, idiosyncratic reactions do not occur in most patients at any dose, but, when they take place they can be fatal. These reactions are characterized by immune reactions and are generally referred to as hypersensitivity, allergic, type B, or type II reactions.

Smith and Obach [10] have proposed that decisions regarding safety testing of metabolites should be based on absolute abundance of the molecules rather than their relative abundance (compared to the parent) as was proposed by MIST or FDA guidelines. This suggestion was based on the consideration that the presence of a metabolite as some percentage of the parent drug does not convey the concentrations to which an animal or target cells are exposed. For example, given equal potencies, exposing an animal to a metabolite present at 1% of the dose of drug A dosed at 100 mg/kg would constitute a greater risk than exposing the same animal to a metabolite present at 50% of drug B dosed at 1 mg/kg. These authors have

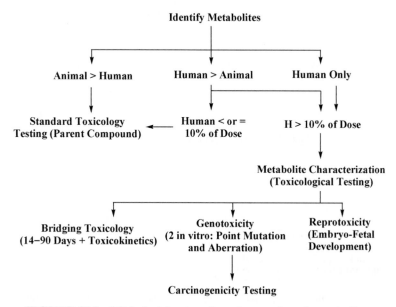

FIGURE 27.2 FDA decision tree for safety testing of metabolites.

proposed a new flowchart for metabolite testing. The reader is encouraged to follow the development of this matter carefully by looking for future FDA guidelines.

It is noteworthy that all of the guidelines or recommendations just discussed require a human study using radiolabeled drugs to conduct thorough metabolite identification and profiling studies before accurate measurements of each circulating metabolite can be assessed.

27.3 HOW ARE METABOLITES GENERATED?

Although many organs are capable of metabolizing xenobiotics in animals, the liver is universally recognized as the major site of drug metabolism. Therefore, it is common to use hepatic subcellular fractions such as microsomes and S9 fractions for the generation of metabolites. Some of the advantages offered by the use of subcellular fractions include relative ease of preparation (Fig. 27.3), ease of storage, commercial availability, relative low cost, flexibility in the manner of use, amenability to high throughput screening, and utility in mechanistic studies with inhibitors. The disadvantages of the use of microsomes and S9 fractions include potential

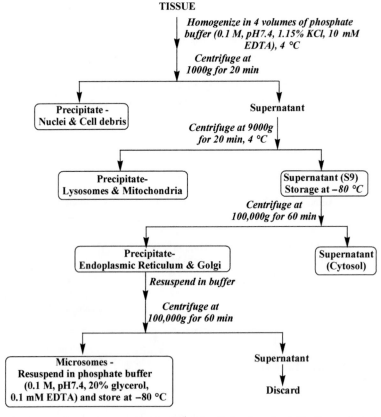

FIGURE 27.3 A scheme for preparation of subcellular fractions. Buffers other than phosphate buffer may be used provided the pH values indicated are observed.

inactivation of some enzymes during preparations (FMOs), loss of cellular compart-mentalization, lack of all cellular enzymes resulting in limited metabolism, and absence of cofactors, which will need to be added or regenerated during the course of an incubation. Consequently, the utility of intact hepatocytes offers a viable and advantagous alternative for generation of hepatic metabolites. When prepared cor-rectly [11], these cells have all their subcellular fractions and compartments intact and functioning, do not require cofactors, will provide sequential metabolism of compounds, and are therefore more representative of *in vivo* metabolism. Addition-ally, hepatocytes are correctly predictive of interspecies differences in drug metabo-lism [12]. The most important factors prohibiting the use of hepatocytes are that it is more complicated to isolate intact fresh hepatocytes than subcellular fractions, it is more costly to procure commercial cryopreserved hepatocytes, and there are limitations associated with cell viability during incubation and freezer storage. It has been recommended that the incubation of hepatocyte suspensions should not exceed 4 hours [12]. It was demonstrated that while this period is sufficiently long to deter-mine metabolic stability and to allow generation of the main metabolites of a test compound, it may be too short to allow generation of some minor, particularly phase II, metabolites [12].

Regardless of which *in vitro* system is used, it is recommended that human bio-logical reagents be utilized in parallel to those from animal species used for phar-macokinetic and efficacy studies. This allows the investigator to quickly determine species differences in metabolite generation and have a chance for an early look into the possibility of formation of metabolites unique to humans. Furthermore, such studies may unravel species differences in rates of clearance and assist in selec-tion of animal species most relevant to the human. Additionally, they assist in determination of whether the metabolic clearance is the cause of rapid clearance in animal species used in PK studies.

In addition to the *in vitro* mixtures, animal matrices are valuable sources of metabolites. These matrices include plasma, urine, bile, feces, and specific tissues. In order to better understand when and how to best utilize these matrices, one must understand the anatomy and physiology of the test subject. Figure 27.4 is a diagram of the anatomical features of an animal as it relates to drug metabolism. As can be observed, after oral administration (left side of the diagram) a drug enters the stomach and is exposed to gastric hydrochloric acid. In humans, the pH of the stomach can be as low as 1 during the fasted state and as high as 5 in the fed state [13]. In animals, varying levels of acidity are observed in different species [14]. The low pH may result in chemical degradation of drugs in the stomach. The basicity of the gastrointestinal tract is elevated going from the stomach to the colon and rectum, where the pH is around 8 [15]. In the small intestine, hydrolytic enzymes secreted by the pancreas may metabolize a drug. The large intestine has a large reservoir of microbial populations, which can perform hydrolytic and reductive biotransformations of the drugs and/or their metabolites. These metabolites, along with any unchanged drug molecules, are excreted in the feces.

The major site of absorption is the small intestine. A drug molecule and/or its metabolites or degradation products can be absorbed through the wall of the small intestine and enter the portal vein. The intestinal epithelial cells, also known as enterocytes, are enzymatically active and can metabolize xenobiotics. Once these molecules enter the portal vein, they are carried to the liver, where further

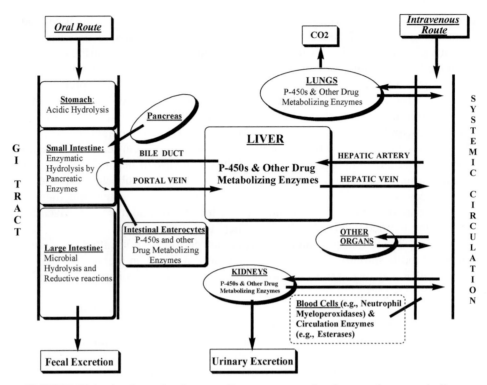

FIGURE 27.4   A schematic of mammalian anatomy as it relates to drug metabolism.

metabolism may take place; a process referred to as "first-pass effect." Some of the unmetabolized drug and/or its metabolites may be secreted into the bile and return to the small intestine via the bile duct. A fraction of these molecules can be reabsorbed through the small intestine wall and enter the portal circulation again, a process referred to as "enterohepatic recirculation." When molecules leave the liver they enter the hepatic vein and move toward the systemic circulation, which in turn carries them to the peripheral tissues and organs. These molecules can go back into the systemic circulation and travel back to the liver and bile duct. Other molecules present in circulation can enter the lung and kidney, both of which are metabolically active organs. In the lung, drug molecules can be converted into metabolites or be extensively metabolized to CO_2 and exhaled. In the kidney, both parent drugs and their metabolites can be filtered out of circulation at the glomerulus or be secreted out by the epithelial cells of the loop of Henle into the urine [13]. These molecules are then excreted in urine (or may be reabsorbed within the loop of Henle). Blood itself is a metabolizing tissue, which has circulating enzymes such as esterases. Additionally, cells such as neutrophils in the blood contain myeloperoxidases capable of metabolizing drugs [16].

In the following sections, examples describe how some of the matrices described earlier may be used in metabolite profiling. In PK and efficacy studies, plasma samples are prepared routinely from serially collected systemic blood. Identification of circulating metabolites in PK studies can prove very valuable in validating the importance of the metabolites identified in *in vitro* studies. Also, by simultaneous monitoring of a parent compound and its circulating metabolites, one may be able to identify pharmacologically active metabolites. This is helpful when there are inconsistencies between maximum plasma concentration and the time to reach that concentration and the maximum efficacy and the time to reach that effect for a drug candidate. Of course, it is important to note that delayed effects are not always due to late forming metabolites and can simply be due to delayed pharmacological effects of a parent molecule. When animals are dually cannulated in the bile duct and portal vein (Fig. 27.4), metabolite profiling of the blood from the portal vein offers a way to differentiate between hepatic and prehepatic (intestinal) metabolism. In these studies, it is imperative to have animals dually cannulated to prevent hepatic metabolites from enterohepatic recirculation via the bile duct (Fig. 27.4).

27.4 WHAT ARE BIOTRANSFORMATION REACTIONS AND HOW DO THEY GENERATE REACTIVE METABOLITES?

Enzymatic reactions responsible for the transformation of xenobiotics to their metabolites are referred to as biotransformation reactions. As mentioned previously, these reactions are generally designed to render xenobiotics more water soluble and therefore more amenable to excretion. The liver is the main site of biotransformation. However, other organs, although usually not to the same extent, are capable of participating in this process. These reactions reduce the half-life of a compound and diminish its oral bioavailability due to the first-pass effect in the liver. Traditionally, biotransformation reactions are grouped into phase I and phase II reactions (Table 27.1).

TABLE 27.1   List of Phase I and II Drug Metabolizing Enzymes

Enzyme	Reaction
Phase I	
Cytochrome P450s (CYP450)	Oxidation and reduction
Monoamine oxidases (MAOs)	Oxidation
Flavin-containing monooxygenases (FMOs)	Oxidation
Alcohol dehydrogenases (ADHs)	Oxidation and reduction
Aldehyde dehydrogenases (ALDHs)	Oxidation and reduction
Xanthine oxidases (XOs)	Oxidation
Epoxide hydrolases (EHs)	Hydrolysis
Carboxylesterases and peptidases	Hydrolysis
Carbonyl (keto) reductases	Reduction
Phase II	
UDP-glucuronosyltransferase	Glucuronidation
UDP-glycosyltransferase	Glycosidation
Sulfotransferase	Sulfation
Methyltransferase	Methylation
Acetyltransferase	Acetylation
Amino acid transferases	Amino acid conjugation
Glutathione-*S*-transferase	Glutathione conjugation
Fatty acid transferases	Fatty acid conjugation

Phase I reactions include hydrolytic, reductive, and oxidative reactions. Esterases, amidases, and epoxide hydrolases are among the hydrolytic enzymes. There are many reductive enzymes such as keto-reductases that catalyze phase I reactions. Finally, oxidative reactions of phase I enzymes are catalyzed by cytochrome P450s, dehydrogenases (i.e., alcohol or aldehyde dehydrogenases), and flavin-containing monooxygenases (FMOs). These highly prevalent oxidative reactions serve to introduce hydroxyl groups on xenobiotics as well as to modify molecules by oxidative N-, S-, and O-dealkylations, which in turn serve to generate free amines, sulfhydryls, and alcohols. A survey of 300 commonly prescribed drugs from multiple therapeutic areas has revealed that cytochrome P450s are responsible for the biotransformation of about half of the marketed drugs [17]. Cytochrome P450s are a superfamily of heme-containing isozymes. They are embedded primarily in the lipid bilayer of the endoplasmic reticulum of liver cells, which are converted into microsomes during homogenization of liver samples. These enzymes have broad substrate specificities and require reduced nicotinamide adenine dinucleotide phosphate (NADPH) as a cofactor. The dominant cytochrome (CYP) isozymes involved in human metabolism of drugs are CYP3A4, CYP2D6, CYP2C9, CYP2C19, CYP1A2, and CYP2E1; ranked according to their order of importance [18]. CYP3A4 were found to be responsible for ~40% of CYP-catalyzed drug metabolism.

Phase II reactions catalyzed by transferases are characterized as conjugation reactions (Table 27.1). These include glucuronidation, sulfation, glutathione and amino acid conjugation, acetylation, and methylation reactions of drugs. Glucuronidation reactions, catalyzed by uridine-diphosphoglucuronosyltransferase or UDPGT (microsomal) using UDP-glucuronic acid (UDPGA) as the endogenous reagent, are the most common phase II reactions. UDPGTs are ubiquitous to most tissues [18]. The net result of this reaction is addition of β-glucuronic acids to alcohols, carboxylic acids, amines, and sulfhydryls. These glucuronides can be deconjugated by β-glucuronidases, which are often used as biochemical tools to free the parent compound during the metabolite identification process. Drug glucuronide conjugates formed in the liver or intestinal enterocytes are excreted into the small intestine after secretion into the bile. Once in the small intestine, these conjugates can be hydrolyzed back to the parent drug by β-glucuronidases secreted into the lumen of the small intestine by the pancreas. The drug molecule can then be reabsorbed (enterohepatic recirculation). The kidney is also a significant site of glucuronidation and is capable of excretion of glucuronides into the urine.

It is not the objective of this chapter to discuss all the biotransformation reactions extensively, as this subject has been reviewed at length in comprehensive review articles [19, 20]. However, a brief overview of this subject is presented to provide the reader with the basic understanding of the subject. Selected examples of phase I biotransformation reaction mechanisms are presented in Fig. 27.5. These general reactions show oxidation of double bonds, heteroatoms, and carbons. Mechanisms of oxidation alpha to heteroatoms like nitrogen, oxygen, and sulfur, which ultimately can lead to cleavage of the carbon–heteroatom bonds, are also depicted. It is worth discussing the reaction mechanism for glucuronidation (Fig. 27.6) because of its prevalence and implication in the development of adverse effects, which will be discussed later. As can be observed, the lone pairs of electrons from an alcohol conduct an SN2 attack on the anomeric carbon of glucuronic acid, which has a phosphoester linkage to the uridinyldiphosphate molecule in UDPGA. This results

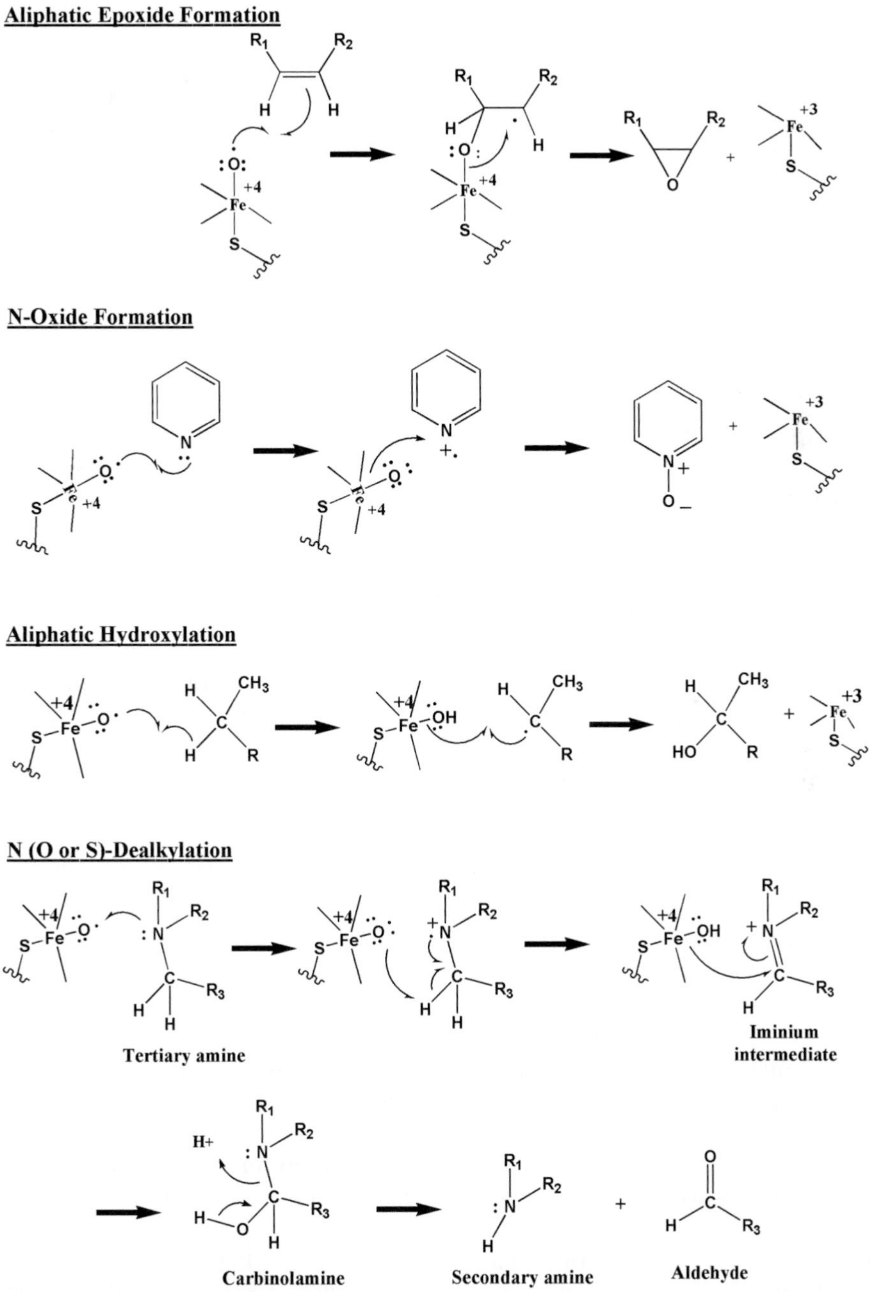

Aliphatic Epoxide Formation

N-Oxide Formation

Aliphatic Hydroxylation

N (O or S)-Dealkylation

Tertiary amine   Iminium
                                                                                intermediate

Carbinolamine   Secondary amine   Aldehyde

FIGURE 27.5   Selected examples of P450 oxidative reaction mechanisms.

in a substitution of the UDP, an inversion of the bond into a β-bond and hence, formation of a β-glucuronide conjugate.

Reactive metabolites have become an increasingly important topic of discussion in recent years due to the adverse effects associated with them. They are the unintended products of what was traditionally referred to as "detoxification pathways"

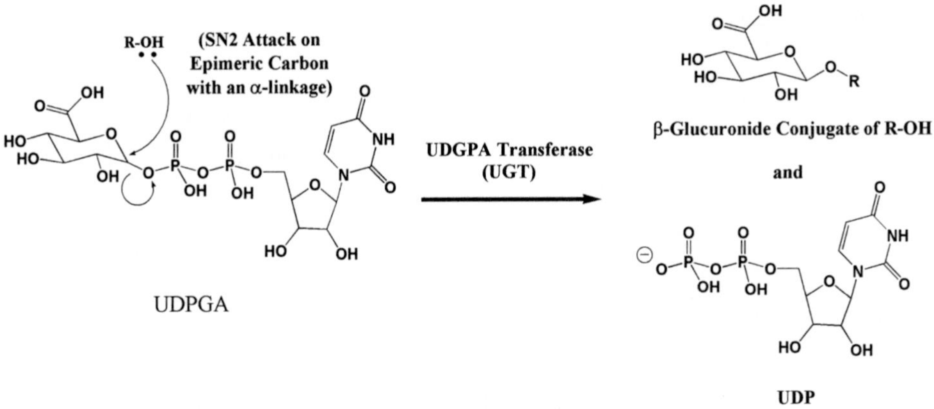

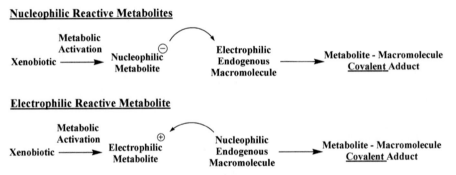

FIGURE 27.6   UDPGA transferase mechanism of glucuronidation. A conjugating nucleophile displaces the uridinyldiphospho moiety of UDPGA by an SN2 attack on the anomeric carbon of glucuronic acid.

Nucleophilic Reactive Metabolites

Xenobiotic →(Metabolic Activation)→ Nucleophilic Metabolite (⊖) ⟶ Electrophilic Endogenous Macromolecule ⟶ Metabolite - Macromolecule Covalent Adduct

Electrophilic Reactive Metabolite

Xenobiotic →(Metabolic Activation)→ Electrophilic Metabolite (⊕) ⟶ Nucleophilic Endogenous Macromolecule ⟶ Metabolite - Macromolecule Covalent Adduct

FIGURE 27.7   Covalent binding to cellular constituents can be conducted by nucleophilic or electrophilic reactions.

[21]. In general, reactive metabolites can be categorized as electrophilic or nucleophilic compounds (Fig. 27.7). After metabolic activation into a nucleophilic compound, a xenobiotic can react with an electrophilic endogenous molecule and form a stable covalent bond. Xenobiotics with a potential to form electrophilic metabolites draw reactions from nucleophilic endogenous molecules and form adducts. In such a way, reactive metabolites can cause enzyme deactivation, lead to off target toxicity, and cause idiosyncratic reactions. As shown in Fig. 27.8, the methylenedioxyphenyl moiety present in many xenobiotics such as Ecstasy (methylenedioxyamphetamine, MDA) can be metabolized to a nucleophilic carbene metabolite, which can covalently bind the heme group within the active site of P450s like CYP2D6, hence resulting in severe toxicity [22]. Demethylation of the methylenedioxy moiety may play a role in the toxicity of such groups due to formation of quinone type intermediates [20, 23]. Aniline is an example of a compound that can be metabolized to form an electrophilic reactive metabolite, namely, a reactive nitrene (Fig. 27.8).

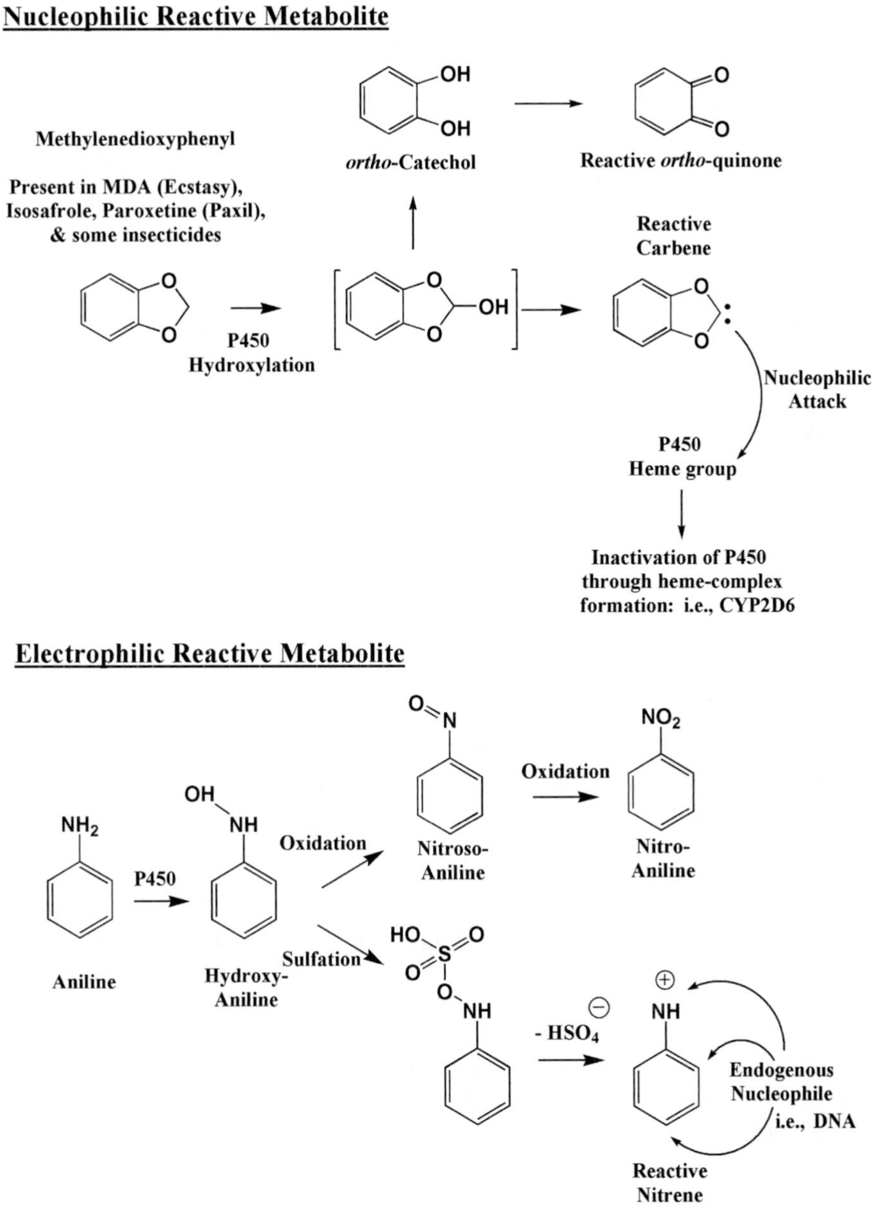

Nucleophilic Reactive Metabolite

Electrophilic Reactive Metabolite

FIGURE 27.8 Selected examples of nucleophilic and electrophilic reactions of reactive metabolites.

Diclofenac, a widely used nonsteroidal anti-inflammatory drug (NSAID), can cause a rare but serious hepatotoxicity [24]. Around four in 100,000 users (180 confirmed cases in the first three years of marketing in the U.S.) of diclofenac users developed severe liver damage with an 8% rate of fatality [24]. Diclofenac contains two masked anilines and a carboxylic acid moiety, all of which provide opportunities for reactive metabolite formation. Figure 27.9 describes biotransformation of the

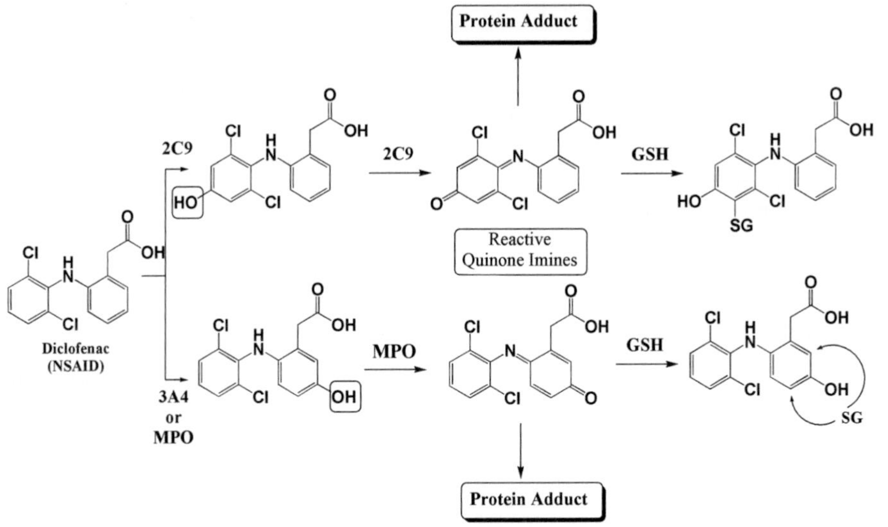

FIGURE 27.9   Potential bioactivation of diclofenac to reactive species.

anilinic groups of diclofenac into electrophilic reactive metabolites capable of binding nucleophilic molecules. As shown, the two aromatic rings can be hydroxylated *para* to the nitrogen by CYP2C9 and CYP3A4 or myeloperoxidases (MPOs). Further metabolism results in the two respective *para*-aminoquinones, which can undergo nucleophilic attacks at *meta* positions to the nitrogen by nucleophiles like glutathione or macromolecules to form covalent adducts. The carboxylic acid moiety on this, as well as many other drugs, is a suitable site for acyl glucuronidation.

A glucuronide conjugate of a carboxylic acid is referred to as an acyl glucuronide. Acyl glucuronides, but not ether glucuronides (of alcohols), have been implicated in irreversible binding of proteins resulting in haptenization and immune reactions. The first documentation of such adduct formation was by Smith et al. [25] using zomepirac, an NSAID with adverse effects, in human plasma and *in vitro* using albumin. The mechanism of toxin formation was described as shown in Fig. 27.10, based on mechanisms previously described for reaction of bilirubin glucuronides [26], glycosylation of hemoglobin [27–29], and albumin [30, 31]. As illustrated in Fig. 27.10, a 1-*O*-acyl glucuronide, which is formed via the mechanism described in Fig. 27.6, can undergo several routes of metabolism. The arrow labeled as 1 shows intramolecular migration of the constituent. During this process the hydroxyl group on C2 of the glucuronic acid substitutes the hydroxyl group of the anomeric carbon (C1) via an SN2 reaction. This process is referred to as "acyl migration" and the acyl group can continue to migrate to the other hydroxyl groups on C3 and C4. The transacylated metabolite, 2-*O*-acyl glucuronide, can exist in two isomeric forms, one of which can undergo a ring opening to yield a reactive aldehyde. Reaction of this aldehyde with an amino group on a protein, referred to as "glycation" of the protein, results in a Schiff base formation. This constitutes a stable covalent linkage of the acyl group to the protein mediated by the glucuronic acid. At this point, the acyl group–protein complex is haptenized and recognizable by the immune system as an antigen. Formation of antibodies against this hapten will be problematic and a

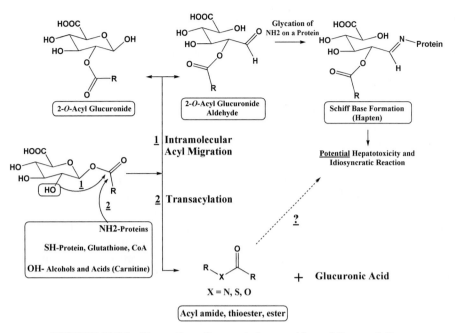

FIGURE 27.10 Formation of an acyl glucuronide and its reactivity.

potential reason for idiosyncratic reactions. Indeed, circulating antibodies against diclofenac–liver protein adducts have been detected in the sera of seven out of seven patients with diclofenac-induced hepatotoxicity [24].

Additionally, the same observation was made in 12 of 20 subjects on diclofenac without hepatotoxicity, and none of the control subjects had this circulating antibody [24]. The other path for an acyl glucuronide metabolism is path 2 in Fig. 27.10. In this case, a nucleophilic moiety such as an amine, sulfhydryl, or hydroxyl group of another molecule will displace the glucuronide moiety to form an acyl amide, thioester, or ester. If these transacylating groups are positioned on macromolecules, haptenization may take place depending on the stability of the covalent bond, this time through a direct linkage of the xenobiotic to a macromolecule.

In order to understand whether reactive metabolites are formed by a drug or drug candidate and to estimate the extent of their formation, elaborate methods have been developed using trapping agents [32]. From a practical standpoint, during the course of drug discovery and development, most compounds with reactive metabolites, if capable of generating significant adducts and adverse effects, will be excluded due to their poor pharmacokinetics (i.e., exposure) or *in vitro* and *in vivo* toxicity. Furthermore, it is difficult to justify eliminating a compound from the discovery process simply based on its ability to form reactive metabolites, unless these data are coupled with toxicity data. This is because there are *in vivo* mechanisms to degrade most covalently bound adducts and prevent adverse effects. Until there are elaborate correlations established to link particular types and levels of adduct formation to incidences of adverse effects and idiosyncratic reactions, the utility of reactive metabolite trapping experiments in the discovery setting is unclear. This is particularly true in most discovery groups because to quantitate the extent of adduct formation, radiolabeled drugs are needed and these generally are not available in the early discovery process. However, trapping experiments may be useful in confirming or removing doubts about specific chemical moieties' ability to generate reactive metabolites if such moieties are associated with toxicity.

27.5   HOW ARE METABOLITES ISOLATED AND IDENTIFIED?

Many techniques are employed for isolation and identification of metabolites. Due to the complexity of matrices that contain metabolites, often one has to use a chromatographic method to separate metabolites from each other and from unrelated chemical entities such as endogenous compounds. In the past, gas or liquid chromatography (GC or LC) was used to accomplish such a task. Analytes were first extracted from the matrices using volatile organic solvents and injected onto a GC column. The compounds of interest eluting off the GC column could be condensed and isolated into cooled vessels and reconstituted in appropriate solvents for the purpose of structural analysis. In the case of liquid chromatography, analytes eluting from the LC column were collected manually or using an automated fraction collector. After evaporation of the LC solvent, analytes of interest were reconstituted into solvents appropriate for structural analysis.

With development of tandem gas chromatography/mass spectrometry (GC/MS), the need for isolation of analytes was eliminated. GC/MS methods for the study of metabolites had a limitation in that the metabolites of interest had to be volatile or had to be derivatized to become volatile enough to elute off a GC column and enter into the mass spectrometer [33]. This added a degree of complexity to metabolism studies, because not only a derivatization step was required, but also the heat used to volatilize the analytes could cause chemical degradation of the analytes. With the advent of tandem liquid chromatography/mass spectrometry (LC/MS), the need for sample collection was alleviated. In LC/MS studies, each analyte eluting from the LC system enters the mass spectrometer for structural analysis. In addition to LC/MS techniques, there are other methods that couple the LC separation to a variety of techniques such as UV, IR, and NMR. The main focus of this discussion is modern LC/MS techniques due to the dominant role of mass spectrometry in metabolite identification.

27.5.1   Mass Spectrometry

The goal of this discussion is to provide the reader with a basic understanding of mass spectrometry as it relates to the identification of metabolites. Therefore, detailed information regarding the architecture of mass spectrometers will not be provided. A mass spectrometer is an instrument designed to distinguish gas-phase ions according to their mass-to-charge (m/z) ratios. Figure 27.11 depicts an oversimplification of an LC/MS instrument. Generally, analytes separated by the LC column enter a chamber referred to as an ion source before entering the high vacuum chamber of a mass spectrometer via a vacuum interface component. The mass analyzer components, as well as the mass detector unit, are placed in a high vacuum chamber to minimize the possibility of intramolecular collisions and to assist in movement of the ions toward the detector. The mass analyzers may be

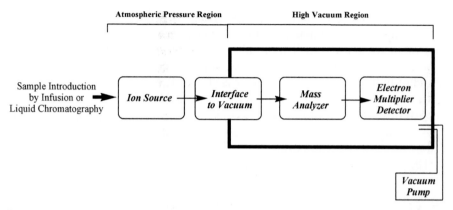

FIGURE 27.11   An oversimplified depiction of the components in a triple-quadrupole mass spectrometer.

operated with electric, magnetic, or both fields. These fields are utilized to move ions to the detector after they enter the high vacuum environment in order to produce a signal. The mass-to-charge ratios (and not just the mass) of ions are responsible for separation of the ions in the electrical and/or magnetic fields.

Ion Generation   Analytes are introduced into a mass spectrometer via an interface called a probe. Details of how an ionization probe operates are not discussed here. It is only pointed out that the analytes suspended in the HPLC solvent pass through a capillary tube within the probe and are introduced into the ion source chamber (discussed later) as a fine mist of droplets. There are several ways in which analytes may be ionized in LC/MS. Atmospheric pressure ionization (API) is a term used commonly to refer to the technique used to generate ions in the ion source and prior to entry into the chambers operated under vacuum. API techniques include electrospray ionization (ESI), atmospheric pressure chemical ionization (APCI), and atmospheric pressure photoionization (APPI). All of these are referred to as soft ionization techniques.

- In the ESI technique, the ions are generated in the mobile phase of the HPLC by adding a proton donor such as acetic or formic acid or a proton acceptor such as ammonium hydroxide. ESI is a solution phase, soft ionization technique used for any type of analyte, regardless of its volatility. With this technique, special attention should be paid to the pK_a of the analyte and the pH of the mobile phase to ensure ionization and to determine whether positive or negative ions will be generated. This in turn determines whether the mass spectrometer should be operated under positive or negative modes. While ESI can be used for most analytes, it seems to be very effective in analysis of polar compounds with large mass ranges. In ESI, the ions are generated in $[M + H]^+$ or $[M - H]^-$ depending on the mode used.
- In the APCI technique, the analytes reach the ion source in a neutral state. They become vaporized within the HPLC mobile phase using temperature and application of a high voltage needle positioned into the corona discharge. This leads

to their gas phase ionization through a complex process. APCI is typically used for analytes of medium to low polarity that have some volatility. This technique is often used with small molecules with molecular weights of up to ~1500 daltons and is extremely robust and not subject to minor changes in buffers and/or buffer strength. As was the case for ESI, APCI can be operated in both positive and negative ion modes.

- APPI is the newest of the three techniques. It is another gas-phase ionization technique, where the ionization is accomplished using a UV light source. The ions are generated in positive mode only and in the form of $[M]^+$ and $[M + H]^+$.

Once the ions are formed they leave the ion source and enter the first vacuum region of the mass spectrometer, commonly referred to as "Interface to Vacuum," through a narrow orifice leading to an ion transfer capillary tube. These ions then move toward the ion guides (quadrupoles 00 and 0 or Q00 and Q0). Ion guides are multipole rod assemblies that operate with radiofrequency (RF) voltage. In this environment, all ions have a stable trajectory and pass through the system while being focused into ion beams on their way to the mass analyzer. All the neutral and oppositely charged ions are pumped away or crash into the surface before the orifice of the capillary tube. Regardless of the type of ionization, the differences in the design and utility of the mass analyzer differentiates different types of mass spectrometers.

Mass Analyzers

Triple Quadrupole   In a triple quadrupole or "triplequad" mass spectrometer, the mass analyzer is divided into three segments, each referred to as a quadrupole or a quad. The reason for the name is that each quadrupole consists of four poles or rods assembled parallel to each other (Fig. 27.12). Rods opposite each other in the quadrupole assembly are considered a pair. Voltages of the same amplitude and polarity are applied to an opposing pair of rods. The voltages applied to the other pair are the same amplitude, but opposite polarity. As the polarity of voltages in each pair of rods oscillates between positive and negative, the ions of interest within each quadrupole are focused and directed toward the detector end of the instrument. In

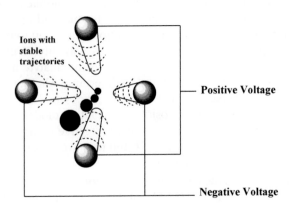

FIGURE 27.12   Movement of ions through a quadrupole.

addition to focusing ions, quadrupoles act as selection devices. The voltages used are of AC and DC nature and because the frequency of the AC voltage is in the radiofrequency range, it is referred to as RF voltage. When selecting for a specific ion, the amplitudes of RF and DC voltages are kept constant, only ions with an m/z that resonate with that particular condition will have stable trajectories to pass through the quadrupole assembly to be detected. All other ions will be destabilized and crash onto the rods and become eliminated. In cases where the RF and DC voltages are ramped up, a process referred to as scanning upward, ions of successively higher m/z ratios will be mobilized and reach the detector through stable trajectories. Therefore the ratio of the RF to DC voltages determines the ability of the mass spectrometer to separate ions of different m/z ratios.

The first and third quads (Q1 and Q3) are mass analyzers, which, depending on the type of experiment, can be configured in a specific manner to detect an ion of interest. The second quad (Q2) is a collision cell filled with an inert gas like argon when conducting collision-induced dissociation (CID) or MS/MS (MS^2) experiments. CID is a transfer of energy to an ion through collision with a neutral molecule (inert gas) resulting in vibration, cleavage, and/or rearrangement of one or more bonds on the ion. The weakest bonds in an analyte cleave first and to a greater extent resulting in fragments. The resulting fragments are used to assemble the structure of the parent ion. One limitation of a triple quad mass spectrometer is that it will not conduct MS experiments beyond MS^2. While for most metabolite identification projects MS^2 data is sufficient in determining general sites of metabolism on a molecule, for a more detailed analysis one may resort to an ion-trap instrument (as described later). Triple quads can be used to conduct several types of experiments. These include full scan, selected ion monitoring, product or daughter ion scan, precursor or parent ion scan, selected or multiple reaction monitoring (SRM or MRM), and constant neutral loss scan.

FULL SCAN MASS SPECTROMETRY   Full scan is an MS^1 experiment, which is used to detect any molecule with an m/z within a certain range in the analyzed sample. A full scan experiment is inclusive of all ionizable molecules in the matrix that enter the mass analyzer and fit the mass range criteria designated by the operator. Figure 27.13 depicts the steps involved in conducting a full scan experiment. As shown in Fig. 27.13, in an MS^1 experiment, Q1 is set to scan the mass range of interest, while Q2 and Q3 are turned off and Q2 does not contain any collision gas. Alternatively, Q1 and Q2 can be turned off while only Q3 is in the scanning mode. The mass range of interest is scanned by ramping RF/DC voltages to select ions from the lowest to highest m/z repeatedly and once every few milliseconds (scan time). Every ion exiting Q1 then gains a clear path through Q2 and Q3 to an electron multiplier detector and its m/z is recorded. In an LC/MS experiment, as analytes are separated by the chromatography column, they enter the mass spectrometer one by one and this, coupled with the fast scanning capability across a mass range, generates a total ion chromatogram (TIC), which includes all ions eluting from the HPLC. The data output obtained from a full scan experiment is a TIC and a mass spectrum associated with each TIC signal (Fig. 27.13). It should be noted that the selected mass range is shown on the x-axis of each mass spectrum.

As was mentioned before, full scan experiments can be used to gather data on all the ionizable compounds in a mixture. Once this process is finished, one can

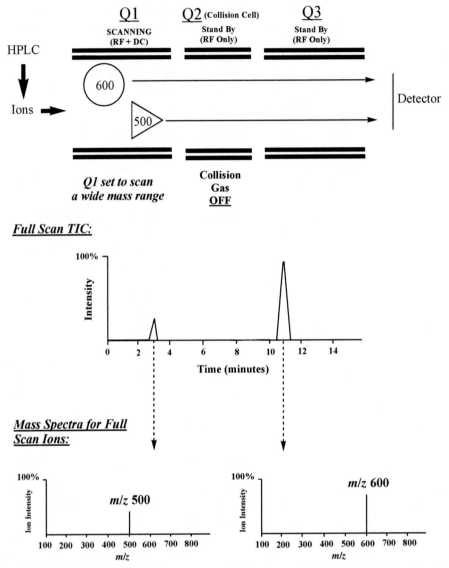

FIGURE 27.13 A schematic of a full scan experiment. All ions pass through the triple quadrupole mass spectrometer to be detected. A full scan TIC and mass spectra are generated.

search for a specific ion (a process referred to as "mass extraction"), to detect the presence of compounds with a specific m/z. The limitation of this experiment is that one cannot distinguish the compound of interest from isobaric compounds because a full scan dataset only provides information on the overall mass of a compound, and not its structural features. In cases when the operator is limited to the use of a single quad mass spectrometer and is unable to perform MS^2 experiments, any TIC peak that shows the m/z of interest may be collected as it elutes from the HPLC and further analyzed by other techniques such as NMR.

SELECTED ION MONITORING   This experiment is useful to detect minute quantities of a known analyte in a complex mixture. Therefore, while it is useful in detection of known metabolites, it is not particularly useful in identification of unknown metabolites. Selected ion monitoring (SIM) or selected ion recording (SIR) is another MS^1 experiment. In contrast to a full scan experiment, where a mass range is scanned repeatedly, in an SIM experiment the mass spectrometer is configured to acquire and record ions with one or a few selected mass-to-charge ratios. SIM is therefore a more sensitive experiment than full scan because all the scan time is used to focus on a specific mass rather than a broad mass range, as was the case for full scan.

PRODUCT OR DAUGHTER ION SCANNING   This MS^2 experiment is useful in understanding the fragmentation pattern of a molecule in the mass spectrometer. In a product ion scanning experiment, a particular ion (parent or precursor) entering Q1 is fragmented through collision with an inert gas in Q2 (collision-induced dissociation, CID) to give rise to its product ions (this utility will be discussed later). In the example presented in Fig. 27.14, the Q1 is set to select only ions with m/z 600 into Q2, while Q2 is filled with the collision gas and Q3 is scanning for a wide mass range (m/z 100–800 as seen on the x-axis of the product ion mass spectrum) selected by the operator to capture all fragments. Therefore, in this example, the ion with m/z 600 passes from Q1 to Q2 (or the collision cell) and fragments. These fragments, m/z 150 and 450, as well as any unfragmented parent ion are detected and captured in the product ion mass spectrum. The product ion TIC will represent the parent ion of m/z 600 detected by Q1 and is linked to the mass spectrum containing the fragment ion masses detected by Q3; in this case 150, 450, and 600.

The intensity of the TIC peak depends on the number of ions with m/z 600 detected in Q1. The intensity of ion signals in the resulting mass spectrum depends on the abundance of each ion after CID. Therefore, in this particular example, the intensity of the TIC depends on how many ions of m/z 600 enter Q1, which is a function of the concentration of the analytes in the sample and its ionization potential. On the other hand, the intensity of the fragment ions in Q3 depends on how well the parent ion fragmented in Q2. By elevating collision energy in Q2, one can completely shatter the ion at m/z 600 and even fragment its product ions at m/z 150 and 450 further into their respective product ions. Respectively, by lowering the collision energy, one will observe more of the parent and less of the product ions in the product ion spectrum. It is recommended to optimize the experimental condition such that around 5–10% of the parent ion is detected in the product ion spectrum to prevent excessive fragmentation.

PRECURSOR OR PARENT ION SCANNING   This experiment is useful in understanding the ions from which a particular fragment originates. In a precursor ion scanning experiment, all the ions produced in the ion source enter Q1 where they are scanned and sequentially transmitted to Q2. After CID in Q2, the product ions enter into Q3 where only the product ion of interest will be selected and transmitted to the detector. In the example given in Fig. 27.15, Q1 is set to scan a wide range of ions (m/z 100–800), and therefore all ions within that range are scanned and transmitted to Q2. CID of all of these ions generates their product ions, which all enter into Q3. However, Q3 is set to scan for a specific product ion of m/z 150. In this case, only one of the two molecules gives rise to that product ion. Generation of product ion

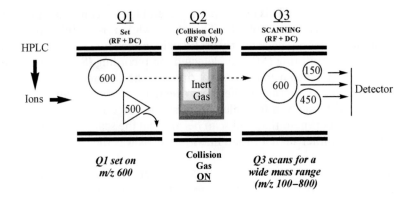

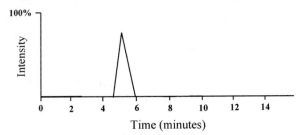

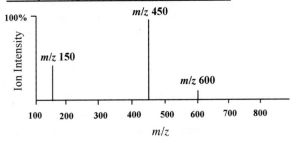

FIGURE 27.14 A schematic of a product or daughter ion scan experiment. Selected ions enter the collision cell and their product ions are detected. A product ion TIC and mass spectra are generated.

m/z 150 is linked to the parent ion with *m/z* 600. The data output of this experiment is a TIC of the precursor ion linked to its mass spectrum. Generally, the choice of which product ion to scan in Q3 depends on a previously conducted MS^2 experiment (i.e., infusion of the parent compound). Ideally, one optimizes the experimental conditions (i.e., collision energy) for the fragment ion of interest and uses the same experimental conditions for conducting the precursor ion scanning experiment. This maximizes the sensitivity of precursor ion detection.

CONSTANT NEUTRAL LOSS SCANNING This MS^2 experiment is useful in detecting conjugates (i.e., glucuronide or sulfate) of known compounds. In a constant neutral

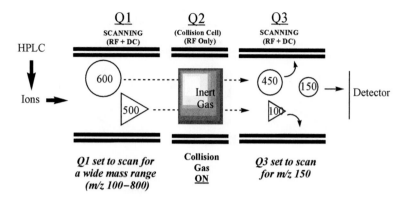

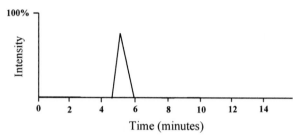

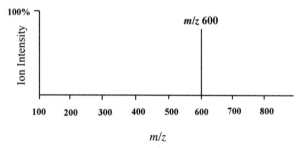

FIGURE 27.15 A schematic of a precursor or parent ion scan experiment. Precursors to selected product ions are determined and precursor TIC and mass spectra are generated.

loss experiment, Q1 and Q3 are linked together and they scan at the same rate, over the same mass range. The respective mass ranges, however, are offset by a mass of a neutral moiety. For example, for detection of a glucuronide conjugate, Q3 will scan 176 atomic mass units below Q1 in order to identify a precursor ion, which after CID in Q2 will give rise to an ion 176 mass units lower than itself. This is indicative of the loss of a glucuronide moiety (from the precursor molecule). In the example depicted in Fig. 27.16, Q1 and Q3 are scanned and only one product ion (m/z 676) is found that is 176 atomic mass units higher than an ion (m/z 500) scanned and transmitted from Q3. The data output of this experiment includes a TIC that shows signals from all parent ions capable of losing m/z 176 and this TIC is linked to the mass spectra of such ions.

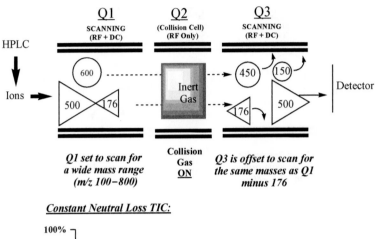

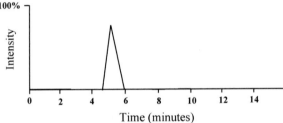

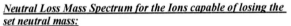

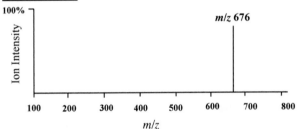

FIGURE 27.16 A schematic of a constant neutral loss scan experiment. Specific precursors to specific product ions are determined. A product ion TIC and mass spectra are generated.

A constant neutral loss is difficult to optimize for detection of unknown conjugated metabolites due to unavailability of synthetic metabolites. In the absence of an optimized method, one risks over- or underfragmenting ions of interest. By using too high of a collision energy, one may not only fragment all of the conjugated metabolite but may also go too far and fragment the product ion (deconjugated ion). By using inadequate levels of collision energy, one may not fragment all of the conjugated metabolites into the product ion. In both cases the sensitivity of constant neutral loss experiments is compromised. Therefore, the operator is left with limited choices. In cases when it is the parent drug itself that has been conjugated, the recommendation is to use a level of collision energy such that minimal fragmentation (~5%) of the parent drug is obtained. In most cases, this is enough energy to tease the conjugated drug apart into the drug, without fragmenting the drug significantly.

SELECTED REACTION MONITORING OR MULTIPLE REACTION MONITORING (MRM)   This MS^2 experiment is very sensitive and useful in detection of trace levels of analytes in a complex mixture. Generally, this experiment is used for quantitation purposes. However, one can potentially use this method to monitor for existence of a particular metabolite if its fragmentation pattern is known. In setting up for an MRM experiment, one must have prior knowledge of the m/z of the molecule of interest and its major fragment resulting from CID of the molecule of interest. This information can be hypothetical or obtained from an infusion experiment prior to the LC/MS experiment utilizing MRM. In an MRM experiment, the intensity of the signal obtained is based on transition of parent m/z to the fragment m/z. In these studies, all the ions produced in the ion source enter Q1, where they are scanned and only the selected parent ion of interest is transmitted to Q2. After CID in Q2, the product or daughter ions enter into Q3, where only the ion of interest will be transmitted to the detector. In the example depicted in Fig. 27.17, the operator has previously determined that the parent molecule (m/z 600) fragments into a major product ion with m/z 150 under the employed experimental conditions. Therefore, the targeted transition will be 600 → 150. During the conduct of the study, all product ions enter Q1 and become scanned to select m/z 600. Only the parent ion with m/z 600 is transmitted to Q2 and fragmented. If and when a product ion of m/z 150 is detected

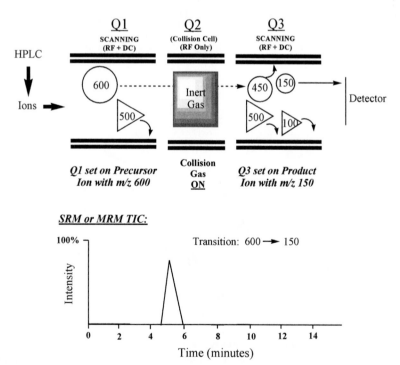

FIGURE 27.17 A schematic of a selected or multiple reaction monitoring (MRM) experiment. A specific ion transition is detected and only a TIC is generated.

by Q3, then a TIC signal representing the transition of 600 → 150 is recorded. All other precursor ions with m/z 600, which do not yield a product ion of 150, are dismissed. As depicted in Fig. 27.17, the output of an MRM experiment is a TIC, which represents a particular ion transition. Mass spectral data are not obtained in an MRM experiment.

Ion Trap   As mentioned before, the differences between mass spectrometers are based mainly on the mass analyzers. Generally, all the steps before the mass analyzer in an ion trap mass spectrometer are similar to those described for triplequads. But there is a fundamental difference between an ion trap and a triple quadruple mass spectrometer. Unlike the experiments performed on triplequads that are tandem in space, experiments conducted on ion traps are tandem in time.

Figure 27.18a simplifies components of a conventional ion trap. After ions enter the trap through the entrance endcap, RF is applied to the ring electrodes to attract or repel the ions. At any one moment the entrance and exit endcaps have an RF of the opposite charge to that of the ring electrodes. This oscillation between opposite

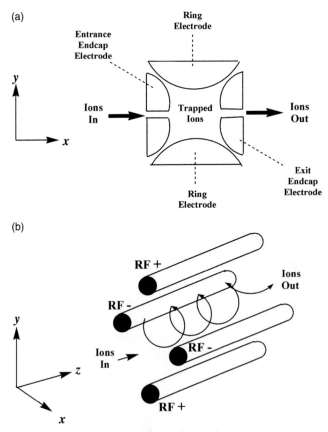

FIGURE 27.18   A schematic of different types of ion trap mass analyzers. (a) A traditional ion trap with a cubic configuration and xy dimensions for ion movement. (b) A linear ion trap with an elongated configuration and xyz dimensions for ion movements.

polarities keeps ions moving around within the trap by being attracted to or rejected by the electrically charged components. Helium gas is used to stabilize the ion movement within the trap and prevent chaotic large orbital motions that result in poor spectral resolution. There are four basic functions in the operation of ion traps and these include ion collection, isolation, excitation, and ejection.

During ion collection, ions enter into the ion trap and are retained there. In the simplest possible type of experiment—a full scan—all ions are trapped, scanned, and ejected to give rise to a spectrum that displays the m/z of all ions that were collected. In ion isolation, all the ions are first collected in the trap as described earlier and then specific RF/DC voltages are applied to eject ions that are not of interest from the trap. This allows only the ion(s) of interest to be retained and transmitted to the detector. This feature can be used for SIM experiments. Also, for the purposes of MS^2 after isolation of the ion of interest, voltages are applied to excite the precursor ion. This occurs by increasing the vibrational energy and its collision with the helium gas in the trap to cause its fragmentation. For an MS^3 experiment of a precursor ion, all the ions are collected and the precursor ion is isolated by ejecting all other ions. The precursor ion is excited to fragment (MS^2), the fragment of interest is isolated by ejecting all other fragments, and the fragment of interest is excited to generate MS^3 fragments. The MS^3 fragments are then scanned and detected.

For all practical purposes, the mechanisms for trapping ions in linear ion traps are similar to the traditional ion traps. The basic difference between the two systems is depicted in Fig. 27.18b. The linear ion trap is made up of a quadrupole and the trapped ions move through the triplequad toward the detector in a corkscrew fashion (z-axis). Therefore, in the linear ion trap, the ions are trapped in the xy plane as well as the z-axis, providing a longer trajectory path to the detector, during which more of the undesirable ions are ejected. This makes linear ion traps more sensitive instruments than their predecessor ion traps.

It is not possible to conduct the MS^2 experiments such as precursor ion, product ion, constant neutral loss scanning, or MRM experiments using ion traps. Ion traps can only conduct full scan and SRM experiments. However, one significant advantage of the ion traps over the triplequad mass spectrometer is their ability to conduct data-dependent acquisition experiments. In this type of experiment, as analytes pass through the HPLC column and into the ion trap, the sequence of events taking place in the ion trap are a full scan followed by an MS^n of any detected ion. This is an extremely powerful technique in that it eliminates the tedious need to first examine the full scan data and then to select ions to study further using MS^n in a different experiment. At the end of each data-dependent acquisition experiment, one can examine the full scan (MS^1) as well as MS^n data from an ion of interest. The inherent difficulty remains to know what ions are drug related and therefore of interest. In order to facilitate identification of drug related material, one may analyze blank samples at the same time and identify TIC signals in the samples that are absent in the blank samples using baseline subtractions. Alternatively, one may conduct a manual search for MS^2 fragments, which are expected to be present in the metabolites of a drug, in the MS^2 spectra obtained during the course of a data-dependent acquisition experiment. In fact, the net result obtained from this manual exercise is equivalent to that of a precursor ion scan experiment conducted on a triplequad.

Another manner by which this type of dataset is useful is to devise a list of hypothetical metabolites based on knowledge of the structure of the parent molecule and potential enzyme reactions responsible for degrading it. This subject requires a considerable level of knowledge of drug metabolizing enzymes and is discussed briefly at a later point. One may then manually search the full scan data for m/z of these potential metabolites and, if found, study the MS^n data that is already obtained in the data-dependent acquisition in detail to decipher its structure. Another potential manner by which one may identify drug related compounds is to use inline UV detection. This method requires that the drug and its metabolites exhibit intense UV absorptivities. Otherwise, utility of this technique in metabolite profiling requires major quantities of the drug and its metabolites in the matrix. Finally, the best method for linking a metabolite to a drug at this time remains the use of radiolabeled drugs and online radiochemical detectors.

Quadrupole Linear Ion Trap   As mentioned previously the triplequad systems have the advantage of conducting experiments such as precursor ion and constant neutral loss scanning as well as MRM experiments for quantitation. However, triplequads cannot perform fragmentations beyond MS^2 for structural analysis. Ion traps can perform MS^n, however, they are not capable of conducting precursor ion, constant neutral loss scanning, and MRM experiments. The Q-Trap^{TM} system is a hybrid of a triple quadrupole and a linear ion trap system. For example, a Q-Trap instrument may be set up to conduct a large set of MRMs and product ion (MS^3) and/or neutral loss scan experiments at the same time. This makes a Q-Trap a very elegant system capable of both quantitation and metabolite identification [34].

Accurate Mass Techniques   Accurate mass refers to good mass accuracy. This is often confused with the concept of "high resolution." The two concepts are not related. It is much easier to obtain good mass accuracy with a high resolution instrument; however, it is possible to have one without the other. Simply put, resolution refers to how well the separation is between two adjacent masses, while accurate mass refers to how precise the mass assignment is for an ion. Therefore it is possible to accurately assign masses to different ions without high resolution; however, to eliminate interference from an isobaric compound one needs to first resolve it from the ion of interest using a high resolution instrument. In order to better understand the power of high resolution mass spectrometers and the utility of accurate mass measurements, one needs to understand the concepts of "mass resolution" and "mass defect."

The term "resolution" in the context of mass spectrometry refers to the ability of the instrument to distinguish between two adjacent peaks (masses) in a mass spectrum. Mass resolution is calculated by dividing the mass of one ion by the difference between that mass and the next higher mass ($R = M/\Delta M$). The higher the resolution of an instrument, the more effectively it distinguishes between two adjacent masses. By rearranging the above formula, one can estimate what adjacent ions may be separated on mass spectrometers of different resolutions ($\Delta M = M/R$). For example, a mass spectrometer with a resolution of 1000 can separate an ion with m/z 400.2000 from another ion only if it is more than 0.4002 amu (ΔM) apart. This means the next highest mass that can be resolved from m/z 400.2000 is m/z 400.6002.

However, a second mass spectrometer with a resolution of 10,000 can separate an ion with m/z 400.2000 from another ion even if it is 0.0400 amu (ΔM) apart. This means the next highest mass that can be resolved from m/z 400.2000 is m/z 400.2400.

Mass defect is the difference between the monoisotopic accurate (exact) mass of an atom and its nominal mass. For example, the monoisotopic accurate mass of oxygen is 15.9949 and its nominal mass is 16. Therefore, the calculated mass defect for oxygen is (15.9949 – 16) or –0.0051. Mass defect of a molecule is the sum total of its atomic mass defects. For example, the mass defect of a molecule with molecular formula $C_8H_{14}N_3O_3$ will be 0.1036 and its accurate and nominal masses will be 200.1036 and 200, respectively. Using a low resolution mass spectrometer, it would not be possible to distinguish $C_8H_{14}N_3O_3$ from $C_8H_{16}N_4O_2$ because they both have the same nominal mass of 200 and exhibit m/z 201.1 (MH^+ in positive ion mode). However, because their atomic composition is different, they each have different mass defects. As mentioned previously, the mass defect of $C_8H_{14}N_3O_3$ is 0.1036 while that of $C_8H_{16}N_4O_2$ is 0.1275. This means that their accurate masses in positive ion mode will be 201.1036 and 201.1275, respectively, and therefore will be separated with the right mass resolution.

Using the formula $R = M/\Delta M$, one can calculate that a high resolution mass spectrometer with a resolution of ~8000 ($M = 201.1036$, $\Delta M = 0.0239$) will be able to separate the two isobaric compounds $C_8H_{14}N_3O_3$ and $C_8H_{16}N_4O_2$ from each other. Assuming that these were unknowns, once distinguished from each other, different molecular formulas could be assigned to these compounds based on their accurate masses. This added feature of high resolution mass spectrometer software provides an investigator with elemental composition of unknown ions and their fragments. This is an extremely powerful tool for metabolite structure assignments of unknowns with a high degree of confidence.

Currently, the more frequently used high resolution mass spectrometers for small molecule structural work include the quadrupole time-of-flight (Q-TOF) [35], the TSQ Quantum AM [36], and the hybrid LTQ/Orbitrap mass spectrometers [37].

27.5.2 LC/NMR

Nuclear magnetic resonance (NMR) spectroscopy has been used widely for structural elucidation of natural products and metabolites [38]. In brief, an NMR instrument includes a strong magnet (up to 800 megahertz) that generates a homogeneous field, a radiofrequency transmitter, a receiver, a recorder, a calibrator, and an integrator. The sample is dissolved in the appropriate deuterated solvent, placed in an NMR tube, suspended in the magnetic field, and spun. The appropriate combinations of radiofrequency and magnetic fields are used to study the environment around ^1H, ^{13}C, ^{15}N, ^{19}F, and other nuclei as well as their relationship to other nuclei in a molecule. This technique is based on absorption of electromagnetic radiation by the sample as a function of the magnetic environment the molecule experiences inside the magnet. A plot of the frequencies of the absorption peaks versus peak intensities is the data output of an NMR experiment [39]. From an NMR plot, information regarding chemical shifts (specific magnetic environment), multiplicity of signals (the interaction between neighboring nuclei), integration of signals, and intramolecular relationships can be extracted. In the case of ^1H-NMR, once protons on an analyte have been characterized using one-dimensional ^{1}H-NMR, two-dimensional NMR experiments such as ^{1}H–^{1}H correlation spectroscopy (COSY) may assist in establishing the relative positions of these protons on a molecule. Positional relationships of protons and carbons can be established by several different types of ^{1}H–^{13}C two-dimensional NMR experiments.

Integration of LC with modern NMR has created a powerful technique for identification of metabolites and without a need for prior isolation. A limitation of this technique is the necessity of using expensive deuterated HPLC solvents and its relative lack of sensitivity. The stop-flow LC system allows for prolonged acquisition of data and in part overcomes the sensitivity issue. Additionally, with the development of solvent suppression softwares to hide signals from protonated solvents and CryoFlowProbes^{TM} to improve sensitivity, the use of NMR has become even more feasible. In fact, with current technology the use of protonated organic modifiers mixed with D_2O and sample sizes as small as 5 μL are possible [38]. Additionally, interfacing LC NMR and MS will provide an even more powerful and complementary technique [40]. For example, chemical moieties such as carboxylic acids that are ^{1}H-NMR silent due to their proton–deuterium exchange are easily detectable by MS. Conversely, closely eluting or even coeluting isomeric or isobaric compounds are likely to be missed by MS but not by NMR [38]. In the arena of drug metabolism, urine after solid-phase extraction and cleanup appears to be the most analyzed matrix using NMR [40]. Bile has presented a challenge due to its content of bile salts, micelles, and detergents [38]. Finally, NMR unlike MS is not a destructive method and the analyzed samples can be retrieved after analysis.

27.5.3   Other Analytical Techniques

Radioactivity   Compounds radiolabeled with ^{3}H or ^{14}C provide excellent and facile means for metabolite detection. This is the most effective method for establishing drug relevance. The radionuclide of choice is ^{14}C because ^{3}H may exchange with water *in vivo* or *in vitro* and create confusion during metabolite profiling. However, because of the lower cost and ease of radiosynthesis, ^{3}H has been employed in metabolism studies, particularly in late stage discovery programs. The decision on the location of the radionuclide on a molecule should be a joint decision among the medicinal chemists, radiochemists, and biotransformation scientists. It is crucial to choose a site on a molecule that is stable and is subject to minimal or no biotransformation reactions. In cases where there is an expectation of cleavage of a molecule due to metabolism, sites on either side of the cleavage may be labeled to ensure the presence of radionuclides in all or most of the metabolites. Radiolabeled drug candidates are generally used during preclinical or clinical development due to the cost of synthesis and the timelines associated with radiosynthesis. The matrices containing these compounds and their metabolites can be analyzed by HPLC while collecting fractions. These fractions can be analyzed on liquid scintillation counters after adding scintillation fluids to reconstruct a radiochromatogram. It is also possible to collect fractions into microplates, dry the solvents under nitrogen, and count the radioactivity on a TopCount microplate counter [41].

Alternatively, an online detection of radioactivity may be employed using a variety of radioactivity detectors to establish a radiochromatogram of the eluting metabolites. HPLC–radiochemical detection requires the use of scintillation fluids for sensitivity. This eliminates the possibility of isolation of radiolabeled metabolites for MS or NMR analysis. It is possible to use online radiochemical detectors that do not utilize scintillation fluid and allow for fraction collection and metabolite isolation. However, this mode of radiodetection is considerably less sensitive than the previous method. A more recent development has been the invention of LC-accurate radioisotope counting (LC-ARC^{TM}). This system uses liquid scintillation fluid and, due to its stop-flow design, it is the most sensitive online mode of radiodetection available. The limit of detection for this method is 5–20 DPM for ^{14}C and 10–40 DPM for ^{3}H, which enables this system to generate thorough metabolite profiles for radiolabeled compounds. It is possible to collect parallel fractions from this instrument that do not contain any scintillation fluids and allow for metabolite isolation. Additionally, it is possible to interface this technology to LC/MS systems [41].

Infrared (IR) Detection   The electromagnetic region between the visible and microwave regions is called infrared radiation. For determination of unknown structures, the region between $4000 \, \text{cm}^{-1}$ and $666 \, \text{cm}^{-1}$ is of the greatest utility [39]. An IR spectrum is characteristic of an entire molecule. However, certain chemical moieties generate the same signals regardless of what molecule they reside on. The presence of specific signals hints at the presence of certain chemical moieties in a molecule but does not provide any information about the structural makeup or architecture of a molecule. This technique may be useful in providing complementary or confirmatory information for structure elucidation of unknowns, as demonstrated in the case study in Section 27.5.5.

Ultraviolet (UV) Detection   Wavelengths in the UV region of the electromagnetic spectrum are expressed in nanometers (nm) and are between 200 and 380 nm. Absorption of UV by a molecule results in the elevation of electrons from ground state orbitals to higher energy orbitals in an excited state [39]. For practical purposes, UV absorption is limited to conjugated unsaturated bonds. Two important factors in UV absorption are the wavelength at which maximal absorption takes place (λ_{max}) and the intensity of absorption (ε, molar absorptivity or extinction coefficient). Both these factors are dependent on the nature of the conjugated unsaturated bonds in a molecule. UV detection of a metabolite in a biological matrix depends on its concentration, intensity of absorption, and presence of interference from other UV active compounds. There are clear examples of studies where UV monitoring of metabolites were helpful in identification of drug related metabolites [42]. However, in other cases, UV detectors are not very informative due to the reasons mentioned previously.

27.5.4   Useful Chemical Modification Techniques

Derivatization reactions may be used to change physicochemical properties of molecules so they behave differently on an HPLC column and/or ionize differently in mass spectrometers. Also, the derivatized analytes may generate informative signals in their mass or NMR spectra. For example, during metabolism of nitrogen- or sulfur-containing compounds, N- or S-oxides may form. By using mass spectrometry alone, one may not be able to decipher whether the site of oxidation was on a carbon

TABLE 27.2   List of Derivatizing Agents

Group	Reaction	Reagent
Hydroxyl	Acetylation	Acetic anhydride/pyridine
	Methylation	Diazomethane
	Dansylation	Dansyl chloride
Amine	Acetylation	Acetic anhydride/pyridine
	Dansylation	Dansyl chloride
Carboxyl	Methylation	Diazomethane, (trimethysilyl)diazomethane, methanol/HCl
	Reduction	Lithium aluminum hydride
N-oxides and S-oxides	Reduction	Titanium trichloride

or a heteroatom within a segment of a molecule. Titanium trichloride (TiCl$_3$) has been used successfully to reduce N-oxides back to amines and establish the position of oxidation on the nitrogen rather than a carbon or even sulfur [43]. The reduction reaction using TiCl$_3$ was found to be efficient even in the presence of biological matrices, which makes this reagent valuable for biotransformation studies. Table 27.2 provides selected reagents that are common for chemical modifications of metabolites. A more comprehensive list of derivatizing reagents has been complied by Knapp [44].

27.5.5   A Case Study

In order to demonstrate the utility of some of the methods discussed earlier, metabolite profiling and identification of the compound in Fig. 27.19 is discussed [45]. In the actual study, this test compound was radiolabeled, and therefore metabolite profiling was performed using a radiochemical detector. Once metabolites of the parent compound were detected using a radiochemical detector, they were studied using LC/MS, NMR, and IR. In the absence of radioactivity, precursor ion scanning of selected fragments of the parent molecule would have determined which analytes were related to the parent compound. The following scenario can address metabolite identification of this compound without the use of radioactivity. First, the fragmentation pattern of the parent compound (m/z 414) is determined by infusing it into the mass spectrometer and conducting an MS^2 experiment. In this case, the product ions were m/z 68, 88, 116, 132, 185, 236, 283, 299, 300, and 386. Figure 27.19a shows a partial interpretation of these fragments. Ions at m/z 299 and 116 represent valuable fragments because they are generated as a result of a fragmentation that divides the molecule into two complementary segments, A and B (Fig. 27.19b). Next, precursor ions to each of the diagnostic product ions (m/z 299 and 116) are found in the biological matrices using precursor ion scans. In this case, a precursor ion scan of the product ion at m/z 116 would yield two TIC signals, both with m/z 414, consistent with that of the parent molecule and an isomer. This indicates that the only molecules in the mixture capable of generating fragments at m/z 116 (segment A) after CID are the parent molecule and its isomer. In contrast, a precursor ion scan of the product ion at m/z 299 would yield seven signals in the precursor ion TIC. This indicates that there are seven chromatographically distinct compounds in the mixture that yield a fragment of m/z 299. This experiment would also provide the

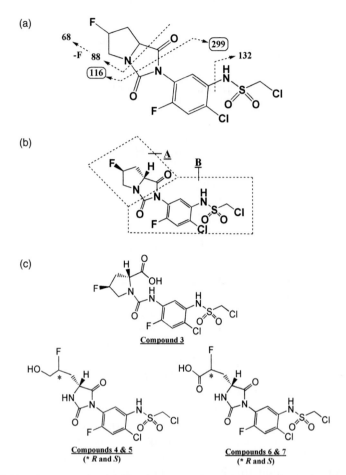

FIGURE 27.19 A case study. (a) The fragmentation pattern of the molecule of interest in a triple quadrupole mass spectrometer. (b) The 116/299 fragmentation results in two diagnostic segments in the molecule. (c) Structures of metabolites 3–7.

m/z associated with each TIC signal. These would be m/z 414 (unmetabolized parent and its isomer), 432 (three of the TIC signals), and 446 (two of the TIC signals). From this we know that there are two compounds with m/z consistent with that of the parent (MH$^+$, m/z 414), three metabolites with m/z 432 (MH$^+$ + 18), and two metabolites with m/z 446 (MH$^+$ + 32).

The next step would be to conduct product ion scans of each of these ions (432 and 446) to obtain fragmentational information on each one. The product ion scans showed that the ions with MH$^+$ at m/z 414 have fragmentation patterns identical to that of the parent molecule. The retention time of the first compound confirmed its identity as the unmetabolized parent compound. Stereochemical considerations (Fig. 27.19) indicated the second compound to be a metabolite resulting from an epimerization of the parent to its diastereomer (later confirmed by use of a synthetic standard). The third compound had an MH$^+$ (m/z 432 or 414 + 18) consistent with a hydrolysis product of the parent. In this metabolite a molecule of water was determined to be added to the hydantoin ring because the product ions of this metabolite included m/z 88 and 134. This indicates that while the fluoropyrrolidine moiety (m/z 88) was still intact, as was the case in the parent molecule, the hydantoin ring system had undergone hydrolysis leading to a ring opening (m/z 134 or 116 + 18). The structure was confirmed with a synthetic standard at a later time. Compounds 4 and 5 also exhibited m/z 434. The product ion scans of both these metabolites were qualitatively identical to each other and different from that of compound 3. The product ion spectra for compounds 4 and 5 showed that segment B was still intact. Therefore a net 18 atomic mass units (amu) had been added to segment A. Also, a CID ion of m/z 414 consistent with the loss of H_2O ($MH^+ - 18$) was observed with both these metabolites, which was indicative of the presence of an alcohol group on these metabolites. However, due to inadequacy of the LC/MS data, the precise position of oxidation on segment A could not be determined using an MS^2 experiment on a quadrupole mass spectrometer. The final structural assignments were based on NMR and IR, as discussed later. Although this was not attempted at the time, this problem could potentially be resolved using an ion trap mass spectrometer by isolating the ion at m/z 134 and conducting further CID experiments on that fragment to obtain secondary and maybe even tertiary diagnostic fragments to enable structural assignments.

Compounds 6 and 7 (m/z 446) also exhibited qualitatively identical mass spectra to each other. As was the case for compounds 4 and 5, both these metabolites lost water after CID. Addition of 32 amu to the parent molecule (or 14 amu to compounds 4 and 5) could have resulted from a net addition of water and a carbonyl group to the parent molecule. However, as for compounds 4 and 5, the precise position of oxidation on segment A could not be determined using an MS^2 experiment and the final structural assignments were based on NMR and IR.

Compounds 4–7 were isolated (20–50 μg) using HPLC for detailed IR and NMR analysis. The IR analysis started by obtaining IR signals on the parent molecule. This work established the diagnostic signals. The IR absorption bands at 1726 and 1785 cm^{-1} were attributed to the hydantoin ring, because five-membered cyclic imide rings generally have two absorption bands in the carbonyl region. Additionally, the ratio of intensities for these absorption bands (A1726/A1785) was 6.6, which was consistent with that of five-membered rings (six-membered rings have a ratio of ~2). These observations were not made for compound 3, where the hydantoin ring was no longer intact. In compounds 4–7, the same hydantoin signals as in the parent compound were observed, indicating that the hydantoin rings were intact and that the site of biotransformation on all of these molecules was on the fluorine-containing pyrrolidine ring.

In compounds 4 and 5, ^{1}H-NMR data supported that segment B of these molecules were intact as previously suggested. Two-dimensional ^{1}H–^{1}H COSY experiments supported a contiguous coupling network of protons. This network extends from the hydantoin proton (ring junction) to the methylene protons on carbon alpha to the fluorine-bearing carbon and the proton geminal to the fluorine. This established that the bonds between carbons in this area were not cleaved. However, the diastereotopic relationship of the methylene protons adjacent to the pyrrolidine nitrogen had been relieved, indicating cleavage of the C—N bond in the pyrrolidine ring and the presence of a hydroxyl group on that carbon. This established compounds 4 and 5 as diastereomeric hydroxyl metabolites, shown in Fig. 27.19c. For compounds 6 and 7, addition of 32 amu could have been due to (1) hydrolytic cleavage of the hydantoin ring followed by oxidation of a carbon on the fluoropyrrolidine ring to a carbonyl; (2) addition of two oxygen atoms to the fluoropyrrolidine ring; or (3) oxidation of the carbon alpha to the fluorine-bearing carbon of a carboxylic acid. The IR data proved that the hydantoin ring was intact and ruled out the first possibility. As was the case for compounds 4 and 5, data from the two-dimensional ^1H–^1H COSY experiments supported a contiguous coupling network of protons from the hydantoin proton to the proton geminal to the fluorine atom. Further examination of the data revealed that the signals due to the methylene protons alpha to the nitrogen in the pyrrolidine ring were lacking. These, along with biosynthetic considerations, led to the conclusion that oxidation of the alcohol groups on compounds 4 and 5 to carboxylic acid had yielded compounds 6 and 7. IR data confirmed the presence of carboxylate moieties on compounds 6 and 7 as shown in Fig. 27.19c.

This study serves as one example of the logical steps involved in structural profiling and identification of a compound. There are numerous such examples in the literature with variations in approach. Readers are encouraged to study these publications to develop a better understanding of this field.

27.6   CONCLUSION

Metabolite profiling and identification is a crucial step in discovery and development of drugs. This activity assists medicinal chemists in designing more metabolically stable and safer drugs, pharmacologists in uncovering active metabolites, and toxicologists in describing potential causative agents for adverse effects. Scientists working in the area of metabolite profiling and identification should keep up with new advances in analytical technologies such as mass spectrometry and NMR. However, it is also imperative that they are well informed on the basic principles of anatomy, physiology, pharmacokinetics, enzymology, and chemistry. This allows for a more comprehensive interpretation of data for their colleagues in medicinal chemistry, pharmacology, and toxicology groups.

ACKNOWLEDGMENT

I would like to extend my sincere gratitude to Ms. Yang Tang, Ms. Samantha Richardson, and Dr. Michael Shirley for their timely assistance in reviewing this chapter.

DEDICATION

With the hope for more extensive discovery of pharmaceutical drugs to alleviate human suffering, I would like to dedicate this chapter to the everlasting memory of my beloved grandmother, Mrs. Kobra Malayeri, whose rich and happy life came to an end in a tragic, painful, and lengthy struggle with cancer on October 13, 2004. She will not be forgotten.

REFERENCES

1. Palani A, Shapiro S, Josien H, Bara T, Clader JW, Greenlee WJ, Cox K, Strizki JM, Baroudy BM. Synthesis, SAR, and biological evaluation of oximino-piperidino-piperidine amides. 1. Orally bioavailable CCR5 receptor antagonists with potent anti-HIV activity. *J Med Chem* 2002;45:3143–3160.

2. Fura A, Su Y-Z, Shu M, Hanson RL, Roongta V, Humphreys WG. Discovering drugs through biological transformation: role of pharmacologically active metabolites in drug discovery. *J Med Chem* 2004;47:1–13.

3. Gad SC. Active drug metabolites in drug development. *Curr Opin Pharmacol* 2003;3:98–100.

4. Baillie TA, Cayen MN, Fouda H, Gerson RJ, Green JD, Grossman SJ, Grossman SJ, Klunk LJ, LeBlanc B, Perkins DG, Shipley LA. Metabolites in safety testing. *Toxicol Appl Pharmacol* 2002;182:188–196.

5. Hastings KL, El-Hage J, Jacobs A, Leighton J, Morse D, Osterberg R. Drug metabolites in safety testing, Letter to the Editor. *Toxicol Appl Pharmocol* 2003;190:91–92.

6. Thompson CD, Barthen MT, Hopper DW, Miller TA, Quigg M. Quantification in patient urine samples of felbamate and three metabolites: acid carbamate and two mercapturic acids. *Epilepsia* 1999;40:769–776.

7. Sladek NE, Doeden D, Powers JF, Krivit W. Plasma concentrations of 4-hydroxycyclophosphamide and phosphoramide mustard in patients repeatedly given high doses of cyclophosphamide in preparation for bone marrow transplantation. *Cancer Treat Rep* 1984;68:1247–1254.

8. Manyike PT, Kharasch ED, Kalhorm TF, Slattery JT. Contribution of CYP2E1 and CYP3A to acetaminophen reactive metabolite formation. *Clin Pharmacol Ther* 2000;67:275–282.

9. Kaplowitz N. Idiosyncratic drug hepatotoxicity. *Nat Rev* 2005;4:489–499.

10. Smith DA, Obach RS. Seeing through the MIST: abundance versus percentage. Commentary on metabolites in safety testing. *Drug Metab Dispos* 2005;33:1409–1417.

11. Lau YY, Sapidov E, Cui X, White RE, Cheng K-C. Development of a novel *in vitro* model to predict hepatic clearance using fresh, cryopreserved, and sandwich-cultured hepatocytes. *Drug Metab Dispos* 2002;30:1446–1454.

12. Gebhardt R, Hengstler JG, Muller D, Glockner R, Buenning P, Laube B, Schmelzer E, Ullrich M, Utesch D, Hewitt N, Ringel M, Hilz BR, Bader A, Langsch A, Koose T, Burger H-J, Maas J, Oesch F. New hepatocyte *in vitro* systems for drug metabolism: metabolic capacity and recommendations for application in basic research and drug development, standard operation procedures. *Drug Metabol Rev* 2003;35:145–213.

13. Guyton AC, Hall JE. *Textbook of Medical Physiology*, 10th ed. Philadelphia: Saunders; 2000.

14. Davies B, Morris T. Physiological parameters in laboratory animals and humans. *Pharm Res* 1993;10:1093–1095.

15. Ritschel WA, Kearns GL. *Handbook of Basic Pharmacokinetics*, 5th ed. Washinton DC: American Pharmaceutical Association; 1999.

16. Zhao CL, Uetrecht JP. Metabolism of ticlopidine by activated neutrophils: implications for ticlopidine-induced agranulocytosis. *Drug Metab Dispos* 2000;28:726–730.

17. Bertz RJ, Granneman GR. Use of *in vitro* and *in vivo* data to estimate the likelihood of metabolic pharmacokinetic interactions. *Clin Pharmacokinet* 1997;32:210–258.

18. Daly AK, Cholerton S, Armstrong M, Idle JR. Genotyping for polymorphisms in xenobiotic metabolism as a predictor of disease susceptibility. *Environ Health Prespect* 1994;102:55–61.

19. Dalvie DK, Kalgutkar AS, Khojasteh-Bakht SC, Obach RS, O'Donnell JP. Biotransformation reaction of five-membered aromatic heterocylic rings. *Chem Res Toxicol* 2002;15:269–299.

20. Kalgutkar AS, Gardner I, Obach RS, Schaffer CL, Callegari E, Henne KR, Mutlib AE, Dalvie DK, Lee JS, Nakai Y, O'Donnell JP, Boer J, Harriman SP. A comprehensive listing of bioactivation pathways of organic functional groups. *Curr Drug Metab* 2005;6: 161–225.

21. Moghaddam MF, Grant DF, Cheek JM, Greene JF, Williamson KC, Hammock BD. Bioactivation of leukotoxins to their toxic diols by epoxide hydrolase. *Nat Med* 1997;3:562–566.

22. Keseru GM, Kolossvary I, Szekely I. Inhibitors of cytochrome P450 catalyzed insecticide metabolism: a rational approach. *Int J Quantum Chem* 1999;73:123–135.

23. Bolton JL, Trush MA, Penning TM, Dryhurst G, Monks TJ. Roles of quinones in toxicology. *Chem Res Toxicol* 2000;13:135–160.

24. Aithal GP, Ramsay L, Daly AK, Sonchit N, Leathart JBS, Alexander G, Kenna JG, Caldwell J, Day CP. Hepatic adducts, circulating antibodies, and cytokine polymorphisms in patients with diclofenac hepatotoxicity. *Hepatology* 2004;39:1430–1440.

25. Smith PC, McDonagh AF, Benet LZ. Irreversible binding of zomepirac to plasma protein *in vitro* and *in vivo*. *J Clin Invest* 1986;77:934–939.

26. McDonagh AF, Palma LA, Lauff JJ, Wu TW. Origin of mammalian biliprotein and rearrangement of bilirubin glucuronides *in vivo* in the rat. *J Clin Invest* 1984;74:763–770.

27. Bunn HF, Gabbay KH, Gallop PM. The glycosylation of hemoglobin: relevance to diabetes mellitus. *Science (Wash DC)* 1987;200:21–27.

28. Koenig RJ, Blobstein SH, Cerami A. Structure of carbohydrate of hemoglobin A_{ic}. *J Biol Chem* 1977;252:2992–2997.

29. Higgins PJ, Bunn HF. Kinetic analysis of the nonenzymatic glycosylation of hemoglobin. *J Biol Chem* 1981;256:5204–5208.

30. Garlick RL, Mazar JS. The principal site of non-enzymatic glycosylation of human serum albumin *in vivo*. *J Biol Chem* 1983;258:6142–6146.

31. Shaklai NR, Garlick RL, Bunn HR. Nonenzymatic glycosylation of albumin alters its conformation and function. *J Biol Chem* 1984;259:3812–3817.

32. Evans DC, Watt AP, Nicoll-Griffith DA, Baillie TA. Drug–protein adducts: an industry perspective on minimizing the potential for drug bioactivation in drug discovery and development. *Chem Res Toxicol* 2004;17:3–16.

33. Bauer E, McDougall J, Cameron BD. The *trans–cis* isomerization of *trans*-4′-(2-hydroxy-3,5-dibromo-benzylamino)cyclohexanol *in vivo* and *in vitro* in different species. *Xenobiotica* 1986;7:625–633.

34. Xia Y-Q, Miller JD, Bakhtiar R, Franklin RB, Liu DQ. Use of a quadrupole linear ion trap mass spectrometer in metabolite identification and bioanalysis. *Rapid Commun Mass Spectrom* 2003;17:1137–1145.

35. Wrona M, Mauriala T, Bateman KP, Mortishire-Smith RJ, O'Connor D. "All-in-one" analysis for metabolite identification using liquid chromatography/hybrid quadrupole time-of-flight mass spectrometry with collision energy switching. *Rapid Commun Mass Spectrom* 2005;19:2597–2602.

36. Jemal M, Ouyang Z, Zhao W, Zhu M, Wells WW. A strategy for metabolite identification using triple-quadruple mass spectrometry with enhanced resolution and accurate mass capability. *Rapid Commun Mass Spectrom* 2003;17:2732–2740.

37. Peterman MS, Duczak N, Kalgutkar AS, Lame ME, Soglia JR. Application of a linear ion trap/orbitrap mass spectrometer in metabolite characterization studies: examination of the human liver microsomal metabolism of the non-tricyclic anti-depressant nefazodone using data-dependent accurate mass measurements. *J Am Soc Mass Spectrom* 2006;17: 363–375.

38. Corcoran O, Spraul M. LC-NMR-MS in drug discovery. *Drug Discov Today* 2003;8:624–631.

39. Silverstein RM, Bassler GC, Morrill TC. *Spectrometric Identification of Organic Compounds*, 4th ed. Hoboken, NJ: Wiley; 1981.

40. Borlak J, Walles M, Elend M, Thum T, Preiss A, Levsen K. Verapamil: identification of novel metabolites in cultures of primary human hepatocytes and human urine by LC-MS^n and LC-NMR. *Xenobiotica* 2003;33:655–676.

41. Nassar A-EF, Parmentier Y, Martinet M, Lee DY. Liquid chromatography–accurate radioisotope counting and microplate scintillation counter technologies in drug metabolism studies. *J Chromatogr Sci* 2004;42:348–353.

42. Shirley MA, Bennani YL, Boehm MF, Breau AP, Pathirana C, Ulm EH. Oxidative and reductive metabolism of 9-*cis*-retinoic acid in the rat. Identification of 13,14-dihydro-9-*cis*-retinoic acid and its taurine conjugate. *Drug Metab Dispos* 1996;24:293–302.

43. Kulanthaivel P, Barbuch RJ, Davidson RS, Yi P, Rener GA, Mattiuz EL, Hadden CE, Goodwin LA, Ehlhardt WJ. Selective reduction of N-oxides to amines: application of drug metabolism. *Drug Metab Dispos* 2004;32:966–972.

44. Knapp DR. *Handbook of Analytical Derivatization Reactions*. Hoboken, NJ: Wiley; 1979.

45. Moghaddam MF, Brown A, Budevska BO, Lam Z, Payne WG. Biotransformation, excretion kinetics, and tissue distribution of an *N*-pyrrolo[1,2-c]imidazolylphenyl sulfonamide in rats. *Drug Metab Dispos* 2001;29:1162–1170.

28

LINKAGE BETWEEN TOXICOLOGY OF DRUGS AND METABOLISM

Ruiwen Zhang and Elizabeth R. Rayburn

University of Alabama at Birmingham, Birmingham, Alabama

Contents

Preclinical Development Handbook: ADME and Biopharmaceutical Properties,
edited by Shayne Cox Gad
Copyright © 2008 John Wiley & Sons, Inc.

28.1   INTRODUCTION

Modern drug therapy relies on better understanding of molecular biology and genetics, the systems biology of diseases, and gene–environment and gene–drug interactions (Fig. 28.1a). In the last two decades, progress has been made in identifying, cloning, sequencing, and characterizing pathogenic genes (foreign and endogenous) important to disease onset and development, leading to novel approaches to drug target validation and to drug discovery and development (Fig. 28.1a). The fast-growing knowledge and technologies of genomics, proteomics, and systems biology are revolutionizing the process of drug discovery and development. For example, increasing numbers of molecular targets (DNA, RNA, and proteins), high-throughput screening technologies, and high-yield chemical syntheses have resulted in ever-increasing numbers of candidate compounds that are available for pharmacology and toxicology testing. In addition, genetic-based therapeutics, such as gene therapy and RNA/DNA-based therapeutics (aptamer, antisense, ribozyme, RNAi, miRNA, etc.), have been challenging the traditional paradigm of pharmacology and toxicology studies of new drugs [1–3].

Although our ability to identify candidate lead compounds with high potency and specificity has largely been improved, many candidate therapeutic agents are prevented from reaching the market due to inappropriate pharmacokinetic/ADME (absorption, distribution, metabolism, and excretion) properties and drug-induced toxicity; both are highly affected by many factors including pathogens, host genes, and drug–environment interactions (Fig. 28.1b). It is desirable that poorly behaved

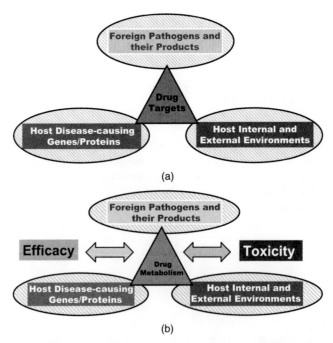

FIGURE 28.1   (a) Drug may target various subjects. (b) Drug metabolism may be affected by various factors.

compounds are removed early in the discovery and early development phases rather than during the more costly late development phases, especially during clinical development. This strategy has been termed "failing early and fast." As a consequence, over the past decades, ADME and toxicity (ADMET) screening studies have been incorporated earlier into the drug discovery phase. The intent of this chapter is to introduce the fundamental ADMET concepts, key tools, reagents, and experimental approaches for predicting human pharmacokinetics and assessing "drug-like" molecules, with an emphasis on the link between toxicology and metabolism (Figs. 28.1b and 28.2a).

Pharmacokinetic (PK) studies, which evaluate the way in which a drug interacts with various barriers within a system, are an integral part of preclinical and clinical drug testing. A typical PK study may be divided into two sections, with respect to the fate of a given drug in the body: *absorption*, the movement of a drug into the bloodstream, and *disposition*, which involves the distribution, metabolism, and excretion of a drug. Preclinical PK studies often provide qualitative and/or quantitative measurements of these events, using various parameters and models to describe the speed, extent, and underlying mechanisms for a chemical entity to enter and remain in various systems/tissues of interest, generally including the plasma and blood cells, body fluids, various host normal tissues such as brain, heart, lungs, liver, kidneys, spleen, bone marrow, and skin, and drug-targeted tissues such as the tumor and infected tissues [4–6]. The related field of pharmacodynamics, which evaluates the effects of a drug and its metabolites on the test system under various physiological and pathological conditions, is often evaluated in tandem with pharmacokinetics. Pharmacodynamic (PD) studies are often carried out with a disease model that mimics the intended human diseases for the test drug and employ various biomarkers to link the biological effects of a drug with its use by various routes of administration under various conditions.

Also of equal importance for drug design are toxicokinetic studies. Toxicokinetics, as the name suggests, provides information on the behaviors and fate of a toxicant/drug in the test systems, with relation to the occurrence and time course of toxic events. While PK and PD studies provide information relative to drug distribution, metabolism, removal, and pharmacological activity, toxicokinetic studies are used to predict the behavior and safety of a compound/drug [7]. Knowing the distribution and especially the speed and extent of metabolism of a drug is helpful in determining its future efficacy and toxicity. Moreover, PK/PD and toxicity/safety studies are a routine part of human clinical trials, and the objectives of preclinical PK/PD and toxicology studies are to predict potential problems earlier in the drug development process. The results of these studies can be extrapolated to give at least a general idea of the likely effects of a particular compound in humans [8]. While still imperfect, numerous *in vitro*, *in vivo*, and *in silico* systems have been developed to evaluate the pharmacokinetics, pharmacodynamics, and toxicity of compounds prior to their use in humans. Of note, there is a trend to move toxicity testing to earlier phases of drug development.

Although typical pharmacology and toxicology studies can give an idea of the distribution and effects of a drug or compound with high predictive value for most cases, unexpected differences in the response to a given drug or compound among various patients have given rise to yet other fields of study—namely, pharmacogenetics, pharmacogenomics, and toxicogenomics—that investigate the effects of genes

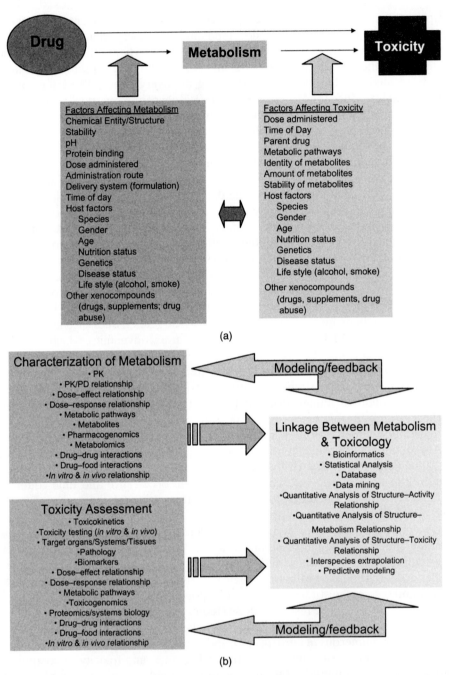

FIGURE 28.2   (a) The linkage between drug metabolism and toxicity. Listed are factors affecting the metabolic and toxic responses to a drug. (b) The framework for studies aiming at the linkage between drug metabolism and toxicity.

of interest on the efficacy and toxicity of a drug or compound, utilizing various technologies in the fields of genetics, genomics, proteomics, and molecular biology [9, 10]. The differential genetic makeup of patients, including differences in the level of gene expression, polymorphisms, and gene deficiencies, can greatly alter the efficacy and toxicity of various therapies [9, 10]. Although many genes and their expression may be involved in various PK/PD and toxicology processes, the majority of pharamcogenomics/pharmacogenetics studies have been focused on genes related to drug metabolism. While differences in expression of the cytochrome P450 enzymes may be the most important factors that affect drug metabolism, there are ever-increasing numbers of various other genes that are shown to determine drug efficacy, metabolism, excretion, and toxicity (discussed in detail in Section 28.2). One of the well-documented cases is dihydropyrimidine dehydrogenase (DPD), a key metabolizing enzyme of 5-fluorouracil, one of the most clinically used anticancer agents. DPD deficiency has clearly been linked to severe 5-fluorouracil toxicity, including death. Pharmacogenetic and pharmacogenomic characteristics of DPD have been well defined by various experimental models, in the general population, and in cancer patients [11].

Another related area of study, metabolomics/metabonomics, has also been gaining recognition in recent years. This area investigates the time-dependent metabolic responses of organisms or physiological systems and the resulting metabolites of chemical entities, foods, and other compounds [12, 13]. The field is of particular interest for preclinical studies because it can be used to determine endpoints for further toxicity studies (clinical chemistry, histopathology, etc.) and to determine potential biomarkers [14–18]. It is also useful for screening purposes in order to eliminate agents with unfavorable profiles while still in early phases of development [19–21]. Because the metabolism of compounds differs based on a number of drug, patient/host, and environmental factors, the relatively new "-dynamics" and "-omics" areas are increasingly important for determining the efficacy and potential risks of new therapeutic agents. Figure 28.2a demonstrates the complexity of the interaction between these factors and their impact on drug metabolism, and thus toxicity.

Figures 28.1 and 28.2 provide a framework for concepts, scientific reasoning, and experimental design of studies aimed at linking drug metabolism and toxicity, the focal point of this chapter. As illustrated in Fig. 28.2b, three major components should be included in these studies: (1) the profile and mechanisms of drug metabolism; (2) the profile and mechanisms of drug toxicity; and (3) the methods and models for linking drug toxicity and metabolism. For drugs that are intended for human use, the major purpose of these preclinical studies should be to predict the potential risks to humans under both pathological and physiological conditions. While there have been significant improvements, there is still a need to develop more predictive models and better computational programs that can facilitate data analysis and extrapolation of the results from experimental models to human patients [22]. Recent progress made in bioinformatics and computational biology will certainly facilitate the fine-tuning of the modeling process and the development of models with better predictive values. The ability to predict the metabolism and toxicity of a compound and their relationship will both improve the results of human clinical trials and the likelihood of success of the new agents.

28.2   DRUG METABOLISM AND ITS ROLE IN TOXICOLOGY

28.2.1   General Principles of Drug Metabolism

As shown in Fig. 28.2a, the drug metabolism process relies on a number of factors. The human body encounters numerous foreign compounds (xenobiotics) during the course of an average day. While some compounds may be consciously taken in, such as food, vitamins, and pharmaceuticals, others, such as pollutants and bacteria with their toxins, are absorbed or consumed because of their ubiquitous presence in the environment.

All of these compounds need to be utilized or removed from the system, and this is accomplished by either metabolism or excretion. Here, we focus on metabolism, more specifically drug metabolism, which is the biotransformation of various drugs to (1) inactive compounds that can readily be excreted from the body or (2) more active compounds that can exert an effect (either positive or negative). Drug metabolism can result in four major outcomes:

1. A decrease in the biological activity of drugs and xenobiotics.
2. An increase in excretion due to the formation of a more water-soluble metabolite.
3. Conversion of a prodrug to an active drug, or conversion of an active drug to a different active compound.
4. Generation of toxic or carcinogenic metabolites.

Which of these processes occurs depends on a variety of factors. While the identity of the agent is the most important, its pharmacokinetics/pharmacodynamics within the human body is a close second. There are several factors that can affect the way that the body responds to xenobiotics.

- *Age.* Infants and children may not have a fully developed system to deal with xenobiotics and may then have different rates of drug metabolism and responses to the compound and toxicities. Older persons also may have differences in their ability to metabolize compounds due to changes that occur to the key metabolic systems, primarily the liver and kidneys.
- *Drug Interactions.* When several drugs are present in the body at the same time, they can cause adverse or unexpected side effects and can cause changes in metabolism. For example, combining two chemotherapeutic agents or a chemotherapeutic agent with an anti-inflammatory agent changes the pharmacokinetics of the chemotherapeutic agents [23, 24]. Common food items can also influence the metabolism of different compounds. It is important to note that there is an increased risk for drug–drug interactions in elderly persons and those who are hospitalized due to their higher frequency of polypharmacy. There is also growing concern over the increase in people who are now more actively self-medicating with over-the-counter agents.
- *Disease States.* Diseases that affect major excretory and metabolic organs (specifically those affecting the liver and kidneys) will change the rate of metabolism of a drug. Also, disease states that involve parenteral feeds can affect the

action and activity of a drug. Moreover, diseases that affect blood flow to various organs will also affect drug metabolism.

- *Occupation.* The occupation of a person in some cases can dictate metabolism. For example, pesticide applicators may have increased drug metabolism because liver enzymes can be induced by chronic exposure to pesticides. For example, exposure of male mice to piperonyl butoxide (PBO), a synergistic active ingredient in pesticides, leads to overexpression of cytochrome P450 genes, such as CYP1A1, CYP2A5, CYP2B9, and CYP2B10 [25].

- *Time of Day.* The expression and types of enzymes and cofactors expressed as well as the speed with which metabolism takes place varies with the host's circadian rhythm. For example, the expression of DPD and dThdPase varies with time in both human patients and experimental animals. This has implications for the metabolism of 5-fluorouracil and its toxicity [26, 27].

- *Genetics.* As mentioned in the Introduction, pharmacogenomics and toxicogenomics are now being studied to determine the metabolism and potential toxic reactions to drugs. Genetics and ethnicity are becoming increasingly recognized for their importance in drug metabolism. For example, one of the major drug metabolic pathways utilizes the cytochrome P450 system, which has several isoforms. One such isoform, CYP2D6, is responsible for metabolizing almost 20–30% [28] of all drugs, and there are about 51 [29] known allelic variants of this isoform.

  In Caucasian individuals with CYP2D6*4 or *5 alleles, 12–21% [29] have problems metabolizing drugs that are substrates for CYP2D6.

  Fifty-one percent [29] of the alleles in the Asian population are the CYP2D6*10 allele, which has a proline substitution for serine at position 34. This leads to the improper folding of the protein, which in turn affects its stability. Patients with this mutation have a reduced ability to metabolize some drugs, such as neuroleptics and antidepressants.

  The CYP2D6*17 allele is seen in about 20–35% [29] of black Africans.

  About 10–16% [29] of the Semitic population (people from Ethiopia, Saudi Arabia, and the Middle East) are ultrarapid metabolizers because they have 2–13 copies of the functional gene, resulting in a very high amount of the enzyme. Individuals with these mutations often do not respond well to neuroleptics and antidepressants because they metabolize the drugs too fast.

28.2.2 Metabolism and Metabolites in Toxicology

Drug metabolism involves various enzymatic pathways and transport systems that can convert xenobiotics to a form that can be more readily excreted. Although the enzymes needed for drug metabolism are present in almost every tissue, the rate at which compounds can be metabolized in a given tissue depends on the amounts and types of metabolic enzymes present in that tissue. Compared to other organs, the liver has very high concentrations of drug-metabolizing enzymes, which are also present in the GI tract, kidneys, lungs, and skin.

While the major function of drug metabolism is to inactivate and eliminate foreign compounds from the body, it can also generate reactive compounds that

TABLE 28.1   Classification of Phase I and Phase II Reactions

Phase I	Phase II
Oxidation	Glucuronidation
Reduction	Sulfation
Hydrolysis	Acetylation
Hydration	Methylation
Dethioacetylation	Glutathione conjugation
Isomerization	Amino acid conjugation
	Fatty acid conjugation
	Condensation

may be harmful. The generation of electrophiles is of particular concern as they can react with cellular components such as DNA and RNA and induce genetic mutations. It is essential to carefully evaluate the advantages and disadvantages of administration prior to the use of any drug. In addition to conventional testing methods (LD_{50} and MTD in animals, and safety evaluations in preliminary human clinical trials), the newer fields of pharmacogenomics, toxicogenomics, and metabolomics are being used to assess the spectrum of metabolites generated and their potential toxicity prior to administration of an agent to human patients.

Drug metabolism generally occurs through two categories of enzymatic reactions: classified as either phase I or phase II reactions. Phase I reactions structurally alter the original compound and are often regarded as ones that prepare a xenobiotic for conjugation in phase II. Phase I reactions include oxidation, reduction, hydrolysis, hydroxylation, dethioacetylation, and isomerization reactions. Phase II reactions, which are catalyzed by enzymes found in hepatocytes, are usually conjugation reactions and involve the addition of a large bulky side group to a compound. In many cases, phase II reactions produce water-soluble and charged metabolites that have reduced biological activity and can readily be excreted in urine or bile. It is worthwhile to note that phase II reactions can precede phase I reactions. For example, the drug isoniazid undergoes phase II metabolism first and results in the formation of an *N*-acetyl conjugate, which can then undergo a phase I hydrolysis reaction [30]. Table 28.1 gives a summary of the phase I and phase II reactions. Figure 28.3 is a scheme that displays the fate of administered drugs.

Drug Metabolism: Effects on Efficacy and Toxicity of the Test Drug

Phase I Reactions   Phase I reactions are carried out by the mixed function oxidase (MFO) system. The most important MFO enzymes include the cytochrome P450s (CYP450). To date, the CYP450 MFO is regarded as the most powerful *in vivo* oxidizing system. This family of monooxygenases can be broken down into the liver microsomal MFO system and adrenal mitochondrial MFO system.

- The liver microsomal MFO system is made up of two components—NADPH cytochrome P450 reductase and cytochrome P450 (CYP450)—which are membrane-bound hemoproteins that use NADPH as a reducing agent and require molecular oxygen as well as FAD and FMN.

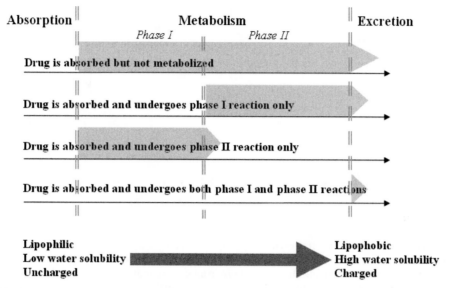

FIGURE 28.3   The fate of administered drugs. Drugs can be absorbed and undergo different fates but ultimately they are all excreted in urine, bile, or feces. As drugs are metabolized, they have decreased lipophilicity, increased water solubility, and increased charge.

- Instead of CYP450 reductase, the adrenal mitochondrial MFO system is made up of an iron–sulfur protein, adrenodoxin, and an adrenodoxin reductase. These two proteins are involved in transferring electrons from NADPH to CYP450 in steroid biosynthesis and bile metabolism. As such, the adrenal MFO system is not a major player in drug metabolism. However, it is important to note that, in the future, it may be necessary to make use of this system for specific agents, particularly to evaluate and optimize drugs that mimic endogenous steroids.

The liver microsomal MFO system catalyzes numerous reactions by transferring electrons from NADPH to CYP450. It does so by activating the iron component of CYP450, enabling the insertion of an oxygen atom into a substrate (drug). A scheme depicting this reaction appears in Fig. 28.4.

NADPH–CYP450 reductase catalyzes nonspecific reactions, and its main role is the transfer of electrons to CYP450 through the use of FAD and FMN. Thus, specificity depends on the different isoforms of the CYP450s. In humans, there are 57 CYP genes and 33 CYP pseudogenes, which can be divided into families and subfamilies. Table 28.2 [35] shows the relative abundance of some of the isoforms and their importance in drug metabolism. Substrate specificity is often hard to assess because one enzyme may be involved in more than one metabolic pathway and one pathway of drug metabolism can involve several different enzymes.

Although the CYP450 catalytic cycle is very important in drug metabolism, it can also create some problems, such as autooxidation. In this process, if the substrate cannot acquire the electrons properly, the system can generate superoxide anions, hydrogen peroxide, or water. This process is of major concern as the CYP450 system has a success rate ranging from 1% to 100%. The production of free radicals can

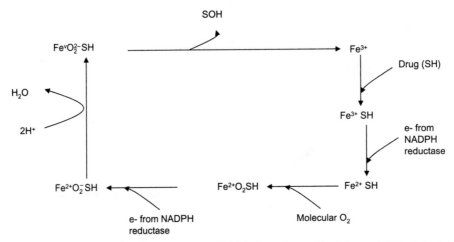

FIGURE 28.4 Drug (here represented by SH) binds to the oxidized form of CYP450, which accepts one electron from NADPH reductase. This reduced form can bind molecular oxygen. Another electron is added and the molecule rearranges to generate the oxidized form of the drug (here SOH), water, and the oxidized form of CYP450.

TABLE 28.2   Different Expression Levels of CYP450 and Their Contributions to Metabolism

Isoform	Percentage of Hepatic CYP450 Content	Isoforms	Percentage Contribution to Metabolism
3A	30	3A 4/5	36
2C	18	2D6	19
1A2	13	2C 8/9	16
2E1	7	1A2	11
2A6	4	2C19	8
2D6	1.5	2E1	4
2B6	0.2	2A6	4
Others	26.3	2B6	3

result in toxicity, and determination of possible reactive oxygen and nitrogen species that can be generated from the drug is important for predicting its toxicity.

Some phase I reactions do not involve the CYP450 MFO system, although these mostly represent reactions of endogenous compounds. However, they can be participants in drug metabolism. Following is a list of these types of reactions.

1. *Oxidations.*
(a) Alcohol oxidation is performed by alcohol dehydrogenase.
(b) Aldehyde oxidation is performed by aldehyde dehydrogenase and aldehyde oxidase.
(c) Xanthine oxidase is concerned with the metabolism of xanthine-containing drugs such as caffeine and allopurinol.

(d) Monoamine oxidase (A and B forms) will oxidatively deaminate primary, secondary, and tertiary amines.

(e) Flavin-containing monooxygenases (FMOs) can oxidize nitrogen-, sulfur-, and phosphorus-containing drugs, by using NADPH and molecular oxygen, in a similar manner as MFOs. However, FMOs will not catalyze the oxidation of negatively charged compounds such as organic acids.

(f) Peroxidase-dependent cooxidation is important in extrahepatic tissues, especially those with low CYP450 levels and activity. In this reaction, peroxidases couple the reduction of hydrogen peroxide and tissue hydroperoxide to the oxidation of other compounds.

2. *Reductions.* Other processes catalyze the reduction of azo compounds, nitro compounds, epoxides, heterocyclic ring compounds, and halogenated hydrocarbons. Examples of such reactions include the reduction of protonsil to triaminobenzene and sulfanilamide, and the successive reductions of nitrobenzene to nitrosobenzene to phenylhydroxylamine to aniline.

3. *Hydrolysis.* The addition of H_2O to compounds such as esters, amides, and carbamates by peptidases, amidases, and esterases results in the generation of new metabolites.

4. *Epoxide Hydrolase.* Epoxide hydrolases catalyze the hydration of epoxides. Since epoxides are known to be reactive species that can bind to DNA and RNA and thus induce mutations, epoxide hydrolase activity serves as a protective measure to decrease toxicity.

Phase II Reactions   As explained previously, phase II reactions usually consist of the addition of a bulky charged group to phase I reaction products to facilitate excretion of drugs. Phase II reactions also involve several enzymes that are capable of catalyzing a wide variety of reactions. Table 28.3 lists phase II reactions, their enzymes, and the functional groups involved.

1. *Glucuronidation.* Glucuronidation involves the addition of UDP glucuronic acid to the substrate and is catalyzed by UDP-glucuronyltransferases (UGTs), which are microsomal membrane-dependent enzymes. It is the main phase II reaction, as UDP glucuronic acid can bind to O, N, C, or S atoms. While UGTs seem to have low specificity in drug metabolism, their specificity increases when dealing with

TABLE 28.3   Summary of Phase II Reactions

Reaction	Enzyme	Functional Group
Glucuronidation	UDP-glucuronyltransferase	—OH, —COOH, —NH$_2$, —SH
Glycosidation	UDP-glycosyltransferase	—OH, —COOH, —SH
Sulfation	Sulfotransferase	—NH$_2$, —SO$_2$NH$_2$, —OH
Methylation	Methyltransferase	—OH, —NH$_2$
Acetylation	Acetyltransferase	—NH$_2$, SO$_2$NH$_2$, —OH, —COOH
Amino acid, glutathione, and fatty acid conjugation and condensation	Glutathione-*S*-transferase	Epoxide, organic halide, —OH, various

endogenous substrates. There are three subfamilies of UGT: UGT1A, UGT2A, and UGT2B, which contain the 15 known isoforms of UGT. While the liver is the main site of glucuronidation, other organs such as the stomach and kidneys have high levels of some UGT isoforms [31]. Drugs that undergo glucuronidation include morphine and codeine.

2. *Sulfation.* Sulfation plays an important role in drug metabolism, especially when phenols and phenol-containing compounds, alcohols, amines, thiols, and some steroids are present. Sulfotransferases (SULTs) catalyze the transfer of a sulfate moiety from 3′-phosphoadenosine 5′-phosphosulfate (PAPS, a cofactor) to the substrate. Since this sulfate moiety has a very low pK_a (~2), sulfate conjugates will be charged at physiologic pH values, making them more water soluble and rapidly excreted. Similar to UGTs, SULTs are mostly found in the liver, as well as extrahepatic organs. It is important to note that the availability of PAPS is a rate-limiting condition of sulfation reactions, and that while there are both membrane-bound and membrane-free forms of SULTs, only the membrane-free forms are involved in drug metabolism. To date, 10 isoforms of cytosolic SULTs have been identified, and all of them have been reported to participate in the activation of procarcinogens. Unstable esters are frequently formed, which can spontaneously rearrange, producing reactive electrophiles capable of binding to DNA and RNA. Drugs that undergo sulfation include ethanol, acetaminophen, dopamine, and minoxidil (Rogaine™).

3. *Acetylation.* Aromatic amines and sulfonamides are the most common substrates for acetylation by *N*-acetyltransferase (NAT). During this process, the acetyl group from acetyl coenzyme A is transferred to the drug substrate, which contains a primary amine, a hydroxyl, or a sulfhydryl group. Unlike glucuronidation and sulfation, acetylation does not produce conjugates that have improved water solubility and excretion. Drugs that undergo acetylation include isoniazid, *p*-aminobenzoic acid, and hydralazine. NATs can be classified as NAT1 or NAT2 and each are regulated independently of the other. Point mutations in NAT2 have been associated with polymorphisms seen in the metabolism of isoniazid, which is often used to identify rapid and slow acetylators. For example, a point mutation at Ile114Thr is often seen in Caucasians but very rarely in Orientals. The latter population has a mutation at nucleotide 857 of NAT2, which results in lower level of active enzyme. Ninety percent of North Africans and 50% of Caucasians are slow acetylators, while 10–30% of the Korean and Japanese populations are slow acetylators [32]. Such genetic polymorphisms will affect the dose response to drugs and increase drug toxicities in slow acetylators.

4. *Methylation.* Drugs that contain O, N, and S atoms can be methylated by methyltransferases, which can be classified into four groups—catechol-*O*-methyltransferase (COMT), phenol-*O*-methyltransferase (POMT), thiopurine *S*-methyltransferase (TPMT), and thiol methyltransferase (TMT). Although the reactions have high substrate specificity, the methyl donor is *S*-adenosyl-methionine (SAM), irrespective of which enzyme is used. Methylation, like acetylation, does not necessarily result in increased water solubility or excretion. Substrates that undergo methylation include histamine, *L*-dopa, and 6-mercaptopurine.

5. *Amino Acid Conjugation.* Drugs that contain a carboxyl group can be conjugated with amino acids in a two-step reaction that requires acyl CoA ligase and amino acid acyltransferase. One of the most important amino acid conjugations is

in bile metabolism. Amino acids such as glycine, glutamine, or taurine (nonprotein amino acid) can be conjugated with their substrates to form products that can be readily excreted in urine [33]. One example of an amino acid conjugation substrate is salicylic acid.

6. *Glutathione Conjugation.* Glutathione S-transferase (GST) catalyzes the conjugation reaction of some drugs with glutathione, which is a tripeptide in which glutamate is bonded to cysteine through the γ-COOH group of glutamate. The other amino acid present in this molecule is glycine. As glutathione (GSH) is a nucleophile, it can bind reactive electrophiles present in the body and thus plays an important protective role. While GSH can spontaneously react with reactive electrophiles, GST can increase the rate of this reaction, as it converts GSH into its active anionic form. Once GSH conjugates have been formed, they undergo other reactions through peptidase and acetylase activities, to mainly produce cysteine and mercapturate conjugates, which can then be excreted in urine. More than 20 GSTs have been discovered and they can be classified as either cytosolic or microsomal [34].

The cytosolic forms are more important for drug metabolism and can participate in conjugation, reduction, and isomerization reactions, while the microsomal forms interact with endogenous substrates. Although concentrations of GSH and GST are relatively high in cells, depletion of GSH can occur, leading to toxicity. For example, high doses of acetaminophen are toxic because the drug covalently binds to GSH and effectively depletes GSH from the system. Acetaminophen bioprocessing usually involves glucuronidation and sulfation reactions, but in high doses, these systems are overloaded and CYP450 starts to process the drug. This produces the toxic metabolite N-acetyl-p-benzoquinone imine (NAPQI) [35], which can attack cellular components. In most cases, NAPQI is eliminated by GSH, but in the case of overdose, there can be a decreased amount of GSH and thus hepatocellular necrosis and death can occur.

Similar to SULTs, NATs, and P450 enzymes, there are also GST polymorphisms. GST has five members (mu, alpha, pi, theta, and sigma). The mu (GSTM1*0) and theta (GSTT1*0) genotypes express a null phenotype, and in individuals with the GSTM1*0 allele (50% of the Caucasian population, ~60% in Chinese and Korean populations), it may indicate a genetic predisposition to lung, colon, and bladder cancers [36–38].

While GSH is usually protective, it has been shown that GST can lead to increased drug resistance to chemotherapeutic agents, possibly through the inhibition of MAP kinase activity and apoptosis [34], which are both mechanisms that are important for the action of many anticancer therapies. TLK199 is a GSH analogue that can produce a GSH inhibitor, TLK117, and thus decrease the effects of GSH on anticancer agents [34].

Drug Metabolism: Effects on Efficacy and Toxicity of Other Drugs   When more than one medication is taken by a patient, there is always a risk that the patient may suffer side effects that are due to the interaction between the different drugs. Drugs may compete for binding sites on plasma proteins or transporters, or can alter the activity of the metabolic enzymes (most notably the CYPs). For example, ketoconazole, used as an antifungal drug, is a potent inhibitor of several CYPs including CYP3A4. When drugs that use CYP3A4, such as anti-HIV viral protease inhibitors, are coadministered with ketoconazole, they cannot be metabolized and their plasma concentration increases, leading to toxicity [39, 40]. Some agents can also induce CYPs in a way to increase their own metabolism or to affect the metabolism of other drugs present in the body. For example, the herbal medicine St. John's wort will induce CYP3A4, leading to increased metabolism of other drugs such as oral contraceptives. The toxicity and efficacy of a drug can also be influenced by diet. For example, when the antihistamine terfenadine was taken with grapefruit juice, it led to arrhythmias. This was due to the fact that grapefruit juice contains furano-coumarins, which are inhibitors of CYP3A4, and terfenadine is a prodrug that requires this specific CYP for bioactivation. Terfenadine levels in the plasma would rise and cause arrhythmias [41].

Toxicokinetics, Toxicodynamics, and Toxicogenomics   In order to predict these types of toxicities, the past few decades have witnessed the exponential expansion of the boundaries of scientific knowledge. Core discoveries, such as DNA and its structure, as well as technical milestones including genetic engineering and initial quantification of cellular processes and their pathways, have been made. Such findings have triggered the evolution of drug evaluation and toxicology from its traditional aspects to one that now includes genetics. These discoveries have led to the development of toxicogenomics, pharmacogenomics, and better ways to study pharmacodynamics and toxicodynamics [42, 43].

In light of the discovery of the multiple enzyme isoforms that are present in metabolic pathways, such as the CYP450s, it is important to consider how genetic diversity plays a role in the metabolism and side effects of xenobiotics. The development of new techniques in the field of toxicogenomics is proving very useful in the elucidation of the genetic components of diseases. For example, by using nucleic acid microarrays, protein chips, and denaturing HPLC (DHPLC), one can identify pathways and mechanisms that are affected by administration of different agents. These methods allow the comparison between multiple nucleic acid sequences and their variants concurrently [42, 43]. This is particularly useful as toxicity is now being recognized as the result of multiple gene interactions, rather than a largely uncharacterized response within the entire body or within certain organ systems [42].

This new trend necessitates the investigation of genetic variability and its relation to phenotypic observations, as well as its importance in drug metabolism and subsequent toxicity. It is clear that toxicogenetics and pharmacogenetics will now play an integral part in drug development and are likely to be increasingly important in the future. Moreover, the use of these strategies by various methods can predict the patient response to treatment, thus helping physicians to select the most appropriate treatment options for individual patients that will improve the efficacy and minimize toxicity of the therapy [42–44].

28.2.3   Examples for Pharmacogenetics and Pharmacogenomics of Therapeutic Drugs

Example 1: 5-Fluorouracil   5-Fluorouracil (5-FU), an antimetabolite of pyrimidine, is commonly used in the treatment of head, neck, breast, ovarian, and gastrointestinal tract cancers [45–47]. However, it is associated with toxicities ranging from stomatitis, diarrhea, skin changes, myelosuppression, and neurological complications [45]. While these symptoms may be observed at standard doses of 5-FU, they have also been shown to be dependent on the dose and schedule of drug administration. A genetic basis to these toxic effects has also been discovered and is thought to be the main cause of the difference in toxicities between patients. The enzyme dihydropyrimidine dehydrogenase is responsible for the catabolism of 5-FU, converting it (about 85% of administered drug) [48] to its inactive and less toxic metabolite, dihydrofluorouracil, and increasing its excretion. 5-FU can also undergo an anabolic pathway, which accounts for its host and tumor toxicity. In patients, the aim is to achieve a balance between the two pathways to limit the amount of toxicity to normal tissues through the catabolic pathway, while not reducing the effects of its anabolic metabolites in tumor cells. However, this balance can be affected in patients who have a partial or complete deficiency of DPD [47]. The dihydropyrimidine dehydrogenase gene (*DPYD*) is known to have 39 alleles [49], and a point mutation at the DPYD*2A allele has been linked to deficiency in DPD [47, 50–52]. It is clear that the alteration in 5-FU metabolism can lead to toxicity to the host. The main factor involved in its toxicity is genetics, emphasizing the need for more accurate risk and safety assessments based on individual patient profiles.

Example 2: Thiopurine Methyltransferase Azathioprine and 6-mercaptopurine (6-MP) are immunosuppressant drugs that are used to treat and prevent reoccurrence of diseases such as acute lymphoblastic leukemia (ALL), inflammatory bowel disease (IBD), ulcerative colitis, rheumatoid arthritis, and organ rejection in transplant patients [53, 54]. The metabolism of these two drugs requires thiopurine methyltransferase (TPMT), which is a cytosolic enzyme that can catalytically methylate these drugs. TPMT has been found to have several alleles that can be used to classify the general population as normal/high, intermediate, and deficient methylators. In Caucasians, this accounts for 90%, 10%, and 0.3–0.6% of the population, respectively [47, 54]. Three main alleles have been linked to deficient methylators, namely, TPMP*20, TPMP*21, and TPMP*22 [54], and these result in a reduction in enzyme activity. Other alleles are also known to be involved in the deficiency (TPMT*2, *3A, *3B, *3C) [47]. This can lead to toxic accumulation of metabolites such as azathioprine and 6-MP along the thiopurine metabolic pathway. Hence, similar to Example 1, patient genetics greatly influence the toxicity of administered drugs.

28.2.4 Examples of the Link Between Toxicology of Drugs and Metabolism

Drug metabolism is vital to the bioactivation, inactivation, and eventual clearance of drugs, but it also represents a major source of toxicity. There are many naturally toxic parent compounds; however, a large portion of therapeutic drugs exert acute or chronic toxic effects only following metabolism. During the drug discovery process, it is important to carefully perform risk and safety assessments of drugs, and to keep in mind issues such as dose-dependent toxicity, species differences with respect to drug action, metabolism and toxicity, and long- and short-term toxicity, as well as reproductive toxicity. In addition to these factors, there are numerous others that affect the potential toxicity of a compound following metabolism. Some of these are listed in Table 28.4.

TABLE 28.4 Examples of Factors that Affect Metabolism and the Subsequent Toxicity of Drugs

Factor	Subclassification	Example
Identity of the compound	Innate toxicity of the parent compound	Vinca alkaloid compounds bind to and disrupt microtubules, resulting in cell cycle arrest [55].
	Presence of toxic constituent atoms or structures	Methoxyflurane releases free inorganic fluorine in the blood, leading to nephrotoxicity [56].
	Generation of free radicals	Many compounds lead to the generation of free radicals following metabolism (e.g., hydroquinones in cigarette tar lead to the production of free radicals and subsequent DNA damage) [57].
	Metabolism/ activation	Prodrugs (e.g., capecitabine) result in different toxicity compared to their parent compound (5-FU) [56].
Polypharmacy	Drug–drug interactions	Warfarin binds to albumin. When phenylbutazone is administered to the same patient, phenylbutazone competes for warfarin's binding site, displacing warfarin and causing the level of free warfarin in the plasma to increase [26].
	Activation or repression of enzyme activity	Drugs can influence the activity of metabolic enzymes, including cytochrome P450s. For example, ketoconazole inhibits CYP3A4. Anti-HIV protease inhibitors are also metabolized by CYP3A4. When the enzyme's activity is repressed, they cannot be metabolized, and their plasma concentration increases [31].
Host status	Genetics and ethnicity	There are 51 known allelic variants of CYP2D6 • 12–21% of Caucasians with CYP2D6*4 or CYP2D6*5 alleles have problems metabolizing 2D6 substrates. • Within the Asian population, the CYP2D6*10 allele leads to improper 2D6 protein folding, reducing the ability to metabolize neuroleptics and antidepressants. • About 10–16% of the Semitic population are ultra-rapid metabolizers because they have 2–13 copies of the functional gene [34].
	Age	Elderly patients have different expression and activity of metabolic enzymes compared to adults, and typically metabolize drugs more slowly [58].
	Concommittant disease	Various disease states can influence metabolism (e.g., cirrhosis, gastrointestinal disorders, hypertension) [59].
Epidemiological factors	Diet	Consumption of grapefruit juice by patients taking the antihistamine terfenadine led to arrhythmias because of high levels of terfenadine in the plasma due to CYP3A4 inhibition by furanocoumarins in the juice [31].
	Occupation	Many occupations can lead to exposure to activators/ repressors of metabolic enzymes (e.g., farmers are likely to experience increased exposure to pesticides) [27].

28.3 METHODS USED IN LINKING DRUG METABOLISM AND TOXICOLOGY

28.3.1 General Principles

As part of the regulatory process, toxicologists face the need for both qualitative and quantitative studies to assess hazardous risks versus benefits of substances that are potentially toxic. Qualitative studies provide the toxicologist with information about the possible hazardous effects of the toxicant via various exposure routes and at various doses. They also provide information about the mode of action, progression of toxic effects, and susceptibility of subjects to the agent [60–63]. To understand the biological factors that affect the dose–response curve, a quantitative relationship among the varying factors must be understood.

Modern toxicology has three key assumptions: (1) toxicity in humans can be predictively modeled in other organisms; (2) selection of an appropriate model is key to accurate prediction in humans; and (3) to understand the relevance to humans, you must understand the strengths and weaknesses of the model selected [60–64]. *In vivo, in vitro*, mathematical, and computer models (*in silico*) are all used to study the effects of metabolism on the toxicity of drugs and xenobiotic compounds. Table 28.5 shows the different methods used to assess the metabolism and toxicity of target drugs and their advantages and disadvantages.

TABLE 28.5 A Summary of the Systems and Methods Used to Evaluate Metabolism and Toxicity, and Their Advantages and Disadvantages

System	Examples	Acquisition	Maintenance	Expense	Human Correlation
In Vivo	Nonhuman primates	Difficult	Difficult	High	High
	Rodents	Easy	Easy	Low	Moderate–high
	Other mammals	Moderate	Moderate	Moderate	Moderate–high
	Nonmammalian models	Easy–moderate	Easy–moderate	Low–moderate	Low–moderate
	Lower animals	Easy	Easy	Low	Low–moderate
In Vitro	Primary cells	Moderate	Moderate–difficult	Low	Moderate (tissue dependent)
	Cancer cells	Easy	Easy–moderate	Low	Moderate (cell and study dependent)
	Isolated organs	Moderate–difficult	Difficult	Moderate	Moderate (cell and study dependent)
	Microsomes	Easy–moderate	Easy–moderate	Low–moderate	Low–moderate
	P450 kits	Easy	Easy	Low–moderate	Low–moderate
In Silico	Scaling	Easy–moderate	Easy–moderate	Low	Moderate (depends on model)
	QSAR	Moderate–difficult	Moderate–difficult	Moderate–high	Moderate, but improving
	PBBK	Moderate–difficult	Moderate–difficult	Moderate–high	Low–moderate, but improving
	BMD	Easy–moderate	Easy–moderate	Moderate–high	Moderate

28.3.2   *In Vivo* Models

In vivo modeling has long been the gold standard in toxicity testing, and extensive *in vivo* studies are still required prior to use of new agents in human clinical trials. *In vivo* models provide the ability to assess the actions or effects of particular drugs and their metabolites in an intact animal before human trials [60–64]. While other research models may provide useful information, only *in vivo* models provide the full picture of the pharmacokinetics, metabolism, and effects of the agent and its metabolites. In order to most effectively use animals for predicting human efficacy and toxicity, it is vitally important that the proper model is chosen.

Nonhuman Primates   Although they are the most closely related (genetically) to humans, nonhuman primates (most often chimpanzees, gibbons, macaques, and baboons) make up only a small percentage of the animals used for biomedical research. However, nonhuman primates are susceptible to many of the same diseases as humans, so primates are used for studies of surgery and diagnostics, as well as for studies of drug efficacy and toxicity of agents that cannot be accurately evaluated in other animals. The most common use for primates is to study new agents for the prevention and treatment of HIV/AIDS.

Nonrodent Mammalian Models   Many models are available for use in biomedical research, each serving to closely model different human systems. While not the most popular models, cats and dogs will continue to play a vital role in biomedical research and for toxicity and PK studies. Because of their similarity with human anatomy and physiology, dogs and cats make excellent models for some diseases and for evaluating toxicity to certain systems. Dogs are especially well suited to studies of compounds with potential cardiotoxicity. They are also frequently used to study renal toxicity of compounds due to their high incidence of kidney disease, and dogs have been a valuable source of preclinical data used to develop novel therapeutic agents [65]. Due to the similarity in anatomy and biochemistry of the cat brain to that of humans, cats have served as important models in the field of neurophysiology and synaptic response. Research using this model has also focused on leukemia, a disease shared by cats and humans, providing information important in understanding immunodeficiency and cancer [66]. Numerous other animals, including mini-pigs and ferrets, are used to study specific types of agents.

Rodent Models   Rodents are the most frequently used model for toxicology testing. Rodents have many advantages that make them valuable as an *in vivo* model system, including their small size, short gestation period, and ease of housing and care. Popular examples include hamsters, rats, and mice. Hamsters provide a model that is relatively free of spontaneous disease but is susceptible to several introduced pathogens. They also have a characteristic cheek pouch that provides an excellent site for the evaluation of proposed carcinogenic agents. Short life spans, rapid reproduction, and a virtual absence of spontaneous disease make the hamster a good model for reproductive toxicology. With gestation time of 15–18 days and a very regular estrus cycle of 4 days, the hamster has the shortest gestation time of all laboratory animals, giving it an advantage over other rodent models [67].

Rats are in the same subfamily as mice, Muridae. The majority of laboratory rats are domesticated varieties of the Norway rat. With their well-defined genetic makeup, this extensively used model has been purpose-bred to be susceptible to specific human diseases, such as hypertension. A wide variety of transgenic and chemically induced rat disease models are also available for laboratory use. Additionally, rats have a ridge that covers the opening of the esophagus, making them unable to vomit. This enables rats to be used for extensive oral/ingestion toxicity studies. Rats are the most commonly used animal to test median lethal doses (LD_{50}).

Disadvantages to the use of rats compared to mice include their size (requiring larger amounts of test compounds compared to mice) and longer life span. Additionally, while the rat genome has been studied extensively, the mouse genome is more well defined. In addition, the rat's blood supply to the heart makes it a poor model for heart-related studies.

The mouse model is the most frequently used model in *in vivo* research. Mouse subspecies origins can be traced back to the beginning of human civilization when mice became commensal with human settlements [68]. Coat color mutations of mice have been noted and recorded for millennia, with widespread domestication of the mouse by the 1700s [68]. Haldane's report in 1915 began the genetic mapping of the mouse. Haldane described the linkage between pink-eye color and albino loci that were later defined as part of mouse chromosome 7. Knowledge of the mouse genome grew slowly over the next 50 years until the discovery of recombinant DNA technology. By 2002, 96% of the mouse genome had been sequenced, leading researchers to even further specialize the mouse model.

There are now a wide variety of mouse models available for evaluating the efficacy and toxicity of compounds for various diseases including cancer, diabetes, lupus, and infectious diseases. Even for just the study of cancer, there are thousands of possible models, including xenograft models (where human tumor cells are injected subcutaneously into immunocompromised animals), syngeneic models (where mouse cancer cells are implanted subcutaneously into normal or immunocompromised mice), transgenic models (with overexpression or targeted knockout of specific gene expression), and chemically induced models (where agents with proven carcinogenic activity are administered to animals in order to determine whether the formation of tumors can be slowed or prevented).

While rabbits are not technically rodents, they are often grouped within the same category. Rabbits have been used at length in biomedical testing as well as in consumer product safety testing. Rabbits are easy to handle, and their large ear veins make blood collection easily accessible. The rabbit, like the rat, does not have the ability to vomit. Extensive evaluations of atherosclerosis and potential therapies for atherosclerosis have been done in rabbits because studies have demonstrated that they develop lesions similar to human fatty streaks when fed a high fat diet [69]. The rabbit model is also often used in irritation testing that is required by law for certain consumer products. Rabbits are also used to evaluate pyrogenicity and muscle irritation by medical devices that are administered parenterally [64].

Guinea pigs were once a very popular subject for scientific research; however, they are used with much less frequency than other rodent models today. While in the past they were used for a variety of studies, including the development of a vaccines and antiviral agents, guinea pigs are now most commonly used to study sensitivity and hypersensitivity to agents for toxicity testing and for studying potential preventive and therapeutic approaches for juvenile diabetes and preeclampsia

[70, 71]. Mice and rats are now used for most of the studies that were previously done in guinea pigs.

Nonmammalian Models   While they are not currently used as a primary model for evaluating new therapeutic agents, fish (especially zebrafish, *Danio rerio*) represent an excellent model for studying embryonic development and exposure to environmental toxicants and are gaining in favor for evaluating pharmaceutical agents [72]. The zebrafish genome is well characterized, and many transgenic and genetically modified fish have been generated [73]. Moreover, it is possible to inject antisense oligonucleotides or siRNA into embryonic fish to generate fish with knocked down genes. Like rodents, the small fish are inexpensive, easy to breed, and relatively easy to maintain. However, given that they are not mammals, they do not represent an accurate translational model for all types of toxicity testing.

Other animals, including avian models (most frequently chickens and embryonic chicks) and frogs (*Xenopus laevis* and other *Xenopus* species) are also frequently used to study embryonic development and gene function [74, 75]. The genetics of these other animals are still being determined (although the *Xenopus* genome has been fairly well characterized), although animals with gene mutations or polymorphisms have been obtained for many species. However, because their genome is not as well characterized as that of other research animals, and because they do not possess some of the anatomical features of mammals, these models are less frequently used for drug development and evaluation.

Finally, lower organisms, including fruit flies (*Drosophila melanogaster*) and roundworms (*Caenorhabitis elegans*) are also being used to study gene function and could provide novel models for toxicity testing. The advantage of these models is that they have been extensively characterized, with the *C. elegans* genome being the first to be completely sequenced, and with all of its cells having been studied and mapped [76, 77]. Drosophila are also frequently subjected to gene manipulation to study gene function and development. Both of these lower organisms are easily bred and maintained in labs and, given their relative simplicity, can facilitate studies of reproductive and developmental toxicity. However, while they represent excellent models for some studies, the use of these models for drug design and evaluation studies is limited.

Despite their many advantages, the use of animals is generally costly, can be controversial, and is not necessarily correlative with human results. Other *in vitro* and computer modeling systems are being used to evaluate the toxicity of compounds and are especially useful for preliminary studies so that fewer animals will be required.

28.3.3   *In Vitro* Models

In addition to the above disadvantages, there are increasing numbers of compounds that need to be screened. Therefore, faster and less expensive models of toxicity evaluation have been established. The use of *in vitro* models for the screening of cytotoxic drugs began in the 1940s with the development of nitrogen mustard derivatives. With the development of chemically defined media in the 1950s, qualitative evaluations in cells grown as monolayers in Petri dishes became easier, and by using protein dyes, dose–response relationships could be determined [78].

Compounds affect cells directly in *in vitro* systems until medium containing compound is removed, allowing observation of direct toxic effects [79]. The advances in *in vitro* methods have allowed for elucidation of many of the mechanisms underlying clinical toxicity. Moreover, in many cases there is a high degree of correlation between the results obtained from animal studies and cell culture studies, providing an alternative to animal models. This allows for both high throughput screening and decreased use of laboratory animals.

The use of *in vitro* models is now generally well accepted as a means of prescreening for toxicity. In early stages, *in vitro* models can assist drug design via permeability (barrier penetration) assays and structure–activity relationships. The preliminary *in vitro* models often are used to decide the fate of compounds and whether they will be selected to continue in the development pipeline.

In vitro toxicity testing can involve everything from bacteria or yeast, to isolated organ preparations or embryos, to cultured human or animal cells. Isolated organ preparations were among the first systems used for *in vitro* toxicity studies. While the data from isolated organ studies may be the most similar to the *in vivo* situation, the nature of these types of studies (require animals, often laborious surgical procedures, and there is often large variation between samples) largely negates their usefulness. Similarly, the use of embryos is labor intensive and not practical for studying anything other than developmental toxicity. Rather, cultured cells (immortalized or isolated and cultured from primary tissue sources) now are the most commonly used model for *in vitro* studies. For example, hepatocytes can be used to evaluate hepatotoxicity, and other cell types (such as endothelial cells or colon cells) can be used to determine whether a drug is likely to enter the bloodstream, to be absorbed by oral administration, or to cross the blood–brain barrier.

28.3.4 Human Cells *In Vitro*

Human Tissues In Vitro   Special consideration must be given to the use of human tissue or primary human cells in *in vitro* modeling. *In vitro* modeling using human tissue could offer valuable preclinical research data and possibly increased safety, but there are still numerous legal and ethical issues involved in the use of human tissues [80, 81]. Improvements in cell culture techniques, along with increasing availability of human tissues, have led to increased use of human primary and immortalized cells in toxicology and pharmacodynamic studies [82]. Human *in vitro* models are being used with physiological models to predict quantitative metabolism, transport, clearance, and pharmacodynamic outcome [82]. The use of human cells may be able to tease apart differences between human responses and animal responses, including differential expression and activity of genes involved in detoxification or in converting drugs to toxic metabolites.

Various methods exist for evaluating the effects of compounds on cells, including methods to evaluate viability (trypan blue staining), proliferation (MTT or MTS assays, BrdUrd incorporation), apoptosis (Annexin-V staining/flow cytometry), and cell cycle progression (propidium iodide staining/flow cytometry) [5, 83]. Due to the ease of isolation of proteins, DNA, and RNA from cells, cell culture also lends itself to evaluation of effects on individual molecular targets. Of particular importance are gene arrays, which allow changes in numerous genes to be observed and quantitated together from a small sample. While the resulting array data are incredibly complex, better statistical methods and data mining software are allowing for inter-pretation of the effects of compounds and metabolites on gene expression, and vice versa.

Primary Cell Cultures   Primary cell cultures are prepared directly from tissue removed from an organism during biopsy or necropsy. As a result, primary cultures have high variability in the types of cells that can grow from a given sample. The well-differentiated heterogeneous nature of primary cell culture allows for it to retain many complex biochemical properties of the tissue of origin [64]. However, cell viability is variable and depends on factors such as damage to the cell mem-brane, cell isolation (anoikis), and the nutrients, growth factors, and hormones avail-able in the media. While heterogeneous cultures are sometimes desirable, more often, single cell types (e.g., B lymphocytes) are required. Many cells can be extracted or purified from heterogeneous samples using gating procedures that eliminate or allow for the passage of cells with expression of certain surface proteins [64]. Other cells can be selected for by the type of container and medium in which they are grown. As a result of individual genetics, the growth kinetics differ between cultures, making results obtained from primary cultures difficult to reproduce. Other com-plications encountered with primary cell lines are their finite life span in culture and the loss of specific cell functions and metabolic capabilities [64].

Permanent and Immortalized Cell Lines   Most *in vitro* systems are established with permanent cell lines, which will grow consistently in culture. Often derived from primary cell line subcultures, permanent cell lines will form continuous diploid or clonal lines that will grow consistently for extended periods of time. Of the popu-lation of diploid cells, at least 75% of the culture will contain the same complement genetic material as the host organism [64]. These cells can typically undergo approxi-mately 40–50 divisions in culture.

Continuous cell lines often originate from tumor cells. Spontaneous or induced transformation (e.g., via infection with Epstein–Barr virus) of a primary cell line results in a cell line that is immortalized. Immortalized cells retain many, but not all, of the characteristics of the primary cells from which they are derived. Transfor-mation can often result in genetic differences from the tissue of origin, including a heteroploid or aneuploid karotype [64]. However, most of the immortalized and tumor-derived cell lines are actually clonal. Clonal cell lines are formed from a genetically homogeneous subline through single cell isolation. Through reisolation and cloning, genetic drift is minimized and the homogeneity of the cell line can be maintained. Via selection media, desirable phenotypes or markers can be selected for. Transformed cells and established tumor cell lines can grow indefinitely and often can grow in suspension since the cells have lost their need for attachment [64].

Cell-Free Systems   Still other *in vitro* systems exist (in addition to cell cultures, and isolated organ or embryo cultures) for evaluating drug metabolism and the presence of potentially toxic metabolites. These typically involve incubation of the target drug with metabolic enzymes or tissues expressing the enzymes. Incubation of a drug with microsomes (isolated vesicles containing metabolic enzymes) can indicate the likely metabolites of the drug [84]. Microsome studies can also be used to assess differences in metabolism of compounds by mutant enzymes or different enzyme isoforms or to assess whether certain compounds activate or repress the activity of the metabolic enzymes [85]. While whole hepatocytes can also be used, isolated microsomes allow for easier examination of the metabolism of a compound by specific enzymes and complexes. However, microsomes do not contain phase II enzymes [86], so results obtained from microsome studies should be considered carefully. In some cases, it may be preferable to use whole hepatocyte preparations, which contain both phase I and II enzymes [86].

To evaluate the effects on particular cytochrome P450 enzymes, or to determine which enzymes metabolize a drug, there are also kits available containing preparations of specific P450 enzymes (available from Human Biologics International, BD Biosciences, Sigma-Aldrich, and others). While not necessarily reflective of what occurs *in vivo*, these kits and microsome preparations are an excellent way to collect preliminary data on likely metabolites of new drugs.

28.3.5 *In Silico* Models

With the advances in technology in the last few decades, the development of *in silico* (computer-based) testing offers a vast array of toxicity testing requiring small sample sizes [87]. While traditional predictive scaling models utilize equations to determine starting and likely maximum doses for more advanced studies, newer *in silico* studies use computer simulations to model the interaction of various compounds with important receptors and to predict efficacy and toxicity. Computer-aided models focus on replacing animal models in toxicity testing through structure-based techniques, quantitative structure–activity relationship (QSAR) methodologies, and PBBK (physiologically based biokinetic) modeling [88]. Preliminary testing has been very promising. QSAR can be used for a wide range of toxicity endpoints including lethality [89–91]. The results of QSAR analysis continue to improve as more compounds are evaluated and can be compared. PBBK can be used to predict toxicity by simulating the kinetic behavior of the compound of interest using available data. Systems biology attempts to use the interaction of the complete system, that is, metabolic, regulatory, signaling, and transport processes. By understanding the interactions between small molecules and their targets, models should be able to better predict toxic effects of test compounds. Besides reducing the number of animals needed in toxicity testing, reliable *in silico* testing could also predict and prevent failure of a compound in later phases of development [90, 91].

Mathematical modeling of toxicity often involves the use of a dose–response model to define the benchmark dose (BMD) that will give a standard response. The user-friendly BMD software is readily available and is a good tool for establishing a reference point/point of departure within an observable dose range [92]. BMD can be applied with as few as two dose groups and one control group, and it makes use of all data points on a dose–response curve.

The major limitation of these alternative models is data reliability. The toxicity predicted through the use of computer simulations is only as accurate as the data used. However, as the state of the science improves through the resolution of dynamic protein structures, more defined metabolic pathways, and characterized genetic variations within the human population, it is likely that *in silico* technology will also improve.

Traditional toxicity testing involved large numbers of animals and it was often impossible to predict the type of toxicity that would result. Current toxicity testing in animals has been greatly streamlined, partly by the use of *in silico* and *in vitro* models to predict possible target organs and useful endpoints. It is likely that as our knowledge of genetics and pharmacogenetics improves, our use of animal models will be further streamlined, and results from the few animal studies that are done will allow more accurate prediction of human toxicity. While it is likely that the number of animals used can be further decreased, it is unlikely that it will ever be possible to completely avoid their use. No other research model can provide investigators with so much information or can reproduce the complex environment found within a living animal.

Fortunately, however, as more data is generated using these various *in vitro, in vivo,* and *in silico* models, it will become easier to develop an understanding of the SARs that exist among different drugs and classes of molecules. This will then facilitate the *in silico* studies, further eliminating the need for using a large number of animals. Combined, all of these technologies will help to ensure that unsafe and ineffective agents do not enter into human clinical trials, thus saving human lives, preserving human quality of life, and guarding the bottom line for the companies developing novel agents.

28.3.6 Predictive Models

Recently, significant progress has been made in predictive toxicology that, from a chemistry perspective, uses a structure–activity relationship (SAR) built on available test data (chemical characteristics, pharmacokinetics, pharmacodynamics, metabolism, toxicity, toxicokinetics, pharmacogenetics, pharmacogenomics, gene profiling, metabolomics, and bioassays) to predict the potential biological activity (e.g., toxicity) of a chemical /drug based solely on its molecular structure and computed properties. Of note, the predictive value of any predictive toxicology approaches that are based on SAR modeling are entirely dependent on and limited by the availability, quality, and quantity of the reference data. In the field of linking metabolism and toxicology, the basic data for SAR modeling include, but are not limited to, the following:

- *In vitro* and *in vivo* toxicology studies
- Characteristics of the chemicals/drugs and their analogues
- *In vitro* and *in vivo* metabolic studies
- *In vivo* and *in vitro* pharmacology screening
- *In vitro* and *in vivo* pharmacology profiling
- Biomarkers/experimental endpoints
- Human accidental exposure studies

Among these data, the following characteristics are particularly important:

- Dose–effect relationship
- Dose–response relationship
- *In vitro/in vivo* relationship

- Therapeutic index/window
- Interspecies scaling

To predict biological activities from chemical structure, there are many computational approaches and programs available; interested readers are directed to several excellent recent reviews [93–96]. Such approaches have proven capabilities when applied to well-defined toxicity endpoints or well-documented metabolic pathways. However, these approaches are less suited to the challenges of global toxicity prediction, that is, for predicting the potential toxicity of structurally diverse chemicals across a wide range of endpoints of regulatory and pharmaceutical concern. In this field, there are several major trends improving the predictive values of the models:

- Large-scale data generation involving more fundamental, interdisciplinary technologies such as systems biology, genomics, proteomics, and metabolomics.
- Increasing public information resources to support these efforts.
- In-depth, well-focused mechanistic studies on chemical biology and toxicology using advanced molecular and genetic approaches (e.g., gene transfer, gene knockout, transgenic animal models) and analytical methods (e.g., real-time quantitative PCR, gene arrays, LC/MS, MS/MS).

Figure 28.5 illustrates a systems approach for SAR modeling to predict the linkage between metabolism and toxicology. The role of bioinformatics (Fig. 28.5)

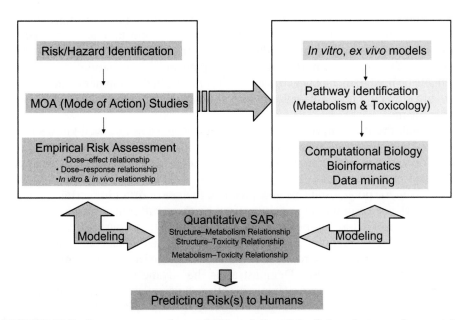

FIGURE 28.5   Systems approaches to SAR modeling of the linkage between drug metabolism and toxicity.

in toxicology data analysis and data mining is critical to SAR modeling, including the following: (1) increasing standardization and digitization of available toxicity data and migration of these data into the public domain; (2) establishing database standards and models that facilitate data integration and mining for both historical and new findings; and (3) linking these toxicology data with chemical structures, leading to hypothesis-driven SAR modeling. Of note, the predictive value of a SAR model should ultimately be confirmed by experimental or clinical data.

28.4 TOXICITY/METABOLISM IN DRUG DEVELOPMENT

28.4.1 Toxicity, Toxicogenomics, and Metabolism

One of the most important steps in preclinical drug development is the evaluation of the metabolism and toxicity of the compound. Many effective drugs fail during toxicity testing. As recent events in the news have shown, the toxicity of compounds is often difficult to predict using traditional toxicity testing. Even extensive animal studies do not give the full picture of toxicity. Moreover, while clinical trials give the most accurate prediction of the response of patients, there are still frequently problems when the new agent is used in a larger population. Depending on the risk–benefit ratio, some toxic agents are still useable, but major toxicity not only costs the pharmaceutical industry time and money that would have been better used for other drugs in the pipeline, but can also result in life-threatening toxicity for patients.

Even when the majority of a population does not experience any major toxicity from a compound, there are genetic variations to important metabolic enzymes (i.e., the cytochrome P450s) that can result in increased or decreased metabolism of a drug, leading to decreased efficacy or increased toxicity. Preclinical testing, including computer modeling, and especially cell culture will be important as more becomes known about the human genome. Pharmacogenomics and toxicogenomics (which study the effect of genes on the efficacy, metabolism, and toxicity of compounds) will likely be used to dictate which agents will continue in development, and whether there are subpopulations of patients who should be cautioned against the use of certain agents.

Although the P450 enzymes may be the most important and well-known metabolic enzymes, there are many others that can affect drug pharmacokinetics and dynamics and can result in otherwise unforeseen toxicity, including examples mentioned in Section 28.2 [50, 54].

While genetic polymorphisms may preclude the use of drugs for certain patients, prior knowledge of potential toxicity caused by these differences can save human lives and ensure that a therapeutic agent can remain in the clinic for other patients. As mentioned, certain mutations within the DPYD gene (which codes for dihydropyrimidine dehydrogenase) result in life-threatening toxicity for patients administered a routine dose of 5-FU. Demonstrating the advances in genetics, molecular biology, and instrumentation, a simple breath test using ^{13}C-labeled uracil was developed that can detect patients who are likely to have DPYD mutations. These patients can be administered alternative therapies while their genotype is confirmed using other methods, such as DHPLC (denaturing HPLC) [97].

28.4.2 "Omics," Toxicology, and Risk Assessment

Being able to predict major toxicity, either for all patients or for certain subsets of patients, could result in saved lives and can lead to a more efficient drug development program. Pharmacogenomics and toxicogenomics can help predict the overall toxicity of compounds and can be used for screening certain subpopulations who may have metabolic differences that could lead to toxicity or inefficacy. In this way, clinical trials and subsequent large-scale use of new agents could be tailored to decrease toxicity and increase efficacy for patients.

Evaluating toxicogenomics and pharmacogenomics is becoming a trend among pharmaceutical companies. For example, Bristol-Myers Squibb started a Department of Applied Genomics in 2001 to evaluate pharmacogenomics and toxicogenomics. Most other major pharmaceutical companies are following suit. Although still in its infancy, pharmacogenomics and toxicogenomics programs have the potential to improve drug development programs by eliminating compounds earlier in the program, allowing more money to be invested in the development of other compounds.

The toxicogenomics "revolution" was sparked by the advent of microarray technology. These arrays utilize small samples of cDNA from cells or tissues to determine the effect of compounds on gene expression [98, 99]. By examining the types of genes that are up- or downregulated by a given compound, it is possible to predict whether a compound might be toxic, and to gain insight into the type of toxicity it causes (e.g., oxidative stress) [99].

Nevertheless, changes at the gene expression level are not necessarily sufficient for assessing the potential risks of new compounds. Often, while there are no changes in gene transcription, there are alterations in protein expression, stability, or activity level. Moreover, different pathways may be activated even while expression levels remain the same. Hence, other "omics" technologies are necessary to more effectively evaluate the effects of a given compound. Proteomics, typically evaluated using two-dimensional (2D) electrophoresis gels (where proteins are separated by charge and then by molecular weight) and mass spectroscopy, can be used to evaluate the expression level and, to a degree, the posttranslational modifications made to numerous proteins. Enzyme assays are usually required to determine the activity of proteins. The newer field of metabolomics (or metabonomics) evaluates the relationship between the genetic profile of an organism/cell and the complement of small molecules present in the plasma/serum or tissues/cells following administration of the agent. Combining all of these "omics" strategies can lead to a more global picture of the response of cells, tissues, or animals to new compounds, can define which genes are important for processing and reacting to the compound, and can be used to predict potential problems with efficacy, resistance, and toxicity.

28.4.3 Future Directions

One of the most exciting outcomes of toxicogenomics is the potential to predict the type of toxicity that may result from administration of a particular agent. Along with this is the ability to determine potential biomarkers that can be used to assess the risk for individual patients. In addition to the already known polymorphisms (i.e., to the cytochrome P450 enzymes), gene and protein expression levels at baseline and following preliminary dosing (using a lower dose of the agent) can be used to determine whether a particular patient is likely to respond to the agent or is especially sensitive to the compound, potentially leading to toxicity. Biomarkers can also be used to detect whether a patient has been exposed to an environmental toxicant [100].

The "omics" studies also present several ethical issues. In addition to perhaps leading to a mandate for more individualized therapy, or at least a screening for polymorphisms in the most common and important metabolic enzymes, there are many other potential applications for "omics" data. For example, toxicogenomics data could be used to predict whether an individual would be more/less sensitive to toxic chemicals. These data could be used to determine which individuals would be allowed to engage in work where exposure could occur [101]. While this type of practice could prevent toxicity due to exposure to common chemicals, it would also constitute a new (and still legal in some states) type of employment discrimination. It may become necessary to pass federal legislation banning discrimination on the basis of genetic information.

On a more basic level, "omics" studies can provide insight into the complex reactions within living organisms. While none of the *in silico*, *in vitro*, or *in vivo* models are currently sufficient for determining the potential metabolites and toxicity of a compound, the addition of pharmacogenomics, toxicogenomics, and metabolomics may result in a more accurate picture of the toxicity of the compound in humans.

In conclusion, while advances have been made in the fields of toxicology, pharmacology, and molecular biology, there is still a lot of work yet to be done in order to make the drug development process faster, easier, and more effective. Study of the toxicity of both the parent compound and its metabolites can be greatly facilitated by examining the interplay between the genome of the experimental model or patient and the agent being administered. Moreover, when the full spectrum of metabolites is known, a more accurate picture of the toxicity and pharmacokinetics of the agent can be derived. With advances in our knowledge about disease processes, new technology, data processing, and statistical analysis, the evaluation of the toxicity of new agents will become faster and more accurate.

ACKNOWLEDGMENTS

We would like to thank Dr. Donald Hill, Ms. Kajal Buckoreelall, Ms. Scharri Ezell, and Ms. Angela Venn for their excellent assistance in preparation of this chapter. The work is partially supported by NIH/NCI grants (R01CA80698, R01CA112029, and R01CA121211) and a DoD Prostate Cancer Research Program grant (W81XWH-06-1-0063).

REFERENCES

1. Rayburn E, Wang H, He J, Zhang R. RNA silencing technologies in drug discovery and target validation. *Lett Drug Des Discov* 2005;2:1–18.
2. Que-Gewirth NS, Sullenger BA. Gene therapy progress and prospects: RNA aptamers. *Gene Ther* 2007;14:283–291.

3. Zhang Z, Wang H, Li M, Rayburn E, Agrawal S, Zhang R. Novel MDM2 p53-independent functions identified through RNA silencing technologies. *Ann NY Acad Sci* 2005;1058:205–214.

4. Walker DK. The use of pharmacokinetic and pharmacodynamic data in the assessment of drug safety in early drug development. *Br J Clin Pharmacol* 2004;58(6):601–608.

5. Wang H, Cai Q, Zeng X, Yu D, Agrawal S, Zhang R. Anti-tumor activity and pharmacokinetics of a mixed-backbone antisense oligonucleotide targeted to RIα subunit of protein kinase A after oral administration. *Proc Natl Acad Sci USA* 1999;96: 13989–13994.

6. Wang H, Rayburn E, Wang W, Kandimalla ER, Agrawal S, Zhang R. Immunomodulatory oligonucleotides as novel therapy for breast cancer: pharmacokinetics, *in vitro* and *in vivo* anti-cancer activity and potentiation of antibody therapy. *Mol Cancer Ther* 2006;5(8):2106–2114.

7. Welling PG. Differences between pharmacokinetics and toxicokinetics. *Toxicol Pathol* 1995;23(2):143–147.

8. Watanabe PG. Toxicokinetics in the evaluation of toxicity data. *Regul Toxicol Pharmacol* 1988;8(4):408–413.

9. Pander J, Gelderblom H, Guchelaar HJ. Insights into the role of heritable genetic variation in the pharmacokinetics and pharmacodynamics of anticancer drugs. *Expert Opin Pharmacother* 2007;8:1197–1210.

10. Goldstein DB, Need AC, Singh R, Sisodiya SM. Potential genetic causes of heterogeneity of treatment effects. *Am J Med* 2007;120(4 Suppl 1):S21–S25.

11. Mattison LK, Johnson MR, Diasio RB. A comparative analysis of translated dihydropyrimidine dehydrogenase cDNA; conservation of functional domains and relevance to genetic polymorphisms. *Pharmacogenetics* 2002;12:133–144.

12. Nicholson JK, Lindon JC, Holmes E. "Metabonomics": understanding the metabolic responses of living systems to pathophysiological stimuli via multivariate statistical analysis of biological NMR spectroscopic data. *Xenobiotica* 1999;29:1181–1189.

13. Thomas CE, Ganji G. Integration of genomic and metabonomic data in systems biology—are we "there" yet? *Curr Opin Drug Discov Dev* 2006;9:92–100.

14. Robertson DG, Reily MD, Baker JD. Metabonomics in preclinical drug development. *Expert Opin Drug Metab Toxicol* 2005;1:363–376.

15. Robertson DG, Reily MD, Sigler RE, Wells DF, Paterson DA, Braden TK. Metabonomics: evaluation of nuclear magnetic resonance (NMR) and pattern recognition technology for rapid *in vivo* screening of liver and kidney toxicants. *Toxicol Sci* 2000;57: 326–337.

16. Nicholls AW, Holmes E, Lindon JC, Shockcor JP, Farrant RD, Haselden JN, Damment SJ, Waterfield CJ, Nicholson JK. Metabonomic investigations into hydrazine toxicity in the rat. *Chem Res Toxicol* 2001;14:975–987.

17. Connor SC, Wu W, Sweatman BC, Manini J, Haselden JN, Crowther DJ, Waterfield CJ. Effects of feeding and body weight loss on the ^{1}H-NMR-based urine metabolic profiles of male Wistar Han rats: implications for biomarker discovery. *Biomarkers* 2004;9: 156–179.

18. Lindon JC, Holmes E, Nicholson JK. Metabonomics in pharmaceutical R&D. *FEBS J* 2007;274:1140–1151.

19. Bailey NJ, Oven M, Holmes E, Nicholson JK, Zenk MH. Metabolomic analysis of the consequences of cadmium exposure in Silene cucubalus cell cultures via ^{1}H NMR spectroscopy and chemometrics. *Phytochemistry* 2003;62:851–858.

20. Griffin JL. Metabonomics: NMR spectroscopy and pattern recognition analysis of body fluids and tissues for characterisation of xenobiotic toxicity and disease diagnosis. *Curr Opin Chem Biol* 2003;7:648–654.

21. Makinen VP, Soininen P, Forsblom C, Parkkonen M, Ingman P, Kaski K, Groop PH, Ala-Korpela M, FinnDiane Study Group. Diagnosing diabetic nephropathy by ^{1}H NMR metabonomics of serum. *MAGMA* 2006;19:281–296.

22. Pelkonen O, Raunio H. *In vitro* screening of drug metabolism during drug development: Can we trust the predictions? *Expert Opin Drug Metab Toxicol* 2005;1:49–59.

23. Posey JA, Wang H, Hamilton J, Delgrosso A, Zhang R, Freda T, Zamboni WC. Phase-I dose escalation and sequencing study of docetaxel and continuous infusion topotecan in patients with advanced malignancies. *Cancer Chemother Pharmacol* 2005;56:182–188.

24. Wang H, Wang Y, Rayburn ER, Hill DL, Rinehart JJ, Zhang R. Dexamethasone as a chemosensitizer for breast cancer chemotherapy: potentiation of the antitumor activity of adriamycin, modulation of cytokine expression, and pharmacokinetics. *Int J Oncol* 2007;30:947–953.

25. Muguruma M, Nishimura J, Jin M, Kashida Y, Moto M, Takahashi M, Yokouchi Y, Mitsumori K. Molecular pathological analysis for determining the possible mechanism of piperonyl butoxide-induced hepatocarcinogenesis in mice. *Toxicology* 2006;228:178–187.

26. Daher GC, Zhang R, Soong S-J, Diasio RB. Circadian variation of pyrimidine catabolizing enzymes in rat liver: possible relevance to 5-fluorodeoxyuridine chemotherapy. *Drug Metab Dispos* 1991;19:285–287.

27. Zhang R, Lu Z, Diasio R, Liu T, Soong S-J. The time of administration of 3'-azido-3'-deoxythymidine (AZT) determines its host toxicity with possible relevance to AZT chemotherapy. *Antimicrob Agents Chemother* 1993;37:1771–1776.

28. Ingelman-Sundberg M. Pharmacogenetics of cytochrome P450 and its applications in drug therapy: the past, present and future. *Trends Pharmacol Sci* 2004;25:193–200.

29. Eichelbaum M, Ingelman-Sundberg M, Evans WE. Pharmacogenomics and individualized drug therapy. *Annu Rev Med* 2006;57:119–137.

30. Sharer JE, Shipley LA, Vandenbranden MR, Binkley SN, Wrighton SA. Comparisons of phase I and phase II *in vitro* hepatic enzyme activities of human, dog, rhesus monkey, and cynomolgus monkey. *Drug Metab Dispos* 1995;23:1231–1241.

31. Fisher MB, Paine MF, Strelevitz TJ, et al. The role of hepatic and extrahepatic UDP-glucuronosyltransferases in human drug metabolism. *Drug Metab Rev* 2001;33:273–297.

32. Zang Y, Zhao S, Doll MA, States JC, Hein DW. The T341C (Ile114Thr) polymorphism of *N*-acetyltransferase 2 yields slow acetylator phenotype by enhanced protein degradation. *Pharmacogenetics* 2004;14:717–723.

33. Rendic S. Summary of information on human CYP enzymes: human P450 metabolism data. *Drug Metab Rev* 2002;34:83–448.

34. http://www.merck.com/mrkshared/mmanual/section22/chapter298/298e.jsp.

35. Hinson JA, Reid AB, McCullough SS, James LP. Acetaminophen-induced hepatotoxicity: role of metabolic activation, reactive oxygen/nitrogen species, and mitochondrial permeability transition. *Drug Metab Rev* 2004;36:805–822.

36. Townsend DM, Tew KD. The role of glutathione-*S*-transferase in anti-cancer drug resistance. *Oncogene* 2003;22:7369–7375.

37. Tukey RH, Strassburg CP. Human UDP-glucuronosyltransferases: metabolism, expression, and disease. *Annu Rev Pharmacol Toxicol* 2000;40:581–616.

38. Landi S. Mammalian class theta GST and differential susceptibility to carcinogens: a review. *Mutat Res* 2000;463:247–283.

39. Giacomini KM, Krauss RM, Roden DM, Eichelbaum M, Hayden MR, Nakamura Y. When good drugs go bad. *Nature* 2007;446:975–977.

40. Dresser GK, Spence JD, Bailey DG. Pharmacokinetic–pharmacodynamic consequences and clinical relevance of cytochrome P450 3A4 inhibition. *Clin Pharmacokinet* 2000;38:41–57.

41. Benton RE, Honig PK, Zamani K, Cantilena LR, Woosley RL. Grapefruit juice alters terfenadine pharmacokinetics, resulting in prolongation of repolarization on the electrocardiogram. *Clin Pharmacol Ther* 1996;59:383–388.

42. Aardema M, MacGregor J. Toxicology and genetic toxicology in the new era of "toxicogenomics": impacts of "-omics" technologies. *Mutat Res* 2002;499:13–25.

43. Waters M, Olden K, Tennant R. Toxicogenomic approach for assessing toxicant-related disease. *Mutat Res* 2003;544:415–424.

44. Thybaud V, Le Fevre AC, Boitier E. Application of toxicogenomics to genetic toxicology risk assessment. *Environ Mol Mutagen* 2007;48:369–379.

45. Diasio RB, Beavers TL, Carpenter JT. Familial deficiency of dihydropyrimidine dehydrogenase: biochemical basis for familial pyrimidinemia and severe 5-fluorouracil-induced toxicity *J Clin Invest* 1998;81:47–51.

46. Lu Z, Zhang R, Diasio RB. Purification and characterization of dihydropyrimidine dehydrogenase from human liver. *J Biol Chem* 1992;267:17102–17109.

47. Gardiner SJ, Begg EJ. Pharmacogenetics, drug-metabolizing enzymes, and clinical practice. *Pharmacol Rev* 2006;58:521–590.

48. Diasio RB, Johnson MR. Dihydropyrimidine dehydrogenase: its role in 5-fluorouracil, clinical toxicity and tumor resistance. *Clin Cancer Res Editorial* 1999;5:2672–2673.

49. Seck K, Riemer S, Kates R, Ullrich T, Lutz V, Harbeck N, Schmitt M, Kiechle M, Diasio R, Gross E. Analysis of the DPYD gene implicated in 5-fluorouracil catabolism in a cohort of Caucasian individuals. *Clin Cancer Res* 2005;11:5886–5892.

50. Lu Z, Zhang R, Diasio RB. Dihydropyrimidine dehydrogenase activity in human peripheral blood mononuclear cells and liver: population characteristics, newly identified deficient patients, and clinical implication in 5-fluorouracil chemotherapy. *Cancer Res* 1993;53:5433–5438.

51. Lu Z, Zhang R, Carpenter JT, Diasio RB. Decreased dihydropyrimidine dehydrogenase activity in population of patients with breast cancer: implication for 5-fluorouracil-based chemotherapy. *Clin Cancer Res* 1998;4:325–329.

52. Gardiner SJ, Begg EJ, Robinson RA. The effect of dihydropyrimidine dehydrogenase deficiency on outcomes with fluorouracil. *Adverse Drug React Toxicol Rev* 2002;21:1–16.

53. www.nlm.nih.gov/medlineplus/druginfo/uspdi/202077.html.

54. Schaeffeler E, Eichelbaum M, Reinisch W, Zanger UM, Schwab M. Three novel thiopurine *S*-methyltransferase allelic variants (*TPMT*20, *21, *22*)—association with decreased enzyme function. *Hum Mutat* 2006;27:976.

55. Jordan MA. Mechanism of action of antitumor drugs that interact with microtubules and tubulin. *Curr Med Chem Anti-Cancer Agents* 2002;2:1–17.

56. Pelusi J. Capecitabine versus 5-FU in metastatic colorectal cancer: considerations for treatment decision-making. *Community Oncol* 2006;3:19–27.

57. Pryor WA. Cigarette smoke radicals and the role of free radicals in chemical carcinogenicity. *Environ Health Perspect* 1997;105:875–882.

58. Hurria A, Lichtman SM. Pharmacokinetics of chemotherapy in the older patient. *Cancer Control* 2007;14:32–43.

59. Rivory LP, Slaviero KA, Clarke SJ. Hepatic cytochrome P450 3A drug metabolism is reduced in cancer patients who have an acute-phase response. *Br J Cancer* 2002;87:277–280.

60. Guengerich FP, MacDonald JS. Applying mechanisms of chemical toxicity to predict drug safety. *Chem Res Toxicol* 2007;20:344–369.

61. Mattes WB. Cross-species comparative toxicogenomics as an aid to safety assessment. Expert *Opin Drug Metab Toxicol* 2006;2:859–874.

62. Seed J, Carney EW, Corley RA, Crofton KM, DeSesso JM, Foster PM, Kavlock R, Kimmel G, Klaunig J, Meek ME, Preston RJ, Slikker W Jr, Tabacova S, Williams GM, Wiltse J, Zoeller RT, Fenner-Crisp P, Patton DE. Overview: using mode of action and life stage information to evaluate the human relevance of animal toxicity data. *Crit Rev Toxicol* 2005;35:664–672.

63. Lu Z, Zhang R, Diasio RB. Comparison of dihydropyrimidine dehydrogenase from human, rat, pig and cow liver: biochemical and immunological properties. *Biochem Pharm* 1993;46:945–952.

64. Gad SC. The mouse ear swelling test (MEST) in the 1990s. *Toxicology* 1994;93:33–46.

65. Niemeyer GP, Welch JA, Tillson M, Brawner W, Rynders P, Goodman S, Dufresne M, Dennis J, Lothrop CD Jr. Renal allograft tolerance in DLA-identical and haploidentical dogs after nonmyeloablative conditioning and transient immunosuppression with cyclosporine and mycophenolate mofetil. *Transplant Proc* 2005;37:4579–4586.

66. Rohn JL, Gwynn SR, Lauring AS, Linenberger ML, Overbaugh J. Viral genetic variation, AIDS, and the multistep nature of carcinogenesis: the feline leukemia virus model. *Leukemia* 1996;10:867–869.

67. Hendry WJ 3rd, Sheehan DM, Khan SA, May JV. Developing a laboratory animal model for perinatal endocrine disruption: the hamster chronicles. *Exp Biol Med* 2002;227:709–723.

68. Mouse Genome Sequencing Consortium, Waterston RH, Lindblad-Toh K, Birney E, et al. Initial sequencing and comparative analysis of the mouse genome. *Nature* 2002;420:520–562.

69. Yanni AE. The laboratory rabbit: an animal model of atherosclerosis research. *Lab Anim* 2004;38:246–256.

70. Gad SC. *Animal Models in Toxicology*, 2nd ed. Philadelphia: Taylor & Francis; 2007, pp 334–402.

71. Reid ME. *The Guinea Pig in Research*. Washington, DC: Human Factors Research Bureau; 1958, pp 62–70.

72. Rubinstein AL. Zebrafish assays for drug toxicity screening. *Expert Opin Drug Metab Toxicol* 2006;2:231–240.

73. http://zfin.org/cgi-bin/webdriver?MIval=aa-ZDB_home.apg.

74. Claudio L, Bearer CF, Wallinga D. Assessment of the US Environmental Protection Agency methods for identification of hazards to developing organisms, Part II: The developmental toxicity testing guideline. *Am J Ind Med* 1999;35:554–563.

75. http://www.xenbase.org/common/.

76. Watts DJ, Strogatz SH. Collective dynamics of "small-world" networks. *Nature* 1998;393:440–442.

77. The *C. elegans* Sequencing Consortium. Genome sequence of the nematode *C. elegans*: a platform for investigating biology. *Science* 1998;282:2012–2018.

78. Dendy PP. The use of *in vitro* methods to predict tumour response to chemotherapy. *Br J Cancer Suppl* 1980;4:195–198.

79. Kikkawa R, Fujikawa M, Yamamoto T, Hamada Y, Yamada H, Horii I. *In vivo* hepato-toxicity study of rats in comparison with *in vitro* hepatotoxicity screening system. *J Toxicol Sci* 2006;31:23–34.

80. Thasler WE, Schlott T, Kalkuhl A, Plan T, Irrgang B, Jauch KW, Weiss TS. Human tissue for *in vitro* research as an alternative to animal experiments: a charitable "honest broker" model to fulfill ethical and legal regulations and to protect research participants. *Altern Lab Anim* 2006;34:387–392.

81. Meslin EM, Quaid KA. Ethical issues in the collection, storage, and research use of human biological materials. *J Lab Clin Med* 2004;144:229–234.

82. MacGregor JT, Collins JM, Sugiyama Y, Tyson CA, Dean J, Smith L, Andersen M, Curren RD, Houston JB, Kadlubar FF, Kedderis GL, Krishnan K, Li AP, Parchment RE, Thummel K, Tomaszewski JE, Ulrich R, Vickers AE, Wrighton SA. *In vitro* human tissue models in risk assessment: report of a consensus-building workshop. *Toxicol Sci* 2001;59:17–36.

83. Wang W, Zhao Y, Rayburn E, Hill D, Wang H, Zhang R. Anti-cancer activity and struc-ture–activity relationships of natural products isolated from fruits of *Panax ginseng*. *Cancer Chemother Pharmacol* 2007;59:589–601.

84. Miners JO, Knights KM, Houston JB, Mackenzie PI. *In vitro–in vivo* correlation for drugs and other compounds eliminated by glucuronidation in humans: pitfalls and promises. *Biochem Pharmacol* 2006;71:1531–1539.

85. Suresh D, Srinivasan K. Influence of curcumin, capsaicin, and piperine on the rat liver drug-metabolizing enzyme system *in vivo* and in vitro. *Can J Physiol Pharmacol* 2006;84:1259–1265.

86. Gomez-Lechon MJ, Castell JV, Donato MT. HepaTocytes—the choice To investigate drug metabolism and toxicity in man: *in vitro* variability as a reflection of *in vivo*. *Chem Biol Interact* 2007;168:30–50.

87. Mayne JT, Ku WW, Kennedy SP. Informed toxicity assessment in drug discovery: systems-based toxicology. *Curr Opin Drug Discov Dev* 2006;9:75–83.

88. Gubbels-van Hal WM, Blaauboer BJ, Barentsen HM, Hoitink MA, Meerts IA, Van der Hoeven JC. An alternative approach for the safety evaluation of new and existing chemicals, an exercise in integrated testing. *Regul Toxicol Pharmacol* 2005;42:284–295.

89. Ekins S, Andreyev S, Ryabov A, Kirillov E, Rakhmatulin EA, Sorokin S, Bugrim A, Nikolskaya T. A combined approach to drug metabolism and toxicity assessment. *Drug Metab Dispos* 2005;34:495–503.

90. Ekins S, Nikolksy Y, Nikolskaya T. Techniques: application of systems biology to absorp-tion, distribution, metabolism, excretion and toxicity. *Trends Pharmacol Sci* 2005;26:202–209.

91. Kruhlak NL, Contrera JF, Benz RD, Matthews EJ. Progress in QSAR toxicity screening of pharmaceutical impurities and other FDA regulated products. *Adv Drug Deliv Rev* 2007;59:43–55.

92. Barlow S, Renwick AG, Kleiner J, Bridges JW, Busk L, Dybing E, Edler L, Eisenbrand G, Fink-Gremmels J, Knaap A, Kroes R, Liem D, Muller DJ, Page S, Rolland V, Schlatter J, Tritscher A, Tueting W, Wurtzen G. Risk assessment of substances that are both geno-toxic and carcinogenic report of an international conference organized by EFSA and WHO with support of ILSI Europe. *Food Chem Toxicol* 2006;44:1636–1650.

93. Duch W, Swaminathan K, Meller J. Artificial intelligence approaches for rational drug design and discovery. *Curr Pharm Des* 2007;13:1497–1508.

94. Norinder U, Bergstrom CA. Prediction of ADMET properties. *Chem Med Chem* 2006;1:920–937.

95. Sardari S, Dezfulian M. Cheminformatics in anti-infective agents discovery. *Mini Rev Med Chem* 2007;7:181–189.

96. Patzel V. *In silico* selection of active siRNA. *Drug Discov Today* 2007;3–4:139–148.

97. Mattison LK, Ezzeldin H, Carpenter M, Modak A, Johnson MR, Diasio RB. Rapid identification of dihydropyrimidine dehydrogenase deficiency by using a novel 2–13C-uracil breath test. *Clin Cancer Res* 2004;10:2652–2658.

98. Nuwaysir EF, Bittner M, Trent J, Barrett JC, Afshari CA. Microarrays and toxicology: the advent of toxicogenomics. *Mol Carcinog* 1999;24:153–159.

99. Pennie WD, Woodyatt NJ, Aldridge TC, Orphanides G. Application of genomics to the definition of the molecular basis for toxicity. *Toxicol Lett* 2001;31:353–358.

100. Sabbioni G, Sepai O, Norppa H, Yan H, Hirvonen A, Zheng Y, Jarventaus H, Back B, Brooks LR, Warren SH, Demarini DM, Liu YY. Comparison of biomarkers in workers exposed to 2,4,6-trinitrotoluene. *Biomarkers* 2007;12:21–37.

101. Weinstein M, Widenor M, Hecker S. Health and employment practices: ethical, legal, and social implications of advances in toxicogenomics. *AAOHN J* 2005;53:529–533.

29

ALLOMETRIC SCALING

WILLIAM L. HAYTON[1] AND TEH-MIN HU[2]

[1]*The Ohio State University, Columbus, Ohio*
[2]*National Defense Medical Center, Taipei, Taiwan*

Contents

Preclinical Development Handbook: ADME and Biopharmaceutical Properties,
edited by Shayne Cox Gad
Copyright © 2008 John Wiley & Sons, Inc.

29.1   INTRODUCTION

29.1.1   Role of Allometric Scaling in Preclinical Development

Allometric scaling is useful in the preclinical drug development phase to project pharmacokinetic parameter values determined experimentally in a few animal species to other species and ultimately to humans. Such projection permits early decisions about the developmental prospects for candidate drugs and forms a basis for selection of drug dosage to provide a desired level of systemic exposure. Projection of human pharmacokinetic parameter values from preclinical animal studies permits calculation of a first dose in humans that achieves a desired systemic exposure. Allometric scaling also plays a quality control function in that failure to observe an expected scaling relationship raises a concern about the validity of pharmacokinetic parameter values on hand or about possibly unusual interspecies variability. The purpose of this chapter is to present allometric scaling techniques in the context of the preclinical drug development process.

29.1.2   Historical Perspectives

Allometry in Biology   The term *allometry* was first coined by Huxley and Teissier [1] in 1936. The *allometric growth* can be described by an algebraic formula, $Y = aM^b$, in which the sizes (Y) of the parts of an organism follow a power law relationship with the overall body mass (M) [1]. While the original concept of allometry was limited to the size-dependent morphological or structural changes within or between species, it has been applied to other size-related attributes, such as biochemical and physiological processes. To date, allometry (or allometric scaling) is often used to denote any size-dependent power law relationship found in biology.

A topic pursued for more than a century is the allometric scaling of metabolic rate across species. Over 160 years ago, Sarrus and Rameaux first recognized the importance of size as a determinant of metabolic rate (MR) (cited by White and Seymour [2]). In 1883 the German scientist Max Rubner [3] described a proportional relationship between MR and body surface area (BSA) in dogs. He then suggested that metabolic rate is proportional to BSA and therefore to body mass (M) to the power of two-thirds, that is, $MR \propto M^{2/3}$, which has been considered as the *surface law*. In 1932 Kleiber [4] concluded that basal metabolic rate was not proportional to surface area, but scaled with an exponent close to three-fourths. Kleiber's finding was later supported by Brody's [5] famous mouse-to-elephant curve. *Kleiber's law* has been generalized as the quarter-power law, which has been considered as ubiquitous and "universal" in biology [6].

Allometry in Pharmacokinetics   While some ponder theories of allometry, biomedical and pharmaceutical scientists face the practical question of how to extrapolate physiological, pharmacological, and toxicological data from animals to humans. In 1949 Adolph [7] listed 34 allometric equations that correlated morphological, physiological, and biochemical parameters with interspecies body mass. For example, creatinine clearance followed the allometric equation with a b value of 0.69 [7]. His quantitative power law relationships suggested overwhelming similarities across species, which formed a biological basis for extrapolation of experimental data from one animal species to another [8]. Adolph's work also had a significant impact on modern development of physiologically based pharmacokinetics ($PBPK$).

Animal scale-up of pharmacokinetics was actively pursued as early as the 1950s. Pinkel [9] proposed the use of body surface area (BSA) as a criterion of drug dosage in cancer chemotherapy, based on the observation of species invariant dose when expressed on a mg/m^2 basis for five antineoplastic agents. Freireich et al. [10] confirmed Pinkel's observation by evaluating the predictive relationship between toxic doses in five adult mammals with adult human data for 18 anticancer drugs. Furthermore, Mellett's [11] analysis of kinetic data for amethopterin and cyclophosphamide in six species, including humans, suggested that an allometric relationship applied for AUC and half-life ($t_{1/2}$).

The concept of scaling pharmacokinetics gained momentum in the early 1970s. Dedrick et al. [12, 13] assumed that pharmacokinetic processes correlated with internal physiological processes and demonstrated that drug concentration profiles in several lab animals were superimposable when a normalization procedure based on the concept of *equivalent time* was adopted. The *equivalent time* was chosen to correlate with body mass to the one-quarter power, based on the similarity principle [14] and the allometric relationship between half-life of methotrexate and body mass of several mammals [13]. This was the first attempt where the similarity principle in biology was applied in animal scale-up of pharmacokinetics [12]. Klotz et al. [15] showed that diazepam plasma clearance was proportional to species body mass to the two-thirds power. Soon thereafter, Weiss et al. [16] detailed the dependence of pharmacokinetic parameters on body mass. They drew the link between pharmacokinetic parameters and body mass by first introducing equations that related pharmacokinetic parameters (hepatic clearance, renal clearance, etc.) to physiological parameters (liver blood flow, GFR, etc.), followed by application of the allometric equations for the physiological parameters. Thus, for a drug eliminated by glomerular filtration, the renal clearance would be $CL_{renal} = GFR = aM^b$, where b was cited as 0.82 [16].

In 1980 Boxenbaum [17] characterized interspecies scaling of liver weight, hepatic blood flow, and antipyrine clearance. A log–log plot of antipyrine intrinsic clearance versus body mass yielded a straight line that well described the data from 10 out of 11 mammalian species, but the human value was a pronounced outlier [17]. The seven fold deviation between estimated and observed human antipyrine intrinsic clearance suggested that extrapolation of human pharmacokinetic parameters from animal data using simple allometry may not generally apply. Later, Boxenbaum [18] introduced maximum life span potential (MLP) into the allometric equation, producing an allometric relationship between intrinsic clearance of antipyrine per MLP and body mass. Boxenbaum's papers drew significant attention and the concept of allometric scaling in pharmacokinetics was well discussed in the 1980s [8, 19–25]. Meanwhile, the suitability of the allometric equation for predicting human pharmacokinetic parameters was further examined [26–29]. Sawada et al. [28] predicted total body clearance, renal clearance, hepatic clearance, volume of distribution, and half-life for six β-lactam antibiotics in humans. Extrapolations were performed using data from mice, rats, rabbits, dogs, and monkeys. For the first time, differences in the plasma protein binding among species was considered an important determinant for the prediction of volume of distribution [28]. Sawada et al. [29] further showed that similarities among animals and humans in tissue distribution of 10 basic drugs failed to produce a successful prediction of the human value. To predict the volume of distribution it was suggested that unbound fraction in plasma (f_{up}) should be included for analysis. In the same period, prediction of human pharmacokinetic parameters using the allometric equation was applied to other antibiotics, such as cephalosporins, monobactams, and macrolides [26, 30].

In the early 1990s an insightful review by Ings [31] heralded a new era for allometry in pharmacokinetics. As this new era began the concept and technique of allometric scaling had become familiar to drug development scientists. But it had also become apparent that the allometric scaling technique was not universally reliable. While for humans the technique sometimes gave acceptable predictions for the pharmacokinetics of those drugs whose elimination was either renal or liver-blood-flow dependent, poor predictions often occurred for low clearance drugs whose elimination was primarily via metabolism. Moreover, the application of the technique was limited to only a few drug classes. These shortcomings contributed to increased research activity in the 1990s. The features of interspecies pharmacokinetic studies in this period include (1) a publication boom focused on interspecies pharmacokinetic scaling for old and new agents and small versus large molecules (proteins); (2) the use of single animal species to extrapolate human pharmacokinetics; (3) the integration of *in vitro* metabolic data into the allometric prediction; (4) the use of the *rule of exponents* along with additional studies of correction factors such as *MLP* and brain weight; and (5) more successful examples of human dose estimation for Phase I studies.

A commentary by Bonate and Howard [32] highlighted an inherent problem faced by those interested in prediction—the uncertainty associated with the prediction. The authors argued that a large bias was associated with publication of predominantly successful allometric scaling attempts, which could lead to a false sense of security with regard to use of allometric scaling to prospectively select dose for a first-time-in-human study. One major problem pointed out by the authors was that prediction intervals are often too wide to be of practical use [32]. By using linear regression and log–log coordinates for prediction, the authors cautioned that an excellent point estimate might not prescribe a good prediction. Moreover, they questioned whether the use of "correction factors" in allometric scaling was appropriate [32, 33].

Hu and Hayton [34] tackled the uncertainty issue in a different way. They carefully analyzed clearance values for 115 xenobiotics from published studies in which at least three species were used for the purpose of interspecies comparison of pharmacokinetics. The allometric exponent for each xenobiotic was calculated along with its confidence interval (*CI*). While it was of interest to note that for each individual drug either 0.67 or 0.75 appeared to be the central tendency of the allometric exponent, the confidence interval of the exponent was often large due to considerable random variability in the clearance values from each species [34].

After so many years of endeavor, it is somewhat discouraging that no matter which allometric method is used for predicting human pharmacokinetic parameters, some drugs will be very poorly predicted. The incorporation of *in vitro* metabolic data improves the prediction performance. Perhaps the most urgent task for the future is to understand what makes certain drugs so unique and how to improve the predictability of these drugs.

29.2   ALLOMETRIC EQUATION

29.2.1   Mathematical Description, $Y = aM^b$

As used here, *scaling* refers to relationships between objects and their representation (e.g., a scale model where 1 cm represents 1 m) or to relationships between elements of a series of similar objects that vary in size only. For example, when geometric bodies such as squares, rectangles, and cubes vary in size, their corresponding linear dimensions differ by a constant ratio. Two geometrically similar rectangles that differ in width by a factor of 2 will differ similarly in length. Length is then said to scale in direct proportion to width, while area scales in direct proportion to the square of width. Geometrically similar bodies are also referred to as *isometric* bodies (*iso* means *equal*).

When bodies are not geometrically similar they are referred to as *allometric* (*allo* means *different*). Characterization of scaling relationships for a series of geometrically dissimilar bodies, for example, mammalian species, is therefore termed *allometric scaling*. For organisms, many aspects of their morphology and physiology change systematically as body mass (M) changes, according to the power function:

$$Y = aM^b \tag{29.1}$$

where a and b are constants, and Y is the particular variable of interest. Because Eq. 29.1 relates so many biological variables to body mass, it has become known as the *allometric equation*. In its logarithmic form, it is

$$\log Y = \log a + b \log M \tag{29.2}$$

Use of the allometric equation for scaling in biology was popularized by Huxley [35]. During the ensuing decades, use of the equation became widespread even though no satisfactory underlying theoretical basis supported its use [7, 36]. The allometric equation was often invoked whenever a linear relationship between log Y and log M was observed. Critics of the nondiscriminatory, routine use of the allometric equation have pleaded for more thoughtful application of the equation, noting that use of the "cookbook approach to study the comparative biology of size has falsely simplified a complex problem" and that "use of the method has been considered equivalent to study of the problem" [37].

The foundations for a theoretical underpinning of the allometric equation were laid by the landmark paper of West, Brown, and Enquist [6], which were strengthened in following years [38, 39]. The paper proposed that organisms utilize a similarly structured material supply network, which provides the common mechanism that underlies the allometric equation and in addition explains the often observed quarter-power (and its multiples) value for the body mass exponent, b. The theory is based on three assumptions: (1) the supply network has "a space-filling fractal-like branching pattern"; (2) "the final branch of the network . . . is a size-invariant unit"; and (3) "the energy required to distribute resources is minimized." An extensive variety of quantifiable biological characteristics conform to the theory, which removes much of the empirical nature of the allometric equation [40].

29.2.2   Interpretation of *a* and *b*

Empirically the values of the body mass coefficient *a* and exponent *b* are simply those that best fit the allometric equation to the particular dataset. The value of *a* is the value of *Y* when the value of *M* equals unity. The *b* value shows the sensitivity of the *Y* value to a change in the *M* value. As is often the case, $b < 1$ and a change in *M* results in a less-than-proportional change in *Y*. In the special case of $b = 1$, *Y* varies in direct proportion to *M*. While Heusner [41] argued that the *a* value is not a constant but rather increases with the size of *M*, applications in scaling pharmacokinetics have generally ignored this possibility.

The *b* value is often interpreted in comparison with the values obtained from simple geometrical relationships; for example, a value of two-thirds that occurs when the variable *Y* is proportional to body surface area rather than body mass [42]. In this regard, the allometric scaling of basal metabolic rate in mammals is of interest as a potential surrogate for the body mass sensitivity of drug metabolism rate. Kleiber [43] proposed for basal metabolism a *b* value of three-fourths, a value that was disputed for several decades, with an alternative value of two-thirds proposed [41, 44–46]. The two-thirds value garnered support from a heat-dissipation mechanism, where it was argued that heat loss is proportional to body surface area and that heat loss is an important constraint that forced its production per unit body mass to decline as body mass increased, in proportion to body surface area. The three-quarters value lacked a compelling mechanistic explanation until the model of West, Brown, and Enquist [6], which convincingly supports the three-fourths value [40].

29.2.3   Using the Allometric Equation

Allometry has been broadly defined as "the study of size and its consequences" [47], and more narrowly described as the specific use of the allometric equation to analyze the body mass influence on quantifiable biological phenomena [37]. In preclinical drug development, the narrow description more aptly applies as the usual problem involves characterization of the association between body mass and quantitative pharmacokinetic and biopharmaceutic parameters—for example, apparent volume of distribution, clearance, half-life, and bioavailability—and using the quantitative association to make predictions. Both inter- and intraspecies applications are possible.

Choice of Species   Preclinical drug development uses laboratory animals to gain insights about the pharmacology and toxicology of candidate drugs. Because animals and human beings show marked congruence in their genome, physiology, and biochemistry, it is hoped that insights obtained from animal studies will be applicable to humans. Dose–response relationships, metabolite profiles, bioavailability properties, pharmacokinetic behaviors, and so forth observed in animal studies are hoped to be predictive for humans. Decades of drug development research have validated the utility of animal studies in preclinical development, and informed the uncertainty involved in extrapolation of animal results to humans, but have also borne witness to marked divergences, which sometimes have been unpredictable and difficult to explain.

Thus, an important and hard-to-answer question is: Which species should be used in preclinical studies? While it is tempting to believe that those species with the closest phylogenetic relationship to humans will be the most reliable for prediction of drug behavior in humans, it has become apparent that substantial differences in metabolic clearance occur between closely related species. Environmental and dietary adaptations are also important determinants that shape quantitative differences (and similarities) in drug behavior among species. In addition, nonscientific considerations such as cost and public acceptance of experimentation with particular species cannot be divorced from the selection of species to be studied. It appears uncontroversial to suggest that test species should be from the Class *Mammalia*, and from the 4000+ members of this class the species most commonly used are rat, dog, rabbit, mouse, and monkey [31] (Table 29.1). While popularity of usage does not necessarily point to the species that provide the best prediction of behavior in humans, there is scant evidence to suggest that alternative species would be better in this regard. A recent review concluded that no animal species consistently shows absorption, distribution, metabolism, and excretion behaviors similar to those of humans [48]. Animals "humanized" by transgenesis may improve this situation [48, 49].

Ideally, the number of test species to use is at least four, particularly if the test animal body mass range does not encompass 70 kg. This recommendation is based on a review of clearance (CL) values for 115 xenobiotics subjected to allometric analysis, where failure to find a statistically significant correlation between log CL and log M occurred for 24 compounds [34]. The correlation failure rate declined as the number of species studied increased: a total of 20 studies used only three species and 16 of those failed to find correlation. The correlation failure rate was dramatically lower for $n \geq 4$: for $n = 4$, five failures to find correlation out of 43 studies; for $n = 5$, 2/31; for $n = 6$, 1/15; and for $n = 7$, 0/6.

TABLE 29.1   Incidence of Use of Animal Species in Scaling Clearance Values for Xenobiotics

Species	Usage (% of 115 Xenobiotics)
Rat	97
Dog	73
Rabbit	62
Mouse	56
Monkey	53
Pig	7.8
Guinea pig	6.1
Sheep	5.2
Hamster	5.2
Baboon	3.5
Chimpanzee	2.6
Cat	2.6
Cow	2.6
Goat	0.9

Source: From Ref. 34, with permission.

While at least four species is optimum, data from fewer species is not unusual and effort has been expended toward development of scaling techniques for this case [50–55]. Allometry using three and even two species was investigated using a 103 nonpeptide xenobiotic training set, along with nonallometric single species approaches to *CL* estimation based on the product of hepatic extraction ratio estimated in animal and human hepatic blood flow [50, 51]. For the 103 drug candidates, volume of distribution (*V*), total body clearance, and mean residence time (*MRT*) were determined from the plasma (serum) concentration–time profile after intravenous (IV) administration in rat, dog, monkey, and human, and it was possible to compare the various prediction techniques using animal data with measured human values. Allometry based on all three animal species, and pairs of species (rat–monkey, rat–dog, and dog–monkey), predicted human *V* and *CL* values within an error of –50% to +100% (exception: dog–monkey pair for *CL*), for about two-thirds of the test compounds, and MRT was predicted within –50% to +100% for about two-thirds of compounds using allometry based on three species and on the rat–dog pair only.

Ideal Body Mass Range   Clearly, the selected species should span a "reasonable range" of body mass values, and if the objective is to scale the animal values to estimate the corresponding human value, it is desirable to include species with *M* values below and above 70 kg. However, resource constraints often make it difficult to study animals larger than 70 kg and very few published studies of pharmacokinetic parameter scaling include species larger than humans (Table 29.1). While pharmacokinetic parameter values frequently conform to the allometric equation, use of a small number of values from experimental animals to prospectively predict human values by extrapolation beyond the range of *M* values is "outright perilous" [36].

It is challenging to state precisely what an appropriate *M* range would be; two orders of magnitude seems reasonable, although not based on theoretical principles. For example, if rat were the smallest species (0.2 kg), then the largest species should be on the order of 20 kg. Also, while it is desirable to avoid extrapolating beyond the *M* value range, it is often necessary to do so, in which case one should minimize the extrapolation. A given error in the extrapolation line would be expected to produce a larger error in the extrapolated value the further the extrapolation. For example, if mouse (0.02 kg) were the smallest species and the largest species were 2 kg, the two-orders-of-magnitude suggestion would be met, but the extrapolated human value would be less certain due to the extrapolation from 2 kg to 70 kg. In this case, the *M* range should be increased to minimize extrapolation.

Optimal Species for Scale-up to Human   Drug development studies mostly utilize species from the mouse–rat–rabbit–monkey–dog group (the standard five) and data are insufficient to fully address this question beyond these five species. Furthermore, only these species have well established background pathology and other species would not be used for toxicology testing even though they might be advantageous for extrapolation of pharmacokinetic behavior to human [31]. As preclinical pharmacokinetic data are usually obtained as part of the toxicology studies, it is pertinent to consider whether some of the five most commonly used species would serve better than the others for prediction of human pharmacokinetic parameter values.

Rat is nearly universally used in preclinical pharmacokinetic studies and its pharmacokinetic parameter values generally relate well to corresponding human values in allometric scaling analyses [51]. A review of the 61 drugs for which CL values were available in human and at least three species showed that qualitatively most of the standard five species were close to the fitted allometric equation line and that the human CL was reasonably predicted most of the time (data used in Ref. 34). Significant deviations were relatively few although more prevalent for rabbit and monkey than for mouse, rat, and dog. On the other hand, in their analysis of a 103 compound dataset, Ward and Smith [50, 51] concluded that monkey was somewhat superior to other species for prediction of human pharmacokinetic parameter values when single species extrapolation was conducted. It therefore appears that none of the standard five species stands out as particularly superior or inferior to the others.

Fitting the Allometric Equation to Data   Approaches that can be used to fit the allometric equation to Y,M data include linear regression of the logarithms of Y and M, and nonlinear least squares or maximum likelihood fitting of the allometric equation to the Y,M data. Both approaches assume that the M values are independent variables and that the error associated with their determination is zero. It is therefore essential to accurately determine the mass (weight) of each animal used for determination of the corresponding Y value, with the associated experimental error being negligible compared with that of the Y value.

While individual Y,M values for each animal could be fitted, it is customary practice to average the values from each species and to fit the allometric equation to the means. On log–log coordinates with a two order of magnitude range for M, individual values for each species cluster close together, and as a practical matter, there is little difference between analysis of individual or lumped data, with regard to the appearance of the plot and the values of a and b.

Avoid application of allometry to M-normalized Y values as this can create spurious correlation [56]. Weighting the Y values is not usually done, probably because the linearized form of the equation is usually fit to log Y, log M points and the magnitude of the range is thereby much reduced. If the equation is fitted directly to Y,M data, a weighting function should be used to prevent the excessive influence of the larger Y values on the a and b values; for example, Y^{-1} or Y^{-2}, or by the reciprocal of the variance of the means. Pertinent statistical characterizations of the goodness of fit should also be calculated and reported; namely, correlation coefficient and its statistical significance, and variance for a and b. Prothero [56] developed by simulation an empirical equation to calculate the standard error (se) for b from the mean percent deviation (PD) of the points about the line, the number (n) of points, and the log of the body mass range (pWR), where WR is M_{max}/M_{min}:

$$se = \frac{0.019(PD)}{pWR \times n^{1/2}} \qquad (29.3)$$

This alternative to the value supplied by standard statistical packages alerts the user to suspect unreliability in the latter when it is smaller than predicted by Eq. 29.3.

29.3 SCALING CLEARANCE

29.3.1 Physiological Basis and Theoretical Considerations

Clearance is generally defined as the proportionality constant that relates the steady-state rate of drug elimination to its concentration in a reference fluid, which is commonly plasma or serum and sometimes whole blood [57]. For expediency plasma concentration (C_p) is used in the following sections with the understanding that it represents the other reference fluids as well. The total body (systemic, plasma) clearance (CL) is a primary pharmacokinetic parameter, often determined experimentally as the ratio of dose to area under the plasma concentration–time profile after IV administration of the dose:

$$CL = \text{Dose} \big/ \int C_p \, dt$$

The total body clearance is the sum of the clearance values contributed by the various organs involved in the elimination of the particular substance. Hepatic clearance (CL_H) is the major contributor to CL of drugs; it contributes more than three-fourths the CL for about 60% of the drugs used in therapeutics [58]. For most hepatically cleared drugs, metabolism is the major mechanism, with biliary excretion of importance for a relatively small number of drugs, usually those that are amphipathic and have molecular weight threshold that differs from species to species in the range 400 ± 100. Renal clearance (CL_R) is a distant second to CL_H in overall importance, being the principal contributor to CL for only about 15% of drugs in current use. For interspecies scaling of CL values it is helpful to know the relative contributions of the liver, kidneys, and other organs to the total body clearance.

Physiologically based models of clearance provide a useful basis for understanding interspecies scaling relationships [16]. These models incorporate the plasma flow (Q) to the clearing organ, the free fraction of drug in the plasma (f_{up}), and the intrinsic activity of the clearance process within the organ (CL_{int}). Each of these components varies among species, and for each there is the possibility that its allometric scaling relationship differs from the others. In the following three sections, expectations for allometric scaling relationships are developed based on relevant physiologically based clearance models.

Hepatic Clearance   Of the several available models of CL_H [57], the well stirred or venous equilibrium model will be used, as other models lead to similar expectations with regard to allometric scaling relationships. The standard representation of the well stirred liver model of CL_H is [59]

$$CL_H = \frac{Q_H f_{up} CL_{int}}{Q_H + f_{up} CL_{int}} \qquad (29.4)$$

CL_{int} here represents the activity of metabolism enzymes or the activity of biliary transport mechanisms.[1] There are two limiting cases, one where $Q_H \gg f_{up} CL_{int}$ (low

---

[1]It may be drug concentration dependent if the metabolism enzyme and/or the transport mechanism are significantly occupied by the drug. This greatly complicates characterization of the pharmacokinetics and thereby the scaling of pharmcokinetic parameter values across species. This situation is not addressed in the present chapter.

extraction case) and the other where $Q_H \ll f_{up}CL_{int}$ (high extraction case). Most drugs fall into the low extraction category and for these $CL_H \cong f_{up}CL_{int}$. The extraction class is readily identified by comparison of the values of CL_H and Q_H; Q_H values are available in the literature [60]. For low extraction drugs the ratio CL_H/Q_H is below 0.25 and for high extraction drugs it is above 0.75. In the low extraction case, interspecies differences in both f_{up} and CL_{int} contribute to interspecies differences in CL_H. To remove the influence of f_{up}, it is recommended that CL_{int} be the hepatic clearance parameter to scale; it is calculated as the ratio CL_H/f_{up}. The human CL_H value is then calculated as the product of the measured human f_{up} and the human CL_{int} predicted by allometric scaling. Interspecies scaling of CL_{int} is problematic; there are examples of high interspecies variability and of a tendency for the predicted human CL_{int} value to substantially exceed the measured value. Predicted human CL_{int} values by allometry applied to animal data should therefore be regarded with appropriate skepticism. Approaches to dealing with this uncertainty are described in Section 29.3.2.

For the high extraction class of compounds, $CL_H \cong Q_H$, and the expectation in allometric scaling is that CL_H would scale as does Q_H; f_{up} is not an issue in this case. Liver blood flow for the standard laboratory animals and humans is well fitted by the allometric equation with the b value being 0.894 [17]. For a high extraction drug therefore, the expectation is that the b value for CL_H would be about 0.9, similar to that for Q_H.

For intermediate extraction drugs (CL_H/Q_H between 0.25 and 0.75), CL_H shows sensitivity to f_{up}, Q_H, and CL_{int}. The influence of f_{up} cannot be removed by scaling CL_H/f_{up} as an f_{up} term remains on the right-hand side of Eq. 29.4. This case is perhaps the most difficult to handle as all three independent determinants can vary in different ways across species, causing CL_H values to vary erratically, the result being no systematic way to scale them.

Renal Clearance   Drug elimination by the kidneys is quantitatively less important than that by the liver; it contributes more than 75% to total clearance for ~15% of drugs used in therapeutics [58]. Renal clearance (CL_R) may be more complex than hepatic clearance as it may involve a combination of glomerular filtration, tubular secretion, tubular reabsorption, and metabolism. Physiological models are available for each process, but their combination is difficult since the processes act in series and are therefore not simply additive. For the filtration component, $f_{up} \times GFR$ is its contribution to CL_R, which may then be reduced due to subsequent tubular reabsorption. The tubular secretion contribution may be modeled along the lines of the well stirred liver model, where Q_R replaces Q_H and represents the postglomerular plasma flow. Tubular reabsorption may also reduce the secretion clearance. Finally, tubular reabsorption of drug from the preurine of the tubule may be passive or involve transporter, and it may be dependent on preurine flow. Clearly, several physiological processes may contribute to the CL_R value; those operative for a particular test compound and their relative contributions are generally only poorly understood at the preclinical stage of development. Nevertheless, CL_R values typically scale relatively well across test animal species and the human CL_R value is typically well predicted by allometric scaling of animal CL_R values. Appropriate adjustments for interspecies differences in f_{up} should be considered; see Role of Protein Binding in Section 29.3.2. For example, both filtered and secreted test sub-

TABLE 29.2   Body Mass Exponent (b) Values for Renal Clearance of Renal Function Test Substances [7]

Test Substance	Renal Clearance by	b
Urea	Filtration	0.72
Inulin	Filtration	0.77
Creatinine	Filtration	0.69
Diodrast	Filtration + secretion	0.89
Hippurate	Filtration + secretion	0.80

stances followed the allometric equation reasonably well, and b values based on measured renal clearance values in rat, rabbit, dog, and human were in the range 0.69–0.89 (Table 29.2) [7]. These substances are little bound (urea, inulin, creatinine) to plasma proteins or highly extracted (diodrast, hippurate) so f_{up} was not a confounding variable.

Total Body Clearance   Total body clearance may be dominated by a single organ and in that case scaling of CL would conform to the expectation for the major pathway. In the event that multiple organs were involved (e.g., liver and kidneys contribute significantly), CL in principle could be a sum of allometric expressions:

$$CL = a_L M^{b_L} + a_R M^{b_R} \tag{29.5}$$

If the b values differed significantly, the relative contribution of each pathway would vary across species and a simple log CL–log M graph would be curved. In practice, b values for the hepatic and renal pathways are not sufficiently different that this behavior is observed, and other pathways generally do not contribute significantly.

29.3.2   Empirical Observations

The following subsections present approaches to the allometric scaling of drug clearance and the performance of each approach as experienced in preclinical drug development. The unembellished application of the allometric equation is considered first and this is followed by a series of modifications aimed at improvement of its performance.

Simple Allometry   A study of the application of Eq. 29.1 to interspecies scaling of drug clearance for 115 xenobiotics in three or more species showed that CL generally followed the allometric equation (Fig. 29.1) (Fig. 3 in Ref. 34). While the equation failed to fit CL values for 24 of the compounds, as indicated by the failure to show a statistically significant correlation, most of the failures could be attributed to use of only three species (see Section 29.2.3, Choice of Species). For 91 compounds, the CL values followed the allometric equation; in most of these cases four or more species were used. From the set of 91 compounds, 68 included humans as

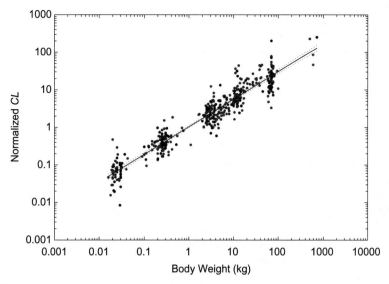

FIGURE 29.1 *CL* values for 91 substances determined in three or more species. Values were normalized by adjustment of all values of *a* to 1 [34].

one of the species. For all but 7 of the 68 compounds, the observed human *CL* value deviated from that predicted by the fitted allometric equation by less than 50%; that is, the measured value was within a range of one-half to twice the predicted value, which is a reasonable marker of precision [52, 55].

This relatively rosy record of success (~90%) has to be tempered by two realities. First, because the human *CL* was included in the fitted datasets, the human *CL* would be expected to lie closer to the predicted value than if it had been omitted from the values used to fit the equation. Second, the data for the various compounds were from the literature, mostly from papers that reported on the allometric scaling of the compound. As negative results are rarely reported, it is not known how often the allometric equation fails to scale *CL* values across species.

Ward and Smith [51] compiled from the literature *CL* values for 103 nonpeptide xenobiotics in rat, dog, monkey, and human after IV administration. Allometric scaling of the three animal species' *CL* values to predict the human *CL* value had a 66% success rate, based on whether the human *CL* was correctly predicted to be in the low, moderate, or high *CL* category, defined as a percentage of hepatic blood flow (<30%, 30–70%, and >70%). The success rate differed across categories, being 80–90% for low *CL* substances and only 30–50% for high *CL* substances.

It might be concluded that allometric scaling of human drug *CL* using three or more animal species is a viable approach. For renally eliminated drugs, the success rate is quite high, particularly when renal elimination is primarily by glomerular filtration, plasma protein binding is low, and tubular reabsorption is minimal. For more complex renal clearance mechanisms, the success rate would tend to decline. For drugs eliminated hepatically, the success rate is not as high as when the kidney is the dominant pathway. There are dozens of hepatic drug metabolism enzymes that across species vary in their activity and substrate selectivity. That along with interspecies variability in the extent of plasma protein binding make the success rates reported above surprisingly high.

To improve the predictive capability of allometry, several embellishments have been proposed. The first to consider is the use of brain weight or maximum life span potential along with M.

Maximum Life Span Potential and Brain Weight   In scaling the CL of extensively metabolized drugs, investigations found early on that the human CL value often fell considerably below the value predicted in animals. Examples include the intrinsic hepatic clearances of antipyrine and phenytoin, which were below the values predicted by application of the allometric equation to animal data by factors of 7 and 4.4, respectively [17]. Compared with other mammals, humans were also noted to have relatively long life spans, and life span was observed to relate to brain weight. As enhanced longevity may necessitate slowed energy consumption, it was thought that drug metabolism rate may also correlate inversely with life span. A quite successful test of this proposition with antipyrine, phenytoin, and clonazepam intrinsic clearances involved allometric scaling of the product of CL_{int} and MLP, the maximum life span potential [18]. This adjustment brought the human CL_{int} values into alignment with the animal values (e.g., antipyrine) (Fig. 29.2).

A variation of this approach is to use brain weight (BW, literature values) as a second independent variable in the simple allometric equation. For example, antipyrine CL_{int} (mL/min) in 15 mammalian species including humans [21] is given by

$$CL_{int} = 0.3865 M^{1.316} BW^{-0.6188} \tag{29.6}$$

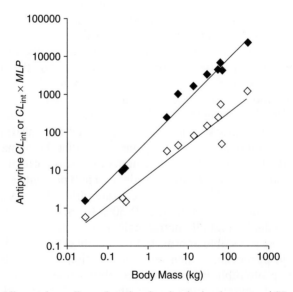

FIGURE 29.2   Allometric scaling of antipyrine intrinsic clearance (CL_{int}) alone ($\diamond$) and after multiplication by MLP ($\blacklozenge$). CL_{int} from Ref. 21 and MLP from Ref. 18. CL_{int} for human and pig moved from below and above the allometric line (lower plot) to be near the allometric line for $MLP \times CL_{int}$ (upper plot).

where M and BW are in kilograms. The coefficient and exponents were determined by fitting the equation to the data using a computer-based algorithm. All 15 calculated CL_{int} values were within -67.4% to $+57.6\%$ of the observed values.

However, not all drugs eliminated by metabolism show overprediction of human clearance upon allometric scaling of animal values; for example, Boxenbaum [18] noted that while some do (antipyrine, benzodiazepines, propranolol), others such as tolbutamide and cyclophosphamide do not. More recent work indicates that human CL values may fall above the allometric line as often as they are below it [34]. Use of MLP or BW generally moves the human CL_{int} value more that it does the values from animals. Thus, the MLP or BW technique would tend to move a human value that was on the simple allometric line to well above the line. As a *prospective* technique to predict human CL_{int}, use of MLP or BW is problematic as the result would be to increase the number of overpredictions as the number of underpredictions was decreased. From the standpoint of first-dose-in-human estimation, this may be undesirable as overprediction of CL would lead to a less conservative first human dose.

The "Rule of Exponents" For prediction of human CL from animal values, Mahmood [61] and Mahmood and Balian [62, 63] examined the predictive capacity of simple allometry, the MLP and BW techniques described in the previous section, and a variant that involved allometric scaling of the $CL \times BW$ product. These studies pointed to the empirical use of the b value obtained from simple allometry to select one of the following methods to predict human CL:

1. For $0.55 < b < 0.75$, use the simple allometric equation.[2]
2. For $0.75 < b < 1.0$, use the MLP technique:

$$CL_{human} = \frac{a70^b}{8.18 \times 10^5} \tag{29.7}$$

    where a and b are obtained from fitting the allometric equation to the product $CL_{animal} \times MLP$ (h), and 8.18×10^5 h is the human MLP.
3. For $b > 1.0$, use

$$CL_{human} = \frac{a70^b}{1.53} \tag{29.8}$$

    where a and b are obtained from fitting the allometric equation to the product $CL_{animal} \times BW$ (kg), and 1.53 kg is the human BW.

This empirical approach based on the b value after simple allometry is known as the *rule of exponents*. For the set of 46 test substances, CL values were available in three or more of mouse, rat, rabbit, guinea pig, goat, monkey, and dog. The predicted human CL was within the range 0.5–2.0 times the observed CL for 33

---

[2]The upper limit (0.75) of the b range was given as 0.70 in Refs. 62 and 63 and as 0.75 in Ref. 61. The 0.75 value was used in this analysis.

substances (72%), and an additional 6 (13%) substances were included in the range 0.2–5.0.

A comprehensive evaluation of the approaches described above for prediction of human CL utilized a 103 compound dataset with CL values determined in rat, dog and monkey [52, 55]. Using the limits 0.5–2.0 for the ratio of predicted to observed CL in humans to define acceptable predictive performance, none of the allometric approaches was particularly successful. Simple allometry with no correction factor performed better (53% of acceptable predicted human CL) than did incorporation of MLP (38%) and BW (45%), and use of the rule of exponents to select among the three approaches (49%). In addition, subsets of test compounds grouped according to physicochemical property ($c \log P$, polar surface area, number of H-bond acceptors, number of rotatable bonds) and route of elimination failed to improve predictive performance. This discouraging analysis suggests that allometry applied to CL values determined in animals will not reliably predict the human CL value. As noted earlier (Section 29.2.3, Choice of Species) use of only three animal species does not provide a robust dataset for projection to other species and the relatively poor performance reported by Nagilla and Ward [52] may reflect in part this constraint.

The search for more reliable techniques to improve the allometric-based approach to prediction of human CL has more recently turned to incorporation of *in vitro* measurements such as activity of hepatic enzymes and plasma protein binding. These efforts are summarized in the following three subsections.

In Vitro *Data for* In Vivo *Prediction* Liver weight follows the allometric equation in mammals with a b value of 0.849 [17], which is similar to that for hepatic blood flow. Thus, in the common mammalian species hepatic blood flow per unit mass of liver is invariant, at about $1.5\,\mathrm{L\,min^{-1}}$ (kg liver)$^{-1}$ and failure to scale CL among species is generally not attributable to liver mass or blood flow issues. It has been known for some time that *in vitro* enzyme kinetic parameters can be quantitatively related to *in vivo* hepatic clearance in a single species. This *in vitro/in vivo* correspondence was first demonstrated in rat by Rane et al. [64]. For seven compounds having a wide range of hepatic extraction ratio, they successfully predicted *in vivo* hepatic extraction ratio from K_M and V_{max} determined in $9000\,g$ supernatant or microsomal preparations along with liver mass and blood flow, and blood free fraction. Others reported similar success [57]. The feasibility of *in vivo* hepatic CL_{int} prediction ($CL_{int} = V_{max}/K_M$) pointed to the potential to use K_M and V_{max} values in animals to predict the human CL_{int}.

A significant problem remained, however. Among the dozens of hepatic enzymes available for xenobiotic metabolism, relatively few are primarily involved in the metabolism of any particular compound. As there are interspecies differences in the relative proportions of the various enzymes and structural differences that can lead to interspecies differences in intrinsic activity and metabolic pathways, it is not so simple a matter to use *in vitro* metabolism parameters determined in laboratory animals to predict CL_{int} in humans [48, 65]. Possible reasons for failure to predict human CL_{int} include nonhepatic metabolism, slow equilibrium between blood and hepatocytes, and involvement of transporters [66]. Recent effort has therefore focused on integration of *in vitro* measures of metabolic activity with *in vivo* CL_{int} values in animals to improve the accuracy of human CL_{int} prediction.

Incorporation of In Vitro Data in Allometry The first successful combination of *in vitro* and *in vivo* data to predict the human CL_{int} took the approach of adjusting each *in vivo* animal clearance (CL_{an}) value by multiplying by the human/animal ratio of *in vitro* V_{max}/K_M [67, 68]. This effectively adjusted each animal CL to the value it would have had if the overall intrinsic activity of drug metabolism enzymes were the same in the test animal and humans on a unit mass basis; that is, CL_{an} could be "humanized" (CL_{an}^h) by the following adjustment:

$$CL_{an}^h = CL_{an} \frac{(V_{max}/K_M)_{human}}{(V_{max}/K_M)_{an}} \qquad (29.9)$$

This adjustment to CL_{an} reduces the problem associated with interspecies differences in metabolism pathways and enzyme activities so that CL_{an}^h values will more likely follow the allometric equation and will also more likely predict the *in vivo* human CL. It is only appropriate for low or intermediate hepatic extraction drugs since for high extraction drugs hepatic blood flow rather than CL_{int} is the principal determinant of CL_H. Because liver size and blood flow scale according to the allometric equation, adjustments for their interspecies differences are unnecessary. At least three animal species should be used.

The *in vitro* V_{max} and K_M values were determined using a hepatic microsome preparation. The impact of inefficiency in the microsomal isolation procedure is minimized if it is similar for all determinations, as assured by simultaneous determination of *in vitro* parameters using the same protocol. Lavé et al. [67] also used an *in vitro* hepatocyte preparation to adjust the *in vivo* CL_{an} with equally good results. For hepatocytes, *in vitro* CL_{int} (volume/10^6 cells) = Dose/$AUC(0-t)$, where $AUC(0-t)$ is the area under the drug concentration–time profile in the hepatocyte suspension over the duration of the incubation. The hepatocyte method for assessment of *in vitro* CL_{int} is the method of choice as it provides the widest array of enzyme activities and generally shows the same metabolite pattern as is seen *in vivo* [69].

Role of Protein Binding Both renal and hepatic clearance may be affected by the degree of plasma binding; namely, when clearance is predominantly composed of low extraction hepatic or active renal tubular secretion clearance, or glomerular filtration. Xenobiotic binding affinity can vary considerably among species, due to differences in the concentration of the particular protein and to differences in the affinity of the xenobiotic for the binding protein [70, 71]. The influence of interspecies variability on the allometric scaling of CL can be reduced by calculation of the "unbound" clearance [72] before the allometric analysis. This adjustment can be added to that shown in Eq. 29.9:

$$CL_{an}^h = CL_{an} \frac{(V_{max}/K_M)_{human}}{(V_{max}/K_M)_{an}} \frac{f_{up,human}}{f_{up,an}} \qquad (29.10)$$

Oral Clearance Clearance determined as Dose/$\int C_p \, dt$ after oral administration of test substance is uncertain due to lack of knowledge about the bioavailability, characterized as the fraction of dose that reaches the systemic circulation, F:

$$CL_{\text{oral}} = \frac{CL}{F} = \frac{Dose}{\int C_p dt} \tag{29.11}$$

Interspecies variability in F due to species-to-species differences in bioavailability (incomplete absorption, presystemic degradation) will be reflected in the apparent oral clearance ($CL_{\text{oral}} = CL/F$) values and will contribute to their scatter around the fitted allometric line. A special case is when $F < 1$ due solely to presystemic hepatic first-pass elimination of the test compound. Here, CL/F is in fact $f_{\text{up}}CL_{\text{int}}$, assuming that $C_p \ll K_M$. For this special case, the adjustments described in Eqs. 29.9 and 29.10 may be carried out and the human CL estimated using the allometric equation. When $F < 1$ for reasons other than hepatic first-pass extraction, there is no adjustment procedure available.

Projections Based on One or Two Species   Lin [48] noted that the per kg rat/ human GFR ratio was 4.8, which is generally found for the rat/human CL_R ratio of renally cleared drugs. He suggested that the human CL_R ($\text{mL}\,\text{min}^{-1}\text{kg}^{-1}$) could therefore be estimated as the rat CL_R ($\text{mL}\,\text{min}^{-1}\text{kg}^{-1}$) divided by 4.8. This seems appropriate since renal clearance is scaled relatively well by the allometric equation.

Ward and Smith [51] examined two-species allometry for estimation of human CL, using 103 test compounds and their CL values determined in rat, dog, monkey, and human. Rat–dog and rat–monkey, but not dog–monkey, pairs provided correct qualitative estimates of human CL category (low, intermediate, or high fraction of hepatic blood flow) with about 60% success. They also investigated calculation of the human CL according to the animal CL expressed as a fraction of liver blood flow multiplied by human liver blood flow:

$$CL_{\text{man}} = \frac{CL_{\text{an}}}{Q_{\text{H,an}}} \times Q_{\text{H,human}} \tag{29.12}$$

While CL was assumed to be primarily hepatic, a check of the 103 test compound list against a database of fraction of dose eliminated in urine (*Goodman and Gilman's the Pharmacological Basis of Therapeutics*, 9th and 10th editions [58]) showed that about one-fourth of the 55 test compounds in the database were predominantly (>50%) eliminated in the urine of humans. Use of Eq. 29.12 makes the tacit assumption that the ratio CL/Q_H is a constant across species, which seems unfounded even when hepatic clearance is the dominant contributor.

29.3.3   Recommended Approach

1. Determine the organ(s) primarily involved in clearance of the test compound. Generally, this will be liver or kidneys with the likelihood of liver being greater.

2. Determine CL after IV administration if possible in a minimum of four lab animal species. Fewer than four will raise the uncertainty considerably in the extrapolated human CL value. CL value for each species should be an average from several animals with interfacility differences minimized. Body mass

should span a range of 100, and the mass of the largest animal should be ~10 kg.

3. If renal clearance is the primary elimination pathway, simple allometry will generally predict the human CL. If f_{up} varies among species, use the unbound clearance in the allometric analysis.

4. If hepatic clearance is the primary elimination pathway, assess whether the clearance is low or high extraction. If the latter, simple allometry will generally predict the human CL.

5. If the primary elimination pathway is hepatic and low extraction, prediction of the human CL by simple allometry has a relatively low probability of success. Use f_{up} and *in vitro* intrinsic clearance measurements in the animals and humans to adjust the *in vivo* animal clearance values prior to allometric analysis.

6. Recognize that the extrapolated human CL value may be far from the true value. Extrapolation is considered successful if it is within a range of one-half to twice the true value.

29.4   SCALING VOLUME OF DISTRIBUTION

29.4.1   Physiological Basis and Theoretical Considerations

Drug distribution is often expressed in terms of the volume of distribution (V_d), which is usually defined as the ratio of drug amount in the body to the plasma (or blood) concentration. It is generally believed that only the unbound drug can freely diffuse across membranes that separate vascular and tissue compartments. Changes in drug protein binding in plasma and tissue can therefore affect drug distribution in the body, which can be described by the following relationship [59]:

$$V_d = V_p + \left(\frac{f_{up}}{f_{ut}} \right) V_t \qquad (29.13)$$

V_p and V_t are the volume of plasma and tissue, respectively, and f_{up} and f_{ut} are the unbound fraction of drug in plasma and tissue, respectively. Considering allometric scaling of V_d, three scenarios are apparent: (1) $V_d \approx V_p$, (2) $V_d \gg V_p$, and (3) $V_d = V_p + V_t$.

When a drug is extensively bound to plasma protein (i.e., $f_{up} \rightarrow 0$), the drug is confined in the vascular space; therefore, $V_d \rightarrow V_p$, which may satisfy condition 1. For a drug that fulfills the first condition, the interspecies scaling of V_d would be expected to follow that of blood volume. Generally, the total blood volume tends to scale across species with the first power of body mass ($M^{0.99}$ [7] and $M^{1.02}$ [73]). Therefore, for drugs with extremely high protein binding in plasma,

$$V_d \approx a M^{1.0} \qquad (29.14)$$

On the other hand, for a drug that is extensively bound to tissue protein (i.e., f_{ut} very small), V_d may be significantly larger than V_p and the second condition may be fulfilled. Usually if $V_d \geq 30\,L$, V_p has only a minor effect on V_d [59]; in this case,

$$V_d \approx \left(\frac{f_{up}}{f_{ut}} \right) V_t \tag{29.15}$$

As indicated in Eq. 29.15, both f_{up} and f_{ut} would affect the magnitude of V_d; therefore, if interspecies variation of protein binding were substantial, it would be difficult to find an allometric relationship for V_d.

When a drug has very low plasma and tissue binding (i.e., f_{up} and $f_{ut} \rightarrow 1$), the V_d of the drug will reflect the volume of total body water (condition 3). Accordingly, the scaling of V_d would correlate with the scaling of the total body water (TBW). The reported b value is 0.89 for the TBW [74]; therefore, for a drug that satisfies condition 3, the allometric relationship could be

$$V_d = aM^{0.89} \tag{29.16}$$

The scaling relationship of the mass (or volume) of the major drug distribution organs could also be indicative for the scaling of V_d. The scaling exponent of major organs ranged from 0.70 to 0.99 [7].

The V_d defined in the compartmental models usually does not represent a real physiological volume; however, it is an important pharmacokinetic parameter for the estimation of clinical loading dose. The rationale behind the scaling of V_d in drug development is at least twofold: (1) the volume of distribution of the central compartment (V_c) can be used to estimate initial plasma concentration, which may serve as an additional indicator for safety/toxicity for first-time dosing in humans; (2) combined with a known CL value, the value of V_c can be used to estimate the half-life, since $t_{1/2} = 0.693(V_d/CL)$. For compounds exhibiting multicompartmental kinetics, other volume terms (V_β, V_{ss}) have also been considered. V_{ss} would be expected to scale according to the principles embodied in Eqs. 29.14–29.16. V_β includes influences of distribution and elimination kinetic parameters and its scaling according to the allometric equation is less certain.

29.4.2   Empirical Observations

Generally, good correlation between body mass and V_c across species is expected. Most reported allometric exponents for V_d scattered about 1.0. Some drugs have b values that deviate significantly from 1.0 [75]. Mahmood [76] showed that V_c can be more accurately predicted than V_β and V_{ss}. It has been suggested that extrapolating V_β or V_{ss} from animal data is of limited significance for the first-time dosing in humans, because both parameters can be estimated later from human data [75]. Obach et al. [77] compared four different methods to predict human V_{ss} and demonstrated that when the allometric method was used, a better prediction was obtained when protein binding was taken into account. The main purpose of predicting V_d was to use the predicted V_d value in combination with a predicted CL value for predicting human $t_{1/2}$, "which is a more meaningful parameter with decision-making impact on the drug discovery and development processes" [77].

Interspecies scaling of V_d has also been applied to protein drugs and the reported allometric exponents were around 1.0. Mordenti [78] analyzed the volume of distribution of five human proteins in humans and laboratory animals as a function of body mass using allometric scaling techniques. The analyses showed that the volume data for each protein were satisfactorily described by an allometric equation. The allometric exponent for V_c ranged from 0.83 to 1.05, and the allometric exponent for V_{ss} ranged from 0.84 to 1.02. In another study, Mordenti [79] reported that the allometric exponents for recombinant human factor VIII were 1.04 and 0.84 for V_c and V_{ss}, respectively.

29.4.3   Limitations and Challenges

Prediction involves uncertainty. To establish a meaningful allometric relationship, it is always desirable to include as many animal species as possible. However, in the real world of drug development, pharmacokinetic data are often obtained from a limited number of preclinical species. It becomes a challenging task to predict any pharmacokinetic parameters when data are only available from two or three species. Mahmood and Balian [80] showed that allometric scaling of V_d from only two species is as predictive as that observed from three or more species. Ward and Smith [50], however, showed a contradictory result, indicating that three-species allometry provided improved quantitative prediction compared with two-species allometry. Moreover, single-species extrapolation has been proposed for making early go/no-go human PK decisions for drug discovery candidates [50, 81]. When the interspecies variation in pharmacokinetics, for a given drug candidate, cannot be understood prospectively, the claim of superiority of any projection based on limited data (i.e., from one to three species) may be futile. In other words, the overall prediction may be equally good or equally bad, depending on how one determines the prediction performance. For estimating volume of distribution, it may imply knowing in advance whether the protein binding (plasma and tissue) of a given drug is likely to be so variable across species. In this regard, the use of *in vitro* binding data may be helpful. Further studies may aim at characterizing the molecular and physicochemical properties of drugs that show high interspecies variability.

29.5   SCALING HALF-LIFE

29.5.1   Rationale and Theoretical Considerations

Half-life is an important pharmacokinetic parameter in that (1) it provides the basis for the selection of dosage regimen and (2) it offers prediction of the time to reach steady-state concentration and of the degree of accumulation. In drug development, the utility of scaling half-life across species lies mainly in predicting the dosing frequency of a lead compound. This is true because a frequently asked question in the compound selection process is: Will compound X be a once daily drug? [77].

Theoretically, half-life can be written

$$t_{1/2} = 0.693\left(\frac{V_d}{CL}\right) \tag{29.17}$$

If one assumes that the V_d scales with $M^{1.0}$ and CL scales as $M^{0.75}$, then the expected scaling relationship would be

$$t_{1/2} = aM^{0.25} \tag{29.18}$$

Practically, there are three ways to predict the half-life in humans: (1) direct extrapolation from animal data using the allometric relationship for half-life, if there is any; (2) indirect prediction using Eq. 29.17, where V_d and CL in humans are predicted *a priori* [63, 77, 82]; and (3) indirect estimation from predicted mean residence time (MRT), using the following relationship [76]:

$$t_{1/2} = 0.693 MRT \tag{29.19}$$

29.5.2   Empirical Observations

Predicting the half-life in humans from animal data is challenging. One study reported that the exponents of the half-life for drugs varied from -0.066 to 0.547, with the average of 0.19 [76]. Riviere et al. [83] conducted an interspecies allometric analysis of the $t_{1/2}$ of 44 drugs across veterinary and laboratory animal species. A total of 11 drugs (25%) showed statistically significant correlations between log $t_{1/2}$ and log M. The exponent b value for this group of drugs ranged from 0.1 to 0.415, with an average of 0.24 ± 0.09. The remaining 33 drugs showed lack of correlation; many of these drugs were low hepatic extraction drugs. Lack of quality data (e.g., narrow body mass range, multiple data sources) may account for the lack of correlation observed with some drugs [83].

29.5.3   Limitations and Challenges

Difficulty in obtaining consistent correlation between $t_{1/2}$ and body mass across species might be due to the fact that $t_{1/2}$ is a hybrid parameter of V_d and CL; that is, both drug distribution and elimination processes determine the value of $t_{1/2}$. Successful prediction of $t_{1/2}$ tended to occur for drugs that are mainly renally excreted and have low protein binding [26]. It would be more difficult to obtain an allometric relationship for drugs that follow complex disposition mechanisms, such as extensive metabolism involving multiple enzymatic systems and high plasma and/or tissue binding. Use of the above-mentioned indirect methods may improve the predictability of $t_{1/2}$. Moreover, the reliability of prediction may be increased by the incorporation of *in vitro* metabolic data [77, 84] and of calculated molecular properties [53]. The main focus of predicting $t_{1/2}$ should be placed on assigning compounds to appropriate dosing regimen categories (e.g., once daily, twice daily), rather than on a precise estimate of $t_{1/2}$ value.

29.6   CONCLUSION

Allometric scaling can be useful in the projection of preclinical pharmacokinetic parameter values to humans. Apparent volume of distribution will generally scale successfully, more so when interspecies differences in plasma protein binding are accounted for. Also, renal clearance generally will scale successfully to humans and accounting for interspecies differences in plasma protein binding will improve the success rate. Scaling metabolic clearance is problematic but progress on incorporation of *in vitro* metabolism parameters and plasma protein binding to adjust animal clearance values for interspecies differences in intrinsic metabolism activity has improved the prospects for successful prediction of human *CL* for compounds cleared primarily by metabolism. In future, transgenic animals with human intrinsic enzyme activities may further improve predictive success.

REFERENCES

1. Huxley JS, Teissier G. Terminology of relative growth. *Nature* 1936;137:780–781.
2. White CR, Seymour RS. Allometric scaling of mammalian metabolism. *J Exp Biol* 2005;208:1611–1619.
3. Rubner N. Ueber den Einfluss der Koerpergroesse auf Stoff und Kraftwechsel. *Z Biol* 1883;19:535–562.
4. Kleiber M. Body size and metabolism. *Hilgardia* 1932;6:315–332.
5. Brody S. *Bioenergetics and Growth*. New York: Reinhold Publishing Corporation; 1945.
6. West GB, Brown JH, Enquist BJ. A general model for the origin of allometric scaling laws in biology. *Science* 1997;276:122–126.
7. Adolph EF. Quantitative relations in the physiological constitutions of mammals. *Science* 1949;109:579–585.
8. Davidson IW, Parker JC, Beliles RP. Biological basis for extrapolation across mammalian species. *Regul Toxicol Pharmacol* 1986;6:211–237.
9. Pinkel D. The use of body surface area as a criterion of drug dosage in cancer chemotherapy. *Cancer Res* 1958;18:853–856.
10. Freireich EJ, Gehan EA, Rall DP, Schmidt LH, Skipper HE. Quantitative comparison of toxicity of anticancer agents in mouse, rat, hamster, dog, monkey, and man. *Cancer Chemother Rep* 1966;50:219–244.
11. Mellett LB. Comparative drug metabolism. *Prog Drug Res* 1969;13:136–169.
12. Dedrick RL. Animal scale-up. *J Pharmacokinet Biopharm* 1973;1:435–461.
13. Dedrick RL, Bischoff KB, Zaharko DS. Interspecies correlation of plasma concentration history of methotrexate (NSC-740). *Cancer Chemother Rep Part 1* 1970;54:95–101.
14. Stahl WR. Similarity analysis of physiological systems. *Perspect Biol Med* 1963;6:291–321.
15. Klotz U, Antonin KH, Bieck PR. Pharmacokinetics and plasma binding of diazepam in man, dog, rabbit, guinea pig and rat. *J Pharmacol Exp Ther* 1976;199:67–73.
16. Weiss M, Sziegoleit W, Forster W. Dependence of pharmacokinetic parameters on the body weight. *Int J Clin Pharmacol Biopharm* 1977;15:572–575.
17. Boxenbaum H. Interspecies variation in liver weight, hepatic blood flow, and antipyrine intrinsic clearance: extrapolation of data to benzodiazepines and phenytoin. *J Pharmacokinet Biopharm* 1980;8:165–176.
18. Boxenbaum H. Interspecies scaling, allometry, physiological time, and the ground plan of pharmacokinetics. *J Pharmacokinet Biopharm* 1982;10:201–227.
19. Boxenbaum H, Ronfeld R. Interspecies pharmacokinetic scaling and the Dedrick plots. *Am J Physiol* 1983;245:R768–R775.

20. Boxenbaum H. Interspecies pharmacokinetic scaling and the evolutionary-comparative paradigm. *Drug Metab Rev* 1984;15:1071–1121.

21. Boxenbaum H, Fertig JB. Scaling of antipyrine intrinsic clearance of unbound drug in 15 mammalian species. *Eur J Drug Metab Pharmacokinet* 1984;9:177–183.

22. Calabrese EJ. Animal extrapolation and the challenge of human heterogeneity. *J Pharm Sci* 1986;75:1041–1046.

23. Mordenti J. Man versus beast: pharmacokinetic scaling in mammals. *J Pharm Sci* 1986; 75:1028–1040.

24. Yates FE, Kugler PN. Similarity principles and intrinsic geometries: contrasting approaches to interspecies scaling. *J Pharm Sci* 1986;75:1019–1027.

25. Hayton WL. Pharmacokinetic parameters for interspecies scaling using allometric techniques. *Health Phys* 1989;57(Suppl 1):159–164.

26. Mordenti J. Forecasting cephalosporin and monobactam antibiotic half-lives in humans from data collected in laboratory animals. *Antimicrob Agents Chemother* 1985;27: 887–891.

27. Swabb EA, Bonner DP. Prediction of aztreonam pharmacokinetics in humans on data from animals. *J Pharmacokinet Biopharm* 1983;11:215–223.

28. Sawada Y, Hanano M, Sugiyama Y, Iga T. Prediction of the disposition of beta-lactam antibiotics in humans from pharmacokinetic parameters in animals. *J Pharmacokinet Biopharm* 1984;12:241–261.

29. Sawada Y, Hanano M, Sugiyama Y, Harashima H, Iga T. Prediction of the volumes of distribution of basic drugs in humans based on data from animals. *J Pharmacokinet Biopharm* 1984;12:587–596.

30. Duthu GS. Interspecies correlation of the pharmacokinetics of erythromycin, oleandomycin, and tylosin. *J Pharm Sci* 1985;74:943–946.

31. Ings RM. Interspecies scaling and comparisons in drug development and toxicokinetics. *Xenobiotica* 1990;20:1201–1231.

32. Bonate PL, Howard D. Prospective allometric scaling: Does the emperor have clothes? *J Clin Pharmacol* 2000;40:665–670; discussion pp 671–676.

33. Mahmood I. Critique of prospective allometric scaling: Does the emperor have clothes? *J Clin Pharmacol* 2000;40:341–344; discussion pp 345–346.

34. Hu TM, Hayton WL. Allometric scaling of xenobiotic clearance: uncertainty versus universality. *AAPS PharmSci* 2001;3:E29.

35. Huxley JS. *Problems of Relative Growth*. London: Methuen; 1932.

36. Schmidt-Nielsen K. *Scaling: Why Is Animal Size So Important?* Cambridge, UK: Cambridge University Press; 1984.

37. Smith RJ. Allometric scaling in comparative biology: problems of concept and method. *Am J Physiol* 1984;246:R152–R160.

38. West GB, Brown JH, Enquist BJ. The fourth dimension of life: fractal geometry and allometric scaling of organisms. *Science* 1999;284:1677–1679.

39. Gillooly JF, Brown JH, West GB, Savage VM, Charnov EL. Effects of size and temperature on metabolic rate. *Science* 2001;293:2248–2251.

40. West GB, Brown JH. The origin of allometric scaling laws in biology from genomes to ecosystems: towards a quantitative unifying theory of biological structure and organization. *J Exp Biol* 2005;208:1575–1592.

41. Heusner AA. Energy metabolism and body size. I. Is the 0.75 mass exponent of Kleiber's equation a statistical artifact? *Respir Physiol* 1982;48:1–12.

42. Gunther B, Morgado E. Dimensional analysis revisited. *Biol Res* 2003;36:405–410.

43. Kleiber M. Body size and metabolic rate. *Physiol Rev* 1947;27:511–541.

44. Feldman HA, McMahon TA. The 3/4 mass exponent for energy metabolism is not a statistical artifact. *Respir Physiol* 1983;52:149–163.

45. Hayssen V, Lacy RC. Basal metabolic rates in mammals: taxonomic differences in the allometry of BMR and body mass. *Comp Biochem Physiol A* 1985;81:741–754.

46. Dodds PS, Rothman DH, Weitz JS. Re-examination of the "3/4-law" of metabolism. *J Theor Biol* 2001;209:9–27.

47. Gould SJ. Allometry and size in ontogeny and phylogeny. *Biol Rev Camb Philos Soc* 1966;41:587–640.

48. Lin JH. Applications and limitations of interspecies scaling and *in vitro* extrapolation in pharmacokinetics. *Drug Metab Dispos* 1998;26:1202–1212.

49. Henderson CJ, Wolf CR. Transgenic analysis of drug-metabolizing enzymes: preclinical drug development and toxicology. *Mol Interv* 2003;3:331–343.

50. Ward KW, Smith BR. A comprehensive quantitative and qualitative evaluation of extrapolation of intravenous pharmacokinetic parameters from rat, dog, and monkey to humans. II. Volume of distribution and mean residence time. *Drug Metab Dispos* 2004;32: 612–619.

51. Ward KW, Smith BR. A comprehensive quantitative and qualitative evaluation of extrapolation of intravenous pharmacokinetic parameters from rat, dog, and monkey to humans. I. Clearance. *Drug Metab Dispos* 2004;32:603–611.

52. Nagilla R, Ward KW. A comprehensive analysis of the role of correction factors in the allometric predictivity of clearance from rat, dog, and monkey to humans. *J Pharm Sci* 2004;93:2522–2534.

53. Jolivette LJ, Ward KW. Extrapolation of human pharmacokinetic parameters from rat, dog, and monkey data: molecular properties associated with extrapolative success or failure. *J Pharm Sci* 2005;74:1467–1483.

54. Ward KW, Nagilla R, Jolivette LJ. Comparative evaluation of oral systemic exposure of 56 xenobiotics in rat, dog, monkey and human. *Xenobiotica* 2005;35:191–210.

55. Nagilla R, Ward KW. Erratum: A comprehensive analysis of the role of correction factors in the allometric predictivity of clearance from rat, dog, monkey to humans. *J Pharm Sci* 2005;94:231–232.

56. Prothero J. Methodological aspects of scaling in biology. *J Theor Biol* 1986;118:259–286.

57. Wilkinson GR. Clearance approaches in pharmacology. *Pharmacol Rev* 1987;39:1–47.

58. Thummel KE, Shen DD. Design and optimization of dosage regimens: pharmacokinetic data. In Limbird LE, Hardman JG, Eds. *Goodman and Gilman's the Pharmacological Basis of Therapeutics*. New York: McGraw-Hill; 2001, pp 1924–2023.

59. Wilkinson GR, Shand DG. Commentary: a physiological approach to hepatic drug clearance. *Clin Pharmacol Ther* 1975;188:377–390.

60. Davies B, Morris T. Physiological parameters in laboratory animals and humans. *Pharm Res* 1993;10:1093–1095.

61. Mahmood I. Interspecies scaling: predicting clearance of anticancer drugs in humans. A comparative study of three different approaches using body weight or body surface area. *Eur J Drug Metab Pharmacokinet* 1996;21:275–278.

62. Mahmood I, Balian JD. Interspecies scaling: predicting clearance of drugs in humans. Three different approaches. *Xenobiotica* 1996;26:887–895.

63. Mahmood I, Balian JD. Interspecies scaling: predicting pharmacokinetic parameters of antiepileptic drugs in humans from animals with special emphasis on clearance. *J Pharm Sci* 1996;85:411–414.

64. Rane A, Wilkinson GR, Shand DG. Prediction of hepatic extraction ratio from *in vitro* measurement of intrinsic clearance. *J Pharmacol Exp Ther* 1977;200:420–424.

65. Calabrese EJ. *Principles of Animal Extrapolation: Predicting Human Responses from Animal Studies*. Chelsea: Lewis Publisher; 1991.

66. Iwatsubo T, Hirota N, Ooie T, Suzuki H, Shimada N, Chiba K, Ishizaki T, Green CE, Tyson CA, Sugiyama Y. Prediction of *in vivo* drug metabolism in the human liver from *in vitro* metabolism data. *Pharmacol Ther* 1997;73:147–171.

67. Lavé T, Schmitt-Hoffmann AH, Coassolo P, Valles B, Ubeaud G, Ba B, Brandt R, Chou RC. A new extrapolation method from animals to man: application to a metabolized compound, mofarotene. *Life Sci* 1995;56:PL473–PL478.

68. Lavé T, Dupin S, Schmitt C, Chou RC, Jaeck D, Coassolo P. Integration of *in vitro* data into allometric scaling to predict hepatic metabolic clearance in man: application to 10 extensively metabolized drugs. *J Pharm Sci* 1997;86:584–590.

69. Lavé T, Coassolo P, Reigner B. Prediction of hepatic metabolic clearance based on interspecies allometric scaling techniques and *in vitro–in vivo* correlations. *Clin Pharmacokinet* 1999;36:211–231.

70. Guarino AM, Anderson JB, Starkweather DK, Chignell CF. Pharmacologic studies of camptothecin (NSC-100880): distribution, plasma protein binding, and biliary excretion. *Cancer Chemother Rep* 1973;57:125–140.

71. Mi Z, Burke TG. Marked interspecies variations concerning the interactions of camptothecin with serum albumins: a frequency-domain fluorescence spectroscopic study. *Biochemistry* 1994;33:12540–12545.

72. Chiou WL, Choi YM. Unbound total (plasma) clearance approach in interspecies pharmacokinetics correlation: theophylline–cimetidine interaction. *Pharm Res* 1995;12: 1238–1239.

73. Stahl WR. Scaling of respiratory variables in mammals. *J Appl Physiol* 1967;48: 1052–1059.

74. Chappell WR, Mordenti J. Extrapolation of toxicological and pharmacological data from animals to humans. In Testa B, Ed. *Advances in Drug Research*, Volume 20. London, UK: Academic Press; 1991, pp 1–116.

75. Mahmood I. Allometric issues in drug development. *J Pharm Sci* 1999;88:1101–1106.

76. Mahmood I. Interspecies scaling: predicting volumes, mean residence time and elimination half-life. Some suggestions. *J Pharm Pharmacol* 1998;50:493–499.

77. Obach RS, Baxter JG, Liston TE, Silber BM, Jones BC, MacIntyre F, Rance DJ, Wastall P. The prediction of human pharmacokinetic parameters from preclinical and *in vitro* metabolism data. *J Pharmacol Exp Ther* 1997;283:46–58.

78. Mordenti J, Chen SA, Moore JA, Ferrailo BL, Green JD. Interspecies scaling of clearance and volume of distribution data for five therapeutic proteins. *Pharm Res* 1991;8: 1351–1359.

79. Mordenti J, Osaka G, Garcia K, Thomsen K, Licko V, Meng G. Pharmacokinetics and interspecies scaling of recombinant human Factor VIII. *Toxico Appl Pharmacol* 1996;4:75–78.

80. Mahmood I, Balian JD. Interspecies scaling: a comparative study for the prediction of clearance and volume using two or more than two species. *Life Sci* 1996;59:579–585.

81. Caldwell GW, Masucci JA, Yan Z, Hageman W. Allometric scaling of pharmacokinetic parameters in drug discovery: can human CL, V_{ss} and $t_{1/2}$ be predicted from *in-vivo* rat data? *Eur J Drug Metab Pharmacokinet* 2004;29:133–143.

82. Bachmann K. Predicting toxicokinetic parameters in humans from toxicokinetic data acquired from three small mammalian species. *J Appl Toxicol* 1989;9:331–338.

83. Riviere JE, Martin-Jimenez T, Sundlof SF, Craigmill AL. Interspecies allometric analysis of the comparative pharmacokinetics of 44 drugs across veterinary and laboratory animal species. *J Vet Pharmacol Ther* 1997;20:453–463.

84. Lavé T, Dupin S, Schmitt M, Kapps M, Meyer J, Morgenroth B, Chou RC, Jaeck D, Coassolo P. Interspecies scaling of tolcapone, a new inhibitor of catechol-*O*-methyltransferase (COMT). Use of *in vitro* data from hepatocytes to predict metabolic clearance in animals and humans. *Xenobiotica* 1996;26:839–851.

30

INTERRELATIONSHIP BETWEEN PHARMACOKINETICS AND METABOLISM

James W. Paxton

The University of Auckland, Auckland, New Zealand

Contents

Preclinical Development Handbook: ADME and Biopharmaceutical Properties,
edited by Shayne Cox Gad
Copyright © 2008 John Wiley & Sons, Inc.

30.1   INTRODUCTION

For most drugs, the magnitude and duration of their pharmacological effect depend on their concentration–time profile within the body. This profile is largely the result of two opposing processes, the rate of drug input into the body and the rate of drug elimination by the body. The study of the time course of drug in the body is termed pharmacokinetics and incorporates the processes of absorption, distribution, metabolism, and excretion (ADME). For most drugs, absorption and distribution determine the speed of onset of drug effect, while metabolism and excretion terminate the action of a drug by removing the active form (with the exception of prodrugs, which undergo biotransformation to the therapeutically active metabolite). The major pharmacokinetic parameters that describe the ADME processes are clearance (CL), volume of distribution (V), elimination half-life $(T_{1/2})$, and bioavailability (F). These pharmacokinetic parameters are key determinants in the design of a suitable dosage regimen, providing information about the magnitude and frequency of dosing (Fig. 30.1).

In drug development, it is estimated that approximately 40% of all new chemical entities (NCEs) fail to become clinically successful drugs due to undesirable pharmacokinetic properties [1–4]. The single greatest factor contributing to inappropriate pharmacokinetics is the process of metabolism. Most drugs are fat/lipid soluble, and metabolism plays a crucial role in their deactivation and the determination of their pharmacokinetic profile. For such drugs, the *in vivo* capacity for metabolism is measured by clearance, which has a major impact on the secondary pharmacokinetic parameters, such as half-life and oral bioavailability. A knowledge of the capacity for the metabolism of an NCE and an understanding of the human metabolism pathways and the enzymes involved have now become key components in the selection of compounds for clinical development. This knowledge is important not only for the optimization of the metabolic stability of the NCE but also to avoid

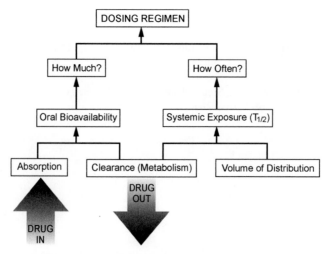

FIGURE 30.1   Relationship between metabolism, pharmacokinetic parameters, and dosing regimen. (Adapted from Ref. 4.)

the likelihood that it is subjected to clinically significant genetic polymorphic metabolism, drug–drug interactions (either by induction or inhibition), or the formation of biologically active or reactive metabolites. This chapter appraises the relationship between metabolism and the resulting pharmacokinetic profile of a drug, and reviews the major factors that may have an impact on a drug's metabolism and may have a detrimental effect on its pharmacokinetics and clinical use.

30.2 IMPORTANT PHARMACOKINETIC PARAMETERS

A basic tenet of pharmacokinetics is that the magnitude of both the desired therapeutic response and/or toxicity of a drug is a function of its concentration in the body [5]. If concentrations are too low at the site of action, therapeutic failure may occur, and conversely, if concentrations are too high, adverse effects and toxicity may result. Thus, successful pharmacotherapy is very often dependent on maintaining the drug concentration within a defined range, known as the *therapeutic range* or *window* [5]. The best place to measure drug concentration presumably would be at the site of action, but most often this is not accessible, being in a tissue such as the brain or the heart, and a blood sample (usually plasma or serum) is used instead. At steady-state conditions when the rate of drug administration is balanced by the rate of drug elimination, the plasma concentration for many drugs is a relatively acceptable index of the concentration at the site of action.

Pharmacokinetics is the study of the drug/metabolite concentration–time profiles resulting from ADME, and the factors that may influence these processes. A knowledge of pharmacokinetics is crucial to determine a rational dosing regimen; that is, how much and how often a drug should be given to achieve the desired therapeutic effect. Rational dosing regimens can be established from several simple pharmacokinetic parameters mainly derived from drug plasma concentration–time curves. The key pharmacokinetic parameters to provide information on dose size and dose frequency are clearance, elimination half-life, and bioavailability. The volume of distribution may also be useful to calculate a loading dose at commencement of treatment in order to more rapidly achieve a particular target concentration. Obviously, the greater the therapeutic index (i.e., the separation of the concentration at which adverse effects appear and the minimum concentration required to produce an effective pharmacological response), the less important is the consideration of a drug's pharmacokinetics and the individualization of the dosage regimen.

30.2.1 Systemic Clearance (CL_P)

Systemic or total plasma clearance (CL_P) is arguably the most important of all pharmacokinetic parameters. Clearance is the most useful parameter for the evaluation of the elimination processes and has the most potential for clinical application. Clearance may be defined as the proportionality constant relating the rate of drug elimination to the plasma concentration (C): thus,

$$CL_P = \text{Elimination rate}/C \qquad (30.1)$$

This equation can be re arranged to give

$$\text{Rate of drug elimination} = CL_P \times C \tag{30.2}$$

Alternatively, the clearance can be defined as the volume of plasma irreversibly cleared of drug per unit time, and usually it has units of L/h or mL/min [5]. Clearance is an index of the capacity for the elimination of an active drug from the body and may involve both metabolism and excretion processes, depending on the physicochemical properties of the drug. For example, a water-soluble drug, such as gentamicin, is eliminated almost entirely unchanged by the kidney, and its clearance will be determined entirely by the ability of the kidney to remove it from the blood flowing through the kidney. However, for most drugs, the total plasma clearance is the sum of clearances by the kidney (CL_R) and liver (CL_H), plus any other route (CL_O), and thus

$$CL_P = CL_R + CL_H + CL_O \tag{30.3}$$

The balance between these processes depends on the relative efficiencies of each process for a particular drug and the drug's physicochemical properties. However, most drugs are relatively lipid soluble (necessary for acceptable oral absorption and tissue distribution), and consequently, metabolism is the major determinant of elimination, usually converting them into inactive and more excretable forms. Thus, for most drugs, hepatic metabolism is the major component of the total plasma clearance.

For any particular organ, the physiological determinants of drug clearance are the organ blood flow, the inherent ability of the organ to extract the drug from the blood, and the extent of binding to plasma proteins and cells. Thus, an equation for the clearance of an eliminating organ, such as the liver, can be derived using the simplest (and most widely employed) model of hepatic clearance (known as the *well-stirred* or *venous equilibrium model*):

$$CL_H = Q_H \times \left[\frac{fu \times CL_{int}}{Q_H + (fu \times CL_{int})} \right] \tag{30.4}$$

where Q_H is the hepatic blood flow, CL_{int} is the intrinsic clearance, and fu is the fraction unbound in blood. This model assumes that the distribution of the drug is so fast in this highly vascular organ that the concentration of the unbound drug in the blood leaving the organ is equal to that within the organ. The full derivation of Eq. 30.4 can be found in Rowland and Tozer [5].

The CL_{int} represents the intrinsic ability of the liver to remove (metabolize) the drug in the absence of any restrictions imposed by protein binding or blood flow to the liver. The term contained in the square brackets of Eq. 30.4 is referred to as the hepatic extraction ratio (ER_H) and is a measure of the efficiency of hepatic removal of drug and may range from 0 (when no drug is extracted) to 1, when the drug is completely removed during a single pass through the liver. Thus, Eq. 30.4 can be simplified to

$$CL_H = Q_H \times ER_H \tag{30.5}$$

Thus, if a drug has a very high intrinsic clearance compared to blood flow, the extraction ratio will tend toward 1, and the drug's hepatic clearance will approach the value of Q_H, the hepatic blood flow (but it can never be greater than this blood flow). Such drugs will exhibit blood-flow-dependent elimination kinetics. In this situation, the liver extraction processes or metabolizing enzymes are so active that the liver removes all, or nearly all, of the drug presented to it. Thus, the actual hepatic clearance is determined by the rate of supply of the drug to the liver, that is, the hepatic blood flow. As nearly all of the drug is already being removed, changes in enzyme activity make little or no difference to clearance. Similarly, protein binding is not important for such drugs as the liver has such high affinity/capacity for the drug that even bound drug can be stripped off the plasma proteins in a single pass through the liver. Thus, the hepatic clearance of a drug such as propranolol, lidocaine, and verapamil, for which the liver has a high metabolic capacity, is limited by hepatic blood flow and is uninfluenced by plasma protein binding [5]. The hepatic clearance of such drugs is relatively insensitive to changes in metabolizing activity brought about by induction or inhibition of hepatic metabolizing enzymes. However, a reduction in the rate of drug transport to the liver, such as a decrease in blood flow in heart failure, for example, would result in a decrease in hepatic clearance [5].

At the other extreme, when a drug's intrinsic clearance is very low compared to blood flow, then the hepatic extraction is low, and Eq. 30.4 for hepatic clearance reduces to

$$CL_H = fu \times CL_{int} \tag{30.6}$$

The hepatic clearance of such drugs is dependent only on enzyme activity and the unbound fraction in the blood. Thus, for a drug such as theophylline, for which the liver has a low metabolic capacity resulting in a low extraction ratio, its hepatic clearance will be affected by a change in enzyme activity but will not be influenced by changes in hepatic blood flow [5]. Thus, the hepatic extraction ratio may be used to roughly divide drugs into three categories: high ($ER_H > 0.7$), intermediate (ER_H 0.3–0.7), and low ($ER_H < 0.3$) extraction ratio drugs. This classification of a NCE is useful in drug development to predict the influence of blood flow, enzyme induction and inhibition, and protein binding on its hepatic clearance and oral bioavailability (see below).

The extraction ratio across any organ may also be defined as the fraction of the drug removed from blood in one passage across that organ and may be determined by measuring the drug concentration in the plasma entering and exiting the organ. For example, ER_H can be calculated using the following equation:

$$ER_H = (C_{in} - C_{out})/C_{in} \tag{30.7}$$

where C_{in} is the drug concentration in the plasma entering the liver, and C_{out} is drug concentration in the plasma exiting the liver.

In biochemical terms, the hepatic intrinsic clearance of a particular drug is a measure of how active the liver drug-metabolizing enzymes are with this drug as a substrate. Using the principles of enzyme kinetics and various *in vitro* enzyme systems (e.g., isolated perfused liver, hepatocytes, liver slices, human microsomes, S9 fraction, and various recombinant enzyme expression systems), it is possible to calculate a value for the *in vitro* intrinsic clearance. For example, using a one-site enzyme model and the Michaelis–Menten equation:

$$\text{Rate of metabolism (elimination)} = (V_{max} \times C)/(K_m + C) \tag{30.8}$$

where V_{max} is the maximal velocity of the reaction, K_m is the substrate concentration at which half maximal velocity is attained, and C is the substrate concentration. When substrate concentration is much less than K_m, Eq. 30.8 reduces to

$$\text{Rate of elimination} = (V_{max}/K_m) \times C \tag{30.9}$$

This ratio of V_{max}/K_m estimated from *in vitro* data can be used as an approximation of the expected *in vitro* intrinsic clearance of a drug and usually has units of µL/min/mg of microsomal protein (if using a microsomal preparation). More recently in drug development, it has become popular to use the "depletion" method and measure the disappearance of an NCE over time in an *in vitro* system, and express this as a disappearance half-life, and then calculate intrinsic clearance from this [6–8]. The *in vitro* intrinsic clearance parameter can then be scaled up to the whole liver using various scaling parameters as suggested by a number of investigators [9, 10]. Furthermore, the latter can be extrapolated to predict an expected *in vivo* hepatic clearance value for that particular drug in humans. This can be done using a number of different models for the liver, including the *dispersion, parallel-tube*, or *well-stirred model*. The latter two are currently most often utilized because of their simpler mathematical basis. They differ from each other with regard to their assumption on how drug concentrations decline within the liver: the *well-stirred* model assumes the concentration to be homogeneous throughout the organ and to be reflected by the outflow concentration; whereas the parallel-tube model considers an exponential decline in drug concentration through the organ. The dispersion model is intermediate between those two with respect to drug mixing within the organ but is mathematically more complex. Further details on these models can be found in Refs. 9–11. In a comprehensive comparison of the three models, Ito and Houston [12] observed minimal differences between the models for the prediction of the *in vivo* hepatic clearance and suggested that the well-stirred model was adequate in a screening process to identify an NCE with a high or low clearance. The extrapolation of *in vitro* data to predict *in vivo* hepatic clearance has been extensively reviewed over recent years [13–15].

Acceptable correlations between *in vitro* and *in vivo* clearance values have been reported for a few lipophilic drugs, demonstrating the utility of these models/methods, but in general the quantitative predictions of *in vivo* clearance from *in vitro* metabolism data using existing models has been poor [11, 16]. It has been suggested that this is due to the lack of understanding of the interplay between the intrahepatocyte concentration and plasma and tissue binding, and the part played by drug influx and efflux by hepatocyte transporters [11]. Also, it is increasingly being recognized that many drugs exhibit "atypical" enzyme kinetics *in vitro* that cannot be adequately modeled by the basic Michaelis–Menten equation [17]. In order to improve the prediction of the relevant *in vivo* pharmacokinetic parameters, more complex models need to be applied to accommodate (1) more complex enzyme kinetics (e.g., autoactivation, substrate inhibition, interactions between several binding sites on the enzyme); (2) incorporation of active transport mechanisms into, and within, the liver; and (3) tissue binding to both blood and liver components. It has been suggested that a physiologically based pharmacokinetic model might be more appropriate, as such models can incorporate more complex physiological and biochemical processes and are capable of predicting drug disposition quantitatively in different tissues in humans [17]. With the increased understanding of the mechanistic processes of ADME from *in vitro* studies, physiologically based pharmacokinetic modeling may prove to be a more valuable tool in the future [18].

In summary, in preclinical drug development, the prediction that a particular NCE has a high hepatic clearance forewarns that (1) it is likely to be subject to flow-dependent elimination (and may require dose reduction in situations of decreased blood flow such as in congestive heart failure), (2) is subject to high first-pass metabolism and thus will have low oral bioavailability (see Section 30.2.2), and (3) it may be more prone to presystemic drug or food metabolism interactions on oral dosing. In contrast, an NCE with a low hepatic clearance is more susceptible to protein binding changes (but note that the unbound concentration does not change, and thus no change in dose rate is required) and changes in metabolizing enzyme activity due to induction or inhibition.

30.2.2 Oral Bioavailability (*F*)

Orally administered drugs must be absorbed and pass sequentially from the gastrointestinal lumen through the gut epithelia and liver, before entering the systemic circulation. The proportion of an orally administered drug that reaches the systemic circulation intact is referred to as its bioavailability. Hence, bioavailability usually refers to the biologically available portion of the drug dose that may exert its pharmacological actions. Oral bioavailability is a function of the fraction of the dose absorbed, and the fraction of the drug that escapes extrusion back into the gut lumen by active efflux transporter systems and/or metabolism by intestinal and liver enzymes. The latter is referred to as the first-pass metabolism. Although metabolism is largely carried out in the liver, for some drugs, such as cyclosporine, there is evidence that a significant amount also occurs in the enterocytes in the gut wall and contributes to the overall first-pass effect [19, 20]. If a large proportion of a drug is metabolized by the epithelial cells of the gut or by the liver before it reaches the systemic circulation, this will result in a low bioavailability, and consequently, a much greater dose must be administered to compensate for this loss. If we assume all the drug is absorbed intact (i.e., fraction absorbed = 1), then the bioavailability (*F*) depends on the fraction escaping the first-pass extraction, and thus

$$F = 1 - ER_{\text{I+H}} \tag{30.10}$$

where $ER_{\text{I+H}}$ represents the combined extraction ratio for the intestines and the liver. If we consider a drug with a low extraction ratio, which is poorly metabolized by the liver (and the gut wall), nearly all the drug escapes the first-pass process, and bioavailability is essentially complete (as long as it is well absorbed from the gut). For example, if 3% of a theoretical drug is extracted by the liver, the resulting bioavailability will be 97%. However, any major alteration in this extraction ratio by induction (e.g., a doubling of ER_{I+H} from 3% to 6%) or inhibition (e.g., ER_{I+H} halved from 3% to 1.5%) will have very little overall effect on bioavailability with a reduction from 97% to 94% on induction, and an increase from 97% to 98.5% with inhibition. Such changes in bioavailability would be insignificant in the clinical situation. In contrast, if a drug has a high ER_{I+H}, most of the dose is extracted on the first pass through the liver, so that only a minor proportion reaches the systemic circulation intact. Thus, although induction or inhibition of the metabolizing enzymes would have only a small effect on ER_{I+H}, it would have a significant effect on the proportion escaping extraction and on the bioavailability. For example, a theoretical drug with a high ER_{I+H} of 90% would have a bioavailability of 10%. However, if induction of the metabolizing enzymes increased this ER_{I+H} to 95%, this would result in the halving of the bioavailability from 10% to 5%. Similarly, if the metabolizing enzymes were inhibited, decreasing the ER_{I+H} to 80%, a doubling of the bioavailability would result. For many drugs, such changes in bioavailability would certainly be considered significant. Thus, for drugs with high extraction ratios, hepatic and intestinal enzyme activity are the major determinants of first-pass metabolism, and consequently their oral bioavailability. (However, note that after intravenous administration, hepatic blood flow is the major determinant of the systemic clearance of high extraction drugs.) After oral administration, the plasma concentrations of high extraction drugs, such as propranolol and verapamil, are more variable, both within and between individuals compared to the plasma concentrations of low ER_H drugs, and small changes in the metabolism capacity can cause large changes in oral bioavailability [5, 20]. Obviously, if an NCE experiences a very high first-pass metabolism (i.e., $ER_{I+H} \approx 1$) after oral administration, an alternative route of administration may have to be found or the molecule redesigned to increase its metabolic stability and reduce its first-pass metabolism.

30.2.3   Volume of Distribution (V)

Along with plasma clearance, the volume of distribution is the other major independent pharmacokinetic parameter. The concept of distribution volume is used to relate the plasma drug concentration to the dose administered (assuming no elimination has occurred), or to the amount of drug in the body. For most drugs, it does not relate to a real physiological or anatomical space, but provides an estimate of the extent of the drug's distribution through body-fluid compartments and its uptake by tissues. A major determinant is the relative avidity of the drug for tissue components as compared to blood. Obviously, the failure of an NCE to distribute to the site of action in a tissue or a cellular compartment *in vivo* will render the compound inactive and necessitate the redesign of the compound to overcome this problem.

Several volume of distribution terms are used in pharmacokinetics and can be determined in a number of ways. The simplest method is to regard the body as a simple one-compartment model and find the plasma concentration at zero time by back extrapolation of the log concentration–time plot after an intravenous (IV) bolus injection. Many drugs and NCEs adhere to this simple model. However, other two- and three-compartment models may be necessary for an adequate description of the concentration–time profile of some drugs. Alternatively, a steady-state volume of distribution term (V_{ss}) can be derived from pharmacokinetic analysis based on statistical moments [21]. The V_{ss} term essentially corresponds to the plasma and tissues volumes in which a drug is distributed when steady-state conditions have been achieved. Further discussion on compartmental and noncompartmental pharmacokinetic approaches can be found in Section 30.3.

The volume of distribution is a useful parameter for determining the size of the loading dose, in order to get to the steady-state situation more rapidly after a constant rate infusion or repetitive dosing, but has no influence on the magnitude of the steady-state concentration achieved. This is solely determined by the rate of drug administration and the systemic clearance. Probably of more importance with regard to desirable pharmacokinetic characteristics is the influence of volume of distribution on a drug's elimination half-life, as discussed next.

30.2.4   Elimination Half-life ($T_{1/2}$)

The elimination half-life ($T_{1/2}$) is defined as the time taken for half the amount of drug present in the body to be eliminated by either metabolism or excretion. It has been suggested that the half-life of an NCE is a more important pharmacokinetic parameter than either plasma clearance or volume of distribution, with regard to guiding decisions in the drug discovery and development process [10]. Half-life is important because it is an indicator of duration of action for many drugs and thus determines how often a drug needs to be administered. Dosing frequency of most drugs depends on how long the active drug remains in the circulation, which is determined by its half-life. With a knowledge of half-life, the dosing frequency required to avoid large fluctuations in plasma concentrations over the dosage interval may be determined. For example, if a drug is rapidly absorbed and is given every half-life, the peak-to-trough concentration ratio will be ~2. However, if the half-life is short (e.g., less than 4 hours) and the drug exhibits a narrow therapeutic index (e.g., twofold), it is often difficult to administer frequently enough to avoid toxicity at the peak concentration, or loss of effect at the low concentrations before the next dose. In addition, significant compliance issues occur with a dosing frequency greater than once or twice a day [22].

For most drugs, the half-life is independent of concentration and is a function of its clearance (assuming first-order elimination kinetics) and volume of distribution as follows:

$$T_{1/2} = 0.7V/CL \qquad (30.11)$$

where 0.7 is an approximation of the natural logarithm of 2.

Manipulation of an NCE's volume of distribution has not commonly been used to achieve a more favorable "longer" half-life. For example, it could be suggested that the volume of distribution might be enhanced by increasing the overall lipophilicity of an NCE, thus leading to a longer half-life. However, this improvement in volume of distribution might be offset by increased metabolism and clearance, as the binding sites of the metabolizing enzymes are generally lipophilic in nature and more readily accept lipophilic substrates. Thus, any gains in $T_{1/2}$ time due to a larger volume of distribution may be canceled out by increased metabolic activity. More commonly in drug development, strategies are employed to enhance metabolic stability by structural modifications of the NCE in order to decrease hepatic clearance, and thus prolong the half-life, and yet maintain the optimal level of potency [23]. A longer half-life should allow lower and less frequent dosing, thus enhancing patient convenience and promoting better compliance. Additional advantages arising from enhanced metabolic stability of the NCE might also include increased oral bioavailability, reduction in the number (and perhaps significance) of possible active metabolites, and lower intra- and interpatient variability in plasma concentration–time profiles (which largely result from differences in metabolic capacity). However, such chemical modifications to improve metabolic stability may in some cases give rise to additional problems with properties such as reduced absorption or increased renal excretion, resulting in a lack of overall improvement in desirable pharmacokinetic properties [24].

An alternative and perhaps easier strategy for reducing dosing frequency for a drug with a short $T_{1/2}$ would be the development of a slow-release formulation [25]. This would slow the rate of drug absorption into the body, so that the magnitude of the concentration fluctuations during a dosing interval would be determined by the absorption rate rather than the elimination rate. A similar approach to lengthen the duration of drug action can make use of a prodrug. The synthesis of a prodrug with a relatively slow metabolic conversion to the active species would result in this conversion step being the rate-determining step in the disappearance of the active species, and would determine its plasma concentration–time profile and thus require less frequent dosing [26].

The elimination half-life of a drug is also useful in predicting the time required to achieve steady-state conditions during a continuous intravenous infusion or repetitive dosing. The maximum effect of many drugs might be expected once this steady-state equilibrium had been achieved during chronic dosing. This is generally accepted to occur after 4–5 half-lives. Similarly, when drug dosing is terminated, it takes 4 half-lives for more than 90% of the drug to be eliminated.

30.3   APPROACHES TO PHARMACOKINETIC ANALYSIS

30.3.1   Compartmental Analysis

The traditional approach to pharmacokinetic analysis involves the use of compartmental analysis, which focuses on the rates of absorption, distribution, and elimination, usually in terms of first-order rate constants (linear kinetics) [27]. This is known as the model-dependent approach. When the exchange of a drug between the plasma and tissue proceeds rapidly compared with the rate of elimination, the whole body may be considered mathematically as a single compartment. This one-compartment model is the simplest model and regards the body as a single, kinetically homogeneous unit, and the decline in plasma concentration after a single bolus intravenous injection can be described by a single exponential function. If the distribution of the drug out of the plasma is so slow that it cannot be disregarded, a model must then be considered, which contains a central compartment and at least one other peripheral compartment. Although these compartments lack physical or anatomical reality, for many drugs, the central compartment may correspond to the plasma or blood volume, together with the extracelular fluid of highly perfused tissues such as the heart, lungs, liver, kidneys, and endocrine glands. It is also presumed that the drug is eliminated solely from this central compartment. Drugs distribute within a few minutes through this compartment and equilibrium between plasma and tissues is rapidly established. The peripheral compartment is then formed by less perfused tissue such as muscle, skin, or adipose tissue into which the drug may enter more slowly. This combined effect of two compartments gives rise to a biphasic concentration–time curve after an intravenous bolus injection, with two distinct linear portions when drawn on a semilog ordinate scale. Although drug disposition to the peripheral compartment is slow, it is usually much faster than the elimination rate of the drug. The two-compartment model may be expanded to contain additional compartments, which can be described mathematically as the sum of as many individual exponential functions as there are relevant compartments. In practical terms, the sensitivity of the available assay technique for the determination of the drug concentration usually allows the definition of a maximum of three compartments. This approach to pharmacokinetic analysis allows mathematical simulations and the prediction of drug concentrations in plasma (representing the central compartment) and in other deep compartments. These models are usually robust for a variety of conditions, such as altered physiological or pathological conditions and during chronic medication [27].

30.3.2 Noncompartmental Analysis

An alternative and perhaps simpler approach to pharmacokinetic analysis is the use of noncompartmental analysis (the model-independent approach), where the drug pharmacokinetic parameters are determined using statistical moments and are derived from relationships involving the area-under-the-zero-moment-curve (AUC) and the area-under-the-first-moment-curve ($AUMC$) of the plasma drug concentration–time curve [27]. No complicated modeling of the disposition of the drug is required, but consequently it lacks the predictive and/or simulative power for drug concentration in the plasma and other tissue compartments [16]. Further discussion and a comparison of these two approaches to pharmacokinetic analysis can be found in Atkinson et al. [21].

30.3.3 Physiologically Based Analysis

Yet another more complex approach to pharmacokinetic analysis involves using physiologically based pharmacokinetic models. This method attempts to take into account the fundamental anatomical and physiological factors (e.g., blood flow to the different organs/tissues, organ uptake and active transport, and tissue binding) that influence drug uptake and disposition [18, 27]. Individual organs or tissue groups are linked in an anatomically correct fashion via the circulatory system, with drug elimination permitted from the relevant organs. This is by far the most realistic view of what is happening to the drug in the body but requires extensive computing power and data inputs (e.g., blood flow, partitioning or tissue binding data for all species). Examples of physiologically based pharmacokinetic models of varying complexity can be found in the review by Gerlowski and Jain [28]. Due to their complexity, these models have only had a limited application to clinical studies to date, but they are expected to have greater importance in the future [17, 27].

30.4   PREDICTING PHARMACOKINETIC PARAMETERS IN HUMANS

As mentioned earlier, very often *in vitro* drug metabolism information in isolation fails to scale up and provide robust predictions of the pharmacokinetics of an NCE in the human population. An alternative strategy for predicting plasma pharmacokinetic parameters of NCEs in humans involves the use of allometric scaling methods plus preclinical animal pharmacokinetic data [29].

30.4.1   Allometric Scaling

Interspecies allometric scaling is based on empirically observed relationships between physiological and biochemical parameters (e.g., basal metabolic rate, creatinine clearance, and cytochrome weight) and body weight among mammals [30]. As pharmacokinetic parameters are a function of biochemical and physiological processes, these have also been shown to scale with body weight across species [31, 32]. This has allowed the prediction of pharmacokinetic parameters, such as CL and V, by using a simple power function of the form

$$Y = aB^n \tag{30.12}$$

where Y is the dependent variable (e.g., clearance) and B is the body weight, with a and n being the allometric coefficient and exponent, respectively. Allometric scaling from preclinical animal studies has proved to be useful for the prediction of the volume of distribution in humans, particularly if plasma protein differences between species are taken into account [33, 34]. However, allometric scaling has not proved to be particularly successful at predicting the hepatic clearance of drugs eliminated mainly by metabolism, especially those with low hepatic clearance. Adjustments to the basic allometric equation using maximum life span potential and brain weight have been proposed, but with limited success [34–36]. More recently, a combination of allometric scaling with *in vitro* human microsomal data has been proposed [36–38]. However, in a recently published study on the comparison of five different models (including allometric scaling with *in vitro* data input) using a dataset of 22 extensively metabolized compounds, Zuegge and colleagues [39] concluded that the most cost-effective and accurate approach for the prediction of hepatic clearance by metabolism was based on *in vitro* data alone, and that the inclusion of *in vivo* preclinical data and allometric scaling did not significantly improve prediction accuracy. They found that the prediction accuracy of the allometric models was at the lower end of all methods compared.

30.4.2   Microdosing

With the development of ultrasensitive analytical technologies (such as accelerator mass spectrometry (AMS), and positron emission tomography (PET)) with the capability of measuring drug and metabolite concentrations in the low picogram to femtogram range, human microdosing has been proposed as a new approach to obtaining crucial human pharmacokinetic data for comparing and selecting drug candidates earlier in their development [40–42]. Both technologies have the necessary sensitivity to follow the fate of trace amounts of radiolabeled drug in the body after very small doses (e.g., 1% of a therapeutic dose, maximally <100 μg), which would be expected to have no biological activity. PET can provide real-time data on the distribution of a radiolabeled drug in the body and its availability at the site of action; whereas AMS combined with high performance liquid chromatography (HPLC) can quantitate extremely low concentrations of a drug and metabolites in body fluids at time intervals after dosing [43]. The essential aim of microdosing studies is to obtain early human pharmacokinetic information for new drug candidates to assist in the candidate selection process, rather than acquiring efficacy or safety data. The major question with regard to human microdosing is whether the pharmacokinetic parameters after microdoses replicate those observed at therapeutic doses. In a small trial of five diverse drugs eliminated by metabolism, Garner [44] reported a 70% correspondence between the pharmacokinetics after a microdose and a therapeutic dose. However, more in-depth studies are required to judge the predictive abilities of microdosing in humans, and whether it will play a significant role in drug development in the future is not known at present. The exquisite sensitivity and specificity of the combination of HPLC and AMS also raises the possibility of the "cocktail" or cassette-dosing approach, where several NCEs are administered simultaneously in microdoses, and their pharmacokinetics are followed concurrently. This allows for a larger number of compounds to be investigated, and more efficient and rapid identification of the compound with the most desirable pharmacokinetics in humans.

30.5 METABOLISM FEATURES THAT MAY CONVEY PHARMACOKINETIC DISADVANTAGES

As previously indicated, metabolism is responsible for determining the major pharmacokinetic parameters of clearance, bioavailability, and half-life for most drugs. These pharmacokinetic characteristics in turn are very important in defining the pharmacological and toxicological profile of an NCE and indicating to drug developers whether favorable pharmacokinetics can be expected in patients. Desirable pharmacokinetics in patients would include a suitable half-life to allow a convenient dosing frequency of once or twice daily, and low hepatic/intestinal metabolism to allow acceptable and reproducible oral bioavailability. However, it is also important to realize that, although the preclinical *in vitro* and *in vivo* data might predict favorable pharmacokinetics in humans, there are a number of factors (discussed later) that may have a significant impact on an NCE's metabolism, leading to undesirable pharmacokinetic characteristics in patients and ultimately compound failure.

30.5.1 Nonlinear Pharmacokinetics

In the preceding discussion on pharmacokinetics, it has been assumed that the disposition systems operating on the drug obey first-order kinetics. This means that clearance, volume of distribution, bioavailability, and elimination half-life are independent of drug concentration (and dose). Under these conditions, drug accumulation is a linear function of dose, and any change in dose rate will produce a proportional change in the steady-state concentration. Some drugs do not have such linear characteristics. The most common cause of nonlinearity is believed to be the limited capacity of certain elimination processes, such as the drug-metabolizing enzyme systems. Most drugs are presented to the metabolizing enzymes at concentrations well below their maximal capacity, and they display first-order kinetics. However, for some drugs to be effective, concentrations are required at sufficiently high levels to cause saturation of the eliminating enzyme system, and the elimination occurs at a constant maximal rate, that is, zero-order kinetics. The anticonvulsant drug phenytoin and ethanol are probably the best known and studied examples of such compounds, where saturation of metabolism occurs with pharmacologically active concentrations [5, 45]. For such compounds, drug elimination rate will depend on the plasma concentration (or the magnitude of the dose), and drug accumulation with repetitive dosing will not be readily predictable. Once saturation of the eliminating system has been reached, the plasma concentration will increase disproportionately with subsequent dosing, and the time required to reach steady state will increase with the increasing half-life. If saturation of the elimination mechanisms is observed at pharmacologically active concentrations in the preclinical development of an NCE, structural modification would be recommended to remove this property, as this compound would be very difficult to use safely in patients, especially if it also had a low therapeutic index.

30.5.2 Drug–Drug Interactions

Drug–drug interactions are a major problem for the pharmaceutical industry and have resulted in drugs being withdrawn after being launched onto the worldwide market [46]. For example, terfenadine (a nonsedating antihistamine used for the treatment of rhinitis) was withdrawn after the occurrence of potentially fatal cardiac arrhythmias due to a substantial increase in its bioavailability when given with ketoconazole or grapefruit juice [46, 47]. Both ketoconazole and grapefruit juice are potent inhibitors of CYP3A4, which is the major enzyme involved in the metabolism of terfenadine and the termination of its activity. Indeed, the most common cause of clinically significant drug–drug interactions is primarily associated with the oxidation reactions catalyzed by the cytochrome P450 (CYP) enzyme family [48]. The CYPs in families 1–3 catalyze the metabolism of approximately 60–70% of all clinically used drugs. Of these, CYP3A4 is probably the most important, as it is involved in the metabolism of half of all drugs. Other important CYP isozymes involved in drug metabolism include CYP1A2, CYP2C9, CYP2C19, and CYP2D6. Inhibition of metabolism usually has a rapid onset and most commonly results in a dramatic increase in plasma concentration and an exaggerated response, with increased risk of toxicity and fatalities in extreme cases. The awareness of these adverse consequences has resulted in the development of a battery of automated screens to identify potent inhibitors of the CYP systems [8]. Some examples of drugs most commonly involved in inhibition of the CYP family include the azole antifungal drugs (e.g., ketoconazole), the quinolone and macrolide antibiotics (e.g., erythromycin), the selective serotonin reuptake inhibitors (e.g., fluoxetine, paroxetine, and fluvoxamine), the antiviral protease inhibitors (e.g., ritonavir and indinavir), and the antiulcer drug cimetidine [49].

The potent inhibition of the CYP enzyme family would be a property to be avoided in the development of an NCE, as it could lead to clinically significant drug–drug interactions. However, the decision to withdraw a drug from the market after evidence of a drug–drug interaction depends on several factors, including the severity of the interaction, the disease being treated, and whether alternative drugs are available. For example, the calcium channel blocker mibefradil, which is a substrate and potent inhibitor of CYP3A4, was withdrawn as there were equally effective drugs available that did not possess this undesirable characteristic. In contrast, a number of protease inhibitors (e.g., indinavir, saquinavir, and ritonavir), which are also potent inhibitors of CYP3A4, were not withdrawn, as there was a lack of effective alternatives in the treatment of HIV infection [50].

Significant drug–drug interactions are not confined to the CYP metabolizing family, as illustrated by the inhibition of dihydropyrimidine dehydrogenase by the antiviral drug sorivudine. Dihydropyrimidine dehydrogenase is a key enzyme in the metabolism (inactivation) of the anticancer drug 5-fluorouracil, and its inhibition by sorivudine caused a reduction in 5-fluorouracil's clearance, leading to elevated concentrations and toxicity. The latter mechanism was believed to have resulted in a number of fatalities in Japan, and consequently sorivudine was withdrawn from the marketplace [51].

Induction of drug-metabolizing enzymes by an NCE may also be problematic in drug development. In contrast to inhibition, induction has a less rapid onset, taking 4–5 days to achieve a peak effect. Most commonly, this results in lower plasma concentrations and treatment failure of comcomitant drugs. Well-known inducing agents include the anticonvulsants (e.g., phenytoin, phenobarbital, and carbamazepine), the antibiotic rifampicin, and the anti-inflammatory agent dexamethasone. Both first-pass metabolism by the intestines and the liver can be dramatically increased by enzyme-inducing agents, resulting in decreased bioavailability and loss of the therapeutic response. The discovery that many compounds induce drug-metabolizing enzymes via an interaction with the nuclear hormone receptors, constitutive androstane receptor (CAR), and the pregnane-X-receptor (PXR) has prompted the development of enhanced throughput systems for identification of CYP inducers, using both PXR radioligand binding assays and also reporter gene technology [52, 53]. The availability of high resolution human PXR ligand-binding domain crystal structures also raises the possibility of *in silico* testing of NCEs for their potential to bind to PXR, as an indication of their induction ability [54].

Drugs likely to be the subject of clinically relevant drug–drug interactions tend to be drugs with a steep concentration–response curve or a narrow therapeutic window [20]. Thus, a relatively small increase in concentration can quickly lead to toxicity, or conversely a decrease can lead to the disappearance of the therapeutic effect. For most drugs, the absence of significant drug–drug interactions may be a crucial determinant of the ultimate clinical success of a drug. Thus, to avoid the potential of drug–drug interactions, it is desirable to develop a new drug candidate that is not a potent CYP inhibitor or inducer, and whose metabolism is not readily inhibited or induced by other drugs. In order to eliminate unfavorable compounds early in development, high throughput *in vitro* systems for identifying drug metabolism pathways, the enzymes involved, and inhibitor/induction potential of new drug candidates are a rapidly evolving area of drug development [8, 55]. However, the information from both induction and inhibition *in vitro* technologies must be integrated with *in silico* approaches to maximize the potential of both [55].

30.5.3 Polymorphic Drug Metabolism

Genetic differences in the expression of many metabolizing enzymes can have an impact on the pharmacokinetic characteristics of a drug in a population of patients and accounts for much of the interindividual variability associated with the efficacy and toxicity of a number of drugs [56]. There are many examples of polymorphisms in genes encoding drug-metabolizing enzymes, which can cause significant differences in drug response within a population (Table 30.1) [57, 58]. As with drug–drug interactions, most information is available for the CYP system, in particular, the polymorphic enzymes CYP2C9, CYP2C19, and CYP2D6, which catalyze the metabolism of approximately 40% of drugs undergoing phase I oxidation [59, 60]. In general, four phenotypes can be identified: poor metabolizers (PMs), who lack the functional enzyme; intermediate metabolizers (IMs), who are heterozygous for one deficient allele or carry two alleles that cause reduced activity; extensive metabolizers (EMs), who have two normal alleles; and ultrarapid metabolizers (UMs), who have multiple gene copies. Thus, the dosing requirement for a drug such as nortriptyline (which is a substrate for CYP2D6), may differ 10–20-fold among individuals. Consequently, using a "standard" dose in a European population would be expected to elicit no response in the 5% of the population who are UMs (due to too rapid metabolism of the drug), and perhaps elicit an adverse reaction in the 7% of the population who are PMs due to excessively high plasma concentrations [58]. The distribution frequency of these CYP2D6 phenotypes differs between ethnic groups. For example, 10% of Spaniards and 29% of Ethiopians have been reported to be UMs for the CYP2D6 polymorphism [61]. Similarly, polymorphisms in CYP2C19 have been shown to have clinical consequences resulting in toxicity, or lack of efficacy with many drugs, including S-mephenytoin, omeprazole, imipramine, and proguanil [58]. Population studies have indicated that CYP2C19 PMs occur in 3–5% of Caucasians and African Americans, 12–23% in most Asian groups, and 38–79% in Polynesian and Micronesian populations [59]. In a Japanese study, patients with peptic or duodenal ulcers were treated with a dual therapy of low dose omeprazole

TABLE 30.1 Examples of Genetic Polymorphisms Influencing Drug Metabolism

Gene[a]	Substrates
CYP2C9	Tolbutamide, diclofenac, warfarin, phenytoin
CYP2C19	Omeprazole, lansoprazole, diazepam, proguanil
CYP2D6	Antidepressants, codeine, β-blockers
CYP2A6	Coumarin
UGT1A1	Irinotecan
NAT2	Isoniazid, sulfonamide
TPMT	6-Mercaptopurine, 6-thioguanine, azathioprine
DPD	5-Fluorouracil
ALDH2	Acetaldehyde

[a]UGT1A1, UDP-glucuronosyltransferase 1A1; NAT2, N-Acetyltransferase 2; TPMT, thiopurine S-methyltransferase; DPD, dihydropyrimidine dehydrogenase; ALDH2, aldehyde dehydrogenase 2.

Source: Adapted from Ref. 56.

and amoxicillin [62]. Cure rates were highly dependent on CYP2C19 phenotype, with only 25% in EMs, rising to 60% in IMs, and 100% in PMs. The high cure rate in PMs was thought to be due to lack of metabolism, resulting in higher omeprazole plasma concentrations and a longer half-life. These examples illustrate some of the problems that arise with drugs that are eliminated mainly by polymorphic enzymes, especially their use in different ethnic populations. This is important for the global perspective of the pharmaceutical industry, and most companies now take the pharmacogenetic aspects of CYP metabolism into account during drug development. Obviously, an NCE that has a high affinity for a polymorphic metabolizing enzyme that plays a major role in its elimination would be less favorable than one that did not display this characteristic [63]. However, as costs decrease, predictive genotyping of patients may be justified for drugs subject to significant polymorphic metabolism, especially those with a narrow therapeutic index. For example, it has been suggested that the prospective use of the UGT1A1 genotype assay would identify patients with the UGT1A1*28 genotype, which is associated with reduced metabolism of SN-38 (the active metabolite of the anticancer drug irinotecan), and increased incidence of significant toxicity [64]. Such genotyping may help to ensure safer and more effective therapy in the future.

30.5.4 Formation of Active/Reactive Metabolites

The rapid and extensive hepatic metabolism of an NCE may lead not only to pharmacokinetic disadvantages but also to issues with the identification of metabolites and evaluation of their biological activity. In general, *in vivo* metabolism leads to the formation of inactive and more readily excretable metabolites, but in some cases, metabolites with potent biological activity or toxic properties are produced, which may influence the outcome of therapy. The function and fate of these metabolites need to be studied, in order to gain a full insight into the potential biological consequences of exposure to the NCE. Metabolism to reactive intermediates is one of the major mechanisms by which drugs exert toxic effects. Despite a huge investment and many years of research, it is still not possible at present to accurately predict the potential for toxicity of a compound that has been shown to undergo metabolic activation [65]. It is important in drug development to investigate the metabolic fate of an NCE and evaluate the biological properties of possible metabolites. The relative merits of current and potential strategies for dealing with metabolite characterization have recently been reviewed by Nassar and Talaat [66]. The advancement of robotic systems using *in vitro* incubations of an NCE with human microsomes, hepatocytes, or liver slices, accompanied by the analysis of metabolites using techniques such as liquid chromatography–mass spectrometry (LC-MS) and/or liquid chromatography–nuclear magnetic resonance (LC-NMR) has made this more applicable in practice. In particular, significant advances in metabolite identification have been achieved using high performance liquid chromatography coupled with various mass analysers, such as triple quadrupole, quadrupole time-of-flight, ion trap, and quadrupole linear ion trap mass spectrometers [67, 68]. However, with the improved sensitivity and efficiency of NMR technology, the complementary nature of NMR and MS in definitive structure identification is being realized, and combined LC-MS-NMR systems will become crucial in the elucidation and confirmation of metabolite identification in the near future. Combined LC-MS-NMR systems are in the midst of an evolutionary phase at present that will lead to greatly improved ability and efficiency in metabolite identification [66]. However, although structural information on metabolites can be a considerable asset for enhancing and streamlining the process of NCE development, in order to eliminate potentially toxic compounds early in the development process, it must be integrated with computational technologies to obtain maximum benefits [66, 69, 70]. Comprehensive databases of metabolism and toxicological information are available, and software packages can indicate possible metabolites and identify structural features that may confer adverse properties to molecules [4, 66, 67]. With the advent of improved algorithms and the availability of ever-increasing computing power, the future of drug metabolism and toxicity prediction is envisaged as an integration of structure–activity relationship models based on compound structure with "pattern" databases of tissue or organ response to drugs, and "systems biology" databases of metabolic pathways, genes, and regulatory networks [71, 72].

30.6   CONCLUSION

For many drugs, metabolism plays a central role in defining the concentration–time profile in the body and, consequently, the magnitude and duration of the biological response. We have only a very limited understanding of the relationships between a molecule's structure and its physicochemical properties and its likely metabolic fate in the body. Drug metabolism may occur in many different tissues in the body and may be catalyzed by a large variety of diverse enzymes, which can be influenced by innumerable factors. The capacity for the metabolism of a compound *in vivo* is usually measured by the hepatic clearance, which is arguably the most important pharmacokinetic parameter, with a major influence on the secondary parameters of half-life and oral bioavailability. Clearance, half-life, and bioavailability are key components in the design of a suitable oral dosage regimen, providing information on the magnitude and frequency of dosing. Thus, metabolism is the single most important factor contributing to inappropriate or undesirable pharmacokinetic characteristics in an NCE. This relationship between an NCE's metabolic profile (rate, extent, and multiplicity of resulting metabolites) and the overall systemic clearance in a patient is extremely complex and provides a formidable challenge for the prediction of this parameter in humans from preclinical *in vitro* human data and animal studies. There are many issues concerning the nonphysiological nature of the *in vitro* screening systems, interspecies differences in metabolizing enzymes and their regulation, the part played by active transporters in tissue distribution, and the complexities of *in vivo* pharmacokinetics and toxicity. Nevertheless, some progress has been made over the past ten years with the development of a more diverse range of investigative tools, including superior technology to measure and identify compounds and their metabolites at extremely low concentrations, the automation and expansion of various *in vitro* screening tests to allow more rapid understanding of the ADME fate of a compound, and *in silico* approaches based on molecular modeling, structure–activity relationships, and metabonomics. To fully realize the potential of these advances, there is the need to integrate these technologies into a single comprehensive environment for drug development. A small amount of progress has been made, but much is yet to be done to attain the ultimate goal of being able to predict human metabolism and pharmacokinetics (and toxicity) based solely on the structure of a novel NCE.

REFERENCES

1. Prentis RA, Lis Y, Walker SR. Pharmaceutical innovation by seven UK-owned pharmaceutical companies (1964–1985). *Br J Clin Pharmacol* 1988;25:387–391.

2. Thompson TN. Early ADME in support of drug discovery: the role of metabolic stability studies. *Curr Drug Metab* 2000;1:215–241.

3. Palmer A. New horizons in drug metabolism, pharmacokinetics and drug delivery. *Drug News Perspect* 2003;16:57–62.

4. Van de Waterbeemd H, Gifford E. ADMET *in silico* modeling: Towards prediction paradise? *Nat Rev* 2003;2:192–204.

5. Rowland M, Tozer TN. *Clinical Pharmacokinetics: Concepts and Applications*, 3rd ed. Baltimore: Williams and Wilkins; 1995, pp 1–184.

6. Bachmann KA, Ghosh R. The use of *in vitro* methods to predict *in vivo* pharmacokinetics and drug interactions. *Curr Drug Metab* 2001;2:299–314.

7. Jones HM, Houston JB. Substrate depletion approach for determining *in vitro* metabolic clearance: time dependencies in hepatocyte and microsomal incubations. *Drug Metab Dispos* 2004;32:973–982.

8. Riley RJ, Grime K. Metabolic screening *in vitro*: metabolic stability, CYP inhibition and induction. *Drug Discov Today: Technol* 2004;1:365–372.

9. Iwatsubu T, Hiroja J, Ooie T, Suzuki H, Shimada N, Chiba K, Ishizaki T, Green CE, Tyson CA, Sugiyama Y. Prediction of *in vivo* drug metabolism in the human liver from *in vitro* metabolism data. *Pharmacol Ther* 1997;73:147–171.

10. Obach SR, Baxter JG, Liston TE, Silber BM, Jones BC, MacIntyre F, Rance DJ, Wastall P. The prediction of human pharmacokinetic parameters from preclinical and *in vitro* metabolism date. *J Pharmacol Exp Ther* 1997;283:46–59.

11. Masimirembwa CM, Bredberg U, Andersson TB. Metabolic stability for drug discovery and development. *Clin Pharmacokinet* 2003;42:515–528.

12. Ito K, Houston JB. Comparison of the use of liver models for predicting drug clearance using *in vitro* kinetic data from hepatic microsomes and isolated hepatocytes. *Pharm Res* 2004;21:785–792.

13. Houston JB, Galetin A. Progress towards prediction of human pharmacokinetic parameters from *in vitro* technologies. *Drug Metab Rev* 2003;35:393–415.

14. Tracy TS, Hummel MA. Modeling kinetic data from *in vitro* drug metabolism enzyme experiments. *Drug Metab Rev* 2004;36:231–242.

15. Ito K, Houston JB. Prediction of human drug clearance from *in vitro* and preclinical data using physiologically based and empirical approaches. *Pharm Res* 2005;22:103–112.

16. Smith DA, van De Waterbeemd H. Pharmacokinetics and metabolism in early drug discovery. *Curr Opin Chem Biol* 1999;3:373–378.

17. Theil F-P, Guentert TW, Haddad S, Poulin P. Utility of physiologically based pharmacokinetic models to drug development and rational drug discovery candidate selection. *Toxicol Lett* 2003;138:29–49.

18. Schmitt W, Willmann S. Physiology-based pharmacokinetic modeling: ready to use. *Drug Discov Today Technol* 2004;1:449–456.

19. Wacher VJ, Salphati L, Benet LJ. Active secretion and enterocytic drug metabolism barriers to drug absorption. *Adv Drug Deliv Rev* 2001;46:89–102.

20. Gibbs MA, Hosea NA. Factors affecting the clinical development of cytochrome P450 3A substrates. *Clin Pharmacokinet* 2003;42:969–964.

21. Atkinson AJ, Daniels CE, Dedrick RL, Grudzinskas CE, Markey SP. *Principles of Clinical Pharmacology*. San Diego: Academic Press; 2001, pp 29, 75–90.

22. Katzung BG. *Basic and Clinical Pharmacology*, 9th ed. New York: Lange Medical Books/McGraw-Hill; 2004, pp 1095–1096.

23. Nassar A-EF, Kamel AM, Clarimont C. Improving the decision-making process in the structural modification of drug candidates: enhancing metabolic stability. *Drug Discov Today* 2004;9:1020–1028.

24. Smith D, Schmid E, Jones B. Do drug metabolism and pharmacokinetic departments make any contribution to drug discovery? *Clin Pharmacokinet* 2002;41:1005–1019.

25. Thombre AG. Assessment of the feasibility of oral controlled release in an exploratory development setting. *Drug Discov Today* 2005;10:1159–1166.

26. Testa B. Prodrug research: futile or fertile. *Biochem Pharmacol* 2004;68:2097–2106.

27. Mathiowitz E. *Encyclopedia of Controlled Drug Delivery*. Hoboken, NJ: John Wiley & Sons; 1999, pp 833–851.

28. Gerlowski LE, Jain RK. Physiology-based pharmacokinetic modeling: principles and applications. *J Pharm Sci* 1983;72:1103–1127.

29. Mahmood I, Balian D. Interspecies scaling: predicting clearance of drugs in humans. Three different approaches. *Xenobiotica* 1996;26:887–895.

30. Davidson IWF, Parker JC, Beliles RP. Biological basis for extrapolation across mammalian species. *Regul Toxicol Pharmacol* 1986;6:211–237.

31. Boxenbaum H. Interspecies scaling, allometry, physiological time, and the ground plan of pharmacokinetics. *J Pharmacokinet Biopharm* 1982;10:201–227.

32. Paxton JW. The allometric approach for interspecies scaling of pharmacokinetics and toxicity of anticancer drugs. *Clin Exp Pharmacol Physiol* 1995;22:851–854.

33. Paxton JW, Kim SN, Whitfield LR. Pharmacokinetic and toxicity scaling of the antitumor agents, amsacrine and a new analog (CI-921) in mice, rats, rabbits, dogs and humans. *Cancer Res* 1990;50:2692–2697.

34. Mahmood I, Balian JD. The pharmacokinetic principles behind scaling from preclinical results to Phase I protocols. *Clin Pharmacokinet* 1999;36:1–11.

35. Boxenbaum H, Fertig JB. Scaling of antipyrine intrinsic clearance of unbound drug in 15 mammalian species. *Eur J Drug Metab Pharmacokinet* 1984;9:177–183.

36. Lavé TL, Coassolo P, Reigner B. Prediction of hepatic metabolic clearance based on interspecies allometric scaling techniques and *in vitro–in vivo* correlations. *Clin Pharmacokinet* 1999;36:211–231.

37. Mahmood I. Prediction of clearance in humans from *in vitro* human liver microsomes and allometric scaling. A comparison study of the two approaches. *Drug Metab Drug Interact* 2002;19:49–64.

38. Keldenich J. Prediction of human clearance (CL) and volume of distribution (VD). *Drug Discov Today Technol* 2004;1:389–395.

39. Zuegge J, Schneider G, Coassolo C, Lave T. Prediction of hepatic metabolic clearance: comparison and assessment of prediction models. *Clin Pharmacokinet* 2001;40:553–563.

40. Aboagye EO, Price PM, Jones T. *In vivo* pharmacokinetics and pharmacodynamics in drug development using positron-emission tomography. *Drug Discov Today* 2001;6: 293–302.

41. Lappin G, Garner RC. Big physics, small doses: the use of AMS and PET in human microdosing of development drugs. *Nat Rev Drug Discov* 2003;2:233–240.

42. Wilding IR, Bell JA. Improved early clinical development through human microdosing studies. *Drug Discov Today* 2005;10:890–894.

43. White INH, Brown K. Techniques: the application of accelerator mass spectrometry to pharmacology and toxicology. *Trends Pharm Sci* 2004;25:442–447.

44. Garner RC. Less is more: the human microdosing concept. *Drug Discov Today* 2005;10: 449–451.

45. Winter ME. *Basic Clinical Pharmackinetics*, 4th ed. Philadelphia: Lippincott Williams & Wilkins; 2004, p 321.

46. Li AP. Screening for human ADME/Tox drug properties in drug discovery. *Drug Discov Today* 2001;6:357–366.

47. Dahan A, Altman H. Food–drug interaction: grapefruit juice augments drug bioavailability—mechanism, extent and relevance. *Eur J Clin Nutr* 2004;58:1–9.

48. Lin JH, Lu AYH. Inhibition and induction of cytochrome P450 and the clinical implications. *Clin Pharmacokinet* 1998;35:361–390.

49. Smith DA, Abel SM, Hyland R, Jones BC. Human cytochrome P450s: selectivity and measurement *in vivo. Xenobiotica* 1998;28:1095–1128.

50. De Maat MMR, Ekhart GC, Huiteman ADR, Koks CHW, Mulder JW, Beijnen JH. Drug interactions between antiretroviral drugs and comedicated agents. *Clin Pharmacokinet* 2003;42:223–282.

51. Okuda H, Ogura K, Kato A, Takubo H, Watabe T. A possible mechanism of eighteen patient deaths caused by interactions of sorivudine, a new antiviral drug, with oral 5-fluorouracil prodrugs. *J Pharmacol Exp Ther* 1998;287:791–799.

52. Waxman DJ. P450 gene induction by structurally diverse xenochemicals: central role of nuclear receptors CAR, PXR and PPAR. *Arch Biochem Biophys* 1999;369:11–23.

53. Willson T, Kliever SA. PXR, CAR and drug metabolism. *Nat Rev Drug Discov* 2002;1: 259–266.

54. Goodwin B, Redinbo MR, Kliewer SA. Regulation of CYP3A gene transcription by the pregnane X receptor. *Annu Rev Pharmacol Toxicol* 2002;42:1–23.

55. Rostami-Hodjegan A, Tucker G. "In silico" simulations to assess the *in vivo* consequences of *in vitro* metabolic drug–drug interactions. *Drug Discov Today Technol* 2004;1: 441–448.

56. Hiratsuka M, Mizugaki M. Genetic polymorphisms in drug metabolising enzymes and drug targets. *Mol Genet Metab* 2001;73:298–305.

57. Pirmohamed M, Park BK. Genetic susceptibility to adverse drug reactions. *Trends Pharmacol Sci* 2001;22:298–305.

58. Ingelman-Sundberg M. Pharmacogenetics of cytochrome P450 and its applications in drug therapy: the past, present and future. *Trends Pharmacol Sci* 2004;25:193–200.

59. Goldstein J. Clinical relevance of genetic polymorphisms in the human CYP2C subfamily. *Br J Clin Pharmacol* 2001;52:349–355.

60. Kirchheiner J, Brockmoller J. Clinical consequences of cytochrome P450–2C9 polymorphisms. *Clin Pharmacol Ther* 2005;77:1–16.

61. Bondy B, Zill P. Pharmacogenetics and psychopharmacology. *Curr Opin Pharmacol* 2004;4:72–78.

62. Furuta T, Ohashi K, Kamata T, et al. Effect of genetic differences in omeprazole metabolism on cure rates for *Helicobacter pylori* infection and peptic ulcer. *Ann Intern Med* 1998;129:1027–1030.

63. Walker DK. The use of pharmacokinetic and pharmacodynamic data in the assessment of drug safety in early drug development. *Br J Clin Pharmacol* 2004;58:601–608.

64. Kiang TKL, Ensom MHH, Chang TKH. UDP-glucuronosyltransferases and clinical drug–drug interactions. *Pharmacol Ther* 2005;106:97–132.

65. Evans DC, Watt AP, Nicoll-Griffith DA, Baille TA. Drug–protein adducts: an industry perspective on minimizing the potential for drug activation in drug discovery and development. *Chem Res Toxicol* 2004;17:3–16.

66. Nasser A-EF, Talaat RE. Strategies for dealing with metabolite elucidation in drug discovery and development. *Drug Discov Today* 2004;9:317–327.

67. Anari MR, Baille TA. Bridging cheminformatic metabolite prediction and tandem mass spectrometry. *Drug Discov Today* 2005;10:711–717.

68. Rossi DT, Sinz MW. *Mass Spectrometry in Drug Discovery*. New York: Marcel Dekker; 2002, pp 271–336.

69. Yu H, Adedoyin A. ADME-Tox in drug discovery: integration of experimental and computational technologies. *Drug Discov Today* 2003;8:852–861.

70. Nasser A-EF, Kamel AM, Clarimont C. Improving the decision-making process in structural modification of drug candidates: reducing toxicity. *Drug Discov Today* 2004;9: 1055–1064.

71. Bugrim A, Nikolskaya T, Nikolsky Y. Early prediction of drug metabolism and toxicity: systems biology and modeling. *Drug Discov Today* 2004;9:127–135.

72. Whittaker PA. What is the relevance of bioinformatics to pharmacology. *Trends Pharmacol Sci* 2003;24:434–439.

31

EXPERIMENTAL DESIGN CONSIDERATIONS IN PHARMACOKINETIC STUDIES

WILLIAM W. HOPE, VIDMANTAS PETRAITIS, AND THOMAS J. WALSH

National Cancer Institute, National Institutes of Health, Bethesda, Maryland

Contents

31.1 Introduction
31.2 Defining the Overall Goal of the Experiments
31.3 Experimental Platforms
31.4 Impact of Drug Measurement on Study Design
31.5 Choosing the Dosage Range and the Number of Dosages Used to Define Pharmacokinetic Relationships
31.6 Sampling Times
    31.6.1 Defining the Number and Timing of Informative Sampling Points
    31.6.2 Peak Concentrations
    31.6.3 When Precisely to Acquire Pharmacokinetic Data
    31.6.4 Optimal Sampling and D-Optimal Design
31.7 Determination of Drug Concentrations in Tissues and Bodily Fluids
31.8 Conclusion
    References

31.1 INTRODUCTION

Pharmacokinetics is the study of the spatial and temporal distribution of drugs. Pharmacokinetic studies are conducted in experimental contexts for two major reasons. The first is to define pharmacokinetic relationships for new drugs that may

Preclinical Development Handbook: ADME and Biopharmaceutical Properties,
edited by Shayne Cox Gad
Copyright © 2008 John Wiley & Sons, Inc.

be beneficial for patients. This process is important for preclinical drug development where one wants to develop candidate molecules with pharmacokinetic profiles that are likely to be favorable for clinical use or that meet predefined developmental targets. A further understanding of the pharmacokinetics in experimental systems is required to obtain prior information before proceeding to human Phase I and II studies. The second reason to conduct pharmacokinetic studies is to further understand the concentration–effect relationships (i.e., pharmacodynamic relationships). For both these purposes, an accurate description of pharmacokinetics is vital in order to obtain appropriate conclusions regarding drug behavior and utility. To achieve this goal, appropriate experimental design is essential.

This chapter outlines some of the issues in the design of experimental models, which enable pharmacokinetic relationships to be established. The objective is to estimate the pharmacokinetic relationships as precisely as possible, at minimum cost, and using the minimum possible number of animals and analytical samples. Although this subject matter is vast, we focus our discussion on antimicrobial pharmacology from which broader principles may be extrapolated.

31.2 DEFINING THE OVERALL GOAL OF THE EXPERIMENTS

The experimental goals and aims will, to a large extent, dictate the design of the pharmacokinetic experiments. One obviously wishes to design the experiment to yield data to address the problems in hand. In this regard, a clear idea as to the overall experimental goal is required. This along with at least some preliminary pharmacodynamic data will determine (1) the concentrations of drug that are likely to induce a pharmacological effect of interest and are therefore relevant for the pharmacokinetic experiments; (2) the length of the experimental period over which one requires pharmacokinetic information; (3) the likely schedules of drug which will be employed; (4) the experimental conditions that will be used (e.g., severity of the model, immune status of the model, or other physiological derangements).

Studying the appropriate dosages and schedules for the right period of time and in the right model are important because (1) the pharmacokinetics may change as a function of dose (i.e., become nonlinear, especially at higher dosages when clearance mechanisms become saturated); (2) one needs to know about the pharmacokinetics over the entire course of the experimental period rather than for a mere fraction; (3) there may be drug accumulation with different schedules of administration, which may have a bearing on the pharmacodynamic relationships; and (4) the pharmacokinetic relationships may be different in different models. The immunological status, model severity, or degree of physiological derangement may significantly alter the pharmacokinetics of any given compound. In the circumstances in which the severity of the model precludes intensive blood sampling, an approach may be to define pharmacokinetic parameters in healthy animals and cross reference data from a select number of informative points from the animals with the disease in question—this is discussed in more detail in Section 31.6.4.

Thus, the experimental conditions used in the pharmacokinetic model should replicate as closely as possible those used to define the exposure–response relationships. Given the cost of pharmacokinetic experiments, a prudent approach is to perform only these experiments when one is reasonably sure of the experimental conditions that will be used for other aspects of the study.

31.3 EXPERIMENTAL PLATFORMS

The design of the pharmacokinetic experiment will vary according to the type of experimental platform. In small animals, such as mice, repeated sampling from a single animal is extremely difficult. In this circumstance, pharmacokinetic data can be acquired by designing a serial sacrifice study, in which a cohort of animals receiving a given dose of drug are sacrificed at predefined time points over the course of the experimental period. Blood from mice can be obtained from a terminal cardiac puncture after the administration of a general anesthetic. Alternatively, while technically more challenging, serial blood samples can be obtained in the same mouse from the saphenous vein or from a retro-orbital puncture. The principal disadvantage of such an approach is the relatively small volume of blood that can be procured from each mouse. The number of mice sacrificed at each time point depends on the confidence with which one wishes to estimate the pharmacokinetic relationships. Usually a minimum of three animals is required at each time point, but four to six may be appropriate if the drug concentrations are likely to be variable, or precise estimates of the pharmacokinetic parameters are required. Using such a design, one has point estimates of measures of central tendency (e.g., mean concentration) and the associated dispersions at each time point for each dose. The observed variance from the replicate samples can be used as a weighting function in the pharmacokinetic modeling process. A similar "serial sacrifice" design obviously applies for other experimental platforms in which the experiment is destroyed in the sampling process.

In larger animals, such as rabbits, or *in vitro* models such as hollow fiber systems, multiple samples may be taken from a single animal or via a sampling port. Clearly, however, there is a limit in terms of the volume of blood that can be drawn from an animal over time; in rabbits, for example, this volume is approximately 7 mL/kg. Studying pharmacokinetics in this manner is similar to intensive pharmacokinetic sampling strategies in humans. The data from such an experimental design can be analyzed in one of two ways: (1) the mean and standard deviation for a group of individual animals receiving a given dose of drug in which blood has been drawn at the same time point can be determined; the analysis in this circumstance is similar to murine models, described above, in which the mean drug concentration can be weighted using the inverse of the observed variance at each observation point; (2) a population methodology can be employed; in this case there is no attempt to calculate the mean and standard deviation of the pharmacokinetic data between groups of rabbits. Rather, the data from each rabbit are modeled on an individual basis. In this case, weighting is assumed to be inversely proportional to the estimated assay variance. This relationship can be established by a regression of the mean values and the corresponding standard deviations of samples of known concentration, which encompass the dynamic range of the assay and which have been run in at least quadruplicate. The principal advantage of this approach is that one is able to obtain estimates for both the central tendencies (mean and median values) and dispersions for the population as a whole, *in conjunction* with an optimal set of pharmacokinetic parameters for each individual animal. Such an approach may be advantageous when one wishes to directly link drug exposure with effect within the same animal. The ability to sample repeatedly from one animal means that fewer large animals are required to establish pharmacokinetic relationships than is the case in smaller animals such as mice. Furthermore, the sacrifice of a larger animal may not be necessary after an appropriate washout period, depending on the compound in question.

31.4 IMPACT OF DRUG MEASUREMENT ON STUDY DESIGN

The practical limitations of drug analysis have an important bearing on the design of experimental pharmacokinetic experiments. Drug levels are most frequently measured using high performance liquid chromatography (HPLC). Other methods such as bioassay or ELISA may be used. Increasingly, however, mass spectrometry is used because of its analytical sensitivity and the possibility of high throughput analysis. One aspect of drug measurement that is critical to the design of pharmacokinetic experiments is the lower limits of detection and quantification. Knowledge of these limits may have an influence on the design of pharmacokinetic experiments in the following ways: (1) there is little point in studying dosages that produce concentrations of drug beneath the limit of detection; (2) as one approaches the limit of quantification, the variance in most analytical assays increases, thus directly influencing the confidence with which the pharmacokinetic parameters can be estimated; and (3) the inability to measure low concentrations of drug may lead to erroneous estimates of the pharmacokinetics of a given drug. This may lead to underestimations of the magnitude of drug exposure that develops following the administration of an otherwise efficacious dose; these concepts are depicted in Fig. 31.1.

If it is clear that the analytical sensitivity of the assay is suboptimal and precludes the ability to accurately describe the pharmacokinetics, then a number of approaches

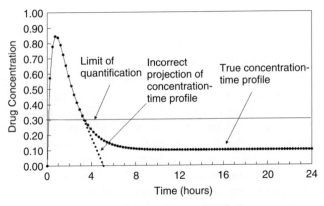

FIGURE 31.1 The impact of the limit of quantification on the ability to accurately describe the terminal phase of distribution. The figure shows the incorrect projection of the concentration–time profile at times beneath the limit of quantification, which leads to an underestimate of total drug exposure.

are possible. First, an attempt can be made to improve the limit of quantification via the optimization of the chosen analytical method (e.g., for HPLC analysis changing the mobile phase, detection settings, or the sample injection volume may improve the analytical sensitivity and the limit of quantification). Second, a more sensitive analytical method can be tried—in the majority of cases this means resorting to mass spectrometry. Third, tissue levels of drug can be measured; such an approach may be particularly useful for drugs that undergo extensive tissue distribution and that also exhibit prolonged mean residence times within tissues. By simultaneously comodeling serum and tissue drug concentrations, one may be able to estimate serum concentrations of drug that are well below the limit of detection. Such an approach is exemplified by a recent paper by Louie and colleagues [1] who were able to obtain accurate estimates of the antifungal agent caspofungin, by comodeling serum and kidney drug concentrations.

31.5 CHOOSING THE DOSAGE RANGE AND THE NUMBER OF DOSAGES USED TO DEFINE PHARMACOKINETIC RELATIONSHIPS

The range of dosages used to determine the pharmacokinetic relationships should encompass those that will be used to define the pharmacodynamic relationships. The importance of studying more than one dose is to determine whether the pharmacokinetics are linear or nonlinear. Following the administration of progressively higher dosages, clearance mechanisms may become saturated, and nonlinear pharmacokinetics will be observed. This is especially important if nonlinear kinetics are observed with dosages that are planned for the pharmacodynamic experiments. Ideally, a minimum of three dosages should be studied, but depending on the drug more may be appropriate.

An insight into whether a drug displays linear pharmacokinetics can be achieved in the following ways: (1) the presence of a linear system can be inferred using the principle of superposition; in this case, the drug concentrations following different dosages divided by the administered dose should be superimposable; (2) there should be a linear relationship between the area under the concentration–time curve (AUC) and the different dosages; (3) the pharmacokinetic parameters determined for each dosage group should not vary significantly from dose to dose; and (4) a more sophisticated method involves fitting and comparing both linear and nonlinear pharmacokinetic models to the entire dataset. A fit of one model compared with another, which is superior in a statistically significant manner, can be used to infer whether the pharmacokinetics are linear or nonlinear. An example of this process applied to human data is illustrated in a study by Lodise and colleagues [2], where an attempt was made to distinguish whether the beta-lactam piperacillin was better accounted for by a linear of nonlinear pharmacokinetic model.

31.6 SAMPLING TIMES

31.6.1 Defining the Number and Timing of Informative Sampling Points

The identification of sampling times is a critical component in the ability to obtain confident estimates of the pharmacokinetic parameters. In general, given the considerable time and resources involved in determining pharmacokinetic relationships, one wishes to sample as little as possible, while still ensuring acceptable estimates of the pharmacokinetic parameters will be obtained. The key in this regard is the identification of informative sampling points. The information content at various time points throughout the dosing interval is not constant. The distribution of information content is a function of the shape of the concentration–time profile of a drug and the structural pharmacokinetic model that is used to obtain parameter estimates. Importantly, the trough concentration, which is frequently used in therapeutic drug monitoring, is the least informative data point for describing pharmacokinetics, since it provides little information regarding the shape of the preceding concentration–time profile. Some idea as to likely informative points can be obtained from prior knowledge of drug behavior, even if acquired in other experimental platforms. Several experiments may be required to fully characterize the concentration–time profile for a drug in early development or to define the pharmacokinetics within a new experimental system. Informative points tend to occur at points of inflection in the concentration–time curve and can be formally identified using optimal design theory (see Section 31.6.4).

31.6.2   Peak Concentrations

Peak concentrations, unlike troughs, tend to be information rich. In order to capture this information, sampling in the immediate period following drug administration is frequently performed. While this approach is standard and useful, there are some important caveats. (1) The use of compartmental pharmacokinetic modeling techniques requires an assumption of full compartmental mixing; this refers to the presence of homogeneous concentrations of drug throughout the compartment in question. The time required for full mixing to occur, even for drugs that are injected intravenously, is not instantaneous. Sampling should be delayed until full mixing is likely to have occurred; this time depends on both the route of administration and the blood circulation time. A balance must be struck between waiting for mixing to occur, but not waiting too long that important information contained within the period immediately following drug administration is lost. (2) Drug concentrations are changing very rapidly in the early period following drug administration. Consequently, relatively small errors in the time of sampling are likely to have a significant impact on the observed plasma drug concentrations. This may be an issue for experimental reproducibility and fitting pharmacokinetic models to the data obtained immediately following drug administration. (3) In attempting to capture peak concentrations, there may be considerable logistical issues in administering drug to a relatively large number of animals, and then sampling 5–15 minutes later. This is especially the case for mice, where the number of animals tends to be high, and blood samples are usually obtained by cardiac puncture. Even in the hands of experienced personnel, the time taken to obtain a blood sample from an individual mouse is approximately 1 minute. Small departures from this demanding schedule may significantly disrupt the ability to obtain samples at the desired times. Thus collecting data immediately following drug administration requires careful planning, organization, and cooperation among co-workers.

31.6.3 When Precisely to Acquire Pharmacokinetic Data

An issue arises as to whether pharmacokinetic relationships should be defined after the initiation of drug administration or at steady state (if the latter is achieved within the study period). There is no universally correct approach, but there are two guiding principles when planning a pharmacokinetic study. (1) An attempt should be made to collect informative data throughout the study period, regardless of the timing. Consequently, it may be appropriate to sample relatively intensively during the early period following drug administration, again at steady state, and at other select informative times between these periods. Such an approach may help to identify the extent of drug accumulation, and any nonlinearities that may appear with repeated drug administration. (2) If sampling occurs after repeated dosing (e.g., following the sixth dose of drug), the determination of the concentration of drug immediately prior to drug administration should be defined (i.e., a prelevel should be drawn). If this data point is not modeled or the preceding dosages are not recorded as inputs into the system, then accurate estimates for the pharmacokinetic parameters will not be obtained—information regarding prior system inputs and initial conditions cannot simply be ignored.

31.6.4 Optimal Sampling and D-Optimal Design

D-optimal design theory has been applied extensively to humans as a means of acquiring informative data. In circumstances in which intensive sampling is not possible (e.g., neonates, patients with critical illness), D-optimal design allows for samples to be drawn at times when system information is near maximal. Such an approach allows confident estimates of the pharmacokinetic parameters using a minimal dataset. Such an approach can also be applied to experimental models, to minimize the number of samples required to be drawn and analyzed. In our laboratory, rabbits with invasive pulmonary aspergillosis (a fungal infection of the lung) are unable to tolerate intensive plasma sampling. An approach successfully employed by us is to acquire a relatively information-rich dataset in healthy animals and use these data to identify a limited number of informative sampling points in infected rabbits, thus allowing the pharmacokinetic parameters to be estimated while minimizing the burden of repeated blood sampling.

Optimal design can be performed using the sample module of the pharmacokinetic program ADAPT II of D'Argenio and Schumitsky [3]. The mean parameter values and the associated standard deviations are entered, along with the dosages of drug and the number of sampling times that are required. The identification of informative sampling times may also be important in other contexts, in which one wishes to ensure or demonstrate that the administration of a drug results in a concentration–time profile that is comparable to what was defined in a previously similar but subtly different model. Examples include the following: (1) ensuring that there is no pharmacokinetic interaction between drugs given in combination; in this circumstance, one may choose a small number of informative sampling times to demonstrate that the drug concentrations are the same as when the drugs are administered in isolation; (2) if there has been a departure from the conditions in which the original pharmacokinetic relationships were defined, but to a degree that is unlikely to have a significant effect on the pharmacokinetics, one may wish to obtain a small number of samples in order to confirm that the concentration–time profiles are similar. For example, the original pharmacokinetic relationships may have been defined in an infection model using a particular strain or species; subsequently, one may wish to study a related species, but the experimental conditions are otherwise identical, and a full pharmacokinetic study may not be justified. In this situation it may be possible to sample at several informative points to ensure that the concentration–time profile is the same.

31.7   DETERMINATION OF DRUG CONCENTRATIONS IN TISSUES AND BODILY FLUIDS

Frequently, an assumption is made that there is a linear relationship between the concentrations of drug in the central compartment and concentrations that develop at the effect site (i.e., the site of the drug receptor). In the majority of cases this is true, meaning that serum and tissue drug concentrations do in fact track one-to-one. This enables the response at the effect site to be described in terms of the concentration–time profile within the central compartment. On occasions, however, a better understanding of drug effect can be obtained by measuring the concentration of drug at the effect site itself. Despite a linear relationship, knowledge of the concentrations at the effect site may be important for the following reasons: (1) the shape of the concentration–time profile may be different in the two compartments and for certain drugs and drug classes this may have a bearing on drug effect; (2) there may be differences in protein binding between the serum and the effect site, which could affect the free fraction of drug available to interact with its receptor; (3) there may be dissociation between the concentration–time profiles because of delayed trafficking of drug to the effect site, resulting in hysteresis and leading to an apparent dissociation between serum drug concentrations and the observed effect; (4) despite a linear relationship between the serum and the effect site, there may be an insufficient concentration of drug to elicit a biological response at the effect site; and (5) there may be unique and unappreciated transport mechanisms from the serum to the effect site—an example of this is the concentration that the macrolide group of antibiotics achieve in the epithelial lining fluid (ELF) of the lung, despite extremely low serum drug concentrations. Thus, on occasions, there may be a requirement to measure the concentration of drug in tissues or bodily fluids in order to link drug concentrations at the effect site and the drug effect itself.

The measurement of tissue drug concentrations is not straightforward. The important issues include the following. (1) Tissue from normal animals (i.e., devoid of drug) is required to generate a standard curve, which is used to determine the concentrations of drug within tissues. Ideally the assay needs to be optimized and validated for each tissue in order to define the limit of quantification. (2) In order to obtain an estimate of the time course (pharmacokinetics) of drug within the tissue compartment, serial sampling (if possible) or serial sacrifice experiments are required. The shape of the concentration–time profile may differ from the serum, meaning that different sampling times from those used in serum may be required. Animals should be serially sacrificed throughout the dosing interval. This means the numbers of animals that are required to determine the pharmacokinetics in tissues may be greater than if serum pharmacokinetics alone are determined. This may have important implications for the cost and feasibility of such a study. (3) One should always bear in mind the complexities of distribution of drug within tissues. The effect of a drug results from an interaction with its receptor, which may only exist within subcompartments. A tissue homogenate, on the other hand, consists of a mixing of all the different compartments within tissue, including the vascular space. This principle is exemplified in a study by Groll et al. [4], where the compartmentalization of intrapulmonary lipid formulations of amphotericin B was characterized in pulmonary alveolar macrophages and epithelial lining fluid. Consequently, drug levels determined from tissue homogenates should be viewed as an approximation of the concentration of drug available to the receptor.

There are a number of additional advantages to simultaneously studying tissue and serum concentrations of drug. The comodeling of serum and tissue data may enable better estimates of pharmacokinetic parameters. A good example of this was provided by Louie et al. [1], who described the pharmacokinetics of the antifungal drug caspofungin in a murine model of invasive candidiasis. Caspofungin is cleared rapidly from the serum and is avidly taken up by tissues. The lower limit of quantification of caspofungin using HPLC is relatively high. The concentrations of drug in the kidney and serum were measured and comodeled. This approach enabled a more accurate estimate of the pharmacokinetics; the caspofungin half-life increased when the serum and tissue data were comodeled. This approach also enabled a circumvention of the problem induced by a relatively high limit of quantification mentioned earlier. Instead of moving to a more sensitive analytical assay to enable a more accurate description of the terminal elimination phase, this was achieved by measuring and comodeling drug concentrations in the kidney. In this circumstance, as drug concentrations in the serum decline beneath the lower limit of quantification, drug is still "seen" returning from peripheral compartments that are acting as a repository of drug (in this case, the kidney).

31.8 CONCLUSION

An accurate description of the pharmacokinetic properties of a drug underpins a further understanding of concentration–effect relationships. The design of pharmacokinetic experiments is critical to ensure that pharmacokinetic relationships can be accurately estimated. If the design of pharmacokinetic experiments is flawed, and the resultant pharmacokinetic models are incorrect, then erroneous conclusions regarding the concentration–effect relationship may result. This chapter summarizes our approach to the design of pharmacokinetic experiments and highlights ways in which pharmacokinetic relationships can be efficiently and accurately estimated.

REFERENCES

1. Louie A, Deziel M, Liu W, Drusano MF, Gumbo T, Drusano GL. Pharmacodynamics of caspofungin in a murine model of systemic candidiasis: importance of persistence of caspofungin in tissues to understanding drug activity. *Antimicrob Agents Chemother* 2005;49: 5058–5068.

2. Lodise TP Jr, Lomaestro B, Rodvold KA, Danziger LH, Drusano GL. Pharmacodynamic profiling of piperacillin in the presence of tazobactam in patients through the use of population pharmacokinetic models and Monte Carlo simulation. *Antimicrob Agents Chemother* 2004;48:4718–4724.

3. D'Argenio DZ, Schumitzky A. *ADAPT II. A Program for Simulation, Identification, and Optimal Experimental Design. User Manual.* Los Angeles: Biomedical Simulations Resource, University of Southern California; 1997. http://bmsr.esc.edu/.

4. Groll AH, Lyman CA, Petraitis V, Petraitiene R, Armstrong D, Mickiene D, Alfaro RM, Schaufele RL, Sein T, Bacher J, Walsh TJ. Compartmentalized intrapulmonary pharmacokinetics of amphotericin B and its lipid formulations. *Antimicrob Agents Chemother* 2006;50:3418–3423.

32

BIOAVAILABILITY AND BIOEQUIVALENCE STUDIES

ALEXANDER V. LYUBIMOV[1] AND IHOR BEKERSKY[2]

[1]*University of Illinois at Chicago, Chicago, Illinois*
[2]*Consultant, Antioch, Illinois*

Contents

Preclinical Development Handbook: ADME and Biopharmaceutical Properties,
edited by Shayne Cox Gad
Copyright © 2008 John Wiley & Sons, Inc.

32.1 INTRODUCTION

The two questions that confront the pharmaceutical scientist during the process of developing a molecule into a drug are "Is it safe?" and "Is it therapeutic?" The question of safety is an important issue that surfaces very early in development; without a clear understanding of what defines safe use, it is difficult, if not impossible, to continue development. Thus, animal toxicology/safety studies are the primary ingredient in any NDA submission. However, such studies are just as important in the conduct of an IND-enabling program, which allows the conduct of the first human clinical studies.

Today, the process of developing a new chemical entity (NCE) into a drug that is approved for marketing follows a well-defined and regulated pathway. The key issues that will determine approval are safety and efficacy in the Phase III trials. In this context, preclinical animal studies provide both the initial and subsequent "windows" on toxicity safety and thus have a direct impact on decisions as to the first clinical trials and on a dosing regimen in such trials. In fact, concerns about safety and efficacy are evaluated throughout the whole drug development process.

In spite of reservations that can be raised about the extrapolation of animal data to humans, toxicology studies provide the best currently available assessments of what can reasonably be expected in humans. The designs obtained from toxicology studies are thus of particular concern since safety predictions based on the data obtained cannot be found to be unwarranted in retrospect. The challenge to the pharmaceutical scientist therefore is to use available "tools" that provide information on toxicity and drug disposition in the animals used in toxicology/safety studies. Regardless of the stage in development, the systemic exposure (e.g., the AUC) is the metric by which the relationship of drug disposition and toxicity is evaluated.

In this context, the inclusion of biopharmaceutics and pharmacokinetics into preclinical development, specifically into the toxicological/safety studies, is a logical step since drug concentration data defines the extent of exposure to drugs.

32.1.1 Rationale for Bioavailability/Bioequivalence (BA/BE) Studies

Bioavailability and bioequivalence are pharmacokinetic (PK) terms that quickly gained importance in the "early" days of the development of pharmacokinetics as a drug development science. As such, their use was primarily targeted to clinical development. Bioavailability is defined in the *Code of Federal Regulations*, Title 21, 320.1 [1] as the rate and extent to which the active ingredient or active moiety is absorbed from a drug product and becomes available at the site of action. For drug products that are not intended to be absorbed into the bloodstream, bioavailability may be assessed by measurements intended to reflect the rate and extent to which the active ingredient or active moiety becomes available at the site of action.

In clinical use, it is not unusual that several dose strengths or different dosage forms (capsules, tablets) are used; therefore a study(ies) is (are) conducted to ascertain that the same plasma concentration time profile is obtained at the different strengths or dosage forms, thus providing the appropriate drug exposure for patient management—that is, bioequivalence. Bioequivalence is often used in clinical trials for comparison of the reference (pioneer) and generic drugs. The *Code of Federal*

Regulations, Title 21, Volume 5 [2] defines bioequivalence as the absence of a significant difference in the rate and extent to which the active ingredient or active moiety in pharmaceutical equivalents or pharmaceutical alternatives becomes available at the site of drug action when administered at the same molar dose under similar conditions in an appropriately designed study. Where there is an intentional difference in rate (e.g., in certain controlled release dosage forms), certain pharmaceutical equivalents or alternatives may be considered bioequivalent if there is no significant difference in the extent to which the active ingredient or moiety from each product becomes available at the site of drug action. This applies only if the difference in the rate at which the active ingredient or moiety becomes available at the site of drug action is intentional and is reflected in the proposed labeling, is not essential to the attainment of effective body drug concentrations on chronic use, and is considered medically insignificant for the drug.

The extent of product bioavailability is estimated by the area under the blood concentration versus time curve (AUC). AUC is most frequently estimated using the linear trapezoidal rule. Other methods for AUC estimation may be proposed and should be accompanied by appropriate literature references during protocol development.

For a single-dose bioequivalence study, AUC should be calculated from time 0 (predose) to the last sampling time associated with quantifiable drug concentration AUC_{0-LOQ}. The comparison of the test and reference product value for this noninfinity estimate provides the closest approximation of the measure of uncertainty (variance) and the relative bioavailability estimate associated with AUC_{0-INF}, the full extent of product bioavailability.

In a multiple-dose study, the AUC should be calculated over one complete dosing interval (AUC_{0-t}). Under steady-state conditions, AUC_{0-t} equals the full extent of bioavailability of the individual dose AUC_{0-INF} assuming linear kinetics. For drugs that are known to follow nonlinear kinetics, the sponsor should consult with the Center for Veterinary Medicine (CVM) to determine the appropriate parameters for the bioequivalence determination [7].

The rate of absorption is estimated by the maximum observed drug concentration (C_{max}) and the corresponding time to reach this maximum concentration (T_{max}). When conducting a steady-state investigation, data on the minimum drug concentration (trough values) observed during a single dosing interval (C_{min}) should also be collected. Generally, three successive C_{min} values should be provided to verify that steady-state conditions have been achieved. To determine a steady-state concentration, the C_{min} values should be regressed over time and the resultant slope should be tested for its difference from zero [7].

Confidence intervals should routinely be used to interpret bioequivalence data. The following bioavailability and bioequivalence standards are usually required:

- The 90% confidence interval of the relative mean AUC of the test reference formulation should be within 80–125%.
- The relative mean measured C_{max} of the test to reference formulation should be within 80–125%.
- The relative mean measured C_{min} of the test to reference formulation should be within 80–125%.

32.1.2   Need and Aim of BA/BE Studies

In preclinical toxicology studies, the selection of the dosage form is not as complicated as for clinical use and this will be addressed subsequently. The issue of doses is of importance as the selection of doses for the various types of toxicology studies is an occult process that involves varying amounts of soft data. However, in order to provide a good prospective assessment/projection regarding safety in humans based on systemic exposure, it is clear that BA/BE principles also apply to animal toxicity studies.

In terms of bioavailability, toxicology studies usually entail three or four dose levels; and BA is "relative" as systemic exposure is evaluated by the linearity (or nonlinearity) of eliminating the kinetic at each dose level and/or as a function of time during the toxicity study. Considering that the dose range in toxicology studies is usually a large multiple of the clinical dose, a relative BA is acceptable in data evaluation of drug concentration and toxic effect(s).

Bioequivalence in preclinical animal studies is a more complex issue and in practical terms applies mostly to dog and primate studies where different oral dosage forms may be evaluated (solutions, capsules of neat drug, galenic tablets) to ensure a maximal drug release profile and thus a definition of the "line" between pharmacology and toxicology.

It is important to know that the drug is bioavailable at the selected route of administration, and that the absence of toxic or pharmacologic effect is real and not just a result of the drug not being absorbed.

In short, both concepts have an application to animal toxicology studies as the exposure needs to be determined and confirmed in order to calculate the animal to human safety margins on which clinical development is dependent.

32.1.3   Role of BA/BE Studies in Drug Development and Nonclinical Studies

As stated earlier, the concepts of BA/BE were first used in clinical development as tools to define a clear and consistent therapeutic use. Considering that the objective of toxicology studies is to demonstrate the toxic potential of the drug across a wide dose range, over varying durations of administration, and across different dosage forms and at least two species, the utility of BA/BE is readily apparent as a means to provide the best prospective assessment of animal safety data in terms of a safe exposure in humans. This is especially true in early stages of development where there is limited exposure/safety data in humans available.

32.1.4   Regulatory Considerations and Guidelines

Bioavailability and/or bioequivalence studies play a key role in the drug development period for both new drug products and their generic equivalents. For both, these studies are also important in the postapproval period in the presence of certain manufacturing changes. The article by Chen et al. [3] reviews the regulatory science of bioavailability and bioequivalence and provides the FDA's recommendations for drug sponsors who intend to establish bioavailability and/or demonstrate bioequivalence for their pharmaceutical products during the developmental process or after approval. Statistic and pharmacokinetic principles of bioavailability and bioequivalence trials are described in Rajaram et al. [4]. This document was prepared as a set of workshop material for the International Congress on Medical and Care Compunetics in June 2004 in Den Hague, The Netherlands.

Toxicokinetics (TK) is the inclusion of pharmacokinetic principles into the toxicology/safety studies conducted in animal species. The objectives of TK are to evaluate drug absorption, distribution, and elimination as a function of dose level; to aid in the selection of realistic dose levels that can be maintained over the duration of the study; to determine the duration of exposure to drug; to determine the effect of chronic drug administration on the absorption and disposition of that drug; and to aid in interpreting and extrapolating the toxicological response in different species.

With few exceptions, toxicology/safety studies are conducted in accordance with the Good Laboratory Practice (GLP) regulations [5]; thus data collection and recording are conducted in a manner that is acceptable to all dossier reviewing regulatory agencies and are subject to verification by a QA unit. In terms of providing commonly acceptable objectives and "suggestions" as to the study design, one can refer to FDA and/or ICH guidelines. A tabulation of these guidelines is presented in Table 32.1. There are no specific preclinical BA/BE in either FDA or ICH guidelines; however, most of the definitions and approaches applicable for preclinical BA/BE studies can be found in two FDA documents: *Bioavailability and Bioequivalence Studies for Oral Administered Drug Products—General Considerations* [6] and *Bioequivalence Guidance*, Center for Veterinary Medicine [7].

32.1.5 Importance of Safety Margins

As stated earlier, the extent of systemic drug exposure in animal toxicology studies is directly correlated to the determination of safety margins to calculate a safe dose in humans. The first human clinical trials are concerned with administering a safe dose without covert toxicity. The challenge is that only animal toxicity/safety data are available. This may now change with the introduction of Phase 0 studies.

A comprehensive approach to the estimation of the human dose from animal data is available [8]. In short, having NOAELs (mg/kg) from animal studies, one can extrapolate a human equivalent dose based on body surface area, from the tables provided in the guidance [8]; a safety factor is chosen and the human equivalent dose is divided by that factor.

The result is the maximum recommended starting dose. A default safety factor of 10 is normally used, and although higher factors provide more flexibility for the strength of the clinical dose, factors lower than 10 do not necessarily mean a clinical hold if other data/information are available as an aid in the assessment of the projected safety in humans. It should be kept in mind that the NOAEL is not a static number and is redetermined as the duration of the toxicology studies becomes longer in keeping with the clinical objectives and study duration. It should also be pointed out that regardless of the place in development, it is important to know the drug release profile from the dosage forms used in the toxicity/safety studies (i.e., the bioavailability) in order to estimate the animal to human safety margins with assurance.

TABLE 32.1   FDA and ICH Guidelines

Agency	Title	Date
FDA	*Bioavailability and Bioequivalence Studies for Oral Drug Products—General Considerations*	March 2003
	Bioequivalence Guidance	9 October 2002
	Exploratory IND Studies	18 January 2006
	Carcinogenicity Study Protocol Submissions	23 May 2002
	Format and Content of the Nonclinical Pharmacology/ Toxicology Section of an Application	1 February 1987
	Immunotoxicology Evaluations of Investigational New Drugs	1 November 2002
	Photosafety Testing	7 May 2003
	Single Dose Acute Toxicity Testing for Pharmaceuticals—Revised	26 August 1996
	Reference Guide for the Nonclinical Toxicity Studies of Antiviral Drugs Indicated for the Treatment of N/A Non-Life Threatening Disease: Evaluation of Drug Toxicity Prior to Phase 1 Clinical Studies	1 February 1989
	Integration of Study Results to Access Concerns About Human Reproductive and Developmental Toxicities	13 November 2002
	Nonclinical Safety Evaluation of Pediatric Drug Products	3 February 2003
	Nonclinical Studies for Development of Pharmaceutical Excipients	18 May 2005
	Statistical Aspects of the Design, Analysis, and Interpretation of Chronic Rodent Carcinogenicity Studies of Pharmaceuticals	8 May 2001
ICH	*M3—Nonclinical Safety Studies for the Conduct of Human Clinical Trials for Pharmaceuticals*	25 November 1997
	S1A—The Need for Long-Term Rodent Carcinogenicity Studies of Pharmaceuticals	1 March 1996
	S1B—Testing for Carcinogenicity in Pharmaceuticals	23 February 1998
	S1C—Dose Selection for Carcinogenicity Studies of Pharmaceuticals	1 March 1995
	S1C(R)—Dose Selection for Carcinogenicity Studies of Pharmaceuticals: Addendum on a Limit Dose and Related Notes	4 December 1997
	S2A—Specific Aspects of Regulatory Genotoxicity Tests for Pharmaceuticals	24 April 1996
	S2B—Genotoxicity: Standard Battery Testing	21 November 1997
	S3A—Toxicokinetics: The Assessment of Systemic Exposure in Toxicity Studies	January 1995
	S4A—Duration of Chronic Toxicity Testing Animals (Rodent and Nonrodent Toxicity Testing)	25 June 1999
	S5B—Detection of Toxicity to Reproduction for Medicinal Products	22 September 1994
	S6—Preclinical Safety Evaluation of Biotechnology Derived Pharmaceuticals	18 November 1997
	S7A—Safety Pharmacology Studies for Human Pharmaceuticals	13 July 2001
	S7B—Safety Pharmacology Studies for Assessing the Potential for Delayed Ventricular Repolarization (QT Interval Prolongation) by Human Pharmaceuticals	14 June 2002 (Draft)
	S8—Immunotoxicity Studies for Human Pharmaceuticals	April 2006

TABLE 32.2   Acronyms and Definitions

Acronym	Definition
BA	Bioavailability means the rate and extent to which the active ingredient or active moiety is absorbed from a drug product and becomes available at the site of action. For drug products that are not intended to be absorbed into the bloodstream, bioavailability may be assessed by measurements intended to reflect the rate and extent to which the active ingredient or active moiety becomes available at the site of action (21 CFR 320.1).
BE	Bioequivalence means the absence of a significant difference in the rate and extent to which the active ingredient or active moiety in pharmaceutical equivalents or pharmaceutical alternatives becomes available at the site of drug action when administered at the same molar dose under similar conditions in an appropriately designed study.
AUC	Area Under the Curve is the integral of drug plasma concentration over a specific time (AUC_t) or to infinity (AUC_{inf}) and is a measure of drug amount absorbed (systemic absorption) into the systemic circulation.
GLP	Good Laboratory Practices Regulation.
PK	Pharmacokinetics.
NDA	New Drug Application.
QA	Quality Assurance.
NOAEL	No-Observed-Adverse-Effect-Level.
MRSD	Maximum Recommended Starting Dose.
HED	Human Equivalent Dose.
TK	Toxicokinetics.
IND	Investigative New Drug Application.
CMC	Controls, Manufacture, and Chemistry.

32.1.6   Definitions

As is the case with many texts, the use of acronyms is a common way to avoid repetitive use of a concept. A partial tabulation of acronyms and definitions of terms that are germane to the present text is presented in Table 32.2.

32.2   IND-TARGETED NONCLINICAL DEVELOPMENT

The filing of an IND is the first step in the drug development process. The IND contains nonclinical pharmacology in animal disease models, toxicology in two animal species of duration that does not exceed the duration of the proposed first clinical trial(s), preliminary ADME data, an Investigators Brochure, protocol synopsis of the proposed clinical trial, and CMC information.

32.2.1   Objective

The objective of the IND is thus to obtain FDA "approval" to proceed with the conduct of the proposed clinical trial, that is, study the molecule in the intended model—humans. Prior to the IND filing it is usual to have a pre-IND meeting with the reviewing division, where what the IND will contain is presented and FDA input is solicited as to its "acceptance." In most cases the first clinical study, being a PK/ tolerance study, is in normal volunteers. However, for some indications this study can be conducted in a small number of patients and be of a short duration. In general, the duration of the toxicology studies, the dose ranges used, the NOAELs obtained, and the safety margins that are estimated determine the final clinical protocol for the initial human study(ies).

32.2.2   Species in IND-Targeted Toxicology Studies

Although it is not our purpose to discuss the format or content of an IND dossier, it is useful to present an outline of the IND to indicate the position and role of nonclinical toxicology studies. A general outline of the IND is given in Table 32.3.

Throughout drug development, toxicology/safety studies are conducted in two species. As most drugs are intended for oral administration, the rat and dog are the primary species used for reasons of availability, costs, and long history of use. However, not all drugs are targeted for oral delivery and other routes (intravenous, dermal, etc.) and species (rabbit for reproductive toxicology, monkey) may be used (Table 32.4). In general, the current climate supports a "minimal" IND as presented in the recent FDA guidance—*Guidance for Industry, Investigators, and Reviewers: Exploratory IND Studies.* This guidance allows sponsors a great deal of flexibility in the IND content and in the toxicity studies required, provided limited human exposure and no therapeutic intent is the objective of the initial clinical trial. Thus,

TABLE 32.3   Outline of an IND

Covering Letter
Questions for the FDA
Section 1: Form 1571
Section 2: Table of Contents
Section 3: Introductory Statement
Section 4: General Investigational Plan
• Clinical Development Plan
• Planned Exposure
• Safety/Estimation of Potential Risk
Section 5: Investigators Brochure
Section 6: Protocol(s)
Section 7: Chemistry, Manufacture and Controls (CMC)
• Drug Substance
• Drug Product
Section 8: Nonclinical Pharmacology and Toxicology
• Overview of the Nonclinical Testing Strategy
• Nonclinical Pharmacology
• Nonclinical Pharmacokinetics and Metabolism
• Toxicology
• Conclusions
• References
• End of Text Tables: Summary Tabulations
• Copies of Literature Cited
• Copies of Final Study Reports

TABLE 32.4   Species and Study Types in an Exploratory IND

Species	Study Type
Mouse	Acute toxicity, subchronic toxicity (2 weeks), genotoxicity (*in vivo* micronucleus)
Rat	Acute toxicity, subchronic toxicity (2 weeks), genotoxicity
Rat	Safety pharmacology—Irwin test, and CNS effects
Rabbit	Reproductive toxicology
Dog	Acute toxicity and subchronic toxicity, safety pharmacology—QT interval prolongation
Monkey	Safety pharmacology-QT interval prolongation

a "go/no go" decision can be reached very early and is based on human, albeit limited, experience. It is important to point out that in case the data supports moving forward in development, the traditional toxicology/safety program must be conducted to continue development.

The species and studies that would be contained in such an IND are outlined below. It should also be pointed out that the route of administration in these studies would be the intended route in the clinic.

Not all of the above studies are conducted for an IND filing, and Table 32.4 presents a "menu" of what can be conducted. In general, acute and subchronic toxicity, the core genotoxicity, and safety pharmacology are required, with the most appropriate species chosen.

32.2.3   Key Elements of IND-Target Development

Throughout all drug development, safety is a factor, perhaps the key factor. The parameters that define safety are presented in the following text. It should be pointed out that as/when development moves forward with the aim of a NSA filing, safety in nonclinical studies continues to be evaluated in studies of longer duration (6 month study in rats, 9 month study in dogs/monkeys, the full panel of reproductive toxicity, carcinogenicity studies in mice and rats). However, the use of toxicokinetics and BA/BE issues remain to support the extent of exposure determinations and data interpretation. Examples of studies/data on file as well as from published reports are presented in the subsequent discussion. In this context it should be pointed out that although numerous studies germane to the present chapter are conducted, the majority are not published—thus the inclusion of data "gleaned" from personal files.

Toxicology/Safety Profile   As shown in Table 32.3, Section 8 of the IND deals with toxicology, and considering that at this time in development, other sections may be rather sparse. As stated earlier, the results of the toxicity studies, in terms of NOAEL and safety margins, are key for the conduct of the first human studies. The other sections provide data that characterize the physicochemical properties of the drug, its stability, and the clinical dosage form for these studies (CMC section); the proposed clinical plan; and the Investigator's Brochure. The toxicological/safety profile is presented in detail and is comprised of nonclinical pharmacology (the rationale for development), nonclinical pharmacokinetics and metabolism, and toxicology. For all of these components, the text contains the elements of study design, results, discussion and conclusions, and summary tabulations of the data obtained. Copies of QA final study reports are also included in the submission.

Extent of Absorption   In practice, the actual (numerical) extent of absorption is not determined in the context of toxicology studies. It is important, however, to demonstrate/ascertain absorption, and this is achieved by the toxicokinetic evaluations; this data is evaluated in a relative, intradose manner and as a function of both dose and time.

Usually the level of absorption (bioavailability) is obtained from the nonclinical PK and ADME studies. Considering that these studies are conducted in the same species and with the same dosage forms as the toxicology studies, the data are thus available to provide a reasonable assessment of the bioavailability of the drug in the toxicity studies, if such an assessment is needed.

An example of a PK study in dogs for bioavailability (relative to an IV injection) of a solution and a solid dosage form (a preliminary clinical capsule) is shown in Fig. 32.1. The plasma concentration–time profiles clearly show a good oral bioavailability of the drug from the solution, whereas it was virtually quantitative from the preliminary capsule considered for the first clinical trials. The use of this capsule for the toxicity safety studies was considered as it would provide the maximum drug release profile and thus clearly define the toxicological profile and the NOAEL.

Assessment of Safety Margins Based on Systemic Exposure   At the IND stage, the primary objective is to provide safety assessments, based on which the first human studies are conducted. These Phase I studies determine single-dose pharmacokinetics/tolerance in normal volunteers with the safe dose obtained in humans from the safety margins calculated from the results of the IND-enabling toxicity studies [9, 10]. A "simple" treatment of safety factor calculations can be derived from the

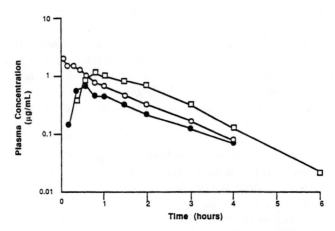

FIGURE 32.1   Mean plasma concentrations of the neuroleptic in dogs following a 5 mg/kg dose intravenously (○), as an oral solution (●), and as a clinical capsule (□). (From I. Bekersky, personal data.)

comprehensive methods presented in the guidance [8]. In brief, one can calculate the human dose expected to result in the same effect seen in the animal studies (HED); the safety margin can be estimated on a mg/kg comparison of doses, using the equation $HED = $ Animal $NOAEL \times (W_{animal}/W_{human})^{0.33}$. This calculation takes into account both the weight and the relative body surface area.

A similar equation uses a "conversion factor" (S) that addresses the issue of body surface area: (S factor) $\times$ ($NOAEL$ dose in mg/kg)/S factor$_{human}$ = Safe dose in humans in mg/kg (the HED). Knowing the extent of systemic exposure (AUC) from toxicokinetic assessments provides an additional level of confidence to the determination of the NOAEL, and thus to the calculation of the safety margins, and in turn, to setting a safe dose for the initial human trials.

Relationship of Absorption to Dosage Form(s) and Route of Administration   The nature of the nonclinical studies that are conducted in drug development depends on the targeted disease, the route of administration in therapeutic use, and the anticipated treatment duration in humans. Thus administration by the oral, intravenous, dermal, inhalation, subcutaneous, and ocular routes in studies ranges from a single dose to a lifetime exposure. As pointed out earlier, although the rat and dog are the most frequently used species, rabbits, mice, mini- and micropigs, and monkeys are also used. The aim is to use the species that are considered to be the most relevant to humans in terms of the intended clinical use.

To discuss and/or present all possible routes of administration is not our intention here. Needless to say, the extent of absorption must be determined relative to a "standard." In this context, examples of some routes of administration are given as illustrative of this principle.

Regardless of species and route of administration, the need is to administer high, but justifiable, doses in order to establish safety margins for human exposure and to determine the target organs of toxicity. Although bioavailability for IV administration is not an issue, it is for other routes of administration. Thus the incorporation of TK into toxicity studies along with assessments of bioavailability ensures not only that the drug is present systemically, but that the extent of systemic exposure is "maximal" in order to obtain the best possible assessment of the toxicological profile.

Oral Administration   The primary route of administration in many, perhaps most, nonclinical toxicity studies is oral; this is due to the fact that that is the "preferred" route of delivery in the marketplace. However, as stated earlier, other routes—intravenous, subcutaneous, inhalation, topical—are also used, both in the marketplace and thus in the preclinical toxicity studies. The absorption in all cases is determined (TK) and the extent estimated by comparison to PK studies; for example, AUC post-IV to AUC from other routes of administration.

The dosage form itself (i.e., "formulation") can have pronounced effects on the absorption and thus on the selection of the dose. Such effects are well described, especially for oral drugs. Some examples from our own studies and the literature are discussed later in several sections of this chapter.

The rat is the species most commonly used with oral administration the route of choice and is the primary rodent utilized in toxicology studies. Oral administration by gavage as a solution or suspension is the most frequently employed dosage form and is used in studies of up to 6–9 months duration. The primary consideration is the choice of vehicle. Solutions in water are chosen if the solubility of the drug is sufficient to deliver the highest dose proposed. For drugs of low or limited solubility, a dispersing agent for use in an aqueous milieu is selected. A vehicle of 0.5% aqueous Tween 80 (i.e., polysorbate 80) has a long history of use for a wide range of drugs. Cellulose and its derivatives (e.g., methyl-, carboxy-), starch, and different natural oils (e.g., corn, sesame) are often used as a vehicle for oral gavage formulations. For studies of greater duration than 9 months (i.e., lifetime carcinogenicity studies), oral drugs are usually administered as an admixture in the diet of the rats.

The absorption in all studies is determined from the TK data and evaluated as to whether the drug release profile from the dosage form is sufficient to define the toxicological profile. An example of mean plasma concentration–time data comparing gavage administration to the administration of a similar dose as a dietary admix to rats is shown in Fig. 32.2. In this example, a composite profile was obtained using three rats per time point using alternate animals. The challenge in rodent studies is the small volume of blood that can be taken; thus an analytical method with a low LOQ is needed. Because of the small amount of blood available, rats are usually alternated through the blood collection time points and in mice blood collection is usually terminal.

Use of the dog, the most commonly utilized nonrodent species, allows a wide range of evaluations of oral dosage forms without the "liability" of limited blood sample volume. An example of comparative absorption profile in dogs is shown in Fig. 32.3, where an equivalent dose was administered as a solution and a formulated capsule. In Fig. 32.4 the absorption profile of a highly lipophilic drug formulated as two different salts of Labrafil (a fatty acid complex used to solubilize drugs) is shown. In both cases, the different absorption profile as a function of the dosage form is clearly demonstrated.

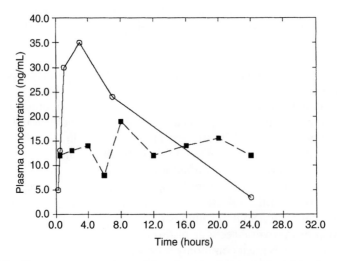

FIGURE 32.2   Plasma concentrations of drug in rats after oral administration as a solution/suspension by gavage (○) and as a dietary admix (■). (From I. Bekersky, personal data.)

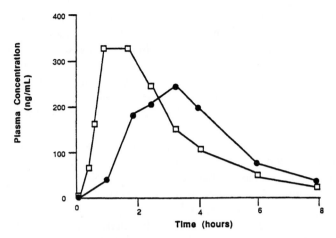

FIGURE 32.3   Mean plasma concentrations of drug in dogs after 20 mg/kg oral administrations as a solution in PEG (□) and a formulated capsule (●). (From I. Bekersky, personal data.)

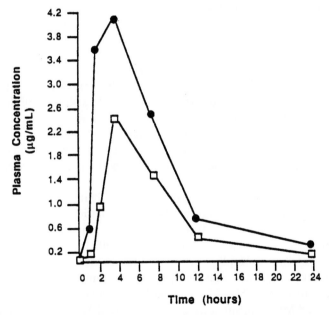

FIGURE 32.4   Mean plasma concentrations of drug in dogs after a 10 mg/kg oral administration of capsules of NMG-Larafil (□) and TEA-Labrafil (●). (From I. Bekersky, personal data.)

Low oral bioavailability of some drugs can be improved by including certain enhancers in drug formulation or special coating of the tablet/capsules. Enhancement of drug bioavailability may be studied in several animal species and can be predictable for humans. Coadministration of compound A and indinavir resulted in a 17-fold increase in oral AUC of compound A in rats due to the inhibition of the metabolism of compound A by indinavir, whereas compound A did not affect indinavir metabolism as indicated by the unchanged indinavir AUC [11]. Similarly, the systemic exposure of compound A in dogs and monkeys was increased substantially following oral coadministration with indinavir by sevenfold and >50-fold, respectively. Enhancement in compound A systemic exposure by indinavir in humans is predicted based on the *in vivo* animal and *in vitro* human studies.

Labrasol was found to improve the intestinal absorption of gentamicin (GM) in rats. Bioavailability of GM in several different formulations containing labrasol was evaluated in beagle dogs [12].

In Wistar rats, 1.0% (w/v) *N*-trimethyl chitosan chloride (quaternized chitosan derivative) solution significantly increased the absorption of the peptide analogue, resulting in a fivefold increase of octreotide bioavailability compared with the controls (octreotide alone). Coadministration of 1.0% (w/v) chitosan hydrochloride did not enhance octreotide bioavailability [13].

In dogs dosed orally, cefoxitin bioavailability increased from 2.4% to 29% with an enteric-coated tablet containing 600 mg PCC, but uncoated tablets containing palmitoyl-DL-carnitine chloride resulted in no improvement of absorption [14]. Glycosylated bile acid analogue was also used in dogs to increase the absorption of gentamicin [15]. The increase in bioavailability depended on the site of administration. Bioavailabilities in controlled and enhanced states, respectively, were 6% and 54% when administered to the ileum, 4% and 23% for jejunal dosing, and 2% and 10% when administered orally.

Dodecylmaltoside (surfactant) increased the colonic absorption of azetirelin 8.7-fold in rats, and increased oral bioavailability in dogs from 15% to 44% when combined with citric acid in an enteric-coated capsule formulation [16]. The extent of absorption enhancement reported ranged from less than twofold to fourfold to fivefold, with maximum bioavailabilities in rats and dogs of approximately 7% and 19%, respectively [17, 18]. Intraduodenal bioavailability of calcein in rats was improved from 2% to 25–37% with microemulsion formulations containing a mixture of caprylic acid or capric acid and their sodium salts, as well as medium chain glycerides [19].

Medium chain glycerides have been delivered orally in several types of formulations. A self-emulsifying w/o microemulsion formulation containing 22% MCG was administered intraduodenally to rats (3.3 mL/kg); the bioavailability of calcein improved from 2.4% to 45%, and the bioavailability of a hydrophilic peptide improved from 0.5% to 27% [20].

To aid delivery to the lower intestine, capsules containing cefmetazole in an MCG solution were enteric coated [21]. Cefmetazole bioavailability in dogs was 65% with the enteric-coated MCG capsules, 21% with uncoated MCG capsules, and 6% with enteric-coated capsules without MCG. Enteric coating of capsules also improved bioavailability of ceftriaxone in monkeys when administered in MCG.

A vehicle containing 1.5% chitosan at pH 6.7 increased the bioavailability of intraduodenally administered buserelin in rats from 0.1% to 5.1% [22]. A 10-fold increase in the oral bioavailability of paclitaxel was observed in mice when coadministered with the P-gp inhibitor SDZ PSC 833 [23]. A similar magnitude of enhanced bioavailability was found in human subjects administered paclitaxel with 15 mg/kg cyclosporin, another P-gp inhibitor [24]. Oral absorption of digoxin in mice was increased by coadministered SDZ PSC 833, and brain concentrations and brain/plasma ratios were also increased by the P-gp inhibitor, raising the possibility that systemic absorption of P-gp inhibitors could alter the pharmacologic and toxic effects of coadministered drugs [25].

Intravenous (IV) Administration   As stated earlier, bioavailability is not an issue for IV administration as the total dose is delivered. However, there are other considerations that impact on the dose size and thus on the safety margins obtained. The IV dosage form must be a solution and thus the physicochemical properties of the drug are taken into consideration. Once the formulation is established, its compatibility with blood must be determined to establish venous and perivenous tolerance. In addition, the duration of injection (or infusion) is evaluated to establish the safety margin; however, it should be stated that this factor may not be applicable to human use because of anatomical and physiological difference.

It goes without saying that in drugs administered intravenously in the clinic, the issue of bioavailability is not a consideration. However, the species used can be an important determinant based on other factors that determine drug disposition. Examples are given in Tables 32.5 and 32.6, showing that the plasma protein binding parameter was the determinant in the selection of the appropriate species for the toxicological evaluations of ceftriaxone, a parenteral cephalosporin antibiotic. At therapeutic plasma concentrations, the extent of protein binding in human plasma is high (90–95%) and is concentration dependent (Table 32.5). The plasma protein binding in animals that were used in nonclinical development is dependent on the species [26]. In baboon plasma, protein binding (Table 32.5) is concentration dependent and the extent of binding is quite similar to that found in human plasma [26]. In dog plasma, however, protein binding is low with no meaningful relationship to drug concentration. Thus the free concentration of cefriaxone varies greatly in human, baboon, and dog over a similar plasma drug concentration range. As a consequence of the plasma protein binding, the pharmacokinetics of ceftriaxone in humans are nonlinear when based on total drug concentration, but linear if based on the free drug concentration (Table 32.6) [26, 27]. This was the case in baboons, whereas in dogs the pharmacokinetics was the same whether based on total or free drug concentration. These differences played a role in the selection of species for the toxicology studies in early development. In this context, the dog was rejected

TABLE 32.5   Protein Binding Profile of Ceftriaxone in Human and Animal Plasma

Drug Concentration (μg/mL)	Human		Baboon		Dog	
	Bound (%)	Free Concentration (μg/mL)	Bound (%)	Free Concentration (μg/mL)	Bound (%)	Free Concentration (μg/mL)
100	92.7	7.3	95.5	4.5	19.6	80.4
200	88.5	23.0	—	—	13.9	172.2
240	—	—	88.5	27.6	—	—
400	78.7	35.2	—	—	7.1	371.6
560	—	—	65.9	190.9	—	—
800	64.2	64.2	—	—	6.9	744.8
1000	—	—	51.7	483.0	—	—

Source: Adapted from Ref. 27.

TABLE 32.6   Pharmacokinetic Parameters for Ceftriaxone in Humans, Dogs, and Baboon Based on Total (T) And Free (F) Drug Concentrations

Species	Dose (mg/kg)	AUC (μg·h/mL)	V (L)	CL_p (mL/min)	t_{frac12} (h)
Human	150	268 (T)10 (F)	7	10	8.6
			192	262	8.6
	1500	1978 (T)103 (F)	9	13	7.8
			162	249	7.6
Baboon	150	1573 (T)288 (F)	4.5	11	6.1
			11.9	66	2.6
	700	3913 (T)1632 (F)	5.7	21	6.5
			13.1	51	1.7
Dog	20	79 (T)68 (F)	3.8	40	1.2
			5.2	52	1.3

Source: Adapted from Refs. 26 and 27.

TABLE 32.7   Absolute Bioavailability of Drug Applied Topically to Rats and Micropigs

Species	Route	Dose	Application Area	AUC (ng·h/mL)	Bioavailabity, F (%)
Rat	IV	1 mg/kg		642	100 %
	Topical	0.5% (500 mg/m²)	10 cm²	68	≤5%
	Topical (abraded)	0.5% (500 mg/m²)	10 cm²	570	62
Micropig	IV	1 mg/kg		3900	100
	Topical	3% (3000 mg/m²)	400 cm²	70	≤1

Source: Adapted from Ref. 28.

based on the different pharmacokinetic profile relative to humans and was replaced by the baboon.

Dermal Administration   From a toxicological end point, there are two factors that are determined in the development of topical drugs: the local toxicity at the site of application and the potential for systemic toxicity. The skin is a semipermeable barrier and absorption into the systemic circulation can thus be anticipated. In this context, the extent of systemic exposure (i.e., bioavailability) is determined following dermal application. This is determined for both intact and excoriated skin, as in clinical use the skin can be broken (such as in atopic dermatitis) with a subsequent effect on systemic exposure.

An example from a recent development of a dermal product is given in Table 32.7 [28]. Absolute bioavailability (relative to the respective IV administration) was ≤5% (rat) and ≤1% (micropig) based on AUC comparisons. Abrading the skin in a rat study increased the bioavailability to approximately 62%. The comparison of the animal data to human IV (1 mg/kg) and topical administration (0.3%, 5000 cm^2 application area) indicated that the absolute bioavailability in atopic dermatitis patients was less than 0.5%. Interestingly, after 8 days of treatment, bioavailability decreased slightly (<0.3%), presumably reflecting an improvement in the integrity of the skin in response to treatment.

The cutaneous bioavailability of topical 2% minoxidil solution was verified in live hairless mice—minoxidil and propylene glycol deposition on the skin surface, epidermis, and dermis from the single-dose *in vivo* study [29]. Percutaneous absorption of the drug appeared to be a very small fraction of the applied dose. The pharmacokinetics of methotrexate (MTX) in rabbit skin and plasma after IV bolus and iontophoretic delivery at different current densities was studied [30]. The systemic absorption of MTX increased proportionally with increased current.

Inhalation and Ocular Administration   These routes, although less frequently used, present challenges and thus warrant discussion. In the rat, the differences of the respiratory tract and the fact that rats breathe through their noses result in an inadequate model for inhalation exposure to humans. A common approach to rat inhalation studies is by exposing the nose of the animal through an opening into a cylinder filled with air containing a known concentration of the drug. Several difficulties are readily apparent: the actual dose administered and the monitoring of the systemic received. In larger animals (dogs, monkeys) inhalation is administered via a nose mask, resulting in a more discreet administration. As in all studies, a blood sampling protocol for TK analysis is included in the study for the assessment of systemic exposure.

Ocular administration is perhaps the most emotive route of administration; toxicity studies are conducted in rats, rabbits, and monkeys, with the monkey frequently used for its similarity in ocular volume to the human eye. As with topical administration, local toxicity is evaluated as well as systemic toxicity if a partitioning from the eye into the systemic circulation is demonstrated.

Preclinical studies are often performed in an attempt to improve bioavailability of nasal or ocular administered drugs. Enhancement of bioavailability of calcitonin formulated with different alkylglycosides following nasal and ocular administration was studied in rats [31]. Enhancement of bioavailability of insulin nanocomplexes in nasal formulation was also studied in rats [32]. Iontophoresis ocular drug delivery and peak concentrations determination were performed for numerous drugs in rabbit studies [33]. Hayden et al. [34] showed that focal delivery of carboplatin using subconjunctival injection or iontophoretic resulted in significantly higher peak concentrations of carboplatin in the choroid, retina, optic nerve, and vitreous body than those obtained after intravenous delivery.

Comparison of the Different Routes of Exposure   Equivalence of different routes of exposure is not apparent and thus comparison of bioavailability or bioequivalence of the drug administered by the different routes of administration is often studied in various animals. This comparison is illustrated in Table 32.8 and Fig. 32.2. Other examples of such studies are presented next.

The pharmacokinetic parameters of midazolam tablets were compared after administration by the sublingual route and intravenous routes in six rabbits to

TABLE 32.8   Biopharmaceutic Parameters of a Drug in the Dog from a Dosage Form Evaluation Study

Dosage Form	C_{max} (μg/mL)	T_{max} (h)	AUC (μg·h/mL)
Intravenous (IV)			10.3
Aqueous solution	1.5	1.4	12.5
Capsule[a]	1.8	1.5	13.7
Tablet[b]	1.2	1.4	10.8
CMC suspension	0.9	1.0	5.7

[a]Soft gelatin capsule with neat drug.
[b]Tablet formulation for use in first clinical trials.

Source: I. Bekersky, personal data.

determine the bioequivalence between these routes [35]. By the sublingual route, midazolam absorption is substantial and fast. The statistical analysis, on data obtained with HPLC, shows no significant difference between pharmacokinetic parameter values calculated after intravenous and sublingual administration (0.5 mg). The absolute bioavailability was close to 100%. 1-Hydroxy-midazolam seems to have a great importance in BZD activity. To estimate the bioequivalence between intravenous and sublingual midazolam administration, it is necessary to take into account the active metabolites.

Brown et al. [36] compare the bioequivalence of the ceftiofur sodium salt in cattle after a single intramuscular (IM) or subcutaneous (SC) dose of 2.2 mg ceftiofur equivalents/kg body weight. The preestablished criterion for equivalence of the $t >$ 0.2 for IM and SC administration was satisfied. The equivalence of $AUC_{0\text{-}LOQ}$ and $t > 0.2$ for IM and SC administration of 2.2 mg ceftiofur equivalent (CE)/kg doses of ceftiofur sodium suggest similar therapeutic efficacy and systemic safety for the two routes of administration.

The pharmacokinetic properties of a long-acting formulation of chloramphenicol were determined in six yearling cattle after a single intravenous (IV) administration (40 mg/kg body weight) and after two sequential subcutaneous (SC) or intramuscular (IM) administrations [37]. The two extravascular routes were studied during a crossover trial for a bioequivalence test. Bioavailability was 19.1% after IM injection and 12.4% after SC administration. The extent of absorption from the two routes did not differ significantly. The rate of absorption was significantly lower after SC application than it was after IM injection. The time necessary for the plasma concentration to exceed 5 μg/mL was the same for the two routes. Thus, IM and SC routes were bioequivalent. In the other study [38], the pharmacokinetics of chloramphenicol were studied in sheep after three single intravenous (IV), intramuscular (IM), and subcutaneous (SC) administrations (30 mg/kg) during a crossover trial for a bioequivalence test. The two routes of absorption were not bioequivalent. Using the kinetic values, multidose regimens to maintain the therapeutic chloramphenicol blood level (5 μg/mL) were proposed: 60 mg/kg every 12 hours for 72 hours for the IM administration and 45 mg/kg for SC administration according to the same regimen. Chloramphenicol residues remained at the injection site, and 400 hours would be necessary to obtain the level of 10 μg/kg. Determination of the creatinine phosphokinase serum values showed that the subcutaneous route induced less damage to muscle than the intramuscular route.

The disposition of spiramycin (a macrolide antibiotic) in plasma and milk after intravenous, intramuscular, and subcutaneous administration was investigated in healthy cows given a single injection of spiramycin at a dose of 30,000 IU/kg by each route [39]. The dose fraction adsorbed after intramuscular or subcutaneous administration was almost 100% and was bioequivalent for the extravascular routes, but the rates of absorption, the maximal concentrations, and the time to obtain them differed significantly between the two routes. Plasma concentrations of doramectin in 40 cattle dosed by subcutaneous (SC) or intramuscular (IM) injection (200 micrograms/kg) were compared to assess the bioequivalence of the two routes of administration [40]. The bioequivalence of the SC and IM formulation has been established.

Pietropaolo et al. [41] performed direct comparisons between injection of myelin basic protein peptide and administration by several nonparenteral routes to determine whether route impacted benefit in the treatment of murine allergic encephalomyelitis, a model for multiple sclerosis. The range of effective peptide doses spanned over 1000-fold, and route of delivery played a major role in determining optimal dose. The oral route of administration was the least effective, requiring at least 50- to 100-fold more antigen than subcutaneous injection, which in turn required at least 10-fold more antigen than delivery of peptide to the lung using an intratracheal instillation. Intratracheal delivery was also considerably more effective than inhalation of peptide and, unlike inhalation, resulted in obvious penetration of delivered material deep into the lung. The increase in therapeutic efficacy did not appear to result from slower systemic delivery of antigen.

Apomorphine (0.5 mg/kg) was administered subcutaneously and percutaneously to rabbit in order to compare the pharmacokinetic data obtained with these two different routes [42]. For the percutaneous administration, an apomorphine gel was prepared by dissolution of apomorphine in a hydroxypropylmethylcellulose gel of medium viscosity. The peak plasma concentration and the area under the curve were significantly greater with the subcutaneous route. The bioequivalence of the percutaneous route was 35% of the subcutaneous administration. One study [43] reports a paradox: the AUC of apomorphine after intravenous injection in rabbits is anomalously lower (statistically significantly) than after subcutaneous injection.

Bergeron et al. [44] examined the effect of route of administration by giving equimolar amounts of two iron chelators—NaHBED and deferoxamine (DFO)—to *Cebus apella* monkeys as either a subcutaneous (SC) bolus or a 20 min intravenous (IV) infusion. By both routes, NaHBED was consistently about twice as efficient as DFO in producing iron excretion. For both chelators at a dose of 150 μmol/kg, SC was more efficient than IV administration.

Acrylamide bioavailability after aqueous gavage was 60–98% and from the diet was 32–44%; however, first-pass metabolism or other kinetic change resulted in much higher (two- to sevenfold) internal exposures to glycidamide (its epoxide metabolite, GA) when compared to the intravenous route. A similar effect on metabolism for GA following oral administration was previously observed under an identical exposure paradigm in mice [45].

32.2.4 Use of Animal Models for the Selection of Dosage Forms for Nonclinical Toxicology Studies

Some of the issues in selecting a dosage form for animal studies have been touched upon previously. Data that is needed prior to the preparation/choosing of a dosage form are solubility, stability, compatibility with excipients, and particle size, keeping in mind that a "maximum" drug release profile is a target.

For rat studies, use of solutions or suspensions administered via gavage has been described previously. Rats are rarely used for comparison of different dosage forms. Of more illustrative value are studies with large animals (dogs, monkeys), as these species allow more flexibility in the kinds of dosage forms administered. An example of a dosage form evaluation study is given in Table 32.8 where three possible dosage forms for toxicology studies (solution, unformulated capsule, and suspension) as well as a gelenic tablet prepared for the initial clinical trials were tested. The data indicate that relative to an IV administration, the solution, capsule, and galenic tablet were acceptable for use in toxicity studies with a drug release profile equal to the IV Bioavailability of the CMC suspension was approximately half of all the other dosage forms tested.

A biopharmaceutic evaluation that involved the drug particle size and several forms of the drug is given in Table 32.9. The drug in question had excellent oral activity although the form available at the time (the free base as an oil) resulted in severe GI toxicity, which was in all probability due to the prolonged presence of unabsorbed drug substance. Capsules containing salts of the drug were then tested, indicating that the acetate salt resulted in the greatest extent of absorption relative to the other two forms. The subsequent availability of the free base in crystalline form allowed the drug to be micronized, and a second study was conducted to evaluate the absorption profile. This study indicated that reducing the particle size by micronization resulted in higher C_{max}, shorter T_{max}, and AUC values that were considerably higher than those in the first study. Interestingly, the more rapid absorption alleviated the GI toxicity found in preliminary studies, in spite of the considerably higher extent of absorption.

The selection of a formulation for nonclinical studies has received a "modest" treatment as being illustrative of the overall study design in the early stages of drug development. In order to attain a maximum drug release profile, in some cases in

TABLE 32.9 Biopharmaceutic Parameters (Mean ±SD) from Two Dosage Form Evaluation Studies

Dosage Form	C_{max} (µg/mL)	T_{max} (h)	AUC (µg·h/mL)
Nonmicronized			
Free base (oil)	1.6 ± 1.4	2.7 ± 1.2	5.9 ± 5.7
Dihydrochloride	3.6 ± 1.9	0.5 ± 0	11.9 ± 5.3
Acetate salt	4.3 ± 1.9	4.0 ± 2.0	18.9 ± 8.0
Micronized			
Free base	8.4 ± 3.5	1.8 ± 0.5	70.2 ± 6.6
Dihydrochloride	4.9 ± 2.4	2.0 ± 1.4	40.8 ± 21.9
Acetate salt	5.8 ± 2.3	2.1 ± 1.4	41.4 ± 21.6

spite of undesirable physicochemical properties, and thus clearly to define the line between pharmacology and toxicology, formulation selection has become part of the overall development of drugs. In many cases, formulation evaluation studies are not part of the toxicology/safety studies but are conducted in parallel throughout development, with the information obtained being integrated into all evaluations. Examples from the literature of studies dealing with factors that impact on bioavailability are given next.

Seven kinds of poorly water-soluble compounds as the model compounds were used to compare the plasma concentration profile of the drug following single oral administration of each compound to rats and beagle dogs as a solution, an oily solution, a suspension (or a powder), and oil/water (O/W) microemulsions [46]. Thus for six kinds of the model compounds, except disopyramide, the solubility was from 340 to 98,000 times that in water, and the AUC values in plasma concentration of the compound were equivalent to that of solution or O/W microemulsion administration, or were increased by 1.5–78 times that of suspension administration.

The bioavailability of a modified rafoxanide oral suspension was compared to the original innovator product and a generic formulation in a single-dose, randomized, parallel design study in sheep [47]. The area under the rafoxanide plasma concentration versus time curve (AUC), AUC extrapolated to infinity, and maximum plasma rafoxanide concentrations (C_{max}) were significantly smaller for both the modified and generic formulations relative to the original product. There were no significant differences between the modified and generic formulations. In terms of the calculated 90% confidence t-intervals of the mean % ratios, the modified and generic formulations were not bioequivalent to the original product, since they were substantially below the accepted range of 80–125%.

32.2.5 Species Differences in Bioavailability

There are many processes that determine bioequivalence of a given drug among species, including absorption from a site of administration; renal, biliary, and intestinal elimination; sequestration (in particular, binding to proteins or other macromolecules); distribution and redistribution; biotransformation; and receptor population density and uniqueness. Short [48] reviewed physiologic and pharmacologic parameters that affect drug distribution, elimination, and metabolism to make comparisons of bioequivalence of drugs between sheep and other ruminants. Interspecies differences are very important for selecting an appropriate species for preclinical studies. The following is a summary of recent literature describing interspecies differences in pharmacokinetics of a wide range of therapeutic agents.

Pharmacokinetics and pharmacodynamics of controlled release gastroretentive dosage forms (CR-GRDF), which improve the bioavailability of medications, were studied for several drugs in rats and dog models [49–52]. The bioavailability of melagatran (active form of ximelagatran) following oral administration of ximelagatran was 5–10% in rats, 10–50% in dogs, and about 20% in humans, with low between-subject variation [53]. The oral bioavailability of levovirin was 29.3% in rats, 51.3% in dogs, and 18.4% in monkeys [54]. Zebularine showed oral bioavailability of 6.7% in mice, 3.1% and 6.1% in rats, and was <1% in monkeys [55].

Extrapolation of pharmacokinetics from animals to humans may be performed based on *in vitro* metabolism studies in hepatocytes. *In vitro* degradation studies of vinpocetine with hepatocytes have shown that the activity of human hepatocytes is about one order of magnitude higher than the activity of dog hepatocytes, and two orders of magnitude higher than that of rat hepatocytes [56]. These differences can explain the differences in bioavailabilities of vinpocetine in the three species (52% in rats, 21.5% ± 19.3% in dogs, and 6.2% ± 1.9% in humans). In dogs and humans, the compound seems to be metabolized exclusively in the liver, whereas in rats extrahepatic metabolism seems also to be important. The *in vivo* clearance predicted from the activity of hepatocytes is in good agreement with the values measured *in vivo* in the case of humans and dogs.

The interspecies absorption, distribution, metabolism, and elimination (ADME) profile of *N*-geranyl-*N'*-(2-adamantyl)ethane-1,2-diamine (SQ109), a new diamine-based antitubercular drug, were characterized after intravenous and oral single administration in rodents and dogs [57]. Based on IV equivalent body surface area dose, the terminal half-life of SQ109 in dogs was longer than that in rodents, reflected by a larger volume of distribution and a higher clearance rate of SQ109 in dogs, compared to that in rodents. The oral bioavailability of SQ109 in dogs, rats, and mice were 2.4–5%, 12%, and 3.8%, respectively. The binding of [^{14}C]SQ109 (0.1–2.5 μg/mL) to plasma proteins varied from 6% to 23% depending on the species (human, mouse, rat, and dog). SQ109 was metabolized by rat, mouse, dog, and human liver microsomes, resulting in 22.8%, 48.4%, 50.8%, or 58.3%, respectively, of SQ109 remaining after a 10 min incubation at 37 °C.

Compound A (potent inhibitor of the hepatitis C virus (HCV) NS5B polymerase) exhibited marked species differences in pharmacokinetics [58]. Plasma clearance was 44 mL/min/kg in rats, 9 mL/min/kg in dogs, and 16 mL/min/kg in rhesus monkeys. Oral bioavailability was low in rats (10%) but significantly higher in dogs (52%) and monkeys (26%). Compound A was eliminated primarily by metabolism in rats, with biliary excretion accounting for 30% of its clearance. Metabolism was mainly mediated by cyclohexyl hydroxylation, with N-deethylation and acyl glucuronide formation constituting minor metabolic pathways. Qualitatively, the same metabolites were identified using *in vitro* systems from all species studied, including humans. The low oral bioavailability of compound A in rats was mostly due to poor intestinal absorption. A series of high affinity GABA(A) agonists showed good oral bioavailability in both rat and dog [59].

The pharmacokinetics of DA-6034 in rats and dogs and the first-pass effect in rats were examined [60]. The low bioavailability (approximately 0.136%) of DA-6034 at a dose of 50 mg/kg in rats could be due to considerable intestinal first-pass effect (approximately 69% of oral dose) and unabsorbed fraction from the gastro-intestinal tract (approximately 30.5%). The clearance of adaphostin (potential anti-cancer agent) from plasma, on a square meter (m^2) basis, was equivalent for mice and rats but more rapid in dogs [61]. Oxytocin antagonist, 2',4'-difluorophenyldike-topiperazine derivative 37, has good bioavailability (46%) in the rat and moderate bioavailability (13–31%) in the dog [62], while 5-chloroindole had good oral bio-availability in both rat and dog [63].

BMS-378806 (prototype of novel HIV attachment inhibitors) exhibited species-dependent oral bioavailability, which was 19–24% in rats and monkeys and 77% in dogs [64]. In rats and monkeys, absorption was prolonged, with an apparent terminal half-life of 2.1 and 6.5 hours, respectively. In rats, linear pharmacokinetics was observed between IV doses of 1 and 5 mg/kg and between PO doses of 5 and 25 mg/kg. The total body clearance was intermediate in rats and low in dogs and monkeys. The steady-state volume of distribution was moderate (0.4–0.6 L/kg), contributing to a short half-life (0.3–1.2 hours) after IV dosing.

The pharmacokinetics and disposition of *N*-(2,6-dichlorobenzoyl)-4-(2,6-dimethoxyphenyl)-L-phenylalanine (TR-14035), a novel a4ss1/a4ss7 antagonist, were investigated in the rat and dog [65]. Results indicated extensive clearance of TR-14035 and low oral bioavailability, 17% and 13% in the rat and dog, respectively, at an oral dose of 10 mg/kg. A species-dependent difference in metabolism was observed. The principal metabolite, *O*-desmethyl TR-14035, observed in rat, dog, and probably human, was further conjugated with sulfate in the rat, but never in dog and human, based on *in vitro* metabolism and *in vivo* metabolite profile studies. Urinary excretion was a minor elimination route, but an interesting species difference was recognized. TR-14035 was reabsorbed from the rat renal proximal tubules and, by contrast, secreted into the tubules in the dog, probably via active transport systems.

Exposure of MGS0028, a potent group II metabotropic glutamate receptor agonist, increased proportionally (1–10 mg/kg PO) in rats, with bioavailability >60% at all doses. However, bioavailability was only approximately 20% in monkeys, and active metabolite was found in relatively high abundance in plasma. In dogs, oral bioavailability was >60%, and the metabolite was not detected. James et al. [66] found that the rat was a better *in vivo* model than the dog for the prediction of human systemic exposure in HIV-1 nonnucleoside reverse transcriptase inhibitors of the diaryltriazine and diarylpyrimidine classes of compounds [67]. The absolute bioavailability of YM466, a new factor Xa inhibitor, was 2.7–4.5% in rats, almost constant regardless of the dose levels investigated, while it was 6.9–24.6% in dogs, indicating nonlinear pharmacokinetics.

The bioavailability of SNI-2011, cevimeline, a novel muscarinic acetylcholine receptor agonist, was approximately 50% and 30% in rats and dogs, respectively. Major metabolites in plasma were both S- and N-oxidized metabolites in rats and only N-oxidized metabolite in dogs, indicating that a large species difference was observed in the metabolism of SNI-2011 [68].

Absolute oral bioavailability of a gavage dose of galantamine was high in rat (77%) and dog (78%). In mice and rats, the bioavailability of galantamine administered via the food was lower than of galantamine administered by gavage [69]. Elimination half-life of galantamine was relatively large in rat and dog and smaller in mouse and rabbit. Galantamine plasma levels after single and repeated administration of 10 mg/kg/day in all species investigated except female rat and rabbit were much higher than mean therapeutic plasma levels of galantamine obtained in humans. The pharmacokinetic profile of galantamine after repeated oral administration in rats was most similar to the profile obtained after repeated administration of 12 mg bid in humans.

Not only species but even a strain within the same species may predispose to pharmacokinetics differences especially when different strains exhibit different metabolism. Systemic exposure to oxycodone and noroxycodone was consistently higher for cytochrome P450 (CYP)2D1/2D2-deficient dark Agouti (DA) rats than for CYP2D1/2D2-replete Sprague–Dawley (SD) rats showing that strain differences predominated over diabetes status [70].

32.3 NDA-TARGETED NONCLINICAL DEVELOPMENT

When the IND is "opened" and the nonclinical and Phase I data are indicative of a "go" decision, the NDA-targeted studies are conducted. Whereas the IND contained acute and subchronic (2 and/or 4 week) toxicology studies, depending on the indication sought, an acceptable NDA will contain chronic toxicity studies in support: 6 month rat, 9 month dog (or monkey), 78 week carcinogenicity study in mice, and 24 month carcinogenicity study in rats. This would be the case for IV, PO, and inhalation drugs. For topical drugs, 52 week photocarcinogenicity and 2 year topical carcinogenicity studies are conducted.

32.3.1 Toxicokinetics in Chronic Toxicity Studies

Considering that the duration of exposure in chronic studies is severalfold that of subchronic studies, it is even more important to assess the extent of exposure. To this end, range-finding studies are conducted to ascertain that the dose range that will be used in the definitive study will provide both a NOAEL and a definition of toxicity. In general, the concepts that have been described previously hold for these studies. Toxicokinetics are an integral part of protocol designs to determine if there are changes with the duration of treatment. It is hoped that the bioavailability of the dosage form has been determined during the pre- and post-IND development, with the assurance of a consistent and demonstrable extent of systemic exposure.

It is worthwhile mentioning that the oral carcinogenicity studies are conducted with the drug administered as a dietary admix. This would require a "bridging study" comparing bioavailability of the dietary admix to a systemic administration to determine the bioavailability. Such studies entail a 5–8 sample profile over 24 hours, whereas the toxicokinetics in the definitive admix studies would consist of a single blood draw, usually at approximately 9 am.

An example of a gavage versus admix comparison using serial sampling is shown in Fig. 32.2; from such data, exposure and bioavailability based on AUC can readily be determined. Single sample monitoring over the course of a chronic study, however, is useful as accumulation or induction over the study time course can be ascertained and such data will be of help in the study evaluation.

32.3.2 Use of Animals to Evaluate the BA/BE of Clinical Dosage Forms

In the early stages of development, it is important to determine whether the dosage form targeted for clinical use has an acceptable level of bioavailability. To evaluate the dosage form in a clinical study is time consuming and costly. In this case, the clinical form was first evaluated in dogs and subsequently in humans. The results are shown in Table 32.10. Compared to IV administrations, the bioavailability of the oral capsule formulation in dog was low (27%), and based on data from ADME studies, the low bioavailability was considered to be due to extensive metabolism. Urinary excretion data indicated that only a small fraction of the dose (0.2–0.3%) was eliminated as the intact drug, with the rest excreted as a hydroxyl metabolite. It was considered that even though the bioavailability was low, the level was sufficient to continue with a clinical study. As shown in Table 32.10, the results in humans were similar: low C_{max} and low bioavailability of the intact drug (approximately

TABLE 32.10   Biopharmaceutic Comparison of a Drug in Dog and Human

Species	Dosage Form	Dose (mg/kg)	C_{max} (µg/mL)	AUC_{inf} (µg·h/mL)	F^a (%)
Dog	Capsule	7.5	0.62	66	27
Human	Tablet	10	0.08	142	37

[a]Relative to IV dose and corrected for dose.

Source: Adapted from Ref. 79.

TABLE 32.11   Comparison of Drug Release Profile of Drug from Similar Dosage Forms in Dog and Human

Species	Dosage Form	Dose (mg/kg)	T_{max} (h)	C_{max} (ng/mL)	AUC (ng·h/mL)
Dog	PEG solution	20	1	320	920
	Captex capsule	20	3	230	928
Human	PEG capsule	0.2	3	446	1524
	Neobee capsule	0.2	4	336	1004

Source: I. Bekersky, personal data.

37%). In this case, the study in dogs indicated a level of oral bioavailability that was acceptable for a clinical evaluation; a clinical study was then conducted with similar results to those found in dogs.

In Table 32.11, an evaluation of several dosage forms in dogs and subsequently in humans is shown. In dogs, there was little difference between the oral formulations tested, although the PEG solution resulted in a more rapid absorption based on T_{max}. In humans, however, the capsules containing PEG formulation appeared to be more bioavailable, an AUC of 1524 ng·h/mL versus an AUC of 1004 ng·h/mL for the Neobee formulation. Capsules containing drug as solution/suspension in PEG were subsequently developed for use in clinical trials.

In another study, preliminary experiments with an antibiotic indicated a low relative bioavailability. Physicochemical considerations suggested that ester analogues represented an approach that could potentially enhance the oral bioavailability of the parent compound. Ester analogues of the drug were synthesized and tested as solutions in dogs. The results are summarized in Table 32.12. Relative to the solution, both esters enhanced the oral bioavailability: 26% of the Bac ester, and 22% of the Piv ester; the bioavailability of the parent drug was 10%. On the basis of these results, both esters were administered to humans with results comparable to those "predicted" by the dog study.

Use of the dog to provide insights pertaining to drug absorption is not restricted to situations where information prospective to the first clinical trials is desired. Even when the clinical trials are well advanced, the dog can be utilized to ascertain a situation that may require reformulation of the clinical dosage form. An example of such a case is given in Table 32.13. The drug was unstable in the presence of oxygen and light and was formulated as a micronized suspension in oil within a soft elastic gelatin (SEG) capsule. On aging, these capsules failed to meet the dissolution speci-

TABLE 32.12   Oral Bioavailability of Drug Analogue Solutions in Dog and Human

Species	Drug Form	Dose (mg/kg)	C_{max} (μg/mL)	AUC (μg·h/mL)	Bioavailability F (%)
Dog	Parent	20	2.6	6.9	10
	Bac ester	20	9.1	18	26
	Piv ester	20	5.5	15	22
Human	Bac ester	5.3	4.4	7	29
	Piv ester	5.3	3.2	6	25

Source: I. Bekersky, personal data.

TABLE 32.13   Biopharmaceutic Evaluation of Potential Clinical Formulations in Dog and Human

Species	Administration	Approximate Dose (mg/kg)	C_{max} (μg/mL)	AUC_{inf} (μg·h/mL)	F^a (%)
Dog	Oral solution	4	3.33	12	
	"New" SEG capsule	4	1.05	4.5	39
	"Aged" SEG capsule[b]	4	1.23	5.5	47
Human	"New" SEG capsule	1	0.26	3.8	60
	"Aged" SEG capsule	1	0.29	3.7	59

[a]Bioavailability relative to respective oral solution and corrected for dose.
[b]"Aged" capsules were stored for 4 years and failed dissolution specifications.

Source: Adapted from Ref. 79.

fications for the product. To determine whether reformulation was required, these "aged" capsules were tested in dogs relative to the identical "new" formulation. In the dog study, no changes in the bioavailability were found due to aging. This was confirmed in a study in humans that gave similar results to those found in the dog study.

The dog can also be used in exploratory research. The drug in question was under development for parenteral delivery only. Oral administration to dogs resulted in very low C_{max} (3–4 μg/mL) with a bioavailability of approximately 4% relative to IV administration. However, since some oral absorption did occur, an exploratory program with dogs was initiated to study the feasibility of developing an oral dosage form for humans. The results are given in Table 32.14. The intraduodenal (ID) and rectal administration to the dog of two exploratory formulations containing an absorption enhancer indicated a significant increase in absorption as indicated by the C_{max} and AUC values. Based on these data, the concept was tested in humans. Although the bioavailability via the different routes in enteral administration was

TABLE 32.14   Biopharmaceutic Parameters of a Drug in Dog and Human Following a Single Administration by Different Routes

Species	Route	Dose	C_{max} (µg/mL)	T_{max} (h)	AUC_{inf} (µg·h/mL)	F (%)
Dog	IV	20 mg/kg	—	—	102	—
	ID[a]	50 mg/kg	47	0.5	82	32
	Rectal	50 mg/kg	28	0.2	24	10
Human	IV	500 mg	—	—	427	—
	ID	500 mg	6	0.16	24	6
	Rectal	500 mg	23	0.75	124	29

[a]ID, intraduodenal.

Source: I. Bekersky, personal data.

reversed in humans when compared to dogs, the potential enteral delivery in humans was ascertained.

32.3.3   Role and Impact of Nonclinical Studies on Clinical Development: Animal to Humans

During Phase I–IIa, factors such as a food effect, gender effect, and pre- and systemic metabolism are determined prior to Phase IIb in order to set/justify dose selection for the pivotal Phase III studies. Nonclinical studies have provided "windows" of information prospectively to the conduct of label–targeted human clinical pharmacology studies; examples are given next.

The bioavailability in beagle dogs and the dissolution rates of cyclandelate from five capsule preparations commercially available in Japan were measured [71]. One of the capsules that showed an extremely low bioavailability in humans also showed the lowest bioavailability in beagle dogs, although the difference in bioavailability with the highest preparation was smaller than in humans. A significant correlation was obtained between the results of the studies in humans and beagles. However, the power of the test using beagles was extremely low in comparison with that in the human study. Food enhanced the bioavailability of cyclandelate from the capsules, having the highest and lowest bioavailability in the fasted state in beagles as observed previously in the human study. The bioinequivalence of the cyclandelate capsules detected in the fasted state disappeared in the fed state in the beagle dog study, while the bioinequivalence still remained in the nonfasted state in human subjects. Thus bioequivalence testing in the fed state led to different results in both species.

Coadministration of food increases the rate and extent of cilostazol absorption [72]. After investigating the effect of concomitant food intake on the bioavailability of two nifedipine-containing modified-release dosage forms, authors concluded that a change from taking Slofedipine XL in the fed to the fasted state might result in increased systemic concentrations of nifedipine [73]. In the dog, food decreased the mean area under the plasma concentration–time curve value of compound LY354740, an analogue of glutamic acid, by approximately 34%, hence decreasing the oral bioavailability of the compound [74].

Concomitant intake of levodopa preparations with banana juice, but not with a commercial banana beverage, caused a drug–food interaction reducing levodopa bioavailability in rats [75]. Mean (±SD) peak concentrations of tepoxalin were significantly higher after feeding of low fat ($1.08 \pm 0.37\,\mu g/mL$) and high fat ($1.19 \pm 0.29\,\mu g/mL$) diets than in fasted dogs ($0.53 \pm 0.20\,\mu g$ /mL), suggesting that feeding improves oral bioavailability [76].

Bioavailability and pharmacokinetics may be gender dependent. Jann et al. [77] showed that gender may be a significant factor in ondansetrons disposition. Gender differences in the pharmacokinetics of DA-6034 were found after intravenous but not an oral administration at a dose of 50 mg/kg to male and female Sprague–Dawley rats [78]. In rats, plasma levels of galantamine were lower in females than in males, whereas in mice, females showed higher levels than males [69]. No gender differences were observed in dogs. Sex difference was also observed in the pharmacokinetics of cevimeline in rats but not in dogs [68].

32.4 CONCLUSION

Toxicology/safety studies in animals are an integral part of any drug development program, the results of which have a direct impact on both the IND and the NDA. The calculations of safety margins for human doses are based on the measurements of systemic exposure (AUC) and the NOAEL in the animal studies. In this context, the inclusion of pharmacokinetics into the conduct/evaluation of animal toxicity studies (toxicokinetics) has become routine. Toxicokinetic evaluations ascertain that a level of systemic absorption was achieved, the intrastudy relationship of this absorption to the doses administered, and absorption changes with the duration of exposure. The inclusion of bioavailability concepts adds the element of quantity, as the level of absorption relative to a standard is obtained. As a maximum drug release profile is desired, in many cases several dosage forms are tested. Thus bioequivalence determinations of several dosage forms intended for toxicology studies provide assurance that the most appropriate dosage form is used. The bioequivalence is also determined to assess equivalence between the routes of administration, species differences, and drug derivatives preference.

Animal studies for bioavailability/bioequivalence are used both prospectively and retrospectively, and depending on the objective and study design, form an animal to human bridge in drug development.

REFERENCES

1. *Code of Federal Regulations*, Title 21, 320.1.
2. *Code of Federal Regulations*, Title 21, Volume 5.
3. Chen ML, Shah V, Patnaik R, Adams W, Hussain A, Conner D, Mehta M, Malinowski H, Lazor J, Huang SM, Hare D, Lesko L, Sporn D, Williams R. Bioavailability and bioequivalence: an FDA regulatory overview. *Pharm Res* 2001;18(12):1645–1650.
4. Rajaram L, Roy SK, Skerjanec A. Bioavailability and bioequivalence trials: statistics & pharmacokinetic principles. *Stud Health Technol Inform* 2004;159–179.

5. Good Laboratory Practice Regulations, Title 21 of the *Code of Federal Regulations*, Part 58, effective 20 June, 1979.

6. *Bioavailability and Bioequivalence Studies for Oral Administered Drug Products—General Considerations*. Washington DC: US FDA; 2003.

7. *Bioequivalence Guidance*, Center for Veterinary Medicine. Washington DC: US FDA; 2002.

8. *Estimating the Maximum Safe Starting Dose in Initial Clinical Trials for Therapeutics in Adult Healthy Volunteers*. Washington DC: US FDA; 2005.

9. *Guidance for Industry, Investigators, and Reviewers: Exploratory IND Studies*. Washington DC: US FDA; 2006 .

10. Freireich EJ, Gehan EA, Rall DP, Schmidt LH, Skipper HE. Quantitative comparison of toxicity of anticancer agents in mouse, rat, hamster, dog, monkey, and man. *Cancer Chemother Rep* 1966:50(4):219–244.

11. Jin L, Chen IW, Chiba M, Lin JH. Interaction with indinavir to enhance systemic exposure of an investigational HIV protease inhibitor in rats, dogs and monkeys. *Xenobiotica* 2003;33(6):643–654.

12. Rama Prasad YV, Eaimtrakarn S, Ishida M, Kusawake Y, Tawa R, Yoshikawa Y, Shibata N, Takada K. Evaluation of oral formulations of gentamicin containing labrasol in beagle dogs. *Int J Pharm* 2003;268(1–2):13–21.

13. Thanou M, Verhoef JC, Marbach P, Junginger HE. Intestinal absorption of octreotide: *N*-trimethyl chitosan chloride (TMC) ameliorates the permeability and absorption properties of the somatostatin analogue *in vitro* and *in vivo*. *J Pharm Sci* 2000;89(7): 951–957.

14. Sutton SC, LeCluyse EL, Engle K, Pipkin JD, Fix JA. Enhanced bioavailability of cefoxitin using palmitoylcarnitine. II. Use of directly compressed tablet formulations in the rat and dog. *Pharm Res* 1993;10:1516–1520.

15. Axelrod HR, Kim JS, Longley CB, Lipka E, Amidon GL, Kakarla R, Hui YW, Weber SJ, Choe S, Sofia MJ. Intestinal transport of gentamicin with a novel, glycosteroid drug transport agent. *Pharm Res* 1998;15:1876–1881.

16. Sasaki I, Tozaki H, Matsumoto K, Ito Y, Fujita T, Murakami M, Muranishi S, Yamamoto A. Development of an oral formulation of azetirelin, a new thyrotropin-releasing hormone (TRH) analogue, using *N*-lauryl-*b*(-D-maltopyranoside as an absorption enhancer. *Biol Pharm Bull* 1999;22:611–615.

17. Aungst BJ, Saitoh H, Burcham DL, Huang S-M, Mousa SA, Hussain MA. Enhancement of the intestinal absorption of peptides and non-peptides. *J Control Release* 1996;41: 19–31.

18. Burcham DL, Aungst BJ, Hussain M, Gorko MA, Quon CY, Huang S-M. The effect of absorption enhancers on the oral absorption of the GPIIb/IIIa receptor antagonist, DMP 728, in rats and dogs. *Pharm Res* 1995;12:2065–2070.

19. Constantinides PP, Welzel G, Ellens H, Smith PL, Sturgis S, Yiv SH, Owen AB. Water-in-oil microemulsions containing medium-chain fatty acids/salts: formulation and intestinal absorption enhancement evaluation. *Pharm Res* 1996;13:210–215.

20. Constantinides PP, Scalart J-P, Lancaster C, Marcello J, Marks G, Ellens H, Smith PL. Formulation and intestinal absorption enhancement evaluation of water-in-oil microemulsions incorporating medium-chain glycerides. *Pharm Res* 1994;11:1385–1390.

21. Sekine M, Terashima H, Sasahara K, Nishimura K, Okada R, Awazu S. Improvement of bioavailability of poorly absorbed drugs. II. Effect of medium chain glyceride base on the intestinal absorption of cefmetazole sodium in rats and dogs. *J Pharmacobio-Dyn* 1985;8:286–295.

22. Lueßen HL, de Leeuw BJ, Langemeÿer WE, de Boer AG, Verhoef JC, Junginger HE. Mucoadhesive polymers in peroral peptide drug delivery. VI. Carbomer and chitosan improve the intestinal absorption of the peptide drug buserelin *in vivo*. *Pharm Res* 1996;13:1668–1672.

23. Van Asperen J, van Tellingen O, Sparreboom A, Schinkel AH, Borst P, Nooijen WJ, Beijnen JH. Enhanced oral bioavailability of paclitaxel in mice treated with the P-glycoprotein blocker SDZ PSC 833. *Br J Cancer* 1997;76:1181–1183.

24. Terwogt JMM, Beijnen JH, ten Bokkel Huinink WW, Rosing H, Schellens JHM. Coadministration of cyclosporin enables oral therapy with paclitaxel. *Lancet* 1998;352: 285.

25. Mayer U, Wagenaar E, Dorobek B, Beijnen JH, Borst P, Schinkel AH. Full blockade of intestinal P-glycoprotein and extensive inhibition of blood–brain barrier P-glycoprotein by oral treatment of mice with PSC833. *J Clin Invest* 1997;100:2430–2436.

26. Popick AC, Crouthamel WG, Bekersky I. Plasma protein binding of ceftriaxone. *Xenobiotica* 1987;17:1139–1145.

27. Patel IH, Kaplan SA. Pharmacokinetic profile of ceftriaxone in man. *Am J Med* 1984; 77:17–25.

28. Bekersky I, Lilja H, Lawrence I. Tacrolimus pharmacology and non clinical studies. FK506 to protopic. *Semin Cutan Med Surg* 2001;20:226–232.

29. Tsai JC, Weiner N, Flynn GL, Ferry JJ. Drug and vehicle deposition from topical applications: localization of minoxidil within skin strata of the hairless mouse. *Skin Pharmacol* 1994;7(5):262–269.

30. Stagni G, Shukla C. Pharmacokinetics of methotrexate in rabbit skin and plasma after iv-bolus and iontophoretic administrations. *J Control Release* 2003;93(3):283–292.

31. Ahsan F, Arnold J, Meezan E, Pillion DJ. Enhanced bioavailability of calcitonin formulated with alkylglycosides following nasal and ocular administration in rats. *Pharm Res* 2001;18(12):1742–1746.

32. Simon M, Wittmar M, Kissel T, Linn T. Insulin containing nanocomplexes formed by self-assembly from biodegradable amine-modified poly(vinyl alcohol)-graft-poly(L-lactide): bioavailability and nasal tolerability in rats. *Pharm Res* 2005;22(11):1879–1886.

33. Eljarrat-Binstock E, Domb AJ. Iontophoresis: a non-invasive ocular drug delivery. *J Control Release* 2006;110(3):479–489.

34. Hayden BC, Jockovich ME, Murray TG, Voigt M, Milne P, Kralinger M, Feuer WJ, Hernandez E, Parel JM. Pharmacokinetics of systemic versus focal carboplatin chemotherapy in the rabbit eye: possible implication in the treatment of retinoblastoma. *Invest Ophthalmol Vis Sci* 2004;45:3644–3649.

35. Odou P, Barthelemy C, Chatelier D, Luyckx M, Brunet C, Dine T, Gressier B, Cazin M, Cazin JC, Robert H. Pharmacokinetics of midazolam: comparison of sublingual and intravenous routes in rabbit. *Eur J Drug Metab Pharmacokinet* 1999;24(1):1–7.

36. Brown SA, Chester ST, Speedy AK, Hubbard VL, Callahan JK, Hamlow PJ, Hibbard B, Robb EJ. Comparison of plasma pharmacokinetics and bioequivalence of ceftiofur sodium in cattle after a single intramuscular or subcutaneous injection. *J Vet Pharmacol Ther* 2000;23(5):273–280.

37. Sanders P, Guillot P, Mourot D. Pharmacokinetics of a long-acting chloramphenicol formulation administered by intramuscular and subcutaneous routes in cattle. *J Vet Pharmacol Ther* 1988;11(2):183–190.

38. Dagorn M, Guillot P, Sanders P. Pharmacokinetics of chloramphenicol in sheep after intravenous, intramuscular and subcutaneous administration. *Vet Q* 1990;12(3):166–174.

39. Sanders P, Moulin G, Guillot P, Dagorn M, Perjant P, Delepine B, Gaudiche C, Mourot D. Pharmacokinetics of spiramycin after intravenous, intramuscular and subcutaneous administration in lactating cows. *J Vet Pharmacol Ther* 1992;15(1):53–61.

40. Nowakowski MA, Lynch MJ, Smith DG, Logan NB, Mouzin DE, Lukaszewicz J, Ryan NI, Hunter RP, Jones RM. Pharmacokinetics and bioequivalence of parenterally administered doramectin in cattle. *J Vet Pharmacol Ther* 1995;18(4):290–298.

41. Pietropaolo M, Olson CD, Reiseter BS, Kasaian MT, Happ MP. Intratracheal administration to the lung enhances therapeutic benefit of an MBP peptide in the treatment of murine experimental autoimmune encephalomyelitis. *Clin Immunol* 2000;95(2):104–116.

42. Durif F, Beyssac E, Coudore F, Paire M, Eschalier A, Aiache M, Lavarenne J. Comparison between percutaneous and subcutaneous routes of administration of apomorphine in rabbit. *Clin Neuropharmacol* 1994;17(5):445–453.

43. Ugwoke MI, Agu RU, Kinget R, Verbeke N. Intravenous versus subcutaneous injections of apomorphine in rabbits: a pharmacokinetic paradox. *Boll Chim Farm* 2003;142(8): 315–318.

44. Bergeron RJ, Wiegand J, Brittenham GM. HBED ligand: preclinical studies of a potential alternative to deferoxamine for treatment of chronic iron overload and acute iron poisoning. *Blood* 2002;99(8):3019–3026.

45. Doerge DR, Young JF, McDaniel LP, Twaddle NC, Churchwell MI. Toxicokinetics of acrylamide and glycidamide in Fischer 344 rats. *Toxicol Appl Pharmacol* 2005;208(3): 199–209.

46. Araya H, Nagao S, Tomita M, Hayashi M. The novel formulation design of self-emulsifying drug delivery systems (SEDDS) type O/W microemulsion I: enhancing effects on oral bioavailability of poorly water soluble compounds in rats and beagle dogs. *Drug Metab Pharmacokinet* 2005;20(4):244–256.

47. Swan GE, Botha CJ, Taylor JH, Mulders MS, Minnaar PP, Kloeck A. Differences in the oral bioavailability of three rafoxanide formulations in sheep. *J S Afr Vet Assoc* 1995;66(4): 197–201.

48. Short CR. Consideration of sheep as a minor species: comparison of drug metabolism and disposition with other domestic ruminants. *Vet Hum Toxicol* 1993;35(Suppl 2): 40–56.

49. Klausner EA, Lavy E, Stepensky D, Friedman M, Hoffman A. Novel gastroretentive dosage forms: evaluation of gastroretentivity and its effect on riboflavin absorption in dogs. *Pharm Res* 2002;19:1516–1523.

50. Klausner EA, Eyal S, Lavy E, Friedman M, Hoffman A. Novel levodopa gastroretentive dosage form: *in vivo* evaluation in dogs. *J Control Release* 2003;88:117–126.

51. Stepensky D, Friedman M, Srour W, Raz I, Hoffman A. Preclinical evaluation of pharmacokinetic–pharmacodynamic rationale for oral CR metformin formulation. *J Control Release* 2001;7:107–115.

52. Hoffman A, Stepensky D, Lavy E, Eyal S, Klausner E, Friedman M. Pharmacokinetic and pharmacodynamic aspects of gastroretentive dosage forms. *Int J Pharm* 2004;277(1–2): 141–153.

53. Eriksson UG, Bredberg U, Hoffmann KJ, Thuresson A, Gabrielsson M, Ericsson H, Ahnoff M, Gislen K, Fager G, Gustafsson D. Absorption, distribution, metabolism, and excretion of ximelagatran, an oral direct thrombin inhibitor, in rats, dogs, and humans. *Drug Metab Dispos* 2003;31(3):294–305.

54. Lin CC, Luu T, Lourenco D, Yeh LT, Lau JY. Absorption, pharmacokinetics and excretion of levovirin in rats, dogs and cynomolgus monkeys. *J Antimicrob Chemother* 2003;51(1): 93–99.

55. Holleran JL, Parise RA, Joseph E, Eiseman JL, Covey JM, Glaze ER, Lyubimov AV, Chen YF, D'Argenio DZ, Egorin MJ. Plasma pharmacokinetics, oral bioavailability, and interspecies scaling of the DNA methyltransferase inhibitor, zebularine. *Clin Cancer Res* 2005;11(10):3862–3868.

56. Szakacs T, Veres Z, Vereczkey L. *In vitro–in vivo* correlation of the pharmacokinetics of vinpocetine. *Pol J Pharmacol* 2001;53(6):623–628.

57. Jia L, Noker PE, Coward L, Gorman GS, Protopopova M, Tomaszewski JE. Interspecies pharmacokinetics and *in vitro* metabolism of SQ109. *Br J Pharmacol* 2006;147(5): 476–485.

58. Giuliano C, Fiore F, Di Marco A, Padron Velazquez J, Bishop A, Bonelli F, Gonzalez-Paz O, Marcucci I, Harper S, Narjes F, Pacini B, Monteagudo E, Migliaccio G, Rowley M, Laufer R. Preclinical pharmacokinetics and metabolism of a potent non-nucleoside inhibitor of the hepatitis C virus NS5B polymerase. *Xenobiotica* 2005;35(10–11):1035–1054.

59. Goodacre SC, Street LJ, Hallett DJ, Crawforth JM, Kelly S, Owens AP, Blackaby WP, Lewis RT, Stanley J, Smith AJ, Ferris P, Sohal B, Cook SM, Pike A, Brown N, Wafford KA, Marshall G, Castro JL, Atack JR. Imidazo[1,2-*a*]pyrimidines as functionally selective and orally bioavailable GABA(A)alpha2/alpha3 binding site agonists for the treatment of anxiety disorders. *J Med Chem* 2006;49(1):35–38.

60. Chung HJ, Choi YH, Choi HD, Jang JM, Shim HJ, Yoo M, Kwon JW, Lee MG. Pharmacokinetics of DA-6034, an agent for inflammatory bowel disease, in rats and dogs: contribution of intestinal first-pass effect to low bioavailability in rats. *Eur J Pharm Sci* 2006;27(4):363–374.

61. Li M, Wang H, Hill DL, Stinson S, Veley K, Grossi I, Peggins J, Covey JM, Zhang R. Preclinical pharmacology of the novel antitumor agent adaphostin, a tyrphostin analog that inhibits bcr/abl. *Cancer Chemother Pharmacol* 2006;57(5):607–614.

62. Borthwick AD, Davies DE, Exall AM, Livermore DG, Sollis SL, Nerozzi F, Allen MJ, Perren M, Shabbir SS, Woollard PM, Wyatt PG. 2,5-Diketopiperazines as potent, selective, and orally bioavailable oxytocin antagonists. 2. Synthesis, chirality, and pharmacokinetics. *J Med Chem* 2005;48(22):6956–6969.

63. Ahmed M, Briggs MA, Bromidge SM, Buck T, Campbell L, Deeks NJ, Garner A, Gordon L, Hamprecht DW, Holland V, Johnson CN, Medhurst AD, Mitchell DJ, Moss SF, Powles J, Seal JT, Stean TO, Stemp G, Thompson M, Trail B, Upton N, Winborn K, Witty DR. Bicyclic heteroarylpiperazines as selective brain penetrant 5-HT6 receptor antagonists. *Bioorg Med Chem Lett* 2005;15(21):4867–4871.

64. Yang Z, Zadjura L, D'Arienzo C, Marino A, Santone K, Klunk L, Greene D, Lin PF, Colonno R, Wang T, Meanwell N, Hansel S. Preclinical pharmacokinetics of a novel HIV-1 attachment inhibitor BMS-378806 and prediction of its human pharmacokinetics. *Biopharm Drug Dispos* 2005;26(9):387–402.

65. Tsuda-Tsukimoto M, Ogasawara Y, Kume T. Pharmacokinetics and metabolism of TR-14035, a novel antagonist of a4ss1/a4ss7 integrin mediated cell adhesion, in rat and dog. *Xenobiotica* 2005;35(4):373–389.

66. James JK, Nakamura M, Nakazato A, Zhang KE, Cramer M, Brunner J, Cook J, Chen WG. Metabolism and disposition of a potent group II metabotropic glutamate receptor agonist, in rats, dogs, and monkeys. *Drug Metab Dispos* 2005;33(9):1373–1381.

67. Lewi P, Arnold E, Andries K, Bohets H, Borghys H, Clark A, Daeyaert F, Das K, de Bethune MP, de Jonge M, Heeres J, Koymans L, Leempoels J, Peeters J, Timmerman P, Van den Broeck W, Vanhoutte F, Van't Klooster G, Vinkers M, Volovik Y, Janssen PA. Correlations between factors determining the pharmacokinetics and antiviral activity of HIV-1 non-nucleoside reverse transcriptase inhibitors of the diaryltriazine and diarylpyrimidine classes of compounds. *Drugs R D* 2004;5(5):245–257.

68. Washio T, Kohsaka K, Arisawa H, Masunaga H. Pharmacokinetics and metabolism of the novel muscarinic receptor agonist SNI-2011 in rats and dogs. *Arzneimittelforschung* 2003;53(1):26–33.

69. Monbaliu J, Verhaeghe T, Willems B, Bode W, Lavrijsen K, Meuldermans W. Pharmacokinetics of galantamine, a cholinesterase inhibitor, in several animal species. *Arzneimittelforschung* 2003;53(7):486–495.

70. Huang L, Edwards SR, Smith MT. Comparison of the pharmacokinetics of oxycodone and noroxycodone in male dark Agouti and Sprague–Dawley rats: influence of streptozotocin-induced diabetes. *Pharm Res* 2005;22(9):1489–1498.

71. Kaniwa N, Ogata H, Aoyagi N, Ejima A, Takahashi T, Uezono Y, Imasato Y. Bioavailability of cyclandelate from capsules in beagle dogs and dissolution rate: correlations with bioavailability in humans. *J Pharmacobiodyn* 1991;14(3):152–160.

72. Bramer SL, Forbes WP. Relative bioavailability and effects of a high fat meal on single dose cilostazol pharmacokinetics. *Clin Pharmacokinet* 1999;37(Suppl 2):13–23.

73. Schug BS, Brendel E, Chantraine E, Wolf D, Martin W, Schall R, Blume HH. The effect of food on the pharmacokinetics of nifedipine in two slow release formulations: pronounced lag-time after a high fat breakfast. *Br J Clin Pharmacol* 2002;53(6):582–588.

74. Johnson JT, Mattiuz EL, Chay SH, Herman JL, Wheeler WJ, Kassahun K, Swanson SP, Phillips DL. The disposition, metabolism, and pharmacokinetics of a selective metabotropic glutamate receptor agonist in rats and dogs. *Drug Metab Dispos* 2002;30(1):27–33.

75. Ogo Y, Sunagane N, Ohta T, Uruno T. Banana juice reduces bioavailability of levodopa preparation. *Yakugaku Zasshi* 2005;125(12):1009–1011.

76. Homer LM, Clarke CR, Weingarten AJ. Effect of dietary fat on oral bioavailability of tepoxalin in dogs. *J Vet Pharmacol Ther* 2005;28(3):287–291.

77. Jann MW, ZumBrunnen TL, Tenjarla SN, Ward ES Jr, Weidler DJ. Relative bioavailability of ondansetron 8-mg oral tablets versus two extemporaneous 16-mg suppositories: formulation and gender differences. *Pharmacotherapy* 1998;18(2):288–294.

78. Yang SH, Bae SK, Kwon JW, Yoo M, Lee MG. Gender differences in the pharmacokinetics of DA-6034, a derivative of flavonoids, in rats. *Biopharm Drug Dispos* 2006;27(1):47–51.

79. Crouthamel WG, Bekersky I. Preclinical evaluation of new drug candidates and drug delivery systems in the dog. In Crouthamel WG, Sarapu AC, Eds. *Animal Models for Oral Drug Delivery in Man: In Vitro and In Vivo Approaches*. Washington DC: American Pharmaceutical Association; 1983, pp 107–123.

33

MASS BALANCE STUDIES

JAN H. BEUMER, JULIE L. EISEMAN, AND MERRILL J. EGORIN
University of Pittsburgh Cancer Institute, Pittsburgh, Pennsylvania

Contents

33.1 INTRODUCTION

A well-designed mass balance study significantly expands information about the pharmacological behavior of an active compound. Among many things, a preclinical

Preclinical Development Handbook: ADME and Biopharmaceutical Properties,
edited by Shayne Cox Gad

mass balance study can elucidate excretory pathways, organ distribution of parent drug and metabolites, and metabolic profiles. Moreover, a preclinical mass balance study can set the stage for its clinical counterpart, the human mass balance study.

Possible Objectives of a Preclinical Mass Balance Study

- Identify the excretory pathways of a drug (in general, urine and feces).
- Assess extent and kinetics of metabolism. Is the compound rapidly metabolized and how fast are the produced metabolites eliminated?
- Assess extent and kinetics of excretion. Is all radioactivity eventually excreted, and how long must excreta be collected?
- Elucidate the metabolic fate of a drug. How many metabolites can be observed and/or identified, and how much of the radioactivity do they account for?
- Assess organ distribution. Does (ir)reversible tissue binding occur, explaining incomplete recovery of radioactivity in excreta? Are there specific organs displaying accumulation?
- Provide information to optimally perform the human mass balance study. Is the choice of the isotope and its position in the molecule correct? Generate metabolite reference compounds and predict the radiation exposure of participants in the human mass balance study.

In general, a "mass balance study" is exactly what the term implies. This study involves the "balancing" of quantities of "mass." The "mass" that leaves the system (parent drug and metabolites excreted by various routes like urine and feces) is "balanced" against the known "mass" that was entered into the system (an amount of parent drug administered to the organism). Since most drugs undergo metabolic conversion before being excreted, a radioisotopically labeled variant of the compound is commonly administered to facilitate the quantitation of the sum of parent drug and metabolites in a variety of biological matrices. We propose the following definition for a mass balance study: "A pharmacokinetic study, aimed at characterizing the metabolic and excretory fate of a compound by collecting and analyzing excreta after administration of the compound, employing an analytical technique that allows tracing and quantitation of the compound and its products in spite of metabolic conversion."

Mass balance studies in their simplest form (as often performed in humans) are usually limited to just this particular balance, the amount that is recovered in excreta after an extended collection period, relative to the amount originally administered. However, contrary to a human mass balance study, a preclinical mass balance study allows the calculation of this mass balance at any given time by quantitating radioactivity present in various organs as well as in excreta. Thus, a preclinical mass balance study can provide information about the whereabouts of drug and metabolites inside and outside the organism at any time. This is the unique trait of the preclinical mass balance.

The relevance of the preclinical mass balance study is not limited to only preparing for the human mass balance study. It provides crucial information for the toxicokinetic evaluation of a compound. Toxicokinetic studies are aimed at integrating pharmacokinetics/metabolism and toxicity in nonclinical safety studies. Good agreement of the pharmacokinetics and metabolism of a drug in a specific animal species and humans increases the validity of the safety studies in this species for clinical safety issues [1–4]. Therefore, when there is close agreement between a specific animal species and humans with regard to excretory pathways and metabolic profile (characteristics that are best investigated by the mass balance study), this species is likely to be a better model for safety studies of the respective drug. The importance of metabolites and interspecies comparison is reflected by the recent distribution of a draft guidance for industry by the Center for Drug Evaluation and Research entitled *Safety Testing of Drug Metabolites* [5], which states the following. "Based on data obtained from *in vivo* and *in vitro* metabolism studies, when the metabolic profile of a parent drug is similar qualitatively and quantitatively across species, we can generally assume that potential clinical risks of the parent drug and its metabolites have been adequately characterized during standard non-clinical safety evaluations" [5]. Identification and pharmacologic characterization of individual metabolites is key in comparing results of preclinical studies with those of human studies [4].

The mass balance study is a unique and complicated study. It generally involves the use of radioisotopes and analysis of radioactivity, parent compound, and metabolites in a variety of matrices. As will be shown, a wealth of information can be gained from a mass balance. Fully exploiting a preclinical mass balance study requires careful design and the use of many techniques. In this chapter, the design of preclinical mass balance studies is addressed. The methodologies and expertise required for the conduct of these studies are provided, and we propose ways to express the results. Examples of the usefulness of mass balance studies in drug development are given and used to illustrate the importance of understanding the data obtained from mass balance studies.

33.2   DEFINITIONS

Mass Balance Study. A pharmacokinetic study, aimed at characterizing the metabolic and excretory fate of a compound by collecting and analyzing excreta after administration of the compound, employing an analytical technique that allows tracing and quantitation of the compound and its products in spite of metabolic conversion.

Total Radioactivity. The radioactivity content of a matrix, which consists of the sum of the parent drug and its metabolites that still contain the radioactive label.

Metabolite. Any compound being produced from the handling of a parent compound in the body.

Radioisotope. An isotope of an element capable of spontaneously emitting energetic particles by the disintegration of its atomic nuclei.

Tracer. The added (radioisotopical) portion of a compound used to follow the course of the metabolic process of that compound.

Specific Activity. A measure of the radioactivity per unit mass of a compound.

Autoradiolysis. Radiolysis of a radioactive material resulting directly or indirectly from its radioactive decay.

33.3 STUDY DESIGN

33.3.1 Timing of a Mass Balance Study

Performing a mass balance study with one or more animal species can be a costly and time-consuming investment. Hence, there needs to be evidence of activity at specified doses and dose schedules, initial toxicity studies must be satisfactory, and pharmacokinetics of unchanged drug should have been established. As will be argued, rational planning of a mass balance study requires knowledge of *in vitro* metabolic profiles of the compound in the species being used in preclinical safety studies and considered for the mass balance study. This will yield the most relevant information for clinical trials. Metabolic studies in animals may be performed in the late phase of the lead optimization [6]. However, even if the compound has already entered clinical trials, a preclinical mass balance can still be of use. If there are differences in (side) effects between humans and animals, these discrepancies may be explained by the *in vivo* metabolic profiles of the species.

33.3.2 Guidelines

Role of a Preclinical Mass Balance Study in Complying with Guidelines for Drug Development   The U.S. FDA [7] and its European counterpart, EMEA [8], have a number of guidelines delineating information that is required to lead a compound through the drug development process. Although there is no guideline specifically for preclinical mass balance studies, a preclinical mass balance study can play a role in obtaining information crucial to drug development. The preclinical mass balance study provides a description of the metabolism of a drug and the contribution of metabolism to overall elimination. This information is crucial in the development of a drug [9]. In determining the maximum recommended starting dose (MRSD) for initial clinical trials from a human equivalent dose, as a default, the most sensitive animal species is used. However, based on differences in absorption, distribution, metabolism, and excretion between species, a different species may be selected, thus increasing the MRSD and reducing the time spent on initial clinical trials [10]. Furthermore, a mass balance study provides the information that is assessed by the (draft) guidance, *Safety Testing of Drug Metabolites* [5].

Performing a Mass Balance Study   In performing a preclinical mass balance study, a number of guidelines and regulations must be followed. As regulations may vary by country, one should refer to the locally applicable institutional guidelines, but these guidelines will generally cover: IACUC, an institutional review board (IRB), working with radioactivity in general and in combination with animals specifically. As always in working with radioactivity, contamination must be minimized by working on absorbents, using disposable tools, and performing sweep tests after every experiment. Surveys with detectors will not suffice because they are not sensitive enough to detect all radioisotopes (including those most commonly used—^{14}C and ^{3}H).

33.3.3 The Radioisotope and Its Position in the Molecule

The choice of radioisotope and its position in the molecule can have a major impact on chemical and metabolic stability and can thus determine the results of a mass balance study. Use of ^{14}C as the radioactive isotope is generally preferable to any other radioisotope. The labeled compound only serves its purpose if it behaves identically to the nonlabeled compound and if the radioisotope is not lost chemically by exchange or during metabolism. Prior knowledge of the metabolism of a compound (from microsomal incubation studies, known analogues, or *in silico* predictions) can assist in determining the optimal radioisotope and its position. Since ideally the same radiolabeled compound is used in both the preclinical and clinical mass balance studies, human metabolic data must be considered as well.

If the studied molecule is large and/or is expected to divide metabolically into two parts, dual labeling may be considered. By labeling one part of the molecule with ^{3}H and the other part with ^{14}C, both parts may be traced independently [11, 12]. Even triple labeling has been reported [13].

Isotopes Several different radioisotopes can be employed to trace the whereabouts of a drug and its metabolites. In choosing the isotope to be used, one should be aware of the type of decay, the decay half-life, and the energy of the emitted particle (see Table 33.1). The type of radiation that is easiest to handle is β^- radiation (electrons). Working with γ-emitters requires use of lead shielding, because the highly energetic γ-radiation easily penetrates solid matter and tissue. Contrary to γ-radiation, the surroundings of a β-source are easily shielded from radiation by a layer of plastic/Plexiglas, and the radiation of, for example, ^{14}C will only penetrate up to 50 cm of air [12]. In addition, detection of β-radiation is readily accomplished by liquid scintillation counting. If a radioisotope has a short half-life, care must be taken to minimize the time between drug preparation and usage in the study or the labeled drug will have degraded. The following formula can be used to calculate the percentage of radioisotope remaining after preparation of a radioisotopically labeled compound:

TABLE 33.1 Radioisotopes Employed in Preclinical Mass Balance Studies [12, 14]

Radioisotope	Type of Decay	Half-life	Energy (MeV)	Comments
^{3}H	$\beta-$	12.3 y	0.019	Easily lost, low energy
^{14}C	$\beta-$	5,730 y	0.156	Long half-life
^{32}P	$\beta-$	14.3 d	1.71	Correction for decay, complicated handling
^{35}S	$\beta-$	87.5 d	0.167	Correction for decay
^{36}Cl	$\beta-$	300,000 y	0.71	Long half-life
^{131}I	$\beta-$	8.0 d	0.80–2.16	Correction for decay
	γ		0.67, 0.77	

$$\% \text{ Remaining} = 100 \cdot \frac{A_t}{A_0} = 100 \cdot (2)^{-(t/t_{1/2})}$$

where A_0 is radioactivity at time $t = 0$, A_t is radioactivity at time t, and $t_{1/2}$ is decay half-life. In addition, quantitated radioactivity levels must be corrected for the time expired between administration and quantitation. The following formula can be used to calculate the activity at $t = 0$ from the radioactivity quantitated at time t:

$$A_0 = A_t \cdot (2)^{(t/t_{1/2})}$$

Given the atomic composition of drug molecules, the most commonly used radio-isotopes are ^{14}C (radiocarbon) and ^{3}H (tritium), although the use of other radioisotopes has been documented [12]. The radiation emitted by ^{14}C is about eightfold more energetic than that of ^{3}H (0.156 MeV versus 0.019 MeV). Thus, quantitation of ^{14}C is easier and suffers less from matrix effects [14]. Even so, the use of ^{3}H may be required when very small amounts of a compound need to be detected, since higher specific activities may be achieved with ^{3}H (29.1 Ci/milliatom) than with carbon (62.4 mCi/milliatom) [12].

Although positron emitters can have their use in investigating drug pharmacology, their generally very short half-life (<2 h) limits their use in mass balance studies [15].

On the rare occasion that a drug contains an element that occurs in the body only at trace levels, the use of a radioisotopically labeled compound may be avoided. For example, metal-containing compounds may be quantitated using element-specific techniques such as atomic absorption spectrometry (AAS), inductively coupled plasma atomic emission spectrometry (ICP-AES), or inductively coupled plasma mass spectrometry (ICP-MS) [16, 17], and fluoro compounds can be traced employing ^{19}F-NMR [18].

Although it would seem obvious that after labeling with the radioisotope the compound must have the same chemical formula, this is not always the case. Occasionally, the disposition of a compound is investigated by substituting with a foreign (radioactive) element [19]. This substitution results in a different compound, and consequently, the new compound likely displays different metabolic and dispositional characteristics.

Chemical Stability   A major disadvantage of using ^{3}H, despite the ease and low costs, is its tendency to be exchanged with hydrogen in aqueous matrices, producing nonlabeled compound and tritiated water. Especially if ^{3}H bonded to heteroatoms or α-positioned relative to a double bonded heteroatom, it is likely to be exchanged [20, 21]. A ^{14}C atom is not likely to be chemically exchanged.

Metabolic Stability   The use of a compound labeled at a chemically stable position does not guarantee that the detected radioactivity adequately represents its metabolism and disposition. The position needs to be metabolically stable as well. For example, positioning a radioisotope in an N-methyl moiety or the side chain part of an ester [22] (although easy to synthesize) will not result in a useful compound to trace metabolites. The radioisotope would quickly be lost by oxidative dealkylation and hydrolysis, respectively [23]. The isotope needs to be positioned in a relatively central part of the compound to enable tracing of its primary metabolites. It is therefore not surprising that the radioisotope is preferentially positioned in an aromatic or alicyclic ring system. Computer-assisted metabolism prediction (CAMP) is available to predict the metabolic stability by means of databases of known metabolic transformations. The suitability of a label may be predicted by *in vitro* (liver microsomal incubation or hepatocytes) testing of the compound [24] or by reviewing the metabolism of analogues. For example, a review of the literature on the metabolism of pyrimidine antimetabolites shows the metabolic loss of the 2-carbon as carbon dioxide, while the 6-carbon is quite stable [25]. Thus, when deciding on the position of the ^{14}C in an investigational pyrimidine compound, the 6-position is preferred over the 2-position.

Kinetic Isotope Effect   Although a radioisotope is in many regards equal to its stable-isotope counterpart, chemically it may still behave slightly differently. Heavier isotopes will form stronger chemical bonds, and thus reaction kinetics (like metabolic conversion) will be affected. This is called the *kinetic isotope effect* [21]. Thus, the radioisotopically labeled compound may well undergo a different metabolism and display a different disposition from the nonlabeled compound. The replacement of hydrogen (^{1}H) with tritium (^{3}H) is a tripling in mass, while the substitution of a carbon atom (^{12}C) with radiocarbon (^{14}C) is only a 17% increase. Therefore, the use of tritiated compounds is more likely to yield results biased by the kinetic isotope effect [21]. However, the kinetic isotope effect is relevant only if the rate-limiting step in the overall metabolic conversion is affected. Generally, cleavage of the carbon–hydrogen bond is the rate-limiting step in the oxidation of aliphatic hydrocarbons. Whether or not this is the case for an aromatic carbon–hydrogen bond depends on the substitution pattern [26]. An example illustrating the kinetic isotope effect is the reduced formation of the genotoxic α-hydroxy metabolite of tamoxifen in rats after exchange of hydrogen for deuterium [27].

33.3.4   Animals

Nonclinical safety testing is usually performed in rats and mice, and a nonrodent mammal [28, 29]. The default rule for starting a first-in-human-study is two mammals, one of which is nonrodent. When dealing with biologicals, species selection will be linked to the presumed mechanism of action and the presence of the target in the available species. In the literature, preclinical mass balance studies are often reported in a rodent species, in dog, and in a primate. However, the choice of species must be a conscious one. Every animal has its own characteristics that influence the metabolic fate of a drug, and the costs and ease of performing the study. Even within species, different strains may have different properties. Inbred strains are the result of several generations of brother × sister mating. Consequently, inbred animals are homozygous at almost all loci, except sex. The genetic homogeneity of present and future generations ensures homogeneity in phenotype and thus more consistent experimental results. Conversely, outbred animals display a more variable genotype and phenotypic behavior.

Metabolic Differences   Ideally, the animal species to use for the preclinical mass balance study is the one showing the highest degree of *in vitro* metabolic concordance with humans. Early identification of human metabolic routes of elimination and metabolites by *in vitro* studies can provide a clear direction for preclinical studies in animals [30, 31]. *In vitro* incubations of the drug with liver slices, hepatocytes, and microsomal and nonmicrosomal fractions can provide useful information to assess this metabolic concordance. It should be noted that these *in vitro* incubations are unable to capture all aspects of the *in vivo* metabolism. First, gastrointestinal, kidney, and lung metabolism and biliary excretion are not assessed in these experiments. Second, phase II metabolism does not necessarily occur in microsomes without addition of the various conjugating moieties, and liver slices have limited enzymatic stability [30].

Obviously, known interspecies differences in metabolism should be taken into account. If the drug has an aromatic amine moiety, it is likely a substrate for *N*-acetyltransferase. Since dogs lack this enzyme [31], to perform a mass balance study with this drug in dogs is not expected to yield information that is relevant to human metabolism, disposition, and safety of this drug. Table 33.2 lists some reported metabolic differences of animal species relative to humans. In addition to drug-metabolizing enzymes being either present or absent in different species, the organ distribution can also vary widely [32]. With the advent of genetically altered animal strains, some of these differences can be diminished, if not eliminated. For example, esterase activity in rodents greatly exceeds esterase activity in humans. Currently, plasma-esterase-deficient mice have become available, providing a better metabolic model for compounds that are a likely substrate for esterases [33, 34].

Animal Size   Animal size has many implications for the mass balance study. A large animal allows repeated blood sampling. It also produces more, more frequent, but likely less concentrated urine that can enable metabolite profiling. On the other hand, large animals are more costly to buy and to keep, are less easily handled,

TABLE 33.2   Some Metabolic Differences of Animal Species Relative to Humans

Species	Enzyme	Effect	Substrates	References
Mouse	Carbonyl reductase	Low activity	Anthracyclines	31
	Carboxylesterase	High activity	Esters, lactones	34
	Deoxycytidine kinase	Low activity (10-fold)	Cytidine analogues	87
Rat	Amidase	High activity	Amides	88
	Carboxylesterase	High activity	Esters, lactones	22, 34
	CYP2C8	Substrate mismatch	Paclitaxel	31
	Cytidine deaminase	Absent	Cytidine analogues	32
	N-acetyltransferase	High activity	Aromatic amines	31
Dog	Cytidine deaminase	Low	Cytidine analogues	89
	N-acetyltransferase	Absent	Aromatic amines	31
All	Microsomal epoxide hydroxylase	Low	Epoxides	90
	UGTs	Negligible	Various, SN38, AZT	31

and require a larger amount of the (radioisotopically labeled) investigational compound.

Age   In general, young but mature adult animals are used for pharmacokinetic studies. Many enzyme activity levels are age dependent. In immature animals, enzyme activity may not have fully developed yet. In older animals, activity of some enzymes may be declining while others may increase. In addition, body composition changes, with an increasing fat percentage over time [35–37]. Most importantly, the results must be comparable with preclinical safety studies, and the age of the animals used in those studies can be used as a guideline.

Sex   Sex can be an important determinant of pharmacokinetic and metabolic parameters in animals [38–42]. Sex-dependent differences may be predicted by *in vitro* studies [43]. However, sex-dependent metabolic differences in humans are less dramatic, even though they may be present [44]. Therefore, the sex of the animals to be used may be determined by the methodology of the preceding safety studies.

Sample Size   The sample size of the study is dependent on the information that needs to be obtained, and it obviously influences costs and logistics. If only an excretory mass balance study is needed, it will suffice to use few animals (three or four should be a minimum), and to collect excreta for a specified time (e.g., until an acceptable portion of the dose has been recovered). However, if the plasma metabolic profile of the compound is to be investigated, serial sampling is required, which is often destructive in smaller animals. A minimum of three or four animals should be used per time point to allow determination of a standard deviation. The number of time points is dependent on whether the investigation of the metabolic profile is more qualitative in nature, or the complete plasma profile of the drug, total radioactivity, and/or metabolites need to be determined. Usually, larger animals are studied in a smaller sample size for both cost and ethical reasons.

Genetically Modified Species   As mentioned earlier with regard to esterase-deficient mice, it is possible to use genetically modified strains of a species in order to better mimic the human metabolic system. However, there is another application for genetically modified strains. Various gene-knockout (KO) and gene-knockin (KI) models have been developed for the mouse, to illustrate the *in vivo* function of a variety of enzymes/efflux pumps, for example, the CYP3A4-KI [45], *mdr1a*(–/–) [46], *mdr1a/b*(–/–) [6, 47], *ABCG2*(–/–) [48], and *SLC22A1*(–/–) [49]. When a mass balance of an IND is performed in these genetically altered strains and their wild-type counterparts, basic information can be obtained pertaining to the excretory function of the efflux pumps. In addition, quantitation of unchanged drug or radioactivity in the organs (especially those known to express efflux pumps like brain, testis, and heart) [47, 50–53] of these animals shows the relevance of efflux pumps to organ disposition. These data can predict possible interactions with other drugs competing for or blocking the efflux pumps. To diminish interspecies differences in substrate specificity of CYP450 enzymes, mice with humanized enzymes are under development [54, 55].

33.3.5   Dosing

Pharmacological Dose   Assuming that the compound and its radioisotopically labeled counterpart behave identically, the pharmacological dose consists of the sum of unlabeled and labeled compound. Usually, the contribution of the radioactive part is negligible relative to the unlabeled amount of drug, hence the use of the term "tracer." However, to obtain a sufficient specific activity (Bq/mg) of a potent (dosed in low amounts), high molecular weight drug, a large fraction of the molecules (e.g., 80% [56]) will actually have to be labeled. To be relevant, the pharmacological dose should be comparable to pharmacological or toxicological relevant doses as established in safety studies. Even if linear pharmacokinetics of the parent compound has been shown, the metabolic disposition may be nonlinear. Therefore, the pharmacological dose should not deviate too much from previously established doses.

Radioactive Dose   The radioactive dose to be used depends on the specific objectives of the study and the sensitivity of the analytical methods. If the objective is to describe plasma and tissue profiles of the parent drug and metabolites (e.g., by HPLC with radioactivity detection), a higher radioactive dose may be required than for merely describing the excretory fate of a drug. The amount of radioactivity required is also dependent on the pharmacokinetic characteristics of the compound.

A literature search for mass balance studies with chemically related compounds and previous pharmacokinetic studies with the compound under investigation can give an impression of what results may be obtained with a certain dose. Next, a pilot study will provide valuable samples to test an analytical method and to assess the adequacy of the radioactive dose.

The radioactive dose is usually expressed in curies (Ci), as opposed to the SI unit of becquerel (Bq). The conversion of these units is $1\,mCi = 37\,MBq$ and $1\,Bq = 60\,DPM$, where DPM means disintegrations per minute. Typical radioactive doses (^{14}C) are approximately $1–2\,\mu Ci$/mouse, $5–20\,\mu Ci$/rat, $5–100\,\mu Ci$/dog, and $40–120\,\mu Ci$/monkey, compared to $100\,\mu Ci$/human. Recently, the use of accelerator mass spectrometry (AMS) was described in a mass balance study in dogs, requiring only $45\,nCi$ of radioactivity [57]. AMS has received attention for its potential use in microdosing humans [58]. Given the complexity of the technique, its use in preclinical mass balance studies will likely be limited.

Dosing Schedule   Most mass balance studies are performed as a single-dose study. However, when single-dose tissue distribution studies suggest that the apparent half-life of the test compound (and/or metabolites) in organs or tissues significantly exceeds the apparent half-life of the elimination phase in plasma and is also more than twice the dosing interval in the toxicity studies, repeated-dose tissue distribution studies may be appropriate [4, 59].

Route of Administration   For the mass balance study to be relevant to clinical practice, the route of administration should mimic the anticipated clinical route of administration as much as possible. For comparative and/or scientific purposes, different routes of administration can be studied as well.

33.4 METHODOLOGY

33.4.1 Dose Administration

Preparation   Parenteral dosing solutions should be prepared under aseptic conditions. Because radioisotopically labeled compounds may not be available as a sterile product, one should be aware of possible bacterial contamination of the dosing solution. Aseptic filtration may be used, but loss of compound by adsorption to the filter unit must be assessed. The dosing solution should be prepared in excess to enable qualitative and quantitative analysis after completion of the study.

Administration   The dose should be administered according to established practice. There are guidelines for maximum volumes that may be administered to animals, which should be followed. Oral administration is usually performed after an overnight fast to assure rapid and reproducible gastrointestinal transit. When dosing multiple groups of animals, stratifying all the animals according to body weight and using one mouse of every stratum per group may achieve a homogeneous weight distribution.

When an infusion device is used, this must be flushed after administration to account for any radioactivity that may have remained in the lines. An organic solvent like methanol may be best suited for this. The amount of radioactivity recovered from the flushing solvent must be subtracted from the calculated dose administered to obtain the actual administered dose [25].

Quality Control   Preclinical studies are usually conducted with a nonstandardized formulation of the compound, if it is formulated at all. This is especially true for a mass balance study, because the isotopically labeled compound is often custom synthesized in one batch [60]. In addition, the dose consists of both the isotopically labeled part and the nonlabeled part.

First, for both nonlabeled drug and tracer, the content needs to be determined. This is essential to assure that a relevant pharmacological dose was administered, and to calculate eventually the recovery of the dose in the excreta. In case of a known, established specific activity, the dose of drug can be determined by taking an aliquot for scintillation counting. Using the specific activity of the compound (Bq/g), one can convert the radioactive content to total drug content.

Second, the purity of the dose needs to be established. Given the incidental production of most radioisotopically labeled compounds, it is likely that the purity is not as high as with standard reference compounds and may even be lower than the declaration of the manufacturer [21]. In addition, the radioisotopically labeled compound is likely to be less stable than the nonlabeled compound. Due to the inherent radioactive nature of the compound, energy is released, producing free radicals, which may increase degradation of the compound, a process called *autoradiolysis*. In solution, ethanol, serum albumin, and ascorbic acid have been reported to slow down autoradiolysis [61–63]. In the literature, the purity of the compound used is often not reported. Yet a purity of at least 95% is essential to perform a mass balance study. Impurities can have different pharmacokinetic characteristics and may be toxic. The radiochromatographic system used for metabolic profiling may be employed as a stability-indicating assay for the compound and, afterwards, the dosing solution. In general (with compounds containing a chromophore), HPLC with UV absorbance or photodiode array UV detection will be able to assess the overall purity of both labeled and nonlabeled compound together.

33.4.2 Sample Collection and Analysis

A mass balance study can consist of merely collecting the excreta after administration of a radiolabeled drug. These studies do not characterize the metabolism, distribution, or disposition of the compound within the body. However, much more information can be obtained from a mass balance study by sampling various matrices in time, as is discussed later.

In general, no stability data are available for the compound and its metabolites in the different matrices (and organs may contain drug-metabolizing enzymes). Consequently, immediate storage at −20 °C or less is advisable, in order to prevent degradation products to be mistakenly identified as metabolites.

Schedule In order to reliably estimate pharmacokinetic parameters, sampling should be adequately planned. In the case of intravenous administration, an early plasma sample is imperative to determine the area under the plasma concentration versus time curve. Thereafter, sampling must be frequent enough to separately characterize the distribution and the elimination phases. The elimination phase is ideally sampled for at least 4 half-lives. In the case of orally administered drugs, frequent plasma sampling should be performed around the expected time of maximum plasma concentration. Sometimes there is no data available to help schedule the sampling. A pilot study in a couple of animals may then be performed to get a rough estimate of the plasma concentration versus time profile, which can also serve to set the required concentration range of the analytical method.

Ideally, excreta are collected until all radioactivity administered has been recovered. However, 100% recovery will usually not be achieved [25]. Under the assumption of instantaneous excretion, 93% of radioactivity will have been excreted after four terminal radioactivity plasma half-lives. Unfortunately, the elimination half-life of radioactivity from plasma is usually not known. Another reported approach uses radioactivity levels in urine and feces for drug and radioactivity [25]. When less than 1% of administered radioactivity is excreted for 2 consecutive days, collection can be stopped. Prolonged collection will not substantially increase recovery. Small animals may be housed together to collect pooled excreta.

Urine Urine is a liquid matrix; it is easily mixed, aliquoted, and quantitatively analyzed. Urine can be collected separately from feces with a metabolic cage (Fig. 33.1). Because urine is often used for qualitative analysis, it needs to be collected on ice in order to halt any degradation processes. To calculate the total excretion of a compound and its metabolites, the volume of urine excreted in the collection period must be accurately established. This can be accomplished by determining the volume with a graduated cylinder or by weighing, but the latter only if the relative density of the urine is near 1. At the end of the collection period, the collection part of the metabolic cage should be washed with a solvent to remove any adsorbed radioactivity from the device. The solvent used for this wash step must be chosen

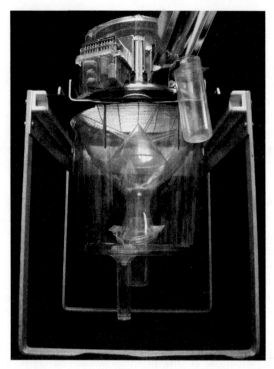

FIGURE 33.1 Metabolic cage for the separate collection of urine (lower left collection cone) and feces (middle collection cone) of rodents.

such that the compound is expected to dissolve easily. The radioactivity found in this wash fluid should be calculated by multiplying the volume of wash solvent that was used (not the volume that was collected) with the concentration of radioactivity. If the investigated compound is known, or suspected, to adsorb to container surfaces, addition of an organic solvent or bovine serum albumin may be considered before subsequent aliquoting and processing.

Feces Feces are collected separately from urine with metabolic cages. They are weighed and then homogenized with a homogenization device to obtain a pipettable, homogeneous matrix. Disposable homogenizer probes are available and may be preferable when processing radioactive samples. Depending on the eventual use of the homogenate (extraction of individual metabolites) and the properties of the compound and its metabolites (solubility, adsorption to container surfaces), homogenization may be done with water, buffer, or bovine serum albumin solution. In general, adsorption to container surfaces will not be an issue with fecal homogenate because the fecal particles will have a high surface area relative to the container surface area. The ratio with which feces are homogenized (varying from 2:1 to 10:1, v/w) will affect pipettability and sensitivity of subsequent analyses. A more dilute homogenate will result in a truly pipettable matrix, with proportionally reduced concentrations of the analytes. More concentrated homogenates may be pipettable, but not accurately so. When determining the radioactivity content, aliquots of homogenate should be weighed. Because feces is a dark-colored matrix, decoloration prior to liquid scintillation counting may be warranted.

Bile   Occasionally, bile is collected to assess the biliary excretion of radioactivity and analytes. Because reabsorption of bile salts is essential for normal bile production (both quantitatively and qualitatively), bile may not be sampled over extended periods of time, that is, longer than 1–2 hours [64, 65]. An elegant but intricate way to deal with this issue is to replenish with blank bile from undosed animals while sampling the bile from the treated animal. Similarly, the contribution of enterohepatic recirculation may be assessed [66].

Blood and Red Blood Cells   Blood must be collected from a site distant from that of administration. This is done to prevent residual dosing solution at the administration site from biasing the concentration of the drawn sample. Next, one can determine total radioactivity in either whole blood or in red blood cells (RBCs) after centrifugation and aspiration of plasma. In combination with plasma radioactivity levels, this allows calculation of the blood/plasma ratio or the RBCs/plasma ratio, respectively. These parameters can be interconverted, but such a conversion requires information about the hematocrit [67].

Because red blood cells and blood can be somewhat viscous, an aliquot should be accurately weighted in a sample vial. Liquid scintillation counting of blood or red blood cells is often difficult due to the intense red color, which necessitates decoloration before liquid scintillation counting. A suitable protocol may be: weighting approximately 150 mg of the red blood cell pellet into a 20 mL scintillation vial; adding 500 μL of tissue solubilizer and 500 μL of water, followed by vortexing and incubating for 10 min at 50 °C; adding 100 μL of 0.1 M EDTA and 200 μL of 30% hydrogen peroxide, followed by vortexing of the sample and incubation at 50 °C for 10 min; finally, 20 mL of scintillation fluid may be added prior to scintillation counting.

Plasma   Plasma can be aspirated after centrifugation of blood. Because it is a relatively colorless matrix, liquid scintillation counting is straightforward. It consists of mixing an aliquot with liquid scintillation fluid followed by counting.

Expired Air   For a number of positions of the radioactive ^{14}C label (e.g., 2-position of pyrimidines, N-methyl), the expiration of radioactivity as $^{14}CO_2$ is predictable [68]. However, it may not be possible to prevent expiration of radioactivity, especially when there is no information about the metabolic fate of a compound or any analogues. When mass balance is not achieved (i.e., a large part of the radioactive dose cannot be accounted for in the total of excreta, organs, and carcass), one must consider the possibility of loss through expiration as $^{14}CO_2$.

Expired air may be sampled by keeping the animals in an airtight chamber with continuous air replacement and leading the expired air through a basic solution, thus precipitating the $^{14}CO_2$ as the nonvolatile carbonate. A sodium hydroxide [12] or 2-methoxyethanol-ethanolamine (2:1) solution [69] can be used to capture the carbon dioxide. Before air is pumped into the chamber it may need to be led through a similar basic solution to eliminate any natural $^{14}CO_2$, thereby reducing the background radioactivity counts. Eventually, the precipitated carbonate is counted for its radioactive content.

Organs A preclinical mass balance study employing a radioisotopically labeled drug is usually conducted when the time course, persistence, and potential accumulation of the drug and/or its metabolites in various parts of the animal body needs to be assessed [4].

After dissection, organs should be weighed and frozen as soon as possible. To obtain a pipettable homogeneous matrix for further analysis, homogenization may be required. If no other measurements than total radioactivity determination are intended, direct tissue solubilization may be considered as a faster and easier sample processing method (see below).

A pipettable organ homogenate may be obtained by homogenizing the organ with 3 parts (v/w) of phosphate-buffered saline pH 7.4, water, or 4% bovine serum albumin. The choice of solvent may be dependent on solubility, stability, and adsorption characteristics of the compound under investigation. In addition, the solvent used may interfere with subsequent analytical or pharmacodynamic assays. A fixed ratio of liquid to organ weight is preferable to a fixed volume per organ because the former will assure identical concentrations of organ constituents like proteins, which may be relevant to solubility, stability, and adsorption.

If organ radioactivity concentrations are to be assessed, it is imperative to sample and homogenize the whole organ, and not to sample parts (of different lobes) of the organ. For example, analyte concentrations are reported to vary significantly within a lobe (52-fold) or between lobes of a single liver (25-fold), likely due to differences in regional structure and blood and lymph flows [70]. On the other hand, it may be necessary to determine intratissue distribution of radioactivity. For example, distribution of radioactivity of an anticancer drug to the viable part of a tumor is relevant, but this information will be lost during homogenization [71]. Tissue autoradiography may be employed to identify such a phenomenon.

The organs of the GI tract can be homogenized after removal of the content or as a whole. By removing the content followed by separate analysis, any radioactivity can be more exactly ascribed to GI content (unabsorbed or excreted radioactivity) and organ radioactivity, respectively. This may be especially relevant with orally administered compounds.

Carcass Oftentimes, the radioactivity in excreta does not account for the complete radioactive dose. A compound or its metabolites may exhibit a long half-life or may irreversibly bind to tissue components, or the radioisotope may get incorporated into endogenous compounds. Therefore, it may be required to assess the amount of residual radioactivity in the carcass. Individual organs are easily homogenized or digested and consequently analyzed for radioactivity. The carcass, however, is less easily processed. It contains remaining organs, muscle, connective tissue, and, most importantly, bone, skin, and fur. In order to achieve a homogenate with a high degree of homogeneity, the carcass (with an appropriate liquid phase) is first processed using a blender. Due to the high collagen content, a higher solvent volume to carcass weight ratio (from 4:1) may have to be used for homogenization to prevent coalescing of the homogenate. Next, a tissue solubilizer or a concentrated sodium hydroxide solution may be used to dissolve the tissues as much as possible (allowing it to stand for several days or applying heating). The latter should be done in closed containers to avoid evaporation of solvents prior to taking an aliquot for scintillation counting.

Digestion, Decoloration, and Oxidation of Samples   A number of problems may be encountered in the processing of samples for radioactivity counting. Homogenization is not suitable for all organs (e.g., bone, skin) and is labor intensive, yet it is less destructive (e.g., determination of proteins, DNA, or individual compounds remains a possibility). Digestion of organs (or homogenate aliquots) with a tissue solubilizer is easy and fast, reduces the color of the sample, but is totally destructive. Lastly, oxidation of samples is destructive and labor intensive, but may be essential for processing nonhomogenizable matrices or determination of ^3H in the presence of ^{14}C.

Digestion of organs or homogenate aliquots can be performed with so-called tissue solubilizers. Although destructive, this methodology can save a lot of time and effort because it may not be necessary to homogenize the sample beforehand. However, too much of these reagents may adversely affect the scintillation counting process, so that care must be taken to minimize the amount required. Manufacturers of these reagents can provide data on amounts required and the effects on the scintillation counting process.

Usually, the color interfering with scintillation counting is caused by iron-containing components of the sample like hemes. Treatment of the sample (homogenate or digested organ) with peroxide is the common method to reduce the color intensity. A suggested method would be taking a 100 µL aliquot of homogenate (3:1, v/w in water), adding 100 µL of 0.1 M EDTA (chelating metal ions, reducing excessive foaming of the hydrogen peroxide), followed by 200 µL of ~30% hydrogen peroxide. Incubation for 10 min at 50 °C will speed up the decoloration reaction. Next, 5–20 mL of liquid scintillation fluid may be added before counting. Variations of peroxides have been described, such as treatment with solubilizer followed by 0.4 mL of benzene saturated with benzoyl peroxide, or bleaching with glacial acetic acid and hydrogen peroxide [72, 73].

A sample oxidizer consists of a coiled platinum wire that can hold the sample. Additives may be applied to optimize the oxidation process. Subsequently, under a continuous oxygen flow, the sample is oxidized by heating the platinum wire using an electric current, and converting the carbon content to carbon dioxide and the hydrogen content to water, leaving nonvolatile components as ashes. The carbon dioxide containing the $^{14}CO_2$ and the water containing the ^3H_2O are trapped separately on adsorption columns and eluted into separate counting vials. Transfer efficiencies of over 95% are usually achieved with this technique. Especially in the case of double labeling of a compound with possible false-positive counts of ^{14}C in the ^3H counts, this technique is very suitable. Before bone is oxidized, it may be pulverized first to increase the surface area available for the oxidation process.

Irrespective of the eventual method used for sample processing, it is essential to determine the end efficiency of the procedure. Adding a known amount of radioactivity to a sample, processing it, and determining the liquid scintillation count easily achieves this. One should also prepare an identical sample without the organ component to establish the influence of the reagents used on the counting process. This may identify the need to use less of the reagents and instead increase the duration of heating the sample. An overall efficiency/accuracy of at least 90% should be aimed for.

Liquid Scintillation Counting For the determination of total radioactivity in samples (the composite of parent drug and metabolites still containing the radioactive label), liquid scintillation counting is often employed [12]. The sample is processed in such a way that it is in a liquid form. An aliquot is mixed with liquid scintillation fluid, a mixture of compounds that are excited by β-radiation and convert the absorbed energy to multiple light pulses. The sample is analyzed by a liquid scintillation counter that converts the light pulses into a number of observed counts per minute (CPM). Because not all the disintegrating nuclei result in a count, the CPM need to be converted to the real number of disintegrations per minute (DPM). The ratio of CPM to DPM is the counting efficiency, which is higher for isotopes with more energetic radiation ($^{32}P > {}^{14}C > {}^{3}H$). Most liquid scintillation counters will be able to determine the counting efficiency of a sample and thus correct the measured count to the actual count. This correction is usually performed by either of two ways. The first is the external standard calibration. A radioactive (γ-) source is placed next to the sample, causing a known amount of additional excitation in the sample. The ratio of the actual counts to the expected counts is a measure of the counting efficiency. The second method is the internal standard calibration. With decreasing efficiency, the signal intensity versus energy distribution shifts to lower energies. Using a prerecorded quench curve, the counting efficiency can be determined from this shift. To maximize the counting efficiency, a sufficiently high scintillation fluid-to-sample ratio must be used (ideally more than 5:1). In addition, the mixture of sample and scintillation fluid must be one homogeneous phase. There are a variety of liquid scintillation fluids available that are suitable for organic, aqueous, and high salt content samples, respectively. Sometimes, especially when the sample is colored, counting efficiency drops, and the correction becomes flawed. This color quenching occurs, in particular, with red samples (blood, liver, kidney, etc.). A suitable sample preparation step involving digestion and decoloration may resolve this problem. Heating of the sample or exposure to sunlight may excite the scintillants (luminescence) and result in an erroneously high count. This can be avoided by letting the samples stand overnight in the dark before counting. The error in the radioactive count is inversely related to the root of the count and the counting time. Increasing the counting time will therefore result in more precise measurements, especially with lower concentrations of radioactivity. In general, a counting time of 5–10 min will suffice. When a double label is used (e.g., labeling a compound simultaneously with both ^{14}C and ^{3}H), the signal of one isotope can cross talk into the signal of the other isotope. The ^{3}H signal will also pick up part of the ^{14}C signal. Adjusting the settings of the liquid scintillation counter and using corrections may yield the separate counts for both isotopes.

33.4.3 Metabolic Profiling

The overview of the metabolism of a drug is often called the *metabolic profile* [25]. Recently, the FDA posted a draft guidance describing the need for safety testing of metabolites representing more than 10% of systemic exposure human [5]. Thus, early preclinical identification of metabolites of potential relevance to humans is key. A mass balance study is well suited to elucidate the metabolic profile of a compound because it employs a radioisotopically labeled compound, enabling detection of the parent drug and its metabolites even if the latter are structurally still unknown. After structural elucidation, metabolites may be tested for their pharmacological and toxicological properties. This is important in drug development because the concentrations of the parent drug and/or its active metabolites may provide an important link between drug exposure and desirable and/or undesirable drug effects. For this reason, the development of sensitive and specific assays for a drug and its key metabolites is critical to the study of metabolism and drug–drug interactions [9]. Next, a discussion is provided of the various matrices, sample pretreatment, chromatographic separation, and detection.

Matrix Selection Ideally, metabolites are identified and quantified in plasma, urine, and feces. A matrix is especially interesting when a large proportion of the radioactivity is not explained by unchanged drug (this proportion consists of metabolites). This requires knowledge of the level of the total radioactivity and the unchanged drug in the matrix. Because the metabolites excreted in one matrix may be qualitatively different from those in another matrix, preferably, metabolic profiling is executed in all of these matrices. In addition, metabolites in a target organ (for activity or toxicity) may be relevant. However, quantification of metabolites can be complicated. Plasma may not be available in sufficient amounts to allow analysis of metabolites after analysis of total radioactivity and unchanged drug, especially when it concerns a small animal. Pooling of samples from individual animals may then be considered. It can be difficult to isolate compounds from feces, impeding metabolic profiling. Urine is a concentrated matrix that is suitable and most commonly used for metabolic profiling.

Sample Pretreatment Conventionally, sample pretreatment is aimed at selective extraction and concentration of one or more specific analytes. However, for metabolic profiling one needs to concentrate all metabolites with their heterogeneous physicochemical characteristics, while reducing matrix-derived interference. Consequently, sample pretreatment for metabolic profiling is usually nonspecific and consists of (1) addition of a water-miscible organic solvent, (2) centrifugation to precipitate salts, proteins, and insoluble matter, (3) concentration or evaporation of the supernatant, and (4) reconstitution in a suitable solvent. The efficiency of each of these steps can be monitored and optimized using radioactivity determinations [74]. Radioactivity lost during evaporation may be explained by volatile metabolites or tritiated water.

Chromatographic Separation The high resolution of high performance liquid chromatography (HPLC) makes it the method of choice over other chromatographic methods such as thin layer chromatography. By applying a shallow gradient elution (e.g., C18 column, 5–90% ACN linear, in 60 min), metabolites of a large polarity range can be separated. The use of a guard column can protect the column from high concentrations of matrix-derived constituents [12]. When subsequent mass spectrometric analysis is considered, mobile phase components should be chosen that are compatible with mass spectrometry (i.e., they should allow adequate ionization of the compounds and must be volatile). In reverse phase chromatography, the parent compound (often less polar than its metabolites) elutes last. The gradient can be designed so that the parent compound elutes at the end of the chromatographic run. An initial run time of 60 min may be necessary to separate all the metabolites, but this may be shortened when the elution times of the metabolites are known and the assay is used more routinely [25].

Detection Techniques   The compounds eluting from the HPLC system may be detected with various techniques, used in parallel or in series. Parallel detection techniques involve splitting the column effluent, thereby reducing sensitivity. However, some techniques are destructive in nature and thus cannot be employed in front of another technique. Because mass balance studies employ radioisotopically labeled compounds, radioactivity detection is the primary technique, unambiguously indicating the presence of metabolites at specific retention times. Ultraviolet absorption, preferably using a photodiode array, can be used to indicate changes in the chromophore. Mass spectrometry can be used to acquire additional structural information or to confirm the presence of a suspected metabolite. Finally, more complicated techniques like nuclear magnetic resonance (NMR) may be utilized, especially when investigating fluorinated compounds. Sometimes the radioactive samples may need to be diluted down to an acceptable level of radioactivity to permit their handling in different laboratory areas.

Radioactivity Detection   Radioactivity detection may be performed either online or offline. Online radioactivity detection is rapid but destructive. It consists of admixing a scintillation fluid with the column effluent (usually in a 3:1, v/v ratio), passing it through a detection cell (a coiled, transparent tube), and recording the counts in time. The mixing of the column effluent with the scintillation fluid excludes any further analytical characterization of the effluent. Furthermore, the online radioactivity counting decreases sensitivity. When employing a flow rate of 1 mL/min, a 3:1 (v/v) ratio of scintillation fluid and a 500 µL detection cell, the residence time of any component in the detection cell is only 7.5 seconds. The offline detection method is more laborious, consisting of fractionation of the column effluent (every 15–60 s). Fractions can be counted for radioactivity, for example, for 5 min each (increasing sensitivity 40-fold relative to offline detection). Offline detection can be performed nondestructively by taking only an aliquot of each fraction for scintillation counting, reserving the residual sample of fractions with high levels of radioactivity for subsequent structural identification. A drawback of the offline radioactivity detection is its labor-intensive nature, precluding rapid sequential sample analysis.

When a more energetic radioisotope is being used (e.g., ^{32}P), it may be possible to detect the radioactivity without using scintillation fluid, by using Çerenkov detection. This allows collection of unadulterated effluent after radioactivity detection [12].

Photodiode Array Detection   Absorption measurement using a photodiode array is a nondestructive detection technique. However, it is nonselective, necessitating comparison of the sample chromatogram with a blank. A shift in the spectrum relative to that of the parent compound indicates a metabolic modification of the chromophore. When applying a gradient elution, the change in mobile phase composition may also cause a shift of the spectrum.

Mass Spectrometry   More qualitative information may be derived from mass spectrometric analysis of selected fractions after offline profiling or after splitting the column effluent. Changes in the mass spectrum relative to the spectrum of the unchanged compound provide structural information. For example, a mass increase of +16 atomic mass units indicates hydroxylation, +42 atomic mass units indicates acetylation, −14 atomic mass units indicates demethylation, and so on. After tentative structural elucidation of a metabolite, the retention time and mass spectrum may be compared to that of a synthetic standard.

Nuclear Magnetic Resonance   If there is a fluorine atom present in the compound, ^{19}F-NMR may be applied to detect, quantitate, and characterize parent compound and metabolites. A large signal for the fluorine ion indicates that the compound is extensively dehalogenated, and those metabolites are thereafter undetectable by ^{19}F-NMR [18]. Although at present quantitation with ^{19}F-NMR is hampered by matrix-related effects [75], in the future, more powerful NMR equipment is expected to improve quantitative application, even as to enable *in vivo* monitoring of drug and metabolite distribution [76].

Additional Characterization   Besides chromatographic separation of a sample and detection of its metabolic constituents, there is more one can do with the samples. Collection of a particular fraction and repeated chromatographic separation may lead to isolation of a metabolite with sufficient purity to allow determination of the full mass spectrum, absorbance spectrum [77], NMR spectrum, and so on.

In addition, incubation with β-glucuronidase and sulfatase can indicate the presence of glucuronide and sulfate conjugates, respectively, of the parent compound or its phase I metabolites. A decrease in peak area indicates the presence of the conjugate, while an increase indicates the corresponding aglycone counterpart [78].

Finally, metabolites obtained from *in vitro* incubations of the compound of interest, that subsequently have been elucidated structurally, should be used as reference compounds.

33.5 RESULTS

There are a number of useful parameters that may be determined from a mass balance:

- Mass balance calculation
    Recovery in urine, feces, air, carcass, and total recovery
    Major excretory pathway
    Ratio of unchanged drug/radioactivity

- Plasma pharmacokinetics (unchanged drug and radioactivity)

  Half-life

  AUC and the unchanged/radioactivity ratio

  C_{max}, T_{max}
- Assessment of absorption

  Unchanged drug AUC_{PO}/AUC_{IV}, bioavailability

  Total radioactivity AUC_{PO}/AUC_{IV}, indication of fraction absorbed
- Organ distribution

  Percentage of radioactivity in organs in time/at end of study

  Drug and metabolite levels in target organs

  Organ to plasma radioactivity levels in time

  Organ AUC to plasma AUC ratios of radioactivity

  Organ radioactivity ratios of genetically modified to wild-type strain
- Metabolic profiling

  Number of metabolites (especially those accounting for >10% of radioactivity)

  Structural information of previously unknown metabolites

  Pharmacokinetic parameters of metabolites

  Obtaining reference compounds

  Concordance in metabolic profile between species

33.5.1 Mass Balance Calculation

The mass balance calculation consists of calculating the amount of radioactivity administered and calculating the amount of radioactivity recovered in urine, feces, and, if applicable, expired air:

Recovery =

Urine	volume (mL)·concentration (DPM/mL)	
Feces	weight (g)·homogenization factor·concentration (DPM/mL)	
Organs	weight (g)·homogenization factor·concentration (DPM/mL)	
Expired	DPM collected as ^{14}C-carbonate	+

Total

                                     divided by   ·100%

Dosed   Volume dosed (mL)·concentration (DPM/mL)

The total expired radioactivity can be calculated by integrating the ^{14}C-expiration rate versus time curve or collecting all the expired air. The relative contributions of feces and urine to the recovery of the dose determine the major excretory pathway.

After stopping collection of the excreta, the animals may be sacrificed, and the radioactivity still deposited in the carcass may (after suitable processing) be determined to increase the percentage of radioactive dose accounted for.

The fraction of radioactivity in urine and/or feces that is represented by unchanged drug is an indication of the importance of metabolism relative to unchanged excretion. However, this requires the availability of an analytical method suited to quantitate unchanged drug in excreta.

33.5.2   Plasma Pharmacokinetics

Although the validity of calculating (pseudo) pharmacokinetic parameters based on total or undiscriminated radioactivity levels has been debated, they may have some, if limited, use [79, 80]. Capturing as much of the area under the plasma radioactivity versus time curve increases the usefulness of pseudopharmacokinetic parameters. If a good fit of the terminal elimination phase is achieved and more than 90% of the $AUC_{0\text{-inf}}$ is captured in the $AUC_{0\text{-last}}$, the exposure to the total of the drug and its products is adequately described, even if theoretically the curve consists of multiple monoexponential functions.

Calculation of a half-life for total radioactivity may be useful when comparing such a value with the half-life of the unchanged drug. A much longer half-life for total radioactivity indicates a potential for underestimating the risk of accumulation of metabolites when solely focusing on parent drug. In addition, a pseudo-half-life for radioactivity may aid in determining the usefulness of continued collection of excreta to maximize recovery in the mass balance study.

The ratio of the AUC of unchanged drug over the AUC of total radioactivity is a measure of the importance of metabolism in the elimination of the drug. If this ratio in plasma is different from the ratio of unchanged drug to total radioactivity as determined in the excreta, this may indicate selective excretion or reabsorption of unchanged drug or metabolites, and degradation or metabolism of the drug after glomerular filtration or biliary excretion, respectively.

Finally, C_{max} and T_{max} should be reported, although they will generally coincide with those of the unchanged drug.

33.5.3   Assessment of Absorption

In the case of orally administered drugs that have an incomplete bioavailability, this may be due to incomplete absorption and/or first-pass metabolism by the intestine and the liver. The use of a radioactively labeled drug can provide a measure of the extent of absorption relative to first-pass. The (dose-corrected) ratio of the oral AUC versus the intravenous AUC of the unchanged drug in plasma yields the overall bioavailability. The ratio of the oral AUC versus the intravenous AUC of the total radioactivity in plasma (or the urinary recovery of radioactivity after oral versus intravenous administration) is an indication of the fraction absorbed [20, 81]. Although sometimes these ratios are used quantitatively, this is not correct. The radioactivity in plasma (or urine) after oral administration may consist of different metabolites compared to the radioactivity after intravenous administration. Therefore, distribution characteristics and excretion routes of the total radioactivity may differ between the administration routes and cannot be directly compared. Proper assessment of the contributions of gut and liver to bioavailability can be assessed by measuring plasma AUC of unchanged drug after oral, intraportal, and intravenous administration, respectively [82].

33.5.4 Organ Distribution

Documenting the organ distribution of radioactivity (and unchanged drug) can be informative.

After stopping the collection of excreta, radioactivity in the organs can complete the mass balance to 100%. Any radioactivity still unaccounted for is likely to have been lost through expiration ($^{14}CO_2$ or ^3H_2O).

Following the radioactivity in organs during the study indicates how quickly drug-related material is taken up by an organ (e.g., target organs where it may exert its intended or side effect) and how quickly it is redistributed and excreted again. For example, the organ distribution of lovastatin radioactivity indicated preferential accumulation of radioactivity in liver, the target organ. Further speciation showed that the active hydroxy-acid metabolite constituted the majority of liver radioactivity [22].

Organ/plasma ratios of radioactivity may be a resultant of physicochemical characteristics (lipophilic drugs will accumulate in fat), the activity of drug transporters, and the retention by irreversible binding or uptake of the radioactive label into endogenous substances. Ratios of organ AUC to plasma AUC may be calculated as a measure of relative exposure. These data may also be used to extrapolate radioactivity dosimetry data for the human mass balance [83, 84]. Retention of radioactivity in organs may reflect tissue binding of metabolites, but it may also be caused by a delayed elimination of metabolites. Upon repeated exposure, this may result in accumulation of metabolites to possibly toxic levels.

Drug concentrations are not routinely measured in red blood cells. The ratio of radioactivity in red blood cells relative to plasma (if the ratio deviates from 1.0) may indicate (active) uptake of drug into red blood cells. Knowledge of drug partitioning into red blood cells is useful, so that drug clearances from blood by organs of elimination may be evaluated relative to organ blood flows [4].

Comparison of organ distribution data between wild-type animals and animals defective in a drug transporter can be informative to predict the effects of drugs when they are combined with known inhibitors of these transporters [52, 53].

33.5.5 Metabolic Profiling

Determining the metabolic profile is important given the frequent occurrence of clinically relevant active metabolites [85]. It also enables identification of interspecies differences in metabolic profiles [46]. Reference compounds of possible metabolites can be obtained from prior *in vitro* studies. The *in vivo* study can then confirm the presence of metabolites observed *in vitro*. Consequently, metabolites observed in the preclinical mass balance study are likely to be seen in the human mass balance study, and, therefore, metabolite reference compounds may be isolated from the urine or feces obtained in the preclinical mass balance study.

Metabolites can be quantitated even before the structure has been elucidated. The radioactivity-peak areas are simply converted to molar amounts using the specific radioactivity of the administered compound. If such quantification is possible with adequate precision and accuracy, even pharmacokinetic parameters of these metabolites can be calculated, as shown with formoterol in humans [86].

The presence of metabolites in urine while absent in plasma or the absence of parent drug in urine while present in plasma may indicate renal metabolism or reabsorption processes [69].

Human metabolites that constitute a quantitatively large part of total radioactivity in urine, feces, or plasma, and metabolites that (based on their chemical structure) are likely to have a pharmacological or toxic effect, should be investigated for safety testing [5]. Based on metabolites observed in the preclinical studies, such investigations may be initiated earlier.

REFERENCES

1. The European Agency for the Evaluation of Medicinal Products. *Note for Guidance on Toxicokinetics: A Guidance for Assessing Systemic Exposure in Toxicology Studies.* The European Agency for the Evaluation of Medicinal Products; 1995. Accessed 3 May 2004.

2. The European Agency for the Evaluation of Medicinal Products. *Note for Guidance on Non-clinical Safety Studies for the Conduct of Human Clinical Trials for Pharmaceuticals.* The European Agency for the Evaluation of Medicinal Products; 2000. Accessed 3 May 2004.

3. Center for Drugs and Biologics, Food and Drug Administration, Department of Health and Human Services. *Guideline for the Format and Content of the Nonclinical Pharmacology/Toxicology Section of an Application.* Center for Drug Evaluation and Research; 1997. Accessed 3 May 2004.

4. Peck CC, Barr WH, Benet LZ, Collins J, Desjardins RE, Furst DE, Harter JG, Levy G, Ludden T, Rodman JH. Opportunities for integration of pharmacokinetics, pharmacodynamics, and toxicokinetics in rational drug development. *Clin Pharmacol Ther* 1992;51(4): 465–473.

5. US Department of Health and Human Services, Food and Drug Administration. *Guidance for Industry—Safety Testing of Drug Metabolites* (draft guidance). Center for Drug Evaluation and Research (CDER): 2005. www.fda.gov/cder/guidance/index.htm. Accessed 16 September 2005.

6. Balani SK, Miwa GT, Gan LS, Wu JT, Lee FW. Strategy of utilizing *in vitro* and *in vivo* ADME tools for lead optimization and drug candidate selection. *Curr Top Med Chem* 2005;5(11):1033–1038.

7. Department of Health and Human Services. US Food and Drug Administration-Center for Drug Evaluation and Research Home Page. http://www.fda.gov/cder/index.html. Accessed 7 January 2006.

8. EMEA. European Medicines Agency–Human Medicines Home Page. http://www.emea. eu.int/index/indexh1.htm. Accessed 8 January 2006.

9. US Department of Health and Human Services, Food and Drug Administration. *Guidance for Industry—In Vivo Drug Metabolism/Drug Interaction Studies—Study Design, Data Analysis, and Recommendations for Dosing and Labeling.* Center for Drug Evaluation and Research (CDER), Center for Biologics Evaluation and Research (CBER); 1999. www.fda.gov/cder/guidance/index.htm. Accessed 16 September 2005.

10. US Department of Health and Human Services, Food and Drug Administration. *Guidance for Industry—Estimating the Maximum Safe Starting Dose in Initial Clinical Trials for Therapeutics in Adult Healthy Volunteers.* Center for Drug Evaluation and Research (CDER); 2005. www.fda.gov/cder/guidance/index.htm. Accessed 9 February 2006.

11. Dalvie D. Recent advances in the applications of radioisotopes in drug metabolism, toxicology and pharmacokinetics. *Curr Pharm Des* 2000;6(10):1009–1028.

12. *Principles and Methods of Toxicology.* Philadelphia: Taylor&Francis; 2001.

13. Fagerholm U, Breuer O, Swedmark S, Hoogstraate J. Pre-clinical pharmacokinetics of the cyclooxygenase-inhibiting nitric oxide donor (CINOD) AZD3582. *J Pharm Pharmacol* 2005;57(5):587–597.

14. Budavari S. *The Merck Index.* Whitehouse Station, NJ: Merck&Co; 1996.

15. Hutchinson OC, Collingridge DR, Barthel H, Price PM, Aboagye EO. Pharmacokinetics of radiolabelled anticancer drugs for positron emission tomography. *Curr Pharm Des* 2003;9(11):917–929.

16. Minami T, Ichii M, Okazaki Y. Comparison of three different methods for measurement of tissue platinum level. *Biol Trace Element Res* 1995;48(1):37–44.

17. Hughes MF, Devesa V, Adair BM, Styblo M, Kenyon EM, Thomas DJ. Tissue dosimetry, metabolism and excretion of pentavalent and trivalent monomethylated arsenic in mice after oral administration. *Toxicol Appl Pharmacol* 2005;208(2):186–197.

18. Desmoulin F, Gilard V, Malet-Martino M, Martino R. Metabolism of capecitabine, an oral fluorouracil prodrug: (19)F NMR studies in animal models and human urine. *Drug Metab Dispos* 2002;30(11):1221–1229.

19. Ferraiolo BL, Moore JA, Crase D, Gribling P, Wilking H, Baughman RA. Pharmacokinetics and tissue distribution of recombinant human tumor necrosis factor-alpha in mice. *Drug Metab Dispos* 1988;16(2):270–275.

20. Pleiss U. [Radioactive-labeled pharmaceutical agents.] Werkzeuge bei der Arzneimittelentwicklung. Radioaktiv markierte pharmazeutische Wirkstoffe. *Pharmazie Zeit* 2005; 34(6):514–519.

21. Dueker SR, Jones AD, Clifford AJ. Protocol development for biological tracer studies. *Adv Exp Med Biol* 1998;445:363–378.

22. Duggan DE, Chen IW, Bayne WF, Halpin RA, Duncan CA, Schwartz MS, Stubbs RJ, Vickers S. The physiological disposition of lovastatin. *Drug Metab Dispos* 1989;17(2): 166–173.

23. Horsmans Y, Saliez A, van d BV, Desager JP, Geubel AP, Pauwels S, Lambotte L. ^{14}C-Propoxyphene demethylation in the rat. An example of differences between liver and intestinal drug-presystemic metabolism. *Drug Metab Dispos* 1997;25(11):1257–1259.

24. Dalvie D. Recent advances in the applications of radioisotopes in drug metabolism, toxicology and pharmacokinetics. *Curr Pharm Des* 2000;6(10):1009–1028.

25. Beumer JH, Beijnen JH, Schellens JH. Mass balance studies, with a focus on anticancer drugs. *Clin Pharmacokinet* 2006;45(1):33–58.

26. Browne TR, Van Langenhove A, Costello CE, Biemann K, Greenblatt DJ. Pharmacokinetic equivalence of stable-isotope-labeled and unlabeled drugs. Phenobarbital in man. *J Clin Pharmacol* 1982;22(7):309–315.

27. Phillips DH, Potter GA, Horton MN, Hewer A, Crofton-Sleigh C, Jarman M, Venitt S. Reduced genotoxicity of [D5-ethyl]-tamoxifen implicates alpha-hydroxylation of the ethyl group as a major pathway of tamoxifen activation to a liver carcinogen. *Carcinogenesis* 1994;15(8):1487–1492.

28. Toxicokinetics: the assessment of systemic exposure in toxicity studies-ICH topic S3A. ICH; 1995. *CPMP/ICH/385/95.* Accessed 9 February 2006.

29. US Department of Health and Human Services, Food and Drug Administration. *Guidance for Industry—M3 Nonclinical Safety Studies for the Conduct of Human Clinical Trials for Pharmaceuticals.* Center for Drug Evaluation and Research (CDER); 1997. www.fda.gov/cder/guidance/index.htm. Accessed 16 September 2005.

30. US Department of Health and Human Services, Food and Drug Administration. *Guidance for Industry—Drug Metabolism/Drug Interaction Studies in the Drug Development Process: Studies In Vitro*. Center for Drug Evaluation and Research, Center for Biologics Evaluation and Research; 1997. www.fda.gov/cder/guidance.htm. Accessed 16 September 2005.

31. Collins JM. Inter-species differences in drug properties. *Chem-Biol Interact* 2001;134(3): 237–242.

32. Camiener GW, Smith CG. Studies of the enzymatic deamination of cytosine arabinoside. I. Enzyme distribution and species specificity. *Biochem Pharmacol* 1965;14(10):1405–1416.

33. Sharkey EM, ONeill HB, Kavarana MJ, Wang H, Creighton DJ, Sentz DL, Eiseman JL. Pharmacokinetics and antitumor properties in tumor-bearing mice of an enediol analogue inhibitor of glyoxalase I. *Cancer Chemother Pharmacol* 2000;46(2):156–166.

34. Morton CL, Iacono L, Hyatt JL, Taylor KR, Cheshire PJ, Houghton PJ, Danks MK, Stewart CF, Potter PM. Activation and antitumor activity of CPT-11 in plasma esterase-deficient mice. *Cancer Chemother Pharmacol* 2005;56(6):629–636.

35. van Bezooijen CF. Influence of age-related changes in rodent liver morphology and physiology on drug metabolism—a review. *Mech Ageing Dev* 1984;25(1–2):1–22.

36. Leakey JE, Cunny HC, Bazare J Jr, Webb PJ, Feuers RJ, Duffy PH, Hart RW. Effects of aging and caloric restriction on hepatic drug metabolizing enzymes in the Fischer 344 rat. I: The cytochrome P-450 dependent monooxygenase system. *Mech Ageing Dev* 1989; 48(2):145–155.

37. Leakey JA, Cunny HC, Bazare J Jr, Webb PJ, Lipscomb JC, Slikker W Jr, Feuers RJ, Duffy PH, Hart RW. Effects of aging and caloric restriction on hepatic drug metabolizing enzymes in the Fischer 344 rat. II: Effects on conjugating enzymes. *Mech Ageing Dev* 1989;48(2):157–166.

38. Czerniak R. Gender-based differences in pharmacokinetics in laboratory animal models. *Int J Toxicol* 2001;20(3):161–163.

39. Witkamp RF, Yun HI, van't Klooster GA, van Mosel JF, van Mosel M, Ensink JM, Noordhoek J, Van Miert AS. Comparative aspects and sex differentiation of plasma sulfamethazine elimination and metabolite formation in rats, rabbits, dwarf goats, and cattle. *Am J Vet Res* 1992;53(10):1830–1835.

40. Witkamp RF, Lohuis JA, Nijmeijer SM, Kolker HJ, Noordhoek J, van Miert AS. Species- and sex-related differences in the plasma clearance and metabolite formation of antipyrine. A comparative study in four animal species: cattle, goat, rat and rabbit. *Xenobiotica* 1991;21(11):1483–1492.

41. Griffin RJ, Godfrey VB, Kim YC, Burka LT. Sex-dependent differences in the disposition of 2,4-dichlorophenoxyacetic acid in Sprague–Dawley rats, B6C3F1 mice, and Syrian hamsters. *Drug Metab Dispos* 1997;25(9):1065–1071.

42. Kato R, Yamazoe Y. Sex-specific cytochrome P450 as a cause of sex- and species-related differences in drug toxicity. *Toxicol Lett* 1992;64–65(Spec No):661–667.

43. Klecker RW, Cysyk RL, Collins JM. Zebularine metabolism by aldehyde oxidase in hepatic cytosol from humans, monkeys, dogs, rats, and mice: influence of sex and inhibitors. *Bioorg Med Chem* 2006;14(1);62–66.

44. Schwartz JB. The influence of sex on pharmacokinetics. *Clin Pharmacokinet* 2003;42(2): 107–121.

45. van Herwaarden AE, Smit JW, Sparidans RW, Wagenaar E, van der Kruijssen CM, Schellens JH, Beijnen JH, Schinkel AH. Midazolam and cyclosporin a metabolism in

transgenic mice with liver-specific expression of human CYP3A4. *Drug Metab Dispos* 2005;33(7):892–895.

46. Marathe PH, Shyu WC, Humphreys WG. The use of radiolabeled compounds for ADME studies in discovery and exploratory development. *Curr Pharm Des* 2004;10(24):2991–3008.

47. Jonker JW, Wagenaar E, van Deemter L, Gottschlich R, Bender HM, Dasenbrock J, Schinkel AH. Role of blood–brain barrier P-glycoprotein in limiting brain accumulation and sedative side-effects of asimadoline, a peripherally acting analgaesic drug. *Br J Pharmacol* 1999;127(1):43–50.

48. Merino G, Jonker JW, Wagenaar E, van Herwaarden AE, Schinkel AH. The breast cancer resistance protein (BCRP/ABCG2) affects pharmacokinetics, hepatobiliary excretion, and milk secretion of the antibiotic nitrofurantoin. *Mol Pharmacol* 2005;67(5):1758–1764.

49. Jonker JW, Wagenaar E, Mol CA, Buitelaar M, Koepsell H, Smit JW, Schinkel AH. Reduced hepatic uptake and intestinal excretion of organic cations in mice with a targeted disruption of the organic cation transporter 1 (Oct1 [Slc22a1]) gene. *Mol Cell Biol* 2001;21(16):5471–5477.

50. Breedveld P, Pluim D, Cipriani G, Wielinga P, van Tellingen O, Schinkel AH, Schellens JH. The effect of Bcrp1 (Abcg2) on the *in vivo* pharmacokinetics and brain penetration of imatinib mesylate (Gleevec): implications for the use of breast cancer resistance protein and P-glycoprotein inhibitors to enable the brain penetration of imatinib in patients. *Cancer Res* 2005;65(7):2577–2582.

51. Schinkel AH, Wagenaar E, Mol CA, van Deemter L. P-glycoprotein in the blood–brain barrier of mice influences the brain penetration and pharmacological activity of many drugs. *J Clin Invest* 1996;97(11):2517–2524.

52. Schinkel AH, Wagenaar E, van Deemter L, Mol CA, Borst P. Absence of the mdr1a P-glycoprotein in mice affects tissue distribution and pharmacokinetics of dexamethasone, digoxin, and cyclosporin A. *J Clin Invest* 1995;96(4):1698–1705.

53. Schinkel AH, Smit JJ, van Tellingen O, Beijnen JH, Wagenaar E, Van DeemTer L, Mol CA, van der Valk MA, Robanus-Maandag EC, te Riele HP. Disruption of the mouse mdr1a P-glycoprotein gene leads to a deficiency in the blood–brain barrier and to increased sensitivity to drugs. *Cell* 1994;77(4):491–502.

54. Gonzalez FJ, Yu AM. Cytochrome P450 and xenobiotic receptor humanized mice. *Annu Rev Pharmacol Toxicol* 2006;46:41–64.

55. Gonzalez FJ. Cytochrome P450 humanised mice. *Hum Genomics* 2004;1(4):300–306.

56. Beumer JH, Rademaker-Lakhai JM, Rosing H, Lopez-Lazaro L, Beijnen JH, Schellens JH. Trabectedin (Yondelis, formerly ET-743), a mass balance study in patients with advanced cancer. *Invest New Drugs* 2005;23(5):429–436.

57. Rickert DE, Dingley K, Ubick E, Dix KJ, Molina L. Determination of the tissue distribution and excretion by accelerator mass spectrometry of the nonadecapeptide ^{14}C-Moli1901 in beagle dogs after intratracheal instillation. *Chem-Biol Interact* 2005;155(1–2):55–61.

58. Lappin G, Garner RC. Big physics, small doses: the use of AMS and PET in human microdosing of development drugs. *Nat Rev Drug Discov* 2003;2(3):233–240.

59. *Pharmacokinetics: Guidance for Repeated Dose Tissue Distribution Studies—ICH Topic S3B*. ICH; 2005. *CPMP/ICH/385/95*.

60. Dent NJ. The inspection of drug metabolism and pharmacokinetic studies. *Qual Assur* 1992;1(3):230–236.

61. *Safe and Secure—A Guide to Working Safely with Radiolabelled Compounds.* Amersham; 2005. http://www1.amershambiosciences.com/applic/upp00738.nsf/vLookupDoc/196245642-A125/$file/Safe_Secure%202003.pdf. Accessed 2 November 2005.

62. Kishore R, Eary JF, Krohn KA, Nelp WB, Menard TW, Beaumier PL, Hellstrom KE, Hellstrom I. Autoradiolysis of iodinated monoclonal antibody preparations. *Int J Radiat Appl Instrum B* 1986;13(4):457–459.

63. Kinuya S, Yokoyama K, Tega H, Hiramatsu T, Konishi S, Yamamoto W, Shuke N, Aburano T, Watanabe N, Takayama T, Michigishi T, Tonami N. Rhenium-186-mercaptoacetyltriglycine-labeled monoclonal antibody for radioimmunotherapy: *in vitro* assessment, *in vivo* kinetics and dosimetry in tumor-bearing nude mice. *Japanese J Cancer Res* 1998;89(8): 870–878.

64. Smit MJ, Temmerman AM, Havinga R, Kuipers F, Vonk RJ. Short- and long-term effects of biliary drainage on hepatic cholesterol metabolism in the rat. *Biochem J* 1990;269(3): 781–788.

65. Accatino L, Hono J, Koenig C, Pizarro M, Rodriguez L. Adaptive changes of hepatic bile salt transport in a model of reversible interruption of the enterohepatic circulation in the rat. *J Hepatol* 1993;19(1):95–104.

66. Nezasa K, Takao A, Kimura K, Takaichi M, Inazawa K, Koike M. Pharmacokinetics and disposition of rosuvastatin, a new 3-hydroxy-3-methylglutaryl coenzyme A reductase inhibitor, in rat. *Xenobiotica* 2002;32(8):715–727.

67. Rowland M, Tozer TN, *Clinical Pharmacokinetics—Concepts and Applications.* Baltimore: Williams & Wilkins; 1995.

68. Mukherjee KL, Heidelberger C. Studies on fluorinated pyrimidines. IX. The degradation of 5-fluorouracil-6-C14. *J Biol Chem* 1960;235:433–437.

69. Melgar MD, Zuleski FR, Malbica JO. Metabolism, disposition, and pharmacokinetics of tracazolate in rat and dog. *Drug Metab Dispos* 1984;12(4):396–402.

70. Lee HJ, Chiou WL. Marked heterogeneity in the intrahepatic distribution of quinidine in rats: implications in pharmacokinetics. *J Pharm Sci* 1990;79(9):778–781.

71. Ings RM, Breen M, Devereux K, Gray AJ, Edwards FE, Lucas C, Briggs M, Robinson BV, Campbell DB. The comparative disposition of [^{14}C]-fotemustine in non-tumourous and tumourous mice. *Cancer Chemother Pharmacol* 1990;27(2):106–110.

72. Tomiyama Y, Brian JE Jr, Todd MM. Cerebral blood flow during hemodilution and hypoxia in rats: role of ATP-sensitive potassium channels. *Stroke* 1999;30(9):1942–1947.

73. Berger H, Sandow J, Heinrich N, Albrecht E, Kertscher U, Oehlke J. Disposition of the ^{3}H-labeled gonadotropin-releasing hormone analog buserelin in rats. *Drug Metab Dispos* 1993;21(5):818–822.

74. Slatter JG, Schaaf LJ, Sams JP, Feenstra KL, Johnson MG, Bombardt PA, Cathcart KS, Verburg MT, Pearson LK, Compton LD, Miller LL, Baker DS, Pesheck CV, Lord RS III. Pharmacokinetics, metabolism, and excretion of irinotecan (CPT-11) following I.V. infusion of [(^{14})C]CPT-11 in cancer patients. *Drug Metab Dispos* 2000;28(4):423–433.

75. Lenz EM, Wilson ID, Wright B, Partridge EA, Rodgers CT, Haycock PR, Lindon JC, Nicholson JK. A comparison of quantitative NMR and radiolabelling studies of the metabolism and excretion of Statil (3-(4-bromo-2-fluorobenzyl)-4-oxo-3*H*-phthalazin-1-ylacetic acid) in the rat. *J Pharm Biomed Anal* 2002;28(1):31–43.

76. Griffiths JR, Glickson JD. Monitoring pharmacokinetics of anticancer drugs: non-invasive investigation using magnetic resonance spectroscopy. *Adv Drug Deliv Rev* 2000;41(1): 75–89.

77. Sparreboom A, Huizing MT, Boesen JJ, Nooijen WJ, van Tellingen O, Beijnen JH. Isolation, purification, and biological activity of mono- and dihydroxylated paclitaxel metabolites from human feces. *Cancer Chemother Pharmacol* 1995;36(4):299–304.

78. Gilbert PJ, Hartley TE, Troke JA, Turcan RG, Vose CW, Watson KV. Application of ^{19}F-n.m.r. spectroscopy to the identification of dog urinary metabolites of imirestat, a spirohydantoin aldose reductase inhibitor. *Xenobiotica* 1992;22(7):775–787.

79. Jansen AB. Total radioactivity half-lives. *Drug Metab Dispos* 1979;7(5):350.

80. Di Carlo FJ. Undifferentiated radioactivity revisited. *Drug Metab Dispos* 1980;8(4): 287–288.

81. Lemaire M, Bodoky A, Heberer M, Niederberger W. Quantification of absorption, intestinal and hepatic first pass effect in a chronic dog model. *Eur J Drug Metab Pharmacokinet* 1991;Spec No 3:132–135.

82. Vachharajani NN, Shyu WC, Shah VR, Barbhaiya RH. Pharmacokinetic assessment of the sites of first-pass metabolism of BMS-181101, an antidepressant agent, in rats. *J Pharm Pharmacol* 1998;50(3):275–278.

83. Dain JG, Collins JM, Robinson WT. A regulatory and industrial perspective of the use of carbon-14 and tritium isotopes in human ADME studies. *Pharm Res* 1994;11(6): 925–928.

84. *Code of Federal Regulations*. Prescription drugs for human use generally recognized as safe and effective and not misbranded: drugs used in research. FDA; 2002. Accessed 3 May 2004.

85. Garattini S. Active drug metabolites. An overview of their relevance in clinical pharmacokinetics. *Clin Pharmacokinet* 1985;10(3):216–227.

86. Rosenborg J, Larsson P, Tegner K, Hallstrom G. Mass balance and metabolism of [(3)H]Formoterol in healthy men after combined i.v. and oral administration-mimicking inhalation. *Drug Metab Dispos* 1999;27(10):1104–1116.

87. Collins JM, Grieshaber CK, Chabner BA. Pharmacologically guided phase I clinical trials based upon preclinical drug development. *J Nat Cancer Inst* 1990;82(16):1321–1326.

88. Uchida T, O'Brien RD. Dimethoate degradation by human liver and its significance for acute toxicity. *Toxicol Appl Pharmacol* 1967;10(1):89–94.

89. Dareer SM, Mulligan LT Jr, White V, Tillery K, Mellett LB, Hill DL. Distribution of [^{3}H]cytosine arabinoside and its products in mice, dogs, and monkeys and effect of tetrahydrouridine. *Cancer Treat Rep* 1977;61(3):395–407.

90. Kitteringham NR, Davis C, Howard N, Pirmohamed M, Park BK. Interindividual and interspecies variation in hepatic microsomal epoxide hydrolase activity: studies with *cis*-stilbene oxide, carbamazepine 10, 11-epoxide and naphthalene. *J Pharmacol Exp Ther* 1996;278(3):1018–1027.

34

PHARMACODYNAMICS

BEOM SOO SHIN, DHAVAL SHAH, AND JOSEPH P. BALTHASAR
University at Buffalo, The State University of New York, Buffalo, New York

Contents

34.1 INTRODUCTION

Pharmacodynamics refers to the study of relationships between drug concentrations and pharmacological effects. The mathematical description of these relationships, through the use of appropriate *pharmacodynamic models*, facilitates the characterization and comparison of candidate drugs, facilitates the rational selection of appropriate dosing regimens, and assists in the investigation and identification of

Preclinical Development Handbook: ADME and Biopharmaceutical Properties,
edited by Shayne Cox Gad
Copyright © 2008 John Wiley & Sons, Inc.

the mechanisms associated with drug action. This chapter is structured to provide an overview and a catalog of mathematical models that may be employed to characterize drug pharmacodynamics. Section 34.2 provides a brief overview of the analysis of pharmacodynamic data, Section 34.3 reviews mathematical models used to relate fixed (e.g., steady-state) drug concentrations to drug effects, and Section 34.4 covers basic and advanced models that relate the time course of drug exposure to the time course of drug effects. Section 34.5 provides a brief summary of the chapter.

34.2   OVERVIEW

Pharmacodynamics can be defined as the study of the relationships between the systemic exposure of drug and its biological action. Upon intravascular or extravascular administration, the drug enters the systemic circulation directly or with an absorption phase. Once the drug reaches the systemic circulation, drug is distributed into various organs and then eliminated by metabolism and excretion. *Pharmacokinetics* refers to the investigation of the rates and extent of drug absorption, distribution, metabolism, and excretion, and *pharmacokinetic models* allow description of the relationship between drug dosing and the time course of drug concentrations in the body. The combination of pharmacokinetic models with pharmacodynamic models, which relate drug exposure to drug response, allows for the characterization and prediction of the relations hips between the timing of drug administration and the time course of drug effects (Fig. 34.1). The main differences between pharmacokinetics and pharmacodynamics are summarized in Table 34.1 [1].

Pharmacological responses are initiated by binding of drug molecule with proteins (e.g., enzymes, receptors) or, in certain cases, DNA. The intensity of the drug response is altered as a function of the administered dose, with a higher receptor–drug binding generally producing a greater response. At a certain point, the response may be saturated and the relationship between drug concentration and response becomes nonlinear. In 1927, Clark [2] first introduced the drug–receptor binding concept into pharmacodynamics. It was suggested that the quantitative effect of acetylcholine was mediated by a receptor-binding process. Clark's occupancy theory was elaborated by Ariens and De Groot [3] and Stephenson [4] and became a fundamental basis for the field of pharmacodynamics. Upon long-term infusion or multiple dosing, drug concentrations in each area of the body will approach a steady state, where concentrations are constant with time. In such cases, drug response may be assumed to be "static" or time invariant. Section 34.3 of this chapter discusses several mathematical models that have been developed to describe static drug concentration–response relationships, including the E_{max} and the sigmoid E_{max} model.

Although static models are useful in some situations, "kinetic" models, which relate the time course of drug concentration to the time course of drug response, provide a much more complete characterization of drug pharmacodynamics, and kinetic models often provide great insight into the underlying mechanisms responsible for drug effects. Kinetic models of drug response are reviewed in Section 34.4. The simplest of the kinetic models, *direct effect models*, assume a direct relationship

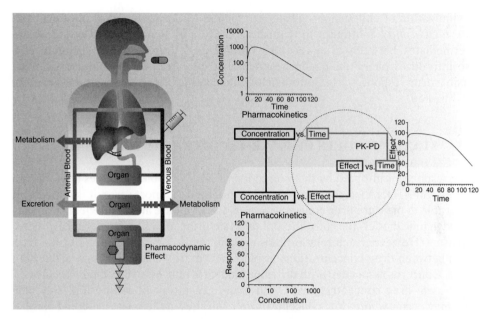

FIGURE 34.1 Representative diagram for relationship between pharmacokinetics and pharmacodynamics. Pharmacokinetics mainly deals with the time course of drug absorption (A), distribution (D), metabolism (M), and elimination (E). Pharmacodynamics deals with the drug effect as a function of drug concentration. Pharmacokinetic and pharmacodynamic (PKPD) modeling combines the two processes to allow prediction and characterization of the time course of drug effects.

TABLE 34.1   Main Differences Between Pharmacokinetics and Pharmacodynamics

Characteristics	Pharmacokinetics	Pharmacodynamics
Broad definition	What body does to the drug	What the drug does to the body
Influence	Affected by interactions throughout the whole body	Affects specific drug receptors/ signaling pathways
Determinants	Typically governed by simple physiologic determinants	Typically determined by complex, nonlinear response and control pathways
Linearity	Typically linear	Typically nonlinear
Initial condition	Baseline concentrations are zero prior to drug dosing	Nonzero baseline response prior to drug dosing

between drug concentrations in plasma and drug response. In many cases, drug responses are delayed relative to the time course of drug concentrations in plasma. Several models have been developed to describe mechanisms responsible for this delay. For example, the *biophase model* assumes that the delay between the time course of drug concentrations in plasma and the time course of drug effect is due to the kinetics of drug distribution to the site of drug action (i.e., the biophase). *Indirect effect models* assume that the delay is related to the production or elimination of endogenous substances related to the observed drug effect, and *transduction models* attempt to describe a cascade of signaling events that act as intermediates between drug–receptor binding and drug response. Section 34.4 also introduces pharmacodynamic models that may be used to characterize irreversible drug responses (e.g., cytotoxicity) and complexities including tolerance and sensitization.

34.3 "STATIC" MODELS OF PHARMACOLOGICAL RESPONSE

Drug response is initiated by the interaction of drug with biomolecules (e.g., receptors, enzymes, DNA) at the biophase. Unfortunately, in most cases, it is difficult or impossible to measure drug concentrations at the biophase and, consequently, pharmacodynamic models typically attempt to relate drug effects to drug concentrations in plasma. However, such relationships are confounded by any disequilibrium that exists between drug concentrations in plasma and drug concentrations at the biophase. Concerns associated with distribution delays may be overcome by the use of *steady-state* drug concentrations. Upon long-term intravenous infusion, a steady state may occur, where drug concentrations in all sites in the body, including plasma and the biophase, remain constant with time. Under these circumstances, a unique, monotonic relationship between drug concentrations in plasma and drug concentrations at the biophase may be assumed. Following administration of drug at a variety of infusion rates, sufficient data may be available to develop relationships between steady state concentrations and the magnitude of drug effect. Due to the nature of the steady state, these relationships may be considered to be time invariant or "static," and these relationships are unable to describe the time course of drug response. This section introduces drug–receptor binding theory and several static pharmacodynamic models, including the E_{max} model, the log-linear E_{max} model, and the sigmoid E_{max} model.

34.3.1 Drug–Receptor Binding

The biological action of a drug is initiated by the interaction of the drug with free receptor, which may be expected to follow the law of mass action:

Drug [D] + Receptor [R]   Drug–receptor
                                 complex [DR]   Effect (E)

R and D represent free receptor and drug; DR and E represent the drug–receptor complex and the effect of drug, respectively. The brackets [ ] signify the representation of molar concentrations. Typically, the following assumptions are made for this equation:

1. The interaction is reversible.
2. The receptor, drug, and drug–receptor complex are in equilibrium.

3. The receptor contains one binding site for the drug.
4. The drug and receptor interact rapidly to form the drug–receptor complex.

At equilibrium,

$$K_D = \frac{[D][R]}{[DR]} \tag{34.1}$$

where K_D is the equilibrium dissociation constant for the drug–receptor complex.

The total concentration of receptor, $[R_T]$, is the sum of bound and free receptors.

$$[R_T] = [R] + [DR] \tag{34.2}$$

By rearranging Eq. 34.2, we have

$$[R] = [R_T] - [DR] \tag{34.3}$$

By substituting Eq. 34.3 into Eq. 34.1, the following equation is obtained:

$$K_D = \frac{([R_T] - [DR]) \times [D]}{[D][R]} = \frac{[R_T][D] - [DR][D]}{[DR]} \tag{34.4}$$

And by Rearranging Eq. 34.4, we have

$$[DR] = \frac{[R_T][D]}{K_D + [D]} \tag{34.5}$$

In 1954, Ariens and De Groot [3] proposed the concept that drug–receptor complex [DR] is linearly proportional to the effect of drug. According to this theory, [DR] can be substituted by effect E, and the total receptor concentration $[R_T]$, which will bind with drug and form [DR], can be represented by the maximum response E_{max}. The steady-state free drug concentration at the biophase [D] is often assumed to be the same as the steady-state free drug concentration in plasma $[C_p]$. Taken together, Eq. 34.5 can be rewritten as follows:

$$E = \frac{E_{max} \times [C_p]}{K_D + [C_p]} \tag{34.6}$$

K_D is in units of concentration (mass/volume). EC_{50} may be defined as the drug concentration associated with the binding of 50% of the drug receptor, where effect is one-half of E_{max} [$E_{max}/2$].

$$\frac{E_{max}}{2} = \frac{E_{max} \times [EC_{50}]}{K_D + [EC_{50}]} \tag{34.7}$$

By rearranging Eq. 34.7, K_D can be represented as the concentration that produces 50% of the maximum response:

$$K_D = EC_{50} \tag{34.8}$$

Equation 34.6 can be rewritten as follows:

$$E = \frac{E_{max} \times [C_p]}{EC_{50} + [C_p]} \tag{34.9}$$

This equation is often referred to as the *maximum effect (E_{max}) model.*

34.3.2 E_{max} Model

The E_{max} model predicts a hyperbolic relationship between concentration and response, where, at low concentrations, the relationship between concentration and response is linear but, as the dose increases, the response becomes saturated and reaches a plateau (Fig. 34.2). As indicated in the simple E_{max} model (Eq. 34.9), drug response will be zero when no drug is present. However, in many cases, the effects produced by endogenous ligands for the receptor may not be differentiated from drug effects, and it is necessary to consider a "baseline" level of response (E_0):

$$E = E_0 + \frac{E_{max} \times [C_p]}{EC_{50} + [C_p]} \tag{34.10}$$

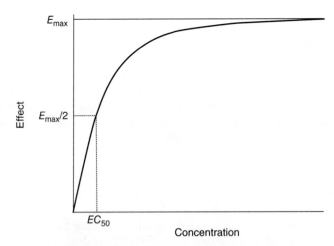

FIGURE 34.2 Typical effect versus concentration relationship predicted by the E_{max} model. At low concentrations, there is a linear relationship between drug concentration and response. As the concentration increases, the drug response pathways become saturated and eventually a plateau is achieved. E_{max} represents the maximal effect of the drug and EC_{50} represents the potency of the drug. EC_{50} is defined as the concentration of drug required to produce 50% of the maximum effect.

where E_0 represents the baseline effect measured in the absence of drug.

In cases where drug inhibits a physiological process, effect may be characterized by rearrangement of the E_{max} model as follows:

$$E = E_0 - \frac{I_{max} \times [C_p]}{IC_{50} + [C_p]} \tag{34.11}$$

In the inhibitory model, the maximum inhibitory response and the concentration that produces 50% of the maximum inhibitory response are regarded as I_{max} and IC_{50} instead of E_{max} and EC_{50}. In certain cases, response is represented as the percentage change of baseline value. Using the percentage change makes the baseline zero and thus a simple E_{max} model (Eq. 34.9) may be applied.

Efficacy, Potency, and Intrinsic Activity   In Fig. 34.2, E_{max} represents the *efficacy* of the drug and EC_{50} represents the *potency* of the drug. The efficacy means the strength of response that is generated by a single receptor [4]. The potency is commonly represented by the EC_{50} value. A smaller EC_{50} value means a higher potency. Figure 34.3 presents effect versus concentration curves for drugs with differing efficacy and potency. In Fig. 34.3a, both drug A and drug B have the same E_{max} value, although drug A has a smaller EC_{50} value compared with drug B. Thus, to reach the same response, a higher concentration is needed for drug B as compared with drug A, indicating that drug A exhibits a higher potency than drug B. In Fig. 34.3b, drug A has a smaller EC_{50} value compared with drug B. However, the E_{max} value of drug B is higher than that of drug A. Thus, drug A has a higher potency but lower efficacy compared with drug B. Another important concept of the E_{max} model is the *intrinsic activity* (ε) introduced by Ariens and De Groot [3]. The intrinsic activity can be presented by a relationship between response and occupancy of receptor. Although biological response is directly proportional to receptor occupancy, drugs with different intrinsic activity will generate different levels of response at any given value of receptor occupancy (e.g., as seen with "full agonists" vs. "partial agonists").

$$\varepsilon = \frac{[DR]}{E} \tag{34.12}$$

Linear Model   At low concentrations of drug, the relationship between concentration and response is assumed to be linear (Fig. 34.4a):

$$E = mC_p + E_0 \tag{34.13}$$

where m represents the slope, which is equivalent to E_{max}/EC_{50}. However, as the concentration increases, the drug receptors will become saturated and eventually the response reaches the E_{max}. Thus, this linearization of the E_{max} model is valid only at low concentrations ($C_p \ll EC_{50}$).

Log-Linear Model   As indicated previously, when plotted on a linear scale, the E_{max} model predicts a hyperbolic relationship between drug concentration and

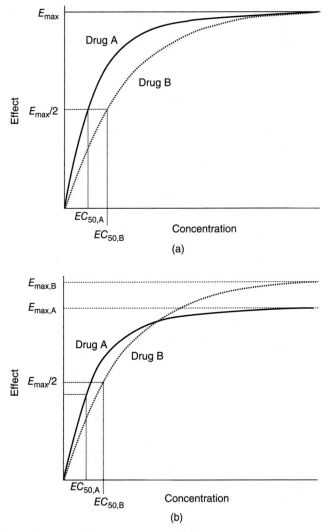

FIGURE 34.3   Influence of E_{max} and EC_{50} on effect versus concentration profiles predicted by the E_{max} model. (a) Drug A and drug B have the same efficacy (E_{max}) but drug A is more potent compared to drug B ($EC_{50,A} < EC_{50,B}$). Thus, to reach the same response, higher concentrations of drug B are needed compared to drug A. (b) Drug A and drug B show different efficacy and different potency. Drug A has a smaller EC_{50} value compared to drug B, and drug A has a smaller E_{max} value compared to drug B. Thus, drug A shows higher potency but less efficacy compared to drug B.

response. However, when plotted using a log scale for drug concentration, the plot becomes sigmoidal (Fig. 34.4b), and a log-linear relationship is found between concentration and response over the range of 20–80% of E_{max}. This relationship may be represented with the following equation:

$$E = m\log(C_p) + b \tag{34.14}$$

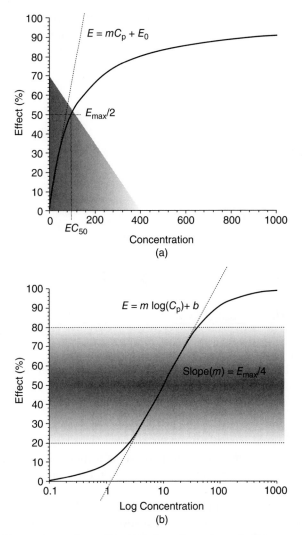

FIGURE 34.4 Comparison of rectilinear and semilog plots of effect versus concentration profiles predicted by the E_{max} model. (a) Plotting effect versus concentration profile on a linear scale provides a hyperbolic relationship between response and drug concentration. At very low concentrations of drug, the relationship between response and concentration can be described as linear and can be represented by the equation $E = mC_p + E_0$, where m is the slope and E_0 is the intercept. (b) Plotting the effect versus concentration profile on a semilog scale, the relationship between response and concentration becomes sigmoidal. Between 20% and 80% of the maximum response, the relationship between response and concentration is linear and may be described by the equation $E = m \log(C_p) + b$, where m is the slope and b is the intercept. The slope of this linear relationship (m) is equal to one-quarter of the maximum response ($E_{max}/4$).

where m and b represent the slope and the intercept, respectively. However, note that in contrast to the linear model, the intercept of the log-linear model does not represent the baseline effect.

The meaning of slope (m) may be derived as follows [5]:

$$\text{Slope} = m = \frac{dE}{d\ln C_p} \tag{34.15}$$

Since C_p can be written as

$$e^{\ln C_p} = C_p \tag{34.16}$$

Eq. 34.9 may be rewritten as

$$E = \frac{E_{max} \times [e^{\ln C_p}]}{EC_{50} + [e^{\ln C_p}]} \tag{34.17}$$

Solving for the slope, or the derivative of E with respect to $e^{\ln C_p}$, we find

$$\frac{dE}{d\ln C_p} = \frac{E_{max}C_p(EC_{50} + C_p) - E_{max}C_p^2}{(EC_{50} + C_p)^2} = \frac{E_{max}EC_{50}C_p}{(EC_{50} + C_p)^2} \tag{34.18}$$

Using Eq. 34.18, the slope at $C_p = EC_{50}$ can be derived as follows:

$$\frac{dE}{d\ln C_p} = \frac{E_{max}EC_{50}^2}{(2EC_{50})^2} = \frac{E_{max}}{4} \tag{34.19}$$

As shown in Eq. 34.19, the slope will increase as a function of E_{max}. Additionally, this derivation allows rapid estimation of E_{max} from the slope of the E versus. $\ln C_p$ relationship.

The major benefit of the linear and log-linear models is, of course, the linearization of the relationship. These linearizations allow characterization of pharmacodynamic relationships with the use of simple linear regression, thereby avoiding the need for more computationally intensive analyses (e.g., nonlinear regression) [6, 7]. Although increased availability of nonlinear regression software has minimized the need for application of linearized models for final analyses of datasets, the linear models remain useful for initial analyses and for estimation of initial parameter values (i.e., to facilitate subsequent nonlinear regression analyses).

34.3.3   Sigmoid E_{max} Model (Hill Equation)

The *sigmoid E_{max} model* was first introduced by Hill to explain the association of oxygen with hemoglobin [8]. Wagner applied this equation to pharmacodynamics in 1968 [9]. Mathematically, this equation is an extension of the E_{max} model by adding the Hill coefficient (n). In the sigmoid E_{max} model, the relationship between receptor and drug can be represented as

Drug $[D_n]$ + Receptor $[R]$ Drug–receptor complex $[D_nR]$ Effect (E)

where R and D represent free receptor and drug, respectively. DR and E represent the drug–receptor complex and effect, and n represents the Hill coefficient. At equilibrium,

$$K_D = \frac{[D]^n[R]}{[D_nR]}$$ (34.20)

Free receptor concentration can be described as

$$[R] = [R_T] - [D_nR]$$ (34.21)

Substituting Eq. 34.21 into Eq. 34.20, we find

$$K_D = \frac{[D]^n[R_T] - [D_nR][D]^n}{[D_nR]}$$ (34.22)

Rearranging Eq. 34.22 in terms of $[D_nR]$, we have

$$[D^nR] = \frac{[R_T][D]^n}{K_D + [D]^n}$$ (34.23)

Using a derivation similar to that employed for the E_{max} model (above), we have

$$E = \frac{E_{max} \times [C_p]^n}{EC_{50}^n + [C_p]^n}$$ (34.24)

The Hill coefficient determines the "steepness" of the effect versus concentration curve. As with the E_{max} model, the response range between 20% and 80% of E_{max} is linear when plotted on semilog axes. If $n = 1$, the curve of the sigmoid E_{max} model is identical with the E_{max} model. When n is greater than 1 $(n > 1)$, the linear portion of the curve becomes steeper. Conversely, if n is less than 1 $(n < 1)$, the linear portion of the curve becomes more shallow. The value of n does not change EC_{50} and E_{max} values and all curves pass through the EC_{50} (Fig. 34.5).

The steepness of the curve can also be represented by the following equation [5]:

$$\frac{dE}{d \ln C_p} = \frac{n E_{max}}{4}$$ (34.25)

In this equation, the linear portion of the slope is directly proportional to the Hill coefficient. Theoretically, the n value reflects cooperativity in drug binding with

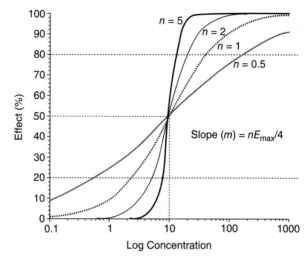

FIGURE 34.5 Effect versus concentration profiles predicted by the sigmoidal E_{max} model. If the Hill coefficient, n, is equal to 1, the curve is identical to that predicted by the E_{max} model. If $n > 1$, then the linear portion of the curve (between 20% and 80% of the maximum response) becomes steeper; and if $n < 1$, the linear portion becomes more shallow. The slope of the linear portion is equal to the Hill coefficient multiplied by one-quarter of the maximum response ($nE_{max}/4$).

specific receptors. In practical terms, the n value is determined by curve fitting and is typically considered as an empirical parameter with no defined physiological meaning. However, attempts have been made to explain the Hill coefficient pharmacologically and mechanistically. In 1994, Hoffman and Goldberg [10] suggested that the Hill coefficient reflected the extent of heterogeneity in drug receptors. They proposed that the statistical distribution of heterogeneity could affect the steepness of the effect versus concentration curve, where more homogeneous receptor populations would be associated with high values of n.

34.4 "KINETIC" MODELS OF PHARMACOLOGICAL RESPONSE

Static pharmacodynamic models are limited to consideration of equilibrium or steady-state conditions and, consequently, static models are unable to describe the time course of pharmacological effect following acute dosing. Evaluation of drug response following acute dosing, particularly where plasma concentrations change rapidly with time, often facilitates the identification of underlying mechanisms associated with drug effect. In this section, "kinetic" models are described that allow characterization of the time course of drug effect. When linked with an appropriate pharmacokinetic model, the combined pharmacokinetic–pharmacodynamic (PKPD) model allows description of the time course of drug effect as a function of the time course of drug administration.

34.4.1 Direct Effect Models

Some drug responses may be characterized as *direct effects*, where interaction of drug and the drug receptor leads to an observed response by direct action of the drug. In practical terms, a drug effect may be categorized as "direct" when all events associated with response proceed very rapidly relative to the kinetics of drug–receptor binding (e.g., consider the vasodilatory and antihypertensive effects of sodium nitroprusside, which appear to be directly and immediately related to the concentrations of sodium nitroprusside in blood). Models appropriate for direct effects are described next.

Levy's Direct Effect Model Following drug administration, the concentration of drug in the body changes with time. Thus, the drug response also changes as a function of time. The first PKPD models, introduced by Gerhard Levy [11, 12], described drugs with direct effects, where it may be assumed that there is no time delay between drug response and drug concentration. Additionally, Levy's initial model assumed rapid equilibration between the drug concentrations in plasma and at the site of action. This model consisted of a one-compartment pharmacokinetic model and log-linear pharmacodynamic model.

Equation 34.26 represents drug concentration as a function of time for a one-compartment model, where k represents a first-order elimination rate constant:

$$\ln C = \ln C_0 - kt \tag{34.26}$$

Equation 34.27 represents the log-linear model, which explains the linear relationship between response and log concentration in the response range between 20% and 80% of E_{max}:

$$E = m \ln C + e \tag{34.27}$$

Equation 34.27 may be rearranged as

$$\ln C = \frac{E - e}{m} \tag{34.28}$$

At the initial concentration, C_0, the effect can be represented by the initial effect, E_0. Thus, another equivalent equation may be derived:

$$\ln C_0 = \frac{E_0 - e}{m} \tag{34.29}$$

By substituting Eqs. 34.28 and 34.29 into Eq. 34.26, the following equation results:

$$\frac{E - e}{m} = \frac{E_0 - e}{m} - kt \tag{34.30}$$

Finally, multiplying each term by m and simplifying yields

$$E = E_0 - kmt \qquad (34.31)$$

Interestingly, the model predicts that pharmacological effect will decline linearly with time, whereas drug concentrations decline exponentially with time (Fig. 34.6) [13]. Although this model only describes the region associated with 20–80% of maximal response, this region includes the entire therapeutic working range for many approved drugs (e.g., theophylline) and, consequently, this simple model has been shown to be extremely useful.

E_{max} *Model* Levy's direct response model only covers the linear range (20–80% of maximum response) of the time course of pharmacodynamic responses. Most time courses of pharmacodynamic profiles consist of linear and nonlinear curves. To obtain a complete profile of the time course of pharmacodynamic responses, the

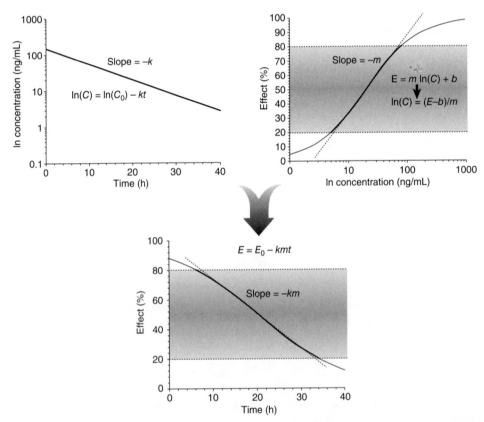

FIGURE 34.6 Levy's direct effect model. This model consists of two functions, one is pharmacokinetics (linear, one-compartment) and the other is pharmacodynamics (log-linear; E_{max} model). Note that the model predicts a linear decline in pharmacologic effect with time despite an exponential decline in drug concentration with time. Effect declines with the slope $(-km)$, reflecting both pharmacokinetics (k) and pharmacodynamics (m).

E_{max} or sigmoid E_{max} model may be linked with appropriate pharmacokinetic models. In Fig. 34.7, the time course of drug concentration and pharmacological response are shown. This decline of drug concentration is predicted from a one-compartment model after intravenous bolus injection (Eq. 34.32) and the pharmacological response curve is predicted by the E_{max} model linked to the one-compartment pharmacokinetic model (Eq. 34.33).

$$C = C_0 e^{-kt} \tag{34.32}$$

$$E = \frac{E_{max} C_0 e^{-kt}}{E_{50} + C_0 e^{-kt}} \tag{34.33}$$

Immediately following intravenous (IV) bolus injection of a drug, the model predicts a small change in the drug response despite a large change in drug concentration. This prediction is due to the saturation of receptors at high drug concentrations. Within the range of 20–80% of the maximum response, the time course of pharmacological response declines linearly as a function of time, which is consistent with Levy's direct effect model. At low concentrations, below the EC_{50}, the drug response declines in parallel with drug concentration as predicted by the log-linear model. The direct effect E_{max} model was first introduced by Wagner in 1968. Using the E_{max} model linked with one-compartment IV bolus injection model, Wagner measured the total response of various dosing intervals by calculating the area under the response–time curve (AUC_E) [9]. He demonstrated that the total response was increased substantially by decreasing the dosing interval from 24 h to

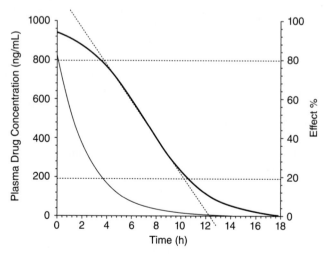

FIGURE 34.7 Predictions of a PKPD model defined with a one-compartment pharmacokinetic model and a direct effect E_{max} pharmacodynamic model. Initially, drug effect shows a plateau despite a large change of concentration, and this is due to the saturation of drug receptors at high drug concentrations. Within the range of 20–80% of maximum response, the time course of pharmacological response declines linearly as a function of time. At concentrations less than EC_{50}, drug response declines in parallel with drug concentration.

12 h (with simulated administration of the same total dose). With further decreases in the dosing interval (to 6 h or 3 h), the response continued to increase, but in smaller increments. As such, this simulation predicted that drug response could be changed by modulation of the dosing regimen, and high drug response may be achieved by dividing doses into smaller quantities given more frequently. This principle has been demonstrated in clinical studies [14, 15] and provides an early demonstration of the use of modeling and simulation to guide the selection of optimal dosing strategies.

Biophase Model   In many cases, the time course of drug effect is delayed relative to the time course of plasma concentrations. This delay between drug effect and concentration may be recognized by comparing the time value associated with maximum plasma concentrations (T_{max}) and the time value associated with maximum effect. Additionally, plotting the effect data versus plasma concentration data will often show a nonunique relationship of effect and concentration, where the same value of drug concentration is associated with two different levels of effect (Fig. 34.8). The plot of effect versus concentration will form a counterclockwise hysteresis loop, where, at a given concentration, the effect value is lower prior to T_{max} relative to effect value observed following T_{max}. Delays in the relationship between drug effect and drug concentration may be explained by several mechanisms. Common causes for delays between effect and plasma concentration include (1) distribution delays between plasma and the site of drug action (i.e., the biophase), (2) indirect effect kinetics, where the delay is related to the time course of production or elimination of an endogenous mediator of effect, (3) delays associated with the formation of an active metabolite, and (4) delays associated with transduction mechanisms. Clockwise hysteresis may also be observed in effect versus plasma concentration plots, where effect at a given concentration decreases with time. Clockwise hysteresis occurs much less frequently than counterclockwise hysteresis, and it is typically associated with the development of pharmacological tolerance [16].

The concept of drug distribution to the biophase was first introduced by Furchgott in 1955 [17], and mathematically described by Segre in 1968. Several years later, Sheiner and co-workers [18] introduced a simple model consistent with first-order drug distribution to the biophase, and this *effect site model* rapidly gained wide use. Figure 34.9 shows a simple effect site PKPD model, where a one-compartment IV bolus injection model is linked with the hypothetical effect site compartment. The differential equations for the rate of change in drug concentration of central and hypothetical effect compartments are

$$\frac{dC_p}{dt} = -k_{el}C_p \qquad (34.34)$$

$$\frac{dC_e}{dt} = k_{1e}C_e - k_{eo}C_e \qquad (34.35)$$

Solving these two differential equations yields

$$C_p = C_0 e^{-kt} \qquad (34.36)$$

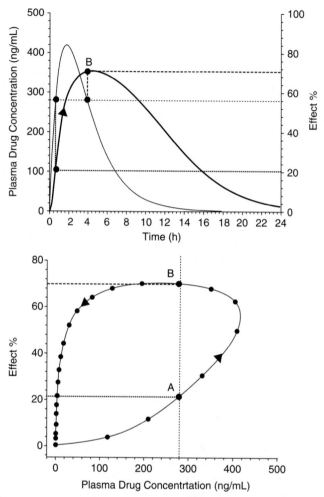

FIGURE 34.8 Counterclockwise hysteresis curve of effect versus plasma drug concentration. In case of delayed response (upper panel), plotting of effect versus plasma concentration will show a counterclockwise hysteresis loop (lower panel). Counterclockwise hysteresis loops show a nonunique relationship of effect and concentration, where a given concentration value is associated with two values of drug effect (note ascending (A) and descending (B) concentrations).

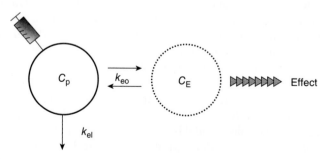

FIGURE 34.9 Biophase model. k_{el} represents the elimination rate constant of drug from the central compartment and k_{eo} represents the rate constant for drug distribution between the central and biophase compartments. (Adapted from Ref. 18.)

$$C_e = \frac{k_{1e}C_0}{k_{eo} - k_{el}}(e^{-kt} - e^{-k_{eo}t}) \tag{34.37}$$

Of note, the effect site model assumes that an insignificant quantity of drug distributes to the biophase and, consequently, the effect site compartment does not influence the plasma pharmacokinetics of the drug. The rate constants k_{1e} and k_{eo} are typically assumed to be identical for model simplification and, with this simplification, Eq. 34.37 may be rewritten as

$$C_e = \frac{k_{eo}C_0}{k_{eo} - k_{el}}(e^{-kt} - e^{-k_{eo}t}) \tag{34.38}$$

In most applications of the effect site model, the drug is assumed to produce a direct effect, which is described through the relationship of the effect site concentration, C_e, and the pharmacological response with an E_{max} or sigmoid E_{max} model.

$$E = \frac{E_{max}C_e}{E_{50} + C_e} \tag{34.39}$$

Distribution delays have also been described in PKPD models by the assumption that the biophase is within a peripheral compartment of a mammillary compartmental pharmacokinetic model [19, 20]. Although these models are quite similar to Sheiner's effect site model, some important differences exist. First, the hypothetical effect site compartment of Sheiner's model is not an actual compartment, and a negligible amount of drug is assumed to distribute to the hypothetical effect compartment. This independency between the hypothetical effect compartment and the pharmacokinetic model provides tremendous flexibility and, consequently, Sheiner's model is much more robust than models assuming that effect occurs in a peripheral pharmacokinetic compartment. Second, mammillary, multicompartment pharmacokinetic models predict that drug concentrations in the central and peripheral compartments decline in parallel; however, the biophase model allows values of k_{eo} that may be much smaller than any of the pharmacokinetic rate constants. This facilitates characterization of the time course of effects that dissipate at a rate much slower than predicted by the plasma clearance of drug (Fig. 34.10). The value of k_{eo} dictates the shape of the hysteresis curve, as shown in Fig. 34.11, and also influences the magnitude of the response, as shown in Fig. 34.12. Due to the assumption of first-order kinetics for entry and loss of drug from the biophase, the effect site model predicts that peak concentrations in the effect compartment will occur at the same time for all doses (i.e., from a given dosage regimen), and the effect site model predicts that all doses will lead to peak effects at the same time (relative to drug administration). Following large doses of drug, the effect will plateau at E_{max} and the effect versus time curve will decline linearly over the range of 20–80% of maximum effect. The biophase model is very robust, and the model has been applied successfully to characterize the delayed pharmacological responses of many drugs [21–24].

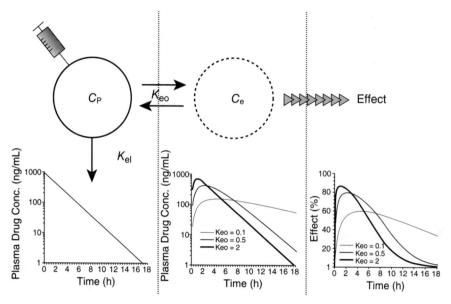

FIGURE 34.10 Simulated time course profile of effect site drug concentration and drug effect as a function of k_{eo}. Higher values of k_{eo} provide a more rapid rise and fall in effect compartment concentrations and responses that are less delayed. Small values of k_{eo}, where $k_{eo} \ll k_{el}$, leads to a "flip-flop" phenomenon where the time course of effect is very protracted relative to the time course of drug concentrations in plasma.

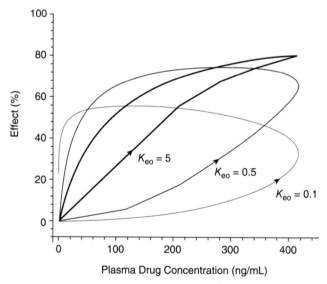

FIGURE 34.11 The impact of k_{eo} on the shape of the hysteresis loop. At high values of k_{eo}, there is rapid equilibration between plasma and effect compartment drug concentrations, and this leads to little delay in the time course of drug effect relative to drug concentration. As k_{eo} approaches infinity, the hysteresis loop collapses.

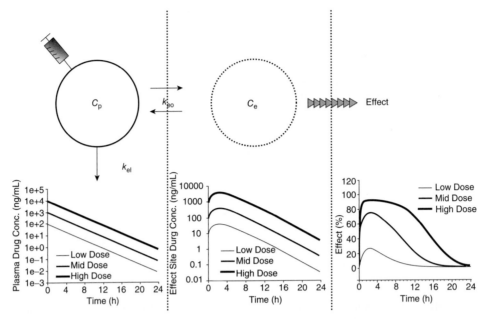

FIGURE 34.12   Biophase model simulations: effect of dose. Drug concentration versus time profiles within the hypothetical effect compartment are delayed relative to plasma concentrations; however, the time associated with peak concentrations in the effect compartment are identical for all doses. At large doses, the plateau in the response profile represents E_{max}, and the magnitude of effect declines linearly in the range of 20–80% of the maximum response.

34.4.2   Indirect Response Models

Following the introduction of the biophase model [18], many investigators used the biophase model to explain time delays in drug response with little thought as to whether the biophase model was mechanistically appropriate for the given application. Given the simple, robust nature of the biophase model, the model provided good characterization of a wide variety of response data; however, in many cases, the model did not allow simultaneous characterization of data from different doses, and the model did not allow accurate, prospective predictions of drug response. One main reason for these difficulties was the application of the biophase model to drugs that achieve effects indirectly, where the measured drug response occurs not as a direct effect, but due to the effect of drug on the production or elimination of endogenous substances associated with the measured response (Fig. 34.13).

Areins introduced the concept of indirect effects in 1964 [25], while Nagashima et al. [7] first applied an indirect effect model for PKPD to explain the effect of warfarin on the time course of prothrombin complex activity. Warfarin is an inhibitor of vitamin K epoxidase, which reduces the vitamin K epoxide to vitamin K. Vitamin K is needed for blood coagulation as a cofactor for carboxylation of clotting factors; thus, inhibition of vitamin K production results in the inhibition of coagulation [26]. Due to the indirect nature of the effect of warfarin on the measured response (coagulation), and due to the time delays associated with the elimination

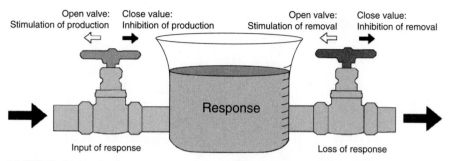

FIGURE 34.13 Indirect effects: impact of changes in the production or elimination of response mediators on the measured response. Stimulation of the production or inhibition of the elimination of response mediators will lead to an increase in the measured response. However, inhibition of input or stimulation of the elimination of response mediators will lead to a decrease in the measured response.

of vitamin K and clotting factors, the time course of warfarin effect is dramatically delayed relative to the time course of warfarin exposure, and this delay was well captured by the indirect effect model of Nagashima et al. [7] Jusko and Ko [27] subsequently developed and elaborated a family of models to allow mechanistically appropriate characterization of four common types of indirect effects.

The conceptual basis for indirect response models is provided in the differential equation

$$\frac{dR}{dt} = k_{in} - k_{out} R \tag{34.40}$$

where R refers to the measured response, k_{in} is the zero-order rate constant for the production of the response, and k_{out} is the first-order rate constant for loss of the response. Under steady-state conditions, the change of response over time becomes zero; thus, the initial response can be represented as follows:

$$R_0 = \frac{k_{in}}{k_{out}} \tag{34.41}$$

After administration of drug, the measured response (R) is changed from the effect of drug (inhibition or stimulation) on the production or dissipation of response, as a function of drug concentration. Four general submodels have been deduced (Fig. 34.14). Models I and II describe the time course of drug response by inhibition of the rate constant associated with production (k_{in}) or dissipation (k_{out}). The inhibitory function includes a parameter, I_{max}, which describes the maximal extent of inhibition; I_{max} is always greater than zero and less than or equal to one ($0 < I_{max} \leq 1$).

$$I(t) = 1 - \frac{I_{max} C_p}{IC_{50} + C_p} \tag{34.42}$$

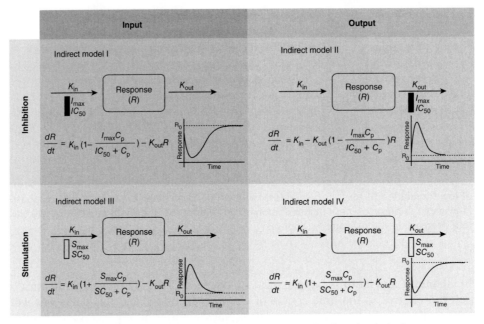

FIGURE 34.14   Basic indirect effect models. Shown are the four basic indirect response submodels (I, II, III and IV), and typical response patterns.

C_p represents the plasma concentration and IC_{50} represents the drug concentration needed to produce 50% of the maximum inhibitory response.

Models III and IV include a stimulation function $S(t)$, which affects the production or dissipation of response.

$$S(t) = 1 + \frac{S_{max}C_p}{SC_{50} + C_p} \qquad (34.43)$$

C_p represents the plasma concentration, SC_{50} represents the drug concentration that produces 50% of the maximum stimulation response, and S_{max} represents the maximum stimulation response. Unlike the inhibitory function $I(t)$, the value of S_{max} is any value greater than zero.

In model I, the rate of change in response over time may be represented by Eq. 29.43, and the results of simulation of drug response after intravenous injection of four different doses are shown in Fig. 34.15.

$$\frac{dR}{dt} = k_{in}\left(1 - \frac{I_{max}C_p}{IC_{50} + C_p}\right) - k_{out}R \qquad (34.44)$$

The "baseline" response, in the absence of drug, is assumed to be equivalent to the steady-state solution provided in Eq. 34.41. Immediately after dosing, plasma drug concentrations are high ($C_p \gg IC_{50}$), and inhibitory function $I(t)$ becomes $(1 - I_{max})$. If $I_{max} = 1$, then the term k_{in} is eliminated, and the decline of the drug response is

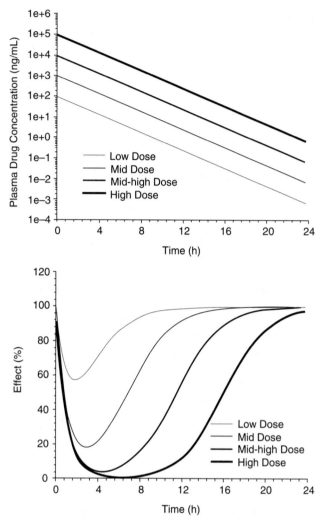

FIGURE 34.15 Simulated profile of the indirect response model I, with four different doses. As the amount of dose increases, indirect response model I predicts an increase an response and an increase in the time associated with maximum effect.

governed solely by the first-order rate of k_{out}. Thus, initial decline in the slope of the ln response versus time profile becomes $-k_{out}$. As plasma concentrations decrease, the inhibitory effect of drug decreases and, eventually, response begins to increase back to the baseline value. The minimum response value may be defined as the peak effect of drug, R_{max}. At R_{max}, the change of drug response with time will equal zero, and Eq. 34.44 may be rearranged to solve for R_{max} as follows:

$$R_{max} = \frac{k_{in}}{k_{out}}\left(1 - \frac{I_{max}C_p}{IC_{50} - C_p}\right) = R_0\left(1 - \frac{I_{max}C_p}{IC_{50} - C_p}\right) \tag{34.45}$$

When $C_p \gg IC_{50}$, the inhibitory function $I(t)$ becomes $(1 - I_{max})$, and Eq. 34.45 can be rewritten as

$$R_{max} = R_0(1 - I_{max}) \quad \text{model I} \tag{34.46}$$

In a similar manner, R_{max} for models II, III, and IV can be shown as follows:

$$\dot{R}_{max} = R_0/(1 - I_{max}) \quad \text{model II} \tag{34.47}$$

$$R_{max} = R_0(1 + S_{max}) \quad \text{model III} \tag{34.48}$$

$$R_{max} = R_0/(1 + S_{max}) \quad \text{model IV} \tag{34.49}$$

After R_{max} has been reached, the response starts to go back to baseline. However, even if the plasma drug concentration is below the IC_{50}, time is needed for reequilibration and to return back to baseline. This is the primary difference from the biophase model. In the biophase model, the delayed response is governed by the rate constant from plasma to biophase, k_{eo}; thus, the time of maximum effect is not affected by dose. However, in indirect response models, higher doses will result in a longer plateau and increase in the time of maximum effect.

Concerning the shape of the time course of the response profile, four subgroup indirect response models can be divided into two groups, with either a downward trend in response (for models I and IV) or an upward trend in response (for models II and III). In assigning an appropriate model, it is reasonable to start with consideration of the shape of the response profile. Additionally, Sharma and Jusko [28] proposed an infusion study, using multiple dosing rates to allow collection of data to assist with model selection. In many ways, the kinetics represented by the indirect response model equation are similar to those associated with IV infusion in a one-compartment pharmacokinetic model. The zero-order rate constant for the production (k_{in}) corresponds to the zero-order infusion rate (K_o), and the first-order rate constant (k_{out}) for loss of the response corresponds to the elimination rate constant of plasma compartment (k_{el}). In the case of infusion, the time to reach steady state ($t_{R_{max}}$) is governed by the elimination rate constant, not the infusion rate. Similarly, in indirect response, the time to reach maximum response is governed by k_{out}. In models I and III, $t_{R_{max}}$ is constant (for all drug infusion rates), since k_{out} is not affected by changes in "input." However, in models II and IV, $t_{R_{max}}$ would change as a function of drug infusion rate, because k_{out} is affected by the administration of drug. As such, appropriate selection of indirect models is facilitated by administration of drug over a range of infusion rates.

34.4.3 Transduction Models

The starting point for a pharmacological response is drug–receptor binding. However, in many cases, generation of pharmacological responses requires subsequent signal transduction events. For example, prednisone, a glucocorticoid hormone, binds to cytosolic receptors. The prednisone–receptor complex is then tranlocated to the nucleus, where the complex binds with DNA, modulating the rate of RNA transcription, protein production, and, finally, protein expression [29]. Such cascading steps for signal transduction require time and lead to delayed responses. Ideally, receptor

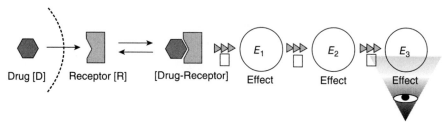

FIGURE 34.16 Transit compartment model for signal transduction. Response starts by drug–receptor binding, but the measured effect is achieved via a signal transduction process. τ represents transit time required for the signal to move from compartment to compartment in the transduction cascade. (Adapted from Ref. 30.)

and gene mediated processes should be included in a PKPD model to explain the delayed responses. However, data associated with each step in the signal transduction cascade is difficult to obtain due to limitations of technical feasibility. Although the delayed response may be due to complicated signal transduction pathways, relatively simple transit compartment models have been applied to successfully describe the time course of associated responses *in vivo* [30]. A representative transit compartment model for the signal transduction process is shown in Fig. 34.16.

As proposed by Ariens and Stephenson, the drug effects may be directly proportional to the concentration of drug–receptor complexes. The initial effective signal in a signal transduction cascade, E^*, may be defined as a function of drug–receptor complexes and the intrinsic efficacy of the drug:

$$E^* = \varepsilon \cdot [DR] \tag{34.50}$$

where ε represents the efficacy of the drug.

The E^* term may be included within any of the direct or indirect effect models described previously. For example, within the E_{max} model,

$$E^* = \frac{E_{max}C_e}{EC_{50} + C_e} \tag{34.51}$$

where C_e represents the free drug concentration at the effect site.

To characterize signal transduction, a cascade of transit compartments is employed:

$$\frac{dE}{dt} = \frac{1}{\tau}(E^* - E) = \frac{1}{\tau}\left(\frac{E_{max}C_e}{EC_{50} + C_e} - E\right) \tag{34.52}$$

where τ represents the transit time.

Additional transit compartments may be employed to allow greater delay and flexibility in the response versus time profile. If the signal transduction process involves three transit compartments, the signal transit step of each transit compartment can be represented by the following series of equations:

$$\frac{dE_1}{dt} = \frac{1}{\tau}(E^* - E_1) = \frac{1}{\tau}\left(\frac{E_{max}C_e}{EC_{50} + C_e} - E_1\right) \tag{34.53}$$

$$\frac{dE_2}{dt} = \frac{1}{\tau}(E_1 - E_2) \tag{34.54}$$

$$\frac{dE_3}{dt} = \frac{1}{\tau}(E_2 - E_3) \tag{34.55}$$

The transit time between each compartment is often assumed to be equal ($\tau = \tau_1 = \tau_2 = \tau_3$). Simulated profiles for each transit compartment, with different transit time values, are shown in Fig. 34.17. As shown in this figure, the response associated with the final transit compartment (E_3) is more delayed compared with the initial transit compartment (E_1). Also, as the transit time (τ) increases, responses become more delayed, and the maximum peak effect is decreased.

Within signal transduction processes, there is opportunity for the amplification or dampening of the signal. Power coefficients may easily be incorporated with transit compartments to account for these effects.

$$\frac{dE_3}{dt} = \frac{1}{\tau}(E_2^\gamma - E_3) \tag{34.56}$$

Simulated data associated with a range of power coefficients are shown in Fig. 34.18 in terms of simulation. For example, if the power coefficient of the last transit compartment is less than 1, the effect is lower than the unity condition. This indicates that effect is suspended between transit compartments E_2 and E_3. Conversely, if the power coefficient of the last transit compartment is greater than 1, the effect is higher than the unity condition. This indicates that effect is amplified between transit compartments E_2 and E_3 [31].

Transit compartment models are typically employed in an empirical manner to allow curve fitting with a minimal number of parameters. However, when detailed mechanistic data are available, this information may easily be added to the structure of the transit compartments to enhance the mechanistic reality of the model [33–35].

34.4.4 Irreversible Effects

Drug effects may be categorized as reversible or irreversible. Examples of irreversible effects include cell killing by action of anticancer or antimicrobial agents, irreversible enzyme inhibition, and formation of covalent drug adducts (e.g., via formation of reactive drug metabolites [1]). PKPD modeling of irreversible effects was introduced by Jusko [36] to explain chemotherapeutic effects.

A typical cell proliferation model of a chemotherapeutic agent is shown in Fig. 34.19a. The representative equation for the growth and death of cells by the action of a drug is

$$\frac{dR}{dt} = k_s \cdot R - k \cdot C \cdot R \tag{34.57}$$

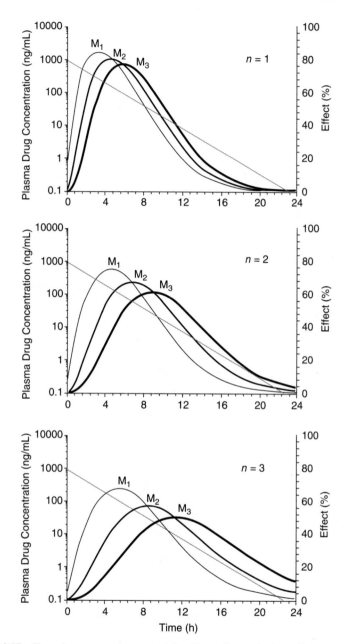

FIGURE 34.17   Transit compartment model: effect of transit time. Response in the final compartment (M_3) is delayed compared to the first effect compartment (M_1). As transit time increases, the response becomes more delayed for all three compartments, and the maximum effect decreases (upper, middle, and lower panels).

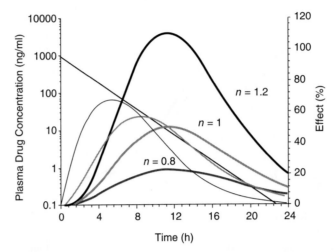

FIGURE 34.18 Transit compartment model: effect of the power coefficient. Higher values of the power coefficient ($\gamma > 1$) will amplify response; conversely, power coefficients below 1 will lead to a dampened response.

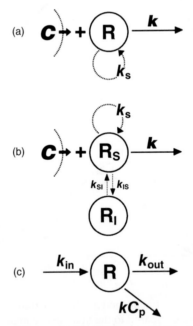

FIGURE 34.19 Representative irreversible effect model for chemotherapeutic agents. **(a)** Cell killing model for the effect of a chemotherapeutic agent. (Adapted from Ref. 36.) **(b)** Phase-specific model of cell killing. k_{SI} and k_{IS} are the rate constants for cell movement between compartments associated with sensitivity to drug and with insensitivity to drug. (Adapted from Ref. 38.) **(c)** Application of an indirect response model within a model for irreversible cell killing. (Adapted from Ref. 40.)

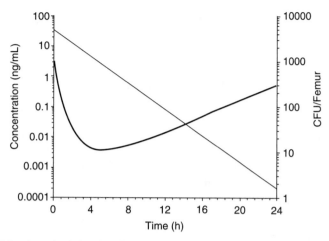

FIGURE 34.20 A typical simulated profile for the effect of a chemotherapeutic agent on cell number. The biphasic profile results from the processes of cell proliferation and drug-induced cell killing.

R represents the number of cells, k_s represents the first-order rate constant for growth rate in the natural condition, and k represents the second-order rate constant for cell killing by the action of drug. This equation includes terms for the natural growth and death of cells by the drug effect; thus, the change in the number of cells as a function of time is represented as a biphasic profile that consists of killing and regrowing phases (Fig. 34.20). The linear term for death of a cell by the drug effect (kC) can be substituted by the E_{max} model as

$$\frac{dR}{dt} = k_s \cdot R - \frac{K_{max}C}{KC_{50}+C} \cdot R \tag{34.58}$$

Using this model, Zhi et al. [37] characterized the effect of piperacillin on the killing and growth kinetic of *Pseudomonas aeruginosa*.

Some chemotherapeutic agents show cell cycle phase-specific effects. To characterize this property, Jusko [38] proposed extension of the cell proliferation model by adding an insensitive cell compartment (Fig. 34.19b):

$$\frac{dR_S}{dt} = k_S \cdot R_S - k \cdot C_S \cdot R_S - k_{SI}R_S + k_{IS}R_I \tag{34.59}$$

$$\frac{dR_I}{dt} = k_{SI}R_S - k_{IS}R_I \tag{34.60}$$

R_I represents the number of insensitive cells and k_{SI} and k_{IS} represent the rate constants for conversion into each cell compartment. The interconversion rate between sensitive and insensitive cells is governed by the rate constants k_{SI} and k_{IS}. Another modified form of this model was successfully applied to describe the pharmacodynamic effect of β-lactam antibiotics in *in vitro* bactericidal kinetics [39].

The modeling of irreversible effect can be extended to the indirect response model (Fig. 34.19c). The typical equation of an indirect response model modified for characterization of an irreversible effect is as follows:

$$\frac{dR}{dt} = k_{in} - k_{out} \cdot R - k \cdot C_p \cdot R \qquad (34.61)$$

Acetyl salicylic acid irreversibly inhibits platelet aggregation, and the turnover time of platelets is 7–10 days; thus, a small amount of aspirin shows a long duration of the antiplatelet effect. Using an irreversible effect model, Yamamoto et al. [40] explained the long duration of the antiplatelet effect of acetyl salicylic acid. The extension of this model with addition of precursor compartment was used to explain the prolonged duration of the effect of omeprazole [41].

34.4.5 Tolerance Models

Repeated or continuous exposure to several drugs such as glyceryl trinitrate, morphine, dobutamine, nicotine, cocaine, and benzodiazepines leads to clockwise hysteresis due to pharmacological tolerance [42]. Tolerance may occur due to desensitization, downregulation of receptor, or depletion of precursor. In the E_{max} model, desensitization and downregulation of drug receptors may be characterized by increasing EC_{50} and decreasing E_{max} as functions of time ($EC_{50} \cdot e^{kt}$, $E_{max} \cdot e^{-kt}$) [43]. In another mathematical model of tolerance, Porchet et al. [44] proposed the time-dependent development of a hypothetical antagonist to the effects of nicotine (Fig. 34.21a). Wakelkamp et al. [45] employed an indirect response model to describe acute tolerance to furosemide. In this model, the observed response was used to drive the production of a "modulator," which antagonized the effect of the drug (Fig. 34.21b). Equations describing this model are

$$\frac{dR}{dt} = k_{in} - k_{out} \cdot \left(1 - \frac{I_{max} \cdot ER}{IC_{50} + ER}\right) \cdot R \cdot (1 + M) \qquad (34.62)$$

$$\frac{dM}{dt} = k_{tol} \cdot R - k_{tol} \cdot M \qquad (34.63)$$

where M represents the modulator response and k_{tol} represents the first-order rate constant of loss and production of modulator responses. Among other models of tolerance is an adaptive pool model presented by Gardmark et al. [46] to describe morphine tolerance.

34.5 CONCLUSION

The relationship between the magnitude and time course of pharmacological response and the time course of drug concentrations is often complex and may be impacted by the time course of drug diffusion to the biophase, the interaction of

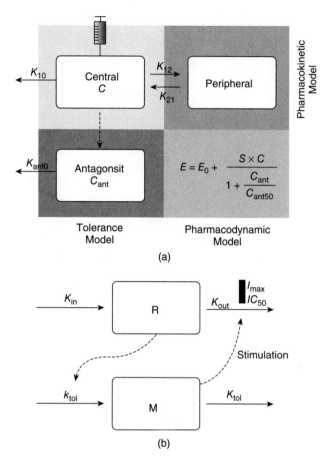

FIGURE 34.21   Representative tolerance models. **(a)** Model for acute tolerance to nicotine effect. Tolerance is generated due to the generation of a hypothetical agent that antagonizes drug effect. (Adapted from Ref. 44.) **(b)** Application of an indirect response model to describe tolerance to furosemide. Tolerance results from generation of a modulator that counteracts the effect of furosemide. (Adapted from Ref. 45.)

drug with endogenous mediators of effect, transduction or signaling events, and the development of pharmacological tolerance or sensitization. The main sequences of drug response are summarized in Fig. 34.22 [47]. As the field of PKPD modeling has progressed, there has been movement from empirical models to models that may be deemed to be more mechanistically appropriate. There is promise that mechanism-based PKPD modeling may accelerate efforts to enhance the therapeutic efficacy and safety of drug therapy, lead to rapid identification of optimal dosing strategies, and assist in testing hypotheses related to the mechanisms responsible for drug action. The catalog of models presented in this chapter offers a starting point for readers interested in using pharmacodynamic analyses to achieve these goals.

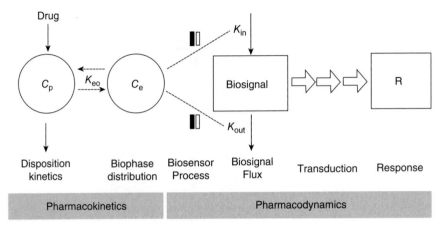

FIGURE 34.22   Pharmacokinetics and pharmacodynamics. This scheme summarizes many of the processes associated with the relationship between the time course of drug administration and the time course of drug response. The time course of response is potentially impacted by drug disposition, drug diffusion to the biophase, interaction of drug with processes associated with the production and elimination of endogenous mediators of response, and signaling pathways associated with the measured drug response. (Adapted from Ref. 47.)

ACKNOWLEDGMENTS

Work on this chapter was supported by Grants AI60687 and CA118213 from the National Institutes of Health. Dr. Beom Soo Shin is supported by a fellowship provided by Pfizer, Inc.

REFERENCES

1. Jusko WJ. In *Course on Pharmacokinetic–Pharmacodynamic Modeling Concepts and Applications*. Buffalo, NY: The State University of New York; 2006.
2. Clark AJ. The reaction between acetyl choline and muscle cells. *J Physiol* 1926;61: 530–546.
3. Ariens EJ, De Groot WM. Affinity and intrinsic-activity in the theory of competitive inhibition. III. Homologous decamethonium-derivatives and succinyl-choline-esters. *Arch Int Pharmacodyn Ther* 1954;99:193–205.
4. Stephenson RP. A modification of receptor theory. *Br J Pharmacol Chemother* 1956;11: 379–393.
5. Levy G. In *Course of Pharmacokinetic–Pharmacodynamic Modeling: Concepts and Applications*. Buffalo, NY: The State University of New York; 1995.
6. McDevitt DG, Shand DG. Plasma concentrations and the time-course of beta blockade due to propranolol. *Clin Pharmacol Ther* 1975;18:708–713.
7. Nagashima R, O'Reilly RA, Levy G. Kinetics of pharmacologic effects in man: the anticoagulant action of warfarin. *Clin Pharmacol Ther* 1969;10:22–35.
8. Hill AV. The possible effects of the aggregation of the molecules of hemoglobin on its dissociation curves. *J Physiol (London)* 1910;61:530–546.

9. Wagner JG. Kinetics of pharmacologic response. I. Proposed relationships between response and drug concentration in the intact animal and man. *J Theor Biol* 1968;20: 173–201.

10. Hoffman A, Goldberg A. The relationship between receptor–effector unit heterogeneity and the shape of the concentration–effect profile: pharmacodynamic implications. *J Pharmacokinet Biopharm* 1994;22:449–468.

11. Levy G. Relationship between elimination rate of drugs and rate of decline of their pharmacologic effects. *J Pharm Sci* 1964;53:342–343.

12. Levy G. Kinetics of pharmacologic effects. *Clin Pharmacol Ther* 1966;7:362–372.

13. Levy G. Pharmacokinetics of succinylcholine in newborns. *Anesthesiology* 1970;32: 551–552.

14. Alvan G, Paintaud G, Wakelkamp M. The efficiency concept in pharmacodynamics. *Clin Pharmacokinet* 1999;36:375–389.

15. Lalonde RL, Pieper JA, Straka RJ, Bottorff MB, Mirvis DM. Propranolol pharmacokinetics and pharmacodynamics after single doses and at steady-state. *Eur J Clin Pharmacol* 1987;33:315–318.

16. Girard P, Boissel JP. Clockwise hysteresis or proteresis. *J Pharmacokinet Biopharm* 1989;17:401–402.

17. Furchgott RF. The pharmacology of vascular smooth muscle. *Pharmacol Rev* 1955;7: 183–265.

18. Sheiner LB, Stanski DR, Vozeh S, Miller RD, Ham J. Simultaneous modeling of pharmacokinetics and pharmacodynamics: application to *d*-tubocurarine. *Clin Pharmacol Ther* 1979;25:358–371.

19. Kramer WG, Kolibash AJ, Lewis RP, Bathala MS, Visconti JA, Reuning RH. Pharmacokinetics of digoxin: relationship between response intensity and predicted compartmental drug levels in man. *J Pharmacokinet Biopharm* 1979;7:47–61.

20. Wagner JG, Aghajanian GK, Bing OH. Correlation of performance test scores with "tissue concentration" of lysergic acid diethylamide in human subjects. *Clin Pharmacol Ther* 1968;9:635–638.

21. Hammarlund-Udenaes M, Paalzow LK, De Lange EC. Drug equilibration across the blood–brain barrier—pharmacokinetic considerations based on the microdialysis method. *Pharm Res* 1997;14:128–134.

22. Collins JM, Dedrick RL. Distributed model for drug delivery to CSF and brain tissue. *Am J Physiol* 1983;245:R303–R310.

23. Wang Y, Welty DF. The simultaneous estimation of the influx and efflux blood–brain barrier permeabilities of gabapentin using a microdialysis-pharmacokinetic approach. *Pharm Res* 1996;13:398–403.

24. Gupta SK, Ellinwood EH, Nikaido AM, Heatherly DG. Simultaneous modeling of the pharmacokinetic and pharmacodynamic properties of benzodiazepines. I: Lorazepam. *J Pharmacokinet Biopharm* 1990;18:89–102.

25. Ariens EJ. *Molecular Pharmacology*. New York: Academic Press; 1964.

26. Whitlon DS, Sadowski JA, Suttie JW. Mechanism of coumarin action: significance of vitamin K epoxide reductase inhibition. *Biochemistry* 1978;17:1371–1377.

27. Jusko WJ, Ko HC. Physiologic indirect response models characterize diverse types of pharmacodynamic effects. *Clin Pharmacol Ther* 1994;56:406–419.

28. Sharma A, Jusko WJ. Characteristics of indirect pharmacodynamic models and applications to clinical drug responses. *Br J Clin Pharmacol* 1998;45:229–239.

29. Boudinot FD, D'Ambrosio R, Jusko WJ. Receptor-mediated pharmacodynamics of prednisolone in the rat. *J Pharmacokinet Biopharm* 1986;14:469–493.

30. Mager DE, Jusko WJ. Pharmacodynamic modeling of time-dependent transduction systems. *Clin Pharmacol Ther* 2001;70:210–216.

31. Sun YN, Jusko WJ. Transit compartments versus gamma distribution function to model signal transduction processes in pharmacodynamics. *J Pharm Sci* 1998;87:732–737.

32. Oosterhuis B, Braat MC, Roos CM, Wemer J, Van Boxtel CJ. Pharmacokinetic–pharmacodynamic Modeling of Terbutaline bronchodilation in asthma. *Clin Pharmacol Ther* 1986;40:469–475.

33. Nichols AI, Boudinot FD, Jusko WJ. Second generation model for prednisolone pharmacodynamics in the rat. *J Pharmacokinet Biopharm* 1989;17:209–227.

34. Sun YN, DuBois DC, Almon RR, Jusko WJ. Fourth-generation model for corticosteroid pharmacodynamics: a model for methylprednisolone effects on receptor/gene-mediated glucocorticoid receptor down-regulation and tyrosine aminotransferase induction in rat liver. *J Pharmacokinet Biopharm* 1998;26:289–317.

35. Xu ZX, Sun YN, DuBois DC, Almon RR, Jusko WJ. Third-generation model for corticosteroid pharmacodynamics: roles of glucocorticoid receptor mRNA and tyrosine aminotransferase mRNA in rat liver. *J Pharmacokinet Biopharm* 1995;23:163–181.

36. Jusko WJ. Pharmacodynamics of chemotherapeutic effects: dose–time-response relationships for phase-nonspecific agents. *J Pharm Sci* 1971;60:892–895.

37. Zhi JG, Nightingale CH, Quintiliani R. Microbial pharmacodynamics of piperacillin in neutropenic mice of systematic infection due to *Pseudomonas aeruginosa*. *J Pharmacokinet Biopharm* 1988;16:355–375.

38. Jusko WJ. A pharmacodynamic model for cell-cycle-specific chemotherapeutic agents *J Pharmacokinet Biopharm* 1973;1:175–200.

39. Yano Y, Oguma T, Nagata H, Sasaki S. Application of logistic growth model to pharmacodynamic analysis of *in vitro* bactericidal kinetics. *J Pharm Sci* 1988;87:1177–1183.

40. Yamamoto K, Abe M, Katashima M, Sawada Y. Pharmacodynamic analysis of antiplatelet effect of aspirin in literature—modeling based on inhibition of cyclooxygenase in the platelet and the vessel wall endothelium. *Jpn J Hosp Pharm* 1996;22:113–141.

41. Abelo A, Eriksson UG, Karlsson MO, Larsson H, Gabrielsson J. A turnover model of irreversible inhibition of gastric acid secretion by omeprazole in the dog. *J Pharmacol Exp Ther* 2000;295:662–669.

42. Gardmark M, Brynne L, Hammarlund-Udenaes M, Karlsson MO. Interchangeability and predictive performance of empirical tolerance models. *Clin Pharmacokinet* 1999;36:145–167.

43. Lalonde RL. In Burton ME, Shaw LM, Schentag JJ, Evans WE, Eds. *Applied Pharmacokinetics & Pharmacodynamics*. Baltimore: Lippincott Williams & Wilkins; 2006, pp 60–81.

44. Porchet HC, Benowitz NL, Sheiner LB. Pharmacodynamic model of tolerance: application to nicotine. *J Pharmacol Exp Ther* 1988;244:231–236.

45. Wakelkamp M, Alvan G, Gabrielsson J, Paintaud G. Pharmacodynamic modeling of furosemide tolerance after multiple intravenous administration. *Clin Pharmacol Ther* 1996;60:75–88.

46. Gardmark M, Karlsson MO, Jonsson F, Hammarlund-Udenaes M. Morphine-3-glucuronide has a minor effect on morphine antinociception. Pharmacodynamic modeling. *J Pharm Sci* 1998;87:813–820.

47. Jusko WJ, Ko HC, Ebling WF. Convergence of direct and indirect pharmacodynamic response models. *J Pharmacokinet Biopharm* 1995;23:5–8.

35

PHYSIOLOGICALLY BASED PHARMACOKINETIC MODELING

HARVEY J. CLEWELL III,[1] MICAELA B. REDDY,[2] THIERRY LAVÉ,[3] AND MELVIN E. ANDERSEN[1]

[1]*The Hamner Institutes for Health Sciences, Research Triangle Park, North Carolina*
[2]*Roche Palo Alto LLC, Palo Alto, California*
[3]*F. Hoffmann-La Roche Ltd., Basel, Switzerland*

Contents

35.1   INTRODUCTION

Pharmacokinetics is the quantitative study of factors that control the time course for absorption, distribution, metabolism, and excretion (ADME) of compounds within the body. Pharmacokinetic (PK) models provide sets of equations that simulate the time courses of compounds and their metabolites in various tissues throughout the body. The interest in PK modeling in pharmacology and toxicology arose from the need to relate internal concentrations of active compounds at their target sites with the doses of the compound given to an animal or human subject. The reason, of course, is a fundamental tenet in pharmacology or toxicology that both beneficial and adverse responses to compounds are related to the free concentrations of active compounds reaching target tissues rather than the amounts of compound at the site of absorption. The relationships between tissue dose and administered dose can be complex, especially in high dose toxicity testing studies, with multiple, repeated daily dosing, or when metabolism or toxicity at routes of entry alter uptake processes for various routes of exposure. PK models of all kinds are primarily a tool to assess internal dosimetry at target tissues for a wide range of exposure situations.

In the 1930s, Teorell [1, 2] provided a set of equations for uptake, distribution, and elimination of drugs from the body. These papers are rightly regarded as providing the first physiological model for drug distribution. However, computational methods were not available to solve the sets of equations at that time. Exact mathematical solutions for distribution of compounds in the body could only be obtained for simplified models in which the body was reduced to a small number of compartments that did not correspond directly with specific physiological compartments. Over the next thirty years, PK modeling focused on these simpler descriptions with exact solutions rather than on developing models more concordant with the structure and content of the biological system itself. These approaches are sometimes referred to as *data-based* compartmental modeling, since the work generally took the form of a detailed collection of time-course blood/excreta concentrations at various doses. Time-course curves were analyzed by assuming particular model structures and estimating a small number of model parameters by curve-fitting. In the earliest of these models, all processes for metabolism, distribution, and elimination were treated as first order (i.e., rates changed in direct proportion to the concentration of the chemical species). Two areas of concern that particularly affected data-based compartmental PK modeling arose in the 1960s and early 1970s: (1) the saturation of elimination pathways and (2) the possibility that blood flow rather than metabolic capacity of an organ might limit clearance. Saturation led to models that were not first order, making it difficult to derive exact solutions to the sets of equations, while blood-flow-limited metabolism in an organ meant that the removal rate constant from a central compartment could not increase indefinitely as the metabolic capacity increased [3].

Scientists trained in chemical engineering and computational methods developed physiologically based pharmacokinetic (PBPK) models for chemotherapeutic compounds [4]. Many of these compounds are highly toxic and have therapeutic efficacy by being slightly more toxic to rapidly growing cells (the cancer cells) than to normal tissues. Initial successes with methotrexate [5] led to PBPK models for other compounds, including 5-fluorouracil [6] and cisplatin [7]. These seminal contributions showed the ease with which realistic descriptions of physiology and relevant pathways of metabolism could be incorporated into PBPK models and paved the way for their more extensive use.

Although PBPK modeling was initially developed in the pharmaceutical industry [8–10], its recent use has primarily been in the area of environmental risk assessment. In the pharmaceutical area, the use of PBPK models was limited in drug development mainly due to the perceived mathematical complexity of the models and the labor-intensive input data required. However, advances in the prediction of hepatic metabolism and tissue distribution from *in vitro* and *in silico* data have made the use of these models more attractive, providing the opportunity to integrate key input data from different sources to not only estimate PK parameters and predict plasma and tissue concentration–time profiles, but also to gain mechanistic insight into the compound's properties. Thus, there is recent evidence of growing interest in applying PBPK models for the discovery and development of drugs [11, 12]. Strategies for PBPK application in drug research are being published [13, 14] and several commercial PBPK simulation tools have recently become available (e.g., GastroPlus™ and PK-Sim®, to name a few).

Some of the inertia to developing PBPK models was also due to the idea that extrapolations were unnecessary since human PK data would eventually be developed in clinical studies. This viewpoint neglects other attributes inherent in PBPK approaches. Some of the capabilities offered by PBPK approaches that have driven their extensive use in environmental risk assessment are: (1) creating models from physiological, biochemical, and anatomical information, entirely separate from collection of detailed concentration time-course curves; (2) evaluating mechanisms by which biological processes govern disposition of a wide range of compounds by comparison of PK results with model predictions; (3) using compounds as probes of the biological processes to gain more general information on the way biochemical characteristics govern the importance of various transport pathways in the body; (4) applying the models in safety assessments; and (5) using annotation of a modeling database as a repository of information on toxicity and kinetics of specific compounds [8]. Due to these perceived advantages, PBPK modeling was adopted as a tool for toxicological investigations and risk assessment in the early 1980s and many advances were made in this area. Recently, PBPK modeling has received new attention from the pharmaceutical industry. Lupfert and Reichel [11] recently wrote:

"The stage is set for a wide penetration of PBPK modeling and simulations to form an intrinsic part of a project starting from lead discovery, to lead optimization and candidate selection, to preclinical profiling and clinical trials."

Here, we present fundamental information necessary to understanding the application of PBPK models in preclinical drug development. Next, we describe the emerging role of PBPK modeling in the pharmaceutical industry in terms of advances in the available tools and increasingly used applications. Additionally, we provide our thoughts on potential applications that have not yet been widely explored. Although some advances have been made in applying PBPK modeling in the development of biotherapeutics (e.g., PBPK modeling for monoclonal antibodies in the mouse [15] and human [16]), this chapter is primarily geared toward small molecules.

35.1.1   Noncompartmental, Compartmental, and PBPK Modeling

Noncompartmental analysis (NCA) is widely used in the pharmaceutical industry for the analysis of single-dose PK (SDPK) data and PK data generated during safety studies. NCA, which involves calculating parameters such as steady-state volume of distribution (V_{ss}), clearance (CL), area under the plasma concentration curve (AUC), and peak plasma concentration (C_{max}) based solely on experimental data (i.e., these calculations are model independent), is a convenient way to understand, tabulate, and compare the PK properties of compounds. NCA results are easy to understand and a standard analysis technique. However, NCA results cannot be used to perform simulations or extrapolate to other exposure conditions. Although it is possible to use NCA parameters in a one-compartment model for performing simulations, this method is not likely to result in accurate predictions of pharmacokinetics.

Classical PK models are less commonly used than NCA calculations, but are used to perform simulations (e.g., use data generated for one experimental design to simulate a different experimental design). For example, a compartment model parameterized with intravenous (IV) SDPK data can be used to simulate an IV infusion study, and compartment modeling can be used to predict steady-state pharmacokinetics from SDPK data. Standard software packages often provide flexible tools for developing one-, two-, and three-compartment models from time-course plasma concentrations and provide statistical tools for discriminating between models. Compartment models require more mathematical skill than NCA but are still easy to use. However, the parameters and compartments in compartment models have no physiological meaning and provide no basis for extrapolating from the conditions of the experimental data used to develop the model.

PBPK models differ from classical PK models in that they include specific compartments for tissues involved in exposure, toxicity, biotransformation, and clearance processes connected by blood flow; compartments and blood flows are described using physiologically meaningful parameters, which allows for interspecies extrapolation by altering the physiological parameters appropriately. As with compartment models, PBPK models can be used to simulate a variety of conditions. Because the models have a mechanistic basis, extrapolation to situations differing from the conditions of the data used to calibrate the model is justifiable [17]. PBPK modeling has been used to great effect for interspecies extrapolation, both among animal models [18] and for predicting human pharmacokinetics based on animal data [13, 19]. The mechanistic basis of PBPK models allows for applications such as understanding species differences in pharmacokinetics, determining if results from different experimental designs are consistent, and exploring possible mechanisms responsible for unexpected or unusual data. These attributes have led to widespread development of PBPK models in recent years [20].

Possibly the primary reason that PBPK models fell out of favor in the pharmaceutical industry is that PBPK models require more than the plasma time-course concentrations that are required by NCA and compartment models. PBPK models require physiological, physicochemical, and biochemical parameters. The physiological, mechanistic basis of the models is both their strength (the mechanistic basis provides exception utility) and their weakness (PBPK models can be expensive and time consuming to construct). However, recent contributions to the literature have demonstrated the effective application of PBPK models using the data normally generated during preclinical development [13, 14, 21, 22]. While NCA and compartment models will always be useful for many routine applications, PBPK modeling can be used for many situations when NCA and compartmental modeling simply cannot be used.

35.1.2   Modeling and Simulation Considerations in the Generation of Drug Metabolism and Pharmacokinetic (DMPK) Data

In preclinical drug development, an array of data is generated to investigate the potential of prospective drug candidates to have drug-like ADME properties in humans (Table 35.1). Preliminary screens tend to have high throughput and quick turnaround times, but less physiological relevance. As increasingly promising compounds are identified, ADME assays with more physiological relevance, but lower throughput and higher cost, are utilized. In the past, the conceptual model underlying preclinical development could be described as a filtering approach. The medicinal chemists would generate many candidates, and as compounds went through an array of screens for pharmacological, DMPK, and toxicological properties, compounds would be slowly eliminated from consideration until only the best compounds (clinical candidates) remained.

More recently, a different paradigm analogous to a cycle has been adopted. Medicinal chemists generate compounds that are tested for pharmacological activity. In parallel or in series, key ADME screening assays are employed to test for known liabilities of a class of compounds. For example, typical primary screens might be for permeability or metabolic stability, but should drug–drug interactions (DDIs) be a key liability for a given chemical class, then the appropriate DDI screen might be chosen as a primary screen, for example, to avoid the key liability of inhibition and/or induction of CYP3A4 by protease inhibitors for HIV [23]. Screening data is fed back to chemists, who go on to design better molecules based on assay results. The best compounds make it through the screening process to undergo more physiologically relevant, more expensive screens. Regardless of the screening cascade determined to be the best choice for a specific pharmacological target, much of the data generated is useful input for PBPK models. However, to ensure that PBPK modeling can be used to best advantage, a modeling strategy should be considered when making data generation choices.

TABLE 35.1 Common Screening Tools Used to Understand ADME Properties in Preclinical Development

Absorption	Distribution	Metabolism	Excretion
Physicochemical properties (calculated and measured)	Protein binding	Stability in biological fluids	Urinary excretion
Solubility	Equilibrium dialysis	Plasma, blood stability	*In vitro* MDCK and HEK
Log *P*	Ultracentrifugation	Gut metabolism	*In situ* isolated, perfused rat kidney
Log *D*	Ultrafiltration	Caco-2 stability	*In vivo* urine measurement
pK_a	Distribution in blood	Intestinal microsomes	Biliary excretion
Polar surface area	Blood-to-plasma ratio	Bile, gut fluids	*In vitro* hepatocytes
Permeability	CNS penetration	Hepatic metabolism	*In situ* isolated, perfused rat liver
Artificial membrane	Permeability assays	Liver microsomes	*In vivo* bile duct cannulated rats or dogs
PAMPA	*In vitro* Caco-2	Hepatocytes	Transporter assays
In vitro models	Transporter assays	Liver S-9, cytosol, slices	
Caco-2 cell line	*In vivo* time-course tissue concentrations, microdialysis, mdr1a +/+, −/− mice	Metabolic pathway	
MDCK cell line		Metabolite ID *in vitro*, *in vivo*, and *in situ*	
P_{eff} with P-gp inhibited	*In vivo* PK	Reaction phenotyping	
In vivo models	Volume of distribution	Recombinant CYPs	
Bioavailability		Liver microsomes with P450	
Portal vein cannulated animals		Inhibition	
Transporter assays		CYP, UGT	
Cell lines		Induction	
Oocytes		PXR	
		Hepatocyte RNA, activity	

The integration of preclinical data is a key to selecting good compounds for clinical development. The most common method for selecting compounds is by eliminating the compounds that fail to meet criteria for DMPK screens, and then picking the best candidate from the remaining compounds based on efficacy and other concerns. But take, for example, a choice between the following compounds: compound A has excellent efficacy in a rat pharmacology bioassay and good bioavailability, but has much higher protein binding in humans than rats, while compound B has good efficacy and good bioavailability, but has protein binding in humans similar to that of rats. Which compound should be chosen to move forward? We suggest integrating all available preclinical data using PBPK modeling, and whenever feasible integrating pharmacology data to develop the PK/PD (PK/pharmacodynamic) relationship, to come up with the most accurate, quantitative interpretation of the dataset and, therefore, the most science-driven selection of the clinical candidate.

35.2 PBPK MODELING FUNDAMENTALS

The basic approach for the development of a PBPK description is illustrated in Fig. 35.1. The process of model development begins with the identification of the compound and effect of concern. Literature evaluation involves the integration of available information about mechanisms of efficacy and/or toxicity, pathways of biochemical metabolism, the nature of the active compound processes involved in absorption, transport, and excretion, tissue partitioning and binding characteristics, and physiological parameters (e.g., tissue weights and blood flow rates) for the species of interest. Using this information, the investigator develops a PBPK model that expresses mathematically a conception of the animal/chemical system. In the

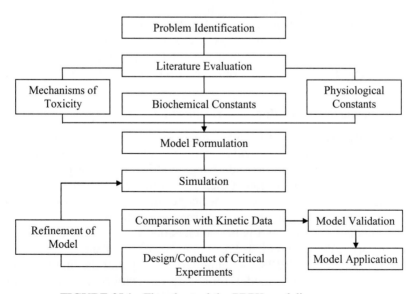

FIGURE 35.1 Flowchart of the PBPK modeling process.

model, the various time-dependent biological processes are described as a system of simultaneous differential equations. A mathematical model of this form can easily be written and exercised using commonly available computer software. The specific structure of the model is driven by the need to estimate the appropriate measure of tissue dose under the various exposure conditions of concern in both the experimental animal and the human. Before the model can be used with confidence, it has to be validated against kinetic information and, in many cases, refined based on comparison with the experimental results. The model itself can frequently be used to help design critical experiments to collect data needed for its own validation.

The chief advantage of a PBPK model over an empirical description is its greater predictive power. Since known physiological parameters are used, a different species can be modeled by simply replacing the appropriate constants with those for the species of interest, or by allometric scaling [18, 24, 25]. Similarly, the behavior for a different route of administration can be determined by adding equations that describe the nature of the new input function.

Since measured physicochemical and biochemical parameters are used, the behavior for a different compound can quickly be estimated by determining the appropriate constants. An important result is the ability to reduce the need for extensive experiments with new compounds. The process of selecting the most informative experimental data is also facilitated by the availability of a predictive PK model. Perhaps the most desirable feature of a physiologically based model is that it provides a conceptual framework for employing the scientific method in which the hypothesis can be described in terms of biological processes, predictions can be made on the basis of the description, and the hypothesis can be revised on the basis of comparison with experimental data.

The trade-off against the greater predictive capability of physiologically based models is the requirement for an increased number of parameters and equations. However, values for many of the parameters, particularly the physiological ones, are already available in the literature [4, 26–30], and *in vitro* techniques have been developed for rapidly determining the compound-specific parameters [31]. An important advantage of PBPK models is that they provide a biologically meaningful quantitative framework within which *in vitro* data can be more effectively utilized [32]. There is even a prospect that predictive PBPK models can someday be developed based almost entirely on data obtained from *in vitro* studies.

35.2.1 Elements of PBPK Model Development

This section explores some of the key issues associated with the development of PBPK models. It is meant to provide a general understanding of the basic design concepts and mathematical forms underlying the PBPK modeling process and is not meant to be a complete exposition of the PBPK modeling approach for all possible cases. It must be understood that the specifics of the approach can vary greatly for different types of compounds and for different applications.

Model building is an art and is best understood as an iterative process in the spirit of the scientific method [33–35]. A number of excellent reviews have been written on the subject of PBPK modeling [20, 36, 37], and the literature includes examples of successful PBPK models for a wide variety of compounds that provide a wealth of insight into various aspects of the PBPK modeling process [20]. These sources should be consulted for further detail on the approach for applying the PBPK methodology in specific cases.

Tissue Grouping   The first aspect of PBPK model development that will be discussed is determining the extent to which the various tissues in the body may be grouped together. Although tissue grouping is really just one aspect of model design, which is discussed in the next section, it provides a simple context for introducing the two alternative approaches to PBPK model development: *lumping* and *splitting*. In the context of tissue grouping, the guiding philosophy in the lumping approach can be stated as: "Tissues that are pharmacokinetically and toxicologically indistinguishable may be grouped together." In this approach, model development begins with information at the greatest level of detail that is practical, and decisions are made to combine physiological elements (tissues and blood flows) to the extent justified by their similarity [38]. The common grouping of tissues into richly (or rapidly) perfused and poorly (or slowly) perfused on the basis of their perfusion rate (ratio of blood flow to tissue volume) is an example of the lumping approach. The contrasting philosophy of splitting can be stated as: "Tissues that are pharmacokinetically or toxicologically distinct must be separated." This approach starts with the simplest reasonable model structure and increases the model's complexity only to the extent required to reproduce data on the compound of concern for the application of interest. Lumping (starting with a large number of compartments and then testing whether they can be combined) requires the greater initial investment in data collection and, if taken to the extreme, could paralyze model development. On the other hand, splitting (starting with a small number of compartments and only increasing complexity if the simple model fails) is more efficient but runs a greater risk of overlooking compound-specific determinants of disposition.

There are two alternative approaches for determining whether tissues are kinetically distinct or can be lumped together. In the first approach, the tissue rate constants are compared. The rate constant (k_T) for a tissue is similar to the perfusion rate except that the partitioning characteristics of the tissue are also considered:

$$k_T = Q_T/(P_T \cdot V_T)$$

where Q_T is the blood flow to the tissue (L/h), P_T is the tissue:blood partition coefficient for the compound, and V_T is the volume of the tissue (L). Thus, the units of the tissue rate constant are the same as for the perfusion rate, L/h, but the rate constant more accurately reflects the kinetic characteristics of a tissue for a particular compound.

The second, less rigorous, approach for determining whether tissues should be lumped together is simply to compare the performance of the model with the tissues combined and separated. The reliability of this approach depends on the availability of data under conditions where the tissues being evaluated would be expected to have an observable impact on the kinetics of the compound. Sensitivity analysis can sometimes be used to determine the appropriate conditions for such a comparison [39].

Model Design Criteria   The alternative approaches to tissue grouping discussed previously are actually reflections of two competing criteria that must be balanced during model design: *parsimony* and *plausibility*. The principle of parsimony simply states that a model should be as simple as possible for the intended application (but no simpler). This "splitting" philosophy is related to that of Occam's razor: "Entities should not be multiplied unnecessarily." That is, structures and parameters should not be included in the model unless they are needed to support the application for which the model is being designed.

There is no easy rule for determining the structure and level of complexity needed in a particular modeling application. The decision of which elements to include in the model structure for a specific compound and application draws on all of the modeler's experience and knowledge of the animal–chemical system. The wide variability of PBPK model design for different compounds can be seen by comparing the diagram of the PBPK model for methotrexate [5], shown in Fig. 35.2, with the diagram for the retinoic acid PBPK model [19], shown in Fig. 35.3.

The desire for parsimony in model development is driven not only by the desire to minimize the number of parameters whose values must be identified, but also by the recognition that as the number of parameters increases, the potential for unintended interactions between parameters also increases. A generally accepted rule of software engineering warns that it is relatively easy to design a computer program that is too complicated to be completely comprehended by the human mind. As a model becomes more complex, it becomes increasingly difficult to validate, even as the level of concern for the trustworthiness of the model should increase.

Countering the desire for model parsimony is the need for plausibility of the model structure. As discussed in Section 35.1, it is the physiological and biochemical realism of PBPK models that gives them an advantage for extrapolation. The

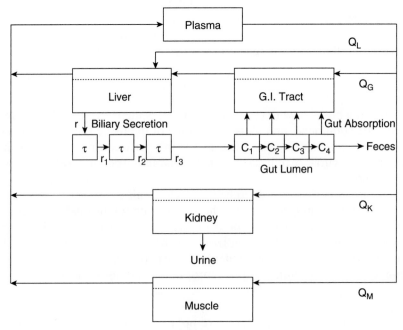

FIGURE 35.2   PBPK model for methotrexate [5].

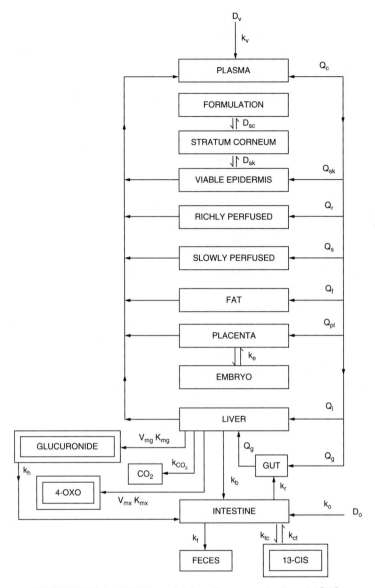

FIGURE 35.3 PBPK model for all-*trans*-retinoic acid [19].

credibility of a PBPK model's predictions of kinetic behavior under conditions different from those under which the model was validated rests to a large extent on the correspondence of the model design to known physiological and biochemical structures. In general, the ability of a model to adequately simulate the behavior of a physical system depends on the extent to which the model structure is homomorphic (having a one-to-one correspondence) with the essential features determining the behavior of that system.

Model Identification   The process of model identification begins with the selection of those model elements that the modeler considers to be minimum essential determinants of the behavior of the particular animal–chemical system under study, from the viewpoint of the intended application of the model. Comparison with appropriate data, relevant to the intended purpose of the model, can then provide insights into defects in the model that must be corrected either by reparameterization or by changes to the model structure. Unfortunately, it is not always possible to separate these two elements. In models of biological systems, estimates of the values of model parameters will always be uncertain, due both to biological variation and experimental error. At the same time, the need for biological realism unavoidably results in models that are "overparameterized"; that is, they contain more parameters than can be identified from the kinetic data the model is used to describe.

Model identification is the selection of a specific model structure from several alternatives, based on conformity of the models' predictions to experimental observations. The practical reality of model identification in the case of biological systems is that regardless of the complexity of the model there will always be some level of "model error" (lack of homomorphism), which will result in systematic discrepancies between the model and experimental data. This model structural deficiency interacts with deficiencies in the identifiability of the model parameters, potentially leading to misidentification of the parameters or misspecification of structures. This most dangerous aspect of model identification is exacerbated by the fact that, in general, adding equations and parameters to a model increases the model's degrees of freedom, improving its ability to reproduce data, regardless of the validity of the underlying structure. Therefore, when a particular model structure improves the agreement of the model with kinetic data, it can only be said that the model structure is "consistent" with the kinetic data; it cannot be said that the model structure has been "proved" by its consistency with the data. In such circumstances, it is imperative that the physiological or biochemical hypothesis underlying the model structure is tested using nonkinetic data.

35.2.2   Elements of Model Structure

The process of selecting a model structure can be broken down into a number of elements associated with the different aspects of uptake, distribution, metabolism, and elimination. This section treats each of these elements in turn.

Storage Compartments   Naturally, any tissues that are expected to accumulate significant quantities of the compound or its metabolites need to be included in the model structure. As discussed earlier, these storage tissues can be grouped together to the extent that they have similar time constants. The muscle tissue in the methotrexate model (Fig. 35.2) is an example of a storage compartment. The generic mass balance equation for storage compartments such as these is

$$dA_T/dt = Q_T \cdot C_A - Q_T \cdot C_{VT}$$

where A_T is the mass of compound in the tissue (mg), C_A is the concentration of compound in the arterial blood reaching the tissue (mg/L), and C_{VT} is the concentration of compound in the venous blood leaving the tissue (mg/L). Thus, this mass balance equation simply states that the rate of change in the amount of compound in the tissue with respect to time (dA_T/dt) is equal to the difference between the rate at which compound enters the tissue and the rate at which compound leaves the tissue. We can then calculate the concentration of the compound in the storage tissue (C_T) from the amount in the tissue and the tissue volume (V_T):

$$C_T = A_T/V_T$$

In PBPK models, it is common to assume *venous equilibration*; that is, that in the time that it takes for the blood to perfuse the tissue, the compound is able to achieve its equilibrium distribution between the tissue and blood. Therefore, the concentration of the compound in the venous blood can be related to the concentration in the tissue by the equilibrium tissue : blood partition coefficient, P_T:

$$C_{VT} = C_T/P_T$$

Therefore, we obtain a differential equation in A_T:

$$dA_T/dt = Q_T \cdot C_A - Q_T \cdot A_T/(P_T \cdot V_T)$$

If desired, we can reformulate this mass balance equation in terms of concentration:

$$dA_T/dt = d(C_T \cdot V_T)/dt = C_T \cdot dV_T/dt + V_T \cdot dC_T/dt$$

If (and only if) V_T is constant (i.e., the tissue does not grow during the simulation), $dV_T/dt = 0$, and

$$dA_T/dt = V_T \cdot dC_T/dt$$

so we have the alternative differential equation:

$$dC_T/dt = Q_T \cdot (C_A - C_T/P_T)/V_T$$

This alternative mass balance formulation, in terms of concentration rather than amount, is popular in the PK literature. However, in the case of models with compartments that change volume over time (e.g., in a model incorporating growth of a single or multiple tissues) it is preferable to use the formulation in terms of amounts in order to avoid the need for the additional term reflecting the change in volume ($C_T \cdot dV_T/dt$).

Depending on the compound, many different tissues can potentially serve as important storage compartments. The use of a fat storage compartment is typically required for lipophilic compounds. The gut lumen can also serve as a storage site for compounds subject to enterohepatic recirculation, as in the case of methotrexate. Important storage sites for metals, on the other hand, can include the kidney, red blood cells, intestinal epithelial cells, skin, bone, and hair [40]. Transport to and from a storage compartment does not always occur via the blood, as was described previously; for example, in some cases the storage is an intermediate step in an excretion process (e.g., hair, intestinal epithelial cells). As with methotrexate, it may also be necessary to use multiple compartments in series, or other mathematical devices, to model plug flow (i.e., a time delay between entry and exit from storage).

Blood Compartment   The description of the blood compartment can vary considerably from one PBPK model to another depending on the role the blood plays in the kinetics of the compound being modeled. In some cases the blood may be treated as a simple storage compartment, with a mass balance equation describing the summation (Σ) of the venous blood flows from the various tissues and the return of the total arterial blood flow (Q_C) to the tissues, as well as any urinary clearance (if, as in the case of glomerular filtration, clearance is described as occurring from the blood compartment):

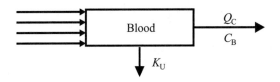

$$dA_B/dt = \sum (Q_T \cdot C_{VT}) - Q_C \cdot C_B - K_U \cdot C_B$$

where A_B is the amount of compound in the blood (mg), Q_C is the total cardiac output (L/h), C_B is the concentration of compound in the blood (mg/L), and K_U is the urinary clearance (L/h). The value for K_U can often be estimated from the unbound fraction in plasma (f_{ub}) and the glomerular filtration rate (GFR), unless active transport processes contribute to renal elimination. An alternative method for estimating human renal clearance based on rat renal clearance and incorporating species-specific physiological differences in GFR has been proposed [13, 41].

Most often, drug concentrations are measured in plasma or serum and not in whole blood; hence, plasma or serum is the reference fluid for the derived PK parameters such as clearances and volumes of distribution. However, whole blood, not plasma or serum, is flowing through the vessels of the human body. Therefore, provided that there is evidence in support of fast equilibration of drug between red blood cells and plasma [42], whole blood rather than plasma is the more appropriate reference fluid for calculating and interpreting clearances and volumes of distribution. For this reason, parameterization of the PBPK model is often performed in terms of blood flows. To compare calculated plasma concentrations to experimental data, the calculated blood concentration must then be divided by the blood-to-plasma ratio (BPR), which is often measured experimentally.

In cases where a compound is not taken up by the red blood cells, plasma flow can be used in place of blood flow in the model [5]. For some compounds, where exchange between plasma and red blood cells is slow compared to tissue perfusion, it may be necessary to model the red blood cells as a storage compartment in communication with the plasma via diffusion-limited transport. Typically, however, exchange between red blood cells and plasma is fast compared to tissue distribution, and the blood can be treated as a single compartment.

If the blood is an important storage compartment for a compound, it may be necessary to carefully evaluate data on tissue concentrations, particularly the richly perfused tissues, to determine whether compound in the blood perfusing the tissue could be contributing to the measured tissue concentration. For other compounds, the amount of compound actually in the blood may be relatively small, in which case only the concentration may be of interest. In this case, instead of having a true blood compartment, a steady-state approximation can be used to estimate the concentration in the blood at any time. Assuming the blood is at steady state with respect to the tissues,

$$dA_B/dt = 0$$

Therefore, solving the blood equation for the concentration:

$$C_B = \sum_T (Q_T \cdot C_{VT})/Q_C$$

Metabolism/Elimination   The liver is frequently the primary site of metabolism for a compound. The following equation is an example of the mass balance equation for the liver in the case of a compound that is metabolized through both saturable and nonsaturable components:

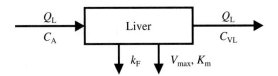

$$dA_L/dt = Q_L \cdot (C_A - C_{VL}) - k_F \cdot C_{Lfree} \cdot V_L - V_{max} \cdot C_{Lfree}/(K_m + C_{Lfree})$$

where Q_L is the total blood flow (arterial and portal) to the liver and C_{Lfree} is the free (unbound) concentration in the liver.

In the equation above, the first term on the right-hand side of the equation represents the mass flux associated with transport in the blood and is essentially identical to the case of the storage compartment described previously. In the case of the liver, however, it should be noted that there are two sources of blood flow: the arterial flow directly to the liver and the portal flow that first perfuses the intestines. When appropriate, these two blood flows can be differentiated in the model (Fig. 35.2 and 35.3).

The second term in the equation above describes metabolism by a linear (first-order) pathway with rate constant k_F (h^{-1}) and the third term represents metabolism by a saturable (Michaelis–Menten) pathway with capacity V_{max} (mg/h) and affinity K_m (mg/L). If it were desired to model a water-soluble metabolite produced by this saturable pathway, an equation for its formation and elimination could also be added to the model:

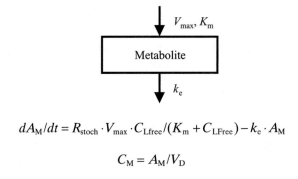

$$dA_M/dt = R_{stoch} \cdot V_{max} \cdot C_{LFree}/(K_m + C_{LFree}) - k_e \cdot A_M$$

$$C_M = A_M/V_D$$

where A_M is the amount of metabolite in the body (mg), R_{stoch} is the stoichiometric fractional yield of the metabolite (unitless) (times the ratio of its molecular weight to that of the parent compound), k_e is the rate constant for the clearance of the metabolite from the body (h^{-1}), C_M is the concentration of the metabolite in the plasma (mg/L), and V_D is the apparent volume of distribution for the metabolite (L).

The definition of free concentration in the liver (C_{Lfree}) in these equations is not as straightforward as it may at first appear. In cases where hepatic clearance is relatively low, the free concentration in the liver is often assumed to be equal to the free (unbound) concentration in the blood; that is, $C_{Lfree} = f_u \cdot C_B$. However, when hepatic clearance is high, the free concentration in the liver can be drawn well below the free concentration in the blood, and such an assumption may be inappropriate. An alternative assumption that is often made is that the free concentration in the liver can be estimated by dividing the total liver concentration by the liver:blood partition coefficient; that is, $C_{Lfree} = C_L/P_L$ [5]. This approximation is particularly useful for compounds whose metabolism is limited by hepatic blood flow at low concentrations. If the intent is to use *in vitro* estimates of the metabolic parameters (V_{max}, K_m, k_f) in the model, then the definition of the *in vivo* free concentration should be consistent with the conditions under which the *in vitro* estimates of intrinsic clearance were obtained. In principle, this could require adjusting for differences in binding between the *in vitro* medium and the tissue *in vivo*, although such adjustments are seldom performed in practice.

Metabolite Compartments   In principle, the same considerations that drive decisions regarding the level of complexity of the PBPK model for the parent compound must also be applied for each of its metabolites, and their metabolites, and so on. As in the case of the parent compound, the first and most important consideration is the purpose of the model. If the concern is a direct parent compound effect and the compound is inactivated by metabolism, then there is no need for a description of metabolism beyond its role in the clearance of the parent compound. The model for methotrexate (Fig. 35.2) is an example of a parent compound model.

If one or more of the metabolites are considered to contribute to the efficacy or toxicity of a compound, it may also be necessary to provide a more complete description of the kinetics of the metabolites themselves. For example, in the case of teratogenicity from all-trans retinoic acid, both the parent compound and several of its metabolites are considered to be toxicologically active; therefore, in developing the PBPK model for this compound it was necessary to include a fairly complete description of the metabolic pathways [19]. Fortunately, the metabolism of xenobiotic compounds often produces metabolites that are relatively water soluble, simplifying the description needed. In many cases, a classical one-compartment description may be adequate for describing the metabolite kinetics. In other cases, however, the description of the metabolite (or metabolites) may have to be as complex as that of the parent compound. If reactive intermediates produced during the metabolism of a compound are responsible for toxicity, a very simple description of the metabolic pathways might be adequate [43].

Target Tissues   Typically, a PBPK model used in drug development applications will include compartments for any target tissues for the efficacy of the compound and could also include target tissues of toxicity if the model is to be used for assessing safety. The target tissue description may in some cases need to be fairly complicated, including such features as *in situ* metabolism, binding, and pharmacodynamic processes in order to provide a realistic measure of biologically effective tissue exposure.

A fundamental issue in determining the nature of the target tissue description required is the need to identify the active form of the compound. A compound may produce an effect directly, through its interaction with tissue constituents, or indirectly, through a metabolite. In the case of toxicity, it is often the metabolism of a compound that leads to undesired effects, either through the production of reactive metabolites during metabolism or due to the toxicity of a circulating metabolite.

The specific nature of the relationship between tissue exposure and response depends on the mechanism, or mode of action, involved. Rapidly reversible effects may result primarily from the current concentration of the compound in the tissue, while longer-term effects may depend on both the concentration and duration of the exposure. Although therapeutic effects are generally due to the administered compound, an active metabolite may extend efficacy or cause undesired side effects or toxicity. In general, the appropriate measure of tissue exposure for a toxic side effect of a compound may be different from the appropriate measure for its therapeutic effect. For example, the therapeutic effect of a drug may depend on the prolonged maintenance of a relatively low concentration sufficient to occupy a receptor in the target tissue, while its toxicity may result from transient, high rates of metabolism in the liver occurring shortly after dosing. In such a case, PBPK modeling of the concentration time course in the liver and target tissue for different dosing routes or regimens might help to maximize the therapeutic index for the compound. For a developmental toxicity, the concentration time course might also have to be convoluted with the window of susceptibility for a particular gestational event. The evaluation of the various modes of action for the beneficial and toxic effects of a compound is the most important step in a PK analysis and a principal determinant of the structure and level of detail that will be required in the PBPK model.

Uptake Routes   Each of the relevant uptake routes for the compound must be described in the model. Often there are a number of possible ways to describe a particular uptake process, ranging from simple to complex. As with all other aspects of model design, the competing goals of parsimony and realism must be balanced in the selection of the level of complexity to be used. The following examples are meant to provide an idea of the variety of model code that can be required to describe the various possible uptake processes.

Intravenous Administration (Bolus Dosing)

$$A_{B0} = Dose \cdot BW$$

where A_{B0} is the amount of compound in the blood at the time of dosing ($t = 0$), *Dose* is the administered dose (mg/kg), and *BW* is body weight (kg).

Intravenous Administration (Infusion)   In the case where a steady-state approximation has been used to eliminate the blood compartment, we have

$$C_B = (Q_L \cdot C_{VL} + \cdots + Q_F \cdot C_{VF} + k_{IV})$$

where

$$k_{IV} = \begin{cases} Dose \cdot BW/t_{IV} & (t < t_{IV}) \\ 0 & (t > t_{IV}) \end{cases}$$

where t_{IV} is the duration of time over which the infusion takes place (h). In this case, the model code must be written with a "switch" to change the value of k_{IV} to zero at $t = t_{IV}$.

Oral Gavage   For a compound that is completely absorbed in the stomach,

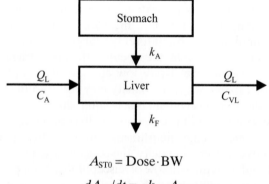

$$A_{ST0} = Dose \cdot BW$$

$$dA_{ST}/dt = -k_A \cdot A_{ST}$$

$$dA_L/dt = Q_L \cdot (C_A - C_L/P_L) - k_F \cdot C_L \cdot V_L/P_L + k_A \cdot A_{ST}$$

where A_{ST0} is the amount of compound in the stomach at the beginning of the simulation, A_{ST} is the amount of compound in the stomach at any given time, and k_A is a first-order rate constant (h^{-1}) describing uptake from the stomach.

For a compound that is incompletely absorbed,

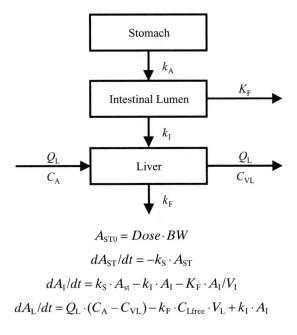

$$A_{ST0} = Dose \cdot BW$$

$$dA_{ST}/dt = -k_S \cdot A_{ST}$$

$$dA_I/dt = k_S \cdot A_{st} - k_I \cdot A_I - K_F \cdot A_I/V_I$$

$$dA_L/dt = Q_L \cdot (C_A - C_{VL}) - k_F \cdot C_{Lfree} \cdot V_L + k_I \cdot A_I$$

where A_I is the amount of compound in the intestinal lumen (mg), k_I is the rate constant for intestinal absorption (h^{-1}), K_F is the fecal clearance (L/h), and V_I is the volume of the intestinal lumen (L).

The rate of fecal excretion of the compound is then

$$dA_F/dt = K_F \cdot A_I/V_I$$

The examples described above are highly simplified descriptions. For example, they describe uptake from the stomach or intestinal lumen directly to the liver, when in fact the uptake is into the tissues of the gastrointestinal (GI) tract with subsequent transport to the liver in the portal blood. While this simplification is adequate in some cases, a more accurate description may be necessary in others, such as when metabolism in the gut tissues is important or portal blood flow could limit uptake. The equations shown above also do not describe biliary excretion or other processes that might be important determinants of the intestinal concentration and fecal excretion of a compound over time. Again, these processes would need to be included in the full model description for compounds where these processes are important [19]. Note also that this simple formulation does not consider the plug flow of the intestinal contents and will not reproduce the delay that actually occurs in the appearance of a compound in the feces. Such a delay could be added using a delay function available in common simulation software, or multiple compartments could be used to simulate plug flow, as shown in the diagram of the methotrexate model (Fig. 35.2).

Although in some cases a simple, first-order model can adequately describe oral absorption, more physiologically representative approaches have been developed and shown to be useful for predicting the fraction absorbed, for example, a compartmental approach such as the ACAT model [44] and a model describing the GI tract as a tube [45]. Simulation of oral absorption using physiologically based models represents another challenge because of the many processes involved such as the release, dissolution, degradation, metabolism, uptake, and absorption of a compound as it transits through the different segments of the digestive tract [46]. Oral absorption simulations require *in vitro* and *in silico* input data such as solubility, permeability, particle size, partition coefficient (log$P$), ionization constant (pK_a), and dose [47, 48].

Inhalation   For compounds that are volatile, it is necessary to describe the exchange of vapor between the lung air and blood in the alveolar region. This is true even if the compound is not administered by inhalation, because exhalation can be an important route of clearance for volatile compounds regardless of the dose route.

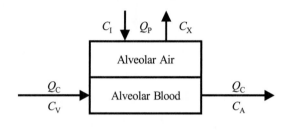

$$dA_{AB}/dt = Q_C \cdot (C_V - C_A) + Q_P \cdot (C_I - C_X)$$

where A_{AB} is the amount of compound in the alveolar blood (mg), C_V is the concentration of compound in the pooled venous blood (mg/L), C_A is the concentration of compound in the alveolar (arterial) blood (mg/L), Q_P is the alveolar (not total pulmonary) ventilation rate (L/h), C_I is the concentration of compound in the inhaled air (mg/L), and C_X is the concentration of compound in the alveolar air (mg/L). Assuming the alveolar blood is at steady state with respect to the other compartments,

$$dA_{AB}/dt = 0$$

Also, assuming lung equilibration (i.e., that the blood in the alveolar region has reached equilibrium with the alveolar air prior to exhalation),

$$C_X = C_A/P_B$$

where P_B is the blood:air partition coefficient.

Substituting into the equation for the alveolar blood and solving for C_A, we have

$$C_A = (Q_C \cdot C_V + Q_P \cdot C_I)/(Q_C + Q_P/P_B)$$

Note that the rate of elimination of the compound by exhalation is just $Q_P \cdot C_X$. The alveolar ventilation rate, Q_P, does not include the "deadspace" volume (the portion of the inhaled air that does not reach the alveolar region) and is therefore roughly 70% of the total respiratory rate. The concentration C_X represents the "end-alveolar" air concentration; in order to estimate the average exhaled concentration (C_{EX}), the deadspace contribution must be included:

$$C_{EX} = 0.3C_I + 0.7C_X$$

PBPK models including more detailed physiological descriptions of inhalation exposures developed to understand toxicological effects of reactive vapors in the nasal cavity have been reviewed [49].

Dermal   A simple model can be used to describe dermal absorption from a constant-concentration vehicle on the skin surface.

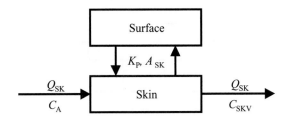

$$dA_{SK}/dt = K_P \cdot A_{SFC} \cdot (C_{SFC} - C_{SK}/P_{SKV})/1000 + Q_{SK} \cdot (C_A - C_{SK}/P_{SKB})$$

where A_{Sk} is the amount of compound in the skin (mg), K_P is the skin permeability coefficient (cm/h), A_{SFC} is the skin surface area (cm^2), C_{SFC} is the concentration of compound on the surface of the skin (mg/L), C_{SK} is the concentration of the compound in the skin (mg/L), P_{SK} is the skin:vehicle partition coefficient (i.e., the vehicle containing the compound on the surface of the skin), Q_{SK} is the blood flow to the skin region (L/h), C_A is the arterial concentration of the compound (mg/L), and P_{SKB} is the skin:blood partition coefficient.

Due to adding this compartment, the equation for the blood in the model must also be modified to add a term for the venous blood returning from the skin ($+Q_{SK} \cdot C_{SK}/P_{SKB}$), and the blood flow and volume parameters for the slowly perfused tissue compartment must be reduced by the amount of blood flow and volume for the skin. Approaches used to include the dermal exposure route in PBPK models have been reviewed [50]. Several reviews discuss the wide variety of available compartment models and provide guidance for choosing among them [51, 52].

Experimental Apparatus   In some cases, in addition to compartments describing the animal–chemical system, it may also be necessary to include model compartments that describe the experimental apparatus in which measurements were obtained.

Distribution/Transport   There are a number of issues associated with the description of the transport and distribution of the compound that must be considered in the process of model design. Discussions of the more common ones are included here.

Diffusion-Limited Transport Most of the PBPK models in the literature are flow-limited models; that is, they assume that the rate of tissue uptake of the compound is limited only by the flow of the compound to the tissue in the blood. While this assumption appears to be reasonable in general, for some compounds and tissues uptake may be diffusion limited. Examples of tissues for which diffusion-limited transport has often been described include the skin, placenta, brain, and fat. The model compartments described thus far have all assumed flow-limited transport. If there is evidence that the movement of a compound between the blood and a tissue is limited by diffusion, a two-compartment description of the tissue can be used with a "shallow" exchange compartment in communication with the blood and a diffusion-limited "deep" compartment that represents the actual tissue:

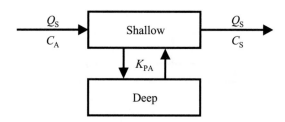

$$dA_S/dt = Q_S \cdot (C_A - C_S) - K_{PA} \cdot (C_S - C_D/P_D)$$
$$dA_D/dt = K_{PA} \cdot (C_S - C_D/P_D)$$

where A_S is the amount of compound in the shallow compartment (mg), Q_S is the blood flow to the shallow compartment (L/h), C_S is the concentration of compound in the shallow compartment (mg/L), K_{PA} is the permeability–area product for diffusion-limited transport (L/h), C_D is the concentration of compound in the deep compartment (mg/L), P_D is the tissue:blood partition coefficient, and A_D is the amount of compound in the deep compartment (mg).

Saturable Tissue Binding When there is evidence that saturable binding is an important determinant of the distribution of a compound into a tissue (such as evidence of dose-dependent tissue partitioning), a simple description of tissue binding can be added to the model. In this description, only free (unbound) compound is considered to be available for transport or clearance at any given moment in time. For example, in the case of saturable binding in the liver,

$$dA_L/dt = V_L \, dC_L/dt = Q_L \cdot (C_A - C_{Lfree}) - k_F \cdot C_{Lfree}$$

where A_L is the total (free plus bound) concentration of the compound in the liver (mg), C_{Lfree} is the concentration of free (unbound) compound in the liver (mg/L), and k_F is the rate constant for metabolism (h^{-1}).

The apparent complication in adding this equation to the model is that the change in the total amount of compound in the tissue (dA_L/dt) is needed for the mass balance, but the determinants of the kinetics are described in terms of the free concentration in the tissue (C_{Lfree}). To solve for free in terms of total, we note that

$$C_L = C_{\text{Lfree}} + C_{\text{Lbound}}$$

where C_{Lbound} is the concentration of bound compound in the tissue (mg/L). We can describe the saturable binding with an equation similar to that for saturable metabolism:

$$C_{\text{Lbound}} = B_m \cdot C_{\text{Lfree}} / (K_d + C_{\text{Lfree}})$$

where B_m is the binding capacity (mg/L) and K_d is the binding affinity (mg/L). Substituting this equation into the previous one, we have

$$C_L = C_{\text{Lfree}} + B_m \cdot C_{\text{Lfree}} / (K_d + C_{\text{Lfree}})$$

Rewriting this equation to solve for the free concentration in terms of only the total concentration would result in a quadratic equation, the solution of which could be obtained with the quadratic formula. However, taking advantage of the iterative algorithm by which these PBPK models are exercised (as will be discussed later), it is not necessary to go to this effort. Instead, a much simpler implicit equation can be written for the free concentration (i.e., an equation in which the free concentration appears on both sides):

$$C_{\text{Lfree}} = C_L / (1 + B_m / (K_d + C_{\text{Lfree}}))$$

In an iterative algorithm, this equation can be solved at each time step using the previous value of C_{Lfree} to obtain the new value! A new value of C_L is then obtained from the mass balance equation for the liver using the new value of C_{Lfree}, and the process is repeated. An underlying assumption for this simple description of tissue binding is that the binding is rapidly reversible compared to the movement or clearance of free compound, such that equilibrium between free and bound chemical can be maintained.

In fact, at least two different computational approaches have been used to describe saturable binding in PBPK models. The concentration of free compound can either be estimated, as described above, from solving a conservation equation for total mass that apportions the total amount of compound between free and bound forms using the equilibrium dissociation constants, K_d, and binding maxima, B_m [53], or it can be estimated by explicitly including both "on" (association) and "off" (dissociation) rate constants, k_a and k_d [54]. In the latter case, the dissociation binding constant (with units of concentration) is the ratio of the two rate constants, k_d/k_a. The advantage of the rate constant approach is that it does not require the assumption that binding is fast compared to transport and clearance.

While these two computational approaches have usually been applied within tissues, they can also be readily applied to binding in blood if the concentrations and affinities of binding proteins are known. However, in most modeling of drugs, protein binding in blood is linear (not saturable at clinically relevant concentrations) and can be characterized by a single parameter, fraction unbound, rather than estimates of concentrations of binding sites and their affinities for binding. Nevertheless, there are cases where protein binding is more appropriately described as a nonlinear process [55]. Alternative descriptions of blood binding will be discussed in more detail in the next section.

Binding in Blood   Protein binding in blood can be a key determinant of drug disposition, affecting compound availability for interaction with therapeutic targets as well as for clearance. A high fraction bound in the blood also gives rise to concerns regarding potential drug–drug interactions that might displace bound drug and produce a transient increase in drug concentrations to potentially toxic levels. Methodologies to estimate drug binding and approaches for the quantitative description of this binding in PK models have been areas of intense interest over the past four to five decades. Consideration of blood binding faces two parallel challenges. First, when drugs are bound in capillary blood, what fraction should be regarded as available for transport into tissue? Second, how does the binding in blood influence blood:tissue partitioning? Historically, these questions have been addressed both in empirical descriptions and in PBPK models, and some care is required to reconcile the different approaches and arrive at a consistent quantitative treatment of blood binding and transport of compound throughout the body in both types of modeling approaches.

In the standard description of clearance of a compound from blood by tissue metabolism, binding in the blood is assumed to be linear and the fraction unbound, f_u, is simply multiplied by the intrinsic clearance, leading to a straightforward relationship:

$$CL = Q_T \cdot f_u \cdot CL_{int}/(Q_T + f_u \cdot CL_{int})$$

In this relationship, the maximal tissue clearance, even with a low fraction unbound, is total tissue blood flow. That is, all of the compound in the blood, whether bound or unbound, becomes available for clearance as long as the intrinsic clearance is sufficiently large. Note that in this description the fraction unbound is not a function of the clearance. In fact, the derivation of this equation rests on the assumption that dissociation of bound compound in the blood is fast compared to the rate of tissue clearance. If the uptake of a compound into the tissue is limited by the rate of dissociation of the compound from binding proteins in the blood, the simple formula above will overestimate its clearance.

In PBPK models, blood concentrations of bound and free compound can be described separately, as discussed in the previous section, and only free compound is generally considered to be available to participate in processes such as diffusion, metabolism, tissue reaction, and intercompartmental transfer. As in the case of tissue binding, the relationship of free to bound concentrations in the blood is generally calculated by knowledge of dissociation binding constants (K_d) and maximum concentrations of binding proteins (B_m), as describe previously. An example of this approach has been described in the case of a PBPK model for estradiol [55]. This approach differs from the simple clearance formula given above in that the fraction unbound can be a nonlinear function of the concentration of the compound in the blood. It shares, however, the assumption that the "on" and "off" rates for binding are fast compared to rates of clearance. The alternative description of binding described in the previous section, which explicitly includes the binding rate constants, would be preferred in cases where this assumption may be violated.

Protein binding in blood is a critical component of drug action and drug efficacy. PK models need to carefully consider the manner in which binding can be introduced into the basic equations and track free concentrations at sites of action or at least within the plasma. Introduction of blood binding in PBPK models raises some conceptual challenges, especially in comparing conventional empirical approaches with PBPK approaches intended to track thermodynamically free concentrations throughout the body. Although simple descriptions are often adequate, careful consideration of the underlying kinetic processes and their relative rates for the compound and tissues of interest is required to assure that a particular modeling approach is appropriate [56].

Tissue : Blood Partitioning   Regardless of the manner in which blood binding is implemented in PBPK models, another challenge arises in describing equilibration between blood and tissues. In general, both the blood and the tissues will contain free and bound forms of the compound. For equilibration, only the free compound in the plasma diffuses across the tissue capillary interface into the tissue, and at equilibrium between blood and tissue, the free concentration in the plasma and the tissue is expected to be equal (except in the case of active transport). However, the equilibrium relationship of the concentrations in tissues compared to the blood or plasma is typically described with empirical partition coefficients based on measurements of total concentrations of the compound. Differential binding in plasma and tissue will therefore influence apparent tissue partitioning.

The relationship between apparent tissue : blood partitioning and binding in blood versus tissue can be straightforwardly described, as long as no other factors affect distribution. Assuming that (1) there is no need to adjust for the effect of clearance, and (2) there is no evidence of active transport of the compound between blood and tissue, the free fraction in the tissue, f_{ut}, can then be estimated:

$$P_{tb} = P_{tp}/BPR = (f_{up}/f_{ut})/BPR$$

where P_{tb} is the tissue : blood partition coefficient, P_{tp} is the tissue : plasma partition coefficient, BPR is the blood to plasma ratio, f_{up} is the fraction unbound in the plasma, and f_{ut} is the fraction unbound in the tissue.
Then

$$f_{ut} = f_{up}/(P_{tb} \cdot BPR)$$

In fact, there are quite a number of different determinants of the apparent partitioning between blood and tissues:

- Partitioning due to lipophilicity
- Plasma binding
- Tissue binding

- Active transport
- Clearance processes
- Blood to plasma ratio (for converting tissue:plasma partitions to tissue: blood)

A measured or estimated partition coefficient may reflect any combination of these factors, and the modeler must be aware of this potential complexity in attempting to use a particular set of data on a compound. For example, if partition coefficients have been estimated from QSAR, they are likely to primarily reflect lipophilic partitioning and may need to be adjusted for differences in binding in plasma and tissues. Alternatively, the model can be designed to separately describe lipophilic partitioning, using the estimated partition coefficients, and binding, based on other data. *In vitro*-derived partition coefficients, on the other hand, may reflect both thermodynamic partitioning and binding, although disruption of the tissue architecture may alter the binding characteristics of the tissue. It is also necessary to ensure that no metabolic clearance of the compound occurs in either blood or tissue during the measurements. *In vivo*-derived partition coefficients may reflect lipophilicity, binding, and active transport, as well as the effect of any clearance processes [57]. Due to this complexity, it may in some cases be preferable to estimate model parameters for tissue partitioning by fitting the *in vivo* blood and tissue concentration data rather than trying to use it directly to calculate "partition coefficients" for the model.

Model Diagram   As described in the previous sections, the process of developing a PBPK model begins by determining the essential structure of the model based on the information available on the compound's toxicity, mechanism of action, and PK properties. The results of this step can usually be summarized by an initial model diagram, such as those depicted in Fig. 35.2 and 35.3. In fact, in many cases a well-constructed model diagram, together with a table of the input parameter values and their definitions, is all that an accomplished modeler should need in order to create the mathematical equations defining a PBPK model. In general, there should be a one-to-one correspondence of the boxes in the diagram to the mass balance equations (or steady-state approximations) in the model. Similarly, the arrows in the diagram correspond to the transport or metabolism processes in the model. Each of the arrows connecting the boxes in the diagram should correspond to one of the terms in the mass balance equations for both of the compartments it connects, with the direction of the arrow pointing from the compartment in which the term is negative to the compartment in which it is positive. Arrows only connected to a single compartment, which represent uptake and excretion processes, are interpreted similarly.

The model diagram should be labeled with the names of the key variables associated with the compartment or process represented by each box and arrow. Interpretation of the model diagram is also aided by the definition of the model input parameters in the corresponding table. The definition and units of the parameters can indicate the nature of the process being modeled (e.g., diffusion-limited vs. flow-limited transport, binding vs. partitioning, saturable vs. first-order metabolism).

35.3 PBPK MODEL IMPLEMENTATION

The purpose of developing a PBPK model is to perform simulations and learn about the system (Fig. 35.1). But first, the model must be parameterized, coded using some type of software package, and tested to make sure it is working properly. Also, sensitivity analysis and other techniques must be used to understand the model and verify that key inputs are known with sufficient accuracy to result in reasonable simulation results.

35.3.1 Model Parameterization

Once the model structure has been determined, it still remains to identify the values of the input parameters in the model.

Physiological Parameters   Estimates of the various physiological parameters needed in PBPK models are available from a number of sources in the literature, particularly for the human, monkey, dog, rat, and mouse [4, 26–30]. Estimates for the same parameter often vary widely, however, due both to experimental differences and to differences in the animals examined (age, strain, activity). Ventilation rates and blood flow rates are particularly sensitive to the level of activity [26, 28]. Data on some important tissues are relatively poor, particularly in the case of fat tissue. Table 35.2 shows typical values of a number of physiological parameters in several species.

Biochemical Parameters   One large barrier to the application of PBPK models in preclinical drug development has been that tissue : plasma partition coefficients (P_{tp}) are too expensive to routinely measure. Partition coefficients can be determined by *in vivo* or *in vitro* measurements [31, 57, 58] or can be estimated from quantitative structure–activity relationship (QSAR) modeling. Perhaps the driving force behind the recent interest in PBPK modeling in the pharmaceutical industry was reported successes in developing methods for *a priori* predictions of P_{tp} values for volatile organic compounds based on their solubilities in the neutral lipid, phospholipid, and water fractions of tissues as estimated using a vegetable oil : water partition coefficient; the necessary tissue composition data has been tabulated for a variety of tissues [59–61]. This approach was eventually extended to using the mechanistic equations for predicting P_{tp} values for drugs [62]. Briefly, these mechanistic equations assume that the drug distributes homogeneously into the tissue and plasma by passive diffusion, where two processes are accounted for: (1) nonspecific binding to lipids estimated from drug lipophilicity data ($\log P$, $\log D$) and (2) specific reversible binding to common proteins present in plasma and tissue estimated from the fraction unbound in the plasma (f_{up}). These P_{tp} values can be used to estimate the volume of distribution [63]. Recent contributions have focused on improving methods for calculating P_{tp} values for moderate-to-strong bases by developing a method incorporating the electrostatic interactions with tissue acidic phospholipids [64] and for acids, very weak bases, neutrals, and zwitterions by incorporating the effect of drug ionization on distribution processes [65].

One of the greatest challenges is typically the characterization of metabolism, which can also make use of both *in vivo* and *in vitro* methods. For compounds

TABLE 35.2   Typical Physiological Parameters for PBPK Models

Species	Mouse	Rat	Monkey	Human
Ventilation				
Alveolar (L/h)[a]	29.0^b	15.0^b	15.0^b	15.0^b
Blood flows				
Total (L/h)[a]	16.5^c	15.0^c	15.0^c	15.0^c
Muscle (fraction)	0.18	0.18	0.18	0.18
Skin (fraction)	0.07	0.08	0.06	0.06
Fat (fraction)	0.03	0.06	0.05	0.05
Liver (arterial) (fraction)	0.035	0.03	0.065	0.07
Gut (portal) (fraction)	0.165	0.18	0.185	0.19
Other organs (fraction)	0.52	0.47	0.46	0.45
Tissue volumes				
Body weight (kg)	0.02	0.3	4.0	80.0
Body water (fraction)	0.65	0.65	0.65	0.65
Plasma (fraction)	0.04	0.04	0.04	0.04
RBCs (fraction)	0.03	0.03	0.03	0.03
Muscle (fraction)	0.34	0.36	0.48	0.33
Skin (fraction)	0.17	0.195	0.11	0.11
Fat (fraction)	0.10^d	0.07^d	0.05^d	0.21
Liver (fraction)	0.046	0.037	0.027	0.023
Gut tissue (fraction)	0.031	0.033	0.045	0.045
Other organs (fraction)	0.049	0.031	0.039	0.039
Intestinal lumen (fraction)	0.054	0.058	0.053	0.053

[a]Scaled allometrically: $QC = QCC \cdot BW^{0.75}$.
[b]Varies significantly with activity level (range: 15.0–40.0).
[c]Varies with activity level (range: 15.0–20.0).
[d]Varies substantially (lower in young animals, higher in older animals).

cleared by hepatic metabolism, intrinsic clearance values determined *in vitro* with hepatocyte or microsomal substrate depletion or kinetic assays are typically used. Many researchers have described physiological methods for scaling hepatocyte and microsome data, including Zuegge et al. [66], Lavé et al. [67], Houston [68], Houston and Carlile [69], Obach [70], and Ito et al. [71]. Recently improved parameters for the physiological scaling of human hepatocyte and microsome data have been published [72].

Allometry   The different types of physiological and biochemical parameters in a PBPK model are known to vary with body weight in different ways [24]. Typically, the parameterization of PBPK models is simplified by assuming standard allometric scaling [28], as shown in Table 35.3, where the scaling factors, b, can be used in the following equation:

$$Y = aX^b$$

where Y is the value of the parameter at a given body weight, X (kg), and a is the scaled parameter value for a 1 kg animal.

TABLE 35.3   Standard Allometric Scaling for Physiologically Based Pharmacokinetic Model Parameters

Parameter Type (units)	Scaling (power of body weight)
Volumes	1.0
Flows (volume per time)	0.75
Ventilation (volume per time)	0.75
Clearances (volume per time)	0.75
Metabolic capacities (mass per time)	0.75
Metabolic affinities (mass per volume)	0
Partition coefficients (unitless)	0
First-order rate constants (inverse time)	−0.25

While standard allometric scaling provides a useful starting point, or hypothesis, for cross-species scaling, it is not sufficiently accurate for some applications. In the case of the physiological parameters, the species-specific parameter values are generally available in the literature [4, 26–30] and can be used directly in place of the allometric estimates. For compound-specific parameters, *in vitro* data for metabolism, distribution, or absorption relevant to the species under consideration are used in most of the cases in preference to allometric estimates. However, allometric scaling might provide first parameter estimates when data is lacking.

Parameter Optimization   In many cases, important parameter values needed for a PBPK model may not be available in the literature. In such cases it is necessary to measure them in new experiments, to estimate them by QSAR techniques, or to identify them by optimizing the fit of the model to an informative dataset. Even in the case where an initial estimate of a particular parameter value can be obtained from other sources, it may be desirable to refine the estimate by optimization. For example, given the difficulty of obtaining accurate estimates of the fat volume in rodents, a more reliable estimate may be obtained by examining the impact of fat volume on the kinetic behavior of a lipophilic compound. Of course, being able to uniquely identify a parameter from a kinetic dataset rests on two key assumptions: (1) that the kinetic behavior of the compound under the conditions in which the data was collected is sensitive to the parameter being estimated, and (2) that other parameters in the model, which could influence the observed kinetics, have been determined by other means and are held fixed during the estimation process. When it is necessary to estimate multiple parameters from *in vivo* PK data, using sensitivity analysis to verify that sufficient data are available and optimizing on individual parameters before performing a global optimization has been recommended [73].

The actual approach for conducting a parameter optimization can range from simple visual fitting, where the model is run with different values of the parameter until the best correspondence appears to be achieved, to use of a quantitative mathematical algorithm. The most common algorithm used in optimization is the least-squares fit. To perform a least-squares optimization, the model is run to obtain a set of predictions at each of the times a data point was collected. The square of the difference between the model prediction and data point at each time is calculated and the results for all of the data points are summed. The parameter being estimated is then modified, and the sum of squares is recalculated. This process is repeated until the smallest possible sum of squares is obtained, representing the best possible fit of the model to the data.

In a variation on this approach, the square of the difference at each point is divided by the square of the prediction. This variation, known as relative least squares, is preferable in the case of data with an error structure that can be described by a constant coefficient of variation (i.e., a constant ratio of the standard deviation to the mean). The former method, known as absolute least squares, is preferable in the case of data with a constant variance. From a practical viewpoint, the absolute least-squares method tends to give greater weight to the data at higher concentrations and results in fits that look best when plotted on a linear scale, while the relative least-squares method gives greater weight to the data at lower concentrations and results in fits that look best when plotted on a logarithmic scale.

A generalization of this weighting concept is provided by the extended least-squares method. In the extended least-squares algorithm, the heteroscedasticity parameter can be varied from 0 (for absolute weighting) to 2 (for relative weighting) or can be estimated from the data. In general, setting the heteroscedasticity parameter from knowledge of the error structure of the data is preferable to estimating it from a dataset.

A common example of identifying PBPK model parameters by fitting kinetic data is the estimation of tissue partition coefficients from experiments in which the concentration of compound in the blood and tissues is reported at various time points. Using an optimization approach, the predictions of the model for the time course in the blood and tissues could be optimized with respect to the data by varying the model's partition coefficients. There is little difference in the strength of the justification for estimating the partition coefficients in this way as opposed to estimating them directly from the data (by dividing the tissue concentrations by the simultaneous blood concentration). In fact, the direct estimates would probably be used as initial estimates in the model when the optimization was started.

A major difficulty in performing parameter optimization results from correlations between the parameters. When it is necessary to estimate parameters that are highly correlated, it is best to generate a contour plot of the objective function (sum of squares) or confidence region over a reasonable range of values of the two parameters [74].

Mass Balance Requirements   One of the most important mathematical considerations during model design is the maintenance of mass balance. Simply put, the model should neither create nor destroy mass. This seemingly obvious principle is often violated unintentionally during the process of model development and parameterization. A common violation of mass balance, which typically leads to catastrophic results, involves failure to exactly match the arterial and venous blood flows in the model. As described previously, the movement of compound in the blood (in units of mass per time) is described as the product of the concentration of compound in the blood (in units of mass per volume) times the flow rate of the blood (in units of volume per time). Therefore, to maintain mass balance, the sum of the blood flows leaving any particular tissue compartment must equal the sum of the blood flows entering the compartment. In particular, to maintain mass balance in the blood compartment (regardless of whether it's actually a compartment or just a steady-state equation), the sum of the venous flows from the individual tissue compartments must equal the total arterial blood flow leaving the heart:

$$\sum Q_T = Q_C$$

Another obvious but occasionally overlooked aspect of maintaining mass balance during model development is that if a model is modified by splitting a tissue out of a lumped compartment, the blood flow to the separated tissue (and its volume) must be subtracted from that for the lumped compartment. Moreover, even though a model may initially be designed with parameters that meet the above requirements, mass balance may unintentionally be violated later if the parameters are altered during model execution. For example, if the parameter for the blood flow to one compartment is increased, the parameter for the overall blood flow must be increased accordingly or an equivalent reduction must be made in the parameter for the blood flow to another compartment. Particular care must be taken in this regard when the model is subjected to sensitivity or uncertainty analysis; inadvertent violation of mass balance during Monte Carlo sampling can lead to erroneous sensitivity results [39].

A similar mass balance requirement must be met for transport other than blood flow. For example, if the compound is cleared by biliary excretion, the elimination of compound from the liver in the bile must exactly match the appearance of compound in the gut lumen in the bile. Put mathematically, the same term for the transport must appear in the equations for the two compartments, but with opposite signs (positive vs. negative). For example, the following equation could be used to describe a liver compartment with first-order metabolism and biliary clearance:

$$dA_L/dt = Q_L \cdot (C_A - C_L/P_L) - k_F \cdot C_L \cdot V_L/P_L - K_B \cdot C_L$$

where K_B is the biliary clearance rate (L/h). The equation for the intestinal lumen would then need to include the term: $+K_B \cdot C_L$.

As a model grows in complexity, it becomes increasingly difficult to assure its mass balance by inspection. Therefore, it is a worthwhile practice to check for mass balance by including an equation in the model that adds up the total amount of compound in each of the model compartments, including metabolized and excreted compound, for comparison with the administered or inhaled dose.

35.3.2 Numerical Solution of Model Equations

The previous sections have focused on the process of designing the PBPK model structure needed for a particular application. At this point the model consists of a number of mathematical equations: differential equations describing the mass balance for each of the compartments and algebraic equations describing other relationships between model variables. The next step in model development is the coding of the mathematical form of the model into a form that can be executed on a computer. There are many options available for performing this process, ranging from programming languages such as Fortran, C, and MatLab to more sophisticated simulation software packages such as acslXtreme and Berkeley Madonna.

Mathematically, a PBPK model is represented by a system of simultaneous ordinary differential equations. Each of the differential equations describes the mass balance for one of the "state variables" (compartments) in the model. There may also be additional differential equations to calculate other necessary model outputs, such as the area under the concentration curve (*AUC*) in a particular compartment, which is simply the integral of the concentration over time. The resulting system of equations is referred to as simultaneous because the time courses of the compound in the various compartments are so interdependent that solving the equations for any one of the compartments requires information on the current status of all the other compartments; that is, the equations for all of the compartments must be solved at the same time. This kind of mathematical problem, in which a system is defined by the conditions at time zero together with differential equations describing how it evolves over time, is known as an *initial value problem*, and matrix decomposition methods can be used to obtain the simultaneous solution.

A number of numerical algorithms are available for solving such problems. They all have in common that they are stepwise approximations; that is, they begin with the conditions at time zero and use the differential equations to predict how the system will change over a small time step, resulting in an estimate of the conditions at a slightly later time, which serves as the starting point for the next time step. This iterative process is repeated as long as necessary to simulate the experimental scenario.

The more sophisticated methods, such as the Gear algorithm (named after the mathematician David Gear, who developed it), use a predictor–corrector approach, in which the corrector step essentially amounts to "predicting backwards" after each step forward, in order to check how closely the algorithm is able to reproduce the conditions at the previous time step. This allows the time step to be increased automatically when the algorithm is performing well, and to be shortened when it is having difficulty, such as when conditions are changing rapidly. However, due to the wide variation of the time constants (response times) for the various physiological compartments (e.g., fat vs. richly perfused), PBPK models often represent "stiff" systems. Stiff systems are characterized by state variables (compartments) with widely different time constants, which cause difficulty for predictor–corrector algorithms. The Gear algorithm was specifically designed to overcome this difficulty. It is therefore generally recommended that the Gear algorithm (or an alternative stiff system solver such as the Rosenbrock method) be used for executing PBPK models.

Regardless of the specific algorithm selected, the essential nature of the solution will be a stepwise approximation. However, all of the algorithms made available in computer software are convergent; that is, they can stay arbitrarily close to the true solution, given a small enough time step. On modern personal computers, even large PBPK models can be run to more than adequate accuracy in a reasonable timeframe.

35.3.3   Model Evaluation

This section discusses various issues associated with the evaluation of a PBPK model. Once an initial model has been developed, it must be evaluated on the basis of its conformance with experimental data. In some cases, the model may be exercised to predict conditions under which experimental data should be collected in order to verify or improve model performance. Comparison of the resulting data with the model predictions may suggest that revision of the model will be required. Similarly, a PBPK model designed for one compound or application may be adapted to another compound or application, requiring modification of the model structure and parameters. It is imperative that revision or modification of a model is conducted with the same level of rigor applied during initial model development, and that structures are not added to the model with no other justification than that they improve the agreement of the model with a particular dataset.

In addition to comparing model predictions to experimental data, model evaluation includes assessing the biological plausibility of the model structures and input parameters, and the resulting confidence that can be placed in extrapolations performed by the model [75]. Both elements of testing the model—kinetic validation and mechanistic validation—are necessary to provide confidence in the model. Unfortunately, there is a temptation to accept kinetic validation alone, particularly when data for mechanistic validation are unavailable. It should be remembered, however, that the simple act of adding equations and parameters to a model will, in itself, increase the flexibility of the model to fit data. Therefore, every attempt should be made to obtain additional experimental data to provide support for the mechanistic hypothesis underlying the model structure.

Model Documentation   In cases where a model previously developed by one investigator is being evaluated for use in a different application by another investigator, adequate model documentation is critical for evaluation of the model. The documentation for a PBPK model should include sufficient information about the model so that an experienced modeler could accurately reproduce its structure and parameterization. Usually the suitable documentation of a model will require a combination of one or more "box and arrow" model diagrams together with any equations that cannot be unequivocally derived from the diagrams. Model diagrams should clearly differentiate blood flow from other transport (e.g., biliary excretion) or metabolism, and arrows should be used where the direction of transport could be ambiguous. All tissue compartments, metabolism pathways, routes of exposure, and routes of elimination should be clearly and accurately presented. All equations should be dimensionally consistent and in standard mathematical notation. Generic equations (e.g., for tissue "i") can help to keep the description brief but complete. The values used for all model parameters should be provided, with units. If any of the listed parameter values are based on allometric scaling, a footnote should provide the body weight used to obtain the allometric constant as well as the power of body weight used in the scaling.

35.3.4 Model Validation

Internal validation consists of the evaluation of the mathematical correctness of the model [34]. It is best accomplished on the actual model code but, if necessary, can be performed on appropriate documentation of the model structure and parameters, as described earlier (assuming, of course, that the actual model code accurately reflects the model documentation). A more important issue regards the provision of evidence for external validation (sometimes referred to as verification). The level of detail incorporated into a model is necessarily a compromise between biological accuracy and parsimony. The process of evaluating the sufficiency of the model for its intended purpose, termed *model verification*, requires a demonstration of the ability of the model to predict the behavior of experimental data different from that on which it was based.

Whereas a simulation is intended simply to reproduce the behavior of a system, a model is intended to confirm a hypothesis concerning the nature of the system. Therefore, model validation should demonstrate the ability of the model to predict the behavior of the system under conditions that test the principal aspects of the underlying hypothetical structure. While quantitative tests of goodness of fit may often be a useful aspect of the verification process, the more important consideration may be the ability of the model to provide an accurate prediction of the general behavior of the data in the intended application.

Where only some aspects of the model can be verified, it is particularly important to assess the uncertainty associated with the aspects that are untested. For example, a model of a compound and its metabolites that is intended for use in cross-species extrapolation to humans would preferably be verified using data in different species, including humans, for both the parent compound and the metabolites. If only parent compound data is available in the human, the correspondence of metabolite predictions with data in several animal species could be used as a surrogate, but this deficiency should be carefully considered when applying the model to predict human metabolism. One of the values of biologically based modeling is the identification of specific data that would improve the quantitative prediction of toxicity in humans from animal experiments.

In some cases it is necessary to use all of the available data to support model development and parameterization. Unfortunately, this type of modeling can easily become a form of self-fulfilling prophecy: models are logically strongest when they fail, but psychologically most appealing when they succeed [33]. Under these conditions, model verification can be particularly difficult, putting an additional burden on the investigators to substantiate the trustworthiness of the model for its intended purpose. Nevertheless, a combined model development and verification can often be successfully performed, particularly for models intended for interpolation, integration, and comparison of data rather than for true extrapolation.

Parameter Verification   In addition to verifying the performance of the model against experimental data, the model should be evaluated in terms of the plausibility of its parameters. This is particularly important in the case of PBPK models, where the parameters generally possess biological significance and can therefore be evaluated for plausibility independent of the context of the model. The source of each model input parameter value should be identified, whether it was obtained from prior literature, determined directly by experiment, or estimated by fitting a model output to experimental data. Parameter estimates derived independently of tissue time course or dose–response data are preferred. To the extent feasible, the degree of uncertainty regarding the parameter values should also be evaluated. The empirically derived *Law of Reciprocal Certainty* states that the more important the model parameter, the less certain will be its value. In accordance with this principle, the most difficult, and typically most important, parameter determination for PBPK models is the characterization of the metabolism parameters.

When parameter estimation has been performed by optimizing model output to experimental data, the investigator must assure that the parameter is adequately identifiable from the data [34]. Due to the confounding effects of model error, overparameterization, and parameter correlation, it is quite possible for an optimization algorithm to obtain a better fit to a particular dataset by modifying a parameter that in fact should not be identified on the basis of that dataset. Also, when an automatic optimization routine is employed, it should be restarted with a variety of initial parameter values to assure that the routine has not stopped at a local optimum. These precautions are particularly important when more than one parameter is being estimated simultaneously, since the parameters in biologically based models are often highly correlated, making independent estimation difficult. Estimates of parameter variance obtained from automatic optimization routines should be viewed as lower bound estimates of true parameter uncertainty since only a local, linearized variance is typically calculated. In characterizing parameter uncertainty, it is probably more instructive to determine what ranges of parameter values are clearly inconsistent with the data than to accept a local, linearized variance estimate provided by the optimization algorithm.

It is usually necessary for the investigator to repeatedly vary the model parameters manually to obtain a sense of their identifiability and correlation under various experimental conditions, although some simulation languages include routines for calculating parameter sensitivity and covariance or for plotting confidence region contours. Sensitivity analysis and Monte Carlo uncertainty analysis techniques can serve as useful methods to estimate the impact of input parameter uncertainty on the uncertainty of model outputs. However, care should be taken to avoid violation of mass balance when parameters are varied by sensitivity or Monte Carlo algorithms, particularly where blood flows are affected.

Sensitivity Analysis   To the extent that a particular PBPK model correctly reflects the physiological and biochemical processes underlying the pharmacokinetics of a compound, exercising the model can provide a means for identifying the most important physiological and biochemical parameters determining the PK behavior of the compound under different conditions [39]. The technique for obtaining this information is known as *sensitivity analysis* and can be performed by two different methods. Analytical sensitivity coefficients are defined as the ratio of the change in a model output to the change in a model parameter that produced it. To obtain a sensitivity coefficient by this method, the model is run for the exposure scenario of interest using the preferred values of the input parameters, and the resulting output (e.g., brain concentration) is recorded. The model is then run again with the value of one of the input parameters varied slightly. Typically, a 1% change is appropriate. The ratio of the resulting incremental change in the output to the change in the input represents the sensitivity coefficient. It is usually more convenient to use log-normalized sensitivity coefficients, which represent the ratio of the fractional change in output to the fractional change in input. For example, if a 1% increase in an input parameter resulted in a 0.5% decrease in the output, the log-normalized sensitivity coefficient would be −0.5. Log-normalized sensitivity coefficients >1.0 in absolute value represent amplification of input error and would be a cause for concern. An alternative approach is to conduct a Monte Carlo analysis, as described below, and then to perform a simple correlation analysis of the model outputs and input parameters. This type of approach is often referred to as *global sensitivity analysis* [76]. Both methods have specific advantages. The analytical sensitivity coefficient most accurately represents the functional relationship of the output to the specific input under the conditions being modeled. The advantage of the global sensitivity analysis is that it also reflects the impact of interactions between the parameters during the Monte Carlo analysis.

Uncertainty and Variability Analysis   Evaluations of the uncertainty and/or the variability associated with the predictions of a PBPK model are often performed using the Monte Carlo simulation approach [77, 78]. In a Monte Carlo simulation, a probability distribution for each of the PBPK model parameters is randomly sampled, and the model is run using the chosen set of parameter values. This process is repeated a large number of times until the probability distribution for the desired model output has been created. Generally, 1000 iterations or more may be required to ensure the reproducibility of the mean and standard deviation of the output distributions as well as the 1st through 99th percentiles. To the extent that the input parameter distributions adequately characterize the uncertainty in the inputs, and assuming that the parameters are reasonably independent, the resulting output distribution will provide a useful estimate of the uncertainty associated with the model outputs. If simulations are performed so that the probability distribution for PBPK model parameters represents the variability expected in the human population, then the Monte Carlo analysis will result in the simulation of pharmacokinetics expected for a population.

In performing a Monte Carlo analysis, it is important to distinguish uncertainty from variability. As it relates to the impact of pharmacokinetics in risk assessment, uncertainty can be defined as the possible error in estimating the "true" value of a parameter for a representative ("average") person. Variability, on the other hand, should only be considered to represent true interindividual differences. Understood in these terms, uncertainty is a defect (lack of certainty), which can typically be reduced by experimentation, and variability is a fact of life, which must be considered regardless of the risk assessment methodology used. An elegant approach for separately documenting the impact of uncertainty and variability is "two-dimensional" Monte Carlo, in which distributions for both uncertainty and variability are developed and multiple Monte Carlo runs are used to convolute the two aspects of overall uncertainty. Unfortunately, in practice, it is often difficult to differentiate the contribution of variability and uncertainty to the observed variation in the reported measurements of a particular parameter.

Due to its physiological structure, many of the parameters in a PBPK model are interdependent. For example, the blood flows must add up to the total cardiac output and the tissue volumes (including those not included in the model) must add up to the body weight. Failure to account for the impact of Monte Carlo sampling on these mass balances can produce erroneous results. In addition, some physiological parameters are naturally correlated, such as cardiac output and respiratory ventilation rate, and these correlations should be taken into account during the Monte Carlo analysis.

Although sophisticated methods of uncertainty analysis can provide valuable information, very simple techniques can also be used as a way to effectively communicate uncertainty. By simply determining the minimum and maximum values of an uncertain but important model parameter, and performing a simulation for a range of values, the impact of that parameter on PK predictions can be illustrated. When predicting human pharmacokinetics based on preclinical data, there is always uncertainty. Quantifying key uncertainties and providing a range of possible outcomes that could all be reasonable based on the current knowledge of the PK properties of the compound will allow for more informed decision-making.

Collection of Critical Data   As with model development, the best approach to model evaluation is within the context of the scientific method. The most effective way to evaluate a PBPK model is to exercise the model to generate a quantitative hypothesis; that is, to predict the behavior of the system of interest under conditions "outside the envelope" of the data used to develop the model (at shorter/longer durations, higher/lower concentrations, different routes, different species, etc.). In particular, if there is an element of the model that remains in question, the model can be exercised to determine the experimental design under which the specific model element can best be tested. For example, if there is uncertainty regarding whether uptake into a particular tissue is flow or diffusion limited, alternative forms of the model can be used to compare predicted tissue concentration time courses under each of the limiting assumptions under various experimental conditions. The experimental design and sampling time that maximize the difference between the predicted tissue concentrations under the two assumptions can then serve as the basis for the actual experimental data collection. Once the critical data has been collected, the same model can also be used to support a more quantitative experimental inference. In the case of the tissue uptake question just described, not only can the *a priori* model predictions be compared with the observed data to test the alternative hypotheses, but the model can also be used *a posteriori* to estimate the quantitative extent of any observed diffusion limitation (i.e., to estimate the relevant model parameter by fitting the data). If, on the other hand, the model is unable to reproduce the experimental data under either assumption, it may be necessary to reevaluate other aspects of the model structure. The key difference between research and analysis is the iterative nature of the former. It has wisely been said, "If we knew when we started what we had to do to finish, they'd call it search, not research."

35.4   GENERIC PBPK MODELS

Despite the clear value of compound-specific PBPK models developed by scientists with experience in kinetic modeling and designed to address kinetic issues specific to that compound, there is also a need for simpler modeling techniques that can readily be applied across diverse compounds by an inexperienced user. The past ten years have seen tremendous advances in the capabilities of generic PBPK models that can simulate pharmacokinetics for humans or preclinical species based on a combination of physicochemical properties and *in vitro* data. The generic PBPK model has recently become an increasingly important tool in assessing DMPK properties in preclinical development. Recent work has demonstrated the value of applying generic PBPK models in early preclinical development [14, 21, 22, 79].

35.4.1   User-Friendly Software Packages Bringing PBPK Modeling to the Nonexpert

The possible benefits from having PBPK software packages available for scientists who are nonmodelers have been a topic of interest for many years. Such a tool would need to meet many criteria to be broadly useful. This tool would need to be user-friendly, fast, flexible, and requiring little mathematical expertise from the user. The import of data into the tool and the export of results from the tool would need to be fast and automatable. The required input would be clearly defined and difficult to enter incorrectly, making consistent use by scientists of varying backgrounds possible. The tool would ideally be applicable through all stages of preclinical through clinical development. The pharmaceutical industry now has many tools that meet some or all of these criteria. Tools using physiology-based whole body models for the simulation of the PK behavior including absorption, distribution, and elimination include GastroPlus™ (Simulations Plus Inc., www.simulations-plus.com), Simcyp (Simcyp, www.simcyp.com), PK-Sim® (Bayer Technology Services, www.pksim.com), MEDICI-PK (AT Computing in Technology GnbH, www.cit-wulkow.de), and Cloe PK® (Cyprotex, www.cyprotex.com).

35.4.2   Recent Advances in Generic PBPK Modeling Tools

GastroPlus, which is well known in the pharmaceutical industry for its capabilities in predicting oral absorption in preclinical species based on the ACAT model, has recently expanded to include the capability of PBPK modeling. In the most recent version, GastroPlus includes a physiological intestinal model for humans in fed and fasted states as well as models for the rat, dog, cynomolgus monkey, and mouse. Several additional modules are available for parameter optimization, for combining the absorption model with physiological and compartmental PK models, and for PD models. The software also includes clinical trial simulation capabilities and a powerful method of performing sensitivity analysis. Although currently only PBPK modules for the rat and human are available, users can create PBPK models for other species themselves by creating input files with appropriate physiological parameters. The performance of GastroPlus to predict absorption was evaluated by Parrott and Lavé [80]. In this study, GastroPlus was compared to iDEA™, another software to predict absorption that is no longer commercially available.

Another tool for predicting human pharmacokinetics, Simcyp (Simcyp Limited, Sheffield, UK), was previously known as a DDI clinical trial simulator but has expanded to include PBPK modeling capabilities. Simcyp utilizes fundamental scaling procedures described by Houston [68] for the prediction of *in vivo* hepatic clearance (CL_H) from *in vitro* metabolism data. These *in vitro* metabolism data can be obtained from individual cytochrome P450s (CYP) in human-expressed recombinant systems. These are used for predicting behavior not only in average individuals but also in whole populations or in special subpopulations. In order to predict drug–drug interactions involving CYP, Simcyp utilizes the relationship between the inhibitor concentration at the active site *in vivo* and the inhibition constant (K_i) determined *in vitro*. Competitive inhibition, induction, and/or mechanism-based inactivation mechanisms can be investigated within this software, according to the principles described by Ito et al. [71] and Tucker et al. [81]. Simcyp not only predicts the mean value but also simulates the extremes in the population by applying a Monte Carlo approach. This software comes with a database of physiological properties for specific populations and of PK information for specific drugs on the market (e.g., the CYP3A4 substrate midazolam, the CYP3A4 inducer rifampicin, and the CYP3A4 inducer and inhibitor ritonavir).

Yet another tool, PK-Sim, developed as a user-friendly tool for PBPK modeling, has PBPK models in the mouse, rat, dog, monkey, and human. In the model, tissue concentrations depend on the blood flow rate to the tissue, the rate of permeation into the tissue, active transport processes into and out of the tissue, and the rate of metabolism within a tissue. Although this detailed description allows significant flexibility and complexity, the user-friendly interface also allows for simple simulations whereby the more complex features are not utilized. In PK-Sim, the GI tract is described as a single tube with physiologically relevant dimensions and spatially varying properties such as pH and surface area. The software has Monte Carlo capabilities, and simulations examining the impact of interindividual variability can be performed using the population PK module. Physiological parameters for people from 0 to 80 years old are provided, allowing simulations of pharmacokinetics in the young and the elderly. Also, the software has the capability of linking PK to PD behavior with a PK/PD module.

In a fresh approach to PBPK modeling, the new software MEDICI-PK was developed using a novel software concept aimed at providing increased flexibility while maintaining user-friendliness. Instead of adopting the traditional approach whereby user-friendliness is made possible by adopting a static model, in MEDICI-PK the system of differential equations is generated automatically when starting a simulation. This software allows for predictions of parent compound and multiple metabolites, and interactions (metabolic and otherwise) between compounds [82]. MEDICI-PK has PBPK modeling capabilities for multiple species (e.g., the human, mouse, and dog) that can be extended by the user, and also contains PD modeling capabilities.

Cloe-PK is a commercial tool aimed at prediction of human pharmacokinetics at the earliest stages of drug discovery [83]. The PBPK model includes 14 organs and tissues, clearance by metabolism and renal excretion, and diffusion-limited uptake in tissues. In each of the organ compartments, the capillary, intracellular, and extracellular spaces are explicitly included. Using *in vitro* and *in silico* data as input, this software can predict human IV and oral *AUC* from clinical trial data within 2-fold and 3.75-fold, respectively (www.cyprotex.com/products/pk_howwell.htm). Studies on the accuracy of the model for predicting PK behavior in the rat and human have been published [21, 22] and illustrate the utility of this software for predicting pharmacokinetics and ranking compounds based on minimal data and *in silico* parameters.

These software packages are exceptionally useful tools, and we expect them to be increasingly used in the pharmaceutical industry. However, their implementation may require a modeling and simulation expert to determine appropriate applications and methods of use and to perform validation exercises to convince the scientists involved with the preclinical development of drugs that the packages do indeed work. Additionally, in-house PBPK expertise and models will still be necessary because these standard tools do not allow the flexibility to simulate every situation that will arise. For example, currently some generic PBPK tools do not yet have the capability to simulate exposures to a parent compound and a metabolite, which could be of interest for simulating the pharmacokinetics of prodrugs or investigating possible PK interactions between the parent and metabolite. Also, generic PBPK software packages have sophisticated capabilities that may require an expert modeler to determine appropriate ways to use (and not misuse) the features (e.g., GastroPlus has the capability of simulating enterohepatic cycling, and PK-Sim can incorporate saturable and nonsaturable metabolism in multiple tissue compartments). In addition, the availability of such tools simplifies the technical use of PBPK models; however, a good understanding of the models and underlying equations is still mandatory in order to guarantee good interpretation of output.

35.5   INTEGRATING PRECLINICAL DATA USING THE PBPK MODEL

Here, we provide examples of how PBPK modeling is a valuable tool in several stages of drug development. During the lead identification (LI) and lead optimization (LO) stages, limited data is available. During the clinical candidate selection, more data is available. Finally, a rich dataset is available prior to entry into humans. The availability of data and issues that arise at each stage dictate the utility of PBPK modeling.

35.5.1   Preclinical Data Useful for PBPK Modeling

Much of the data typically generated in the preclinical development process used to characterize key aspects of ADME can be used in PBPK model development (Table 35.1). The first information generated includes *in silico* parameters (e.g., polar surface area, pK_a, and $\log P$ values are calculated). Metabolic stability studies (e.g., in microsomes or hepatocytes) are often considered critical to determine if hepatic metabolism is a major route of elimination and if first-pass metabolism might result in unacceptably low bioavailability [84, 85]. Screens for permeability and solubility are often implemented early in the process. Plasma protein binding might be measured to determine if a compound will have a sufficient free concentration for therapeutic efficacy [86]. The blood-to-plasma ratio, *BPR*, might be measured to provide a rational basis for the appropriate biological fluid for assay (e.g., blood or plasma) and to aid in interpreting PK data [42]. Also, screens specific to a disease area might be implemented. For example, a P-glycoprotein (P-gp) screen might be used to determine if a compound will be able to penetrate the central nervous system.

Single-dose pharmacokinetic (SDPK) studies in a rodent species might be performed to determine if a compound has drug-like PK properties and adequate bioavailability. Later studies might include SDPK studies in a nonrodent species. Hepatocyte or microsomal clearance data can be scaled to estimate the *in vivo* metabolic clearance in preclinical species and humans [70, 87]. The scaled clearance in preclinical species can be compared to clearance in SDPK studies to determine if hepatic metabolism is a major route of elimination in preclinical species. If the clearance seen in SDPK studies is higher than the clearance scaled from hepatocyte or microsome data, urine and/or bile might be collected in SDPK studies to provide additional information on mechanisms of clearance.

These studies provide pharmaceutical scientists with qualitative information on the potential human PK behavior of a compound. Using PBPK modeling, the results of the various preclinical assays can be integrated to provide a quantitative prediction of human pharmacokinetics [88]. During preclinical development, DMPK data are constantly being generated. Therefore, the human PK projection will change as more information becomes available. A PBPK model can act as a repository of current information and is easily updated when new PK or PD data becomes available. An important feature of PBPK models is that they can be used to determine the key data that should be generated.

35.5.2 Lead Identification and Optimization Stages

Drug discovery is increasingly "data rich" with high throughput chemistry generating numerous compounds that are rapidly screened for pharmacological and PK properties. Determination of *in vivo* pharmacokinetics is considerably more costly and slower than *in vitro* screening, and so there is interest in optimizing resources by using simulation to prioritize compounds. Physiologically based pharmacokinetics can be used at this stage to prioritize compounds prior to *in vivo* experimentation—getting an estimate of the expected PK profile of new drug candidates in humans and providing some mechanistic understanding of the compound's properties and of the relevance of the assays used in the screening strategy.

Because of the mechanistic basis of PBPK models, when they do not adequately describe animal PK data, this means that a biological phenomenon affecting pharmacokinetics has not been included in the model and is not represented by the assays used to screen the compounds. Therefore, if a PK issue for a promising compound becomes apparent, PBPK modeling allows you to determine which mechanisms are consistent with the observed data. This information can be used to guide further experimentation to arrive more rapidly at the desired information. Understanding pharmacokinetics in preclinical species using PBPK modeling can also provide a scientific basis for determining which preclinical species are most relevant to humans, thereby improving the scientific rationale of the selected screening strategy.

The emerging technology of generic PBPK modeling has been shown in recent studies to have potential as a valuable tool for assessing the pharmacokinetics of compounds in the early stages of drug development. For example, recent papers reported studies on applying generic PBPK modeling to predict rat pharmacokinetics [21] and human pharmacokinetics [22] following IV administration of test compound. These studies were conducted to evaluate the commercial PBPK modeling package Cloe PK [83]. The PBPK model included 14 organs and tissues, clearance by metabolism and renal excretion, and diffusion-limited uptake in tissues. For these rat and human models, model input included molecular weight, octanol/water partitioning, octanol/water distribution coefficient at a pH of 7.4, hepatic intrinsic metabolic clearance, and the unbound fraction in plasma. Model development involved the use of a training dataset consisting of 82 compounds for the rat model and 69 compounds for the human model. After the models were developed, they were tested using data from test datasets consisting of 134 compounds in the rat and 18 compounds in the human. Using this approach to rank compounds and select the 25% most likely to have the best exposure (i.e., AUC) resulted in 61% of the best compounds being selected, which is a 2.4-fold improvement over random selection [21]. Brightman et al. [22] concluded that "the generic PBPK model is potentially a powerful and cost-effective tool for predicting the mammalian pharmacokinetics of a wide range of organic compounds, from readily available *in vitro* inputs only."

In a similar study, Parrott et al. [79] studied applying generic PBPK modeling to predict rat pharmacokinetics following IV or PO administration of test compound. This rat PBPK model included 11 tissue compartments and clearance by metabolism in the liver; uptake in tissues was assumed to be perfusion limited. GastroPlus was used to simulate oral absorption. For this model, the necessary input included structure-based predictions of lipophilicity, ionization, and protein binding, intrinsic clearance based on rat hepatocyte data, experimentally measured aqueous solubility, and artificial membrane permeability. To improve the prediction of AUC following oral administration of compounds, particularly for compounds with $\log P > 4$, it was necessary to use solubility in simulated intestinal fluid since aqueous solubility apparently underestimates *in vivo* solubility for highly lipophilic compounds. Parrott et al. [79] noted that "overall, this evaluation shows that generic simulation may be applicable for typical drug-like compounds to predict differences in PK parameters of more than twofold based upon minimal measured input data." The authors recommend that, for applying the method for new series of compounds outside the range of the training dataset, the model be verified for several compounds before it is generally applied.

35.5.3   Clinical Candidate Selection

PBPK modeling has a great potential to assist clinical candidate selection where numerous factors must be considered and data related to the pharmacokinetics and pharmacodynamics of a compound needs to be combined and compared in a rational way. This potential was illustrated by Parrott et al. [14], who demonstrated the use of PBPK modeling to select the best compound from among five candidates for the clinical lead. The preclinical data for the five candidates was integrated and the efficacious human doses and associated internal exposures were estimated. For this calculation, the PBPK models were linked to an E_{max} PD model so that the dose resulting in a 90% effect could be identified. This example showed that the PBPK approach facilitates a sound decision on the selection of the optimal molecule to be progressed by integrating the available information and focusing the attention onto the expected properties in human. Importantly, the method can include estimates of variability and uncertainty in the predictions to verify that decisions are based on significant differences between the compounds.

35.5.4   Supporting Entry into Humans

After a clinical candidate has been selected, the first-in-human (FIH) dose must be selected. There are many ways of selecting the FIH dose. For example, in therapeutic areas other than oncology, FIH dose estimates can be determined by multiplying the no-observed-adverse-effect-level (NOAEL) from preclinical toxicology studies by a safety factor, by using human data for a similar compound when they are available, or by using a PK model based on preclinical data to determine the dose that will result in a systemic exposure identified as therapeutic based on preclinical pharmacology data [89]. When this last approach is adopted, it is often referred to as performing a human PK extrapolation.

The first step of the human PK extrapolation is to identify the internal measure of exposure (e.g., the C_{min}, C_{max}, or AUC) believed to be efficacious in humans based on pharmacology data. Next, a human PK model for IV exposures is developed based on all preclinical data. This PK model can be developed in many ways, including PBPK modeling [13]. The oral exposure route is added to the human IV PK model. Again, there are many ways to model oral absorption, for example, by using an empirical first-order oral absorption rate constant or using the physiological ACAT model. Finally, once the model is developed, the dose that will result in the therapeutic exposure is determined. The estimated efficacious dose and other information (e.g., the C_{min}, C_{max}, $AUC(0–24\,h)$, CL, V_{ss}, $t_{1/2}$) are reported. PK projections can be based on a single or repeated (e.g., steady-state) exposure. At this stage it is important to understand the uncertainty of the FIH dose estimate.

Uncertainty can be illustrated by presenting a range of results (e.g., dose, AUC) from different models, or a range of results for different values of a key parameter that is not known with great certainty. If uncertainty is too great, additional experiments can be designed to aid in narrowing the possible values of key parameters. If uncertainty is extensive and cannot be reduced with additional experimentation, it is perhaps better to simply state that uncertainty is too great to predict human pharmacokinetics than to report a human PK projection that is not likely to be correct. PBPK modeling can be used as a tool to understand the quantitative impact of uncertainty from key knowledge gaps and also helps to minimize uncertainty due to species differences in PK properties.

In its best form, the human PK extrapolation is an integration of all preclinical data (e.g., *in vivo* data for the rodent and nonrodent, and *in vitro* data in the corresponding preclinical species as well as human) to provide a scientifically defensible estimate (extrapolation) of the likely pharmacokinetics of a compound in humans. Luttringer et al. [90] recently examined the ability of PBPK modeling to predict human pharmacokinetics based on preclinical species, using epiroprim as a test compound due to significant species differences in its PK properties. By incorporating information on species differences in PK properties from *in vitro* studies (e.g., in protein binding, the blood-to-plasma ratio, and intrinsic clearance in hepatocytes), PBPK modeling was able to reduce the uncertainty inherent in interspecies extrapolation and to provide a better prediction of human pharmacokinetics than allometric scaling or by direct scaling of hepatocyte data.

Recently, Jones et al. [13] reported similar results in a comparison between empirical and physiologically based approaches for the human PK extrapolation. Human pharmacokinetics of 19 compounds that had entered into humans was predicted using Dedrick plot analysis and PBPK modeling. A strategy for predicting human pharmacokinetics by focusing on methods for understanding the effects of absorption, distribution, and elimination from a physiological perspective was

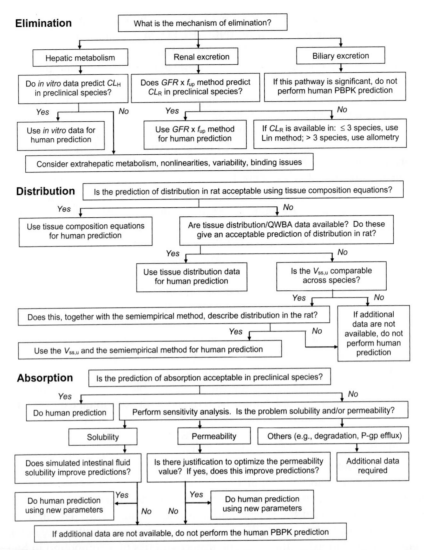

FIGURE 35.4 A strategy for applying PBPK modeling to predict human pharmacokinetics prior to FIH. CL_H, hepatic clearance; CL_R, renal clearance; f_{up}, unbound fraction in plasma; *GFR*, glomerular filtration rate; QWBA, quantitative whole-body autoradiography; $V_{ss,u}$, steady-state volume of distribution of unbound drug. (Adapted from Ref. 13.)

developed (Fig. 35.4). The ability of PBPK modeling to predict pharmacokinetics in preclinical species was tested, and the human pharmacokinetics was only predicted if the model could predict pharmacokinetics in preclinical species. Based on this criterion, for 70% of the 19 compounds included in the study, a human PK prediction could be made. Jones et al. [13] noted: "The prediction accuracy for these compounds in terms of the percentage of compounds with an average-fold error of <2-fold was 83%, 50%, 75%, 67%, 92% and 100% for apparent oral clearance (CL/F), apparent volume of distribution during terminal phase after oral administration

(V-z/F), terminal elimination half-life (t1/2), peak plasma concentration (C-max), area under the plasma concentration-time curve (AUC) and time to reach C-max (t(max)), respectively." Simulated plasma concentrations and PK parameters were compared with human data so that the accuracy of the prediction methods could be assessed. The human PK data were more accurately predicted by the PBPK modeling approach than by the empirical approach. Using the strategy proposed by Jones et al. [13], the model development guides the strategy for gathering the data necessary for a complete understanding of likely human PK behavior.

Poor predictions with PBPK models are often a result of incomplete knowledge resulting in processes not correctly incorporated into the model (e.g., for biliary clearance and enterohepatic recirculation there are limited options for quantitatively predicting the effects on human pharmacokinetics). For such situations, an alternative method of performing the human PK extrapolation (e.g., allometric scaling) might seem attractive. However, allometric scaling is based on the assumption that clearance is proportional to $BW^{0.75}$ and that steady-state volume of distribution is proportional to BW^1 due to physiological properties (i.e., the same physiological properties that are incorporated in PBPK models). If PBPK modeling does not appear to be a good method for a compound, there is no reason to believe that allometric scaling or other empirical methods will work either. Additionally, developing methods for including increasingly complex PK mechanisms (e.g., first-pass metabolism and transporters in the gut, EH cycling, biliary excretion, and multiple pathways of elimination) is an active area of research, and methods for predicting human pharmacokinetics even with PK complications will soon be possible.

35.6 EXAMPLES OF THE USE OF PBPK MODELING IN DRUG DEVELOPMENT

In this section, two examples are provided of successful PBPK models for drugs that have been developed in the past: methotrexate (a cancer therapeutic) and all-*trans*-retinoic acid (a cancer therapeutic and skin treatment). Two areas in which PBPK modeling will become increasingly important in the future are then discussed: evaluation of PK variability and modeling of pharmacodynamics.

35.6.1 Methotrexate

The PBPK model for methotrexate (MTX) provides an excellent example of the iterative nature of the process of developing a PBPK model for a drug. The stated rationale for the approach used was "basing the model, as much as possible, on established, independently verifiable, physiological concepts" [5]. For the initial model development [91], a single IV dose of 3 mg/kg, which falls in the range of clinical treatment levels, was evaluated in CDF-1 male mice. Key observations regarding the behavior of the kinetic data included an unusually large initial drop in the plasma MTX concentration, indicating rapid uptake, tissue localization, and excretion (MTX is not metabolized extensively in mice). A subsequent asymptotic leveling of the concentration curves for all tissues was taken as evidence for zero-order uptake of MTX from the gut. A rapid early increase in the concentration of

MTX in the small intestine, with a peak gut lumen:plasma concentration ratio of about 100, demonstrated the importance of enterohepatic recycling.

Based on these observations, an initial MTX model was developed that included five compartments: plasma, muscle, liver, kidneys, and GI tract tissue/lumen [91]. The authors also derived reduced model structures with three compartments (plasma/body, liver, gut lumen) or two compartments (plasma/body plus gut lumen) to expedite solution of the associated system of equations. Flow-limited transport was assumed in all versions of the model, except as described below. The model incorporated a time-delay term to account for bile transport and holding time. Biliary clearance rates were estimated by bile duct cannulation experiments. To account for GI travel time and fecal excretion delays, time-delay functions were also applied in the gut lumen. Renal clearance was determined by comparison of the integrated plasma concentration data with cumulative urinary excretion data. Plasma protein binding was estimated at 25%. Comparison of experimental data and model predictions showed good agreement in general, although the model overpredicted gut lumen concentrations for times less than 60 minutes, probably due to the simple time-delay description of biliary transport.

In order to refine their initial model, Bischoff et al. [5] studied a variety of dose levels of MTX in several species, including humans. The additional data reproduced the initial data's features of (1) a rapid drop in MTX plasma concentrations and a corresponding increase in gut lumen concentrations, indicating the importance of tissue uptake and biliary secretion; (2) a peak gut lumen:plasma ratio of approximately 100; and (3) linear binding of MTX in tissues as plasma concentrations increased above 0.1 µg/mL, indicating nonlinear binding at low concentrations. The authors speculated that this phenomenon was probably due to strong binding to dihydrofolate reductase.

A revised PBPK model (Fig. 35.2) was developed to describe the more extensive data. Renal clearance of MTX was determined by comparing the time integral of plasma concentration with cumulative urine formation after intraperitoneal (IP) or IV administration. Tissue:plasma equilibrium ratios were derived from constant infusion experiments and/or the portion of the IV pulse injection curve after initial redistribution. Constant tissue:plasma equilibrium ratios at high concentrations indicated linear binding, while at lower concentrations, equilibrium ratios were represented by the sum of linear nonspecific binding and strong binding (presumed to be associated with dihydrofolate reductase).

An important feature of the revised model was its use of multicompartment submodels for biliary secretion and GI transport (Fig. 35.2). The original model used a mathematical time-delay (step function) to simulate bile formation and secretion from the liver. The abrupt introduction of bile into the GI tract lumen at the delay time caused the model to overshoot the data in this time period. In the revised model, biliary secretion was represented by a three-compartment submodel in which a series of discrete compartments was able to produce a smoother "S-shaped" bile concentration efflux curve.

MTX transit through the GI tract was modeled using an approach similar to that used for biliary secretion. Due to the tubular flow nature of the gut lumen, an assumption of uniform mixing would not predict the correct time course for concentrations appearing in the feces. Therefore, the GI tract was divided into four distinct regions with the feces exiting from the last compartment. An assumption of zero-order absorption from the GI tract that was adequate for the single-dose level described in the initial modeling was not adequate for the wider range of dose levels investigated in the follow-up study. The revised model therefore provided for both saturable and nonsaturable GI tract absorption. In the absence of detailed data indicating otherwise, absorption characteristics were assumed to be the same for all regions, but specific location-dependent absorption characteristics could be included using this approach.

Comparison of model predictions and experimental data demonstrated that a single model structure was able to describe MTX distribution and excretion reasonably well for the mouse, rat, dog, and human, using species-specific parameters. The greatest uncertainty in the model was in the kinetics describing intestinal absorption. The authors concluded that GI tract absorption was not readily saturable, and both saturable and nonsaturable absorption should be included in the model. Based on the observed kinetic behavior at very low doses, the authors concluded that strong, saturable nonlinear binding occurred in the liver and kidney, probably related to binding with dihydrofolate reductase.

35.6.2 All-*trans*-Retinoic Acid

A PBPK model for all-*trans*-retinoic acid (ATRA; tretinoin) was developed in order to provide a coherent description of the absorption, distribution, metabolism, and excretion of the compound and its metabolites across species and routes of administration [19]. The goal of developing such a model was to provide a more biologically relevent dose measure than administered dose for assessing the human teratogenic risk from ATRA.

The PBPK model developed for ATRA provided a full physiological description for ATRA, with compartments for plasma, liver, gut, intestinal lumen, fat, skin, richly perfused tissues, slowly perfused tissues, placenta, and embryo (Fig. 35.3). Both oxidation (to the 4-oxo derivative) and glucuronidation of ATRA were described with saturable kinetics. Conversion to the 13-*cis* isomer (13-*cis*-RA; isotretinoin) and the subsequent metabolism of that compound were also included (not shown). Simpler compartmental descriptions were used for the metabolites, since there was no evidence that they preferentially partitioned into any of the body tissues. A third metabolic pathway, side chain oxidation producing CO_2, was also included. Oral uptake was described by zero-order stomach emptying and first-order uptake from the intestinal lumen. Dermal uptake was described by a two-compartment model, with compartments representing the stratum corneum and viable epidermis. Distribution was assumed to be flow limited except for dermal uptake and transplacental transfer, which were assumed to be diffusion limited. Excretions into urine and feces were modeled as first-order processes, with all chemicals being excreted in the feces and only glucuronides being excreted in the urine. Enterohepatic recirculation of ATRA and its metabolites was also described.

The physiological parameters for adult animals were obtained from Brown et al. [30]. Gestational parameters were based on previous modeling of rats [92, 93]. Partition coefficients were based on distribution studies with mice [94] and with a human placenta [95]. The ATRA volume of distribution calculated using these partitions, 1.1 L/kg, agrees with measured values. Biliary excretion was adjusted on the basis of data from rats with exteriorized bile ducts [96, 97]. The metabolic

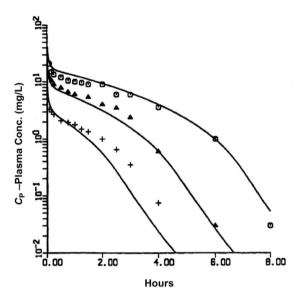

FIGURE 35.5   Simulation of plasma concentration of all-*trans*-retinoic acid in the plasma of nonhuman primates following intravenous (IV) dosing at 5, 2.5, and 1 mg/kg.

parameters were adjusted using data for IV administration of ATRA in rats [97] and monkeys [98], as well as from metabolite measurements [96, 99]. A key difference in the metabolism of ATRA across species is the predominance of the oxidative pathway in the rodent [96, 97], in contrast with the predominance of the glucuronide pathway in the primate [99].

The PBPK model for IV dosing of ATRA in the monkey (Fig. 35.5) was scaled allometrically to predict the kinetics for oral dosing of human leukemia patients with 1.1 mg/kg ATRA [100]. The only parameters adjusted in this extrapolation were those describing the rate of oral uptake. All other parameters were calculated from those for the monkey. The resulting model provided an excellent description of the kinetics for humans with oral dosing (Fig. 35.6). It was also able to reproduce the observed kinetics for total radioactivity following topical administration of ATRA (Fig. 35.7). In contrast to the kinetic data, which could only provide an estimate of total exposure to ATRA plus its metabolites, the PBPK model was able to provide separate estimates of internal exposure to ATRA and its active and inactive metabolites. An important result of the modeling was to demonstrate that the low dose rate associated with dermal exposure results in high efficiency clearance of ATRA to its inactive glucuronide metabolites, as opposed to oral dosing, where the higher dose rate leads to a greater proportion of active oxidative metabolites.

The model was used to simulate oral clinical dosing with ATRA, as well as minimal teratogenic doses of ATRA in the primate and rodent. Based on literature data on the teratogenic potential of the various chemical species, the most appropriate dose surrogate could be either C_{max} or AUC for the total concentration of active retinoids (ATRA + 4-oxo-ATRA + 13-*cis*-RA + 4-oxo-13-*cis*-RA). The glucuronides are not included in this dose measure since they do not cross the placenta. On

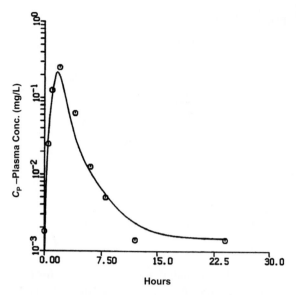

FIGURE 35.6 Simulation of all-*trans*-retinoic acid concentration in plasma of human subject receiving an oral dose of 1.1 mg/kg.

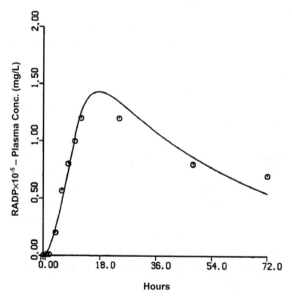

FIGURE 35.7 Simulation of total radiation in plasma following topical treatment of human subject with 50 micrograms of all-*trans*-retinoic acid.

the other hand, based on activity at retinoic acid receptors it could be argued that the most appropriate dose surrogate could be the peak concentration or area under the curve for ATRA alone. In either case, maternal plasma levels were used as a surrogate for fetal levels, based on evidence from animal studies that concentrations achieved in maternal and fetal plasma are similar. The calculated

E 35.4 Comparison of Dose Surrogates for Retinoic Acid Teratogenicity

	Route	Dose (mg/kg)	All-*trans*-Retinoic Acid C_{max} (ng/mL)	All-*trans*-Retinoic Acid *AUC* (ng·h/mL)	Total Active Retinoids C_{max} (ng/mL)	Total Active Retinoids *AUC* (ng·h/mL)	Total Retinoids C_{max} (ng·eq/mL)
Minimal teratogenic doses (all-*trans*-RA)							
Mouse	Oral	4.0	1,048	1,852	2,681	12,658	3,107
Rat	Oral	2.5	943	2,029	1,918	13,554	2,051
Monkey	Oral	5.0	1,830	3,714	2,294	5,962	4,983
Clinical doses (human)							
ATRA	Oral	1.1	218	695	264	1,088	1,237
13-*Cis*	Oral	1.1	654[a]	3,154[a]	1,033	7,103	1,148

[a]Reflects concentration of 13-*cis*-RA rather than all-*trans*-RA.

dose surrogates, as well as the estimated peak plasma level for total retinoids (which includes the glucuronides), for several species are shown in Table 35.4.

One test of a useful dose surrogate is that similar values should be calculated at similar effect levels across species. For a minimal teratogenic effect, all of the dose surrogates in Table 35.4 (including administered dose) are within a factor of 2–3 across species. The most consistent dose surrogate is the C_{max} for total active retinoids, which is essentially constant across species. Based on this dose measure, the internal exposure of patients receiving oral ATRA treatment for cancer is below the threshold for teratogenic effects by about a factor of 7–10. However, this comparison assumes that the maternal plasma concentration profile is representative of fetal exposure. If one takes into consideration the longer period of organogenesis in the human (around 35 days) as compared to the rodent (around 10 days) and assumes, as a worst case, fetal exposure at the maximum maternal concentration throughout the entire period, the margin of safety could be as low as 2–3. It is of interest that the kinetics of 13-*cis*-RA in the human are considerably different from those of ATRA. 13-*cis*-RA has a much longer half-life than ATRA in the human and oxidation, rather than glucuronidation, is the dominant form of metabolism. The calculated plasma concentrations and *AUC* values for total active retinoids following oral treatment with 13-*cis*-RA are in the same range as those causing teratogenic effects in animals. This result is consistent with the observation of teratogenic effects associated with the human use of 13-*cis*-RA (isotretinoin, Table 35.4). This PBPK model was used by the FDA in its evaluation of the safety of a topical skin treatment containing ATRA.

35.6.3 Future Directions

Interindividual Variability Because of the heterogeneity of the human population, it is generally expected that there will be a broad range of responses to the biological effects of drugs. This heterogeneity is produced by interindividual variations in physiology, biochemistry, and molecular biology, reflecting both genetic and environmental factors, and results in differences among individuals in the biologically effective tissue dose associated with a given administered dose (pharmacokinetics) as well as in the response to a given tissue dose (pharmacody-namics). Often it is possible to distinguish specific classes of individuals, such as infants or the elderly, who appear to be more susceptible to a specific effect. PBPK modeling provides the capability to quantitatively describe the potential impact of PK factors on the variability of individual response. Because the parameters in a PBPK model have a direct biological correspondence, they provide a useful frame-work for determining the impact of observed variations in physiological and bio-chemical factors on the population variability in dosimetry.

For example, PBPK models can be used to determine the impact of differences in key metabolism enzymes, whether due to multiple genotypic expression, such as polymorphisms, or just due to normal variation in enzyme activities within the general population. Other potential modulators of sensitivity that can be addressed quantitatively with a PBPK model include physical condition, level of activity, disease states, age, hormonal status, and interactions with other chemicals and drugs. In each case, the PBPK model provides a quantitative structure for determining the effect of these various factors on the relationship between the administered dose and the internal (biologically effective) target tissue exposure. When coupled with Monte Carlo analysis, the PBPK model provides a method to assess the quantitative impact of these sources of variability on individual response (as opposed to average population response) by comparing model predicted internal doses over the distri-bution of individual parameter values.

It is useful to consider the total variability among humans in terms of three con-tributing sources: (1) the variation across a population of "normal" individuals at the same age (e.g., young adults); (2) the variation across the population resulting from their different ages (e.g., infants or the elderly); and (3) the variation resulting from the existence of subpopulations that differ in some way from the "normal" population (e.g., due to genetic polymorphisms). A fourth source of variability, health status, should also be considered. To the extent that the variation in physio-logical and biochemical parameters across these population dimensions can be elu-cidated, PBPK models can be used together with Monte Carlo methods to integrate their effects on the *in vivo* kinetics of a compound and predict the resulting impact on the distribution of responses (as represented by target tissue doses) across the population.

There has sometimes been a tendency in drug development to use information on the variability of a specific parameter, such as the *in vitro* activity of a particular enzyme, as the basis for expectations regarding the variability in dosimetry for *in vivo* exposures. However, whether or not the variation in a particular physiological or biochemical parameter will have a significant impact on *in vivo* dosimetry is a complex function of interacting factors. In particular, the structures of physiological and biochemical systems frequently involve parallel processes (e.g., blood flows, metabolic pathways, excretion processes), leading to compensation for the variation in a single factor. Moreover, physiological constraints may limit the *in vivo* impact of variability observed *in vitro*. For instance, high affinity intrinsic clearance can result in essentially complete metabolism of all the compound reaching the liver in the blood; under these conditions, variability in amount metabolized *in vivo* would be more a function of variability in liver blood flow than variability in metabolism *in vitro*. Thus, it is often true that the whole (the *in vivo* variability in dosimetry) is less than the sum of its parts (the variability in each of the PK factors).

The overall PK variability across a population is a function of many compound-specific, genetic, and physiological factors. Due to the complex interactions among these factors, speculation regarding the extent of population variability on the basis of the observed variation in a single factor can be highly misleading. Analysis using PBPK modeling and Monte Carlo techniques provides a more reliable approach for estimating population PK variability. PBPK modeling can also be useful in a more qualitative sense, to determine whether there is reason for concern regarding a particular age-group that might be more sensitive due to PK differences. Similar analyses can be performed to determine whether exposure during special life stages, such as gestation or lactation, represents a significant concern.

Modeling of Pharmacodynamics   The growing popularity of the PBPK modeling approach represents a movement from simpler kinetic models toward more biologically realistic descriptions of the determinants that regulate disposition of drugs in the body. To a large extent, the application of these PBPK models to study the time courses of compounds in the body is simply an integrated systems approach to understanding the biological processes that regulate the delivery of drugs to target sites. Many PBPK models integrate information across multiple levels of organization, especially when describing interactions of compounds with molecular targets, such as reversible binding of ligands to specific receptors, as in the case of methotrexate binding to dihydrofolate reductase [5, 101]. In such cases, the PBPK models integrate molecular, cellular, organ level, and organism-level processes to account for the time courses of compounds, metabolites, and bound complexes within organs and tissues in the body. The system under scrutiny in PBPK models is more the integrated physiological system, appropriate enough for a discipline defined as physiologically based modeling.

The main goal of PBPK models is quite simple—to predict the target tissue dose of compounds and their metabolites at target tissues and, in some cases, to describe interactions in target tissues. PBPK models once developed are extensible. They can be used to extrapolate to various other conditions because of their biological fidelity. While the goal in applying these models is to predict dosimetry, it is important to remember that the overall goal of using PBPK modeling in efficacy and safety assessment with drugs is broader than simply estimating tissue dose, regardless of the level of detail provided in the interactions of compounds with tissue constituents. The goal in the larger context is to understand the relationship between dose delivered to target tissues and the biological sequelae of the exposure of target tissues to compounds. The specific steps that lead from these dose metrics to tissue, organ, and organism-level responses have usually been considered part of the pharmacodynamic (PD) process. In general, PD models used in drug evaluation have been more empirical, utilizing simple effect compartments correlated with blood or tissue concentrations of active compound. Another inexorable development will be expansion of the systems approaches into the PBPD arena. This latter area will represent a systems biology approach for describing perturbations of biological systems by compounds and the exposure/dose conditions under which these perturbations become sufficiently large to pose significant health risks or sufficiently large to achieve specific therapeutic outcomes.

The systems biology approach (Fig. 35.8) focuses on normal biological function and the perturbations associated with exposure to compounds. Perturbations of

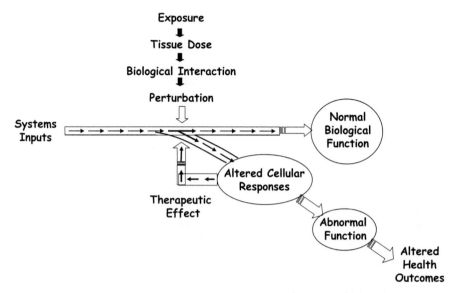

FIGURE 35.8 Diagram of the approach for understanding the pharmacological and toxicological effects of compounds in terms of their interaction with the biological system. The horizontal axis represents the biological component of the interaction, and the vertical axis represents the chemical component. Drugs can both restore altered biological function (efficacy) and produce altered function (toxicity).

biological processes by compounds lead to either adverse responses (toxicity) or restoration of normal function to a compromised tissue (efficacy). The effects of compounds, whether for good or ill, can best be described by PBPK approaches linked through PBPD models of responses of cellular signaling networks. Toxicity and efficacy are then defined by an intersection of compound action with the biological system. Toxicology and pharmacology are disciplines at the interface of chemistry/pharmacokinetics (primarily embedded in the vertical component) and biology/pharmacodynamics (primarily captured by the horizontal chain). Clearly, the main differences in the next generation of systems approaches in PK and PD modeling will be the increasingly detailed descriptions of biology afforded by new technologies and the expansion of modeling tools available for describing the effects of compounds on biological signaling processes.

35.7 CONCLUSIONS AND FUTURE PERSPECTIVES

It is ironic that PBPK modeling of drugs now appears to lag behind modeling of environmental contaminants [102], since the concept of PBPK modeling was first described in the context of drug disposition, in the seminal work of Teorell [1, 2]. In the pharmaceutical industry, noncompartmental "model-free" PK analyses are the standard practice, despite the fact that these methods are useful only for summarizing the characteristics of a dataset (e.g., volume of distribution, mean retention time, terminal half-life) and do not provide the advantages inherent in PBPK modeling (hypothesis testing, prediction, etc.). Their principal advantages are that they are rapid and inexpensive to perform.

However, in recent years there has been increasing pressure on the pharmaceutical industry to accelerate the drug development process, and PBPK modeling has repeatedly been identified as one of the technologies that could prove useful to this end [12, 102–104]. Because the collection of ADME data on a drug is a required element of drug development, much of the data necessary for developing a PBPK model is often available. The PBPK model offers the opportunity to make better use of these data, by serving as a structured repository for quantitative information on the compound, a conceptual framework for hypothesis testing, and a quantitative platform for prediction.

The rapid development of computational chemistry [105], genomics [106], and high throughput screening [107] has brought increasing attention to the discovery phase of drug development, including growing interest in "discovery toxicology" [108]. PBPK modeling can play a complementary role to two other technologies that are finding increasing use in drug discovery: QSAR analysis and genomics. QSAR can be used to estimate compound-specific parameters for the PBPK model, while genomic data can provide mode of action insights that drive model structure decisions. In this scenario, the PBPK model provides a quantitative biological framework for integrating the physicochemical characteristics of the drug candidate, together with *in vitro* data on its ADME and toxicity, within the constraints of the fundamental physiological and biochemical processes governing compound behavior *in vivo*. This approach is particularly effective when used consistently during drug development, because the information gained from modeling of previous candidate compounds can greatly facilitate model development for new compounds with similar structures or properties.

As the drug development process proceeds, the model can be iteratively informed and refined on the basis of the data being collected, and in turn the model can serve as a platform for *in silico* hypothesis testing and experimental design. As the model becomes more robust, it can also be employed for extrapolation (e.g., selection of first human dose) and for simulation (e.g., Monte Carlo analysis for design of clinical trials). The physiological structure of the PBPK model makes it a perfect platform for conducting evaluations of alternative dosing methods and regimens, and for investigating the impact of genetic-, age-, and disease-related differences in physiology and metabolism on drug kinetics. Of particular importance, by using a PBPK model the pharmacodynamic effects of a drug can be investigated more directly, relating the effects to the concentration in the tissue (e.g., the brain) where the compound interacts with the biological system, rather than attempting to elucidate a potentially indirect relationship with a concentration in the central (e.g., plasma) compartment. By obtaining quantitative information on the dose–responses for both the efficacy and toxicity of the compound, the PBPK model can be exercised to evaluate the potential to increase the efficacy/toxicity ratio of the drug through manipulation of dose rate and dose route using novel drug delivery systems. These and other attributes of PBPK models for organizing and interpreting diverse datasets, with the specific goals of understanding efficacy and toxicity, are reviving interest in applying these tools in drug development and evaluation [109–113]. The availability of increasingly sophisticated tools that can make predictions even with early preclinical data will encourage increasing application of PBPK modeling in preclinical development.

ACKNOWLEDGMENTS

The authors thank Dr. Carl Brown, Dr. Werner Rubas, and Dr. Phil Worboys for reviewing the manuscript for this chapter and providing valuable discussion and insight.

REFERENCES

1. Teorell T. Kinetics of distribution of substances administered to the body. I. The extravascular mode of administration. *Arch Int Pharmacodyn* 1937;57:205–225.
2. Teorell T. Kinetics of distribution of substances administered to the body. I. The intravascular mode of administration. *Arch Int Pharmacodyn* 1937;57:226–240.
3. Andersen ME. Saturable metabolism and its relation to toxicity. *Crit Rev Toxicol* 1981;9:105–150.
4. Bischoff KB, Brown RG. Drug distribution in mammals. *Chem Eng Prog Symp Ser* 1966;62(66):33–45.
5. Bischoff KB, Dedrick RL, Zaharko DS, Longstreth JA. Methotrexate pharmacokinetics. *J Pharm Sci* 1971;60:1128–1133.
6. Collins JM, Dedrick RL, Flessner MF, Guarino AM. Concentration dependent disappearance of fluorouracil from peritoneal fluid in the rat: experimental observations and distributed modeling. *J Pharm Sci* 1982;71:735–738.
7. Farris FF, Dedrick RL, King FG. Cisplatin pharmacokinetics: applications of a physiological model. *Toxicol Lett* 1988;43:117–137.
8. Andersen ME, Yang RSH, Clewell HJ, Reddy MB. Introduction: a historical perspective of the development and application of PBPK models. In Reddy MB, Yang RSH, Clewell HJ III, Andersen ME, Eds. *Physiologically Based Pharmacokinetic Modeling: Science and Applications*. Hoboken, NJ: John Wiley & Sons; 2005, pp 1–18.
9. McMullin TS. Drugs. In Reddy MB, Yang RSH, Clewell HJ III, Andersen ME, Eds. *Physiologically Based Pharmacokinetic Modeling: Science and Applications*. Hoboken, NJ: John Wiley & Sons; 2005, pp 273–296.
10. Pott O'Brien W. Antineoplastic agents. In Reddy MB, Yates RSH, Clewell HJ III, Andersen ME, Eds. *Physiologically Based Pharmacokinetic Modeling: Science and Applications*. Hoboken, NJ: John Wiley & Sons; 2005, pp 297–317.
11. Lupfert C, Reichel A. Development and application of physiologically based pharmacokinetic-modeling tools to support drug discovery. *Chem Biodiversity* 2005;2:1462–1486.
12. Nestorov I. Whole body pharmacokinetic models. *Clin Pharmacokinet* 2003;42:883–908.
13. Jones HM, Parrott N, Jorga K, Lave T. A novel strategy for physiologically based predictions of human pharmacokinetics. *Clin Pharmacokinet* 2006;45:511–542.
14. Parrott N, Jones H, Paquereau N, Lavé T. Application of full physiological models for pharmaceutical drug candidate selection and extrapolation of pharmacokinetics to man. *Basic Clin Pharmacol Toxicol* 2005;96:193–199.

15. Baxter LT, Zhu H, Mackensen DG, Jain RK. Physiologically-based pharmacokinetic model for specific and nonspecific monoclonal-antibodies and fragments in normal-tissues and human tumor xenografts in nude-mice. *Cancer Res* 1994;54:1517–1528.

16. Baxter LT, Zhu H, Mackensen DG, Butler WF, Jain RK. Biodistribution of monoclonal-antibodies—scale-up from mouse to human using a physiologically-based pharmacokinetic model. *Cancer Res* 1995;55:4611–4622.

17. Aarons L. Editors' view. Physiologically based pharmacokinetic modeling: a sound mechanistic basis is needed. *Br J Clin Pharm* 2005;60(6):581–583.

18. Dedrick RL, Bischoff KB. Species similarities in pharmacokinetics. *Fed Proc* 1980; 39:54–59.

19. Clewell HJ, Andersen ME, Wills RJ, Latriano L. A physiologically based pharmacokinetic model for retinoic acid and its metabolites. *J Am Acad Dermatol* 1997;36: S77–S85.

20. Reddy MB, Yang RSH, Clewell HJ III, Andersen ME, Eds. *Physiologically Based Pharmacokinetic Modeling: Science and Applications*. Hoboken, NJ: John Wiley & Sons; 2005.

21. Brightman FA, Leahy DE, Searle GE, Thomas S. Application of a generic physiologically based pharmacokinetic model to the estimation of xenobiotic levels in rat plasma. *Drug Metab Dispos* 2006;34:84–93.

22. Brightman FA, Leahy DE, Searle GE, Thomas S. Application of a generic physiologically based pharmacokinetic model to the estimation of xenobiotic levels in human plasma. *Drug Metab Dispos* 2006;34:94–101.

23. Malaty LI, Kuper JJ. Drug interactions of HIV. Protease inhibitors. *Drug Safety* 1999;20:147–169.

24. Adolph EF. Quantitative relations in the physiological constitutions of mammals. *Science* 1949;109:579–585.

25. Dedrick RL. Animal scale-up. *J Pharmacokinet Biopharm* 1973;1:435–461.

26. Astrand P, Rodahl K. *Textbook of Work Physiology*. New York: McGraw-Hill; 1970, pp 157–160, 206–211.

27. International Commission on Radiological Protection (ICRP). Report of the Task Group on Reference Man. ICRP Publication 23; 1975, pp 228–237, 280–285, 325–327.

28. Environmental Protection Agency (EPA). Reference physiological parameters in pharmacokinetic modeling. EPA/600/6–88/004. Washington, DC: Office of Health and Environmental Assessment; 1988.

29. Davies B, Morris T. Physiological parameters in laboratory animals and humans. *Pharm Res* 1993;10:1093–1095.

30. Brown RP, Delp MD, Lindstedt SL, Rhomberg LR, Beliles RP. Physiological parameter values for physiologically based pharmacokinetic models. *Toxicol Indust Health* 1997;13(4):407–484.

31. Jepson GW, Hoover DK, Black RK, McCafferty JD, Mahle DA, Gearhart JM. A partition coefficient determination method for nonvolatile chemicals in biological tissues. *Fundam Appl Toxicol* 1994;22:519–524.

32. Clewell HJ. Coupling of computer modeling with *in vitro* methodologies to reduce animal usage in toxicity testing. *Toxicol Lett* 1993;68:101–117.

33. Yates FE. Good manners in good modeling: mathematical models and computer simulations of physiological systems. *Am J Physiol* 1978;234:R159–R160.

34. Carson ER, Cobelli C, Finkelstein L. *The Mathematical Modeling of Metabolic and Endocrine Systems. Model Formulation, Identification, and Validation*. Hoboken, NJ: John Wiley & Sons; 1983, pp 23–45, 113–127, 217–231.

35. Rescigno A, Beck JS. Perspectives in pharmacokinetics. The use and abuse of models. *J Pharmacokinet Biopharm* 1987;15(3):327–344.

36. Himmelstein KJ, Lutz RJ. A review of the application of physiologically based pharmacokinetic modeling. *J Pharmacokinet Biopharm* 1979;7:127–145.

37. Gerlowski LE, Jain RK. Physiologically based pharmacokinetic modeling: principles and applications. *J Pharm Sci* 1983;72:1103–1126.

38. Nestorov IA, Aarons LJ, Arundel PA, Rowland M. Lumping of whole-body physiologically based pharmacokinetic models. *J Pharmacokinet Biopharm* 1998;26(1):21–46.

39. Clewell HJ, Lee T, Carpenter RL. Sensitivity of physiologically based pharmacokinetic models to variation in model parameters: methylene chloride. *Risk Anal* 1994;14: 521–531.

40. Campain J. Metals and inorganic compounds. In Reddy MB, Yang RSH, Clewell HJ III, Andersen ME, Eds. *Physiologically Based Pharmacokinetic Modeling: Science and Applications*. Hoboken, NJ: John Wiley & Sons; 2005, pp 239–270.

41. Lin JH. Applications and limitations of interspecies scaling and *in vitro* extrapolation in pharmacokinetics. *Drug Metab Dispos* 1998;26:1202–1212.

42. Hinderling PH. Red blood cells: a neglected compartment in pharmacokinetics and pharmacodynamics. *Pharmacol Rev* 1997;49:279–295.

43. Andersen ME, Clewell HJ, Gargas ML, Smith FA, Reitz RH. Physiologically-based pharmacokinetics and the risk assessment for methylene chloride. *Toxicol Appl Pharmacol* 1987;87:185–205.

44. Agoram B, Woltosz WS, Bolger MB. Predicting the impact of physiological and biochemical processes on oral drug bioavailability. *Adv Drug Deliv Rev* 2001;50(Suppl 1): S41–S67.

45. Willmann S, Schmitt W, Keldenich J, Dressman JB. A physiologic model for simulating gastrointestinal flow and drug absorption in rats. *Pharm Res* 2003;20:1766–1771.

46. Semino G, Lilly P, Andersen ME. A pharmacokinetic model describing pulsatile uptake of orally-administered carbon tetrachloride. *Toxicology* 1997;117(1):25–33.

47. Chaturvedi PR, Decker CJ, Odinecs A. Prediction of pharmacokinetic properties using experimental approaches during early drug discovery. *Curr Opin Chem Biol* 2001;5(4): 452–463.

48. Cai H, Stoner C, Reddy A, Freiwald S, Smith D, Winters R, Stankovic C, Surendran N. Evaluation of an integrated *in vitro–in silico* PBPK (physiologically based pharmacokinetic) model to provide estimates of human bioavailability. *Int J Pharm* 2006;308(1–2): 133–139.

49. Dennison JE, Andersen ME. Reactive vapors in the nasal cavity. In Reddy MB, Yang RSH, Clewell HJ III, Andersen ME, Eds. *Physiologically Based Pharmacokinetic Modeling: Science and Applications*. Hoboken, NJ: John Wiley & Sons; 2005, pp 375–387.

50. Reddy MB. PBPK modeling approaches for special applications: dermal exposure models. In Reddy MB, Yang RSH, Clewell HJ III, Andersen ME, Eds. *Physiologically Based Pharmacokinetic Modeling: Science and Applications*. Hoboken, NJ: John Wiley & Sons; 2005, pp 375–387.

51. McCarley KD, Bunge AL. Pharmacokinetic models of dermal absorption. *J Pharm Sci* 2001;90(11):1699–1719.

52. Roberts MS, Anissimov YG, Gonsalvez RA. Mathematical models in percutaneous absorption (Reprinted from *Percutaneous Adsorption* 1999;3–55). *J Toxicol-Cutaneous Ocular Toxicol* 2001;20:221–270.

53. Andersen ME, Mills JJ, Gargas ML, Kedderis L, Birnbaum LS, Neubert D, Greenlee WF. Modeling receptor-mediated processes with dioxin: implications for pharmacokinetics and risk assessment. *Risk Anal* 1993;13(1):25–36.

54. Kohn MC, Lucier GW, Clark GC, Sewall C, Tritscher AM, Portier CJ. A mechanistic model of effects of dioxin on gene expression in the rat liver. *Toxicol Appl Pharmacol* 1993;120(1):138–154.

55. Plowchalk DR, Teeguarden J. Development of a physiologically based pharmacokinetic model for estradiol in rats and humans: a biologically motivated quantitative framework for evaluating responses to estradiol and other endocrine-active compounds. *Toxicol Sci* 2002;69(1):60–78.

56. Mendel CM. The free hormone hypothesis: distinction from the free hormone transport hypothesis. *J Androl* 1992;13(2):107–116.

57. Lam G, Chen M, Chiou WL. Determination of tissue to blood partition coefficients in physiologically-based pharmacokinetic studies. *J Pharm Sci* 1982;71(4):454–456.

58. Lin JH, Sugiyama Y, Awazu S, Hanano M. *In vitro* and *in vivo* evaluation of the tissue-to-blood partition coefficients for physiological pharmacokinetic models. *J Pharmacokinet Biopharm* 1982;10(6):637–647.

59. Pelekis M, Poulin P, Krishnan K. An approach for incorporating tissue composition data into physiologically based pharmacokinetic models. *Toxicol Ind Health* 1995;11:511–522.

60. Poulin P, Krishnan K. A biologically-based algorithm for predicting human tissue—blood partition coefficients of organic chemicals. *Hum Exp Toxicol* 1995;14:273–280.

61. Poulin P, Krishnan K. An algorithm for predicting tissue:blood partition coefficients of organic chemicals from *n*-octanol:water partition coefficient data. *J Toxicol Environ Health* 1995;46:117–129.

62. Poulin P, Theil FP. *A priori* prediction of tissue:plasma partition coefficients of drugs to facilitate the use of physiologically-based pharmacokinetic models in drug discovery. *J Pharm Sci* 2000;89:16–35.

63. Poulin P, Theil F. Prediction of pharmacokinetics prior to *in vivo* studies. 1. Mechanism-based prediction of volume of distribution. *J Pharm Sci* 2002;91:129–156.

64. Rodgers T, Leahy D, Rowland M. Physiologically based pharmacokinetic modeling 1: Predicting the tissue distribution of moderate-to-strong bases. *J Pharm Sci* 2005;94:1259–1276.

65. Rodgers T, Rowland M. Physiologically based pharmacokinetic modelling 2: Predicting the tissue distribution of acids, very weak bases, neutrals and zwitterions. *J Pharm Sci* 2006;95:1238–1257.

66. Zuegge J, Schneider G, Coassolo P, Lavé T. Prediction of hepatic metabolic clearance—comparison and assessment of prediction models. *Clin Pharmacokinet* 2001;40:553–563.

67. Lavé T, Coassolo P, Reigner B. Prediction of hepatic metabolic clearance based on interspecies allometric scaling techniques and *in vitro in vivo* correlations. *Clin Pharmacokinet* 1999;36:211–231.

68. Houston JB. Relevance of *in-vitro* kinetic-parameters to *in-vivo* metabolism of xenobiotics. *Toxicol In Vitro* 1994;8:507–512.

69. Houston JB, Carlile DJ. Prediction of hepatic clearance from microsomes, hepatocytes, and liver slices. *Drug Metab Rev* 1997;29:891–922.

70. Obach RS. Prediction of human clearance of twenty-nine drugs from hepatic microsomal intrinsic clearance data: an examination of *in vitro* half-life approach and nonspecific binding to microsomes. *Drug Metab Dispos* 1999;27:1350–1359.

71. Ito K, Iwatsubo T, Kanamitsu S, Nakajima Y, Sugiyama Y. Quantitative prediction of *in vivo* drug clearance and drug interactions from *in vitro* data on metabolism, together with binding and transport. *Annu Rev Pharmacol Toxicol* 1998;38:461–499.

72. Barter ZE, Bayliss MK, Beaune PH, Boobis AR, Carlile DJ, Edwards RJ, Houston JB, Lake BG, Lipscomb JC, Pelkonen OR, Tucker GT, Rostami-Hodjegan A. Scaling factors for the extrapolation of *in vivo* metabolic drug clearance from *in vitro* data: reaching a consensus on values of human microsomal protein and hepatocellularity per gram of liver. *Curr Drug Metab* 2007;8:33–45.

73. Reddy MB, Andersen ME, Morrow PE, Dobrev ID, Varaprath S, Plotzke KP, Utell MJ. Physiological modeling of inhalation kinetics of octamethylcyclotetrasiloxane in humans during rest and exercise. *Toxicol Sci* 2003;72:3–18.

74. Blau GE, Neely WB. Dealing with uncertainty in pharmacokinetic models using SIMU-SOLV. In *Drinking Water and Health*, Vol. 8. Washington, DC: National Research Council; 1987, pp 185–207.

75. Cobelli C, Carson ER, Finkelstein L, Leaning MS. Validation of simple and complex models in physiology and medicine. *Am J Physiol* 1984;246:R259–R266.

76. Gueorguieva I, Nestorov IA, Rowland M. Reducing whole body physiologically based pharmacokinetic models using global sensitivity analysis: diazepam case study. *J Pharmacokinet Pharmacodyn* 2006;33(1):1–27.

77. Clewell HJ. The use of physiologically based pharmacokinetic modeling in risk assessment: a case study with methylene chloride. In Olin S, Farland W, Park C, Rhomberg R, Scheuplein L, Starr T, Wilson J, Eds. *Low-Dose Extrapolation of Cancer Risks: Issues and Perspectives*. Washington, DC: ILSI Press; 1995.

78. Clewell HJ, Andersen ME. Use of physiologically-based pharmacokinetic modeling to investigate individual versus population risk. *Toxicology* 1996;111:315–329.

79. Parrott N, Paquereau N, Coassolo P, Lavé T. An evaluation of the utility of physiologically based models of pharmacokinetics in early drug discovery. *J Pharm Sci* 2005;94: 2327–2343.

80. Parrott N, Lavé T. Prediction of intestinal absorption: comparative assessment of GASTROPLUS (TM) and IDEA (TM). *Eur J Pharm Sci* 2002;17:51–61.

81. Tucker GT, Houston JB, Huang SM. Optimizing drug development: strategies to assess drug metabolism/transporter interaction potential—toward a consensus. *Pharm Res* 2001;18:1071–1080.

82. Telgmann R, von Kleist M, Huisinga W. Software supported modelling in pharmacokinetics. *CompLife* 2006;216–225.

83. Leahy DE. Integrating *in vitro* ADMET data through generic physiologically based pharmacokinetic models. *Expert Opin Drug Metab Toxicol* 2006;2:619–628.

84. Lavé T, Dupin S, Schmitt C, Valles B, Ubeaud G, Chou RC, Jaeck D, Coassolo P. The use of human hepatocytes to select compounds based on their expected hepatic extraction ratios in humans. *Pharm Res* 1997;14:152–155.

85. Thompson TN. Early ADME in support of drug discovery: the role of metabolic stability studies. *Curr Drug Metab* 2000;1:215–241.

86. Poggesi I. Predicting human pharmacokinetics from preclinical data. *Curr Opin Drug Discov Dev* 2004;7:100–111.

87. Riley RJ, McGinnity DF, Austin RP. A unified model for predicting human hepatic, metabolic clearance from *in vitro* intrinsic clearance data in hepatocytes and microsomes. *Drug Metab Dispos* 2005;33:1304–1311.

88. Poulin P, Theil FP. Prediction of pharmacokinetics prior to *in vivo* studies. II. Generic physiologically based pharmacokinetic models of drug disposition. *J Pharm Sci* 2002;91:1358–1370.

89. Reigner BG, Blesch KS. Estimating the starting dose for entry into humans: principles and practice. *Eur J Clin Pharmacol* 2002;57:835–845.

90. Luttringer O, Theil F-P, Poulin P, Schmitt-Hoffmann AH, Guentert TW, Lavé T. Physiologically based pharmacokinetic (PBPK) modeling of disposition of epiroprim in humans. *J Pharm Sci* 2003;92:1990–2007.

91. Bischoff KB, Dedrick RL, Zaharko DS. Preliminary model for methotrexate pharmacokinetics. *J Pharm Sci* 1970;59:149–154.

92. Fisher JW, Whittaker TA, Taylor DH, Clewell H III, Andersen ME. Physiologically based pharmacokinetic modeling of the pregnant rat: a multiroute exposure model for trichloroethylene and its metabolite, trichloroacetic acid. *Toxicol Appl Pharmacol* 1989;99: 395–414.

93. O'Flaherty EJ, Scott W, Schreiner C, Beliles RP. A physiologically based kinetic model of rat and mouse gestation: disposition of a weak acid. *Toxicol Appl Pharmacol* 1992;112:245–256.

94. Kalin JR, Starling ME, Hill DL. Disposition of all-*trans*-retinoic acid in mice following oral doses. *Drug Metab Dispos* 1981;9:196–201.

95. Asai M, Faber W, Neth L, di Sant'Agnese PA, Nakanishi M, Miller RK. Human placental transport and metabolism of all-*trans*-retinoic acid *in vitro*. *Placenta* 1991;12: 367–368.

96. Zile MH, Inhorn RC, DeLuca HF. Metabolites of all-*trans*-retinoic acid in bile: identification of all-*trans*- and 13-*cis*-retinoyl glucuronides. *J Biol Chem* 1982;257:3537–3543.

97. Swanson BN, Frolik CA, Zaharevitz DW, Roller PP, Sporn MB. Dose-dependent kinetics of all-*trans*-retinoic acid in rats. Plasma levels and excretion into bile, urine, and faeces. *Biochem Pharmacol* 1981;30:107–113.

98. Adamson PC, Balis FM, Smith MA, Murphy RF, Godwin KA, Poplack DG. Dose-dependent pharmacokinetics of all-*trans*-retinoic acid. *JNCI* 1992;84:1332–1335.

99. Kraft JC, Slikker W Jr, Bailey JR, Roberts LG, Fischer B, Wittfoht W, Nau H. Plasma pharmacokinetic and metabolism of 13-*cis*- and all-*trans*-retinoic acid in the cynomolgus monkey and the identification of 13-*cis*- and all-*trans*-retinoyl–glucuronides. *Drug Metab Dispos* 1991;19:317–324.

100. Muindi JRF, Frankel SR, Huselton C, DeGrazia F, Garland WA, Young CW, Warrell RP Jr. Clinical pharmacology of oral all-*trans* retinoic acid in patients with acute promyelocytic leukemia. *Cancer Res* 1992;52:2138–2142.

101. Dedrick RL. Pharmacokinetic and pharmacodynamic considerations for chronic hemodialysis. *Kidney Int* 1975;7(Suppl 2):S7–S15.

102. Rowland M, Balant L, Peck C. Physiologically based pharmacokinetics in drug development and regulatory science: a workshop report (Georgetown University, Washington, DC, 29–30, May 2002). *AAPS PharmSci* 2004;6(1):E6.

103. Peck CC, Barr WH, Benet LZ, Collins J, Desjardins RE, Furst DE, et al. Opportunities for integration of pharmacokinetics, pharmacodynamics, and toxicokinetics in rational drug development. *J Pharm Sci* 1992;81(6):605–610.

104. Charnick SB, Kawai R, Nedelman JR, Lemaire M, Niederberger W, Sato H. Perspectives in pharmacokinetics. Physiologically based pharmacokinetic modeling as a tool for drug development. *J Pharmacokinet Biopharm* 1995;23:217–229.

105. Jorgensen WL. The many roles of computation in drug discovery. *Science* 2004;303(5665): 1813–1818.

106. Ricke DO, Wang S, Cai R, Cohen D. Genomic approaches to drug discovery. *Curr Opin Chem Biol* 2006;10(4):303–308.

107. Lahoz A, Gombau L, Donato MT, Castell JV, Gomez-Lechon MJ. *In vitro* ADME medium/high-throughput screening in drug preclinical development. *Mini Rev Med Chem* 2006;6(9):1053–1062.

108. van de Waterbeemd H, Gifford E. ADMET *in silico* modelling: towards prediction paradise? *Nat Rev Drug Discov* 2003;2(3):192–204.

109. Blesch KS, Gieschke R, Tsukamoto Y, Reigner BG, Burger HU, Steimer JL. Clinical pharmacokinetic/pharmacodynamic and physiologically based pharmacokinetic modeling in new drug development: the capecitabine experience. *Invest New Drugs* 2003; 21(2):195–223.

110. Lin JH, Lu AYH. Role of pharmacokinetics and metabolism in drug discovery and development. *Pharmacol Rev* 1997;49:403–449.

111. Lin J, Sahakian DC, de Morais SMF, Xu JJ, Polzer RJ, Winter SM. The role of absorption, distribution, metabolism, excretion and toxicity in drug discovery. *Curr Top Med Chem* 2003;3:1125–1154.

112. Poulin P, Schoenlein K, Theil FP. Prediction of adipose tissue:plasma partition coefficients for structurally unrelated drugs. *J Pharm Sci* 2001;90:436–447.

113. Theil FP, Guentert TW, Haddad S, Poulin P. Utility of physiologically based pharmacokinetic models to drug development and rational drug discovery candidate selection. *Toxicol Lett* 2003;138:29–49.

36

MATHEMATICAL MODELING AS A NEW APPROACH FOR IMPROVING THE EFFICACY/TOXICITY PROFILE OF DRUGS: THE THROMBOCYTOPENIA CASE STUDY

Zvia Agur,[1,2] Moran Elishmereni,[1] Yuri Kogan,[1] Yuri Kheifetz,[1] Irit Ziv,[2] Meir Shoham,[2] and Vladimir Vainstein[1,2]

[1]*Institute for Medical Biomathematics (IMBM), Bene-Ataroth, Israel*
[2]*Optimata Ltd., Ramat-Gan, Israel*

Contents

Preclinical Development Handbook: ADME and Biopharmaceutical Properties,
edited by Shayne Cox Gad
Copyright © 2008 John Wiley & Sons, Inc.

36.1   INTRODUCTION

Despite recent innovations, many life-threatening diseases still lack effective treatments. In March 2004, the U.S. Food and Drug Administration (FDA) agency issued a major report that identifies both the problems and the potential solutions for bringing more breakthroughs in medical science to patients, as quickly and efficiently as possible. The report looks at the development processes for drugs, biologics, and medical devices and calls for a joint effort of industry, academic researchers, product developers, patient groups, and the FDA to identify key problems and to develop solutions: "A new product development toolkit—containing powerful new scientific and technical methods such as computer-based predictive models . . . is urgently needed to improve predictability and efficiency along the critical path from laboratory concept to commercial product" [1]. The role of the present chapter is to demonstrate how the science of biomathematics can be harnessed for improving the solution of safety issues in the critical path of drug development, in general, and in the transition from the preclinical phases to Phase I, in particular.

36.1.1   Biomathematics and Its Use for Rationalizing Drug Treatment Strategies: A Short History

A new synthesis of ecology and "hard" biology, called biomathematics, emerged in the second half of the 20th century in the scientific community. Its role was to rationalize complex biological processes. Thus, in contrast to experimental biologists, who work at the microscopic cellular level and develop analytical tools that are analogous to the still camera in photography, biomathematicians develop formulae, which effectively animate these shots, allowing us to understand the dynamics of the complex process we are investigating. Biomathematics has enabled the development of a range of new theories dealing with significant problems of disease progression and control, hitherto beyond the reach of "snapshot", experimental biology.

But in spite of these efforts, until recently the biomedical research community was unanimous in viewing biological systems as too complex to enable accurate retrieval by mathematical models. This declarable mistrust in the power of biomathematics left the biomedical sciences lagging behind other sciences, as an immature sequel of experimental observations. In recent years, the somewhat disillusioned postgenomic era has rediscovered biological complexity, renaming it "system biology." It seems that, finally, biomathematicians are becoming legitimate and almost beloved children of the scientific community.

In the 1980s, notions from population dynamics have been used by Agur and colleagues to develop relatively simple formulae describing the growth patterns of interwoven populations of healthy and cancerous cells, formulae that have resulted in new drug regimens where the toxicity of chemotherapy has been significantly reduced [2, 3, 63]. The power of mathematics here was to prove the universality of the theoretical results and therefore to justify and encourage collaboration with cancer research experimentalists. The latter not only verified the theory in the laboratory, but also pinpointed the feasibility and strength of the theory-to-lab arrow [4, 5].

In the above mentioned mathematical models, populations are subjected to a loss process due to randomly occurring environmental disturbances, which are effective only during a portion of the life cycle. The models are studied over a large range of time scales of the environmental change and for different degrees of variance in the system parameters. Analysis shows that the expected survival time of the population has a strong nonmonotonic dependence on the relation between the duration of the disturbance-resistant life stages and the periodicity of the environmental disturbance. This effect, termed *resonance phenomenon*, was found at integer and fractional multiple of this relation. Interestingly, persistence in all harshly varying environments is shown to depend on the degree of resonance in the environmental and population processes [2, 6–8, 64].

The universality of the resonance phenomenon, and its implication that the frequency of environmental disturbances determines population growth, seemed to offer attractive possibilities for the control of cancer. Thus, Agur and colleagues have shown, both theoretically and experimentally, how the resonance phenomenon could be employed for choosing cytotoxic drug regimens that allow discrimination between different target cell populations. More specifically, it was asserted that one could determine the period of drug pulses, so as to maximize the elimination of malignant cells and, at the same time, to minimize the destruction of drug-susceptible host cells.

In the first stage, it was necessary to investigate the generality of the resonance phenomenon for the dynamics of different host cell populations. To allow analytical tractability, and hence parameter-independent conclusions, deliberately crude mathematical models of the cancer patient were constructed, making simplified assumptions that both tumor and target host tissues are cells that vary only in cell-cycle parameters. The spatial arrangement of these cells was hence ignored. The interest was focused on comparing the overall behavior of the tumor to that of the host target tissues under different chemotherapy regimens of cell-cycle phase-specific drugs, and on finding regimens that are selective to cancer cells. The conviction was that only a simplified model can clarify the underlying properties of the biomedical scenario. Model analysis showed that the resonance phenomenon is valid when considering drug-induced myelotoxicity and tumor progression. Specifically, the mathematical analysis suggested that the efficacy/toxicity ratio of cell-cycle phase-specific drugs would be maximized at an integer or fractional multiple of the mean cycle time of the host target populations (this being denoted the *Z-method*). This applies either when mean cancer cell-cycle parameters differ from those of the target host cell population, or when those are similar but the variation in the distribution of their cell cycle is larger [3, 9, 10].

It seemed mandatory, already at this level of qualitative understanding of the system, to carefully examine the plausibility of applying the Z-method to cancer and host cells. To this end, a series of laboratory experiments was launched, first examining the effect of drug-pulsing rhythm on cell proliferation, *in vitro*, and then checking how varying the pulsing rhythm of different drugs will affect disease progression on the level of the whole organism.

Applying an antimetabolite chemotherapeutic drug, cytarabine (ara-C), to lymphoma cells *in vitro*, it was experimentally shown that when total drug dose and total treatment duration were kept constant, drug schedules exerting significantly higher cell growth were those possessing periodicity that was an integer multiple of the average population cell-cycle time, as evaluated by rates of DNA synthesis. In equivalent *in vivo* experiments, mice were treated by short ara-C pulses, having different distributions of the interdosing intervals, including stochastically determined periodicity. Toxicity was evaluated by spleen weight, differential peripheral blood measurements, kinetic measurements of bone marrow cell proliferation (with bromodeoxiuridine labeling and flow cytometry analysis), and by overall animal survival. Results of these trials proved the superiority of the Z-method in controlling cell proliferation. In particular, it was shown that when the interdosing interval is an exact multiple of the intermitotic time of bone marrow stem and progenitor cells, cell-cycle kinetics are less affected, myelotoxicity is minimal, and survival time of tumor-bearing mice is maximal [3–5, 11].

The above experiments demonstrate that regimens employing a drug period, which coincides with the inherent periodicity of bone marrow cells, protect the bone marrow rather well, leading to increased life expectancy of cancer-bearing mice. In contrast, other regimens, notably those employing intervals that are randomly distributed around the same mean periodicity, are extremely toxic. In general, this work is a proof of the concept that by using a rational drug scheduling, based on the Z-method, it is feasible to control drug toxicity exerted on the bone marrow of cancer-bearing mice, while at the same time delaying their tumor progression. This conclusion has been further supported under more realistic and complex tumor growth models [12, 13] and under physiologically based mathematical models of human hematopoiesis [14].

The above described mathematical models added important new insights on drug treatment strategies, by considering fundamental effects on cellular dynamics. Yet, to enable mathematical tractability, drug-related characteristics were treated very simplistically. For this reason, only qualitative conclusions can be drawn from these model analyses. Now that the proof of concept has been provided, the models are becoming increasingly instrumental in planning concrete treatment strategies. To this end, modeling of the underlying pathological and physiological processes in a patient is wedded with the detailed relevant pharmacokinetics (PK) and pharmacodynamics (PD) [15, 65]. By uniting in one framework the pharmacological properties of the drug with the dynamic properties of the cells in the target tissues, one obtains an improved understanding of how the timing of drug administration—the interdosing interval, drug fractionation, and other aspects of treatment scheduling—may affect the patient. Biomathematics has the power of integrating the vast biomedical and pharmaceutical knowledge into a concise formal language, which enables intensive calculations of the outcomes of complex processes. These calculations, being by far more comprehensive and accurate than any human intuition can be, justify their use for rational treatment design at any stage of the critical path, especially when partial preclinical results collected in several species are to be used for predicting the human response.

36.1.2   Aims of This Chapter

In this chapter, we discuss the application of mathematical modeling tools to elucidate the hematological disorder thrombocytopenia in different animal species, and to accurately describe the efficacy and safety of the thrombocytopenia-alleviating drugs, thrombopoietin and interleukin-11. Model validation in mice, monkeys, and humans, by the use of diverse experimental information, is discussed, as well as the use of animal models for predicting human safety and for improving patient treatment.

36.2   THROMBOPOIESIS

Any mathematical model describing a biological process is based on a verbal model of the process, that is, on an algorithm concisely describing its essential physiological "flow." We devote this section to a brief presentation of the verbal model of thrombopoiesis, and to the subsequent description of a mathematical model, constituting the essence of platelet development.

36.2.1   Biology

Platelets are components of the hematopoietic system, being the nucleus-lacking derivatives of megakaryocytes (MKs). Platelets function primarily in processes of thrombus formation and vascular repair, but also have roles in natural immunity and metastatic tumor biology. Platelet counts in healthy humans average 150–400 billion cells per liter of blood, a homeostasis that is crucial to maintain. Low counts may lead to severe hemorrhage, renal failure, and other disorders, while high counts indicate poor prognosis with respect to cardiovascular diseases and malignancies. Thrombopoiesis, the formation of blood platelets, has been studied for the last century, although critical advances in our understanding of the unique processes that accompany it are only of the last decade. We refer the reader to Fig. 36.1 for an illustration of the process and to the literature for a more elaborate description [16–19].

Normal platelet formation begins with bone marrow progenitors of the lineage, which descend from hematopoietic stem cells and proliferate in response to certain growth factors. The next stages in the sequence involve the immature forms of MKs (promegakaryoblasts and megakaryoblasts), which then develop into larger, mature MKs. As the cells mature into MKs, they gradually lose their ability to divide but

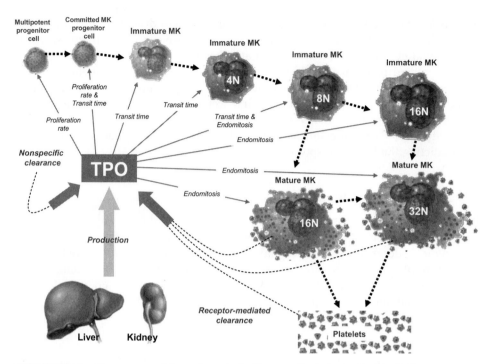

FIGURE 36.1   The process of thrombopoiesis. Uncommited progenitors in the bone marrow (hematopoietic stem cells) proliferate and develop into commited progenitors of the mega-karyocyte (MK) lineage, which further develop into immature forms of MKs (promegakaryo-blasts and megakaryoblasts). These then develop into larger, mature MKs. Maturation of cells is coupled with loss of the mitotic ability, but endomitosis and polyploidy are main-tained until the early stages of MK fragmentation and systemic distribution of platelets. Thrombopoietin (TPO), derived from the liver and kidney constitutively, is a primary media-tor of the platelet formation process and is sequestered by platelets and MKs, as well as nonspecifically.

maintain the function of DNA synthesis, thereby undergoing endomitosis and attaining a polyploid state. Finally, MK fragmentation occurs, resulting in release of platelets, first to bone marrow sinusoids and then to the systemic circulation. Radio-labeling studies indicate that the amount of platelets normally consumed by hemo-stasis is very small and constant. The highly regulated process of platelet consumption is induced by their adhesion to von Willebrand factor (vWF) and extracellular matrix components of damaged blood vessel wall underlying the endothelium. Fol-lowing platelet adhesion, a clot is formed and the vessel wall is recovered. With a life span of approximately 10 days, unconsumed platelets that senesce are removed by macrophages of the reticuloendothelial system, mostly in the spleen.

Thrombopoietin (TPO), a glycoprotein produced by the liver and kidney consti-tutively and by the bone marrow upon demand, is characterized as the primary regulator of platelet formation. Although the focus was set on TPO in the late 1960s, it was successfully cloned only in 1992. TPO acts in all stages of thrombopoiesis, its receptors being expressed on each cell type in the lineage. Interestingly, systemic and bone marrow levels of TPO are inversely correlated to platelet numbers: due to high affinity platelet-bearing TPO receptors, increased amounts of platelets result in high internalization of TPO, forming successful autoregulation of the thrombopoiesis. Slightly less significant cytokines, namely, the interleukins 3, 6, 11, and stem cell factor (SCF), stromal cell-derived factor 1 (SDF-1), and granulocyte macrophage colony-stimulating factor (GM-CSF), were also identified as modulators in normal platelet formation, each acting in different developmental phases, and some acting in synergy with others. Studies indicate that surrounding tissue, comprised of fibroblasts, endothelial cells, and macrophages, is also capable of augmenting thrombopoiesis, although these environmental factors are not thought to be critical since platelets are easily produced also *in vitro*.

The manipulation of molecular and genetic techniques in the last two decades has greatly boosted the understanding of biological pathways and mechanisms involved in platelet formation. Nonetheless, at the current stage, the regulation of thrombopoiesis, the central molecular components taking part in it, and their significance for therapeutic intervention in platelet-associated illnesses are yet to be clarified.

36.2.2 Mathematical Modeling

Although the intricacies of thrombopoiesis are far from being fully elucidated, current knowledge enabled the verbalization and subsequently the mathematical formalization of a basic thrombopoiesis-describing model. Schematized in Fig. 36.2, and elaborated elsewhere, the model divides the entire thrombopoietic lineage into 17 compartments. Every compartment, except for the first, is represented by time-dependent age distribution, where the number of cells is given as a function of discrete age (time spent in the compartment) and time. The number of cells in the first compartment is a function of time only. There are six groups of compartments in the model, in accordance with the above-mentioned structure of the thrombopoietic lineage. The subdivision of the six groups is as follows: (1) one compartment of lineage-uncommitted progenitors (UCP), (2) one compartment of lineage-committed progenitors (CP), (3) six compartments of endomitotic progenitors (EP), (4) four compartments of developing progenitors (DP), (5) four compartments of MKs, and (6) one compartment of blood-circulating platelets.

The first compartment, UCP, refers to all bone marrow hematopoietic progenitor cells that can differentiate into more than one line (e.g., pluripotent stem cells, CFU-GEMM). We assume one homogeneous UCP population, as its division into various subpopulations is not feasible, since kinetic data regarding the various subpopulations of the UCP compartment (i.e., rates of proliferation, maturation, and self-renewal) is rather scarce. In our model, cells of this compartment proliferate at a certain rate (α_{UCP}) and differentiate into MKs or other precursors. Based on previous studies showing that the probabilities of stem cell differentiation into any given hematopoietic lineage are constant, it was assumed that a fixed proportion of mature uncommitted progenitor cells flows into the thrombopoietic lineage (φ_{UCP}). Apoptotic cell death may have a significant effect on cell numbers in the proliferating compartments. Thus, we included its effect together with the effect of cell proliferation in the total amplification of cell number in a specific compartment. Since no information is currently available concerning apoptosis in the nonproliferating MK compartments, this issue was disregarded in these compartments.

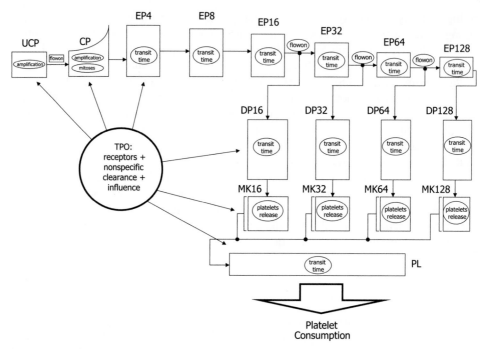

FIGURE 36.2   A scheme of the thrombopoiesis mathematical model. The model consists of 17 compartments, which can be grouped into six clusters: (1) one compartment of lineage-uncommitted stem cell progenitors (UCP), (2) one compartment of lineage-committed progenitors (CP), (3) six compartments of endomitotic progenitors (EP) of ploidies 4N, 8N, 16N, 32N, 64N, and 128N, (4) four compartments of developing progenitors (DP) of ploidies 16N, 32N, 64N, and 128N, (5) four compartments of megakaryocytes (MKs) of ploidies 16N, 32N, 64N, and 128N, and (6) one compartment of individual, blood-circulating platelets. Relevant key parameters included in the kinetic calculations of the different compartments are amplification rate, flow-on fraction (flowon), transit time, and rate of platelet release. The arrows indicate the direction of intercompartmental cell flow.

The CP compartment stands for an age distribution of progenitor cells already committed to the thrombopoietic lineage, but still capable of proliferation. The compartment is characterized by a transit time (τ_{CP}) and a number of mitoses (N_m). The latter represents the average number of possible cell divisions at that stage. This number may be noninteger, considering that certain cells can be quiescent and undergo fewer mitoses than others. Cells leaving CP enter the first of the six EP compartments, which comprises cells that have lost proliferation ability and yet are not sufficiently mature to release platelets. Thus, this subgroup of compartments, namely, EP4, EP8, EP16, EP32, EP64, and EP128, are formed according to the biologically known sequence of cells of the MK lineage bearing ploidy of 4N, 8N, 16N, 32N, 64N, and 128N, respectively. These endomitotic precursors cannot divide but continue endomitosis. The cells that enter the EP4 compartment are of ploidy 2N, at the exit they have ploidy 4N, and so on for subsequent EP compartments. It is assumed that MKs can release platelets only after reaching the 16N-ploidy phase. Hence, to arrive at platelet production in our model, the EP16 compartment must be entered. After cells spend their designated transit time (τ_{EP}) in an EP compartment, they can move to the next EP compartment. Fractions of cells that continue endomitosis after moving through EP16, EP32, or EP64 are designated φ_{EP16}, φ_{EP32}, and φ_{EP64}, respectively, where in normal conditions $\varphi_{EP64} = 0$.

Alternatively, cells at the EP16, EP32, or EP64 stage may stop the endomitotic process by entering the relevant DP compartment, which is represented by four subgroups of cells. DP cells of 16N, 32N, 64N, and 128N ploidy increase their cytoplasmic contents prior to platelet production. Cells that have stopped endomitosis after exiting EP16 compartment enter into DP16; cells that have stopped endomitosis after exiting EP32 compartment enter into DP32, and so forth. After spending a certain amount of time (τ_{DP}) in the DP compartment, cells pass to the corresponding MK compartment. The four subcompartments of this stage signify cells capable of releasing platelets. MK16 compartment receives cells exiting from DP16, MK32 receives cell exiting from DP32, and so on. As in previous compartments, here too the cells are distributed over age (time spent in the compartment), yet there is no predefined transit time. Instead, the new cells entering MK are assumed to have some initial releasing capacity, indicating the number of potential platelets, or total platelets volume, to be released until the cell is exhausted. This capacity is assumed to be larger for cells of larger ploidy. Cells release platelets continuously, and their releasing capacity is consumed until it drops to zero, thereupon disappearing from the compartment.

The last compartment, PL, represents platelet counts distributed by age (time spent in blood after the release). Distribution of mean platelet volume (MPV) is also computed in order to allow calculations of platelet degradation. The platelets are readily consumed by the body in an age-independent manner, and in terms of volume (platelet number multiplied by MPV). There is also a maximal life span for old platelets, so that all nonconsumed platelets disappear upon reaching a maximal age (denoted by τ_{PL}). New platelets appear at every time step, as released by MK cells. This release is also described in terms of volume, and at every time step the amount and MPV are evaluated for the new platelets, taking into account the relative contributions of MK cells of different ploidies.

The formal description of the cellular compartments is supplemented by the model for the endogenous TPO, which regulates the dynamics of the process. A one-compartment PK model for TPO, with a constant production and a linear nonspecific clearance, is applied. In addition, there is an alternative, specific clearance of TPO, achieved through the consumption by the cells (receptor binding and internalization). To include this in the model, distributions of receptors per cell in all the line-committed compartments (CP and the groups that follow) are incorporated. Formulae are constructed for receptor numbers distributed over cell age. Receptors, constantly produced by the cells, excluding platelets that have no nucleus, bind free TPO and are internalized. To reflect the nonspecific clearance of TPO, Michaelis–Menten behavior is assumed for TPO-receptor kinetics.

The major stabilizing feedback in the model is exerted via the effects of TPO on the cells throughout the lineage. Kinetic parameters of the model's compartments are functions of TPO concentrations. In the UCP compartment, the amplification rate is an increasing function of the TPO concentration. Similarly, the number of mitoses in the CP compartment is an increasing function of TPO. In contrast, the transit times in CP, EP, and DP, and the EP flow-on (fraction of cells that continue endomitosis) are decreasing functions of the TPO concentration. Finally, the MPV of released platelets (and consequenty the loss of cell volume) is an increasing function of the TPO concentration in the MK compartments. For all the dependencies listed above, sigmoid functions with saturation for large values of TPO concentration are used. In addition to this feedback, a TPO-independent feedback on cell proliferation in the model, or a "crowding effect," is included as well. The amplification rate in UCP and the number of mitoses in CP are decreasing functions of cell numbers in these compartments, respectively. This represents internal regulation of cell proliferation in these stages. Such functions are also assumed to have a sigmoid form.

The model is mathematically formalized according to the above description, using discrete difference equations. The variables of the model (e.g., cell numbers) are represented as functions of discrete time points, with a certain step Δt. The set of the model equations describes the recursive calculation of the system state for the current time point, using the state of the system at previous time points. For the specific clearance model, steady-state approximations are used, as these processes are on a much faster time scale than all the rest of the model. The model is simulated using a C++ code, and its parameters are estimated either directly from experimental measurements or by fitting the model to the published experimental data. The validation of the model is further described in Section 36.5.

36.3   THROMBOCYTOPENIA

Setting the essential rules for depicting thrombopoiesis, as explained in Section 36.2, it is possible to evaluate not only the homeostatic behavior of the system but also its irregularities. Diversion from normal steady-state thrombopoiesis can arise from various reasons and can have several physiological consequences. In this section, we discuss some of the main mechanisms leading to low platelet count, termed thrombocytopenia (TP). Both current and future therapeutic avenues will be illustrated.

36.3.1   Pathophysiology

The concise summary of TP pathophysiology, presented in this section, is based on extensive reviews of this pathology in the current hematology literature [16, 20, 21]. The clinical significance of TP, characterized by a blood platelet count of less than 150,000 cells per microliter, stems from the major role of platelets in the process of normal hemostasis. Low platelet counts lead to diminished ability of hemostasis and, consequently, increased bleeding propensity. Yet there are important exceptions to this rule. First, clinically significant bleeding occurs regularly only when the amount of platelets decreases below 10,000–20,000/μL. Second, exact clinical manifestation of this disorder depends on the underlying pathophysiological mechanisms. While TP induced by low platelet production leads to increased risk of bleeding, TP caused by excessive platelet consumption may result in an elevated risk of thromboembolism.

TP can be caused by one or more of the following mechanisms (elaborated in the following section): (1) decreased platelet production, (2) increased sequestration of platelets, or (3) their accelerated destruction. TP induced by the first mechanism, impaired production of platelets, accompanies a variety of bone marrow pathologies. Congenital hereditary decreased production TP, one of these cases, is very rare. It can be caused by malfunctioning TPO receptor signaling (e.g., amegakaryocytic TP) or by impaired MK fragmentation into mature platelets. The more common syndrome is acquired decreased production TP. This form of TP can be a result of pathological bone marrow infiltration in hematopoietic malignancies (leukemias and lymphomas) or in massive metastases of extramedullary solid tumors. Alternatively, this could occur in myelodysplastic syndromes and vitamin B_{12} deficiency, when intrinsic maturation defects arise in the early hematopoietic progenitors, with involvement of 1–3 hematopoietic lines. Extrinsic inhibitors of hematopoietic progenitor proliferation, such as (1) cytotoxic drugs (anticancer chemotherapy), (2) circulating autoantibodies to MKs (immune thrombocytopenic purpura, systemic lupus erythematosus, etc.), (3) proinflammatory cytokines (sepsis), or (4) various viral infections (EBV, CMV, HIV, etc.), can induce this TP form as well.

Increased sequestration TP, the second mechanism, is a common finding in splenomegaly of any cause. A frequent consequence of splenic enlargement is increased pressure in the portal vein, which causes draining of blood from the spleen into the liver. This syndrome, referred to as portal hypertension, is present in a variety of chronic liver diseases and in cases of portal vein thrombosis due to hypercoagulation states. In portal hypertension, increased sequestration is often the only cause of TP. Other diseases with splenomegaly generally produce TP of a combined etiology. For example, splenomegaly is associated with conditions of leukemia and lymphoma, in which bone marrow infiltration results in decreased platelet production. Similar combinations of TP mechanisms appear in several infectious disorders (e.g., brucellosis and visceral leishmaniasis) and inflammatory diseases (e.g., Felty's syndrome and systemic juvenile rheumatoid arthritis).

Pathologically accelerated platelet destruction (the third mechanism of TP) can be induced by either increased consumption or physical factors. Physical platelet destruction occurs upon increased blood shear stress near valvular and intravascular prosthetic devices. There are varying disorders of increased platelet consumption by pathological uncontrolled coagulation. Thrombotic thrombocytopenic purpura (TTP) and hemolytic uremic syndrome (HUS) are associated with thrombosis, rather than bleeding, despite low platelet count. Recent progress in TTP research reveals that the underlying pathology involves decreased or absent function of a protease known as a disintegrin and metalloproteinase with a thrombospondin type 1 motif, member 13 (ADAMTS13), responsible for specific cleavage of vWF. As a consequence, large multimers of vWF are formed, and they initiate bouts of platelet adhesion and activation. Conversely, pathogenesis of HUS is incompletely understood. Since this disorder appears typically after certain bacterial infection, it is assumed that cross-reactive antibodies are responsible for platelet activation in this syndrome. Disseminated intravascular coagulation (DIC), distinct from the latter two disorders by its simultaneous induction of both thrombosis and bleeding, is a common feature of several severe illnesses including overwhelming sepsis, poisoning due to snake bites, amniotic fluid embolism, and fat embolism. The pathogenesis of DIC includes uncontrolled activation of intravascular coagulation pathways, leading to increased platelet consumption.

Accelerated destruction TP can also be attributed to immunological disorders. The most recognized disorder of this type is immune (idiopathic) thrombocytopenic purpura (ITP). The underlying pathology consists of formation of autoantibodies against specific platelet surface antigens. Platelets covered with autoantibodies are effectively and prematurely destroyed by the phagocytes of the reticuloendothelial system. In the minority of cases, presence of autoantibodies to MKs is also suspected, which results in TP of mixed etiology—both decreased production and accelerated destruction. Other diseases with autoimmune platelet destruction include systemic lupus erythematosus and antiphospholipid antibody syndrome. Drug-induced immune TP was observed upon the use of many exogenous factors, including heparin, gold, antibiotics, and anti-inflammatory drugs. In these cases, antibodies are formed against the complex of a drug with platelet surface antigens. In heparin-induced TP, thrombotic complications are common (similar to those in TTP), since antibodies lead to excessive platelet activation in addition to increased clearance.

To examine the risk of TP in new drugs, or in yet to be tried drug regimens, the PK and PD of the drug should be simulated superimposed on a mathematical model of the underlying TP mechanism. However, how to determine the specific TP mechanism in each particular case is a very challenging task. While certain clues can be received from the patient's medical history, physical examination, and peripheral blood smear, bone marrow biopsy is frequently required in order to evaluate the number of MKs. Low numbers are indicative of decreased production, while increased numbers are associated with accelerated destruction. Some cases remain undefined, even after thorough laboratory investigation and manipulation of extensive tools. The type of TP guides further clinical workup for specific underlying pathology as well as possible treatment options.

36.3.2 Current Therapy

In light of the different mechanisms for TP, treatment is diverse and highly dependent on the underlying cause. Generally, we can divide current therapy into treatments directed against pathophysiological mechanisms, and symptomatic treatment of TP-induced bleeding/thrombosis. In the majority of the cases, platelet counts do not drop below 10,000–20,000 per microliter of blood, so that serious bleeding complications do not develop. Treatment of the underlying causes includes withdrawal of the offending stimulus (e.g., discontinuation of an immunogenic drug), removal of vWF complexes by plasma exchange in TTP, replacement of mechanical prosthesis by a biological one, and specific treatment of malignancies and infections.

It is imperative to identify accelerated platelet destruction by the reticuloendothelial system, for which splenectomy and/or administration of intravenous immunoglobulins (IVIGs) is indicated in refractory cases. Splenectomies lead to decreased autoantibody production and remove a large fraction of phagocytes responsible for platelet destruction. IVIGs, on the other hand, saturate antibody-binding receptors on the phagocytes and suppress their interaction with antibody-covered platelets and MKs. Therefore, theoretically, IVIGs should be more effective in cases of MK-specific antibodies. This hypothesis, however, has not been examined clinically, due to technical difficulties in identifying antibody specificity in particular patients. Importantly, neither a splenectomy nor IVIG therapy is effective in cases of direct complement-mediated antibody toxicity to platelets and MKs.

Symptomatic treatment of TP-associated bleeding disorders consists mainly of transfusion of donor platelets. Platelet transfusions are commonly used, with approximately 9 million units yearly applied in the United States alone. Although repeated platelet transfusions may aid in preventing bleeding, they can transmit both viral and bacterial infections and can cause alloimmunization, which requires HLA-matched donors. Health care costs and inconvenience to patients also pose a concern. Furthermore, this treatment must be repeated on a regular and frequent basis, due to the short half-life of donor platelets (3–4 days), and since the underlying causes of TP are left untreated. Platelet transfusions are of especially low efficacy in immunologically mediated TP that involve an even shorter platelet half-life.

36.3.3 Novel Cytokine Therapy

Over the past fifteen years, attempts to find new therapies to replace platelet transfusions in the treatment of thrombocytopenic disorders have naturally been focused on the growth factors involved in normal thrombopoiesis (see Section 36.2). Interleukin-11 (IL-11), discovered in 1990 to be a thrombopoietic growth factor secreted from bone marrow stromal cells, was the first candidate for this purpose. The genetically engineered form of this protein, recombinant human IL-11 (rhIL-11), was evaluated for treatment in patients with nonmyeloid malignancies that suffered from chemotherapy-induced thrombocytopenia and did, in fact, produce a dose-dependent increase in platelets. RhIL-11, approved in 1997 for prevention of severe drug-induced thrombocytopenia, is currently the only cytokine licensed in the United States for this purpose. However, with its only modest thrombopoietic activity and its use often associated with intolerable side effects, IL-11 has not satisfied the demands for an efficacious thrombopoietic agent to be applied in the clinical setting [22–24].

In light of the central role of TPO in the proliferation and survival of MKs and increased platelet production, its potential to replace standard platelet transfusion therapy and improve platelet harvesting efficacy in donors seems even greater than that of IL-11 [22, 25]. Recombinant human TPO (rhTPO) has been examined for exogenous application in patients with primary thrombocytopenic disorders, as well as for treatment of chemotherapeutically induced myelosuppression in cancer patients. However, Phase I studies with rhTPO in healthy individuals remain disappointing. In a trial that was aimed at improving platelet yields in donors, some of them developed immune-mediated TP due to appearance of autoantibodies to native TPO. Evaluation of rhTPO therapy has also encountered difficulties due to delayed peak platelet response and neutralizing antibodies formed against the pegylated molecule. It is believed that most complications are caused by significant antigenic differences between the native and recombinant TPO proteins. As a result, this molecule currently remains in its developmental stage and is not yet approved. Small TPO analogues and synthetic TPO-derived agents are currently being developed to bypass immunogenicity-related problems [26–34].

Mathematical modeling of thrombopoiesis (as described in Section 36.2) and drug-induced TP (as will be shown in Section 36.6) can aid in disentangling disease dynamics and in deciphering pathophysiological mechanisms underlying the disease. In particular, mathematical models of TPO-affected thrombopoiesis and of IL-11-induced side effects enable one to propose improved treatment schedules for both drugs, obtaining maximum efficacy and substantially improved safety (see Sections 36.4 and 36.5). In turn, preclinical validation of these improved regimens can give new hope for clinical application of these cytokines in their multiple arenas.

36.4   MODELING DRUG EFFECTS ON THROMBOPOIESIS

Innovative cytokine-based therapeutics of IL-11 and TPO (see Section 36.3) developed for application in thrombopoiesis-related syndromes and for efficiently harvesting donor platelets have been extensively studied in the last decade or so. Yet, even today, toxicity-related limitations of each of these molecules prevent their clinical applicability. The following section is dedicated to mathematical models focusing on both beneficial and detrimental consequences of these therapeutic avenues, and on the manner by which such models may be used to suggest improved treatment strategies.

36.4.1   Toxicity Modeling: Interleukin-11 (IL-11)

Although IL-11 has been approved for treating drug-induced TP for almost a decade, its induction of intolerable toxic effects has impeded its therapeutic use. The cytokine has been shown to elicit a wide range of side effects, mainly associated with blood volume expansion (BVE). These include complications of various grades of edema, anemia, pleural effusion, and cardiac arrhythmia [23].

An initial and generalized perspective on this issue required a mathematical model of IL-11-induced BVE. However, the definitive mechanism underlying IL-11-mediated water accumulation is yet to be discovered, and the incomplete data [23, 35] restrict the possibility to produce a concrete and reliable model for this problem. Instead, a novel biomathematical approach was developed so that not one but several mathematical models, each representing an alternative mechanism for BVE following IL-11 therapy, were devised and evaluated [36]. The underlying assumption here was that by concurrently simulating multiple models, which formally describe alternative mechanisms, but all producing the same fluid-retentive behavior, it is possible to faithfully depict this effect despite the obscurity of the actual mechanism and related data. Accordingly, convergence of all models to yield unified BVE dynamics was the characteristic by which their success and predictive ability was measured. Furthermore, since the range of different models that capture the behavior of stable biological systems (e.g., body water homeostasis) is assumed to be relatively narrow, the chances of arriving at a reliable model was considered even greater in the drug-afflicted BVE setting [36].

Three closely related biologically based models were constructed using ordinary differential equations (ODEs) and standard Michaelis–Menten kinetics. The models incorporated basic water regulation properties (blood volume, pressure, and vascular compartments) and endocrinal feedback effects (compartments for BVE-upregulating and BVE-downregulating hormones), together with the IL-11-induced perturbation of the system. Notably, a short-term neuronal influence or long-term permanent structural changes were not considered, restricting the modeling to the therapeutic time scale. The variation between the different models was expressed in (1) the component directly affected by IL-11, being either blood volume or blood vessels, and (2) the components affected by the endocrinal hormones, being both vessels and volume (full effect) or only volume (partial effect). Thus, model 1 assumes IL-11-induced vessel enlargement and full endocrinal feedback; model 2 assumes IL-11-induced volume expansion and full endocrinal function; and model 3 assumes IL-11-induced volume expansion and partial endocrinal function. The models were identical in all other assumptions.

Dynamics of subcutaneously administered IL-11 were represented by a one-compartment PK model, with first-order absorption from the external tissue. IL-11 concentrations in the tissue (I_T) and plasma (I_P) are given by

$$\dot{I}_T = -c_1 I_T \tag{36.1}$$

and

$$\dot{I}_P = f c_1 I_T - c_2 I_P \tag{36.2}$$

where $I_T (t = 0)$ is the administered IL-11 concentration and $I_P (t = 0) = 0$. The coefficient c_1 denotes the rate of drug transport from the primary tissue to the plasma, c_2 is the drug clearance rate, and the fraction of transferred drug, an indicator of bioavailability, is f.

Blood pressure was described by considering its classical correlation to heart rate, stroke volume, and systemic vascular resistance. As heart rate variability was disregarded in experiments, and an inverse relationship between vascular resistance and vascular capacity was assumed, blood pressure was described to be a function of blood volume and the vascular capacity (expressed in terms of vessel surface):

$$P(t) = \left(\frac{V(t)}{S(t)^{3/2}} \right)^{n_0} \tag{36.3}$$

The function $P(t)$ is blood pressure at time t, $S(t)$ denotes overall vessel surface at time t, $V(t)$ is blood volume at time t, and n_0 is a parameter. Steady-state values of pressure and overall vessel surface and volume were given by P_{st}, S_{st}, and V_{st}, respectively.

Dynamics of the BVE-upregulating hormones (H_U) and the BVE-downregulating hormones (H_D) were subjected to blood pressure variations and were therefore given by

$$\dot{H}_U = \alpha_1 g(P_{st} - P(t)) - d_1 H_U(t) \tag{36.4}$$

and

$$\dot{H}_D = \alpha_2 g(P(t) - P_{st}) - d_2 H_D(t) \tag{36.5}$$

respectively. The description is general and does not refer to hormonal concentrations per se, but rather to effects associated with endocrinal deviations. In Eqs. 36.4 and 36.5, formation rates (α_1, α_2) and degradation rates (d_1, d_2) of the endocrinal effects were taken as constants, and blood pressure deviations from steady state allowed formation of each factor using the function

$$g(x) = \begin{cases} x & \text{if} \quad x > 0 \\ 0 & \text{if} \quad x \leq 0 \end{cases}$$
(36.6)

The vascular structure was described in two-dimensional units, for example, by relating to the average surface of the inner endothelium layer of blood vessels. IL-11-induced vessel surface enlargement (in model 1) and H_U-induced vasoconstriction or H_D-induced vasodilation (in models 1 and 2) were described by biologically compatible nonlinear functions. As described earlier, model 3 does not enable vascular resizing in response to IL-11 or hormones. All three models, however, incorporate simple intrinsic feedback effects to vessel steady state in blood vessel dynamics. Thus, the equations for models 1, 2, and 3 are given by Eqs. 36.7, 36.8, and 36.9, respectively:

$$\dot{S} = \frac{\beta_0 (I_P(t))^{r_0}}{k_0 + (I_P(t))^{r_0}} - \frac{\beta_1 (H_U(t))^{r_1}}{k_1 + (H_U(t))^{r_1}} + \frac{\beta_2 (H_D(t))^{r_2}}{k_2 + (H_U(t))^{r_2}} + \beta_3 (S_{st} - S(t))$$
(36.7)

$$\dot{S} = -\frac{\beta_1 (H_U(t))^{r_1}}{k_1 + (H_U(t))^{r_1}} + \frac{\beta_2 (H_D(t))^{r_2}}{k_2 + (H_U(t))^{r_2}} + \beta_3 (S_{st} - S(t))$$
(36.8)

and

$$\dot{S} = \beta_3 (S_{st} - S(t))$$
(36.9)

Vascular modification rates in response to IL-11, H_U, and H_D are denoted as β_0, β_1 and β_2, respectively, and β_3 is the coefficient of direct vessel surface regulation. Parameters k_0, k_1, k_2 and r_0, r_1, r_2 are positive.

Volume dynamics were initially characterized by water absorption–excretion differences. Absorption rates were assumed not to deviate from steady-state values, whereas excretion rates were taken as susceptible to (1) systemic blood pressure deviations, known to specifically act on renal water excretion, and (2) the IL-11-induced effects. The function of blood volume was therefore described by the difference between absorption rates, which were constant (A_{st}), and excretion rates, which were set as the pressure-related difference between normal steady-state excretion (E_{st}) and the excretion in the IL-11 scenario (E_{drug}):

$$\dot{V} = A_{st} - \left(\frac{P(t)}{P_{st}}\right)^{n_1} (E_{st} - E_{drug}(t))$$
(36.10)

The power coefficient n_1 sets the strength of the dependence of the volume changes on the pressure variation. Assuming equal steady-state absorption and excretion rates ($A_{st} = E_{st}$) under normal conditions, Eq. 36.10 turns into

$$\dot{V} = E_{st}\left(1 - \left(\frac{P(t)}{P_{st}}\right)^{n_1}\right) + \left(\frac{P(t)}{P_{st}}\right)^{n_1} (E_{drug}(t))$$
(36.11)

Excretion of volume in the therapeutic scenario (i.e., the term E_{drug}) was assumed to be affected by the hormones in all three models. As described above, in models 2 and 3 it was additionally assumed that the drug directly influences volume excretion. Both of these effects (IL-11 and hormone mediated) were assumed to be nonlinear and were introduced into the volume dynamics given in Eq. 36.11. For model 1, this gave

$$\dot{V} = E_{\text{st}}\left(1 - \left(\frac{P(t)}{P_{\text{st}}}\right)^{n_1}\right) + \left(\frac{P(t)}{P_{\text{st}}}\right)^{n_1}\left(\frac{\gamma_1(H_{\text{U}}(t))^{q_1}}{m_1 + (H_{\text{U}}(t))^{q_1}} - \frac{\gamma_2(H_{\text{D}}(t))^{q_2}}{m_2 + (H_{\text{D}}(t))^{q_2}}\right) \quad (36.12)$$

while for models 2 and 3, this gave

$$\dot{V} = E_{\text{st}}\left(1 - \left(\frac{P(t)}{P_{\text{st}}}\right)^{n_1}\right) + \left(\frac{P(t)}{P_{\text{st}}}\right)^{n_1}\left(\frac{\gamma_0(I_{\text{P}}(t))^{q_0}}{m_0 + (I_{\text{P}}(t))^{q_0}} + \frac{\gamma_1(H_{\text{U}}(t))^{q_1}}{m_1 + (H_{\text{U}}(t))^{q_1}} - \right.$$
$$\left. \frac{\gamma_2(H_{\text{D}}(t))^{q_2}}{m_2 + (H_{\text{D}}(t))^{q_2}}\right) \quad (36.13)$$

The IL-11-, H_{U}-, and H_{D}-afflicted rates of water excretion are denoted γ_0, γ_1, and γ_2, respectively. Parameters m_0, m_1, m_2, and q_0, q_1, q_2 are positive constants.

Subsequent calibration of the models was accomplished by obtaining and utilizing data from a human study of IL-11 safety, and their predictive ability was evaluated under different regimens of IL-11 therapy. These stages of the work are further described in Section 36.5.

36.4.2   Efficacy Modeling: Thrombopoietin (TPO)

As illustrated in Section 36.3, platelet deficiencies hamper the development of improved therapeutic regimens for hematology and oncology patients, as well as in their clinical management [22, 27]. The possible use of TPO to abrogate these disorders has also been debated (Section 36.3). The PK of rhTPO therapy was mathematically modeled in terms of ODEs and solved numerically using the Euler method. This extension was simulated in conjunction with the thrombopoiesis model described in Section 36.2 (see also Refs. 37 and 38). The independent PK model for rhTPO was similar in its structure to that of endogenous TPO, although the kinetic parameters were assumed to be different. The reason for this lies in the fact that exogenously administered synthetic molecules have been shown to differ from the endogenous analogues in a number of characteristics [32]. The model extension also assumes competitive binding of TPO and rhTPO to cell receptors. When describing the PD of the drug, its effects were considered similar to those of the endogenous protein, the latter already existing in the model. Parameter calibration of the model, as well as its retrospective and prospective validation in different species, is detailed in Section 36.5.

36.4.3   Modeling Combination Therapy: Chemotherapy and TPO Support

The consideration of TPO as a potential candidate for alleviating chemotherapy-induced TP in patients with malignant disorders (see Section 36.3) introduces the issue of combination therapy. The addition of TPO to a cytotoxic-drug-affected scenario, allowing restoration of the damaged thrombopoietic system, can be described via minor manipulation of the basic mathematical model. To do this, one should take into account the effect of chemotherapeutic drugs on the thrombopoietic lineage. Chemotherapy nonspecifically damages all dividing cells, particularly progenitor cells of the thrombopoietic lineage. These targets are represented by the UCP and CP compartments of the TPO model (Section 36.2). Accordingly, the model assumes that the cytotoxic drug eliminates dividing cells in a concentration-dependent manner and, possibly (depending on the drug), in a cell-cycle phase-specific manner. The model incorporates the PK of the drug, to obtain the time course of drug concentrations in blood and bone marrow. Subsequently, a PD model for this drug is applied: the apoptosis probability of a dividing cell is calculated as a function of its position in the cycle and of the current drug concentration.

After constructing such a model and validating it, drug developers and treating physicians can explore the unlimited space of possible conjugate treatments, in which the side effects of chemotherapy are suppressed by use of exogenous TPO. The model allows examining different treatment regimens, predicting their possible outcomes, and selecting the best possible treatment strategies, while avoiding adverse effects, such as those observed in clinical trials of TPO. This identification of improved treatment strategies can be done for the general population, as well as on a patient-specific basis, the latter requiring the specific model parameters of the treated patient, which can be evaluated using the individual platelet profiles post drug intervention.

36.5 USING THE VALIDATED MODEL FOR PREDICTING IMPROVED DRUG EFFICACY/TOXICITY PROFILE

As explained in Section 36.3, clinical evaluation of IL-11 and TPO was obstructed due to safety problems. It was therefore imperative to investigate the mathematical models of TPO-mediated thrombopoiesis and IL-11-induced fluid retention (Sections 36.2 and 36.4), in order to suggest how to overcome the limitations involved in the development of these drugs. We show in this section how species-specific model parameters can be evaluated and the means by which retrospective and prospective validation of the mathematical models is achieved. Thereafter we discuss model use for predicting improved chemotherapy and supportive administration regimens.

36.5.1 Model Validation by Retrospective Human Study Results: IL-11 and TPO

Since modeling IL-11-mediated BVE has employed the specially developed multiple modeling approach (see Section 36.4), the previously depicted diverse models are considered validated and of predictive capability only upon their arrival at unified volume dynamics. The study therefore consisted of two essential steps: experimentally based calibration and parallel assessment of model simulation-derived BVE behavior. These procedures are described next [36].

In the first stage, model parameters were successfully calibrated to retrospectively retrieve clinically evaluated blood volume measurements following daily IL-11 administration of 25 μg/kg doses to healthy volunteers for a week [35]. The data

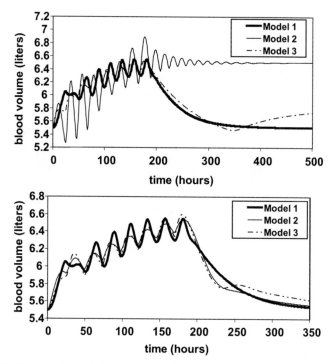

FIGURE 36.3   Comparison of alternative mathematical models for BVE dynamics follow-ing calibration by results of a clinical IL-11 study. Blood volume (liters) measured during one week of IL-11 therapy (7 daily doses of 25 µg/kg) was taken from a previous study in healthy humans. Three models, calibrated with data from either the therapeutic days (upper panel) or both the therapeutic and post-therapeutic windows (lower panel), were simulated under the described experimental treatment schedule. (Data adapted from Ref. 36.)

that served for approximation were collected during the first week, that is, within the therapeutic time frame. However, subsequent simulations of the models under the same regimen failed to generate unified behavior of BVE dynamics (Fig. 36.3, upper panel). In contrast, when simulations were preceded by calibration of the models using data from stages both within therapy (the first week) and up to one month following treatment termination, the output dynamics were highly similar between the models (Fig. 36.3, lower panel). In fact, the observed high correlation between the numbers of experimental points used for model calibration, and the models' increased similarity (data not shown), strengthened the possibility that by using more data points, model similarity and thus reliability and clinical predict-ability can be improved.

In the second stage of the work, the predictability of the models was evaluated in a wider therapeutic spectrum. The models were simulated under IL-11 treatment strategies of various durations, various interdosing intervals, and various dose inten-sities, where model-derived dynamics were again compared to assess the model robustness in portraying BVE dynamics. Highest values of similarity between models, as shown by the difference index, were observed when the average IL-11 dose per day of the tested treatment was close to that of the experimental treatment

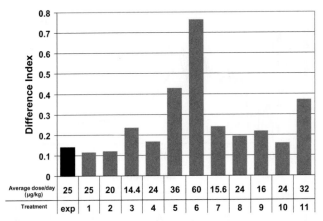

Average dose/day (µg/kg)	25	25	20	14.4	24	36	60	15.6	24	16	24	32
Treatment	exp	1	2	3	4	5	6	7	8	9	10	11

FIGURE 36.4 Model-derived BVE dynamics in therapeutic regimens that are close to experimental schedules in average dose per day values. Model simulations under the experimental schedule (treatment exp) and other regimens of various durations, doses, and inter-dosing intervals (treatments 1–11), following calibration with clinical measurements, are compared using the difference index. (Data adapted from Ref. 36.)

of daily 25 µg/kg doses (see Fig. 36.4 as an example). This suggests that in this example of an obscure toxicity mechanism, one can trust the model-derived BVE predictions for various IL-11 treatments, provided their average daily dose of IL-11 is in proximity to that used in the original clinical experiment.

The mathematical method applied in the case of IL-11 shows that given preliminary experimental data from various stages of therapy, beginning at phases within the therapeutic window and ending at the recuperated steady state, the different models reliably predict dynamics of water retention within a certain span of IL-11-administration strategies. Considering the recommended IL-11 levels (10–100 µg/kg/day), and the above model-derived conclusions, clinical studies evaluating BVE within concentrations of 10, 20, 30, . . . µg/kg/day are required to form a complete predictability frame of BVE within all relevant treatment scenarios. This would then allow appraisal of the clinical applicability of each of these IL-11 therapy schedules, as well as others.

As in the above-presented process of IL-11 model evaluation, clinical information was used for the TPO case. A thrombopoiesis computational model was designed on the basis of the mathematical description of TPO-induced thrombopoiesis (elaborated in Sections 36.2 and 36.4), to enable simulation and evaluation of *in vivo* platelet formation and to suggest therapeutic TPO regimens of improved efficacy and reduced immunogenicity [38]. The computer model was adjusted and validated for murine, simian, and human cases, as will be elaborated later.

Currently, human validation of the thrombopoiesis computer model is possible only in retrospective, as the drug has not yet undergone the appropriate regulatory procedures enabling human administration. To retrospectively validate the model, it was calibrated using a set of biologically realistic parameter values, so that homeostatic behavior (i.e., a normative count of 320,000 platelets/µL blood) was retrieved in untreated conditions. Next, simulation of the computerized model under

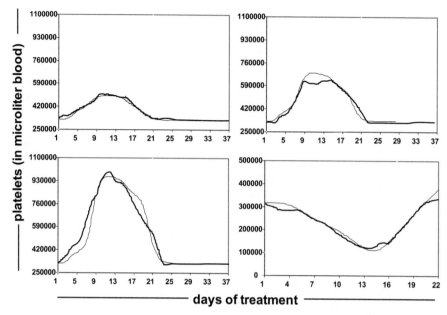

FIGURE 36.5   Model predictions of platelet profiles in patients treated by TPO and chemotherapy compared to clinical results. Average platelet counts in human patients are plotted, following a single IV bolus rhTPO administration of 0.3 μg/kg (upper left panel), 1.2 μg/kg (upper right panel), or 2.4 μg/kg (lower left panel), or an IV infusion of doxorubicin for 3 days, the total dose being 90 mg/m² (lower right panel). Simulation-generated curves are shown by thick lines; clinical results are shown by thin lines.

recombinant human TPO (rhTPO) administration was carried out. Data from a clinical trial [39], which included PK information (i.e., rhTPO concentration in blood) and accurate platelet counts in response to different TPO dosages, served the calibration process: three patients were assigned to a single IV bolus administration of each of the four dosages 0.3, 0.6, 1.2, or 2.4 μg/kg. The three platelet count curves for each dosage were averaged and a single parameter set, which enabled the model to accurately retrieve platelet dynamics observed under the various treatment regimens, as shown in Fig. 36.5, was identified. This parameter set was determined as the representative for the "average patient."

While TPO therapies pose many questions, such as its effects on elevated platelet counts in clonal thrombocytosis, the opposite problem, namely, that of reduced platelet counts, introduces equally significant challenges. Since TP is a common dose-limiting side effect of cancer chemotherapeutics, as discussed in Sections 36.3 and 36.4, accurate predictions of the chemotherapeutically reduced platelet dynamics are of importance when planning treatments. To allow predicting the effect of cytotoxics on thrombopoiesis in individual patients, the average "Virtual Patient" was tested for its ability to retrieve the outcomes of a standard chemotherapeutic treatment by doxorubicin. The model was successfully calibrated in reference to clinical published experimental data [40], as shown by Figure 36.5 (lower right panel) and improved TPO regimens were suggested. Prospective validation of the generality and clinical predictability of the model is warranted. A different biomathematical approach, elaborated in Section 36.7, uses data from human and animal cell cultures and from preclinical studies that are available in the pharmaceutical industry, in order to develop therapeutic strategies with minimal suppression of thrombopoiesis.

In conclusion, the thrombopoiesis computer model was successfully calibrated to accurately retrieve relevant clinical information reflecting TPO therapy, as well as chemotherapy, but it is yet to undergo prospective human validation. Importantly, the models described here for different thrombopoietic growth factors are each targeted toward opposing aspects of therapy: while the IL-11 mathematical model attempts to define the toxicity associated with drug-induced alleviation of TP, the computerized TPO model is aimed at accurately predicting the direct beneficial results of such therapy on platelet restoration.

36.5.2 Model Validation in Prospective Animal Trials: TPO Applied to the Virtual Mouse and Virtual Monkey

To use the model predictions for clinical decision making, one must still substantiate the superiority of the model-suggested improved TPO regimens. This task must be carried out in animals first, not only due to safety issues, but also because typically in such cases, the agent in question is not yet approved for the treatment of patients. Once a proof of concept in animals is provided for its power to suggest improved regimens, the model can become instrumental during the clinical phases of drug development, for avoiding excessive and unnecessary toxicity and for reducing the number of patients in Phase I of the clinical development. These steps are expected to pave the road for routine clinical use of the computer-based prediction tool.

The underlying assumption in this work was that improved TPO schedules are those employing the smallest drug doses required to achieve the desired efficacy. This assumption is based on a biomathematical study that examined the effect of dose intensities on drug immunogenicity. Results of this work suggest that for a given immunoreactive system, there exists a critical drug dose for which the relevant immunogenic threshold is expected to be exceeded, thus affecting patient health [41].

To validate the model's predictions in preclinical experiments with BALB/c mice and rhesus monkeys, the thrombopoiesis model was calibrated to reflect murine or simian thrombopoiesis. This was achieved by using literature-derived data. The species-adapted models, Virtual Mouse and Virtual Monkey, were subsequently used to adjust the improved TPO treatment to the species in question and test this treatment in animal experiments. This work is described in Ref. 38.

Parameter calibration of the thrombopoiesis computer model was performed for fine-tuning the model to accurately describe thrombopoiesis in each species. This work involved definition of a biologically realistic range of values for each parameter in murine thrombopoiesis [28, 42–47] and simian thrombopoiesis [22, 48–54], which were then entered as the initial parameter values, subsequently to be fine-tuned according to the specific tested population. Ability of the model to retrieve platelet profiles in each animal group was then tested.

Next, the prediction accuracy of the thrombopoiesis computer model was validated in mice. Specifically, by simulating the model it was predicted that platelet counts, similar to those achieved with the accepted TPO administration schedule, can also be generated under different schedules of appreciably reduced TPO doses (Fig. 36.6, upper panel). Hence, two different administration regimens were

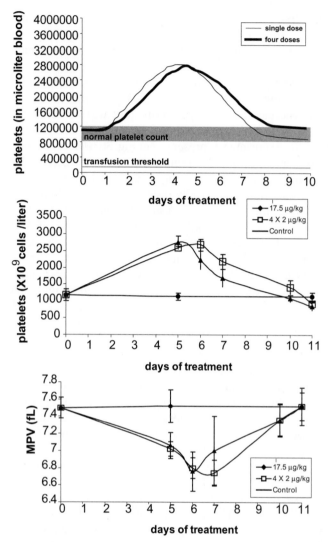

FIGURE 36.6   Model predictions of platelet profiles in mice treated by TPO as compared to experimental results. (Upper panel) The thrombopoiesis model-generated predictions indicating similar efficacy in platelet formation between a "conventional" single-dose TPO treatment of 17.5 μg/kg, and a model-suggested reduced TPO treatment of four daily doses of 2 μg/kg each, comprising only 10–45% of the standard regimen. Experimental results of platelet formation (middle panel) and MPV measurements (lower panel) following conventional rmTPO therapy (black diamonds) and the alternative therapy (white squares) in mice, according to the above schedules, validate the model predictions. Treatments are initiated at day 0. Average ± SD of five mice are shown, per each entry. (Data adapted from Refs. 37 and 38.)

experimentally applied to mice clustered in two experimental arms, and their subsequent responses were compared. Mice of the first arm (A) received a standard regimen consisting of a single injection of 17.5 µg/kg recombinant murine TPO (rmTPO), which was well below the reported saturating level [42]. The second arm (B) tested the model-generated proposition that the same platelet yields can be obtained in mice receiving a total dose of 8 µg/kg rmTPO, divided over four equal daily injections, whereas the null hypothesis here was that a significantly smaller total dose of rmTPO would be less efficient in elevating the platelet counts.

The results of the experiments, presented in Fig. 36.6 (middle panel), clearly show that the platelet profile of arm A (a regimen of one 17.5 µg/kg rmTPO injection) is similar to the profile of arm B (applying a regimen of four daily 2 µg/kg rmTPO doses). The differences are statistically insignificant, as evaluated by the Student's t-test. The average profiles of both arm A and B peaked at fairly the same time (day 5 vs. day 6, respectively) and at similar mean platelet counts of $2741 \pm 193 \times 10^9$/L and $2685 \pm 164 \times 10^9$/L, respectively. The latter schedule resulted in a slightly extended thrombocytosis. MPV, known to decrease in platelet production induced by low dose TPO in mice [55], was compared between arm A and arm B as well (Fig. 36.6, lower panel). Results show that the familiar phenomenon of MPV reduction also occurred similarly in both groups. Once again, arm A had preceded arm B in reaching its nadir by about 24 hours (6.76 fL on day 6, vs. 6.74 fL on day 7, respectively). Specific adverse effects were not observed following either treatment.

In order to evaluate in rhesus monkeys the efficacy of the treatment regimen, already validated in mice, we first checked the ability of the simian thrombopoiesis model to predict individual monkey responses to different TPO treatments. Next, the simian response to the model-suggested schedule was simulated and the resulting predictions were compared with the platelet counts that were experimentally obtained under the model-suggested schedule.

To this end, model parameters were first evaluated to fit the empirical platelet profile of a single rhesus monkey. The quantitatively adequate simulations of thrombopoiesis response to treatment were apparent from their resemblance to the empirical results (Fig. 36.7). This calibrated model was further validated in several other monkeys, each receiving a different drug schedule (see schedule in Fig. 36.8, top panel).

Results in Fig. 36.9 demonstrate that the model predictions run remarkably close to the empirical data points. Note that as the platelet counts were monitored in these monkeys only once weekly, a mismatch is introduced into the comparison between the empirical results and the daily predicted counts. Thus, there is no reason to assume that the peaks in the predicted responses on days that were not tested empirically did not actually take place.

36.5.3 Predicting the Optimal TPO Efficacy/Toxicity Ratio in Monkeys

Once verified, the Virtual Rhesus model was simulated for identifying an improved TPO administration regimen. The model-based regimen was then evaluated for verifying its improved efficacy and safety profile. This was done in two monkeys (see Fig. 36.8, bottom panel). The resulting elevation in platelet counts peaked at 1700–

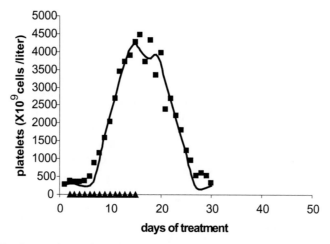

FIGURE 36.7 Comparison of model predictions to empirical data of TPO therapy in a rhesus monkey. Daily experimental measurements (rectangles) are shown as well as model simulations (solid line) of platelet counts of one monkey treated by TPO. Fourteen daily doses of 5 µg/kg TPO were applied, administration days marked by triangles. (Data adapted from Refs. 37 and 38.)

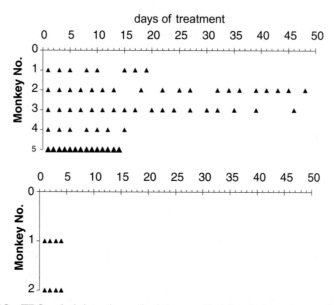

FIGURE 36.8 TPO administration schedules applied in simians for model validation. (Upper panel) Five different schedules, comprising various combinations of 5 µg/kg doses of recombinant full-length rhesus monkey TPO (each dose indicated by triangles), were individually applied to the studied monkeys. (Lower panel) Model-suggested TPO schedules (also using doses of 5 µg/kg) applied to two monkeys.

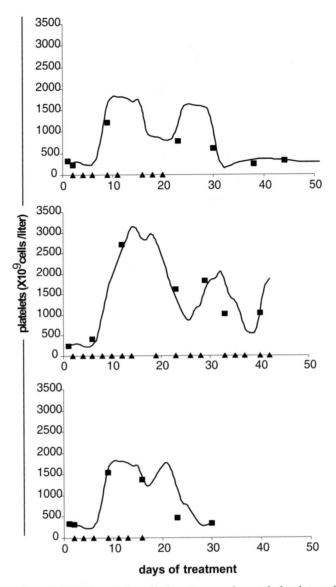

FIGURE 36.9   Comparison of model predictions to experimental platelet profiles of rhesus monkeys under various TPO treatment schedules. Three monkeys (upper, middle, and lower panels) were subjected to individual TPO regimens, consisting of multiple dosing treatments of 5 μg/kg TPO, administration days marked by triangles. Experimental measurements of platelet counts in blood were performed weekly or biweekly (squares) and are plotted against model simulations (solid line).

2400×10^9/L following each treatment cycle. The results of a second cycle of the same treatment were similar to those of the first one in showing no neutralizing antibodies. Only when the dosing cycle was applied for the third time were low antibody titers detectable, which did not jeopardize TPO's efficacy and did not result in decreased platelet counts. The individual empirical responses of the two monkeys

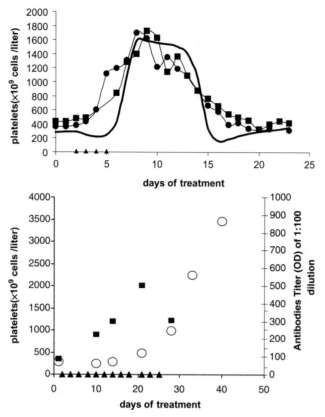

FIGURE 36.10 Superiority of the model-suggested TPO treatment schedule validated in rhesus monkeys, as compared to other regimens. (Upper panel) Empirical platelet profiles of monkeys under the model-suggested TPO regimen of four daily 5μg/kg doses (solid squares and circles) are plotted; administration days are marked by triangles. (Lower panel) Antibody titer and platelet profiles of a monkey undergoing an arbitrary treatment by 12 TPO doses.

to the first treatment cycle are shown in Fig. 36.10 (top panel) (to be compared with a highly immunogenic response of a monkey who underwent another TPO treatment, Fig. 36.9, bottom panel).

These results show that the model-predicted administration regimen of smaller TPO doses with an interval of 24 hours yields platelet counts that are equal in effect to the more than double dose regimen, administered as a bolus injection. This experiment joins previous *in vivo* experiments with other drugs in verifying a mathematical theory discussed in Section 36.1.1, which essentially suggests that treatment efficacy can be decisively influenced by modulating the interdosing interval according to the internal cell kinetics. The monkey experiment supports the model prediction of an equally efficient and nonimmunogenic treatment, if dose is fractionated by an appropriate dosing interval. Importantly, this schedule, adopted for improving safety of TPO administered for platelet harvesting in monkeys, has been in use for the last five years or so. No adverse effects have been associated with this model-suggested treatment.

In general terms, the experimental results in both animal species supported and validated the predictions of the mathematical model that more efficacious treatment with TPO can be implemented. Although intuitively it may not seem beneficial for the patient to replace a single injection by multiple doses, it is clearly of significance for safety considerations.

The computerized mathematical model is capable of successfully predicting treatment scenarios not yet tested experimentally, as well as of identifying safer regimens. This tool is expected to be of aid in suggesting improved drug strategies for an individual or for a patient population. Human trials are necessary for testing the suggested improved TPO strategies, possibly in conjunction with chemotherapy.

36.6   USING THE THROMBOPOIESIS MODEL FOR PREDICTING AN UNKNOWN ANIMAL TOXICITY MECHANISM

Several pathophysiological mechanisms can account for drug-induced TP (see Section 36.3), and the actual underlying mechanism in each particular case can have important therapeutic implications. Yet, no easily applicable noninvasive laboratory tests are available for distinguishing between the different mechanisms for TP. In this section, we describe the manner by which mathematical modeling can help in understanding the dynamics and etiology of drug-induced TP.

A monoclonal antibody-based drug, developed against a platelet-unrelated antigen and currently under preclinical evaluation, was found to possess cross-reactive effects eliciting severe TP in monkeys. Despite routine laboratory testing and histological examination of bone marrow of affected monkeys, the drug's mechanism for inducing TP has not been elucidated. In an attempt to decipher the underlying mechanism, we used the mathematical model for TPO-regulated thrombopoiesis [37, 38], which was previously formed (as described in Section 36.2) and validated *in vivo* (as depicted in Sections 36.4 and 36.5). This model was extended to include the effect of the drug on MKs and platelets. Since the mechanism is still unknown, several biologically plausible alternatives were examined. Antibodies can exert their effect either by antibody-assisted phagocytosis or by complement-mediated direct toxicity [56]. In the first mechanism, antibody-covered platelets or platelet-forming MKs would be efficiently removed by macrophages that bear specific antibody-recognizing receptors. In the latter case, platelet-bound antibodies activate the complement pathway that leads to cell membrane perforation and cell destruction (Fig. 36.11).

Mathematical implementation of both antibody-mediated killing mechanisms into the PD-extended model was performed as follows. For complement-mediated toxicity, an "accumulated hits" model, according to which each platelet suffers from cumulative damage ("hits") induced by antibody-mediated complement binding, was suggested. Upon accumulation of a certain number of "hits," the platelet is permanently damaged. The resulting probability density function, $P(t)$, describing a fraction of platelets with a given number of "hits" in time t postexposure, is given by the gamma function

$$P(t) = \frac{(\alpha t)^m e^{-\alpha t} \alpha}{m!}$$

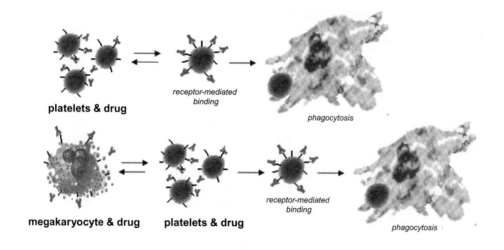

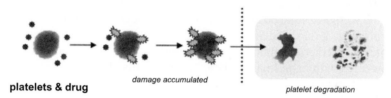

FIGURE 36.11 The "phagocytosis" putative mechanism and the "hits" putative mechanism of drug-induced thrombocytopenia. In the "phagocytosis" mechanism (upper panel), drug molecules bind to platelet and megakaryocyte surface antigens, leading to their phagocytosis by the reticuloendothelial system. In the "hits" mechanism (lower panel), drug molecules bind to platelet surface antigens, leading to complement activation and direct destruction of the cells.

where m is the number of hits needed for platelet destruction, and α is the rate of hit formation. The rate of hits is given by a linear function of the antibody concentration in blood:

$$\alpha = aX + b$$

where X is antibody concentration, and a and b are parameters.

For the case of antibody-mediated phagocytosis, the "phagocytosis" model, it was assumed that the rate of platelet "capture" by macrophages has a Hill's function form, depending on the number of antibodies that are bound to the platelet's surface. This is described as follows:

$$B(i) = \frac{B_{max} i^z}{K^z + i^z}$$

where $B(i)$ is the rate of capture of platelets that possess i bound antibodies, and K and z are parameters. Since binding and dissociation of antibodies from the platelet surface are stochastic processes, the distribution of platelets with respect to the number of bound antibodies, V_i, was explicitly calculated, so that the rate of antibody-induced platelet elimination is given by

$$R = \sum_i V_i B_i$$

Antibodies can act against mature platelets, bone marrow-derived MKs, or both. Hence, several combinations of these suggested drug-toxicity mechanisms were implemented in the extended model. Retrospective results of real-life experiments in a number of individual rhesus monkeys [37, 38] were used for comparison with the simulated outcomes of these various alternative models. For each combination, the PD-associated parameters of the extended model were adjusted to best fit to these experimental results. Only one of the combinations was expected to consistently retrieve experimental data, and thus be identified as the preferable mechanism underlying this antibody-mediated TP. Systemic platelet profiles in individual monkeys following administration of multiple or single doses of the drug were compared with the best-fit profiles produced by models with different drug effect mechanisms (Fig. 36.12). The analysis of these simulations indicated that the "hits" model failed to predict dynamics of the drug-induced TP, while the "phagocytosis" model coincided with experimental data. Model results also show that by assuming toxicity to both platelets and MKs, rather than to just platelets, more precise predictions can be yielded.

We conclude that the developed computerized thrombopoiesis model superimposed by mathematical models for putative toxicity mechanisms can retrieve adverse thrombocytopenic effects recorded empirically in simians. Different models of drug-toxicity mechanisms yield different profiles of blood platelets, yet the antibody-mediated phagocytosis of platelets and MKs seems the most plausible mechanism of the drug-induced TP in this situation. In this manner, mathematical modeling can help decipher the underlying mechanisms of other disorders.

36.7 TRANSITION TO PHASE I

Drug development is a costly and time-consuming endeavor, due to its requirement for enormous collections of data concerning the efficacy and safety of the proposed drug. The ability to extrapolate toxicity and efficacy data from animal to human is therefore of great importance for efficiently advancing development of pharmaceuticals. Yet, despite the efforts invested in this direction, and the great advances achieved in recent years, extrapolation of data from animals to humans is still considered unreliable [57–59]. In this section, we provide a detailed description of an algorithm, which in conjunction with data from cell cultures and animal experiments, can be used for the modeling of clinically stimulated (drug-induced) TP in humans, and we show how this method enables good clinical predictability of this disorder.

As discussed in Section 36.3, TP can result from therapeutic intervention, such as anticancer chemotherapy. The mathematical model of thrombopoiesis, described in Section 36.2, was used as a basic model for retrieving clinical cytotoxic drug-

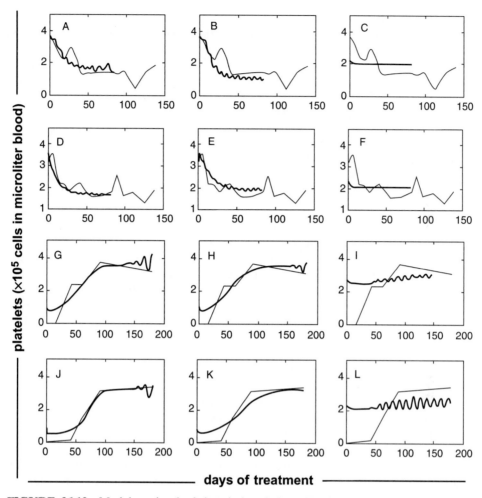

FIGURE 36.12 Model retrieval of drug-induced thrombocytopenia in rhesus monkeys. Platelet dynamics derived from experiments in four monkeys, receiving a treatment of multiple doses (A–F) or a single high dose (G–L) of the drug. The effects of each treatment on the monkey's platelet profile were simulated by the three mathematical models of alternative drug-toxicity mechanisms. Model predictions were then statistically compared with the experimental results. Simulation results are for the "phagocytosis" model assuming that the drug targets platelets alone (left column panels), for the "phagocytosis" model assuming that the drug targets both platelets and megakaryocytes (middle column panels), or for the "hits" model assuming that the drug targets only platelets (right column panels). Panels A–C, D–F, G–I, and J–L correspond to data from each of the four monkeys. Empirical data (thin lines) is shown versus simulation-derived dynamics (thick lines).

induced TP. Yet to obtain a reasonable approximation of the predicted toxicity in humans, based on preclinical data, additional assumptions and simplifications are required. These are detailed next.

First, translation of drug PD from the preclinical to the clinical stage is necessary. One must consider (1) differences between *in vitro* and *in vivo* data and

(2) differences between PD parameters of different species. Both variation types involve built-in inaccuracies. With respect to the comparison between *in vitro* and *in vivo* experiments, a few issues must be taken into account. Cells *in vitro* are more sensitive to a drug, and thus more susceptible to drug-induced apoptosis. They have higher mitotic indices due to less contact inhibition and are usually exposed to constant levels of drug concentration over time. Cells in the physiological, whole-organism context, however, are of lower sensitivity to a drug; the surrounding microenvironment, consisting of high proliferating and less drug-susceptible cells, provides a constant influx of healthy cells into the total pool, thereby limiting the damage caused by the drug [60]. Differences in exposure to growth factors between the two experimental settings exist as well. Drug sensitivity differs not only between *in vitro* and *in vivo* settings, but also in various species, which may differ in size of cells, mitotic indices of various compartments and differential stages of cells, apoptotic indices, transit times, and sensitivity to hormones [61].

In order to replicate clinical use of the drug, the basic mathematical model is extended to incorporate an additional formula for the drug PD. It is assumed that bone marrow cells are exposed to systemic drug concentration at any time, as the tissue is highly vascularized. The model also assumes that cells at different developmental stages, denoted by a subscript X (e.g., UCP, CP, EP), are of diverse sensitivity to the drug. The functional relation between the concentration of the cytotoxic drug in blood (CD_{bl}) and the cytotoxic effect (CE) is given by the equation

$$CE_X(t) = f(CD_{bl}(t)) \tag{36.14}$$

where CE_X denotes the fraction of bone marrow thrombopoietic cells of a differentiation stage X, eliminated following exposure to CD_{bl} at time t ($CD_{bl}(t)$). The dependence is represented by function f, where $0 \le f(CD_{bl}(t)) \le 1$ for any t.

Most cytotoxic drugs target mitotic phases of the cell cycle and are thereby more harmful to proliferating, rather than resting, cells. Accordingly, by further subdividing the model compartments into cell-cycle phases (G0-G1 and S-G2-M subcompartments), a more accurate prediction of drug toxicity can be obtained. For example, in the above model, representation of UCP and CP compartments (see Section 36.2) uses cell-cycle length instead of amplification rate. This allows us to calculate, not only the total number of cells remaining at every time point after drug application but also the number of cells at every age and cell-cycle phase. In EP compartments, the age and the position in the endomitotic cycle are synchronized; thus there is no need for additional distribution. The rest of the compartments, consisting of nondividing cells, are not considered susceptible to the standard cytotoxic drug and are therefore not subdivided in this manner. Cytotoxic drugs that selectively target these stages can be addressed after subdivision of those compartments. In this complex form of the model, parameters (e.g., compartments, sizes, transit times) are evaluated differently for all the species examined, while the model equations themselves retain the same structure.

Following adaptation of the model equations to include the PD of the drug, parameters are calibrated using the available experimental information. Preclinical toxicity data to be used by the model consist of the platelet measurements over time in one animal of a chosen species (S), which has shown (in previous *in vitro* studies) higher sensitivity to the drug than other species. Various sets of data are obtained for a wide range of drug doses, so that different thrombocytopenic responses, from low toxicity to grade 3–4 toxicities, are considered.

The model also exploits data from cell culture assays. For example, for the estimation of the cytotoxic drug concentration, the model uses IC_{20}, IC_{50}, and IC_{90} (the concentrations of the drug leading to inhibition of 20%, 50%, and 90% of *in vitro* cell growth, respectively, as compared to untreated cells). These are obtained from toxicity tests of the platelet lineage-committed bone marrow cells (the CFU-Meg assay), in both human and species S-derived cells [62]. In the complex form of the model, one may also use experimental tools of cell-cycle analysis, such as standard cell-sorting assays.

Based on this data, three functions f (Eq. 36.14), denoted as $f_{\text{inVitroHu}}$, f_{inVitroS}, and f_{inVivoS} for human cell cultures, species S cell cultures, and preclinical S species studies, respectively, can be evaluated. In estimating the function f_{inVivoS}, it is necessary to consider only the drug's killing effect on bone marrow cells of compartment X, the depletion of which is mainly responsible for platelet nadir (see Eq. 36.14). X is identified by the time of the nadir after drug application, taking into account the transit times of the different bone marrow compartments. As a first approximation, only one compartment X of drug-sensitive cells is assumed.

The parameters of function f in the clinical scenario (f_{inVivoHu}), which cannot be estimated as in the other three cases due to lack of data, are thereby calculated according to their counterparts. First, it is assumed that between different species, there is a linear relation between the drug killing effect observed *in vivo* and *in vitro* (i.e., the $f_{\text{inVivo}}/f_{\text{inVitro}}$ ratio is constant between diverse species). The function f_{inVivoHu} is thereby obtained by shifting the IC values on the concentration axis according to this relation, using the *in vitro* data of IC_{50} ($IC_{50\text{inVitroHu}}$) and IC_{90} ($IC_{90\text{inVitroHu}}$). The relation itself is found by comparing the *in vitro* and *in vivo* data for species S. Then the shift of f_{inVivoS} to f_{inVivoHu} on the concentration axis for IC_{50} is computed by the equation

$$IC_{50\,\text{inVivoHu}} = \frac{IC_{50\,\text{inVivoS}} \cdot IC_{50\,\text{inVitroHu}}}{IC_{50\,\text{inVitroS}}} \tag{36.15}$$

The same method can be applied for IC_{90}.

The last step requires simulations of the model with the human parameters, under different regimens, applying the f_{inVivoHu} effect on the same type of bone marrow cells as in species S. The clinical toxicity profile of the drug—that is, the induction and severity of drug-induced TP in humans—is therefore predictable. Importantly, this estimation is a first approximation and a safety factor should be considered prior to initiation of clinical trials.

36.8 CONCLUSION

- Mathematical models are instrumental in increasing the understanding of intricate drug–patient interactions. Specifically, a mathematically based method, termed the Z-method, has been devised for increasing the efficacy/toxicity ratio of chemotherapeutics. The method suggests that safety of cell-cycle-specific drugs can be increased by resonating drug-pulsing with the internal periodicity of target host cells replication. Experimental verification of the Z-method in mice provides a proof-of-concept for the utility of biomathematics in drug development.

- Increasing model complexity, a prerequisite for the quantitative precision of its conclusions, was performed in order to provide a practical tool for predicting drug effects on platelet counts. To this end, thrombopoiesis models of various mammal species have been developed. Models of TPO supportive treatment have been prospectively validated in mice and monkeys.

- Toxicity effects of IL-11 therapy and chemotherapy have been modeled and various drug regimens were tested. Model validation under data limitation has been examined and the need to collect patient's recovery data has been emphasized. The range of the treatment schedules under which the models could reliably predict the outcomes of drug therapy under obscured biological knowledge has been defined.

- The thrombopoiesis model has been employed for suggesting TPO administration schedules, which would maximize drug safety while maintaining its efficacy. Dose fractionation, having a well-calculated, species-dependent dosing interval, preserves drug effect on platelet counts, yet reduces its immunologic adverse effects below the clinically relevant threshold.

- The above schedule, adjusted by the murine thrombopoiesis model, was validated in mice for efficacy. The monkey-adjusted schedule derived from simulations of the simian thrombopoiesis model, was validated in rhesus monkeys for both efficacy and toxicity. Now the human model may be employed for improving safety of TPO mimetics and other thrombocytopenia-alleviating drugs.

- To the best of our knowledge, this is the first instance of a mathematical model generating quantitative predictions, the precision of which was validated in the preclinical setting.

- The thrombopoiesis model can be used, in conjunction with alternative mathematical models, for deciphering unknown drug-toxicity mechanisms in different species. This can be achieved by comparing preclinical study results with the simulated drug-affected platelet profiles, generated for different models of putative drug-toxicity mechanisms.

- In order to facilitate the transition from preclinical studies to Phase I, the mathematical models for the effect of investigational drugs on different animal species can be adapted accordingly and simulated in the human patient model for predicting parameters, the early estimation of which can economize Phase I clinical trials.

REFERENCES

1. FDA White Paper on Innovation and Stagnation in Drug Industry, Challenges and Opportunities on the Clinical Paths to New Medical Products, March 2004.
2. Agur Z. The effect of drug schedule on responsiveness to chemotherapy. *Ann NY Acad Sci* 1986;504:274–277.
3. Agur Z, Arnon R, Schechter B. Reduction of cytotoxicity to normal tissues by new regimes of cell-cycle phase-specific drugs. *Math Biosci* 1988;92:1–15.

4. Agur Z, Arnon R, Sandak B, Schechter B. The effect of the dosing interval on myelotoxicity and survival in mice treated by cytarabine. *Eur J Cancer* 1992;28A(6/7):1085–1090.

5. Ubezio P, Tagliabue G, Schechter B, Agur Z. Increasing 1-beta-D-arabinofuranosylcytosine efficacy by scheduled dosing interval based on direct measurement of bone marrow cell kinetics. *Cancer Res* 1994;54:6446–6451.

6. Agur Z. Persistence in uncertain environments. In Freedman HI, Strobeck C, Eds. *Population Biology, Lecture Notes in Biomathematics*. Heidelberg: Springer-Verlag; 1982, pp 125–132.

7. Agur Z. Randomness, synchrony and population persistence. *J Theor Biol* 1985;112: 677–693.

8. Agur Z, Deneubourg JL. The effect of environmental disturbances on the dynamics of marine intertidal populations. *Theor Population Biol* 1985;27(1):75–90.

9. Cojocaru L, Agur Z. A theoretical analysis of interval drug dosing for cell-cycle-phase-specific drugs. *Math Biosci* 1992;109:85–97.

10. Kheifetz Y, Kogan Y, Agur Z. Long-range predictability in models of cell populations subjected to phase-specific drugs: growth-rate approximation using properties of positive compact operators. *Math Models Methods Appl Sci* 2006;16(7):1–18.

11. Agur Z, Arnon R, Sandak B, Schechter B. Zidovudine toxicity to murine bone marrow may be affected by the exact frequency of drug administration. *Exp Hematol* 1991; 19:364–368.

12. Arakelyan L, Vainstein V, Agur Z. A computer algorithm describing the process of vessel formation and maturation, and its use for predicting the effects of anti-angiogenic and anti-maturation therapy on vascular tumor growth. *Angiogenesis* 2002;5:203–214.

13. Ribba B, Alarcon T, Marron K, Maini PK, Agur Z. Doxorubicin treatment efficacy on non-Hodgkin's lymphoma: computer model and simulations. *Bull Math Biol* 2005;67: 79–99.

14. Vainstein V, Ginosar Y, Shoham M, Ranmar D, Ianovski A, Agur Z. The complex effect of granulocyte on human granulopoiesis analyzed by a new physiologically-based mathematical model. *J Theor Biol* 2005;234(3):311–327.

15. Agur Z, Ziv I, Shohat R, Wick M, Webb C, Hankins D, Arakelyan L, Sidransky D. Using a novel computer technology for tailoring targeted and chemotherapeutic drug schedules to the individual patient. *First AACR International Conference on Molecular Diagnostic in Cancer Therapeutic Development. Chicago IL*, 2006.

16. Hoffman R, Benz EJ, Shattil SJ, Furie B, Cohen HJ, Silberstein LE, McGlave P. *Hematology*, 3rd ed. London: Churchill Livingstone; 2000.

17. Kaushansky K. The molecular mechanisms that control thrombopoiesis. *J Clin Invest* 2005;115:3339–3347.

18. Kaushansky K. Lineage-specific hematopoietic growth factors. *N Engl J Med* 2006; 354:2034–2045.

19. Schulze H, Shivdasani RA. Mechanisms of thrombopoiesis. *J Thromb Haemost* 2005; 3:1717–1724.

20. Cines DB, Bussel JB, McMillan RB, Zehnder JL. Congenital and acquired thrombocytopenia. In *Hematology, the American Society of Hematology Education Program Book*: 2004, pp 390–406.

21. McCrae KR, Bussel JB, Mannucci PM, Cines DB. Platelets: an update on diagnosis and management of thrombocytopenic disorders. In *Hematology, the American Society of Hematology Education Program Book*: 2001, pp 282–305.

22. Demetri GD. Targeted approaches for the treatment of thrombocytopenia. *Oncologist* 2001;6(Suppl 5):15–23.

23. Schwertschlag US, Trepicchio WL, Dykstra KH, Keith JC, Turner KJ, Dorner AJ. Hematopoietic, immunomodulatory and epithelial effects of interleukin-11. *Leukemia* 1999; 13(9):1307–1315.

24. Tepler I, Elias L, Smith JW 2nd, Hussein M, Rosen G, Chang AY, Moore JO, Gordon MS, Kuca B, Beach KJ, Loewy JW, Garnick MB, Kaye JA. A randomized placebo-controlled trial of recombinant human interleukin-11 in cancer patients with severe thrombocytopenia due to chemotherapy. *Blood* 1996;87(9):3607–3614.

25. Haznedaroglu IC, Goker H, Turgut M, Buyukasik Y, Benekli M. Thrombopoietin as a drug: biologic expectations, clinical realities, and future directions. *Clin Appl Thromb/ Hemost* 2002;8:193–212.

26. Basser R. The impact of thrombopoietin on clinical practice. *Curr Pharm Design* 2002; 8(5):369–377.

27. Elting LS, Rubenstein EB, Martin CG, Kurtin D, Rodriguez S, Laiho E, Kanesan K, Cantor SB, Benjamin RS. Incidence, cost, and outcomes of bleeding and chemotherapy dose modification among solid tumor patients with chemotherapy-induced thrombocytopenia. *J Clin Oncol* 2001;19:1137–1146.

28. Kaushansky K, Lin N, Grossman A, Humes J, Sprugel KH, Broudy VC. Thrombopoietin expands erythroid, granulocyte-macrophage, and megakaryocytic progenitor cells in normal and myelosuppressed mice. *Exp Hematol* 1996;24:265–269.

29. Li J, Yang C, Xia Y, Bertino A, Glaspy J, Roberts M, Kuter DJ. Thrombocytopenia caused by the development of antibodies to thrombopoietin. *Blood* 2001;98(12):3241–3248.

30. Vadhan-Raj S. Recombinant human TPO: clinical experience and *in vivo* biology. *Semin Hematol* 1998;35:261–268.

31. Vadhan-Raj S. Clinical experience with recombinant human thrombopoietin in chemotherapy-induced thrombocytopenia. *Semin Hematol* 2000;37(2 Suppl 4):28–34.

32. Vadhan-Raj S. Recombinant human thrombopoietin in myelosuppressive chemotherapy. *Oncology (Williston Park)* 2001;15(7 Suppl 8):35–38.

33. Vadhan-Raj S, Cohen V, Bueso-Ramos C. Thrombopoietic growth factors and cytokines. *Curr Hematol Rep* 2005;4(2):137–144.

34. Wolff SN, Herzig R, Lynch J, Ericson SG, Greer JP, Stein R, Goodman S, Benyunes MC, Ashby M, Jones DV Jr, Fay J. Recombinant human thrombopoietin (rhTPO) after autologous bone marrow transplantation: a phase I pharmacokinetic and pharmacodynamic study. *Bone Marrow Transplant* 2001;27(3):261–268.

35. Dykstra KH, Rogge H, Stone A, Loewy J, Keith JC Jr, Schwertschlag US. Mechanism and amelioration of recombinant human interleukin-11 (rhIL-11)-induced anemia in healthy subjects. *J Clin Pharmacol* 2000;40(8):880–888.

36. Kheifetz Y, Elishmereni M, Horowitz S, Agur Z. Fluid-retention side-effects of the chemotherapy-supportive treatment interleukin-11: mathematical modelling as affected by data availability. *Comput Math Methods Med* 2006;7(2–3):71–84.

37. Skomorovski K, Agur Z. A new method for predicting and optimizing thrombopoietin (TPO) therapeutic protocols in thrombocytopenic patients and in platelet donors [abstract]. *Hematol J* 2001;1(Suppl 1):185.

38. Skomorovski K, Harpak H, Ianovski A, Vardi M, Visser TP, Hartong S, Van Vliet H, Wagemaker G, Agur Z. New TPO treatment schedules of increased safety and efficacy: preclinical validation of a thrombopoiesis simulation model. *Br J of Haematol* 2003; 123(4):683–691.

39. Vadhan-Raj S, Murray LJ, Bueso-Ramos C, Patel S, Reddy SP, Hoots WK, Johnston T, Papadopolous NE, Hittelman WN, Johnston DA, Yang TA, Paton VE, Cohen RL, Hellmann SD, Benjamin RS, Broxmeyer HE. Stimulation of megakaryocyte and platelet

production by a single dose of recombinant human thrombopoietin in patients with cancer. *Ann Intern Med* 1997;126:673–681.

40. Vadhan-Raj S, Patel S, Bueso-Ramos C, Folloder J, Papadopolous N, Burgess A, Broemeling LD, Broxmeyer HE, Benjamin RS. Importance of predosing of recombinant human thrombopoietin to reduce chemotherapy-induced early thrombocytopenia. *J Clin Oncol* 2003;21:3158–3167.

41. Castiglione F, Selitser V, Agur Z. The analyzing hypersensitive to chemotherapy in a cellular automata model of the immune system. In Preziosi L. Ed. *Cancer Modelling and Simulation*. Boca Raton, FL: CRC Press; 2003.

42. Arnold JT, Daw NC, Stenberg PE, Jayawardene D, Srivastava DK, Jackson CW. A single injection of pegylated murine megakaryocyte growth and development factor (MGDF) into mice is sufficient to produce a profound stimulation of megakaryocyte frequency, size, and ploidization. *Blood* 1997;89:823–833.

43. Ebbe S, Stohlman F. Megakaryocytopoiesis in the rat. *Blood* 1965;26:20–35.

44. Luoh S, Stephanich E, Solar G, Steinmetz H, Lipari T, Pestina TI, Jackson CW, de Sauvage FJ. Role of the distal half of the c-Mpl intracellular domain in control of platelet production by thrombopoietin *in vivo. Mol Cell Biol* 2000;20:507–515.

45. Schermer S. *Blood Morphology of Laboratory Animals*. Philadelphia: FA Davis Co; 1967.

46. Siegers MP, Feinendegen LE, Lahiri SK, Cronkite EP. Relative number and proliferation kinetics of hemopoietic stem cells in the mouse. *Blood Cells* 1979;5:211–236.

47. Ulich TR, del Castillo J, Senaldi G, Cheung E, Roskos L, Young J, Molineux G, Guo J, Schoemperlen J, Munyakazi L, Murphy-Filkins R, Tarpley JE, Toombs CF, Kaufman S, Yin S, Nelson AG, Nichol JL, Sheridan WP. Megakaryocytopoiesis: the prolonged hematologic effects of a single injection of PEG-rHuMGDF in normal and thrombocytopenic mice. *Exp Hematol* 1999;27:117–130.

48. De Serres M, Yeager RL, Dillberger JE, Lalonde G, Gardner GH, Rubens CA, Simkins AH, Sailstad JM, McNulty MJ, Woolley JL. Pharmacokinetics and hematological effects of the pegylated thrombopoietin peptide mimetic GW395058 in rats and monkeys after intravenous or subcutaneous administration. *Stem Cells* 1999;17:316–326.

49. Farese AM, Hunt P, Boone T, MacVittie TJ. Recombinant human megakaryocyte growth and development factor stimulates thrombopoiesis in normal nonhuman primates. *Blood* 1995;86:54–59.

50. Harker LA, Hunt P, Marzec UM, Kelly AB, Tomer A, Hanson SR, Stead RB. Regulation of platelet production and function by megakaryocyte growth and development factor in nonhuman primates. *Blood* 1996;87:1833–1844.

51. Harker LA, Marzec UM, Hunt P, Kelly AB, Tomer A, Cheung E, Hanson SR, Stead RB. Dose–response effects of pegylated human megakaryocyte growth and development factor Of platelet production and function in nonhuman primates. *Blood* 1996;88: 511–521.

52. Neelis KJ, Hartong SC, Egeland T, Thomas GR, Eaton DL, Wagemaker G. The efficacy of single-dose administration of thrombopoietin with coadministration of either granulocyte/macrophage or granulocyte colony-stimulating factor in myelosuppressed rhesus monkeys. *Blood* 1997;90:2565–2573.

53. Sola MC, Christensen RD, Hutson AD, Tarantal AF. Pharmacokinetics, pharmacodynamics, and safety of administering pegylated recombinant megakaryocyte growth and development factor to newborn rhesus monkeys. *Pediatr Res* 2000;47:208–214.

54. Wagemaker G, Hartong SC, Neelis KJ, Egeland T, Wognum AW. *In vivo* expansion of hemopoietic stem cells. *Stem Cells* 1998;16(Suppl 1):185–191.

55. Kabaya K, Akahori H, Shibuya K, Nitta Y, Ida M, Kusaka M, Kato T, Miyazaki H. *In vivo* effects of pegylated recombinant human megakaryocytes growth and development factor on hematopoiesis in normal mice. *Stem Cells* 1996;14:651–660.

56. Janeway CA, Travers P, Walport M, Shlomchik M. *Immunobiology*, 6th ed. New York: Garland Science; 2005.

57. Al-Dabbagh SG, Smith RL. Species differences in oxidative drug metabolism: some basic considerations. *Arch Toxicol Suppl* 1984;7:219–231.

58. Kararli TT. Comparison of the gastrointestinal anatomy, physiology, and biochemistry of humans and commonly used laboratory animals. *Biopharm Drug Dispos* 1995;16(5): 351–380.

59. Lin JH. Species similarities and differences in pharmacokinetics. *Drug Metab Dispos* 1995;23(10):1008–1021.

60. Phillips RM, Bibby MC, Double JA. A critical appraisal of the predictive value of *in vitro* chemosensitivity assays. *J Nat Cancer Inst* 1990;82:1457–1468.

61. Harker LA, Finch CA. Thrombokinetics in man. *J Clin Invest* 1969;48:963–974.

62. Ratajczak J, Machalinski B, Samuel A, Pertusini E, Majka M, Czajka R, Ratajczak MZ. A novel serum free system for cloning human megakaryocytic progenitors (CFU-Meg). The role of thrombopoietin and other cytokines on bone marrow and cord blood CFU-Meg growth under serum free conditions. *Folia Histochem Cytobiol* 1998;36(2) 61–66.

63. Agur Z. Population dynamics in harshly varying environments; evolutionary, ecological and medical aspects. In Hallam TG, Gross LJ, Levin SA, Eds. *Mathematical Ecology*. River Edge, NJ: World Scientific; 1988, pp 440–454.

64. Agur Z. Resonance and anti-resonance in the design of chemotherapeutic protocols. *J Theor Biol* 1998;1:237–245.

65. Vainstein V, Ginosar Y, Shoham M, Ianovski A, Rabinovich A, Kogan Y, Selitser V, Ariad S, Chan S, Agur Z. Clinical validation of a physiologically-based computer model of human granulopoiesis and its use for improving cancer therapy by doxorubicin and granulocyte colony-stimulating factor (G-CSF). *Annual Meeting American Society of Hematology (ASH), Orlando, FL*, 2006.

37

REGULATORY REQUIREMENTS FOR INDs/FIH (FIRST IN HUMAN) STUDIES

SHAYNE COX GAD

Gad Consulting Services, Cary, North Carolina

Contents

Preclinical Development Handbook: ADME and Biopharmaceutical Properties,
edited by Shayne Cox Gad
Copyright © 2008 John Wiley & Sons, Inc.

37.1   INTRODUCTION

The safety of pharmaceutical agents, medical devices, and food additives is the toxicology issue of the most obvious and longest-standing concern to the public. A common factor among the three is that any risk associated with a lack of safety of these agents is likely to affect a very broad part of the population, with those at risk having little or no option as to undertaking this risk. Modern drugs are essential for life in today's society, yet there is a consistent high level of concern about their safety.

This chapter examines the regulations that establish how the safety of human pharmaceutical products is evaluated and established in the United States and the other major international markets prior to initial trials in human beings harmonization requirements between countries has proceeded markedly over the last fifteen years [1].

37.2   OVERVIEW OF U.S. REGULATIONS

37.2.1   Regulations: General Considerations

The U.S. federal regulations that govern the testing, manufacture, and sale of pharmaceutical agents are covered in Chapter 1, Title 21 of the *Code of Federal Regulations* (21 CFR). These comprise nine 6 in. × 8 in. (printing on both sides of the pages) volumes that stack 8 in. high. This title also covers foods, veterinary products, and cosmetics. As these topics will be discussed elsewhere in this book, here we briefly review those parts of 21 CFR that are applicable to human health products and medicinal devices [2].

Of most interest to a toxicologist working in this arena would be Chapter 1, Subchapter A (parts 1–78), which cover general provisions, organization, and so on. The Good Laboratory Practices (GLPs) are codified in 21 CFR 58.

Table 37.1 is a checklist of required data to support the development of a drug (in the general case), as well as the expected time to conduct each study through to an audited draft report.

General regulations that apply to drugs are in Subchapter C (Parts 200–299). This covers topics such as labeling, advertising, commercial registration, manufacture, and distribution. Of most interest to a toxicologist would be a section on labeling (Part 201, Subparts A–G, which covers Sections 201.1 through 201.317 of the regulations) as much of the toxicological research on a human prescription drug goes toward supporting a label claim. For example, specific requirements on content and format of labeling for human prescription drugs are covered in Section 201.57. Directions for what should be included under the "Precautions" section of a label are listed in Section 201.57(f). This included Section 201.57(f)(6), which covers categorization of pregnancy risk, and the reliance upon animal reproduction studies in making these categorizations are made quite clear. For example, a drug is given a

TABLE 37.1 General Case Safety Evaluation Requirements [3][a]

Test Requirement (if Approval Sought as Pharmaceutical Ingredient)	Time[b]
Initial Clinical Trial/IND Requirements	
Regulatory Status as a Pharmaceutical Component	
1. Acute toxicity in rodents	6 weeks
2. Acute toxicity in nonrodents	6 weeks
3. Acute parenteral toxicity in rodents	6 weeks
4. Genotoxicity: mutagenicity (bacterial)	4 weeks
5. Genotoxicity: *in vitro* clastogenicity	6 weeks
6. Genotoxicity: *in vivo*	4 weeks
7. Safety pharmacology: CV-hERG[c]	4 weeks
8. Safety pharmacology: CV-Purkinje fiber[c]	4 weeks
9. Safety pharmacology: CV *in vivo*	6 weeks
10. Safety pharmacology: CNS (FOB/Irwin)	4 weeks
11. Safety pharmacology: respiratory—rodent	6 weeks
12. Pivotal/repeat dose in rodents	3–4 months
13. Pivotal/repeat dose in nonrodents	3–4 months
14. Pyrogenicity (if parenteral)	2 weeks
15. Local irritation: ocular	1 month
16. Local irritation: dermal	1 month
17. Immunotoxicity[c]	4 weeks
18. Pivotal/repeat dose in rodents[c]	9 months
19. Pivotal/repeat dose in nonrodents[c]	9 months
20. Reproductive/developmental[c]	6 months
21. Tumorigenicity/carcinogenicity[c]	30 months

[a]All studies described must be performed under GLP.
[b]From study start to draft report.
[c]Not required prior to investigational new drug/first-in-human (IND/FIH) studies but recommended.

Pregnancy Category B if "animal reproduction studies have failed to demonstrate a risk to the fetus." The point here is not to give the impression that the law is most concerned with pregnancy risk. Rather, we wish to emphasize that much basic toxicological information must be summarized on the drug label (or package insert). This section of the law is quite detailed as to what information is to be presented and the format of the presentation. Toxicologists working in the pharmaceutical arena should be familiar with this section of the CFR.

37.2.2 Regulations: Human Pharmaceuticals

The regulations specifically applicable to human drugs are covered in Subchapter D, Parts 300–399. The definition of a new drug is covered in Part 310(g): "A new drug substance means any substance that when used in the manufacture, processing or packaging of a drug causes that drug to be a new drug but does not include intermediates used in the synthesis of such substances."

The regulation then goes on to discuss "newness with regard to new formulations, indications, or in combinations." For toxicologists, the meat of the regulations can be found in Section 312 (INDA) and Section 314 (applications for approval to market a new drug or antibiotic drug or NDA). The major focus for a toxicologist working in the pharmaceutical industry is on preparing the correct toxicology "packages" to be included to "support" these two types of applications. (The exact nature of these packages is covered later.)

In a nutshell, the law requires solid scientific evidence of safety and efficacy before a new drug will be permitted in clinical trials or (later) on the market. The INDA (covered in 21CFR 310) is for permission to proceed with clinical trials on human subjects. Once clinical trials have been completed, the manufacturer or "sponsor" can then proceed to file an NDA (covered in 21 CFR 314) for permission to market the new drug.

As stated in Section 321.21: "A sponsor shall submit an IND if the sponsor intends to conduct a clinical investigation with a new drug . . . [and] shall not begin a clinical investigation until . . . an IND . . . is in effect." Similar procedures are in place in other major countries. In the United Kingdom, for example, a Clinical Trials Certificate (CTC) must be filed or a CTX (clinical trial exemption) obtained before clinical trials may proceed. Clinical trials are divided into three phases, as described in Section 312.21. Phase I trials are initial introductions into healthy volunteers primarily for the purposes of establishing tolerance (side effects), bioavailability, and metabolism. Phase II clinical trials are "controlled studies . . . to evaluate effectiveness of the drug for a particular indication or disease." The secondary objective is to determine common short-term side effects; hence, the subjects are closely monitored. Phase III studies are expanded clinical trials. It is during this phase that the definitive, large-scale, double-blind studies are performed.

The toxicologist's main responsibilities in the IND process are to design, conduct, and interpret appropriate toxicology studies (or "packages") to support the initial IND and then design the appropriate studies necessary to support each additional phase of investigation. Exactly what may constitute appropriate studies are covered elsewhere in this chapter. The toxicologist's second responsibility is to prepare the toxicology summaries for the (clinical) investigator's brochure (described in Section 312.23(a)(8)(ii)). This is an integrated summary of the toxicological effects of the drug in animals and *in vitro*. The U.S. Food and Drug Administration (FDA) has prepared numerous guidance documents covering the content and format of INDs. It is of interest that in the *Guidance for Industry* [4] an in-depth description of the expected contents of the Pharmacology and Toxicology sections was presented. The document contains the following self-explanatory passage: "Therefore, if final, fully quality-assured individual study reports are not available at the time of IND submission, an integrated summary report of toxicological findings based on the unaudited draft toxicologic reports of the completed animal studies may be submitted."

If unfinalized reports are used in an initial IND, the finalized report must be submitted within 120 days of the start of the clinical trial. The sponsor must also prepare a document identifying any differences between the preliminary and final reports, and the impact (if any) on interpretation.

Thus, while the submission of fully audited reports is preferable, the agency does allow for the use of incomplete reports.

Once an IND or CTC/X is opened, the toxicologists may have several additional responsibilities. First, to design, conduct, and report the additional tests necessary to support a new clinical protocol or an amendment to the current clinical protocol (Section 312.20). Second, to bring to the sponsor's attention any finding in an ongoing toxicology study in animals "suggesting a significant risk to human subjects, including any finding of mutagenicity, teratogenicity or carcinogenicity," as described

TABLE 37.2   Composition of Standard Investigational New Drug Application (INDA)[a]

1. IND cover sheets (form FDA-1571)
2. Table of contents
3. Introductory statement
4. General (clinical) investigation plan
5. (Clinical) investigators brochure
6. (Proposed) clinical protocol(s)
7. Chemistry, manufacturing, and control information
8. Pharmacology and toxicology information (includes metabolism and pharmacokinetic assessments done in animals)
9. Previous human experience with the investigational drug
10. Additional information
11. Other relevant information

[a]Complete and thorough reports on all pivotal toxicological studies must be provided with the application.

in 21 CFR 312.32. The sponsor has a legal obligation to report such findings within 10 working days. Third, to prepare a "list of the preclinical studies . . . completed or in progress during the past year" and a summary of the major preclinical findings. The sponsor is required (under Section 312.23) to file an Annual Report (within 60 days of the IND anniversary date) describing the progress of the investigation. INDs are never "approved" in the strict sense of the word. Once filed, an IND can be opened 30 days after submission, unless the FDA informs the sponsor otherwise. The structure of an IND is outlined in Table 37.2.

If the clinical trials conducted under an IND are successful in demonstrating safety and effectiveness (often established at a Pre-NDA meeting, described in 21 CFR 312.47(b)(2)), the sponsor can then submit an NDA. Unlike an IND, the NDA must be specifically approved by the FDA. The toxicologist's responsibility in the NDA/Marketing Authorization Application (MAA) process is to prepare an integrated summary of all the toxicology and/or safety studies performed and be in a position to present and review the toxicology findings to the FDA or its advisory bodies. The approval process can be exhausting, including many meetings, hearings, and appeals. The ground rules for all of these are described in Part A of the law. For example, all NDAs are reviewed by an "independent" (persons not connected with either the sponsor or the FDA) Scientific Advisory Panel, which will review the findings and make recommendations as to approval. MAAs must be reviewed by and reported on by an expert recognized by the cognizant regulatory authority. Final statutory approval in the United States lies with the Commissioner of the FDA. It is hoped that few additional studies will be requested during the NDA review and approval process. When an NDA is approved, the FDA will send the sponsor an approval letter and will issue a Summary Basis of Approval (SBA)(312.30), which is designed and intended to provide a public record on the FDA's reasoning for approving the NDA while not revealing any proprietary information. The SBA can be obtained through Freedom of Information and can provide insights into the precedents for which types of toxicology studies are used to support specific types of claims.

37.2.3 Regulations: Environmental Impact

Environmental Impact Statements, while once important only for animal drugs, must now accompany all MDAs. This assessment must also be included in the Drug Master File (DMF). The procedures, formats, and requirements are described in 21 CFR 2531. This requirement has grown in response to the National Environmental Policy Act, the heart of which required that federal agencies evaluate every major action that could affect the quality of the environment. In the INDs, this statement can be a relatively short section claiming that relatively small amounts will post little risk to the environment. The EEC has similar requirements for drug entities in Europe, although data requirements are more strenuous. With NDAs, this statement must be more substantial, detailing any manufacturing and/or distribution process that may result in release into the environment. Environmental fate (e.g., photohydrolysis) and toxicity (e.g., fish, daphnia, and algae) studies will be required. While not mammalian toxicology in the tradition of pharmaceutical testing, preparing an environmental impact statement will clearly require toxicological input. The FDA has published a technical bulletin covering the tests it may require [5].

37.2.4 Regulations: Antibiotics

The NDA law (safety and effectiveness) applies to all drugs, but antibiotic drugs were treated differently until the passage of FDAMA in 1997. Antibiotic drugs had been treated differently by the FDA since the development of penicillin revolutionized medicine during World War II. The laws applicable to antibiotic drugs were covered in 21 CFR 430 and 431. Antibiotics such as penicillin or doxorubicin are drugs derived (in whole or in part) from natural sources (such as molds or plants), which have cytotoxic or cytostatic properties. They were treated differently from other drugs as the applicable laws required a batch-to-batch certification process. Originally passed into law in 1945 specifically for penicillin, this certification process was expanded by the 1962 amendment (under Section 507 of the Food, Drug, and Cosmetic Act) to require certification of all antibiotic drugs, meaning that the FDA would assay each lot of antibiotic for purity, potency, and safety. The actual regulations were covered in 21 CFR Subchapter D, Parts 430–460 (over 600 pages), which describes the standards and methods used for certification for all approved antibiotics. Section 507 was repealed by FDAMA (Section 125). As a result of the repeal of Section 507, the FDA is no longer required to publish antibiotic monographs. In addition, the testing, filing, and reviewing of antibiotic applications are now handled under Section 505 of the Act like any other new therapeutic agent. The FDA has published a guidance document to which the reader is referred for more details [6, 7].

37.2.5 Regulations: Biologics

Biological products are covered in Subchapter F, Parts 600–680. As described in 21 CFR 600.3(h), "biological product means any virus, therapeutic serum, toxin, antitoxin or analogous product applicable to the prevention, treatment or cure of diseases or injuries of man." In other words, these are vaccines and other protein products derived from animal sources. Clearly, the toxicological concerns with such products are vastly different from those involved with low molecular weight synthetic molecules. There is little rational basis, for example, for conducting a one year, repeated dose toxicity study with a vaccine or a human blood product. The FDA definition for safety with regard to these products is found in 21 CFR 603.1(p): "Relative freedom from harmful effect to persons affected, directly or indirectly, by a product when prudently administered." Such safety consideration has more to do with purity, sterility, and adherence to good manufacturing standards than with the toxicity of the therapeutic molecule itself. The testing required to show safety is stated in the licensing procedures 21 CFR 601.25(d)(1): "Proof of safety shall consist of adequate test methods reasonably applicable to show the biological product is safe under the prescribed conditions." Once a license is granted, each batch or lot of biological product must be tested for safety, and the methods of doing so are written into the law. A general test for safety (i.e., required in addition to other safety tests) is prescribed using guinea pigs as described in Section 610.11. Additional tests are often applied to specific products. For example, 21 CFR 630.35 describes the safety tests required for measles vaccines, which includes tests in mice and *in vitro* assays with tissue culture. Many new therapeutic entities produced by biotechnology are seeking approval as biologics with the results being FDA approval of a Product License Application (PLA). Table 37.3 presents general guidance for the basis of deciding if an individual entity falls under the Center for Drug

TABLE 37.3   Product Class Review Responsibilities

Center for Drug Evaluation and Review

Natural products purified from plant or mineral sources
Products produced from solid tissue sources (excluding procoagulants, venoms, blood
  products, etc.)
Antibiotics, regardless of method of manufacture
Certain substances produced by fermentation
  Disaccharidase inhibitors
  HMG-CoA inhibitors
Synthetic chemicals
  Traditional chemical synthesis
  Synthesized mononuclear or polynuclear products including antisense chemicals
Hormone products

Center for Biologics Evaluation and Review

Vaccines, regardless of manufacturing method
In vivo diagnostic allergenic products
Human blood products
Protein, peptide, and/or carbohydrate products produced by cell culture (other than
  antibiotics and hormones)
Immunoglobulin products
Products containing intact cells or microorganisms
Proteins secreted into fluids by transgenic animals
Animal venoms
Synthetic allergens
Blood banking and infusion adjuncts

Evaluation and Research (CDER) or the Center for Biologic Evaluation and Research (CBER) authority for review.

The International Conference on Harmonization has published its document *S6 Preclincial Safety Evaluation of Biotechnology-Derived Pharmaceuticals*. The FDA (both the Center for Drug Evaluation and Research, and the Center for Biologics Evaluation and Research jointly) has published the document as a *Guidance for Industry* [8, 9].

A current list of regulatory documents available by email (including the most recent PTCs, or points to consider) can be found at DOC_LIST@A1.FDA.GOV.

37.2.6   Regulations Versus Law

A note of caution must be inserted here. The law (the document passed by Congress) and the regulations (the documents written by the regulatory authorities to enforce the laws) are separate documents. The sections in the law do not necessarily have numerical correspondence. For example, the regulations on the NDA process is described in 21 CFR 312, but the law describing the requirement for an NDA process is in Section 505 of the FDCA. Because the regulations rather than the laws themselves have a greater impact on toxicological practice, greater emphasis is placed on regulation in this chapter. For a complete review of FDA law, the reader is referred to the monograph by Food and Drug Law Institute [2].

Laws authorize the activities and responsibilities of the various federal agencies. All proposed laws before the U.S. Congress are referred to committees for review and approval.

37.3   ORGANIZATIONS REGULATING DRUGS IN THE UNITED STATES

The agency formally charged with overseeing the safety of drugs in the United States is the FDA. It is headed by a commissioner who reports to the Secretary of the Department of Health and Human Services (DHHS) and has a tremendous range of responsibilities. Drugs are overseen primarily by the CDER (although some therapeutic or health care entities are considered biologics and are overseen by the corresponding CBER). Figure 37.1 presents the organization of CDER. The organization of CBER is shown in Fig. 37.2.

Most of the regulatory interactions of toxicologists are with the two offices of Drug Evaluation, which have under them a set of groups focused on areas of therapeutic claim (cardiorenal, neuropharmacological, gastrointestinal and coagulation, oncology and pulmonary, metabolism and endocrine, antiinfective and antiviral). Within each of these are chemists, pharmacologists/toxicologists, statisticians, and clinicians. When an INDA is submitted to the offices of Drug Evaluation, it is assigned to one of the therapeutic groups based on its area of therapeutic claim. Generally, it will remain with that group throughout its regulatory approval "life." INDs, when allowed, grant investigators the ability to go forward into clinical (human) trials with their drug candidate in a predefined manner, advancing through various steps of evaluation in human (and in additional preclinical or animal studies)

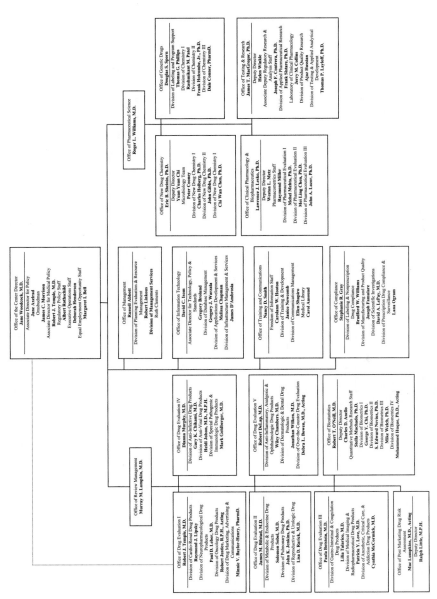

FIGURE 37.1 Organizational chart for CDER.

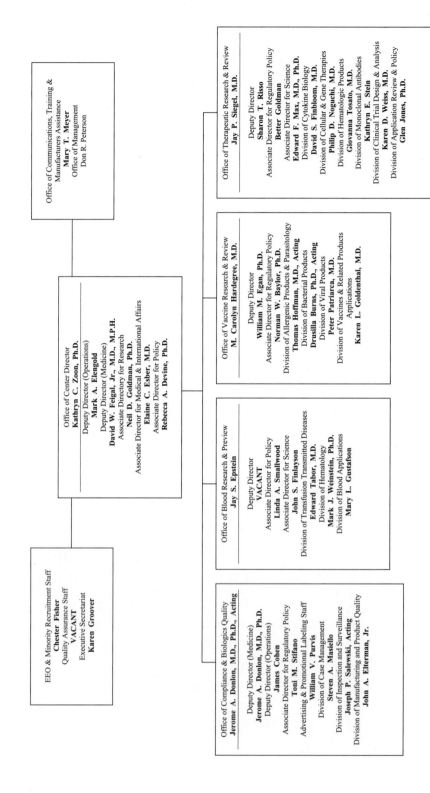

FIGURE 37.2 Organizational chart for CBER.

until an NDA can be supported, developed, and submitted. Likewise for biological products, the PLA or other applications (INDA, IND) are handled by the offices of Biological Products Review of the CBER.

For drugs, there is at least one nongovernmental body that must review and approve various aspects—the USP (United States Pharmacopeia, established in 1820)—which maintains (and revises) the compendia of the same name, as well as the National Formulary, which sets drug composition standards [10]. This volume sets forth standards for purity of products in which residues may be present and tests for determining various characteristics of drugs, devices, and biologics.

37.4   PROCESS OF PHARMACEUTICAL PRODUCT DEVELOPMENT AND APPROVAL

Except for a very few special cases (treatments for life-threatening diseases such as cancer or AIDS), the safety assessment of new drugs as mandated by regulations proceeds in a rather fixed manner. The IND is filed to support this clinical testing. An initial set of studies (typically, studies of appropriate length by the route intended for humans are performed in both a rodent (typically rat) and a nonrodent (usually a dog or a primate)) are required to support Phase I clinical testing. Such Phase I testing is intended to evaluate the safety ("tolerance" in clinical subjects), pharmacokinetics, and general biological effects of a new drug and is conducted in normal volunteers (almost always males).

Successful completion of Phase I testing allows, with the approval of the FDA, progression into Phase II clinical testing. Here, selected patients are enrolled to evaluate therapeutic efficacy, dose ranging, and more details about the pharmacokinetics and metabolism. Longer-term systemic toxicity studies must be in conformity with the guidelines that are presented in the next section. Once a sufficient understanding of the actions, therapeutic dose response, and potential risk-to-benefit ratio of the drug is in hand (once again, with FDA approval), trials move into Phase III testing.

Phase III tests are large, long, and expensive. They are conducted using large samples of selected patients and are intended to produce proof of safety and efficacy of the drug. Two studies providing statistically significant proof of the claimed therapeutic benefit must be provided. All the resulting data from preclinical and clinical animal studies are organized in a specified format in the form of an NDA, which is submitted to the FDA.

By the time that Phase III testing is completed, some additional preclinical safety tests must also generally be in hand. These include the three separate reproductive and developmental toxicity studies (Segments I and III in the rat, and Segment II in the rat and rabbit) and carcinogenicity studies in both rats and mice (unless the period of therapeutic usage is intended to be very short). Some assessment of genetic toxicity will also be expected.

The ultimate product of the pharmaceutical toxicologist will thus generally be the toxicology summaries of the IND and NDA (or PLA). For medical devices, the equivalents are the IDE and Product Development Notification (PDN). Data required to support each of these documents is specified in a series of guidelines, as discussed later.

Acceptance of these applications is contingent not only upon adherence to guidelines and good science, but also to GLPs.

37.5 TESTING GUIDELINES

37.5.1 Toxicity Testing: Traditional Pharmaceuticals

Although the 1938 Act required safety assessment studies, no consistent guidelines were available [11]. Guidelines were first proposed in 1949 and published in the *Food, Drug and Cosmetic Law Journal* that year [12]. Following several revisions, these guidelines were issued as *The Appraisal Handbook* in 1959. While never formally called a guideline, it set the standard for preclinical toxicity test design for several years. The current basic guidelines for testing required for safety assessment in support of the phases of clinical development of drugs were first outlined by Goldenthal [13, 14] and later incorporated into a 1971 FDA publication entitled *FDA Introduction to Total Drug Quality* [15].

37.5.2 General or Systematic Toxicity Assessment

Table 37.4 presents an overview of the current FDA toxicity testing guidelines for human drugs. Table 37.5 presents the parallel ICH guidelines [16], which are now largely supplanting the FDA guidelines. They are misleading in their apparent simplicity, however. First, each of the systemic toxicity studies in these guidelines must be designed and executed in a satisfactory manner. Sufficient animals must be used to have confidence in finding and characterizing any adverse drug actions that may be present. In practice, as the duration of the study increases, small doses are administered and larger numbers of animals must be employed per group. These two features—dosage level and group size—are critical to study designs. Table 37.6 presents general guidance on the number of animals to be used in systemic studies.

Note that for novel chemical structures, the FDA may still require 12 month nonrodent toxicity studies.

The protocols discussed thus far have focused on general or systemic toxicity assessment. The agency and, indeed, the lay public have a special set of concerns with reproductive toxicity, fetal/embryo toxicity, and developmental toxicity (also called *teratogenicity*). Collectively, these concerns often go by the acronyms *DART* (developmental and reproductive toxicity) or *RTF* (reproduction, teratogenicity, fertility). Segment II studies are more designed to detect developmental toxicity. Only pregnant females are dosed during the critical period of organogenesis. Generally, the first protocol DART test (exclusive of range-finding studies) is a Segment I study of rats in fertility and general reproductive performance. This is generally done while the drug is in Phase II clinical trials. Alternatively, many companies are now performing the Segment II teratology study in rats before the Segment I study because the former is less time and resource intensive. One or both should be completed before including women of child-bearing potential in clinical trials. The FDA requires teratogenicity testing in two species—a rodent (rat or mouse) and the rabbit. The use of the rabbit was instituted as a result of the finding that thalidomide was a positive teratogen in the rabbit but not in the rat. On occasion, when a test

TABLE 37.4 Synopsis of General Guidelines for Animal Toxicity Studies for Drugs

Category	Duration of Human Administration	Clinical Phase	Subacute or Chronic Toxicity	Special Studies
Oral or parenteral	Several days Up to 2 weeks	I, II, III, NDA IIIII, NDA	Two species; 2 weeks Two species; 4 weeksTwo species; up to 4 weeks Two species; up to 3 months	For parenterally administered drugs
	Up to 3 months	I, IIIIINDA	Two species; 4 weeksTwo species; 3 months Two species; up to 6 months	Compatibility with blood where applicable
	Six months to unlimited	I, IIIIINDA	Two species; 3 months Two species; 6 months or longer Two species; 9 months (nonrodent) and 6 months (rodent) +Two rodent species for CA; 18 months (mouse) May be replaced with an allowable transgenic mouse study; 24 months (rat)	
Inhalation (general anesthetics)		I, II, III, NDA	Four species; 5 days (3h/day)	
Dermal	Single application	I	One species; single 24 hour exposure followed by 2 week observation	Sensitization
	Single or short-term application	II	One species; 20 day repeated exposure (intact and abraded skin)	
	Short-term application	III	As above	
	Unlimited application	NDA	As above, but intact skin study extended up to 6 months	
Ophthalmic	Single application	I		Eye irritation tests with graded doses
	Multiple applications	I, II, IIINDA	One species; 3 weeks daily applications, as in clinical use One species; duration commensurate with period of drug administration	
Vaginal or rectal	Single application Multiple applications	II, II, III, NDA	Two species; duration and number of applications determined by proposed use	Local and systematic toxicity after vaginal or rectal application in two species
Drug combinations	(4)	III, III, NDA	Two species; up to 3 months	Lethality by appropriate route, compared to components run concurrently in one species

1279

TABLE 37.5 Duration of Repeated Dose Toxicity Studies to Support Clinical Trials and Marketing[a]

Duration of Clinical Trials	Minimum Duration of Repeated Dose Toxicity Studies[b]		Duration of Clinical Trials	Minimum Duration of Repeated Dose Toxicity Studies[c]	
	Rodents	Nonrodents		Rodents	Nonrodents
Single dose	2 weeks[d]	2 weeks	Up to 2 weeks	1 month	1 month
Up to 2 weeks	2 weeks[d]	2 weeks	Up to 1 month	3 months	3 months
Up to 1 month	1 month	1 month	Up to 3 months	6 months	3 months
Up to 6 months	6 months	6 months[b]	>3 months	6 months	Chronic[d]
>6 months	6 months	Chronic[b]			

[a]In Japan, if there are no Phase II clinical trials of equivalent duration to the planned Phase III trials, conduct of longer duration toxicity studies is recommended. [b]Data from 6 months of administration in nonrodents should be available before the initiation of clinical trials longer than 3 months. Alternatively, if applicable, data from a 9 month nonrodent study should be available before the treatment duration exceeds that which is supported by the available toxicity studies.

[c]The table also reflects the marketing recommendations in the three regions except that a chronic nonrodent study is recommended for clinical use >1 month.

[d]In the United States, as an alternative to 2 week studies, single-dose toxicity studies with extended examinations can support single-dose human trials.

TABLE 37.6 Numbers of Animals per Dosage Group in Systemic Toxicity Studies

Study Duration (per sex)	Rodents (per sex)	Nonrodents
2–4 weeks	5	3
13 weeks	20[a]	6
26 weeks	30	8
Chronic	50	10
Carcinogenicity	60[b]	Applies only to contraceptives
Bioassays		Applies only to contraceptives

[a]Starting with 13 week studies, one should consider adding animals (particularly to the high dose) to allow evaluation of reversal of effects.

[b]In recent years there have been decreasing levels of survival in rats on 2 year studies. What is required is that at least 20–25 animals/sex/group survive at the end of the study. Accordingly, practice is beginning to use 70 or 75 animals per sex, per group.

article is not compatible with the rabbit, teratogenicity data in the mouse may be substituted. There are also some specific classes of therapeutics (e.g., the quinalone antibioticsexample) where Segment II studies in primates are effectively required prior to product approval. Both should be completed before entering Phase III clinical trials. The most complicated of the DART protocols—Segment III—is generally commenced during Phase III trials and should be part of the NDA. There are differences in the different national guidelines (as discussed later with international considerations) regarding the conduct of these studies. The large multinational drug companies try to design their protocols to be in compliance with as many of the guidelines as possible to avoid duplication of testing while allowing the broadest possible approval and marketing of therapeutics.

37.5.3 Genetic Toxicity Assessment

Genetic toxicity testing generally focuses on the potential of a new drug to cause mutations (in single-cell systems) or other forms of genetic damage. The tests, generally short in duration, often rely on *in vitro* systems and generally have a single endpoint of effect (point mutations, chromosomal damage, etc.). It is of interest that the FDA has no standard or statutory requirement for genetic toxicity testing but generally expects to see at least some such tests performed and will ask for them if the issue is not addressed. If one performs such a study, any data collected, of course, must be sent to the FDA as part of any INDA, PLA, or NDA. These studies have yet to gain favor with the FDA (or other national regulatory agencies) as substitutes for *in vivo* carcinogenicity testing. However, even with completed negative carcinogenicity tests, at least some genetic toxicity assays are generally required. Generally, pharmaceuticals in the United States are evaluated for mutagenic potential (e.g., the Ames' Assay) or for chromosomal damage (e.g., the *In Vivo* Mouse Micronucleus Test). In general, in the United States, pharmaceutical companies apply genetic toxicity testing in the following fashion:

- *As a Screen.* An agent that is positive in one or more genetic toxicity tests may be more likely than one that is negative to be carcinogenic and therefore may not warrant further development.
- *As an Adjunct.* An agent that is negative in carcinogenicity testing in two species and also negative in a genetic toxicity battery is more likely than not to be noncarcinogenic in human beings.
- *To Provide Mechanistic Insight.* For example, if an agent is negative in a wide range of genetic toxicity screens but still produces tumors in animals, then one could hypothesize that an epigenetic mechanism was involved.

While not officially required, the FDA does have the authority to request, on a case-by-case basis, specific tests it feels may be necessary to address a point of concern. A genetic toxicity test could be part of such a request. In general, therefore, companies deal with genetic toxicity (after "screening") on a case-by-case basis, dictated by good science. If more than a single administration is intended, common practice is to perform the tests prior to submitting an IND.

37.5.4 Toxicity Testing: Biotechnology Products

As mentioned, the regulation of traditional pharmaceuticals (small molecules such as aspirin or digitalis) and biologicals (proteins such as vaccines and antitoxins derived from animal sources) have very different histories. See Section 37.2.5. Until 1972, the NIH (or its forerunning agency, the Hygienic Laboratory of the Department of the Treasury) was charged with the responsibilities of administering the Virus Act of 1902. With the passage of the Food and Drug Laws of 1906, 1938, and 1962, there was recurring debate about whether these laws applied or should apply to biologicals. This debate was resolved when the authority for the regulation of biologics was transferred to the FDA's new Bureau of Biologics (now the CBER) in 1972. Since then, there appears to have been little difference in the matter of regulation for biologics and pharmaceuticals. The FDA essentially regulates biologics as described under the 1902 act, but then uses the rule-making authority granted under the Food and Drug Act to "fill in the gaps."

The Bureau of Biologics was once a relatively "sleepy" agency, primarily concerned with the regulation of human blood products and vaccines used for mass immunization programs. The authors of the 1902 law could hardly have foreseen the explosion in biotechnology that occurred in the 1980s. New technology created a welter of new biological products, such as recombinant-DNA-produced proteins (e.g., tissue plasminogen activator), biological response modifiers (cytokinins and colony-stimulating factors), monoclonal antibodies, antisense oligonucleotides, and self-directed vaccines (raising an immune response to self-proteins such as gastrin for therapeutic reasons). The new products raised a variety of new questions on the appropriateness of traditional methods of evaluating drug toxicity that generated several points-to-consider documents [17–19]. For the sake of brevity, this discussion focuses on the recombinant DNA proteins. Some safety issues have been raised over the years [20]:

- The appropriateness of testing a human-specific peptide hormone in nonhuman species.
- The potential that the peptide could break down due to nonspecific metabolism, resulting in products that had no therapeutic value or even a toxic fragment.
- The potential sequelae to an immune response (formation of neutralizing antibodies, provoking an autoimmune or a hypersensitivity response), and pathology due to immune precipitation and so on.
- The presence of contamination with oncogenic virus DNA (depending on whether a bacterial or mammalian system was used on the synthesizing agent) or endotoxins.
- The difficulty interpreting the scientific relevance of response to supraphysiological systemic doses of potent biological response modifiers.

The intervening last few years have shown that some of these concerns were more relevant than others [21]. The "toxic peptide fragment" concern, for example, has been shown to be without merit. The presence of potentially oncogenic virus DNA and endotoxins is a quality assurance concern and is not truly a toxicological problem. Regardless of the type of synthetic pathway, all proteins must be synthesized in compliance with Good Manufacturing Practices. Products must be as pure as possible, not only free of rDNA but also free of other types of cell debris (endotoxin). Batch-to-batch consistency with regard to molecular structure must also be demonstrated using appropriate methods (e.g., amino acid). The regulatory thinking and experience over the last fifteen years has come together in the document *S6 Preclincial Safety Evaluation of Biotechnology-Derived Pharmaceuticals* prepared by the International Conference on Harmonization. The FDA (both the Center for Drug Evaluation and Research, and the Center for Biologics Evaluation and Research jointly) has published the document as a *Guidance for Industry* [5, 6]. The document intended to provide basic guidance for the preclinical evaluation of biotechnology-derived products, including proteins and peptides, produced by cell culture using rDNA technology, but did not cover antibiotics, allergenic extracts, heparin, vitamins, cellular drug products, vaccines, or other products regulated as biologics. Items covered are summarized as follows [22]:

Test Article Specifications. In general, the product that is used in the definitive pharmacology and toxicology studies should be comparable to the product proposed for the initial clinical studies.

Animal Species/Model Selection. Safety evaluation should include the use of relevant species, in which the test article is pharmacologically active due, for example, to the expression of the appropriate receptor molecule. These can be screened with *in vitro* receptor binding assays. Safety evaluation should normally include two appropriate species, if possible and/or feasible. The potential utility of gene knockout and/or transgenic animals in safety assessment is discussed.

Group Size. No specific numbers are given, but it does state that a small sample size may lead to failure to observe toxic events.

Administration. The route and frequency should be as close as possible to that proposed for clinical use. Other routes can be used when scientifically warranted.

Immunogenicity. It has also been clearly demonstrated in the testing of rDNA protein products that animals will develop antibodies to foreign proteins. This response has been shown to neutralize (rapidly remove from circulation) the protein, but no pathological conditions have been shown to occur as a sequelae to the immune response. Bear in mind, however, that interleukins have powerful effects on immune response, but these are due to their physiological activity and not to an antigen–antibody response. The first has to do with "neutralizing antibodies." That is, is the immune response so great that the test article is being removed from circulation as fast as it is being added? If this is the case, does long-term testing of such a chemical make sense? In many cases, it does not. The safety testing of any large molecule should include the appropriate assays for determining whether the test system has developed a neutralizing antibody response. Depending on the species, route of administration, intended therapeutic use, and development of neutralizing antibodies (which generally takes about 2 weeks), it is rare for a toxicity test on an rDNA protein to be longer than 4 weeks duration. However, if the course of therapy in humans is to be longer than 2 weeks, formation of neutralizing antibodies must be demonstrated or longer-term testing performed. The second antigen–antibody formation concern is that a hypersensitivity response will be elicited. Traditional preclinical safety assays are generally adequate to guard against this if they are 2 weeks or longer in duration and the relevant endpoints are evaluated.

Safety Pharmacology. It is important to investigate the potential for unwanted pharmacological activity in appropriate animal models and to incorporate monitoring for these activities in the toxicity studies.

Exposure Assessment. Single- and multiple-dose pharmacokinetics, toxicokinetics, and tissue distribution studies in relevant species are useful. Proteins are not given orally; demonstrating absorption and mass balance is not typically a primary consideration. Rather, this segment of the test should be designed to determine half-life (and other appropriate pharmacokinetic descriptor parameters), the plasma concentration associated with biological effects, and potential changes due to the development of neutralizing antibodies.

Reproductive Performance and Developmental Toxicity Studies. These will be dictated by the product, clinical indication, and intended patient population.

Genotoxicity Studies. The S6 document states that the battery of genotoxicity studies routinely conducted for traditional pharmaceuticals are not appropriate for biotechnology-derived pharmaceuticals. In contrast to small molecules, genotoxicity testing with a battery of *in vitro* and *in vivo* techniques of protein molecules has not become common U.S. industry practice. Such tests are not formally required by the FDA but, if performed, have to be reported. They are required by European and Japanese regulatory authorities. This has sparked a debate as to whether or not genotoxicity testing is necessary or appropriate for rDNA protein molecules. It is the author's opinion that such testing is, scientifically, of little value. First, large protein molecules will not easily penetrate the cell wall of bacteria or yeast, and (depending on size, charge, lipophilicity, etc.) penetration across the plasma lemma of mammalian cells will be highly variable. Second, if one considers the well-established mechanism(s) of genotoxicity of small molecules, it is difficult to conceive of how a protein can act in the same fashion. For example, proteins will not be metabolized to be electrophilic active intermediates that will crosslink guanine residues. In general, therefore, genotoxicity testing with rDNA proteins is a waste of resources. It is conceivable, however, that some proteins, because of their biological mechanism of action, may stimulate the proliferation of transformed cells. For example, it is a feasible hypothesis that a colony-stimulating factor could stimulate the proliferation of leukemic cells (it should be emphasized that this is a hypothetical situation, presented here for illustrative purposes). Again, this is a question of a specific pharmacological property, and such considerations should be tested on a case-by-case basis.

Carcinogenicity Studies. These are generally inappropriate for biotechnology-derived pharmaceuticals; however, some products may have the potential to support or induce proliferation of transformed cells ... possibly leading to neoplasia. When this concern is present, further studies in relevant animal models may be needed.

These items are covered in greater detail in the S6 guidance document and in a review by Ryffel [23].

So, given the above discussion, what should the toxicology testing package of a typical rDNA protein resemble? Based on the products that have successfully wound their way through the regulatory process, the following generalizations can be drawn.

- The safety tests look remarkably similar to those for traditional tests. Most have been done on three species: the rat, the dog, or the monkey. The big difference has to do with the length of the test. It is rare for a safety test on a protein to be more than 13 weeks long.

- The dosing regimens can be quite variable and at times very technique intensive. These chemicals are almost always administered by a parenteral route—normally intravenously or subcutaneously. Dosing regimens have run the range from once every 2 weeks for an antihormone "vaccine" to continuous infusion for a short-lived protein.

- As reviewed by Ryffel [24], most side effects in humans of a rDNA therapy may be predicted by data from experimental toxicology studies, but there are exceptions. IL-6, for example, induced a sustained increase in blood platelets and acute phase proteins, with no increase in body temperature. In human trials, however, there were increases in temperature.

- The S6 document also mentions monoclonal antibody products. Indeed, many of the considerations for rDNA products are also applicable to monoclonal antibodies (including hybridized antibodies). With monoclonal antibodies, there is the additional concern of crossreactivity with nontarget molecules.

As mentioned, the rapid development in the biotechnology industry has created some confusion as to what arm of the FDA is responsible for such products. In October 1992, the two major reviewing groups, CBER and CDER, reached a series of agreements to explain and organize the FDA's position on products that did not easily fall into its traditional classification schemes. CDER will continue to have responsibility for traditional chemically synthesized molecules as well as those purified from mineral or plant sources (except allergenics), antibiotics, hormones (including insulin and growth hormone), most fungal or bacterial products (disaccharidase inhibitors), and most products from animal or solid human tissue sources. CBER will have responsibility for products subject to licensure (BLA), including all vaccines, human blood or blood-derived products (as well as drugs used for blood banking and transfusion), immunoglobulin products, products containing intact cells, fungi, viruses, proteins produced by cell culture or transgenic animals, and synthetic allergenic products. This situation was further simplified by the introduction of the concept of *well-characterized biologics*. When introduced during the debate on FDA reform in 1996, the proposed section of S-1447 stated that "biological products that the secretary determines to be well-characterized shall be regulated solely under the Federal Food, Drug and Cosmetic Act." Under this concept, highly purified, well-characterized therapeutic rDNA proteins would be regulated by CDER, regardless of therapeutic target [25].

37.5.5 Toxicity/Safety Testing: Cellular and Gene Therapy Products

Human clinical trials of cellular and gene therapies involve administration to patients of materials considered investigational biological, drug, or device products. Somatic cell therapy refers to the administration to humans of autologous, allogenic, or xenogenic cells, which have been manipulated or processed *ex vivo*. Gene therapy refers to the introduction into the human body of genes or cells containing genes foreign to the body for the purposes of prevention, treatment, diagnosing, or curing disease.

Sponsors of cellular or gene therapy clinical trials must file an Investigational New Drug Application (INDA) or in certain cases an Investigational Device Exemption (IDE) with the FDA before initiation of studies in humans. It is the responsibility of the Center of Biologics Evaluation and Research (CBER) to review the application and determine if the submitted data and the investigational product meet applicable standards. The critical parameters of identity, purity, potency, stability, consistency, safety, and efficacy relevant to biological products are also relevant to cellular and gene therapy products.

In 1991, the FDA first published *Points to Consider* in *Human Somatic Cell and Gene Therapy* [18]. At this time virtually all gene therapies were retroviral and were prepared as *ex vivo* somatic cell therapies. This was subsequently reviewed by Kessler et al. [26]. While the data for certain categories of information such as the data regarding the molecular biology were defined in previous guidance documents relating to recombinant DNA products, the standards for preclinical and clinical development were less well defined. Over the past five years, the field has advanced to include not only new vectors but also novel routes of administration. The *Points to Consider in Human Somatic Cell Therapy and Gene Therapy* [27] has thus been recently amended to reflect both the advancements in product development and more importantly the accumulation of safety information over the past five years.

FDA regulations state that the sponsor must submit, in the IND, adequate information about pharmacological and toxicological studies of the drug including laboratory animals or *in vitro* studies on the basis of which the sponsor has considered that it is reasonably safe to conduct the proposed clinical investigation. For cellular and gene therapies, designing and conducting relevant preclinical safety testing has been a challenge to both the FDA and the sponsor. For genes delivered using viral vectors, the safety of the vector system per se must be considered and evaluated.

The preclinical knowledge base is initially developed by designing studies to answer fundamental questions. The development of this knowledge base is generally applicable to most pharmaceuticals, as well as biopharmaceuticals, and includes data to support (1) the relationship of the dose to the biological activity, (2) the relationship of the dose to the toxicity, (3) the effect of route and/or schedule on activity or toxicity, and (4) identification of the potential risks for subsequent clinical studies. These questions are considered in the context of indication and/or disease state. In addition, there are often unique concerns relative to the specific category or product class.

For cellular therapies, safety concerns may include development of a database from studies specifically designed to answer questions relating to growth factor dependence, tumorigenicity, local and systemic toxicity, and effects on host immune responses including immune activation and altered susceptibility to disease. For viral-mediated gene therapies, specific questions may relate to the potential for overexpression of the transduced gene, transduction of normal cells/tissues, genetic transfer to germ cells and subsequent alterations to the genome, recombination/rescue with endogenous virus, reconstitutions of replication competence, potential for insertional mutagenesis/malignant transformation, altered susceptibility to disease, and/or potential risk(s) to the environment.

To date, cellular and gene therapy products submitted to the FDA have included clinical studies indicated for bone marrow marking, cancer, cystic fibrosis, AIDS, and inborn errors of metabolism and infectious diseases. Of the current active INDs, approximately 78% have been sponsored by individual investigators or academic institutions and 22% have also been industry sponsored. In addition to the variety of clinical indications the cell types have also been varied. Examples include tumor infiltrating lymphocytes (TILs) and lymphocyte activated killer (LAK) cells, selected cells from bone marrow, and peripheral blood lymphocytes (e.g., stem cells, myoblasts, tumor cells), and encapsulated cells (e.g., islet cells and adrenal chromaffin cells).

Cellular Therapies   Since 1984 the CBER has reviewed close to 300 somatic cell therapy protocols. Examples of the specific categories include manipulation, selection, mobilization, tumor vaccines, and other.

Manipulation—autologous, allogenic, or xenogenic cells that have been expanded, propagated, manipulated, or had their biological characteristics altered *ex vivo* (e.g., TIL or LAK cells; islet cells housed in a membrane).

Selection—products designed for positive or negative selection if autologous or allogenic cells are intended for therapy (e.g., purging of tumor from bone marrow, selection of CD34+ cells).

Mobilization—*in vivo* mobilization of autologous stem cells intended for transplantation.

Tumor vaccines—autologous or allogenic tumor cells that are administered as vaccine (e.g., tumor cell lines, tumor cell lysates, primary explant). This group also includes autologous antigen presenting cells pulsed with tumor-specific peptides or tumor cell lysates.

Other—autologous, allogenic, and xenogenic cells that do not specifically fit the above; this group includes cellular therapies such as extracorporeal liver assist devices.

Gene Therapies   The types of vectors that have been used, or proposed, for gene transduction include retrovirus, adenovirus, adeno-associated viruses, other viruses (e.g., herpes, vaccinia), and plasmid DNA. Methods for gene introduction include *ex vivo* replacement, drug delivery, and marker studies and others and *in vivo*, viral vectors, plasmid vectors, and vector producer cells.

Ex Vivo

Replacement—cells transduced with a vector expressing a normal gene in order to correct or replace the function of a defective gene.

Drug delivery—cells transduced with a vector expressing a gene encoding a therapeutic molecule that can be novel or native to the host.

Marker studies—cells (e.g., bone marrow, stem cells) transduced with a vector expressing a marker or reporter gene used to distinguish it from other similar host tissues.

Other—products that do not specifically fit the above (e.g., tumor vaccines in which cells are cultured or transduced *ex vivo* with a vector).

In Vivo

Viral vectors—the direct administration of a viral vector (e.g., retrovirus, adeno-virus, adeno-associated virus, herpes, vaccinia) to patients.

Plasmid vectors—the direct administration of plasmid vectors with or without other vehicles (e.g., lipids) to patients.

Vector producer cells—the direct administration of retroviral vector producer cells (e.g., murine cells producing HTK vector) to patients.

Preclinical Safety Evaluation   The goal of preclinical safety evaluation includes the recommendation of an initial safe starting dose and safe dose-escalation scheme in humans, identification of potential target organ(s) of toxicity, identification of appropriate parameters for clinical monitoring, and identification of "at risk" patient population(s). Therefore, when feasible, toxicity studies should be performed in relevant species to assess a dose-limiting toxicity. General considerations in study design include selection of the model (e.g., species, alternative model, animal model, or disease), dose (e.g., route, frequency, and duration), and study endpoint (e.g., activity and/or toxicity).

The approach to preclinical safety evaluation of biotechnology-derived products, including novel cellular and gene therapies, has been referred to as the *case-by case* approach. This approach is science-based, data-driven, and flexible. The major distinction from past practices from traditional pharmaceuticals is that the focus is directed at asking specific questions across various product categories. Additionally, there is a consistent reevaluation of the knowledge base to reassess real or theoretical safety concerns and hence reevaluation of the need to answer the same questions across all product categories. In some cases there may even be conditions that may not need specific toxicity studies: for example, when there is a strong efficacy model that is rationally designed to answer specific questions and/or there is previous human experience with a similar product with respect to dose and regimen.

Basic Principles for Preclinical Safety Evaluation of Cellular and Gene Therapies (Biotechnology-Derived Products in General)

- Use of product in animal studies that is comparable or the same as the product proposed for clinical trial(s).
- Adherence to basic principles of GLP to ensure quality of the study including a detailed protocol prepared prospectively.
- Use of the same or similar route and method of administration as proposed for clinical trials (whenever possible).
- Determination of appropriate doses delivered based on preliminary activity obtained from both *in vitro* and *in vivo* studies (i.e., finding a dose likely to be effective and not dangerous, a no observed adverse effect level, and a dose-causing dose-limiting toxicity).

- Selection of one or more species sensitive to the endpoint being measured (e.g., infections or pathologic sequelae) and/or biological activity or receptor binding.
- Consideration of animal model(s) of disease as better to assess the contribution of changes in physiologic or underlying physiology to safety and efficacy.
- Determination of effect on host immune response.
- Localization/distribution studies—evaluation of target tissue, normal surrounding tissue, and distal tissue sites and any alteration in normal or expected distribution, and local reactogenicity.

Additional Considerations for Cellular Therapies

- Evaluation of cytopathogenicity.
- Evaluation of signs of cell transformation/growth factor dependence—effect on animal cells, normal human cells, and cells prone to transform easily.
- Determination of alteration in cell phenotype, altered cell products, and/or function.
- Tumorigenicity.

Additional Considerations for Gene Therapies

- Determination of phenotype/activation state of effector cells.
- Determination of vector/transgene toxicity.
- Determination of potential transfer to germ line.
- *In vitro* challenge studies—evaluation of recombination or complementation, potential for "rescue" for subsequent infection with wild-type virus.
- Determination of persistence of cells/vector.
- Determination of potential for insertional mutagenesis (malignant transformation).
- Determination of environmental spread (e.g., viral shedding).

37.6 TOXICITY TESTING: SPECIAL CASES

On paper, the general case guidelines for the evaluation of the safety of drugs are relatively straightforward and well understood. However, there are also a number of special case situations under which either special rules apply or some additional requirements are relevant. The more common of these are summarized next.

37.6.1 Oral Contraceptives

Oral contraceptives are subject to special testing requirements. These have recently been modified so that in addition to those preclinical safety tests generally required, the following are also required [28]:

- A 3 year carcinogenicity study in beagles (this is a 1987 modification in practice from earlier FDA requirements and the 1974 publication).
- A rat reproductive (Segment I) study including a demonstration of return to fertility.

37.6.2   Life-Threatening Diseases (Compassionate Use)

Drugs to treat life-threatening diseases are not strictly held to the sequence of testing requirements because the potential benefit on any effective therapy in these situations is so high [29]. In the early 1990s, this situation applied to AIDS-associated diseases and cancer. The development of more effective HIV therapies (protease inhibitors) has now made cancer therapy more the focus of these considerations. Although the requirements for safety testing prior to initial human trials is unchanged, subsequent requirements are flexible and subject to negotiation and close consultation with the FDA's Division of Oncology (within CDER) [29, 30]. The more recent thinking on anticancer agents has been reviewed by DeGeorge et al. [31]. The preclinical studies that will be required to support clinical trials and marketing of new anticancer agents will depend on the mechanism of action and the target clinical population. Toxicity studies in animals will be required to support initial clinical trials. These studies have multiple goals: (1) determine a starting dose for clinical trials, (2) identify target organ toxicity and assess recovery, and (3) assist in the design of clinical dosing regimens.

The studies should generally confirm to the protocols recommended by the National Cancer Institute, as discussed by Greishaber [32]. In general, it can be assumed that most antineoplastic cytotoxic agents will be highly toxic. Two studies are essential to support initial clinical trials (IND phase) in patients with advanced disease. These are studies of 5–14 days in length, but with longer recovery periods. A study in rodents is required that identifies those doses that produce either life-threatening or non-life-threatening toxicity. Using the information from this first study, a second study in nonrodents (generally the dog) is conducted to determine if the tolerable dose in rodents produces life-threatening toxicity. Doses are compared on a mg/m^2 basis. The starting dose in initial clinical trails is generally one-tenth of that required to produce severe toxicity in rodents (STD10) or one-tenth the highest dose in nonrodents that does not cause severe irreversible toxicity. While not required, information on pharmacokinetic parameters, especially data comparing the plasma concentration associated with toxicity in both species, is very highly regarded. Special attention is paid to organs with high cell-division rates—bone marrow, testes, lymphoid tissue, and GI tract. As these agents are almost always given intravenously, special attention needs to be given relatively early in development to intravenous irritation and blood compatibility study. Subsequent studies to support the New Drug Application will be highly tailored, depending on the following:

- Therapeutic indication and mechanism of action.
- The results of the initial clinical trials.
- The nature of the toxicity.
- Proposed clinical regimen.

Even at the NDA stage, toxicity studies with more than 28 days of dosing are rarely required. While not required for the IND, assessment of genotoxicity and developmental toxicity will need to be addressed. For genotoxicity, it will be important to establish the ratio between cytotoxicity and mutagenicity. *In vivo* models (e.g., the mouse micronucleus test) can be particularly important in demonstrating the lack of genotoxicity at otherwise subtoxic doses. For developmental toxicity, ICH stage C–D studies (traditionally known as Segment II studies for teratogenicity in rat and rabbits) will also be necessary.

The emphasis of this discussion has been on purely cytotoxic neoplastic agents. Additional considerations must be given to cytotoxic agents that are administered under special circumstances: those that are photoactivated, delivered as liposomal emulsions, or delivered as antibody conjugates. These types of agents will require additional studies. For example, a liposomal agent will need to be compared to the free agent and a blank liposomal preparation. There are also studies that may be required for a particular class of agents. For example, anthracyclines are known to be cardiotoxic, so comparison of a new anthracycline agent to previously marketed anthracyclines will be expected.

In addition to antineoplastic, cytotoxic agents, there are cancer therapeutic or preventative drugs that are intended to be given on a chronic basis. This includes chemopreventatives, hormonal agents, and immunomodulators. The toxicity assessment studies on these will more closely resemble those of more traditional pharmaceutical agents. Chronic toxicity, carcinogenicity, and full developmental toxicity (ICH A–B, C–D, E–F) assessments will be required. For a more complete review, the reader is referred to DeGeorge et al. [31].

37.6.3 Optical Isomers

The FDA (and other regulatory agencies, as reviewed by Daniels et al. [33]) has become increasingly concerned with the safety of stereoisomeric or chiral drugs. Stereoisomers are molecules that are identical to one another in terms of atomic formula and covalent bonding, but differ in the three-dimensional projections of the atoms. Within this class are those molecules that are nonsuperimposable mirror images of one another. These are called enantiomers (normally designated as *R*- or *S*-). Enantiometric pairs of a molecule have identical physical and chemical characteristics except for the rotation of polarized light. Drugs have generally been mixtures of optical isomers (enantiomers), because of the difficulties in separating the isomers. It has become apparent in recent years, however, that these different isomers may have different degrees of both desirable therapeutic and undesirable toxicologic effects. Technology has also improved, to the extent that it is now possible to perform chiral-specific syntheses, separations, and/or analyses. It is now highly desirable from a regulatory [29, 30, 34, 35] basis to develop a single isomer unless all isomers have equivalent pharmacological and toxicologic activity. The FDA has divided enantiometric mixtures into the following categories:

- Both isomers have similar pharmacologic activity, which could be identical, or they could differ in the degree of efficacy.
- One isomer is pharmacologically active, while the other is inactive.
- Each isomer has completely different activity.

During preclinical assessment of an enantiometric mixture, it may be important to determine to which of these three classes it belongs. The pharmacological and toxicological properties of the individual isomers should be characterized. The pharmacokinetic profile of each isomer should be characterized in animal models with regard to disposition and interconversion. It is not at all unusual for each enantiomer to have a completely different pharmacokinetic behavior.

If the test article is an enantiomer isolated from a mixture that is already well characterized (e.g., already on the market), then appropriate bridging guides need to be performed which compare the toxicity of the isomer to that of the racemic mixture. The most common approach would be to conduct a subchronic (3 month) and a Sement II type teratology study with an appropriate "positive" control group that received the racemate. In most instances, no additional studies would be required if the enantiomer and the racemate did not differ in toxicity profile. If, on the other hand, differences are identified, then the reasons for this difference need to be investigated and the potential implications for human subjects need to be considered.

37.6.4 Special Populations: Pediatric and Geriatric Claims

Relatively few drugs marketed in the United States (approximately 20%) have pediatric dosing information available. Clinical trials had rarely been done specifically on pediatric patients. Traditionally, dosing regimens for children have been derived empirically by extrapolating on the basis of body weight or surface area. This approach assumes that the pediatric patient is a young adult, which simply may not be the case. There are many examples of how adults and children differ qualitatively in metabolic and/or pharmacodynamic responses to pharmaceutical agents. In their review, Schacter and DeSantis [36] state that "the benefit of having appropriate usage information in the product label is that health care practitioners are given the information necessary to administer drugs and biologics in a manner that maximizes safety, minimizes unexpected adverse events, and optimizes treatment efficacy. Without specific knowledge of potential drug effects, children may be placed at risk. In addition, [in] the absence of appropriate proscribing information, drugs and biologics that represent new therapeutic advances may not be administered to the pediatric population in a timely manner." In response to the need for pediatric information, the FDA had developed a pediatric plan. This two-phase plan called first for the development of pediatric information on marketed drugs. The second phase focused on new drugs. The implementation of the plan was to be coordinated by the Pediatric Subcommittee of the Medical Policy Coordinating Committee of CDER. The Pediatric Use Labeling Rule was a direct result of phase 1 in 1994 [7]. Phase 2 resulted in 1997 from a proposed rule entitled *Pediatric Patients: Regulations Requiring Manufacturers to Assess the Safety and Effectiveness of New Drugs and Biologics*. Soon after this rule was proposed, the FDA Modernization Act of 1997 was passed. FDAMA contained provisions that specifically addressed the needs and requirements for the development of drugs for the pediatric population.

The FDAMA bill essentially codified and expanded several regulatory actions initiated by the FDA during the 1990s. Among the incentives offered by the bill, companies would be given an additional six months of patent protection for performing pediatric studies (clinical trials) on already approved products. In fact, the

FDA was mandated by FDAMA to develop a list of over 500 drugs for which additional information would produce benefits for pediatric patients. The FDA is supposed to provide a written request for pediatric studies to the manufacturers [37].

In response to the pediatric initiatives, the FDA has published policies and guidelines and conducted a variety of meetings. CDER has established a web site (http//www.fda.gov/cder/pediatric), which lists three pages of such information. Interestingly, the focus has been on clinical trials, and almost no attention has been given to the preclinical toxicology studies that may be necessary to support such trials. There are three pages of documents on the pediatric web site. None appear to address the issue of appropriate testing. This is a situation that is just now being addressed and is in a great deal of flux.

In the absence of any guidelines from the FDA for testing drugs in young or "pediatric" animals, one must fall back on the maxim of designing a program that makes the most scientific sense. As a guide, the FDA designated levels of postnatal human development and the approximate equivalent ages (in the author's considered opinion) in various animal models are given in Table 37.7. The table is somewhat inaccurate, however, because of differences in the stages of development at birth. A rat is born quite underdeveloped when compared to a human being. A one-day old rat is not equivalent to a one-day old full-term human infant. A four-day old rat would be more appropriate. In terms of development, the pig may be the best model of those listed; however, one should bear in mind that different organs have different developmental schedules in different species.

Table 37.7 can be used as a rough guide in designing toxicity assessment experiments in developing animals. In designing the treatment period, one needs to consider not only the dose and the proposed course of clinical treatment, but also the proposed age of the patient, and whether or not an equivalent dosing period in the selected animal model covers more than one developmental stage. For example, if the proposed patient population is human infants, initiating a toxicity study of the new pharmaceutical agent in 3-day-old rats is not appropriate. Furthermore, if the proposed course of treatment in adult children is 2 weeks, it is unlikely that this would cross over into a different developmental stage. A 2-week treatment initiated in puppies, however, might easily span two developmental stages. Thus, in designing an experiment in young animals, one must carefully consider the length of the treatment period, balancing the developmental age of the animal model and the proposed length of clinical treatment. Where appropriate (infant animals), one needs to also assess changes in standard developmental landmarks, (e.g., eye opening, pinae eruption, external genitalia development) as well as the more standard

TABLE 37.7 Comparison of Postnatal Development Stages

Stage	Human	Rat	Dog	Pig
Neonate	Birth to 1 month	Birth to 1 week	Birth to 3 weeks	Birth to 2 weeks
Infant	1 month to 2 years	1–3 weeks	3–6 weeks	2–4 weeks
Child	2–12 years	3–9 weeks	6 weeks to 5 months	4 weeks to 4 months
Adolescent	12–16 years	9–13 weeks	5–9 months	4–7 months
Adult	Over 16 years	Over 13 weeks	Over 9 months	Over 7 months

indicators of target organ toxicity. The need for maintaining the experimental animals past the dosing period, perhaps into sexual maturity, to assess recovery or delayed effects needs also to be carefully considered.

To summarize, the current status of assessment of toxicity in postnatal mammals, in response to the pediatric initiatives covered in FDAMA, is an extremely fluid situation. One needs to carefully consider a variety of factors in designing the study and should discuss proposed testing programs with the appropriate office at the CDER.

Drugs intended for use in the elderly, like those intended for the very young, may also have special requirements for safety evaluation, but geriatric issues were not addressed in the FDAMA of 1997. The FDA has published a separate guidance document for geriatric labeling [7]. As was the case with pediatric guidance, this document does not address preclinical testing. With the elderly, the toxicological concerns are quite different from the developmental concerns associated with pediatric patients. With the elderly, one must be concerned with the possible interactions between the test article and compromised organ function. The FDA had previously issued a guidance for examining the clinical safety of new pharmaceutical agents in patients with compromised renal and/or hepatic function [38]. The equivalent ICH guideline (S5A) was issued in 1994. Whether this type of emphasis will require toxicity testing in animal models with specifically induced organ insufficiency remains to be seen. In the interim, we must realize that there is tacit evaluation of test article-related toxicity in geriatric rodents for those agents that undergo 2 year carcinogenicity testing. As the graying of America continues, labeling for geriatric use may become more of an issue in the future.

37.6.5 Orphan Drugs

The development of sophisticated technologies, coupled with the rigors and time required for clinical and preclinical testing, has made pharmaceutical development very expensive. In order to recoup such expenses, pharmaceutical companies have tended to focus on therapeutic agents with large potential markets. Treatment for rare but life-threatening diseases have been "orphaned" as a result. An orphan product is defined as one targeted at a disease that affects 200,000 or fewer individuals in the United States. Alternatively, the therapy may be targeted for more than 200,000 but the developer would have no hope of recovering the initial investment without exclusivity. The Orphan Drug Act of 1983 was passed in an attempt to address this state of affairs. Currently applicable regulations were put in place in 1992 [39]. In 1994, there was an attempt in Congress to amend the Act, but it failed to be passed into law. The current regulations are administered by the Office of Orphan Product Development (OPD). The Act offers the following incentives to encourage the development of products to treat rare diseases:

- Seven years exclusive market following the approval of a product for an orphan disease.
- Written protocol assistance from the FDA.
- Tax credits for up to 50% of qualified clinical research expenses.
- Available grant to support pivotal clinical trials.

As reviewed by Haffner [40], other developed countries have similar regulations.

The ODA did not change the requirements of testing drug products. The nonclinical testing programs are similar to those used for more conventional products. They will undergo the same FDA review process. A major difference, however, is the involvement of the OPD. A sponsor must request OPD review. Once OPD determines that a drug meets the criteria for orphan drug status, it will work with the sponsor to provide the assistance required under the Act. The ODA does not review a product for approval. The IND/NDA process is still handled by the appropriate reviewing division (e.g., Cardiovascular) for formal review. The Act does not waive the necessity for submission of an IND and for the responsibility of toxicological assessment. As always, in cases where there is ambiguity, a sponsor may be well served to request a pre-IND meeting at the appropriate division to discuss the acceptability of a toxicology assessment plan.

37.6.6   Botanical Drug Products

There is an old saying, "What goes around, comes around," and so it is with botanicals. At the beginning of the 20th century, most marketed pharmaceutical agents were botanical in origin. For example, aspirin was first isolated from willow bark. These led the way in the middle part of the century, for reasons having to do with patentability, manufacturing costs, standardization, selectivity, and potency. The dawning of the 21st century has seen a grass-roots return to botanical preparations (also sold as herbals or dietary supplements). These preparations are being marketed to the lay public as "natural" supplements to the nasty synthetic chemicals now proscribed as pharmaceutical products. In 1994, the Dietary Supplement Health and Education Act was passed, which permitted the marketing of dietary supplements (including botanicals) with limited submissions to the FDA [33]. If a producer makes a claim that an herbal preparation is beneficial to a specific part of the body (e.g., enhanced memory), then it may be marketed after a 75 day period of FDA review but without formal approval. On the other hand, if any curative properties are claimed, then the botanical will be regulated as a drug and producers will be required to follow the IND/NDA process. In 1997 and 1998 combined, some 26 INDs were filed for botanical products [41].

The weakness in the current regulation has to do with its ambiguity. The line between a beneficial claim and a curative claim is sometimes difficult to draw. What is the difference, for example, between an agent that enhances memory and one that prevents memory loss? Given the number of products and claims hitting the shelves every day, this situation will probably demand increased regulatory scrutiny in the future.

37.7   INTERNATIONAL PHARMACEUTICAL REGULATION AND REGISTRATION

37.7.1   International Conference on Harmonization

The International Conference on Harmonization (ICH) of Technical Requirements for Registration of Pharmaceuticals for Human Use was established to make the drug-regulatory process more efficient in the United States, Europe, and Japan. The U.S. involvement grew out of the fact that the United States is party to the General Agreement on Tariffs and Trade, which included the Agreement on Technical Barriers to Trade, negotiated in the 1970s, to encourage reduction of nontariff barriers to trade [42]. The main purpose of the ICH is, through harmonization, to make new medicines available to patients with a minimum of delay. More recently, the need to harmonize regulation has been driven, according to the ICH, by the escalation of the cost of R&D. The regulatory systems in all countries have the same fundamental concerns about safety, efficacy, and quality, yet sponsors had to repeat many time-consuming and expensive technical tests to meet country-specific requirements. Secondarily, there was a legitimate concern over the unnecessary use of animals. Conference participants include representatives from the drug-regulatory bodies and research-based pharmaceutical industrial organizations of three regions: the European Union, the United States, and Japan, where over 90% of the world's pharmaceutical industries are located. Representation is summarized in Table 37.8. The biennial conference has met four times, beginning in 1991, rotating between sites in the United States, Europe, and Japan.

The ICH meets its objectives by issuing guidelines for the manufacturing, development, and testing of new pharmaceutical agents that are acceptable to all three major parties. For each new guideline, the ICH Steering Committee establishes an expert working group with representation from each of the six major participatory ICH bodies. So far, the ICH has proposed or adopted over 40 safety, efficacy, and quality guidelines (listed in Table 37.9) for use by the drug-regulatory agencies in the United States, Europe, and Japan. The guidelines are organized under broad categories: the "E" series having to do with clinical trials, the "Q" series having to do with quality (including chemical manufacturing and control as well as traditional GLP issues), and the "S" series having to do with safety. Guidelines may be obtained from the ICH secretariat, c/o of IFPMA, 30 rue de St.-Jean, PO Box 9, 1211 Geneva 18, Switzerland, or may be downloaded from a web site set up by Ms. Nancy McClure (http://www.mcclurenet.com/index.html). They are also published in the *Federal Register*. The guidelines of the "S" series will have the most impact on

TABLE 37.8   ICH Representation

Country/Region	Regulatory[a]	Industry[a]
European Union	European Commission (2)	European Federation of Pharmaceutical Industries Associations (2)
Japan	Ministry of Health, Labor and Welfare (2)	Japanese Pharmaceutical Manufacturers Association (2)
United States	Food and Drug Administration (2)	Pharmaceutical Research and Manufacturers of America (2)
Observing organizations	World Health Organization, European Free Trade Area, Canadian Health Protection Branch	International Federation of Pharmaceutical Manufacturers Associations (2): also provides the secretariat

[a]( ) = number of representatives on the ICH Steering Committee.

TABLE 37.9 International Conference on Harmonization Guidelines

Reference	Guideline	Date Issued
E1	The Extent of Population Exposure to Assess Clinical Safety	Oct 94
E2A	Clinical Safety Data Management: Definitions and Standards for Expedited Reporting	Oct 94
E2B(M)	Maintenance of the Clinical Safety Data Management including: Data Elements for Transmission of Individual Case Safety Reports	Nov 00
E2B(R)	Revision of the E2B(M) ICH Guideline on Clinical Safety Data Management Data Elements for Transmission of Individual Case Safety Reports	May 05
E2C	Clinical Safety Data Management: Periodic Safety Update Reports for Marketed Drugs	Nov 96
E2D	Post-Approval Safety Data Management: Definitions and Standards for Expedited Reporting	Nov 03
E2E	Pharmacovigilance Planning	Nov 04
E3	Structure and Content of Clinical Study Reports	Nov 95
E4	Dose Response Information to Support Drug Registration	Mar 94
E5	Ethnic Factors in the Acceptability of Foreign Clinical Data	Feb 98
E6	Good Clinical Practice: Consolidated Guideline; Notice of Availability	May 96
E6A	GCP Addendum on Investigator's Brochure	Mar 95
E6B	GCP: Addendum on Essential Documents for the Conduct of a Clinical Trial	Oct 94
E7	Studies in Support of Special Populations: Geriatrics	Jun 93
E8	Guidance on General Considerations for Clinical Trials; Notice	July 97
E9	Draft Guideline on Statistical Principles for Clinical Trials; Notice of Availability	Feb 98
E10	Choice of Control Group and Related Issues in Clinical Trials	July 00
E11	Clinical Investigation of Medicinal Products in the Pediatric Population	July 00
E12A	Principles for Clinical Evaluation of New Antihypertensive Drugs	Mar 00
E14	Clinical Evaluation of QT/QTc Interval Prolongation and Proarrhythmic Potential for Non-Antiarrhythmic Drugs	May 05
M2	Electronic Transmission of Individual Case Safety Reports Message Specification	Nov 00
M3	Non-Clinical Safety Studies for the Conduct of Human Clinical Trials for Pharmaceuticals	July 97
M4	Organization of the Common Technical Document	Oct 05
M5	Data Elements and Standards for Drug Dictionaries	May 05
Q1A(R)	Stability Testing of New Drug Substances and Products (2nd Revision)	May 03
Q1B	Photostability Testing of New Drug Substances and Products	Nov 96
Q1C	Stability Testing for New Dosage Forms	Nov 96
Q1D	Bracketing and Matrixing Designs for Stability Testing of Drug Substances and Drug Products	Feb 02
Q1E	Evaluation of Stability Data	Feb 03
Q1F	Stability Data Package for Registration Applications in Climatic Zones III and IV	Feb 03
Q2A	Validation of Analytical Procedures: Definitions and Terminology	Oct 94
Q2B	Validation of Analytical Procedures: Methodology	Nov 96
Q3A(R)	Impurities in New Drug Substances Revised Guideline	Feb 02

TABLE 37.9 *Continued*

Reference	Guideline	Date Issued
Q3B(R)	Impurities in New Drug Products Revised Guideline	Feb 03
Q3C	Impurities: Guideline for Residual Solvents	July 97
Q3C(M)	Impurities: Guideline for Residual Solvents (Maintenance)	Sept 02
Q5A	Viral Safety Evaluation of Biotechnology Products Derived from Cell Lines of Human or Animal Origin	Mar 97
Q5B	Quality of Biotechnological Products: Analysis of the Expression Construct in Cells Used for Production of r-DNA Derived Protein Products	Nov 95
Q5C	Q5C: Quality of Biotechnological Products: Stability Testing of Biotechnological/Biological Products	Nov 95
Q5D	Q5D: Derivation and Characterisation of Cell Substrates Used for Production of Biotechnological/Biological Products	July 97
Q5E	Comparability of Biotechnological/Biological Products Subject to Changes in Their Manufacturing Process	Nov 04
Q6A	Specifications: Test Procedures and Acceptance Criteria for New Drug Substances and New Drug Products: Chemical Substances	Oct 99
Q6B	Specifications: Test Procedures and Acceptance Criteria for Biotechnological/ Biological Products	May 99
Q7A	Good Manufacturing Practice Guide for Active Pharmaceutical Ingredients	Nov 00
Q8	Pharmaceutical Development	Nov 05
Q9	Quality Risk Management	Nov 05
S1A	Guideline on the Need for Carcinogenicity Studies of Pharmaceuticals	Nov 95
S1B	Draft Guideline on Testing for Carcinogenicity of Pharmaceuticals	July 97
S1C	Dose Selection for Carcinogenicity Studies of Pharmaceuticals	Oct 94
S1C(R)	Guidance on Dose Selection for Carcinogenicity Studies of Pharmaceuticals: Addendum on a Limit Dose and Related Notes; Availability; Notice	July 97
S2A	Genotoxicity: Guidance on Specific Aspects of Regulatory Genotoxicity Tests for Pharmaceuticals	Jul 95
S2B	Genotoxicity: A Standard Battery for Genotoxicity Testing of Pharmaceuticals; Availability; Notice	July 97
S3A	Toxicokinetics: Guidance on the Assessment of Systemic Exposure in Toxicity Studies	Oct 94
S3B	Pharmacokinetics: Guidance for Repeated Dose Tissue Distribution Studies	Oct 94
S4	Single Dose Toxicity Testing; Revised Guidance	Aug 96
S4A	Duration of Chronic Toxicity Testing in Animals (Rodent and Non-Rodent Toxicity Testing)	Sept 98
S5A	Detection of Toxicity to Reproduction for Medicinal Products	Jun 93
S5B(M)	Maintenance of the ICH Guideline on Toxicity to Male Fertility: An Addendum to the Guideline on Detection of Toxicity to Reproduction for Medicinal Products	Nov 95
S6A	Guidance on Preclinical Safety Evaluation of Biotechnology-Derived Pharmaceuticals; Availability	Nov 97
S7A	Safety Pharmacology Studies for Human Pharmaceuticals	Nov 00
S7B	The Nonclinical Evaluation of the Potential for Delayed Ventricular Repolarization (QT Interval Prolongation) by Human Pharmaceuticals	May 05
S8	Immunotoxicology Studies for Human Pharmaceuticals	Sept 05

toxicologists. The biggest changes having to do with toxicological assessment are summarized next.

Carcinogenicity Studies   Carcinogenicity studies are covered in Guidelines S1A, S1B, and S1C. The guidelines are almost more philosophical than they are technical. In comparison to the EPA guidelines, for example, the ICH guidelines contain little in the way of concrete study criteria (e.g., the number of animals, the necessity for clinical chemistry). There is discussion on when carcinogenicity studies should be done, whether two species are more appropriate than one, and how to set dosages on the basis of human clinical PK data. The following major changes are being wrought by these guidelines:

- Only one 2 year carcinogenicity study should generally be required. Ideally, the species chosen should be the one most like humans in terms of metabolic transformations of the test article.
- The traditional second long-term carcinogenicity study can be replaced by a shorter-term alternative model. In practical terms, this guideline is beginning to result in sponsors conducting a 2 year study in the rat and a 6 month study in an alternative mouse model, such as the P53 or the TG.AC genetically manipulated mouse strains.
- In the absence of target organ toxicity with which to set the high dose at the maximally tolerated dose, the high dose can be set at the dose that produces an area under the curve (AUC). This is 25-fold higher than that obtained in human subjects.

Chronic Toxicity   Traditionally, chronic toxicity of new pharmaceuticals in the United States was assessed in studies of 1 year duration in both the rodent and the nonrodent species of choice. The European view was that studies of 6 months are generally sufficient. The resulting guideline (S4A) was a compromise. Studies of 6 months duration were recommended for the rodent, as rodents would also be examined in 2 year studies. For the nonrodent (dog, nonhuman primate, and pig) studies of 9 months duration were recommended.

Developmental and Reproductive Toxicity   This was an area in which there was considerable international disagreement and the area in which the ICH has promulgated the most technically detailed guidelines (S5A and S5B). Some of the major changes include the following:

- The traditional Segment I, II, and III nomenclature has been replaced with different nomenclature, as summarized in Table 37.10.
- The dosing period of the pregnant animals during studies on embryonic development (traditional Segment II studies) has been standardized.
- New guidelines for fertility assessment (traditional Segment I) studies have shortened the premating dosing schedule (e.g., in male rats from 10 weeks to 4 weeks). There has been an increased interest in assessment of spermatogenesis and sperm function.

TABLE 37.10 Comparison of Traditional and ICH Guidelines for Reproductive and Developmental Toxicology

Traditional Protocol	Stages Covered	ICH Protocol	Dosing Regimen
Segment I (rats)	A. Premating to conception B. Conception to implantation	Fertility and early embryonic development, including implantation	Males: 4 weeks premating, mating (1–3 weeks), plus 3 weeks postmating Females: 2 weeks premating, mating through day 7 of gestation
Segment II (rabbits)	C. Implantation to closure of hard palate D. Closure of hard palate to the end of pregnancy	Embryo–fetal development	Female rabbits: day 6 to day 20 of pregnancy

Study Title	Termination	Endpoints: In-life	Endpoints: Postmortem
Fertility and early embryonic development, including implantation	Females: day 13–15 of pregnancy Males: day after completion of dosing	Clinical signs and mortality Body weights and feed in-take Vaginal cytology	Macroscopic exam + histological exam of gross lesions Collection of reproductive organs for possible histology Quantitation of corpora lutea and implantation sites Seminology (count, motility, and morphology)
Embryo–fetal development		Clinical signs and mortality Body weights and changes Feed in-take	Macroscopic exam + histological exam of gross lesions Quantitation of corpora lutea and implantation sites Fetal body weights Fetal abnormalities
Pre- and postnatal development, including maternal function		Clinical signs and mortality Body weights and changes Feed in-take Duration of pregnancy Parturition	Macroscopic exam + histological exam of gross lesions Implantation Abnormalities (including terata) Live/dead offspring at birth Pre- and postweaning survival and growth (F_1) Physical development (F_1) Sensory functions and reflexes (F_1) Behavior (F_1)

- The new guidelines allow for a combination of studies in which the endpoints typically assessed in the traditional Segment II and Segment III studies are now examined under a single protocol.

For a more complete review of the various study designs, the reader is refereed to the review by Manson [43].

While they were not quite as sweeping in approach as the aforementioned guidelines, a toxicologist working in pharmaceutical safety assessment should become familiar with all the other ICH guidelines in the S series.

In an interesting recent article, Ohno [44] discussed not the harmonization of nonclinical guidelines, but the need to harmonize the timing of nonclinical tests in relation to the conduct of clinical trials. For example, there are regional differences in the inclusion of women of childbearing potential in clinical trials. In the United States, including women in such trials is becoming more important, and therefore evaluation of embryo–fetal development will occur earlier in the drug development process than in Japan. Whether or not such timing or staging of nonclinical tests becomes part of an ICH guideline in the near future remains to be established.

37.7.2   Other International Considerations

The United States is the single largest pharmaceutical market in the world. But the rest of the world (particularly but not limited to the second and third largest markets, Japan and the European Union) represents in aggregate a much larger market, so no one develops a new pharmaceutical for marketing just in the United States. The effort at harmonization (exemplified by the International Conference on Harmonization, or ICH) has significantly reduced differences in requirements for these other countries, but certainly not obliterated them. Although a detailed understanding of their regulatory schemes is beyond this chapter, the bare bones and differences in toxicology requirements are not.

European Union   The standard European Union toxicology and pharmacologic data requirements for a pharmaceutical include the following

- Single-dose toxicity
- Repeat-dose toxicity (subacute and chronic trials)
- Reproduction studies (fertility and general reproductive performance, embryotoxicity, and peri/postnatal toxicity)
- Mutagenic potential (*in vitro* and *in vivo*)
- Carcinogenicity
- Pharmacodynamics
  Effects related to proposed drug indication
  General pharmacodynamics
  Drug interactions
- Pharmacokinetics
  Single dose
  Repeat dose

    Distribution in normal and pregnant animals

    Biotransformation

- Local tissue tolerance
- Environmental toxicity

In general, the registration process in the European Union allows one to apply to either an overall medicines authority or to an individual national authority. Either of these steps is supposed to lead to mutual recognition by all the individual members.

Japan   In Japan, the Ministry of Health, Labor and Welfare is the national regulatory body for new drugs [45].

    The standard LD_{50} test is no longer a regulatory requirement for new medicines in the United States, the European Union, or Japan. The Japanese guidelines were the first to be amended in accordance with this agreement, with the revised guidelines becoming effective in August 1993. The Japanese may still anticipate that single-dose (acute) toxicity studies should be conducted in at least two species, one rodent and one nonrodent (the rabbit is not accepted as a nonrodent). Both males and females should be included from at least one of the species selected: if the rodent, then a minimum of 5 per sex; if the nonrodent, at least 2 per sex. In nonrodents, both the oral and parenteral routes should be used, and normally the clinical route of administration should be employed. In nonrodents, only the intended route of administration need be employed; if the intended route of administration in humans is intravenous, then use of this route in both species is acceptable. An appropriate number of doses should be employed to obtain a complete toxicity profile and to establish any dose–response relationship. The severity, onset, progression, and reversibility of toxicity should be studied during a 14 day follow-up period, with all animals being necropsied. When macroscopic changes are noted, the tissue must be subjected to histological examination.

    Chronic and subchronic toxicity studies are conducted to define the dose level, when given repeatedly, that causes toxicity, and the dose level that does not lead to toxic findings. In Japan, such studies are referred to as repeated-dose toxicity studies. As with single-dose studies, at least two animal species should be used, one rodent and one nonrodent (rabbit not acceptable). In rodent studies, each group should consist of at least 10 males and 10 females; in nonrodent species, 3 of each sex are deemed adequate. Where interim examinations are planned, however, the numbers of animals employed should be increased accordingly. The planned route of administration in human subjects is normally explored. The duration of the study will be dictated by the planned duration of clinical use (Table 37.11).

    At least three different dose groups should be included, with the goals of demonstrating an overtly toxic dose and a no-effect dose, and establishing any dose–response relationship. The establishment of a nontoxic dose within the framework of these studies is more rigorously adhered to in Japan than elsewhere in the world. All surviving animals should also be necropsied, either at the completion of the study or during its extension recovery period, to assess reversal of toxicity and the possible appearance of delayed toxicity. Full histological examination is mandated on all nonrodent animals used in a chronic toxicity study; at a minimum, the highest-

TABLE 37.11 Determination of Duration of Studies

Duration of Dosing in Toxicity Study	Duration of Human Exposure
2 weeks	Single dose or repeated dosage not exceeding 12 days
1 month	Single dose or repeated dosage not exceeding 4 weeks
3 months	Repeated dosing exceeding 1 week and to a maximum of 12 weeks
6 months (rodent)	Repeated dosing exceeding 13 weeks and to a maximum of lifetime
9/12 months[a] (nonrodent)	Repeated dosing exceeding 6 months or where this is deemed to be appropriate

[a]Where carcinogenicity studies are to be conducted, the Koseisho had agreed to forego chronic dosage beyond 6 months.
Source: New Drugs Division Notification No. 43, June 1992.

dose and control groups of rodents must be submitted to a full histological examination.

While the value of repeated-dose testing beyond 6 months has been questioned [46], such testing is a regulatory requirement for a number of agencies, including the U.S. FDA and the Koseisho. In Japan, repeated-dose testing for 12 months is required only for new medicines expected to be administered to humans for periods in excess of 6 months [47]. At the First International Conference on Harmonization held in Brussels, the consensus was that 12 month toxicity studies in rodents could be reduced to 6 months where carcinogenicity studies are required. While not yet adopted in the Japanese guidelines, 6 month repeated-dose toxicity studies have been accepted by the agencies of all three regions. Japan—like the European Union—accepts a 6 month duration if accompanied by a carcinogenicity study. The United States still requires a 9 month nonrodent study.

With regard to reproductive toxicology, as a consequence of the first ICH, the United States, European Union, and Japan agreed to recommend mutual recognition of their respective current guidelines. A tripartite, harmonized guideline on reproductive toxicology has achieved ICH Step 4 status and should be incorporated into the local regulations of all three regions soon [48]. This agreement represents a very significant achievement that should eliminate many obstacles to drug registration.

Preclinical Male Fertility Studies   Before conducting a single-dose male volunteer study in Japan, it is usually necessary to have completed a preclinical male fertility study (Segment I) that has an in-life phase of 10 or more weeks (i.e., 10 weeks of dosing, plus follow-up). Although government guidelines do not require this study to be completed before Phase I trials begin, the responsible Institutional Review Board or the investigator usually imposes this condition. Japanese regulatory authorities are aware that the Segment I male fertility study is of poor predictive value. The rat, which is used in this study, produces a marked excess of sperm. Many scientists therefore believe that the test is less sensitive than the evaluation of testicular weight and histology that constitute part of the routine toxicology assessment.

Female Reproductive Studies   Before entering a female into a clinical study, it is necessary to have completed the entire reproductive toxicology program, which consists of the following studies:

- Segment 1: Fertility studies in the rat or mouse species used in the Segment 2 program.
- Segment 2: Teratology studies in the rat or mouse, and the rabbit.
- Segment 3: Late gestation and lactation studies in a species used in the Segment 2 studies.

Such studies usually take approximately 2 years. Although the U.S. regulations state the need for completion of Segments 1 and 2, and the demonstration of efficacy in male patients, where appropriate, before entering females into a clinical program, the current trend in the United States is toward relaxation of the requirements to encourage investigation of the drug both earlier and in a larger number of females during product development. Growing pressure for the earlier inclusion of women in drug testing may encourage selection of this issue as a future ICH topic. The trend in the United States and the European Union toward including women earlier in the critical program has not yet been embraced in Japan, however.

The three tests required in Japan for genotoxicity evaluation are a bacterial gene mutation test, *in vitro* cytogenetics, and *in vivo* tests for genetic damage. The Japanese regulations state these tests to be the minimum requirement and encourage additional tests. Currently, Japanese guidelines do not require a mammalian cell gene mutation assay. Harmonization will likely be achieved by the Koseisho recommending all four tests, which will match requirements in the United States and European Union. At present, this topic is at Step 1 in the ICH harmonization process. The mutagenicity studies should be completed before the commencement of Phase II clinical studies.

Guidelines presented at the second ICH are likely to alter the preclinical requirements for registration in Japan; they cover toxicokinetics and when to conduct repeated-dose tissue distribution studies. The former document may improve the ability of animal toxicology studies to predict possible adverse events in humans; currently, there are no toxicokinetic requirements in Japan, and their relevance is questioned by many there. Although there is general agreement on the registration requirement for single-dose tissue distribution studies, implementation of the repeated-dose study requirement has been inconsistent across the three ICH parties.

37.7.3   Safety Pharmacology

Japan was the first major country to require extensive pharmacological profiling on all new pharmaceutical agents as part of the safety assessment profile. Prior to commencement of initial clinical studies, the drug's pharmacology must be characterized in animal models. In the United States and Europe, these studies have been collectively called safety pharmacology studies. For a good general review of the issues surrounding safety pharmacology the reader is referred to Hite [1]. The Japanese guidelines for such characterizations were published in 1991 (New Drugs Division Notification No. 4, January 1991). They include the following:

- Effects on general activity and behavior.
- Effects on the central nervous system.
- Effects on the autonomic nervous system and smooth muscle.
- Effects on the respiratory and cardiovascular systems.
- Effects on the digestive system.
- Effects on water and electrolyte metabolism.
- Other important pharmacological effects.

In the United States, pharmacological studies in demonstration of efficacy have always been required, but specific safety pharmacological studies have never been required. Special situational or mechanistic data would be requested on a case-by-case basis. This is a situation that is changing. In the United States the activities of the Safety Pharmacology Discussion Group, for example, have helped bring attention to the utility and issues surrounding safety pharmacology data. In 1999 and 2000, the major toxicological and pharmacological societal meetings had symposia on safety pharmacological testing. Many major U.S. pharmaceutical companies are in the process of implementing programs in safety pharmacology. The issue has been taken up by the ICH and the draft guideline is currently at the initial stages of review. This initial draft (Guideline S7) includes core tests in the assessment of CNS, cardiovascular, and respiratory function. Studies will be expected to be performed under GLP guidelines.

37.8 CONCLUSION

In summary, we have touched upon the regulations that currently control the types of preclinical toxicity testing done on potential human pharmaceuticals. This chapter has reviewed the history, the law, the regulations themselves, the guidelines, and common practices employed to meet regulatory standards.

REFERENCES AND SUGGESTED READING

1. Hite M. Safety pharmacology approaches. *Int J Toxicol* 1997;16:23–31, 37.7.3.
2. FDLI. *Compilation of food and drug laws, Vol. I–III and supplement.* Washington, DC: FDLI; 1995–1998.
3. Gad SC. *Drug Safety Evaluation.* Hoboken, NJ: John Wiley & Sons; 2002.
4. Lumpkin M. *Guidance for Industry: Content and Format of Investigational New Drug Applications* (INDs) *for Phase 1 Studies of Drugs, Including Well-characterized, Therapeutic, and Biotechnology-Derived Products.* 1995. http://www.fda.gov/cder/guidance/phase1.pdf.
5. FDA. *Environmental Assessment Technical Assistance Handbook.* NTIS No. PB87-175345; 1987.
6. *Annual Report of the Pharmaceutical Research and Manufacturer Association* (Priority #2: Improved FDA Regulation of Drug Development). 1998.
7. *Guidance for Industry: Content and Format for Geriatric Labeling (Draft Guidance).* 1998. http://www.fda.gov/cder/guidance/2527dft.pdf.

8. *Guidance for Industry and Reviewers: Repeal of Section 507 of the Federal Food, Drug and Cosmetic Act.* 1997. http://www.fda.gov/cder/guidance/index.htm.

9. *Points to Consider in the Manufacture and Testing of Monoclonal Antibody Products for Human Use.* 1997. http://www.fda.gov/cber/cberftp.html.

10. *United States Pharmacopeia XXIV* and *National Formulary 19.* Philadelphia, PA: USP; 2000.

11. Anderson O. *The Health of a Nation; Harvey Wiley and the Fight for Pure Food.* Chicago: University of Chicago; 1988.

12. Burns J. Overview of safety regulations governing food, drug and cosmetics. In Homberger F, Ed. *The United States in Safety and Evaluation and Regulation of Chemicals 3: Interface Between Law and Science.* New York: Karger; 1983.

13. Goldenthal E. Current view on safety evaluation of drugs. *FDA Papers* May 1968; 13–18.

14. Blakeslee D. Thalidomide, a background briefing. *JAMA HIV/AIDS Information Center Newsline.* 1998. http://www.ama-assn.org/special/hiv/newsline/briefing/briefing.htm.

15. FDA. *Introduction to Total Drug Quality.* Washington, DC: US. Government Printing Office; 1971.

16. ICH. *Non-Clinical Safety Studies for the Conduct of Human Clinical Trials for Pharmaceuticals.* 2000.

17. *Points to Consider in the Production and Testing of New Drugs and Biologicals Produced by Recombinant DNA Technology.* Washington, DC: FDA; 1985.

18. *Points to Consider in Human Somatic Cell Therapy and Gene Therapy.* Washington, DC: FDA; 1991.

19. *Points to Consider in the Characterization of Cell Lines Used to Produce Biologicals.* Washington, DC: FDA; 1993.

20. Wessinger J. Pharmacologic and toxicologic considerations for evaluating biologic products. *Reg Tox Pharmacol* 1989;10:255–263.

21. Hayes T, Ryffel B. Symposium in writing: safety considerations of recombinant protein therapy; introductory comments. *Clin Immunol Immunother* 1997;83:1–4.

22. Buesing, Mary McSweegan. Submitting biologics applications to the Center for Biologics Evaluation and Research Electronically. *Drug Inf J* 1999;33:1–15.

23. Ryffel B. Safety of human recombinant proteins. *Biomed Environ Sci* 1997;10:65–71.

24. Ryffel B. Unanticipated human toxicology of recombinant proteins. *Arch Toxicol Suppl* 1996;18:333–341.

25. Well-Characterized Biologics Would Be Regulated Under FD&C Act By Kassebaum FDA Reform Bill. *-F-D-C Reports (pink sheets)* 1996;58:11–12.

26. Kessler D, Siegel J, Noguchi P, Zoon K, Feidon K, Woodcock J. Regulation of somatic-cell therapy and gene therapy by the Food and Drug Administration. *N Engl J Med* 1993;329:1169–1173.

27. *Points to Consider in Human Somatic Cell Therapy and Gene Therapy.* Washington, DC: FDA; 1996.

28. Berliner VR. US Food and Drug Administration requirements for toxicity testing of contraceptive products. In Briggs MH, Diczbalusy E, Eds. *Pharmacological Models in Contraceptive Development. Acta Endocrinol (Copenhagen)* 1974;185:240–253.

29. FDA. Investigational new drug, antibiotic, and biological drug product regulations, procedures for drug intended to treat life-threatening and severely debilitating illnesses. *Fed Reg* 1988;53(No. 204, 198):41516–41524.

30. FDA. Good Laboratory Practices, *CFR* 21 Part 58, Apr 1988.

31. DeGeorge J, Ahn C, Andrews P, Bower M, Giorgio D, Goheer M, Lee-Yam D, McGuinn W, Schmidt W, Sun C, Tripathi S. Regulatory considerations for the preclinical development of anticancer drugs. *Cancer Chemother Pharmacol* 1998;41:173–185.

32. Grieshaber C. Prediction of human toxicity of new antineoplastic drugs from studies in animals. In Powis G, Hacker M, Eds. *The Toxicity of Anticancer Drugs*. New York: Pergamon Press; 1991, pp 10–24.

33. Daniels J, Nestmann E, Kerr A. Development of stereoisomeric (chiral) drugs: a brief review of the scientific and regulatory considerations. *Drug Inf J* 1997;639–646.

34. FDA. Perspective on development of stereoisomers. *AAPS*, 16 May 1988.

35. FDA's Policy Statement for the Development of New Stereoisomeric Drugs. 1992. http://www.fda.gov/cder/guidance/stereo.htm.

36. Schacter E, DeSantis P. Labeling of drug and biologic products for pediatric use. *Drug Inf J* 1998;32:299–303.

37. Hart C. Getting PSArt the politics and paperwork of pediatric drug studies. *Modern Drug Discov* 1999;2:15–16.

38. CDER. Guideline for the study of drugs likely to be used in the elderly. *FDA*, Nov 1989.

39. Orphan Drug Regulations 21 CFR PART 316. 1992. http://www.fda.gov/orphan/about/odreg.htm.

40. Haffner M. Orphan drug development—international program and study design issues. *Drug Inf J* 1998;32:93–99.

41. Wu K-M, DeGeorge J, Atrachi A, Barry E, Bigger A, Chen C, Du T, Freed L, Geyer H, Goheer A, Jacobs A, Jean D, Rhee H, Osterburg R, Schmidt W, Farrelly J. Regulatory science: a special update from the United States Food and Drug Administration. Preclinical issues and status of investigations of botanical drug products in the United States. *Toxicol Lett* 2000;111:199–202.

42. Barton B. International Conference on Harmonization—good clinical practices update. *Drug Inf J* 1998;32:1143–1147.

43. Manson J. Testing of pharmaceutical agents for reproductive toxicity. In Kimmel C, Buelke-Sam J, Eds. *Developmental toxicology*. New York: Raven Press; 1994; pp 379–402.

44. Ohno Y. Harmonization of the timing of the non-clinical tests in relation to the conduct of clinical trials. *J Control Release* 1999;62:57–63.

45. Currie WJC. *New Drug Approval in Japan*. Waltham, MA: Parexel; 1995.

46. Lumley CE, Walker SE. An international appraisal of the minimum duration of chronic animal toxicity studies. *Hum Exp Toxicol* 1992;11:155–162.

47. Yakuji Nippo, Ltd. *Guidelines for Toxicity Study of Drugs Manual*. Tokyo: Yakuji Nippo Ltd; 1994.

48. ICH. *International Conference on Harmonization Safety Steps 4/5 Documents*. Buffalo Grove, IL: Interpharm Press; 1997.

38

DATA ANALYSIS

Jayesh Vora[1] and Pankaj B. Desai[2]

[1] *PRTM Management Consultants, Mountain View, California*
[2] *University of Cincinnati Medical Center, Cincinnati, Ohio*

Contents

38.1 INTRODUCTION AND SCOPE

Pharmacokinetic analysis of systemic (or blood or plasma) concentration–time data, or amount excreted in urine over various time intervals, represents a critical activity in the preclinical development of drug candidates. This chapter describes the common methods for analysis of such data in support of drug development efforts, with an emphasis on nonclinical drug discovery and development. Theoretical principles underlying pharmacokinetic data analysis are presented elsewhere in other chapters of this volume.

Preclinical Development Handbook: ADME and Biopharmaceutical Properties,
edited by Shayne Cox Gad
Copyright © 2008 John Wiley & Sons, Inc.

Concentration–time or urinary excretion data are typically analyzed to generate estimates of bioavailability, clearance, apparent volume of distribution, and fraction of dose converted to a specific metabolite. These parameters are vital for determination of appropriate dose(s), administration route(s), and dosing regimens in preclinical efficacy and toxicology studies.

Noncompartmental or compartmental methods are generally employed to perform these analyses [1, 2]. At their core, noncompartmental methods, based on statistical moment theory, require estimation of the area under the concentration–time curve. Compartmental methods assume that the body is composed of a series of compartments, even though such compartments have no physiologic relevance, with first-order (concentration-independent) transfer or elimination rate constants between compartments. A one-compartment model, for instance, depicts the body as a single, homogeneous unit, with first-order elimination.

Many modern software applications are available for rapid, reliable, and pharmacokinetic analyses by noncompartmental or compartmental methods (e.g., Win-Nonlin®, Kinetica®, PKAnalyst®, NCOMP) [3].

This chapter discusses noncompartmental methods of pharmacokinetic analysis with primary emphasis on data analysis following intravenous and oral dosing. This chapter is meant to provide an introductory discussion on pharmacokinetic data analysis with a few "hands-on" examples. A comprehensive discussion of all current and emerging pharmacokinetic data analysis techniques is documented in several excellent books [1–5].

38.2   SYSTEMIC CONCENTRATION–TIME PROFILES AND URINARY EXCRETION

38.2.1   Single Intravenous Dose

Following a single intravenous bolus administration, the test article (or drug) is assumed to instantaneously mix within the components of the circulating blood (red and white cells, plasma water, and plasma proteins). Concentration of drug in blood is then gradually diluted through distribution to tissues and organs. Concurrently, the drug may be metabolized or degraded by circulating enzymes (such as esterases) or by metabolic enzymes in the liver (or lungs) or may be excreted unchanged in urine through the kidneys. This complex combination of distribution, degradation, metabolism, and excretion results in a gradual decline in blood or systemic concentrations of drug over time. Whereas individual processes may not be generally discernible, their combination is generally evident as a monoexponential decline in systemic concentrations of drug over time. In instances when one or more processes are relatively slow, a multiexponential decline in systemic concentrations over time is evident. In any event, the apparent terminal monoexponential portion of concentration–time profile is assumed to represent elimination of drug from systemic circulation. A schematic of monoand multiexponential systemic concentration–time profiles following intravenous administration of a drug is depicted in Fig. 38.1.

The complex interplay between distribution and elimination processes observed in systemic circulation following an intravenous dose is also reflected in urine. As the systemic concentration of drug declines, the corresponding amount of unchanged

(a)

(b)

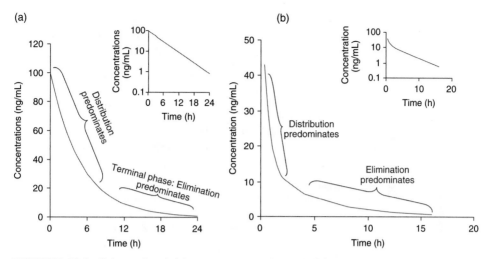

FIGURE 38.1 Schematic of (a) monoexponential and (b) multiexponential concentration–time curves following a single intravenous dose of a drug. (Inset: Semilog concentration–time plot.)

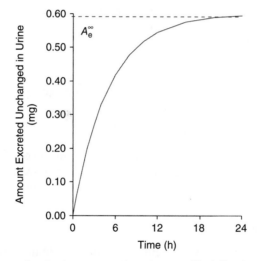

FIGURE 38.2 Schematic of urinary excretion–time profile following a single intravenous dose of a drug.

(unmetabolized) drug excreted in urine increases, reaching a maximum value referred to as the maximum amount of drug excreted unchanged in urine (A_e^∞). In cases when systemic concentration of an administered drug cannot be determined due to inaccessibility of appropriate sampling sites (such as in pediatric or infant patients), measurement of urinary excretion serves as a convenient tool for determination of corresponding pharmacokinetic parameters. A schematic of the urinary excretion–time profile of an intravenously administered drug is presented below in Fig. 38.2. This approach to pharmacokinetic characterization is utilized even for

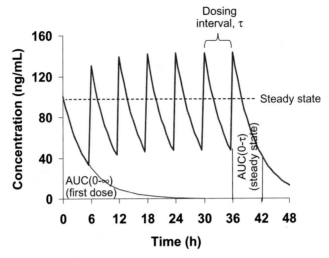

FIGURE 38.3 Schematic of systemic concentration–time profile following multiple intra-venous administration of a drug.

agents that are fully metabolized and some of the metabolites excreted in urine. The reader is referred to the literature for further discussions [5].

38.2.2 Multiple Intravenous Doses

Multiple drug administration generally results in increasing systemic exposure when concentrations from prior doses are not completely eliminated, reaching "steady-state" levels (Fig. 38.3). Such an increase in systemic exposure is commonly referred to as *accumulation*.

  If additional doses are administered following "almost complete" elimination of prior doses then accumulation is minimal. The implications of accumulation (or lack thereof) are discussed elsewhere in this book and in the literature [5].

38.2.3 Single Oral Dose

Following an oral (or other nonparenteral) route of administration, the drug must be released from its dosage form and be absorbed from the site of administration into the systemic circulation. Distribution, degradation, metabolism, and excretion processes occur in parallel with drug absorption. At least initially, absorption rate predominates over other processes, resulting in increasing systemic concentrations of drug with time. As the amount of dose remaining to be absorbed declines at the site of administration, the rate of absorption declines and systemic concentrations reach a peak before declining thereafter in mono- or multiexponential fashion with time, as described previously. A schematic of systemic concentration–time profile following oral (or nonparenteral) administration is presented in Fig. 38.4. As dis-cussed earlier, urinary excretion–time profiles provide an additional window into the absorption, distribution, and elimination processes following oral administration of a drug.

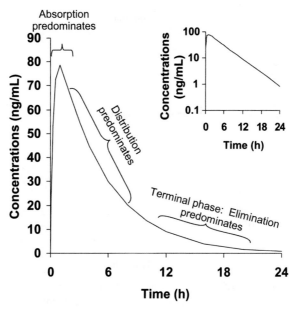

FIGURE 38.4   Schematic of monoexponential concentration–time curve following a single oral (or nonparenteral) dose of a drug. (Inset: Semilog concentration–time plot.)

38.2.4   Other Routes of Administration

The test article may be administered to animals and humans during drug development by a number of other routes, including subcutaneous, intraperitoneally, and transdermally. Such routes result in systemic concentration–time profiles that mimic those following oral dosing (Fig. 38.4). Each includes absorption of the test article from the site of administration to systemic circulation with concurrent distribution, metabolism, and elimination processes. In such cases, drug absorption depends on the amount of administered dose remaining at the administration site. As the amount of administered dose decreases with time, the absorption rate declines as well. Such an absorption process is referred to as *first-order absorption*.

In contrast to changing absorption rates over time, a *zero-order* drug administration maintains constant rate of absorption. Such constant absorption rate is generally achieved by a constant rate intravenous infusion or through osmotic pumps. Typically, drugs with narrow therapeutic window (i.e., low safety margins) are administered in this fashion. Systemic concentrations increase steadily, reaching "steady state" when the rate of drug "input" equals the rate of drug "output" (i.e., removal of drug from systemic circulation). Once the infusion is terminated (or drug delivery device, such as an osmotic pump, is removed), systemic concentrations decline in exponential manner, reflecting either the mono- or multiexponential characteristics described earlier. A schematic of systemic concentration–time profile following a constant rate infusion is presented in Fig. 38.5.

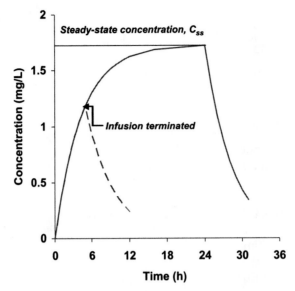

FIGURE 38.5 Schematic of systemic concentration–time profile following intravenous infusion of drug. Infusion was terminated (a) prior to achievement of steady state or (b) following steady state.

38.3 PHARMACOKINETIC ANALYSIS

Pharmacokinetic analysis of systemic concentration–time data is typically initiated by noncompartmental methods resulting, at least initially, in estimation of the apparent terminal elimination half-life ($t_{1/2}$) and area under the concentration–time curve (AUC) (systemic exposure). The terminal elimination rate constant is calculated from the slope of the terminal $\log_{10}$(concentration)–time data:

$$\text{Terminal elimination rate constant, } k_e = -Slope \times 2.303 \qquad (38.1)$$

where, $Slope$ is the slope of the terminal portion of $\log_{10}$(concentration)–time data

$$\text{Terminal elimination half-life, } t_{1/2} = \frac{0.693}{k_e} \qquad (38.2)$$

AUC values are generally estimated using the trapezoidal rule, which is the sum of the area of all trapezoids between two sampling points. The area of the curve beyond the last sampling point is estimated using the ratio of the corresponding concentration value and the terminal elimination rate constant.

$$AUC(0-t_{\text{last}}) = \sum_{t=0}^{t_n} \frac{(C_{n-1}+C_n)}{2} \cdot (t_n - t_{n-1}) \qquad (38.3)$$

$$AUC(0-\infty) = AUC(0-t_{\text{last}}) + AUC_{\text{terminal}} \qquad (38.4)$$

where

$$AUC_{\text{terminal}} = \frac{C_{\text{last}}}{k_e} \qquad (38.5)$$

38.3.1   Example 1: Intravenous Dosing

Following an intravenous dose of 1 mg of Drug X to human volunteers, blood samples were collected for 24 hours. Plasma concentration–time data are summarized in Table 38.1.

Elimination $t_{1/2}$ and AUC Values   The terminal elimination rate constant (k_e) and terminal elimination half-life ($t_{1/2}$) may be estimated by examination of $\log_{10}$(concentration)–time profile to identify the terminal elimination phase and estimate the slope of the corresponding line (Eq. 38.1) (Table 38.2).

The application of Eqs. 38.3–38.5 for estimation of AUC values is exemplified in Table 38.3.

Clearance, Mean Residence Time, and Volume of Distribution   Estimation of apparent terminal half-life ($t_{1/2}$) and AUC values is directly useful in estimation of other key pharmacokinetic parameters, such as clearance (CL), mean residence time (MRT), and volume of distribution (V_{ss}).

$$\text{Systemic clearance } (CL) = \frac{Dose_{\text{IV}}}{AUC(0-\infty)} \qquad (38.6)$$

TABLE 38.1   Plasma Concentration–Time Profile Following a Single Intravenous Dose of 1 mg Drug X to Human Volunteers

Time (h)	Plasma Concentration (ng/mL)
0	100
0.0833	98.3
0.167	96.7
0.25	95.1
0.5	90.5
1	81.9
2	67.0
3	54.9
4	44.9
6	30.1
8	20.2
10	13.5
12	9.07
16	4.08
20	1.83
24	0.82

TABLE 38.2   Estimation of Apparent Terminal Elimination Rate Constant and Half-life Following a Single Intravenous Dose of 1 mg of Drug X to Human Volunteers

Time (h)	Plasma Concentration (ng/mL)	$\log_{10}$(Concentration)
0	100	
0.0833	98.3	
0.167	96.7	
0.25	95.1	
0.5	90.5	
1	81.9	
2	67.0	
3	54.9	
4	44.9	
6	30.1	
8	20.2	
10	13.5	
12	9.07	0.958
16	4.08	0.610
20	1.83	0.263
24	0.823	−0.0846

Slope = −0.0869
k_e (Eq. 38.1) = 0.2 h^{-1}
$t_{1/2}$ (**Eq. 38.2**) = **3.46 h**

TABLE 38.3   Estimation of Area Under Plasma Concentration–Time Curve (AUC) Following a Single Intravenous Dose of 1 mg Drug X to Human Volunteers

(1) Time (h)	(2) Plasma Concentration (ng/mL)	(3) $\dfrac{(C_{n-1}+C_n)}{2}$	(4) $(t_n - t_{n-1})$	(5) AUC Value of Each Trapezoid (Column 3 × Column 4)	(6) Cumulative AUC Values $[AUC(0-t_{last})]$
0	100	99.2	0.0833	8.26	8.26
0.0833	98.3	97.5	0.0833	8.13	16.4
0.167	96.7	95.9	0.0833	7.99	24.4
0.25	95.1	92.8	0.25	23.2	47.6
0.5	90.5	86.2	0.5	43.1	90.7
1	81.9	74.5	1	74.5	165
2	67.0	61.0	1	61.0	226
3	54.9	49.9	1	49.9	276
4	44.9	37.5	2	75.1	351
6	30.1	25.2	2	50.3	401
8	20.2	16.9	2	33.7	435
10	13.5	11.3	2	22.6	458
12	9.07	6.57	4	26.3	484
16	4.08	2.95	4	11.8	496
20	1.83	1.33	4	5.31	501
24	0.823				

$AUC(0-t_{last})$ (Eq. 38.3) = 501 ng·h/mL
$AUC_{terminal}$ (Eq. 38.5) = 4.11 ng·h/mL
$AUC(0-\infty)$ (**Eq. 38.4**) = **505 ng·h/mL**

$$\text{Mean residence time } (MRT) = \frac{AUMC}{AUC} \qquad (38.7)$$

where $AUMC$ is the area under the first-moment time curve, calculated in similar fashion to AUC, using the following formula:

$$AUMC = \left\{ \sum_{t=0}^{t_n} \frac{(t_{n-1} \cdot C_{n-1} + t_n \cdot C_n)}{2} \cdot (t_n - t_{n-1}) \right\} + \left\{ \frac{C_{last} \cdot t_{last}}{k_e} + \frac{C_{last}}{k_e^2} \right\} \qquad (38.8)$$

The apparent volume of distribution at steady state (V_{ss}) is the product of CL and MRT after a single intravenous dose of a drug:

$$V_{ss} = CL \cdot MRT \qquad (38.9)$$

For Drug X, clearance is calculated using Eq. 38.6:

$$CL = 1\,mg/(505\,ng \cdot h/mL) = 1979\,mL/h$$

Calculation of MRT requires estimation of $AUMC$ (Eq. 38.8) as illustrated in Table 38.4.

TABLE 38.4   Estimation of Area Under First-Moment Time Curve ($AUMC$)

(1)	(2)	(3)	(4)	(5)	(6)	(7)
	Plasma				$AUMC$	Cumulative
	Concentration	$t \cdot C$ (Column 1	$\dfrac{(t_{n-1}C_{n-1} + t_n C_n)}{2}$		(Column 4 ×	$AUMC$
Time (h)	(ng/mL)	× Column 2)		$(t_n - t_{n-1})$	Column 5)	Values
0	100	0	4.10	0.0833	0.341	0.341
0.0833	98.3	8.20	12.2	0.0833	1.01	1.35
0.167	96.7	16.1	20.0	0.083	1.66	3.02
0.25	95.1	23.8	34.5	0.250	8.63	11.6
0.5	90.5	45.2	63.6	1	31.8	43.4
1	81.9	81.9	108	1	108	151
2	67.0	134	149	1	149	301
3	54.9	165	172	1	172	473
4	44.9	180	180	2	360	833
6	30.1	181	171	2	342	1176
8	20.2	162	148	2	297	1472
10	13.5	135	122	2	244	1717
12	9.07	109	87.0	4	348	2065
16	4.08	65.2	50.9	4	204	2269
20	1.83	36.6	28.2	4	113	2381
24	0.823	19.8				

$$AUMC\,(0\text{–}t_{last}) = 2381$$
$$(C_{last} \cdot t_{last})/k_e = 98.7$$
$$C_{last}/k_e^2 = 20.6$$
$$AUMC(0\text{–}\infty)\ \textbf{(Eq. 38.8)}$$
$$= \textbf{2501\,ng \cdot h}^2\textbf{/mL}$$

Therefore, using Eq. 38.7, mean residence time (*MRT*) is calculated as

$$MRT = 2501/505 = 4.95\,\text{h}$$

The apparent volume of distribution at steady state, V_{ss}, is calculated using Eq. 38.9:

$$V_{ss} = CL \cdot MRT = (1979\,\text{mL/h}) \cdot 4.95\,\text{h} = 9797\,\text{mL}$$

Urinary Excretion   Assume that urine samples were collected over various time intervals following a single intravenous dose of Drug X. The volume of urine collected over each interval was recorded and the corresponding concentration of unchanged Drug X was determined, as summarized in Table 38.5.

These apparent terminal elimination half-life ($t_{1/2}$) values as well as the fraction of dose excreted unchanged in urine (f_e) may be estimated by plotting the excretion rate (dA_e/dt) against the "midpoint" of sample collection (t_{midp}) (Fig. 38.6, Table 38.6). The theoretical basis for this derivation is beyond the scope of this chapter and is exhaustively discussed in the literature [2, 3, 5].

$$\log \frac{A_e}{dt} = \log(f_e \cdot Dose) - \frac{k_e t}{2.303} \tag{38.10}$$

where f_e, is the fraction of administered dose excreted unchanged in urine.

$$Slope = -k_e/2.303$$

$$t_{1/2} = 0.693/k_e = 3.46\,\text{h}$$

The intercept of the semilogarithmic plot provides an estimate of the fraction of administered dose excreted unchanged in urine at infinity ($f_e \cdot Dose$), 0.123 mg.

TABLE 38.5   Urinary Concentration of Unchanged Drug Following Single Intravenous Administration of 1 mg Drug X to Healthy Volunteers

Time Interval (h)	Urine Volume (mL)	Concentration in Urine (ng/mL)
0–0.5	100	571
0.5–1	74	698
1–2	88	1012
2–4	150	884
4–6	170	523
6–8	250	238
8–12	340	196
12–16	500	59.9
16–20	520	25.9
20–24	450	13.4

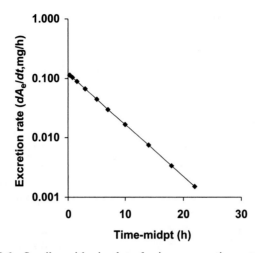

FIGURE 38.6   Semilogarithmic plot of urinary excretion rate versus t_{midpt}.

TABLE 38.6   Urinary Excretion Analysis Following Intravenous Administration of 1 mg Drug X to Healthy Volunteers

(1) Time Interval (h)	(2) Urine Volume (mL)	(3) Concentration in Urine (ng/mL)	(4) Amount Excreted in Urine (A_e, mg) (Column 2 × Column 3)	(5)[a] t_{midpta}	(6)[b] dA_e/dt
0–0.5	100	571	0.0571	0.25	0.114
0.5–1	74	698	0.0517	0.75	0.103
1–2	88	1012	0.0890	1.5	0.0890
2–4	150	884	0.133	3	0.0663
4–6	170	523	0.0889	5	0.0444
6–8	250	238	0.0596	7	0.0298
8–12	340	196	0.0667	10	0.0167
12–16	500	59.9	0.0300	14	0.00749
16–20	520	25.9	0.0135	18	0.00337
20–24	450	13.4	0.00605	22	0.00151

[a]t_{midpt} is the midpoint of the urine collection interval.
[b]dA_e/dt is calculated as $(dA_{e(n+1)} - dA_e n)/(t_{n+1} - t_n)$.

Multiple Intravenous Dosing   For a drug following *linear* (dose- or concentration-independent) *pharmacokinetics*, AUC values at steady state equal those following the first dose:

$$AUC(0-\tau)_{\text{steady state}} = AUC(0-\infty)_{\text{first dose}} \qquad (38.11)$$

where τ is the dosing interval. $AUC(0-\tau)_{\text{steady state}}$ is calculated using the trapezoidal rule as illustrated in Table 38.1.

TABLE 38.7 Estimation of Pharmacokinetic Parameters Following a Single 1mg Oral Dose to Human Volunteers

(1) Time (h)	(2) Plasma Concentration (ng/mL)	(3) Log_{10} (Concentration)	(4) $\dfrac{(C_{n+1} + C_n)}{2}$	(5) $(t_{n+1} + t_n)$	(6) AUC Value of Each Trapezoid	(7) $t \cdot C$	(8) $(t_{n-1}C_{n-1} - t_n C_n)/2$	(9) AUMC Values
0	0		1.29	0.0833	0.107	0	0.107	0.00896
0.0833	2.58		3.78	0.0833	0.315	0.215	0.523	0.0436
0.167	4.99		6.12	0.0833	0.510	0.832	1.321	0.110
0.25	7.24		10.2	0.25	2.55	1.81	4.19	1.05
0.5	13.1		17.4	0.5	8.68	6.56	14.1	7.04
1	21.6		25.6	1	25.6	21.6	40.3	40.3
2	29.5		30.1	1	30.1	59.1	75.6	75.6
3	30.7		29.7	1	29.7	92.0	103	103
4	28.7		25.3	2	50.6	115	123	246
6	21.9		18.7	2	37.4	131	128	255
8	15.5		13.1	2	26.1	124	115	230
10	10.6		8.91	2	17.8	106	96.3	193
12	7.20	0.857	5.23	4	20.9	86.4	69.2	277
16	3.26	0.513	2.36	4	9.44	52.1	40.7	163
20	1.46	0.166	1.06	4	4.25	29.3	22.5	90.2
24	0.658	-0.182				15.8		

$Slope = -0.0866$
$k_e = 0.199\,h^{-1}$
$t_{1/2} = \mathbf{3.48\,h}$

$AUC(0 - t_{last}) = 264$
$C_{last}/k_e = 3.30$
$AUC(0 - \infty) = \mathbf{267\,ng \cdot h/mL}$
$F = \mathbf{52.9\%}$

$AUMC(0 - t_{last}) = 1682$
$(C_{last} \cdot t_{last})/k_e = 79.2$
$C_{last}/k_e^2 = 16.6$
$AUMC(0 - \infty) = \mathbf{1778\,ng \cdot h^2/mL}$
$MRT = \mathbf{0.150\,h}$

TABLE 38.8   Implications of Pharmacokinetic Data Analyses on Drug Discovery and Development

Key Pharmacokinetic Information	Methodological Approach	Drug Discovery and Development Implication
Systemic exposure and peak systemic concentrations	Analysis of systemic concentration–time profile: determination of the area under the curve (AUC) and C_{max}	Potential correlation with drug response (efficacy and/or toxicity)
Rate of drug absorption	Analysis of systemic concentration–time profile: time to C_{max} (T_{max})	Choice of an appropriate route of administration and drug formulation
Systemically available fraction of administered dose	Bioavailability assessment	Choice of an appropriate route of administration and dose
Presystemic or first-pass elimination following oral dosing	Comparison of nonparenteral AUC, and other routes such as portal administration with AUC after intravenous administration	Factors affecting bioavailability
Drug persistence in the body	Apparent terminal elimination half-life ($t_{1/2}$)	Frequency of drug administration and designing "acceptable" dosing regimen
Drug accumulation following multiple dosing (parenteral or nonparenteral)	Analysis of systemic concentration–time profiles at steady state	Relationship of the drug levels to pharmacologically relevant drug levels (therapeutic window)
Route of drug clearance	Rate and extent of urinary excretion and extent of drug metabolism (including *in vitro* methodologies)	Factors affecting drug elimination; extent of intersubject variability in drug disposition; and drug–drug interactions

38.3.2   Example 2: Oral Dosing

The plasma concentration–time data following a single oral dose of 1 mg Drug X is summarized in Table 38.7. Apparent terminal elimination $t_{1/2}$, AUC values, CL, and MRT values are calculated as indicated in Eqs. 38.1–38.2. The corresponding calculations are included in Table 38.7. The maximum plasma concentration (C_{max}) and time to reach C_{max} (T_{max}) are generally determined by observation. Therefore, in this instance,

$$C_{max} = 30.7\,\text{ng/mL}$$

$$T_{max} = 3\,\text{h}$$

Oral bioavailability is defined by the following equation:

$$F(\%) = \frac{AUC_{\text{oral}}/Dose_{\text{oral}}}{AUC_{\text{IV}}/Dose_{\text{IV}}} \qquad (38.12)$$

38.4   IMPLICATIONS OF PHARMACOKINETICS ON DRUG DISCOVERY AND DEVELOPMENT

This chapter describes the typical data analysis methodologies used to characterize the pharmacokinetics of a drug following single or multiple intravenous or oral dosing using systemic (plasma) concentration–time and urinary excretion–time data. The implications of such analyses on drug discovery and development are summarized in Table 38.8.

REFERENCES

1. Gibaldi M, Perrier D. *Pharmacokinetics*, 2nd ed. New York: Marcel Dekker; 1982.
2. Boroujerdi M. *Pharmacokinetics: Principles and Application*. New York: McGraw-Hill; 2002.
3. Bourne DWA. Pharmacokinetic Software Resource. http://www.boomer.org/pkin/soft. html. Accessed on 26 February 2007.
4. Gabrielsson J, Weiner D. *Pharmacokinetic and Pharmacodynamic Data Analysis, Concepts and Applications*, 3rd ed. Stockholm, Sweden: Swedish Pharmaceutical Press; 2001.
5. Rowland M, Tozer TN. *Clinical Pharmacokinetics: Concepts and Applications*, 3rd ed, Baltimore: Lippincott Williams & Wilkins; 1995.

INDEX

Preclinical Development Handbook: ADME and Biopharmaceutical Properties,
edited by Shayne Cox Gad
Copyright © 2008 John Wiley & Sons, Inc.